Multimodality Imaging for Transcatheter Aortic Valve Replacement

James K. Min • Daniel S. Berman
Jonathon Leipsic
Editors

Multimodality Imaging for Transcatheter Aortic Valve Replacement

Springer

Editors
James K. Min
Weill Cornell Medical College
NewYork-Presbyterian Hospital
New York, NY
USA

Daniel S. Berman
Departments of Imaging and Medicine
Cedars-Sinai Medical Center
Cedars-Sinai Heart Institute
David Geffen UCLA School of Medicine
Los Angeles, CA
USA

Jonathon Leipsic
Division of Cardiology
Department of Radiology
University of British Columbia
St. Paul's Hospital
Vancouver
British Columbia
Canada

ISBN 978-1-4471-7189-8 ISBN 978-1-4471-2798-7 (eBook)
DOI 10.1007/978-1-4471-2798-7
Springer London Heidelberg New York Dordrecht

Printed on acid-free paper

Springer is part of Springer Science+Business Media (www.springer.com)

Acknowledgments

To my parents, for inspiration.

–James K. Min

To my parents for their love and support, to my children for the joy and laughter and to my wife Karly for giving meaning to my life.

–Jonathon Leipsic

Contents

Contributors

Shikhar Agarwal, MD, MPH, CPH Department of Cardiovascular Medicine, Cleveland Clinic, Cleveland, OH, USA

Hatem Alkadhi, MD, MPH Insitute of Diagnostic and Interventional Radiology, University Hospital Zurich, Zurich, Switzerland

Alexandra Almonacid, MD Interventional Cardiology Clinical Services, Beth Israel Deaconess Medical Center, Boston, MA, USA

Departments of Internal Medicine (Cardiovascular Division) and Radiology, Beth Israel Deaconess Medical Center, Boston, MA, USA

Department of Anesthesia, Banner Good Samaritan Medical Center, Phoenix, AZ, USA

Chesnal D. Arepalli, MD (DNB) Department of Radiology and Imaging Sciences, Division of Cardiothoracic Imaging, Emory University School of Medicine, Atlanta, GA, USA

Reza Arsanjani, MD Division of Cardiology, Department of Medicine, Cedars-Sinai Medical Center, David Geffen UCLA School of Medicine, Los Angeles, CA, USA

Vinayak Bapat, FRCS, CTh Department of Cardiothoracic Surgery, Guys and St. Thomas' Hospital, London, UK

Israel M. Barbash, MD Department of Interventional Cardiology, Washington Hospital Center, Washington, DC, USA

Department of Cath Lab, Washington Hospital Center, Washington, DC, USA

Adam Berger, MBBS, MPH Department of Medical Imaging, St. Paul's Hospital UBC, Vancouver, BC, Canada

Division of Cardiology, Department of Radiology, University of British Columbia, St. Paul's Hospital, Vancouver, BC, Canada

Daniel S. Berman, MD Departments of Imaging and Medicine, Cedars-Sinai Medical Center, Cedars-Sinai Heart Institute, David Geffen UCLA School of Medicine, Los Angeles, CA, USA

Theodore Blake, BSc, MD, FRCPC Department of Radiology, Stanford University Hospital, Palo Alto, CA, USA

Department of Radiology, Stanford University School of Medicine, Stanford, CA, USA

Gerald S. Bloomfield, MD, MPH Department of Medicine, Duke University Medical Center, Durham, NC, USA

Division of Cardiovascular Medicine, Duke University Medical Center, Durham, NC, USA

Duke Clinical Research Institute, Durham, NC, USA

Mathew Brooks, MD, MBBS, FRACP Department of Cardiology, Royal Melbourne Hospital, Melbourne, VIC, Australia

Piotr P. Buszman, MD, PhD The Skirball Center for Cardiovascular Research, Cardiovascular Research Foundation, Orangeburg, NY, USA

American Heart of Poland, Center for Cardiovascular Research and Development, Katowice, Poland

Blase A. Carabello, MD Department of Medicine, Center for Heart Valve Disease, St. Luke's Episcopal Hospital, Baylor College of Medicine, Houston, TX, USA

Department of Medicine, The W.A. "Tex" and Deborah Moncrief, Jr., Baylor College of Medicine, Medical Care Line Executive, Veterans Affairs Medical Center, Houston, TX, USA

Department of Medicine, Veterans Affairs Medical Center, Houston, TX, USA

Jorge Castellanos, MD, MPP Department of Cardiology, Cedars Sinai Medical Center, Los Angeles, CA, USA

Tarun Chakravarty, MD Department of Cardiology, Cedars-Sinai Heart Institute, Cedars-Sinai Medical Center, Los Angeles, CA, USA

Anson Cheung, MD Department of Cardiovascular Surgery, St. Paul's Hospital, Vancouver, BC, Canada

Benoit Daneault, MD, FRCPC Department of Medicine, Centre Hospitalier Universitaire de Sherbrooke, Université de Sherbrooke, Sherbrooke, QC, Canada

Pamela S. Douglas, MD Department of Medicine, Duke University Medical Center, Durham, NC, USA

Division of Cardiovascular Medicine, Duke University Medical Center, Durham, NC, USA

Duke Clinical Research Institute, Durham, NC, USA

Jean G. Dumesnil, OQ, MD, FRCPC, FACC, FASE (Hon) Department of Cardiology, Quebec Heart and Lung Institute, Laval University, Quebec, QC, Canada

Danny Dvir, MD Department of Interventional Cardiology, Washington Hospital Center, Washington, DC, USA

Department of Interventional Cardiology, MedStar Washington Hospital Center, Washington, DC, USA

Mark R. Dweck, MD, PhD Centre for Cardiovascular Science, University of Edinburgh, Edinburgh, UK

David P. Faxon, MD Cardiovascular Division, Department of Medicine, Brigham and Women's Hospital, Harvard Medical School, Boston, MA, USA

Gudrun Feuchtner, MD Department of Radiology, Innsbruck Medical University, Innsbruck, Austria

Dominik Fleischmann, MD Department of Radiology, Stanford University School of Medicine, Stanford, CA, USA

Gregory P. Fontana, MD Department of Cardiothoracic Surgery, Lenox Hill Heart and Vascular Institute-North Shore/LIJ Health System, New York, NY, USA

Melanie Freeman, MBBS, FRACP Department of Cardiology, St. Paul's Hospital, Vancouver, BC, Canada

George Gellert, MD Interventional Cardiology Clinical Services, Beth Israel Deaconess Medical Center, Boston, MA, USA

Departments of Internal Medicine (Cardiovascular Division) and Radiology, Beth Israel Deaconess Medical Center, Boston, MA, USA

Department of Anesthesia, Banner Good Samaritan Medical Center, Phoenix, AZ, USA

Philippe Généreux, MD Department of Cardiology, Cardiovascular Research Foundation, Columbia University Medical Center, New York, NY, USA

Departement de Cardiologie D'Intervention, Hôpital du Sacré-coeur de Montréal, Université de Montréal, Montréal, QC, Canada

Subha Ghosh, MD Department of Radiology, Wexner Medical Center, Ohio State University, Columbus, OH, USA

Daniel Grafstein, MD Department of Medical Imaging, St. Paul's Hospital, UBC, Vancouver, BC, Canada

Juan F. Granada, MD The Skirball Center for Cardiovascular Research, Cardiovascular Research Foundation, Orangeburg, NY, USA

Ronen Gurvitch, MD, MBBS, FRACP Department of Cardiology, Royal Melbourne Hospital, Melbourne, VIC, Australia

Cameron John Hague, MD, FRCPC Department of Radiology, St. Paul's Hospital, Vancouver, BC, Canada

Rebecca T. Hahn, MD, FACC, FASE Department of Medicine, Columbia University Medical Center, New York-Presbyterian Hospital, New York, NY, USA

Pei-Hsiu Huang, MD Cardiovascular Division, Department of Medicine, Brigham and Women's Hospital, Harvard Medical School, Boston, MA, USA

Brian G. Hynes, MB Department of Interventional Cardiology and Structural Heart Disease, Quebec Heart and Lung Institute, Laval University, Quebec City, QC, Canada

Vladimir Jelnin, MD Department of Cardiology, Lenox Hill Heart and Vascular Institute-North Shore/LIJ Health System, New York, NY, USA

Hasan Jilaihawi, MD, MRCP Department of Cardiology, Cedars-Sinai Heart Institute, Cedars-Sinai Medical Center, Los Angeles, CA, USA

Samir Kapadia, MD, FACC Department of Interventional Cardiology, Sones Cardiac Catheterization Laboratories, Interventional Cardiology Fellowship Program, Cleveland Clinic, Cleveland, OH, USA

Mark J. Kearns, BSc, MD Department of Cardiovascular Surgery, St. Paul's Hospital, Vancouver, BC, Canada

Chad Kliger, MD, MS Department of Cardiology, Lenox Hill Heart and Vascular Institute-North Shore/LIJ Health System, New York, NY, USA

Susheel K. Kodali, MD Department of Interventional Cardiology, Columbia University Medical Center, New York, NY, USA

Amar Krishnaswamy, MD Department of Cardiovascular Medicine, Cleveland Clinic, Cleveland, OH, USA

Elena Ladich, MD Department of Cardiovascular Pathology, CVPath Institute Inc, Gaithersburg, MD, USA

Eric Larose, DVM, MD, FRCPC, FAHA Department of Cardiology, Institut universitaire de cardiologie et de pneumologie de Québec (IUCPQ), Québec, QC, Canada

Faculté de médecine, Université Laval, Québec City, QC, Canada

Jonathon Leipsic, MD, FRCPC, FSCCT Division of Cardiology, Department of Radiology, University of British Columbia, St. Paul's Hospital, Vancouver, BC, Canada

Martin B. Leon, MD Department of Medicine, Columbia University Medical Center, New York-Presbyterian Hospital, New York, NY, USA

Department of Cardiology, Cardiovascular Research Foundation, Columbia University Medical Center, New York, NY, USA

Stamatios Lerakis, MD, FACC, FAHA Division of Medicine, Radiology and Imaging Sciences, Department of Cardiology, Emory University School of Medicine, Atlanta, GA, USA

Department of Biomedical Engineering, Emory University and Georgia Institute of Technology, Atlanta, GA, USA

Diana Litmanovich, MD Department of Radiology, Beth Israel Deaconess Medical Center, Boston, MA, USA

Departments of Internal Medicine (Cardiovascular Division) and Radiology, Beth Israel Deaconess Medical Center, Boston, MA, USA

Department of Anesthesia, Banner Good Samaritan Medical Center, Phoenix, AZ, USA

Raj Makkar, MD, FACC Department of Cardiology, Cedars-Sinai Heart Institute, Cedars-Sinai Medical Center, Los Angeles, CA, USA

James K. Min, MD, FACC, FSCCT Weill Cornell Medical College, NewYork-Presbyterian Hospital, New York, NY, USA

Sean Moore, BS Department of Internal Medicine, Wexner Medical Center at the Ohio State University, Columbus, OH, USA

Jeffrey W. Moses, MD Department of Medicine, Columbia University Medical Center, New York, NY, USA

Robert R. Moss, MD Department of Cardiology, St. Paul's Hospital, Vancouver, BC, Canada

Mastataka Nakano, MD Department of Cardiovascular Pathology, CVPath Institute Inc, Gaithersburg, MD, USA

David E. Newby, MD, PhD Centre for Cardiovascular Science, University of Edinburgh, Edinburgh, UK

Alper Ozkan, MD Department of Cardiovascular Medicine, Cleveland Clinic, Cleveland, OH, USA

Jean-Michel Paradis, MD Department of Interventional Cardiology, Columbia University Medical Center, New York, NY, USA

Philippe Pibarot, DVM, PhD, FACC, FAHA, FASE, FESC Department of Cardiology, Institut Universitaire de Cardiologie et de Pneumologie de Québec, Québec Heart and Lung Institute, Québec, QC, Canada

Augusto D. Pichard, MD, FACC Department of Interventional Cardiology, Washington Hospital Center, Washington, DC, USA

Department of Cardiology, Georgetown University Medical School, MedStar Washington Hospital Center, Washington, DC, USA

Fabian Plank, MD Department of Radiology, Innsbruck Medical University, Innsbruck, Austria

Jeffrey J. Popma, MD Interventional Cardiology Clinical Services, Beth Israel Deaconess Medical Center, Boston, MA, USA

Departments of Internal Medicine (Cardiovascular Division) and Radiology, Beth Israel Deaconess Medical Center, Boston, MA, USA

Department of Anesthesia, Banner Good Samaritan Medical Center, Phoenix, AZ, USA

Rohan Poulter, MD, MBBS, MRCP(UK), FRACP Division of Cardiology, Vancouver General Hospital, Vancouver, BC, Canada

Subha V. Raman, MD, MSEE Department of Cardiovascular Medicine, Ohio State University, Columbus, OH, USA

Josep Rodés-Cabau, MD Department of Interventional Cardiology and Structural Heart Disease, Quebec Heart and Lung Institute, Laval University, Quebec City, QC, Canada

James H.F. Rudd, MD, PhD Division of Cardiovascular Medicine, University of Cambridge, Addenbrooke's Hospital, Cambridge, UK

Carlos E. Ruiz, MD, PhD Department of Cardiology, Lenox Hill Heart and Vascular Institute-North Shore/LIJ Health System, New York, NY, USA

Zainab Samad, MD, MBBS, MHS Department of Medicine, Duke University Medical Center, Durham, NC, USA

Department of Medicine/Radiology, Duke University, Durham, NC, USA

Lowell F. Satler Department of Interventional Cardiology, Washington Hospital Center, Washington, DC, USA

Paul Schoenhagen, MD Departments of Cardiovascular Medicine and Radiology, Imaging Institute and Heart and Vascular Institute, Cleveland Clinic, Cleveland, OH, USA

Yasmin Siddiqui, BA, DO, MPH, MD Department of Internal Medicine, Wexner Medical Center at the Ohio State University, Columbus, OH, USA

Robert J. Siegel, MD, FACC, FASE Department of Cardiology, Cedars Sinai Medical Center, Los Angeles, CA, USA

Christopher R. Thompson, MD, CM, FRCPC (Cardiology) Division of Cardiology, Department of Medicine, St. Paul's Hospital Cardiac Echo Lab and the University of British Columbia, Vancouver, BC, Canada

E. Murat Tuzcu, MD Department of Cardiovascular Medicine, Cleveland Clinic, Cleveland, OH, USA

Renu Virmani, MD Department of Cardiovascular Pathology, CVPath Institute Inc, Gaithersburg, MD, USA

Ron Waksman, MD, FACC Department of Interventional Cardiology, Washington Hospital Center, Washington, DC, USA

Department of Cardiology, MedStar Washington Hospital Center, MedStar Heart Institute, Georgetown University, Washington, DC, USA

John G. Webb, MD, FRCPC, FACC Department of Cardiology, St. Paul's Hospital, Vancouver, BC, Canada

Wm. Guy Weigold, MD, FACC, FSCCT Department of Interventional Cardiology, Washington Hospital Center, Washington, DC, USA

Department of Interventional Cardiology, MedStar Washington Hospital Center, Washington, DC, USA

Miriam L. Wheeler, MB, ChB, FRACP Division of Cardiology, St. Paul's Hospital Cardiac Echo Lab and the University of British Columbia, Vancouver, BC, Canada

Alexander Bruce Willson, MBBS (Hons), MPH, FRACP Division of Cardiology, Department of Radiology, University of British Columbia, St. Paul's Hospital, Vancouver, BC, Canada

Department of Cardiology, Nambour General Hospital, Nambour, QLD, Australia

David A. Wood, MD, FRCPC Division of Cardiology, St. Paul's and Vancouver General Hospital, Diamond Health Care Centre (Cardiology – Level 9), Vancouver, BC, Canada

Why We Need This Book

1

James K. Min, Jonathon Leipsic, and Daniel S. Berman

Over the last decade, remarkable innovations in transcatheter technologies have led to the rapid development of an array of minimally invasive therapies that have challenged conventional treatment paradigms. Amongst these, none is as remarkable or as potentially disruptive as transcatheter aortic valve replacement (TAVR). An archetype of "bench-to-bedside" medicine, the origins of TAVR spanned the expertise of visionary clinicians to engineers to researchers to imagers. The theme underpinning the foundation of TAVR—that of a multidisciplinary approach to its development—persists in its application. From the landmark effort of Cribier who, in 2002, reported the first successful implantation of a transcatheter aortic valve, we have consistently witnessed a team approach to the execution of this complex procedure—bringing together a diverse group of experts to optimize patient outcomes. It is perhaps, in large part, due to this that we have observed an unprecedented growth in the scientific evidence, iterative technological advances, and utilization of TAVR that has surpassed even the most optimistic of observers.

At the time of writing of this text, more than 60,000 TAVR procedures have been performed worldwide, along with two large-scale randomized controlled trials demonstrating a heretofore unparalleled reduction in mortality for inoperable patients with severe valvular disease. Even amongst high-risk individuals, TAVR has proven an effective alternative compared to conventional surgical aortic valve replacement, thus raising a bar of equipoise as to which method should be considered the standard of care. We will, in the near-term future, undoubtedly witness the completion of numerous additional randomized trials and multicenter observational studies for newer transcatheter aortic valves, which are being developed by at least ten other companies. These trials and registries—coupled with differences in valve technologies—will teach us lessons that will affect the procedural success of TAVR and improve the outcomes of our patients in a manner that is simply unforeseeable.

Similar to the multidisciplinary approach to TAVR performance, the pre-, peri-, and post-procedural imaging assessment of patients undergoing TAVR requires multiple imaging modalities. The convergence of different types of imaging specialists to support TAVR has encouraged the use of an array of imaging tools—including transthoracic and transesophageal echocardiography, multidetector computed tomography, magnetic resonance imaging, catheter-based angiography, and dynamic rotational angiography. Our initial intent in the development of this text was to address the imaging needs associated with TAVR. We hope that we have achieved this goal and that this text affords the imaging physician a comprehensive understanding of the pathophysiology of aortic stenosis, the history and evidence supporting the use of TAVR, and an integrated approach to the indications, procedural aspects, and pitfalls of imaging in TAVR. We further hope that the reader will also gain an appreciation of which tests may offer advantages over others in specific situations and a stepwise method to harvest all the essential information provided by these imaging tests.

In the course of structuring this text, we solicited the input from an assembly of authorities in the field—ranging from proceduralists and pathologists to investigators and imagers. In doing so, we observed a consistent theme wherein vital information related to TAVR imaging often appeared in chapters formulated by even nonimagers. With this, we

J.K. Min, MD, FACC, FSCCT (✉)
Weill Cornell Medical College, NewYork-Presbyterian Hospital, New York, NY, USA
e-mail: jkm2001@med.cornell.edu

D.S. Berman, MD
Departments of Imaging and Medicine, Cedars-Sinai Medical Center, Cedars-Sinai Heart Institute David Geffen UCLA School of Medicine, Los Angeles, CA, USA

J. Leipsic, MD, FRCPC, FSCCT
Division of Cardiology, Department of Radiology, University of British Columbia, St. Paul's Hospital, Vancouver, BC, Canada

J.K. Min et al. (eds.), *Multimodality Imaging for Transcatheter Aortic Valve Replacement*, DOI 10.1007/978-1-4471-2798-7_1, © Springer-Verlag London 2014

gained an even greater appreciation of the central role of multimodality diagnostics in the successful performance of TAVR and that these concepts extend beyond imaging for TAVR but apply simply to the principles of TAVR itself. Thus, the present text represents a more far-reaching one that we had initially conceived, and we believe that it is the better for it.

As imagers ourselves, we are appreciative of the opportunity to support the diagnostics associated with this breakthrough technology. And we feel privileged to be part of the TAVR team.

James K. Min
Jonathon Leipsic
Daniel S. Berman

2 Transcatheter Aortic Valve Implantation: Review of Current Evidence

Philippe Généreux and Martin B. Leon

Abstract
Symptomatic severe aortic stenosis (AS) has a poor prognosis when treated medically and inevitably leads to an insidious functional deterioration, heart failure, and death [1]. Surgical aortic valve replacement (SAVR) is the current standard of care and is an accepted method to alleviate symptoms and prolong survival. For an array of reasons, approximately 30 % do not undergo SAVR [2]. However, since Dr. Alain Cribier pioneered the first transcatheter aortic valve replacement (TAVR) procedure in 2002 [3], this relatively new technique has been used extensively in over 40 countries accumulating to >50,000 implantations [4–19]. With results from the randomized PARTNER trial [20], TAVR has emerged as the standard of care for extremely high-risk or "inoperable" patients and is a valid alternative to surgery for selected high-risk but "operable" patients with symptomatic AS [21]. Currently, two different TAVR devices are widely available and used: the balloon-expandable Edwards SAPIEN Transcatheter Heart Valve (Edwards Lifesciences, Irvine, CA) and the self-expanding Medtronic CoreValve™ (Medtronic, Minneapolis, MN). Both devices received CE Mark approval for European commercial sale in 2007, and the Edwards SAPIEN valve received FDA pre-market approval in the USA in November 2011.

Keywords
Technology innovation • Registries • Clinical outcomes • TAVR • Paravalvular regurgitation

P. Généreux, MD
Department of Cardiology, Cardiovascular Research Foundation, Columbia University Medical Center, 111 East 59th street 18th Floor, New York, NY 10022, USA

Departement de Cardiologie D'Intervention, Hôpital du Sacré-Coeur de Montréal, Université de Montréal, Montréal, QC, Canada
e-mail: pgenerevx@crf.org

M.B. Leon, MD (✉)
Department of Medicine, Columbia University Medical Center, New York-Presbyterian Hospital, 161 Fort Washington Avenue, Herbert Irving Pavilion, 6th Floor, New York, NY 10032, USA

Department of Cardiology, Cardiovascular Research Foundation, Columbia University Medical Center, 111 East 59th street 18th Floor, New York, NY 10022, USA
e-mail: ml2398@columbia.edu, mleon@crf.org

Abbreviations

AS	Aortic stenosis
EuroSCORE	European System for Cardiac Operative Risk Evaluation
I-REVIVE	Initial Registry of Endovascular Implantation of Valves in Europe trial
PARTNER	Placement of Aortic Transcatheter Valves
RECAST	Registry of Endovascular Critical Aortic Stenosis Treatment trial
REVIVAL	Percutaneous Endovascular Implantation of Valves trial
REVIVE	Registry of Endovascular Implantation of Valves in Europe trial

J.K. Min et al. (eds.), *Multimodality Imaging for Transcatheter Aortic Valve Replacement*, DOI 10.1007/978-1-4471-2798-7_2, © Springer-Verlag London 2014

SAVR	Surgical aortic valve replacement
SOURCE	SAPIEN Aortic Bioprosthesis European Outcome
STS	Society of Thoracic Surgeons
TA	Transapical
TAVR	Transcatheter aortic valve implantation
TF	Transfemoral
TRAVERCE	The initial multicenter feasibility trial for TA-AVI
VARC	Valve Academic Research Consortium

Introduction

Symptomatic severe aortic stenosis (AS) has a poor prognosis when treated medically and inevitably leads to an insidious functional deterioration, heart failure, and death [1]. Surgical aortic valve replacement (SAVR) is the current standard of care and is an accepted method to alleviate symptoms and prolong survival. For an array of reasons, approximately 30 % do not undergo SAVR [2]. However, since Dr. Alain Cribier pioneered the first transcatheter aortic valve replacement (TAVR) procedure in 2002 [3], this relatively new technique has been used extensively in over 40 countries accumulating to >50,000 implantations [4–19]. With results from the randomized PARTNER trial [20], TAVR has emerged as the standard of care for extremely high-risk or "inoperable" patients and is a valid alternative to surgery for selected high-risk but "operable" patients with symptomatic AS [21]. Currently, two different TAVR devices are widely available and used: the balloon-expandable Edwards SAPIEN Transcatheter Heart Valve (Edwards Lifesciences, Irvine, CA) and the self-expanding Medtronic CoreValve™ (Medtronic, Minneapolis, MN). Both devices received CE Mark approval for European commercial sale in 2007, and the Edwards SAPIEN valve received FDA pre-market approval in the USA in November 2011.

Initial Experience

First-In-Man, Initial Reports, and Feasibility Studies

Cribier and coworkers performed the first TAVR in an inoperable patient in 2002 using a transseptal antegrade approach and a balloon-expandable aortic valve prosthesis, demonstrating the feasibility of percutaneous valve implantation [3]. The antegrade approach was further explored [22], coinciding with the first-in-man retrograde experience of a self-expanding prosthesis (CoreValve™) [23]. Larger series quickly followed, with early experiences of small initiatives using both the balloon-expandable Cribier valve (Edwards Lifesciences Inc.) and the self-expandable CoreValve™ system [9, 19]. The devices showed a procedural success rate of about 80 %.

After demonstration of successful promise from these single-center experiences, several larger multicenter feasibility studies were initiated first in Europe and later in the USA [6, 24–26]. These studies demonstrated that TA and TF TAVR in high-risk patients was feasible and could be performed with a high procedural success rate and a 30-day mortality of 10–15 % (Table 2.1).

Registries (Table 2.2)

Edwards Registries

Several large European and Canadian registries have been published, showing excellent short- and midterm results after TAVR using both the TF and TA devices [12, 15]. The largest registry reported to date is the SOURCE (SAPIEN Aortic Bioprosthesis European Outcome) registry [17, 18]. Overall, 1,038 patients were enrolled at 32 European centers and were treated with either a TF ($n = 463$) or TA approach ($n = 575$). Patients treated by TA had more comorbidities at baseline than TF patients, resulting in a significantly higher

Table 2.1 Multicenter feasibility studies

Study	Enrollment	Number of patients	Approach	Device	Procedural success	30-day mortality
I-REVIVE/RECAST [6]	2003–2005	26	Transseptal	Edwards SAPIEN	85 % (22/26)	16.7 % (6/36)
		7	TF	Edwards SAPIEN	57 % (4/7)	
Grube et al. [9]	2005–2007	86	TF	CoreValve	74 % (64/86)	11.6 % (10/86)
TRAVERCE [26]	2006–2008	168	TA	Edwards SAPIEN	95.8 % (161/168)	14.9 % (25/168)
REVIVAL [24, 25]	2006–2008	40	TA	Edwards SAPIEN	100 % (40/40)	12.5 % (7/40)
	2005–2006	55	TF	Edwards SAPIEN	87 % (48/55)	7.3 % (4/55)

TF transfemoral, *TA* transapical

Table 2.2 Clinical outcomes after TAVR according to access site and device type

Major published data											
Authors	Type of study	Number of patients	STS (%)	Logistic EuroSCORE (%)	Follow-up (months)	Procedural success rate (%)	Mortality 30-day (%)	Mortality 1-year (%)	Major access complications 30-day (%)	Stroke 30-day (%)	Need for new PPM (%)
Edwards SAPIEN: TF											
Lefevre et al. [12]	Registry	61	11.3	25.7	12	95.4	8.2	21.3	16.4	3.3	1.8
Eltchaninoff et al. [8]	Registry	95	17.4	25.6	1	98.3[a]	8.4	–	6.3	4.2	5.3
Himbert et al. [11]	Registry	51	15.0	25.0	12	90.0	8.0[b]	19.0	12.0	6.0	6.0
Rodes-Cabau et al. [15]	Registry	162	9.0	–	24	90.5	9.5	25.0	13.1	3.0	3.6
Thomas et al. [17, 18]	Registry	463	–	14.5	1	95.2	6.3	18.9	22.9	2.4	6.7
Leon et al. [20]	RCT	179	11.2	26.4	12	–	5.0[c]	30.7[c]	16.2	6.7[d]	3.4
Bosmans et al. [4]	Registry	99	–	29.0	12	97.0	6.0	18.0	–	2.0	4.0
Smith et al. [21]	RCT	244	11.7	29.1	12	–	3.3[c]	22.2[c]	14.0	3.7[d]	3.7
Edwards SAPIEN: TA											
Walther et al. [26]	Feasibility study	168	–	27.0	12	95.8	15.0	37.0	1.2	2.0	2.3
Svensson et al. [25]	Feasibility study	40	13.4	35.5	6	87.5	17.5	–	–	5.0	–
Lefevre et al. [12]	Registry	69	11.3	33.8	12	96.4	18.8	50.7	5.8[e]	1.5	3.8
Eltchaninoff et al. [8]	Registry	71	18.4	26.8	1	98.3[a]	16.9	–	5.6[f]	2.8	5.6
Himbert et al. [11]	Registry	24	18.0	28.0	12	100	16.0[b]	26.0	8.0	0	4.0
Rodes-Cabau et al. [15]	Registry	177	10.5	–	1	96.1	11.3	22.0	13.0[f]	1.7	6.2
Thomas et al. [17, 18]	Registry	575	–	16.3	1	95.7	10.3	27.9	4.7	2.6	7.3
Bosmans et al. [4]	Registry	88	–	33.0	12	97.0	14.0	37.0	–	8.0	6.0
Smith et al. [21]	RCT	104	11.8	29.8	12	–	3.8[c]	29.0[c]	3.8	6.8	3.9
D'Onofrio et al. [7]	Registry	504	11.0	26.3	24	99.0	8.3	18.8	–	3.0	5.4
Medtronic CoreValve™: TF											
Tamburino et al. [16]	Registry	663	–	23.0	12	98.0	5.4	15.0	2.0	2.5[g]	17.4
Bosmans et al. [4]	Registry	133	–	25.0	12	98.0	11.0	22.0	–	4.0	22.0
Grube et al. [10]	Registry	86	–	21.6	1	88.0	12.0	–	–	10.0	–
Piazza et al. [14]	Registry	646	–	23.1	1	97.2	8.0	–	1.9	1.9	9.3
Eltchaninoff et al. [8]	Registry	66	21.3	24.7	1	98.3[a]	15.1	–	7.5	4.5	25.7
Petronio et al. [13]	Registry	460	–	19.4	6	98.4	6.1	11.4	2.0	1.7	16.1
Buellesfeld et al. [5]	Registry	126[h]	–	23.0	24	72.6	15.2	28.1	–	9.6	26.2

(continued)

Table 2.2 (continued)

Major published data

Authors	Type of study	Number of patients	STS (%)	Logistic EuroSCORE (%)	Follow-up (months)	Procedural success rate (%)	Mortality 30-day (%)	Mortality 1-year (%)	Major access complications 30-day (%)	Stroke 30-day (%)	Need for new PPM (%)
Medtronic CoreValve™: SC											
Eltchaninoff et al. [8]	Registry	12	21.0	24.6	1	98.3[a]	8.3	–	8.3	0	25.0
Bosmans et al. [4]	Registry	8	–	25.0	12	98.0	11.0	0	–	4.0	22.0
Petronio et al. [13]	Registry	54	–	25.3	6	100	0	6.7	0	1.9	18.5
Zahn et al. [29][i]	Registry	697	–	20.5	1	98.4	12.4	–	19.5	2.8	39.3[j]

TAVR transcatheter aortic valve implantation, *TF* transfemoral, *TA* transapical, *SC* subclavian, *STS* Society of Thoracic Surgeons, *EuroSCORE* European System for Cardiac Operative Risk Evaluation, *RCT* randomized controlled trial, *PPM* permanent pacemaker

[a]Global procedural success rate including Edwards SAPIEN TF, Edwards SAPIEN TA, and Medtronic CoreValve TF and subclavian was 98.3 %

[b]In-hospital mortality

[c]Intention-to-treat mortality rate

[d]Major and minor stroke

[e]Vascular-related complications

[f]Apex-related complications

[g]1 year

[h]124 patients received a TF approach and two an SC approach

[i]Outcomes reported together: 566 (81.2 %) Medtronic CoreValve™ TF, 22 (3.2 %) Medtronic CoreValve™ SC, 106 (15.2 %), Edwards SAPIEN TF

[j]Medtronic CoreValve™ 42.5 %, Edwards SAPIEN 22 %

EuroSCORE (29.1 % vs. 25.7 %; $P<0.001$). Procedural success was 95.2 and 92.7 %, and 30-day mortality was 6.3 and 10.3 % in the TF and TA populations, respectively. The major limitations of this registry were that more than 70 % of the enrolling centers had no prior experience with TAVR and all adverse events were site-reported without core lab analysis. In early 2011, 1-year results were published, demonstrating a 1-year survival of 76.1 % overall, 72.1 % for TA and 81.1 % for TF patients. Among the surviving patients, 73.5 % were NYHA class I or II [17].

CoreValve™ Registries

A number of large dedicated CoreValve registries have been reported [14, 16]. Promising 3-year results were recently reported by Ussia et al. [27], and although not yet published, the results of the ADVANCE CoreValve™ registry were presented recently [28]. ADVANCE represents a 100 % monitored "real-world" experience, with a core laboratory and an independent clinical event committee adjudicating events. The registry included 1,015 patients from 44 experienced (>40 prior procedures) centers between March 2010 and July 2011. The mean logistic EuroSCORE was 19.2 %. At 30 days and 6 months, the rate of all-cause mortality was 4.5 and 12.8 %, respectively, with cardiac mortality of 3.4 and 8.4 %, respectively. ADVANCE provides insights into contemporary TAVR data of experienced operators and is a benchmark for comparing outcomes.

Mixed National Registries

In 2011, results from four mixed CoreValve™ and Edwards European national registries have been reported, mostly using the TF and TA routes (Table 2.2) [4, 8, 29, 30]. Overall, patients included in these registries were at high risk according to surgical risk models, mean EuroSCORE 18–30 %. These registries showed 1-year survival rates ranging between 71.9 and 81.6 %. The UK registry reported the longest follow-up; survival was 73.7 % at 2 years [30]. Several of these national initiatives performed access-route comparisons and reported that survival was generally higher in patients treated through the TF route [4, 30]. However, it should be noted that a transfemoral-first approach is often advocated, which may introduce selection bias and an unequal comparison between the two access routes [31].

Recently, the largest registry to date was reported by the FRANCE 2 investigators [32]. They included 3,195 patients treated between January 2010 and December 2011 at 34 centers. The registry reflects contemporary real-life use of available TAVR devices in patients at high surgical risk; the Edwards SAPIEN and the Medtronic CoreValve™ devices were used in, respectively, 66.9 and 33.1 %. The transfemoral approach was most widely used (74.6 %), followed by transapical (17.8 %), subclavian (5.8 %), and 1.8 % by a non-femoral non-apical approach. Procedural success rate was 96.9 % and 1-year survival in patients was 76.0 %.

Randomized Trials

Completed Trials

While registry reports are of crucial value to assess "real-world" use of TAVR, more rigorous assessments are available from the first multicenter, randomized clinical PARTNER trials (Placement of Aortic Transcatheter Valves; ClinicalTrials.gov Identifier: NCT00530894) (Fig. 2.1) [20, 21]. As the first of two parallel trials completed, the results of PARTNER IB showed that TF TAVR was superior to standard therapy in patients not deemed candidates for surgery [20]. The primary endpoint of all-cause mortality was markedly reduced by 46 % ($P<0.001$). Recently reported 2-years outcomes showed continued encouraging results (Fig. 2.2a) [33]. At 2 years, the primary endpoint of all-cause mortality was reduced from 67.6 % in the standard treatment arm to 43.3 % in the TAVR arm ($P<0.001$).

The PARTNER cohort IA compared TAVR to SAVR and met its non-inferiority endpoint: the all-cause 1-year mortality in the TAVR group was non-inferior to the SAVR group (24.2 % vs. 26.8 %; $P=0.44$; $P=0.001$ for non-inferiority) [21]. Some concerns were raised with regard to early neurologic events that were higher by TAVR as compared to SAVR at 30 days (5.5 % vs. 2.4 %; $P=0.04$) and 1 year (8.3 % vs. 4.3 %; $P=0.04$). Although the recently published 2-year results revealed that stroke rates were similar for TAVR and SAVR during 1 and 2 years with a hazard ratio of 1.22 (95 % CI 0.67–2.23, $P=0.52$), the issue of stroke warrants further investigation and should not be underestimated (Fig. 2.2b, c) [34]. The rate of the composite of all-cause death and stroke was encouragingly similar after TAVR (37.1 %) and SAVR (36.4 %) at 2 years ($P=0.85$).

Ongoing Trials

In the USA, a randomized trial is currently ongoing to evaluate the safety and efficacy of the Medtronic CoreValve™ in the treatment of severe symptomatic AS in patients at high or extreme risk for SAVR (ClinicalTrials.gov Identifier: NCT01240902). The trial consists of two arms. Patients in a high-risk arm will be randomized between SAVR and TAVR; the primary endpoint consists of all-cause mortality at 1 year.

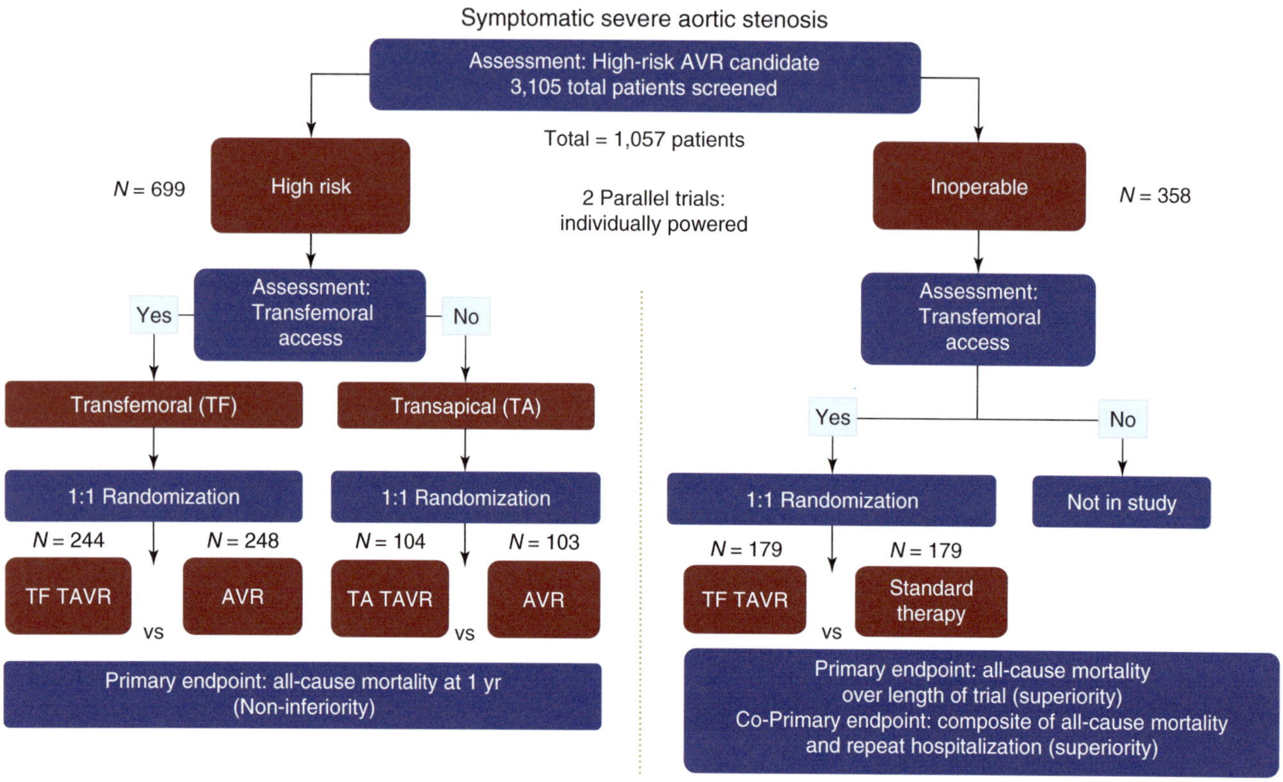

Fig. 2.1 PARTNER trial I design

An extreme risk arm will function as an observational arm in which a composite of all-cause mortality and major stroke is the primary endpoint.

As a sequel to the PARTNER I trial, a second randomized trial (PARTNER II) is currently ongoing. It was designed to investigate the performance and outcomes after TAVR with the next-generation Edwards SAPIEN XT valve, model 9300TFX, as well as the new low-profile 18-Fr NovaFlex™ delivery catheter in patients deemed non-operable (ClinicalTrials.gov Identifier: NCT01314313) (Fig. 2.3). Given the results of the control arm in PARTNER IB, it has been judged that a study comparing TAVR against a "medical management" control group is no longer ethical [35]. Consequently, an "old device" versus "new device" non-inferiority trial was designed. Enrolment was initiated in January 2011, and it is anticipated that primary endpoint results will be published mid-2013.

In Denmark, a phase 2 randomized trial evaluating TAVR in patients ≥70 years of age started enrollment in December 2009 (ClinicalTrials.gov Identifier: NCT01057173). The trial will randomize a total of 280 patients to TAVR ($n = 140$) and SAVR ($n = 140$). The primary endpoint is the composite of all-cause death, myocardial infarction, and stroke at 1 year and is scheduled to be completed late 2013.

In an attempt to expand the indication of TAVR to lower-risk patients, the PARTNER IIA trial will be randomizing patients between TAVR with the SAPIEN XT valve and SAVR in intermediate-risk patients (ClinicalTrials.gov Identifier: NCT01314313) (Fig. 2.3). Similarly, the prospective randomized, international SURTAVR trial will randomize 1,900 intermediate-risk patients between TAVR with the Medtronic CoreValve™ and SAVR at approximately 80 centers throughout the USA, Canada, Europe, and Australia (ClinicalTrials.gov Identifier: NCT01586910).

Alternative Access Sites

Like the TA approach, a subclavian approach allows patients with unfavorable iliofemoral anatomy or extensive disease to be treated with TAVR. Petronio et al. reported a series of 54 patients, showing a procedural success rate of 100 %, a procedural mortality of 0 %, a 30-day mortality of 0 %, and a 6-month mortality of 9.4 % [13]. No specific vascular complications for subclavian access were reported. The subclavian approach is usually performed with the self-expanding CoreValve™ system and can be fully percutaneous [36].

Recently, a transaortic approach with direct access to the ascending aorta through an anterior minithoracotomy has been advocated. Access is gained through a J-shaped partial upper sternotomy or using a small right thoracotomy through

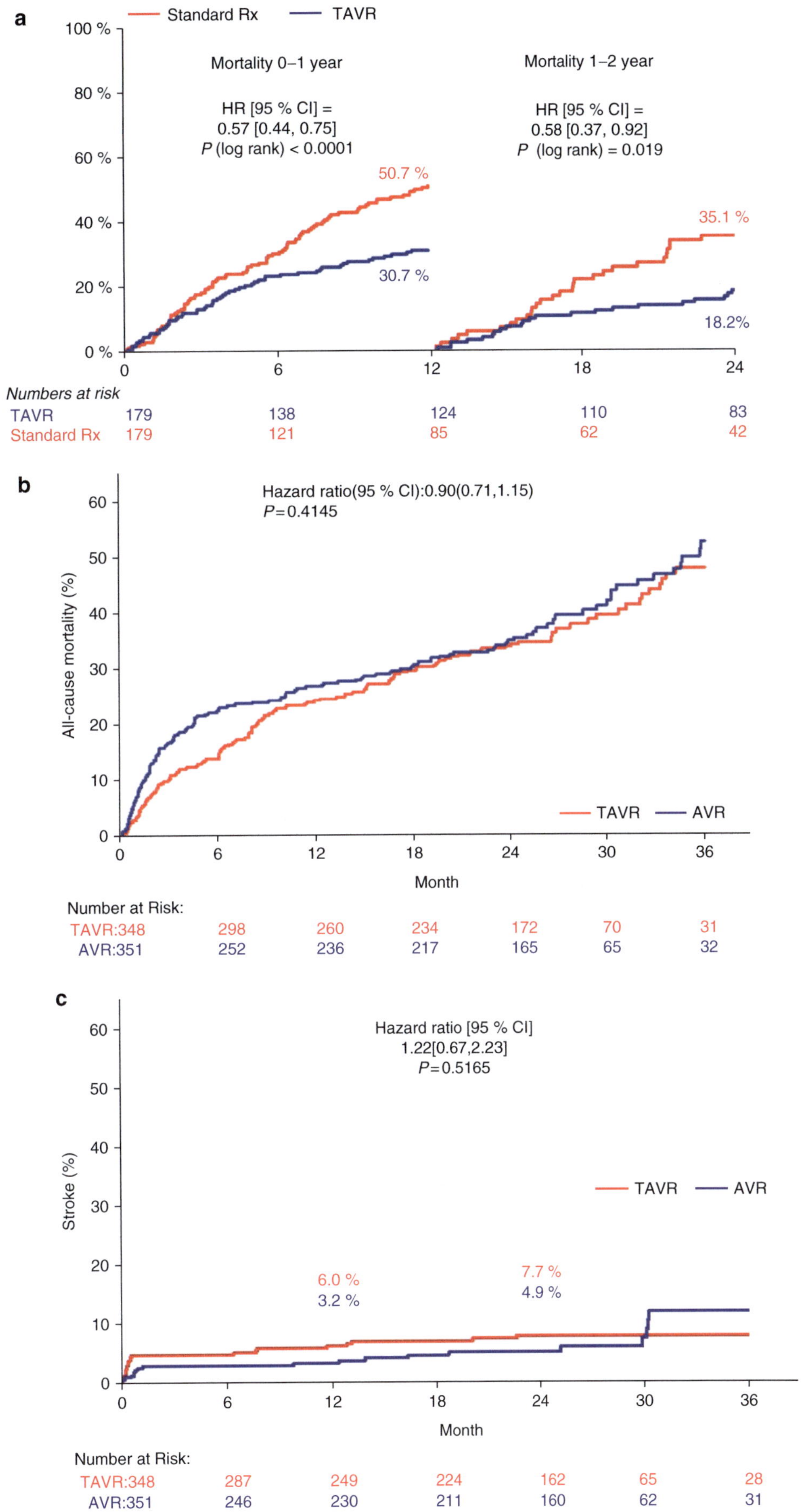

Fig. 2.2 (**a**) A 2-year with 1-year landmark analysis of all-cause mortality Kaplan-Meier curve in PARTNER trial cohort 1B (Reprinted with permission from Leon and colleagues and Makkar and colleagues [20, 33]). (**b**) A 2-year all-cause mortality Kaplan-Meier curve in PARTNER trial cohort 1A (Adapted with permission from Kodali and colleagues [34]). (**c**) A 2-year stroke Kaplan-Meier curve in PARTNER trial cohort 1A (Adapted with permission from Kodali and colleagues [34])

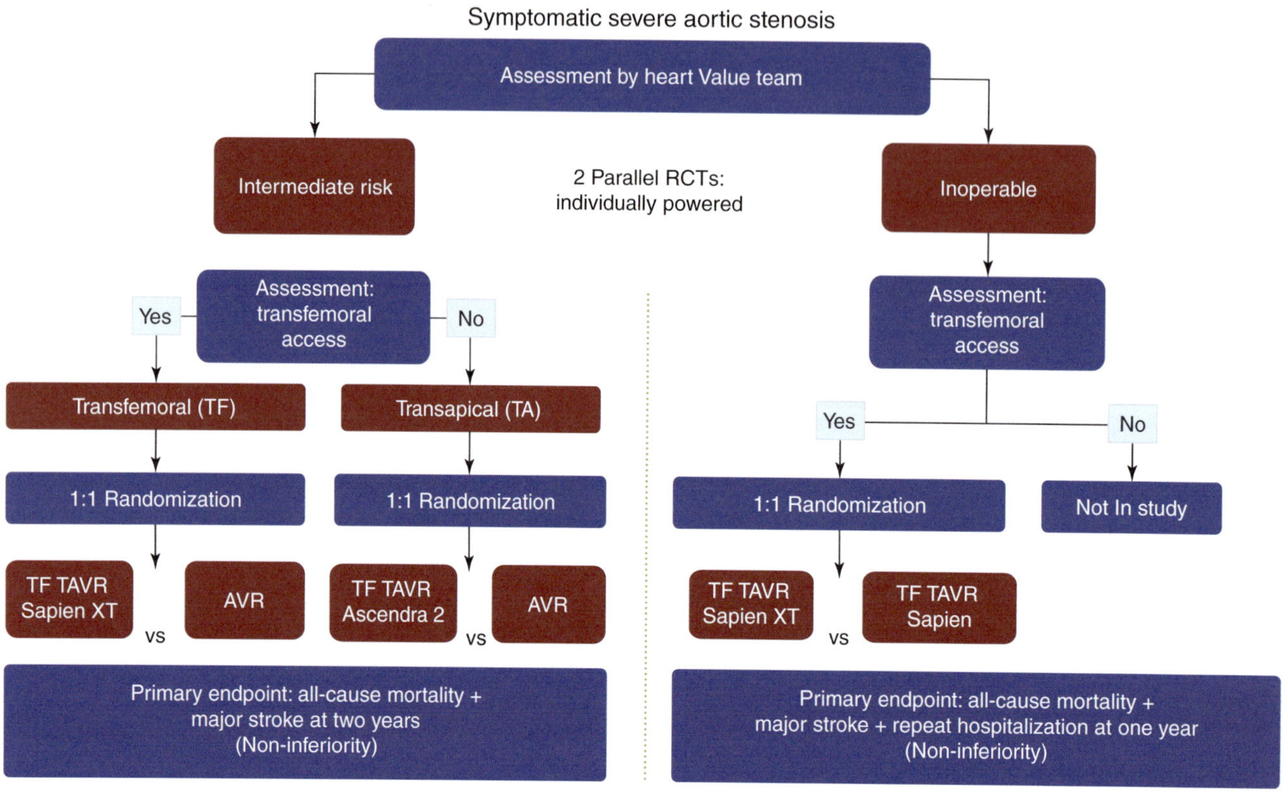

Fig. 2.3 PARTNER trial 2 design

the intercostal space. Avoidance of LV apical injury or inadequate healing along with reduction in postoperative pain and its associated impairment of respiratory dynamics are potential advantages of this novel approach. Encouraging results have been published from small series using both devices [37, 38]. It may be suitable for patients with unfavorable iliofemoral and subclavian anatomy or in whom a TA approach is considered too risky, such as is the case in severe chest deformities, respiratory compromise, or severely reduced ejection fraction.

Valve-In-Valve for Failing Bioprostheses

Since 2007 when the first TAVR was implanted in a failing surgical aortic bioprosthesis in order to avoid redo surgery, interest in this concept has grown and the feasibility and safety has been examined [39, 40]. Piazza and colleagues published a series of 20 patients (mostly TA, 16/20) and reported successful implantation in 18 of 20 patients and in-hospital mortality in 3 patients [41]. Notably, transcatheter heart valves have also been implanted in failing mitral prostheses or even in mitral annuloplasty rings and failing tricuspid prostheses, expanding the potential use of devices originally developed for the aortic position [42, 43].

Valve Durability and Hemodynamic Performance

TAVR has demonstrated excellent immediate and short-term durability of the prosthesis that is comparable to SAVR, with efficacy sustained to at least 3 years [14, 15, 18, 20, 27, 34, 44]. Present data demonstrates that transcatheter heart valves have greater valve areas and lower gradients than surgical bioprostheses (Fig. 2.4) [45], which could reduce the prevalence of prosthesis-patient mismatch [46]. For both the Edwards SAPIEN and Medtronic CoreValve™, there was no evidence of structural or nonstructural valvular deterioration, stent fracture, deformation, or valve migration.

Specific Complications

First-generation devices for TAVR were carefully examined for and demonstrated a non-negligible rate of complications. While newer technologies, improved devices, and more appropriate patient selection and screening—paired with growing operators' experience—have shown reduced occurrence of such complications, they still warrant vigilant attention. Importantly, the original VARC recommendations and the recent publication of the updated VARC-II definitions represent a collaborative effort to improve and facilitate

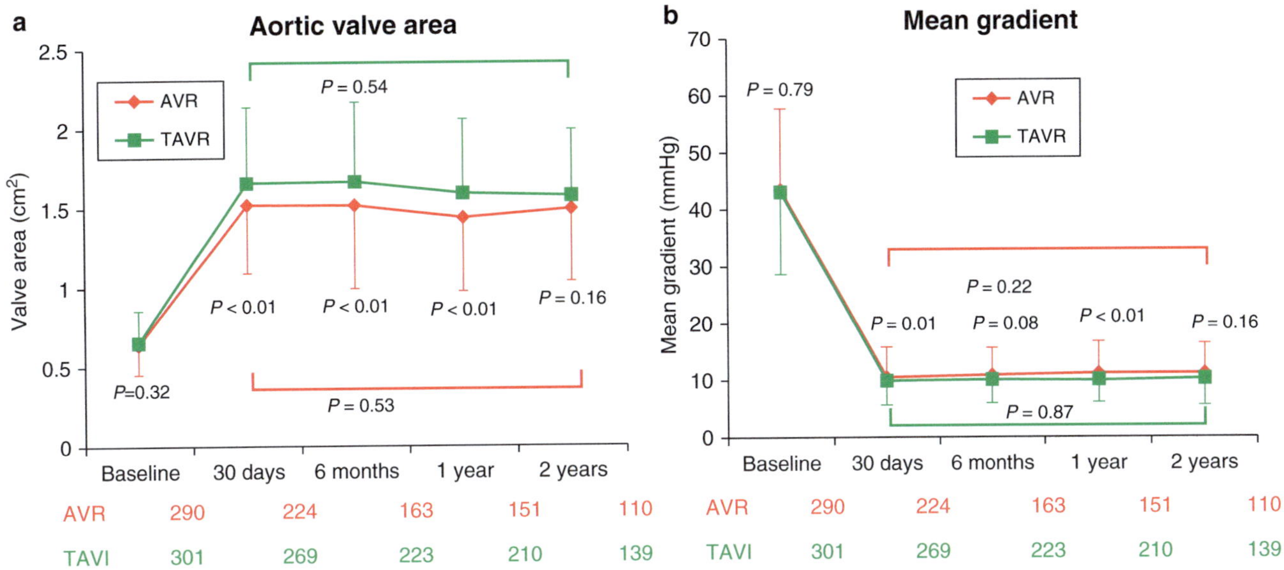

Fig. 2.4 Two-year time trends in hemodynamics after TAVR versus SAVR (Adapted with permission from Kodali and colleagues [34])

identification, report, and adjudication of events post-TAVR and will ensure uniformity and comparability of future published reports [47, 48].

Stroke

Depending on the definition used, reported incidence of stroke in the current literature varies between 1.7 and 8.4 % [8, 13–15, 18, 20, 21]. Neurologic events may occur at different time points during the procedure and may be related to several factors: manipulation of a wire and/or large-diameter catheter through the aortic arch, positioning of the device, calcific embolization during balloon aortic valvuloplasty, and inadequate blood flow to the brain during rapid pacing and device deployment [49, 50]. Moreover, the patient population currently undergoing TAVR consists of very elderly patients in whom the incidence of atrial fibrillation and atherosclerotic disease is high, thus increasing the risk of periprocedural cerebrovascular events [20, 51, 52]. While stroke clearly manifests in clinical symptoms, recent studies have shown "silent" new cerebral ischemia on diffusion-weighted magnetic resonance imaging in up to 70 % of patients [53–55]. Although rarely associated with clinical events, the long-term consequences of these phenomena are unknown.

Initially it was anticipated that stroke associated with TAVR occurred during the procedure, but in-depth analysis of stroke demonstrated a continuous hazard extending beyond the early phase [56]. This hazard was thought to be higher after TAVR in comparison with SAVR. However, recent data showed that while the difference is significant in the first 30 days, the late hazard is similar between TAVR and SAVR [34]. The differential timing of stroke related to TAVR and SAVR warrants further investigation.

Presently, known predictors of early neurological events with TAVR include a prior neurological event, more severe atherosclerotic burden, and smaller valve area. Factors predictive of a constant hazard phase over follow-up include more advanced functional disability, previous stroke, and TA access [56]. The role of atrial fibrillation as a potential mechanism of stroke after TAVR has been emphasized in two recent reports, showing a four times increased risk of stroke [57, 58]. Further work is needed to determine the clinical significance of these findings. Several embolic protection devices are under investigation. Early reports are encouraging, and it is hoped that future use of these devices will lead to a decrease in silent and clinical neurological events after TAVR [59].

Vascular Complications

Vascular complications have been an important limitation of TAVR performed via TF access using first-generation devices. The use of large-diameter catheters and the high-risk characteristics of the current treated population explain the high incidence. Small vessel diameter, severe atherosclerotic disease, bulky calcification, tortuosity, sheath-to-vessel diameter ratio >1.05, and female gender were the main determinants of vascular complications after TF TAVR [60, 61]. The incidence of major vascular complications using the first-generation Edwards SAPIEN system (introducer sheath of 23 and 26 Fr, outer diameter 8.38 and 9.14 mm) varied between 8.3 and 23 % [15, 18, 20, 61–63] and between 1.9 and 14 % [13, 14, 63, 64] using the CoreValve™ system

(18-Fr introducer sheath, outer diameter 7 mm). An association between the occurrence of major vascular complications and survival has been demonstrated by several groups [15, 20, 61–63]. With the use of the latest-generation TAVR systems—with a lower profile 16-Fr introducer sheath—innovative endovascular technique [65, 66], and experienced operators, the rates of major vascular complications have been significantly reduced and have been reported as low as 1 % [67].

Conduction Disturbances

Multiple reports have shown conduction disturbances post-TAVR [68–70]. It is generally accepted that the self-expandable CoreValve™ system, because of the higher and longer-lasting radial forces as well as the deeper implantation site in the left ventricle outflow tract, has a higher rate of pacemaker requirement than the Edwards SAPIEN system. A recent meta-analysis reported that about 28.9 % (23–36 %) of patients implanted with the CoreValve™ valve and 4.9 % (4–6 %) of patients implanted with the Edwards SAPIEN valve will require a new permanent pacemaker [71]. However, it is important to note that the rates reported in the literature have varied greatly. Variations in clinical skill and experience, as well as threshold for pacemaker implantation among physicians, may explain the discrepancy in pacemaker insertion rates in current published series.

Persistent new left bundle branch block has been shown to be the most prevalent ECG finding post-TAVR, being present in up to 55 and 20 % at 1 month after implantation of the CoreValve™ or Edwards SAPIEN valve, respectively [70, 72]. A recent report suggests that this complication is not benign, being an independent predictor of mortality after TAVR, with implantation of the CoreValve™ prosthesis the strongest predictor of new left bundle branch block post-TAVR [73].

Right bundle branch block, low implantation of the prosthesis, small annulus diameter compared to implanted valve size, complete AV block at the time of the procedure, and CoreValve™ device have also been shown to be potential predictors of complete AV block post-TAVR [74, 75]. Recent data suggests that not only bradyarrhythmic events are important for the prediction of post-TAVR pacemaker requirement but that the occurrence of new tachyarrhythmias, such as atrial fibrillation, also portends an important prognostic importance after TAVR [57].

Paravalvular Regurgitation

Significant transvalvular regurgitation is rare after TAVR. However, paravalvular regurgitation, due to incomplete annular sealing, is common. Some degree of paravalvular aortic regurgitation is reported in 80–96 % of cases. In most cases, the degree of regurgitation is trivial or mild. Grade ≥2+ regurgitation is observed in 7–24 % of patients [20, 44, 76–78].

Data from the PARTNER trial shows that significant paravalvular regurgitation ≥2+ is much more prevalent after TAVR than after SAVR (12 % vs. 0.9 %, $P < 0.001$) [21]. During follow-up, regurgitation is more often reduced rather than increased after TAVR (Fig. 2.5a) [27, 34, 44]. Nevertheless, its clinical importance has been emphasized in several reports where grade ≥2+ regurgitation has shown to be an independent predictor of short- and long-term mortality (Fig. 2.5b) [16, 34, 79, 80].

Predictors of ≥1+ paravalvular leakage for the Edwards SAPIEN device have been found to be larger annulus size, height, male sex, age, and cover index ≤8 % (cover index = 100 × [prosthesis diameter − TEE annular diameter size]/prosthesis diameter). In a study, no AR of at least moderate degree was observed with a cover area >8 % [76]. For the CoreValve™ system, greater angle of the left ventricular outflow tract is associated with an increased risk of significant regurgitation, while a depth of 10 mm of the device in relation to the noncoronary cusp is associated with a decreased likelihood of AR [81].

Coronary Obstruction and Myocardial Injury

Coronary obstruction of the left main or the ostium of the right coronary artery is a rare but potentially fatal event [82]. This phenomenon may occur if a calcified native leaflet is displaced over a coronary ostium [83] or if the valve frame or the sealing cuff is positioned directly over a coronary origin. Coronary obstruction may occur either at the time of balloon valvuloplasty or during the TAVR procedure itself. Factors that increase the risk of coronary obstruction include an unusually bulky native leaflet (adjacent to a coronary ostium), a low origin of the coronary ostium (often defined as <12 mm from the basal leaflet insertion as assessed by multidetector computed tomography), a shallow sinus of Valsalva (offering less room for the native leaflet), an oversized prosthesis, and a high prosthesis implantation. Anecdotal cases have reported acute coronary obstructions, most of which were successfully managed by immediate percutaneous angioplasty or bypass surgery [82, 84–86]. Careful evaluation by echocardiography or multidetector CT is invaluable for avoidance of this complication.

Myocardial injury associated with an elevation in cardiac markers following TAVR procedures is common and numerous potential etiologies may explain these occurrences. Specifically, myocardial injury may be caused by some degree of myocardial tissue compression caused by the device itself, global ischemia instigated by short

a

Post procedure	2-Year: None	Trace	Mild	Moderate	Severe
None	17	8	6	1	0
Trace	24	12	11	1	0
Mild	3	10	34	5	0
Moderate	2	1	5	3	0
Severe	0	0	0	0	0

b

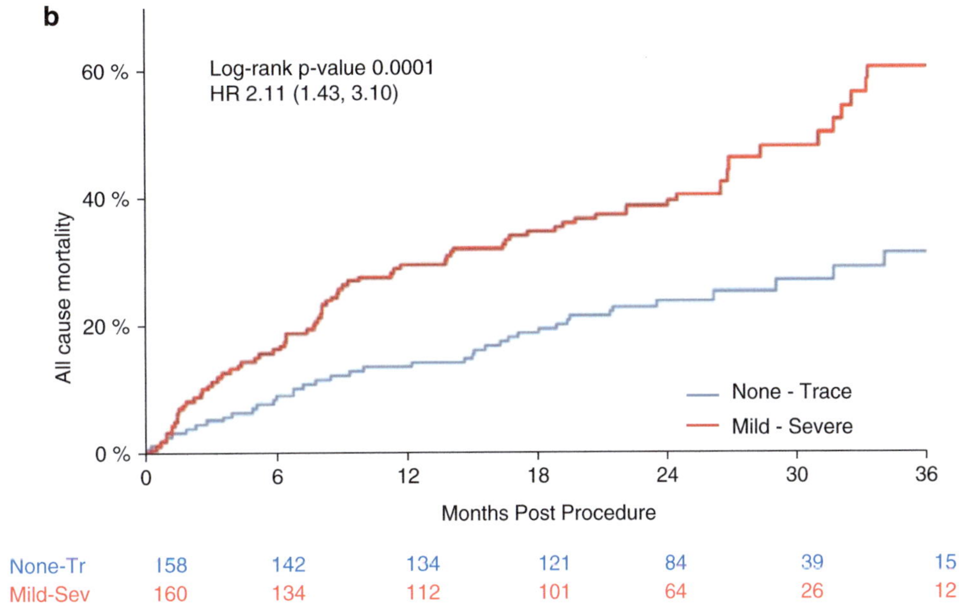

Fig. 2.5 (**a**) Change in paravalvular leak severity over 2-years follow-up (Reproduced with permission from Kodali and colleagues [34]). (**b**) Impact of paravalvular leak on 2-year all-cause mortality (Adapted with permission from Kodali and colleagues [34])

episodes of severe hypotension, or myocardial damage produced by the apical puncture and passage of the large catheter through the ventricular apex when the TA route is employed. Interestingly, transient ST elevations, mostly in the anterior and lateral leads, have been described post-TA TAVR immediately after the procedure in about 20 % of patients and are probably related to incision and suturing of the apex [69]. Rodés-Cabau et al. showed that TAVR is associated with some degree of cardiac troponin T rise above the upper normal limit in 97 % of TF patients and in 100 % of TA patients [87]. After multivariate adjustment, a greater elevation of cardiac troponin T was an independent predictor of mortality at 9 months as well as a factor correlated with less improvement in left ventricular ejection fraction.

Acute Kidney Injury (AKI)

Several reports have focused on AKI, and significant injury (RIFLE ≥2) has been reported with an incidence of approximately 7–8 % [71]. Many of these studies were consistent in identifying blood transfusions as a predictor of AKI, but other factors are associated as well. These features include baseline presence of hypertension, chronic obstructive pulmonary disease, chronic kidney disease, previous myocardial infarction, and the logistic EuroSCORE [88, 89]. The occurrence of AKI has been identified as an independent predictor of in-hospital [89] and late (≥1 year) mortality [88].

Other Complications

Other acute complications, less frequent but potentially lethal, have been described after TAVR, including aortic rupture [90], aortic dissection [91], periaortic hematoma [92], ventricular or aortic embolization of the valve [93], and tamponade [94]. Mitral valve apparatus damage resulting in severe acute mitral regurgitation has also been reported, especially with the TA approach [95]. Not unexpectedly, endocarditis has been described anecdotally [96, 97]. Acute structural valve failure, including prosthesis rupture or malfunctioning leaflet ("frozen leaflet"), is a rare but possible complication after TAVR.

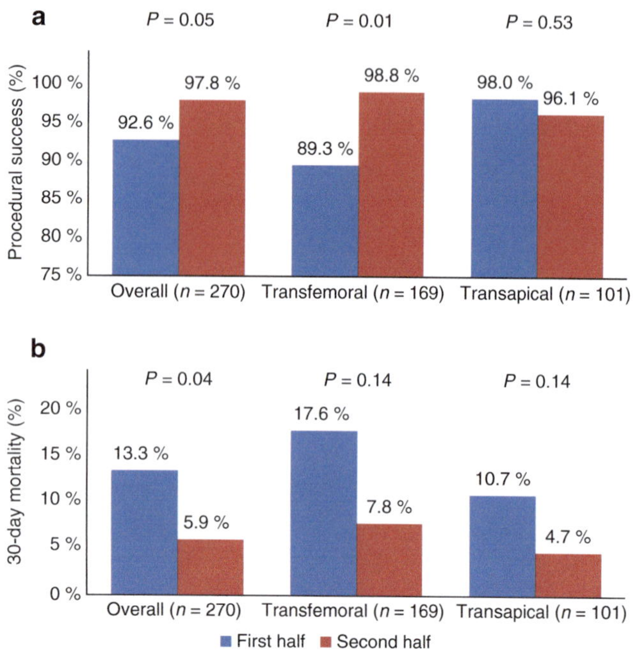

Fig. 2.6 (**a**, **b**) The effect of the learning curve on procedural success (**a**) and 30-day mortality (**b**) after TAVR (Data from Gurvitch and colleagues [98])

Learning Curve

Understanding the importance of patient selection, utilizing better anatomical screening to clarify both the aortic root and iliofemoral geometry, and the development of new devices have led to notable improvements in TAVR outcomes over time. A report highlighting the importance of the learning curve in 270 patients showed that procedural experience was an independent predictor of 30 day survival [98]. Furthermore, the procedural success rate has significantly increased (Fig. 2.6) [98, 99], which has been associated with significantly reduced contrast volumes and radiation doses [100]. With these improvements, overall procedural complications have declined [101].

Conclusions

Currently, SAVR remains the standard of care for most patients with symptomatic severe aortic stenosis. However, with the emergence of several large-scale real-world registries and pivotal PARTNER randomized trials, TAVR has become a viable alternative for patients in whom surgical risk is prohibitive as well as a realistic choice for selected operable patients in whom the risk of either mortality or morbidity is "high." While initial reports confirmed the feasibility and safety of TAVR, observational registries and completed randomized trials have been limited by the use of older-generation devices, enrollment of small numbers of patients, an early learning curve of TAVR operators, self-reported outcomes, and the use of nonstandardized endpoints. While vascular complications and bleeding are declining as TAVR technology improves and continues to miniaturize, stroke and residual paravalvular leak remain important challenges. Embolic protection devices, improved delivery systems, and restriction of the procedure to high-volume centers with a well-trained TAVR heart team offer potential solutions. Improvement of the current technology combined with adoption of standardized definitions [47, 48] for important clinical endpoints will enable meaningful comparisons and future well-conducted randomized trials.

Conflicts of Interest Philippe Généreux has received consulting fees/honoraria from Edwards Lifesciences. Martin B. Leon is a nonpaid member of the Scientific Advisory Boards of Edwards Lifesciences and Medtronic Vascular.

References

1. Ross Jr J, Braunwald E. Aortic stenosis. Circulation. 1968;38 (1 Suppl):61–7.
2. Bach DS, Siao D, Girard SE, Duvernoy C, McCallister Jr BD, Gualano SK. Evaluation of patients with severe symptomatic aortic stenosis who do not undergo aortic valve replacement: the potential role of subjectively overestimated operative risk. Circ Cardiovasc Qual Outcomes. 2009;2(6):533–9.
3. Cribier A, Eltchaninoff H, Bash A, Borenstein N, Tron C, Bauer F, et al. Percutaneous transcatheter implantation of an aortic valve prosthesis for calcific aortic stenosis: first human case description. Circulation. 2002;106(24):3006–8.
4. Bosmans JM, Kefer J, De Bruyne B, Herijgers P, Dubois C, Legrand V, et al. Procedural, 30-day and one year outcome following CoreValve or Edwards transcatheter aortic valve implantation: results of the Belgian national registry. Interact Cardiovasc Thorac Surg. 2011;12(5):762–7.
5. Buellesfeld L, Gerckens U, Schuler G, Bonan R, Kovac J, Serruys PW, et al. 2-year follow-up of patients undergoing transcatheter aortic valve implantation using a self-expanding valve prosthesis. J Am Coll Cardiol. 2011;57(16):1650–7.
6. Cribier A, Eltchaninoff H, Tron C, Bauer F, Agatiello C, Nercolini D, et al. Treatment of calcific aortic stenosis with the percutaneous heart valve: mid-term follow-up from the initial feasibility studies: the French experience. J Am Coll Cardiol. 2006;47(6):1214–23.
7. D'Onofrio A, Rubino P, Fusari M, Salvador L, Musumeci F, Rinaldi M, et al. Clinical and hemodynamic outcomes of "all-comers" undergoing transapical aortic valve implantation: results from the Italian Registry of Trans-Apical Aortic Valve Implantation (I-TA). J Thorac Cardiovasc Surg. 2011;142(4):768–75.
8. Eltchaninoff H, Prat A, Gilard M, Leguerrier A, Blanchard D, Fournial G, et al. Transcatheter aortic valve implantation: early results of the FRANCE (FRench Aortic National CoreValve and Edwards) registry. Eur Heart J. 2011;32(2):191–7.
9. Grube E, Laborde JC, Gerckens U, Felderhoff T, Sauren B, Buellesfeld L, et al. Percutaneous implantation of the CoreValve self-expanding valve prosthesis in high-risk patients with aortic valve disease: the Siegburg first-in-man study. Circulation. 2006;114(15):1616–24.

10. Grube E, Schuler G, Buellesfeld L, Gerckens U, Linke A, Wenaweser P, et al. Percutaneous aortic valve replacement for severe aortic stenosis in high-risk patients using the second- and current third-generation self-expanding CoreValve prosthesis: device success and 30-day clinical outcome. J Am Coll Cardiol. 2007;50(1):69–76.
11. Himbert D, Descoutures F, Al-Attar N, Iung B, Ducrocq G, Detaint D, et al. Results of transfemoral or transapical aortic valve implantation following a uniform assessment in high-risk patients with aortic stenosis. J Am Coll Cardiol. 2009;54(4):303–11.
12. Lefevre T, Kappetein AP, Wolner E, Nataf P, Thomas M, Schachinger V, et al. One year follow-up of the multi-centre European PARTNER transcatheter heart valve study. Eur Heart J. 2011;32(2):148–57.
13. Petronio AS, De Carlo M, Bedogni F, Marzocchi A, Klugmann S, Maisano F, et al. Safety and efficacy of the subclavian approach for transcatheter aortic valve implantation with the CoreValve revalving system. Circ Cardiovasc Interv. 2010;3(4):359–66.
14. Piazza N, Grube E, Gerckens U, den Heijer P, Linke A, Luha O, et al. Procedural and 30-day outcomes following transcatheter aortic valve implantation using the third generation (18 Fr) corevalve revalving system: results from the multicentre, expanded evaluation registry 1-year following CE mark approval. EuroIntervention. 2008;4(2):242–9.
15. Rodes-Cabau J, Webb JG, Cheung A, Ye J, Dumont E, Feindel CM, et al. Transcatheter aortic valve implantation for the treatment of severe symptomatic aortic stenosis in patients at very high or prohibitive surgical risk: acute and late outcomes of the multicenter Canadian experience. J Am Coll Cardiol. 2010;55(11):1080–90.
16. Tamburino C, Capodanno D, Ramondo A, Petronio AS, Ettori F, Santoro G, et al. Incidence and predictors of early and late mortality after transcatheter aortic valve implantation in 663 patients with severe aortic stenosis. Circulation. 2011;123(3):299–308.
17. Thomas M, Schymik G, Walther T, Himbert D, Lefevre T, Treede H, et al. One-year outcomes of cohort 1 in the Edwards SAPIEN Aortic Bioprosthesis European Outcome (SOURCE) registry: the European registry of transcatheter aortic valve implantation using the Edwards SAPIEN valve. Circulation. 2011;124(4):425–33.
18. Thomas M, Schymik G, Walther T, Himbert D, Lefevre T, Treede H, et al. Thirty-day results of the SAPIEN aortic Bioprosthesis European Outcome (SOURCE) Registry: A European registry of transcatheter aortic valve implantation using the Edwards SAPIEN valve. Circulation. 2010;122(1):62–9.
19. Webb JG, Chandavimol M, Thompson CR, Ricci DR, Carere RG, Munt BI, et al. Percutaneous aortic valve implantation retrograde from the femoral artery. Circulation. 2006;113(6):842–50.
20. Leon MB, Smith CR, Mack M, Miller DC, Moses JW, Svensson LG, et al. Transcatheter aortic-valve implantation for aortic stenosis in patients who cannot undergo surgery. N Engl J Med. 2010; 363(17):1597–607.
21. Smith CR, Leon MB, Mack MJ, Miller DC, Moses JW, Svensson LG, et al. Transcatheter versus surgical aortic-valve replacement in high-risk patients. N Engl J Med. 2011;364(23):2187–98.
22. Cribier A, Eltchaninoff H, Tron C, Bauer F, Agatiello C, Sebagh L, et al. Early experience with percutaneous transcatheter implantation of heart valve prosthesis for the treatment of end-stage inoperable patients with calcific aortic stenosis. J Am Coll Cardiol. 2004;43(4):698–703.
23. Grube E, Laborde JC, Zickmann B, Gerckens U, Felderhoff T, Sauren B, et al. First report on a human percutaneous transluminal implantation of a self-expanding valve prosthesis for interventional treatment of aortic valve stenosis. Catheter Cardiovasc Interv. 2005;66(4):465–9.
24. Kodali SK, O'Neill WW, Moses JW, Williams M, Smith CR, Tuzcu M, et al. Early and late (one year) outcomes following transcatheter aortic valve implantation in patients with severe aortic stenosis (from the United States REVIVAL trial). Am J Cardiol. 2011; 107(7):1058–64.
25. Svensson LG, Dewey T, Kapadia S, Roselli EE, Stewart A, Williams M, et al. United States feasibility study of transcatheter insertion of a stented aortic valve by the left ventricular apex. Ann Thorac Surg. 2008;86(1):46–54; discussion -5.
26. Walther T, Kasimir MT, Doss M, Schuler G, Simon P, Schachinger V, et al. One-year interim follow-up results of the TRAVERCE trial: the initial feasibility study for trans-apical aortic-valve implantation. Eur J Cardiothorac Surg. 2011;39(4):532–7.
27. Ussia GP, Barbanti M, Petronio AS, Tarantini G, Ettori F, Colombo A, et al. Transcatheter aortic valve implantation: 3-year outcomes of self-expanding CoreValve prosthesis. Eur Heart J. 2012;33(8):969–76.
28. Wood S. TAVR registry updates ADVANCE the field, raise hopes for lower stroke rates. 2012. http://www.theheart.org/article/1374163.do.
29. Zahn R, Gerckens U, Grube E, Linke A, Sievert H, Eggebrecht H, et al. Transcatheter aortic valve implantation: first results from a multi-centre real-world registry. Eur Heart J. 2011;32(2):198–204.
30. Moat NE, Ludman P, de Belder MA, Bridgewater B, Cunningham AD, Young CP, et al. Long-term outcomes after transcatheter aortic valve implantation in high-risk patients with severe aortic stenosis: the U.K. TAVR (United Kingdom Transcatheter Aortic Valve Implantation) Registry. J Am Coll Cardiol. 2011; 58(20):2130–8.
31. Kappetein AP, Head SJ, Treede H, Reichenspurner H, Mohr FW, Walther T. What is the evidence allowing us to state that transcatheter aortic valve replacement via the femoral artery is a more attractive option compared to transapical valve replacement? EuroIntervention. 2011;7(8):903–4.
32. Gilard M, Eltchaninoff H, Iung B, Donzeau-Gouge P, Chevreul K, Fajadet J, et al. Registry of transcatheter aortic-valve implantation in high-risk patients. N Engl J Med. 2012;366(18):1705–15.
33. Makkar RR, Fontana GP, Jilaihawi H, Kapadia S, Pichard AD, Douglas PS, et al. Transcatheter aortic-valve replacement for inoperable severe aortic stenosis. N Engl J Med. 2012;366(18):1696–704.
34. Kodali SK, Williams MR, Smith CR, Svensson LG, Webb JG, Makkar RR, et al. Two-year outcomes after transcatheter or surgical aortic-valve replacement. N Engl J Med. 2012;366(18):1686–95.
35. Head SJ, Kaul S, Bogers AJ, Kappetein AP. Non-inferiority study design: lessons to be learned from cardiovascular trials. Eur Heart J. 2012;33(11):1318–24.
36. Van Mieghem NM, Luthen C, Oei F, Schultz C, Ligthart J, Kappetein AP, et al. Completely percutaneous transcatheter aortic valve implantation through transaxillary route: an evolving concept. EuroIntervention. 2012;7(11):1340–2.
37. Bapat V, Khawaja MZ, Attia R, Narayana A, Wilson K, Macgillivray K, et al. Transaortic transcatheter aortic valve implantation using Edwards SAPIEN valve: a novel approach. Catheter Cardiovasc Interv. 2012;79(5):733–40.
38. Latsios G, Gerckens U, Grube E. Transaortic transcatheter aortic valve implantation: a novel approach for the truly "no-access option" patients. Catheter Cardiovasc Interv. 2010;75(7):1129–36.
39. Wenaweser P, Buellesfeld L, Gerckens U, Grube E. Percutaneous aortic valve replacement for severe aortic regurgitation in degenerated bioprosthesis: the first valve in valve procedure using the Corevalve Revalving system. Catheter Cardiovasc Interv. 2007; 70(5):760–4.
40. Gurvitch R, Cheung A, Ye J, Wood DA, Willson AB, Toggweiler S, et al. Transcatheter valve-in-valve implantation for failed surgical bioprosthetic valves. J Am Coll Cardiol. 2011;58(21):2196–209.
41. Piazza N, Bleiziffer S, Brockmann G, Hendrick R, Deutsch MA, Opitz A, et al. Transcatheter aortic valve implantation for failing surgical aortic bioprosthetic valve: from concept to clinical application and evaluation (part 2). JACC Cardiovasc Interv. 2011;4(7): 733–42.

42. Cerillo AG, Chiaramonti F, Murzi M, Bevilacqua S, Cerone E, Palmieri C, et al. Transcatheter valve in valve implantation for failed mitral and tricuspid bioprosthesis. Catheter Cardiovasc Interv. 2011;78(7):987–95.
43. de Weger A, Ewe SH, Delgado V, Bax JJ. First-in-man implantation of a trans-catheter aortic valve in a mitral annuloplasty ring: novel treatment modality for failed mitral valve repair. Eur J Cardiothorac Surg. 2011;39(6):1054–6.
44. Gurvitch R, Wood DA, Tay EL, Leipsic J, Ye J, Lichtenstein SV, et al. Transcatheter aortic valve implantation: durability of clinical and hemodynamic outcomes beyond 3 years in a large patient cohort. Circulation. 2010;122(13):1319–27.
45. Clavel MA, Webb JG, Pibarot P, Altwegg L, Dumont E, Thompson C, et al. Comparison of the hemodynamic performance of percutaneous and surgical bioprostheses for the treatment of severe aortic stenosis. J Am Coll Cardiol. 2009;53(20):1883–91.
46. Head SJ, Mokhles MM, Osnabrugge RL, Pibarot P, Mack MJ, Takkenberg JJ, et al. The impact of prosthesis-patient mismatch on long-term survival after aortic valve replacement: a systematic review and meta-analysis of 34 observational studies comprising 27 186 patients with 133 141 patient-years. Eur Heart J. 2012; 33(12):1518–29.
47. Leon MB, Piazza N, Nikolsky E, Blackstone EH, Cutlip DE, Kappetein AP, et al. Standardized endpoint definitions for transcatheter aortic valve implantation clinical trials: a consensus report from the Valve Academic Research Consortium. Eur Heart J. 2011;32(2):205–17.
48. Kappetein AP, Head S, Généreux P, et al. Updated standardized endpoint definitions for transcatheter aortic valve replacement: the VARC-2 consensus document. J Am Coll Cardiol. 2012;60(15): 1438–54. In press.
49. Drews T, Pasic M, Buz S, Unbehaun A, Dreysse S, Kukucka M, et al. Transcranial Doppler sound detection of cerebral microembolism during transapical aortic valve implantation. Thorac Cardiovasc Surg. 2011;59(4):237–42.
50. Szeto WY, Augoustides JG, Desai ND, Moeller P, McGarvey ML, Walsh E, et al. Cerebral embolic exposure during transfemoral and transapical transcatheter aortic valve replacement. J Card Surg. 2011;26(4):348–54.
51. Karalis DG, Quinn V, Victor MF, Ross JJ, Polansky M, Spratt KA, et al. Risk of catheter-related emboli in patients with atherosclerotic debris in the thoracic aorta. Am Heart J. 1996;131(6):1149–55.
52. Kronzon I, Tunick PA. Aortic atherosclerotic disease and stroke. Circulation. 2006;114(1):63–75.
53. Ghanem A, Muller A, Nahle CP, Kocurek J, Werner N, Hammerstingl C, et al. Risk and fate of cerebral embolism after transfemoral aortic valve implantation: a prospective pilot study with diffusion-weighted magnetic resonance imaging. J Am Coll Cardiol. 2010;55(14):1427–32.
54. Kahlert P, Knipp SC, Schlamann M, Thielmann M, Al-Rashid F, Weber M, et al. Silent and apparent cerebral ischemia after percutaneous transfemoral aortic valve implantation: a diffusion-weighted magnetic resonance imaging study. Circulation. 2010;121(7): 870–8.
55. Rodes-Cabau J, Dumont E, Boone RH, Larose E, Bagur R, Gurvitch R, et al. Cerebral embolism following transcatheter aortic valve implantation: comparison of transfemoral and transapical approaches. J Am Coll Cardiol. 2011;57(1):18–28.
56. Miller DC, Blackstone EH, Mack MJ, Svensson LG, Kodali SK, Kapadia S, et al. Transcatheter (TAVR) versus surgical (AVR) aortic valve replacement: occurrence, hazard, risk factors, and consequences of neurologic events in the PARTNER trial. J Thorac Cardiovasc Surg. 2012;143(4):832–43.e13.
57. Amat-Santos IJ, Rodes-Cabau J, Urena M, Delarochelliere R, Doyle D, Bagur R, et al. Incidence, predictive factors, and prognostic value of new-onset atrial fibrillation following transcatheter aortic valve implantation. J Am Coll Cardiol. 2012;59(2):178–88.
58. Nuis RJ, Van Mieghem NM, Schultz CJ, Moelker A, van der Boon RM, van Geuns RJ, et al. Frequency and causes of stroke during or after transcatheter aortic valve implantation. Am J Cardiol. 2012; 109(11):1637–43.
59. Nietlispach F, Wijesinghe N, Gurvitch R, Tay E, Carpenter JP, Burns C, et al. An embolic deflection device for aortic valve interventions. JACC Cardiovasc Interv. 2010;3(11):1133–8.
60. Hayashida K, Lefevre T, Chevalier B, Hovasse T, Romano M, Garot P, et al. Transfemoral aortic valve implantation new criteria to predict vascular complications. JACC Cardiovasc Interv. 2011;4(8): 851–8.
61. Généreux P, Webb JG, Svensson LG, Kodali SK, Satler L, Fearon WF, Davidson CJ, Eisenhauer AC, Makkar RR, Bergman G, Babaliaros V, Bavaria JE, Velazquez OC, Williams MR, Hueter I, Xu K, Leon MB. Vascular complications after TAVR: insights from the PARTNER trial. J Am Coll Cardiol. 2012;60(12):1043–52. In press.
62. Ducrocq G, Francis F, Serfaty JM, Himbert D, Maury JM, Pasi N, et al. Vascular complications of transfemoral aortic valve implantation with the Edwards SAPIEN prosthesis: incidence and impact on outcome. EuroIntervention. 2010;5(6):666–72.
63. Tchetche D, Dumonteil N, Sauguet A, Descoutures F, Luz A, Garcia O, et al. Thirty-day outcome and vascular complications after transarterial aortic valve implantation using both Edwards SAPIEN and Medtronic CoreValve bioprostheses in a mixed population. EuroIntervention. 2010;5(6):659–65.
64. Van Mieghem NM, Nuis RJ, Piazza N, Apostolos T, Ligthart J, Schultz C, et al. Vascular complications with transcatheter aortic valve implantation using the 18 Fr Medtronic CoreValve System: the Rotterdam experience. EuroIntervention. 2010;5(6):673–9.
65. Genereux P, Kodali S, Leon MB, Smith CR, Ben-Gal Y, Kirtane AJ, et al. Clinical outcomes using a new crossover balloon occlusion technique for percutaneous closure after transfemoral aortic valve implantation. JACC Cardiovasc Interv. 2011;4(8):861–7.
66. Hayashida K, Lefevre T, Chevalier B, Hovasse T, Romano M, Garot P, et al. True percutaneous approach for transfemoral aortic valve implantation using the Prostar XL device: impact of learning curve on vascular complications. JACC Cardiovasc Interv. 2012; 5(2):207–14.
67. Toggweiler S, Gurvitch R, Leipsic J, Wood DA, Willson AB, Binder RK, et al. Percutaneous aortic valve replacement vascular outcomes with a fully percutaneous procedure. J Am Coll Cardiol. 2012;59(2):113–8.
68. Bleiziffer S, Ruge H, Horer J, Hutter A, Geisbusch S, Brockmann G, et al. Predictors for new-onset complete heart block after transcatheter aortic valve implantation. JACC Cardiovasc Interv. 2010; 3(5):524–30.
69. Gutierrez M, Rodes-Cabau J, Bagur R, Doyle D, DeLarochelliere R, Bergeron S, et al. Electrocardiographic changes and clinical outcomes after transapical aortic valve implantation. Am Heart J. 2009;158(2):302–8.
70. Piazza N, Onuma Y, Jesserun E, Kint PP, Maugenest AM, Anderson RH, et al. Early and persistent intraventricular conduction abnormalities and requirements for pacemaking after percutaneous replacement of the aortic valve. JACC Cardiovasc Interv. 2008;1(3):310–6.
71. Généreux P, Head SJ, Van Mieghem NM, Kodali S, Kirtane AJ, Xu K, et al. Clinical outcomes after transcatheter aortic valve replacement using Valve Academic Research Consortium definitions: a weighted meta-analysis of 3,519 patients from 16 studies. J Am Coll Cardiol. 2012;59:2317–26.
72. Godin M, Eltchaninoff H, Furuta A, Tron C, Anselme F, Bejar K, et al. Frequency of conduction disturbances after transcatheter implantation of an Edwards SAPIEN aortic valve prosthesis. Am J Cardiol. 2010;106(5):707–12.
73. Houthuizen P, Van Garsse LA, Poels TT, de Jaegere P, van der Boon RM, Swinkels BM, et al. Left bundle branch block induced by

transcatheter aortic valve implantation increases risk of death. Circulation. 2012;126(6):720–8.
74. Erkapic D, Kim WK, Weber M, Mollmann H, Berkowitsch A, Zaltsberg S, et al. Electrocardiographic and further predictors for permanent pacemaker requirement after transcatheter aortic valve implantation. Europace. 2010;12(8):1188–90.
75. Ferreira ND, Caeiro D, Adao L, Oliveira M, Goncalves H, Ribeiro J, et al. Incidence and predictors of permanent pacemaker requirement after transcatheter aortic valve implantation with a self-expanding bioprosthesis. Pacing Clin Electrophysiol. 2010;33(11): 1364–72.
76. Detaint D, Lepage L, Himbert D, Brochet E, Messika-Zeitoun D, Iung B, et al. Determinants of significant paravalvular regurgitation after transcatheter aortic valve: implantation impact of device and annulus discongruence. JACC Cardiovasc Interv. 2009;2(9):821–7.
77. Godino C, Maisano F, Montorfano M, Latib A, Chieffo A, Michev I, et al. Outcomes after transcatheter aortic valve implantation with both Edwards-SAPIEN and CoreValve devices in a single center: the Milan experience. JACC Cardiovasc Interv. 2010;3(11): 1110–21.
78. Rajani R, Kakad M, Khawaja MZ, Lee L, James R, Saha M, et al. Paravalvular regurgitation one year after transcatheter aortic valve implantation. Catheter Cardiovasc Interv. 2010;75(6):868–72.
79. Abdel-Wahab M, Zahn R, Horack M, Gerckens U, Schuler G, Sievert H, et al. Aortic regurgitation after transcatheter aortic valve implantation: incidence and early outcome. Results from the German transcatheter aortic valve interventions registry. Heart. 2011;97(11):899–906.
80. Gotzmann M, Pljakic A, Bojara W, Lindstaedt M, Ewers A, Germing A, et al. Transcatheter aortic valve implantation in patients with severe symptomatic aortic valve stenosis-predictors of mortality and poor treatment response. Am Heart J. 2011;162(2): 238–45.e1.
81. Sherif MA, Abdel-Wahab M, Stocker B, Geist V, Richardt D, Tolg R, et al. Anatomic and procedural predictors of paravalvular aortic regurgitation after implantation of the Medtronic CoreValve bioprosthesis. J Am Coll Cardiol. 2010;56(20):1623–9.
82. Gogas BD, Zacharoulis AA, Antoniadis AG. Acute coronary occlusion following TAVR. Catheter Cardiovasc Interv. 2011;77(3): 435–8.
83. Saia F, Marrozzini C, Marzocchi A. Displacement of calcium nodules of the native valve as a possible cause of left main occlusion following transcatheter aortic valve implantation. J Invasive Cardiol. 2011;23(5):E106–9.
84. Kukucka M, Pasic M, Dreysse S, Hetzer R. Delayed subtotal coronary obstruction after transapical aortic valve implantation. Interact Cardiovasc Thorac Surg. 2011;12(1):57–60.
85. Stabile E, Sorropago G, Cioppa A, Cota L, Agrusta M, Lucchetti V, et al. Acute left main obstructions following TAVR. EuroIntervention. 2010;6(1):100–5.
86. Walther T, Falk V, Kempfert J, Borger MA, Fassl J, Chu MW, et al. Transapical minimally invasive aortic valve implantation; the initial 50 patients. Eur J Cardiothorac Surg. 2008;33(6):983–8.
87. Rodes-Cabau J, Gutierrez M, Bagur R, De Larochelliere R, Doyle D, Cote M, et al. Incidence, predictive factors, and prognostic value of myocardial injury following uncomplicated transcatheter aortic valve implantation. J Am Coll Cardiol. 2011;57(20):1988–99.
88. Nuis RJ, Van Mieghem NM, Tzikas A, Piazza N, Otten AM, Cheng J, et al. Frequency, determinants, and prognostic effects of acute kidney injury and red blood cell transfusion in patients undergoing transcatheter aortic valve implantation. Catheter Cardiovasc Interv. 2011;77(6):881–9.
89. Bagur R, Webb JG, Nietlispach F, Dumont E, De Larochelliere R, Doyle D, et al. Acute kidney injury following transcatheter aortic valve implantation: predictive factors, prognostic value, and comparison with surgical aortic valve replacement. Eur Heart J. 2010;31(7):865–74.
90. Aminian A, Lalmand J, El Nakadi B. Perforation of the descending thoracic aorta during transcatheter aortic valve implantation (TAVR): an unexpected and dramatic procedural complication. Catheter Cardiovasc Interv. 2011;77(7):1076–8.
91. Gerber RT, Osborn M, Mikhail GW. Delayed mortality from aortic dissection post transcatheter aortic valve implantation (TAVR): the tip of the iceberg. Catheter Cardiovasc Interv. 2010;76(2): 202–4.
92. Généreux P, Reiss GR, Kodali SK, Williams MR, Hahn RT. Periaortic hematoma after transcatheter aortic valve replacement: description of a new complication. Catheter Cardiovasc Interv. 2012;79(5):766–76.
93. Tay EL, Gurvitch R, Wijeysinghe N, Nietlispach F, Leipsic J, Wood DA, et al. Outcome of patients after transcatheter aortic valve embolization. JACC Cardiovasc Interv. 2011;4(2):228–34.
94. Lange R, Bleiziffer S, Piazza N, Mazzitelli D, Hutter A, Tassani-Prell P, et al. Incidence and treatment of procedural cardiovascular complications associated with trans-arterial and trans-apical interventional aortic valve implantation in 412 consecutive patients. Eur J Cardiothorac Surg. 2011;40(5):1105–13.
95. Masson JB, Kovac J, Schuler G, Ye J, Cheung A, Kapadia S, et al. Transcatheter aortic valve implantation: review of the nature, management, and avoidance of procedural complications. JACC Cardiovasc Interv. 2009;2(9):811–20.
96. Head SJ, Dewey TM, Mack MJ. Fungal endocarditis after transfemoral aortic valve implantation. Catheter Cardiovasc Interv. 2011;78(7):1017–9.
97. Piazza N, Marra S, Webb J, D'Amico M, Rinaldi M, Boffini M, et al. Two cases of aneurysm of the anterior mitral valve leaflet associated with transcatheter aortic valve endocarditis: a mere coincidence? J Thorac Cardiovasc Surg. 2010;140(3):e36–8.
98. Gurvitch R, Tay EL, Wijesinghe N, Ye J, Nietlispach F, Wood DA, et al. Transcatheter aortic valve implantation: lessons from the learning curve of the first 270 high-risk patients. Catheter Cardiovasc Interv. 2011;78(7):977–84.
99. Grube E, Buellesfeld L, Mueller R, Sauren B, Zickmann B, Nair D, et al. Progress and current status of percutaneous aortic valve replacement: results of three device generations of the CoreValve Revalving system. Circ Cardiovasc Interv. 2008;1(3): 167–75.
100. Alli OO, Booker JD, Lennon RJ, Greason KL, Rihal CS, Holmes Jr DR. Transcatheter aortic valve implantation: assessing the learning curve. JACC Cardiovasc Interv. 2012;5(1):72–9.
101. Nuis RJ, van Mieghem NM, van der Boon RM, van Geuns RJ, Schultz CJ, Oei FB, et al. Effect of experience on results of transcatheter aortic valve implantation using a Medtronic CoreValve System. Am J Cardiol. 2011;107(12):1824–9.

Transcatheter Aortic Valve Replacement: Current Evidence from Large Multicenter Registries

3

Shikhar Agarwal and Samir Kapadia

Abstract

Background: Surgical aortic valve replacement (SAVR) has been considered as a standard of care for treatment of severe symptomatic aortic stenosis (AS). Transcatheter aortic valve replacement (TAVR) has emerged as an attractive alternative for treatment of severe AS in high-risk patients. Despite several large multicenter registries, only one randomized trial (PARTNER) has been published. In the following section, we have summarized the safety and efficacy data from the large multicenter registries.

Results: Although there was a significant degree of heterogeneity in estimates from various registries, the current data have established a reasonable degree of safety and efficacy of TAVR in treatment of severe AS. The 30-day mortality rate ranged from 5.6 % to 13.8 % across the registries. One-year mortality rate ranged from 14.9 % to 36.9 % across all multicenter registries. Besides mortality, the section also reviews incidence rates of several endpoints including myocardial infarction, stroke, conduction abnormalities, arrhythmias and so on. Notably, the 30-day stroke incidence ranged between 1.2 to 4.4 % across the multicenter registries, which was considerably lower than that observed in the PARTNER trial.

Conclusions: TAVR has demonstrated a great degree of promise in treatment of severe symptomatic AS, with favorable short-term and medium-term outcomes. The data from the available multicenter registries has clearly demonstrated that patient selection would be the key to cost-effective utilization of this revolutionary technology.

Keywords

Multicenter registries • Transcatheter aortic valve replacement • Mortality • Permanent pacemaker • Aortic stenosis • Aortic regurgitation • Stroke • Edwards SAPIEN • CoreValve

Introduction

Degenerative aortic stenosis (AS) is one of the most commonly acquired valvular heart diseases in aging adults [1]. Its prevalence has been estimated to be approximately 4 % in individuals aged 80 years or more [1]. Due to increases in life expectancy over the last few decades, the absolute number of patients with degenerative AS continues to increase. In patients with symptomatic AS, surgical aortic valve replacement (SAVR) has been the treatment of choice for over 4 decades. SAVR has been associated with significant improvement in the long-term prognosis as well as quality of life in patients with severe symptomatic AS [2]. The

S. Agarwal, MD, MPH, CPH (✉)
Department of Cardiovascular Medicine,
Cleveland Clinic, 9500 Euclid Avenue, Desk J3-5,
Cleveland, OH 44195, USA
e-mail: agarwas@ccf.org, dr.shikhar.agarwal@gmail.com

S. Kapadia, MD, FACC
Department of Interventional Cardiology,
Sones Cardiac Catheterization Laboratories,
Interventional Cardiology Fellowship Program, Cleveland Clinic,
9500 Euclid Avenue, Desk J2-3, Cleveland, OH 44195, USA
e-mail: kapadis@ccf.org

J.K. Min et al. (eds.), *Multimodality Imaging for Transcatheter Aortic Valve Replacement*,
DOI 10.1007/978-1-4471-2798-7_3, © Springer-Verlag London 2014

overall mortality for isolated SAVR ranges from 2.5 to 4.0 % [3–5]. However, it is estimated that roughly 30–60 % of the elderly patients with symptomatic AS are deemed at "high risk" for conventional SAVR [5–7] and often are denied surgical therapy for this as well as an array of other reasons. In addition, the operative risk of SAVR in octogenarians and nonagenarians has been estimated to be 4.9–9.6 %, which is significantly higher than the baseline operative risk in younger patients [8]. In the presence of multiple medical comorbidities, the operative risk in some patients is estimated to be in excess 50 %, and this population is typically defined as inoperable [8–11].

Due to the fact that a large proportion of high-risk surgical candidates were historically denied SAVR, minimal-access AVR has been developed to mitigate the risk associated with open sternotomy and other complexities associated SAVR. Rapid advancements in transcatheter technology have led to the innovation of transcatheter aortic valve replacement (TAVR). The first human TAVR was performed by Cribier and colleagues in 2002 [12]. Since then, there has been a rapid surge in the utilization of TAVR to treat high-risk patients with severe symptomatic AS. The rapid worldwide dissemination of this disruptive technique carries the hazard that patients that are candidates for conventional surgical AVR would be treated percutaneously. The "off-label" use of TAVR has been estimated to be as high as 67 % in some centers [13].

The multicenter randomized controlled *Placement of Aortic Transcatheter Valves* (PARTNER) trial has demonstrated similarity of surgical AVR and TAVR with respect to mortality, reduction in symptoms, and improvement in valve hemodynamics, up to 2 years of follow-up [14]. While robust clinical evidence emanating from rigorously conducted randomized trials is a cornerstone of premarket conformity assessment processes, it is of paramount importance to recognize the shortcomings of these premarket clinical assessments. The follow-up periods are relatively short; the study populations are preselected and are prone to selection biases. Further, the initial sites for any large-scale device clinical trial typically comprise large academic centers with meticulous oversight. Upon approval of TAVR devices—wherein less-experienced sites begin to perform TAVR and devices are used outside of specific trial inclusion and exclusion criteria—numerous important clinical insights become available. Specifically, the relatively small patient numbers in premarket investigations do not allow detection of rare or infrequent complications or those that occur upon long-term follow-up. Thus, as a part of a continuous quality initiative process, it is vital for any beginning TAVR program to institute a program of routine post-marketing surveillance for identification of long-term outcomes and risks associated with the use of new technology.

As formal post-marketing surveillance programs are instituted, outcome data from multicenter and/or international registries will become increasingly important. The observational studies are generally independent from industry and independently funded. Since these multicenter registries are largely driven by the scientific interests of participating hospitals, there has been an increase in the willingness of large tertiary care centers to participate and contribute information related to experience and outcomes. Many countries including the USA have instituted mandatory reporting of patients undergoing TAVR, which further renders the collected data robust and comprehensive.

Available Devices

Currently, there are two device types available for TAVR: balloon-expandable Edwards valve (Edwards Lifesciences, USA) and the self-expanding CoreValve system (Medtronic, Inc, USA). The first two generations of the Edwards valve (Cribier-Edwards and Edwards SAPIEN) comprised three leaflets of equine and bovine pericardium, respectively, mounted in a stainless steel frame. The valves were implanted using 22 and 24 Fr delivery catheters. The Edwards SAPIEN XT is a third generation of the balloon-expandable Edwards valve, which consists of a tri-leaflet bovine pericardial valve mounted in a cobalt chromium frame. The SAPIEN XT valve is available in 20, 23, 26, and 29 mm sizes and is implanted using 18 Fr (for the 20 and 23 mm valves), 19 Fr (for the 26 mm valve), or 22 Fr (for the 29 mm valve) delivery catheter and sheath systems. With expandable sheath systems, the sheath sizes are even smaller as compared to before.

The first-generation CoreValve system consisted of a self-expanding nitinol frame with bovine pericardial heart valve and was implanted using a 25 Fr delivery catheter and sheath system. The second generation of the CoreValve system consisted of three leaflets of porcine pericardium seated higher in the nitinol frame to provide true supra-annular placement. Finally, the current third generation of the CoreValve system differs slightly from the previous version in the sealing skirt (fabricated from three separate pieces instead of one), to facilitate uniform tissue thickness and improved valve profile. The valve is available in 26, 29, and 31 mm sizes and is implanted using an 18 Fr delivery catheter and sheath system.

Definition of Outcomes

The introduction of new technology is expected to follow a standard evidence-based "bench to bedside" transition pathway, starting with preclinical testing and advancing to clinical investigations. Unfortunately, the explosive growth of TAVR has created a "clinical data conundrum" wherein an enormous body of evidence has accrued before the optimal organization and interpretation of clinical data in a uniform manner. Due to disparate nature of the outcome definitions between treating centers, thoughtful assessment of study outcomes has been rendered difficult and inter-study comparisons are ambiguous. Interventional cardiology has a tradition of well-defined clinical endpoint definitions and recently has incorporated a consensus process to standardize key endpoint definitions by convening an Academic Research Consortium (ARC) among the Academic Research Organizations (ARO) from the USA and Europe and joined by the representatives from the US Food and Drug Administration (FDA) and the industry sponsors [15, 16]. This process has demonstrated the power of effectively managed international collaboration of academic centers, US FDA, and the industry in establishing consensus clinical endpoint definitions, thereby improving the quality of clinical research.

In the spirit of ARC mission statement, the Valve Academic Research Consortium (VARC) was organized comprising ARO, independent experts, the US FDA, and medical device manufactures. The goals of VARC were to pool the expertise of interventional cardiologists, noninvasive cardiologists, cardiothoracic surgeons, clinical trialists, and other specialists—including echocardiographers, vascular specialists, and neurologists—to arrive at a consensus for selecting appropriate clinical endpoints reflecting device, procedures, and patient-related safety and effectiveness. In addition, VARC aimed to achieve consensus for standardizing definitions for single and composite clinical endpoints [17]. Importantly, the first consensus document was intended as a "road map" to facilitate the standardization of future TAVR and other aortic valve research, rather than as a guideline statement [17].

Table 3.1 outlines the consensus definitions of important clinical endpoints, which are of major significance in assessment of safety and efficacy of TAVR. All-cause mortality is an important outcome, which is considered objective as well as pragmatic from the standpoint of ascertainment and adjudication. However, the use of only all-cause mortality to assess the efficacy of TAVR in high-risk AS patients may be misleading, as a significant proportion of deaths may be unrelated to the device or to the procedure. Due to a significant proportion of AS patients with coexisting coronary artery disease (CAD), VARC has proposed a more centrist approach to defining acute myocardial infarction (MI) [18]. VARC defines periprocedural MI as an acute ischemic event with evidence of clinically significant myocardial necrosis, occurring within 72 h of the valve implantation. Acute ischemic events occurring after 72 h are considered as spontaneous MI and are defined according to universal MI guidelines [15]. Strokes are of major concern during and after TAVR, which may occur due to embolic phenomena, aortic dissection, prolonged hypotension, or hemorrhagic complications in the setting of anticoagulants and/or antiplatelet agents. All strokes are classified as major or minor depending on the modified Rankin score at 90 days. A major stroke is defined as a neurological event resulting in modified Rankin score ≥2 at 90 days. Stroke with modified Rankin score <2 at 90 days is considered to be a minor stroke. Transient ischemic attack (TIA) is defined as the complete resolution of neurological symptoms within 24 h without evidence of tissue injury on neuroimaging. For the purposes of clinical trials, VARC advocates that only major strokes should be

Table 3.1 Consensus definitions of clinical endpoints per Valve Academic Research Consortium (VARC)

Mortality	Any death due to approximate cardiac cause (e.g., MI, cardiac tamponade, worsening heart failure)
	Unwitnessed death and death of unknown cause
	All procedure-related deaths, including those related to complication of the procedure or treatment for a complication of the procedure
	Death caused by noncoronary vascular conditions of the cerebrovascular disease, pulmonary embolism, ruptured aortic aneurysm, dissecting aneurysm, or other vascular disease
Periprocedural myocardial infarction (<72 h)	New ischemic symptoms (e.g., chest pain or shortness of breath) or new ischemic signs (e.g., ventricular arrhythmias, new or worsening heart failure, new ST segment changes, hemodynamic instability, or imaging evidence of new loss of viable myocardium or new wall motion abnormality)
	Elevated cardiac biomarkers (preferably CK-MB) within 72 h after the index procedure, consisting of two or more post-procedure samples that are >6–8 h apart with a 20 % increase in the second sample and a peak value exceeding 10× the 99th percentile upper reference limit (URL) or peak value exceeding 5× the 99th percentile URL with the new pathological Q waves in at least two contiguous leads
Spontaneous myocardial infarction (>72 h)	Detection of rise and/or fall of cardiac biomarkers (preferably troponin) with at least one value above the 99th percentile URL, together with evidence of myocardial ischemia with at least one of the following:
	(a) ECG changes indicative of new ischemia (new ST-T changes or new left bundle branch block)
	(b) New pathological Q waves in at least two contiguous leads
	(c) Imaging evidence of new loss of viable myocardium or new wall motion abnormality
	Sudden unexpected cardiac death, involving cardiac arrest, often with symptoms suggestive of myocardial ischemia, and accompanied by presumably new ST elevation, or new left bundle branch block, and/or evidence of fresh thrombus by coronary angiography and/or at autopsy, but death occurring before blood samples could be obtained or at a time before the appearance of cardiac biomarkers in the blood
	Pathological findings of an acute myocardial infarction

(continued)

Table 3.1 (continued)

Stroke	Rapid onset of focal global neurological deficit with a change in level of consciousness or hemiplegia or hemiparesis or numbness or sensory loss affecting one side of the body or dysphagia or aphasia or hemianopia or amaurosis fugax or other neurological signs or symptoms consistent with stroke Duration also focal or group of neurological deficit ≥24 h or <24 h, if therapeutic interventions were performed (e.g., Thrombolytic therapy, or intracranial angioplasty) or available new imaging documents a new hemorrhage or infarct or the more logical deficit results in death No readily identifiable non-stroke cause for the clinical presentation (e.g., brain tumor, trauma, infection, hypoglycemia, peripheral lesion, pharmacological influences) Confirmation of the diagnosis by at least one of the following: (a) Neurology or neurosurgical specialist (b) Neuroimaging procedure (MR or CT scan or cerebral angiography) (c) Lumbar puncture (i.e., spinal fluid analysis diagnostic of intracranial hemorrhage)
Acute kidney injury	Change in serum creatinine (up to 72 h) compared to baseline 1. Stage I: increase in serum creatinine to 150–200 % (1.5–2× increase compared with baseline) or increase of ≥0.3 mg/dL 2. Stage II: increase in serum creatinine to 200–300 % (2–3× increase compared with baseline) or increase between >0.3 and <4.0 mg/dL 3. Stage III: increase in serum creatinine to ≥300 % (>3× increase compared with baseline) or serum creatinine of ≥4 mg/dL with an acute increase of at least 0.5 mg/dL. Patients receiving renal replacement therapy are considered to meet stage III criteria irrespective of other criteria
Life-threatening/ disabling bleeding	Fatal bleeding OR Bleeding in a critical area are organ, such as intracranial, intraspinal, intraocular, pericardial necessitating pericardiocentesis, or intramuscular with compartment syndrome Bleeding causing hypovolemic shock or severe hypotension requiring vasopressors or surgery Overt source of bleeding with drop in hemoglobin of ≥5 g/dL or whole blood or PRBC transfusion ≥4 units
Major bleeding	Overt bleeding either associated with a drop in hemoglobin level of at least 3 g/dL or requiring transfusion of 2 or 3 units of PRBC AND Does not meet criteria for life-threatening or disabling bleeding
Minor bleeding	Any bleeding worthy of clinical mention (e.g., access site hematoma) that does not qualify as life-threatening, disabling, or major
Major vascular complications	Any thoracic aortic dissection Access site or access-related vascular injury (dissection, stenosis, perforation, rupture, arteriovenous fistula, pseudoaneurysm, hematoma, irreversible nerve injury, or compartment syndrome) leading to either death, need for significant blood transfusions (≥4 units), unplanned percutaneous or surgical intervention, or irreversible end-organ damage (e.g., hypogastric artery occlusion causing visceral ischemia and spinal artery injury causing neurological impairment) Distal embolization (non-cerebral) from a vascular source requiring surgery or resulting in amputation or irreversible end-organ damage
Minor vascular complications	Access site or access-related vascular injury (dissection, stenosis, perforation, rupture, arteriovenous fistula or pseudoaneurysm requiring compression or thrombin injection therapy, or hematoma requiring transfusion of ≥2 but <4 units) not requiring unplanned percutaneous or surgical intervention and not resulting in irreversible end-organ damage Distal embolization treated with embolectomy and/or thrombectomy and not resulting in amputation or irreversible end-organ damage Failure of percutaneous access site closure resulting in interventional (e.g., stent graft) or surgical correction and not associated with death, need for significant blood transfusions (≥4 units), or irreversible end-organ damage

considered as an important safety endpoint; however, all neurological events (strokes or TIAs) should be reported as adverse events. Currently, these definitions are considered by many to be in flux, and there is increasing consensus to move away from TIA and focus on all strokes as a hard endpoint.

Vascular complications and bleeding-related events are considered important safety endpoints in TAVR. The use of large sheaths in a predominantly elderly population has led to non-negligible rates of major vascular complications during TAVR [19]. Of note, "access site" is defined as any location (arterial or venous) traversed by a guide wire, catheter, or a sheath (including the left ventricular apex and the aorta). "Access-related" complications are defined as any adverse clinical events that could possibly be associated with any of the access sites used during the procedure.

Besides the solitary endpoints discussed above, VARC proposes three composite endpoints (Table 3.2). "Device success" is an intra-procedural composite endpoint; "combined safety endpoint" is a composite endpoint up to 30 days; and "combined efficacy endpoint" is a composite endpoint at 1 year or longer.

Table 3.2 Consensus definition of composite endpoints per Valve Academic Research Consortium (VARC)

Outcome	Definition
Device success	Successful vascular access, delivery, and deployment of the device and successful retrieval of the delivery system
	Correct position in the proper anatomical location
	Intended performance of the prosthetic heart valve (aortic valve area greater than 1.2 cm^2 and mean aortic valve gradient <20 mmHg or peak velocity <3 m/s, without moderate or severe prosthetic valve aortic regurgitation)
	Only one valve implanted in the proper anatomical location
Combined safety endpoint (at 30 days)	All-cause mortality
	Major stroke
	Life-threatening (or disabling) bleeding
	Acute kidney injury stage III (including renal replacement therapy)
	Periprocedural MI
	Major vascular complication
	Repeat procedure for valvular dysfunction (surgical or interventional therapy)
Combined efficacy endpoint (at 1 year or longer)	All-cause mortality (after 30 days)
	Failure of current therapy for aortic stenosis, requiring hospitalization for symptoms or valve-related or cardiac decompensation
	Prosthetic heart valve dysfunction (aortic valve area less than 1.2 cm^2 and mean aortic valve gradient ≥20 mmHg or peak velocity ≥3 m/s, or moderate or severe prosthetic valve aortic regurgitation)

Table 3.3 Characteristics of multicenter registries of transcatheter aortic valve replacement

Author/publication year	Registry	*N*	Period of study	Number of centers	Edwards valve (*n*)	Core Valve (*n*)	Transfemoral approach (%)	Transapical approach (%)	Other approaches (%)
Gilard/2012	FRANCE 2	3,195	1/2010–10/2011	34	2,107	1,043	2,361 (73.9)	567 (17.7)	267 (8.4)
Rodes-Cabau/2010	Canadian	339	1/2005–6/2009	6	339	0	167 (49.2)	172 (50.8)	0
Lefevre/2011	PARTNER-EU	130	4/2007–1/2008	9	130	0	61 (46.9)	69 (53.1)	0
Meredith/2011	Australia New Zealand	118	8/2008–7/2010	10	0	118	113 (95.8)	0	5 (4.2)
Moat/2011	UK-TAVI	870	12/2007–12/2009	25	410	452	599 (68.9)	271 (31.1)	
Bosmans /2010	Belgian	328	Till 4/2010	15	187	141	232 (70.8)	88 (26.8)	8 (2.4)
Eltchaninoff/2010	FRANCE	244	2/2009–7/2009	16	166	78	161 (66.0)	71 (29.1)	12 (4.9)
Thomas/2010	SOURCE	1,038	11/2007–1/2009	34	1,038	0	463 (44.6)	575 (55.4)	0
Piazza/2008	Multiple European countries	646	4/2007–4/2008	51	0	646	NR	NR	NR
Zahn/2010	German	697	1/2009–12/2009	22	109	588	644 (92.4)	26 (3.7)	27 (3.9)
Tamburino/2011	Italian	663	6/2007–12/2009	14	0	663	599 (90.3)	0	64 (9.7)

Multicenter Registries of TAVR

TAVR was introduced to clinical practice in 2002 by the commercial use of the Edwards valve, with the CoreValve available for use beginning 2007. The earliest experience with the Edwards valve was reported in the Canadian registry comprising experience between 2005 and 2009 and the *SAPIEN Aortic Bioprosthesis European Outcome* (*SOURCE*) registry comprising experience between 2007 and 2009 [20, 21]. The earliest experience with the CoreValve was reported in the multicenter expanded evaluation registry comprising experience between 2007 and 2008 [22]. To date, several multicenter registries of TAVR have been assembled and described [20–30], with a large majority of them reported from several European countries. These registries provide the results after commercialization of the available devices and reflect "real-world" experience worldwide. Despite the "real-world" effectiveness data provided by these registries, there are several important limitations that should be kept in mind. Most of the registry data is derived from hospital-reported data to a central agency. The data are compiled in a retrospective fashion and thus are prone to biases inherent to observational cohort studies, such as selection and ascertainment biases. In most circumstances, the outcomes are not adjudicated by a central agency, and source documentation is not verified, leading to heterogeneity in definitions as well as interpretation of clinical scenarios.

Table 3.3 describes the characteristics of 11 large representative registries that have been described in the literature. The number of participating centers range from nine centers in the PARTNER-EU registry [24] to 51 centers in the multicenter expanded evaluation registry [22]. Of these 11 registries, 3 have exclusively described CoreValve experience [22, 25, 30], 3 have exclusively described Edwards valve experience [20, 21, 24], and the rest have reported combined experiences with both valves [23, 26–29]. Transfemoral approach to TAVR has been reported as the favored approach in most registries and was adopted in 46.9–95.8 % of all reported cases. In the current era, most centers adopt a "transfemoral first" selection policy, with the criteria for a non-transfemoral approach based on the multidisciplinary team's consideration of several factors including degree of calcification, size, tortuosity, and atheroma burden of the aortoiliofemoral arterial system. In recent years, there has been an emphasis on the establishment of "global TAVR" program (comprising of both transfemoral and non-transfemoral approaches), which would allow for the treatment of more than three-fourths of the patients who are denied SAVR [31].

Table 3.4 demonstrates the baseline characteristics of patients included in individual multicenter registries. The mean age in all registries was consistently greater than 80 years, and the proportion of males varied from 44.0 to 59.3 %. There was a significant heterogeneity in the risk profile of patients in various registries. The lowest risk profile was reported in the Australian New Zealand registry reporting a mean (SD) logistic EuroSCORE of 18.4 (11.9)% [25]. In addition to this registry, the UK-TAVI registry also had similar risk profile patients with a median (interquartile range) logistic EuroSCORE of 18.5 (11.7–27.9)% [26]. On the contrary, the other registries had a mean logistic EuroSCORE of >20. The highest risk patients were reported in the PARTNER-EU registry with a mean (SD) logistic EuroSCORE of 30.0 (13.7 %) [24]. With the due consideration of the logistic EuroSCORE in the decision making for TAVR, it is important to remember that a large proportion of patients are refused for surgical AVR and undergo TAVR on the basis of risk factors like porcelain aorta or frailty, neither of which are a part of traditional surgical risk calculators. The prevalence of CAD varied from 41.3 % in the FRANCE registry to 69.0 % in the Canadian registry [20, 28]. Similarly, the history of stroke or cerebrovascular accidents was present in 7.2–22.7 % of the included subjects. Majority of the patients included in the multicenter registries were reported to be symptomatic. The proportion of patients with reported class 3 or class 4 New York Heart Association (NYHA) symptoms varied from 65.5 % in the Italian registry to 90.9 % in the Canadian registry [20, 30].

Procedural Success

The procedural success in the representative registries has varied from 88.5 to 98.4 % (Fig. 3.1). There are potential explanations for the wide range of procedural success across various registries. One primary explanation is the differences in definition of "procedural success" across the various registries. Secondly, these registries represent different time periods in the development of TAVR technology. The

Table 3.4 Characteristics of included patients in various registries

Registry/*N*	Mean (SD) age (years)	Males (%)	Mean (SD) logistic EuroSCORE	Mean (SD) STS score	Prevalence of CAD (%)	Prevalence of stroke (%)	NYHA Class III/ IV (%)	Mean (SD) aortic valve area (cm^2)	Mean (SD) transaortic gradient	Mean (SD) LVEF
FRANCE 2/3,195	82.7 (7.2)	51.0	21.9 (14.3)	14.4 (11.9)	47.9	10.0	75.9	0.7 (0.2)	48.1 (16.5)	53.2 (14.1)
Canadian/339	81.0 (8.0)	44.8	–	9.8 (6.4)	69.0	22.7	90.9	0.6 (0.2)	46.0 (17.0)	55.0 (14.0)
PARTNER-EU/130	82.1 (5.5)	44.6	30.0 (13.7)	11.6 (6.5)	60.0	–	84.6	0.6 (0.2)	47.3 (18.9)	52.8 (16.1)
Australia New Zealand/118	82.3 (7.7)	59.3	18.4 (11.9)	5.6 (2.7)	–	–	83.9	0.7 (0.2)	50.6 (16.2)	57.8 (13.0)
UK-TAVI/870	81.9 (7.1)	52.4	18.5 (11.7–27.9)[a]	–	47.6	–	77.0	–	–	–
Belgian/328	83.0 (6.0)	54.0	28.0 (16.0)	–	58.0	15.0	79.0	0.6 (0.2)	49.0 (16.0)	55.0 (14.0)
FRANCE/244	82.3 (7.3)	56.6	25.6 (11.4)	18.9 (12.8)	41.3	10.2	74.5	0.7 (0.2)	46.0 (16.0)	51.0 (14.0)
SOURCE/1,038	81.1 (6.9)	44.6	27.6 (15.6)	–	51.9	–	–	–	–	–
European registry/646	81.0 (6.6)	46.1	23.1 (13.8)	–	56.8	7.4	82.4	0.6 (0.2)	49.4 (13.9)	51.5 (13.9)
German/697	81.4 (6.3)	44.2	20.5 (13.2)	–	60.5	8.2	87.2	0.6 (0.2)	47.0 (37–60)[a]	52.1 (15.0)
Italian/663	81.0 (7.3)	44.0	23.0 (13.7)	–	48.3	7.2	65.5	0.6 (0.2)	51.8 (17.0)	52.1 (25.5)

[a]Median (interquartile range)

patients included in the registries representing the initial TAVR experience and the use of very early versions of transcatheter valve delivery systems have expectedly reported lower success rates. In addition, the learning curve phenomenon likely exerts a negative influence on the procedural success rates. Most of the contemporary registries describe pooled outcomes from all aspects of the learning phase, including patient selection and imaging as well as procedural finesse and development of bailout strategies. However, in the more recent experience with more contemporary valve and delivery systems, the procedural success rates as well as the post-procedural efficacy rates have seemed to improve significantly. The outlook for TAVR-related outcomes and procedural success appears optimistic with improved iterations of the technology with an anticipated improvement in long-term survival rates in the coming years.

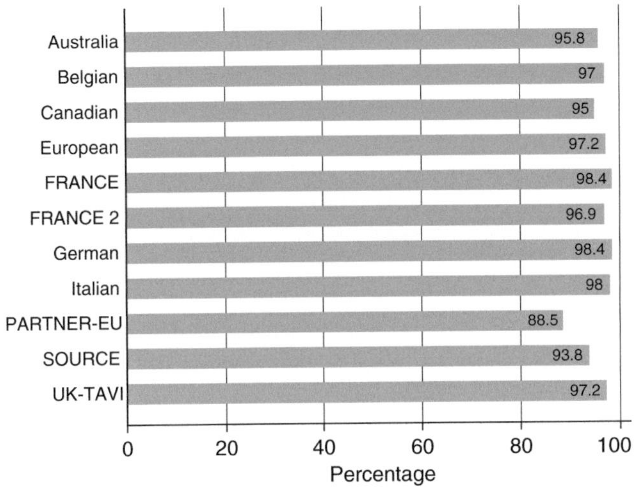

Fig. 3.1 Procedural success across various registries

Mortality

The incidence of all-cause mortality and cardiovascular-related mortality across various multicenter registries is demonstrated in Table 3.5. The 30-day all-cause mortality rates ranged from 5.6 to 13.8 % in the representative registries. The lowest 30-day all-cause mortality rates were encountered in the Australian New Zealand registry (5.6 %) and the Italian registry (5.9 %) [25, 30], while the highest 30-day all-cause mortality rates were observed in the PARTNER-EU registry (13.8 %) and the FRANCE registry (12.7 %) [24, 28]. It should be noted that the 30-day mortality rates documented in a large majority of the registries compare favorably to the contemporary surgical reports of high-risk patients undergoing surgical AVR [32]. The estimated mortality among octogenarians undergoing SAVR is approximately 6.1–9.3 % [9, 33–35]. Since the patients undergoing TAVR as a part of multicenter registries are those that are often denied surgical AVR, it remains difficult to directly compare the effectiveness of these two procedures against each other. A comparison of moderate-risk patients

Table 3.5 All-cause mortality and cardiovascular mortality across various registries

Registry/*N*	30 days	6 months	1 year	>1 year
	All-cause mortality			
FRANCE 2/3,195	9.7	18.6	24.0	–
Canadian/339	10.6	–	22.1[a]	–
PARTNER-EU/130	13.8	26.9	36.9	–
Australia New Zealand/118	5.6	10.5	–	–
UK-TAVI/870	7.1	–	21.4	2 years: 26.3
Belgian/328	11.3	–	24.1	–
FRANCE/244	12.7	–	–	–
SOURCE/1,038	8.5	–	–	–
European registry/646	8.0	–	–	–
German/697	12.4	–	–	–
Italian/663	5.9	–	14.9	2 years: 30.3 3 years: 34.8
	Cardiovascular mortality			
FRANCE 2/3,195	7.0	11.7	14.3	–
Canadian/339	9.4	–	–	–
PARTNER-EU/130	11.5	–	24.6	–
Australia New Zealand/118	5.6	7.1	–	–
Belgian/328	6.1	–	8.5	–
European registry/646	5.9	–	–	–
Italian/663	–	–	11.2	2 years: 12.1 3 years: 13.5

[a]Median follow-up: 8 months

amenable to TAVR or SAVR—with two parallel nested registries for patients suitable for only TAVR or surgical AVR in PARTNER II—will be useful in understanding the true effect of each procedure.

The 6-month mortality rates following TAVR have been reported in three registries: Australia New Zealand (10.5 %), FRANCE 2 (18.6 %), and PARTNER-EU (26.9 %) [24, 25, 28]. The 1-year mortality rates varied from 14.9 % reported in the Italian registry to 36.9 % in the PARTNER-EU registry [24, 30]. Only two registries have published data for follow-up longer than 1 year [26, 36]. The 2-year mortality rate was observed to be 26.3 and 30.3 % in the UK-TAVI and the Italian registries, respectively [26, 30]. The 3-year mortality rate has been reported to be 34.8 % in the Italian registry [36]. These data may be of little surprise given the high-risk profile of the included subjects that have undergone TAVR in these registries.

The distribution of cardiovascular-related deaths in these large-scale registries is of particular interest (Table 3.5). A large majority of all deaths occurring within 30 days period after TAVR have been related to procedural cardiovascular deaths (5.6–11.5 %). However, this proportion of majority shifts rather quickly, with a significant proportion of all deaths occurred due to non-cardiovascular causes at 1-year follow-up. For example, in the FRANCE 2 registry, the incidence of all-cause mortality and non-cardiovascular mortality at 1 year was reported to be 24.0 and 9.7 %, respectively [23]. Similarly, in the Belgian registry, about 65 % of all deaths at 1-year follow-up were attributable to non-cardiovascular causes [27]. The results are equally striking at the 2- and 3-year follow-up reported in the Italian registry [36]. Roughly 60 % of the all deaths occurring at 2- and 3-year follow-up intervals were attributable to non-cardiovascular causes [36]. Most of these patients die as a result of comorbidities or secondary to conditions associated with advanced age. In accordance with the 2008 European position statement on TAVR—which stated that this procedure should not be performed on patients with a life expectancy <1 year—enhanced patient selection is needed for approximately half of all considered patients who may imminently die due to non-cardiovascular causes [37]. In the future, one crucial task will be to identify a patient population that is likely to derive the most advantage from application of TAVR technology, in the perspective of long-term efficacy and cost-effectiveness.

In an analysis performed by Ussia et al., no significant differences in cardiovascular mortality were observed between the moderate-risk and the high-risk cohorts, although a significant difference was noted in the non-cardiovascular mortality in the high-risk population [36]. These findings indirectly suggest that the application of TAVR technology to lower-risk groups may demonstrate improved cardiovascular survival and quality of life with an added advantage of a lower non-cardiovascular-related mortality.

Several studies have identified pre-procedural variables, which may be useful in predicting short-term as well as long-term mortality. The SOURCE registry identified that patients with logistic EuroSCORE between 30 and 35 were significantly more likely to die at 30 days, when compared to those with lower scores [21]. Although the logistic EuroSCORE is a strong predictor of short-term and medium-term post-TAVR mortality, it tends to overestimate the mortality in most patients undergoing TAVR [38–40]. The findings may suggest a relative lack of utility of this scoring system in uniformly predicting risk and outcomes in patients undergoing TAVR and confirm the need for more sophisticated and procedure-specific (rather than generic) scoring systems. Generally, baseline cardiovascular factors like low ejection fraction, pulmonary hypertension, and severe mitral regurgitation along with periprocedural complications seem to have a major role in short-term mortality and mortality occurring during 1-year follow-up [19]. However, noncardiac comorbidities, like chronic obstructive pulmonary disease, chronic kidney disease, and liver disease, are important predictors of mortality during the follow-up period, rather than of the acute mortality [19]. Interestingly, the Canadian registry demonstrated similar 30-day mortality rates in frail patients as compared to the rest of the study group. In addition, the procedural and short-term mortality rates were similar between patients with and without porcelain aorta in this registry [20].

Several recent studies have identified that the degree of post-implant aortic regurgitation (AR) was an important predictor of the 1-year mortality [23, 26]. This is an important observation and requires further systematic assessment. Whether the degree of AR is responsible for an early mortality or is merely a marker for adverse outcomes is not currently clear.

Myocardial Infarction and Stroke

Table 3.6 demonstrates the incidence of MI and stroke in the various registries. The incidence of MI at 30 days has ranged from 0 to 4.6 % across the registries. The intermediate-term incidence of MI in the registry cohort has been observed to be between 1.2 and 6.2 %. This generally wide variability in the MI rates stems from the lack of uniformity in the definition of periprocedural MI among the various TAVR registries.

Strokes during and after TAVR may occur due to embolic phenomena, ensuing (or preexisting) atrial fibrillation, aortic dissection, prolonged hypotension, or hemorrhagic complications in the setting of anticoagulants and/or antiplatelet agents. Although the transcranial Doppler studies have demonstrated that cerebral emboli may occur at any time during TAVR, most have been shown to occur during positioning and implantation of valve prosthesis [41, 42]. This clearly

Table 3.6 Incidence of myocardial infarction and stroke at 30-day and long-term follow-up in the various registries

	Myocardial infarction		Stroke	
Registry/*N*	30 days	Follow-up	30 days	Follow-up
FRANCE 2/3,195	–	1 year: 1.2	–	1 year: major (2.3), minor (1.8)
Canadian/339	1.2	–	2.3	–
PARTNER-EU/130	4.6	6 months: 6.2 1 year: 6.2	2.3	6 months: 5.4 1 year: 6.9
Australia New Zealand/118	–	–	1.7	–
UK-TAVI/870	1.3	–	4.1	–
Belgian/328	–	–	Stroke: 4.4 TIA: 0.9	–
FRANCE/244	–	–	3.6	–
SOURCE/1,038	–	–	2.6	–
European registry/646	0.6	–	1.9	–
German/697	0.3[a]	–	2.8[a]	–
Italian/663	0[a]	1 year: 1.2 3 years: 1.2	1.2[a]	1 year: 2.6 3 years: 3.9

[a]Only procedural rates available. 30-day event rate was not available

indicates that embolization of valve particles from the native calcified aortic valve leaflets might be an important mechanism for cerebral embolization during TAVR. A few studies have demonstrated the feasibility of using embolic protection devices during TAVR [43]. The safety and efficacy of these devices in prevention of cerebral embolic events during TAVR procedures remains to be definitively established. The randomized PROTAVI trial has recently been started in Europe and will help us understand the effect of emboli protection devices in decreasing cerebrovascular pathology detected by MRI.

The 30-day stroke rate across the various registries has ranged between 1.2 and 4.4 %. A few registries have reported stroke rates upon medium-term follow-up. The FRANCE 2 registry reported that the incidence of major and minor strokes at 1-year follow-up was 2.3 and 1.8 %, respectively [23]. Similarly, the Italian CoreValve registry reported the incidence of stroke to be 2.6 and 3.9 % at 1- and 3-year follow-up, respectively [30, 36]. The PARTNER-EU registry reported a slightly higher rate of stroke than the FRANCE 2 and the Italian registries (6 months, 5.4 %; 1 year, 6.9 %) [24]. Although the incidence rate of major stroke is largely consistent between several European registries, there appears to be a discrepancy in the rates between the registry data and the randomized PARTNER trial data [14]. In the cohort A of the PARTNER trial, there was a higher rate of major stroke reported and almost 40 % of the neurological events occurred between 1 month and 1 year of follow-up [14]. There are several possible explanations for these discrepant findings [14]. Firstly, the prevalence of preexisting cerebrovascular disease (almost 30 %) in the PARTNER trial could play a role in the higher incidence of stroke in the trial as compared to the registry data. Secondly, the devices used were first-generation devices and may have been responsible for somewhat higher stroke rates. Thirdly, the diagnosis of stroke was adjudicated by CEC in the PARTNER trial as compared to cardiologists and anesthesiologists assessing neurological function after TAVR in most registries. This may result in underestimation of clinically relevant neurological events in the registry-derived data. Magnetic resonance imaging-based studies have demonstrated cerebral perfusion defects in approximately 70–80 % of the patients undergoing TAVR [44]. Although the majority of these patients are asymptomatic from a neurological standpoint, the MRI and clinical findings nevertheless highlight the need for a systematic assessment of neurological function including cognitive abilities [44].

Arrhythmias, Conduction Abnormalities, and Pacemaker Implantation

Arrhythmias and conduction abnormalities are important concerns after TAVR. Although supraventricular and ventricular arrhythmias have been observed after TAVR at varying frequencies, they are also encountered in roughly 20–30 % of patients after SAVR. Thus, any valid comparison of frequency of arrhythmias between the two strategies would need to include a careful analysis of post-therapy arrhythmias [45]. These findings are of particular relevance as the occurrence of new-onset left bundle branch block after SAVR has been associated with an increased risk of death and subsequent life-threatening arrhythmias during follow-up [46, 47]. New-onset intraventricular conduction abnormalities, particularly the new-onset left bundle branch block, are encountered frequently after TAVR (7–18 % after Edwards valve implantation; 30–83 % after CoreValve implantation) [45, 48–52]. Direct mechanical injury of the left bundle branch and the inflammation due to the stent prosthesis are likely

Table 3.7 Pacemaker implantation after transcatheter aortic valve replacement stratified by valve type

	Edwards valve		CoreValve	
Registry/*N*	30 days	Follow-up	30 days	Follow-up
FRANCE 2/3,195	–	1 year: 11.5	–	1 year: 24.2
Canadian/339	4.9	–	–	–
PARTNER-EU/130	2.3	6 months: 3.1 1 year: 3.1	–	–
Australia New Zealand/118	–	–	40.0	–
UK-TAVI/870	7.4	–	24.4	–
Belgian/328	5.0	–	22.5	–
FRANCE/244	5.4	–	25.6	–
SOURCE/1,038	7.0	–	–	–
European registry/646	–	–	9.3	–
German/697	22.0	–	42.5	–
Italian/663	–	–	17.4	1 year: 19.1

offenders to the conduction system. However, the implications of a new-onset left bundle branch block after TAVR upon long-term adverse outcomes are not well understood.

In several instances, the conduction system abnormalities arising as a result of prosthetic valve placement necessitate the implantation of permanent pacemaker. Table 3.7 demonstrates the incidence of permanent pacemaker implantation in the Edwards valve and CoreValve cohorts. At 30-day follow-up period, the incidence of permanent pacemaker implantation in the Edwards valve cohort and the CoreValve cohort was observed to be 2.3–22.0 % and 9.3–42.5 %, respectively. Among the Edwards valve cohorts, all registries except the German registry reported 30-day pacemaker implantation rate less than 10 % [28]. On the other hand, among the CoreValve cohorts, all registries except the multicenter expanded evaluation registry and the Italian registry reported pacemaker implantation rate greater than 20 %. Among the Edwards valve cohorts, the 1-year pacemaker implantation rate was reported to be 3.1 % in the PARTNER-EU registry and 11.5 % in the FRANCE 2 registry [23, 24]. Among the CoreValve cohorts, the 1-year pacemaker implantation rate was reported to be 19.1 % in the Italian registry and 24.2 % in the FRANCE 2 registry [23, 30].

Among procedural variables, the use of CoreValve system and the deeper (ventricular) implantation of the valve prosthesis have been identified as the most important variables predicting the need for permanent pacemaker implantation [19]. It has been speculated that the nitinol frame of the CoreValve system exerts a higher radial strength on the ventricular septum as compared to the stainless steel or cobalt chromium frame of the Edwards valve, leading to an increased risk of damage to the conduction system. To date, the impact of permanent pacemaker implantation on long-term outcomes has been poorly explored in patients undergoing TAVR. Experience from the surgical series has suggested that permanent pacemaker implantation does not significantly add to long-term mortality [53]. Cost-effective analyses are needed to elucidate the long-term impact of pacemaker implantation in patients undergoing TAVR.

Vascular Complications and Other Adverse Events After TAVR

Table 3.8 demonstrates the vascular complications and bleeding events that may arise after TAVR. There is a significant heterogeneity in the definition and classification of bleeding and vascular complications among these studies. The VARC recommends classification of bleeding events as life-threatening, major and minor bleeding events (Table 3.1). The life-threatening and major bleeding event rates have ranged between 3.2 % in the Italian CoreValve registry and 8.5 % in the PARTNER-EU registry [24, 30]. The incidence of major and minor vascular complications has ranged between 1.9–13.3 % and 4.6–10.4 %, respectively, across the various registries.

Unfortunately, the list of possible complications after TAVR is rather long. Depending on the design characteristics and the final implant position, the prosthetic transcatheter aortic valve comes in close contact with several structures including anterior mitral leaflet, intervalvular fibrosa, ventricular septum, aortic annulus, aortic sinuses, aortic root, coronary arteries, and the conduction system. Collectively, all these structures that are contiguous with the prosthetic aortic valve are called as the "aortic valvar complex." Due to its proximity, the prosthetic transcatheter aortic valve may exert untoward effects on any of these structures resulting in adverse clinical consequences. Table 3.9 lists the incidence of several important complications that have been observed after TAVR.

Major complications resulting in conversion of the TAVR to a surgical AVR occurred in 0.4–2.7 % of the cases. Coronary ostial obstruction—especially of the left main coronary artery—is encountered in 0–1.2 % of the cases undergoing TAVR. Coronary obstruction occurs due to displacement of the native aortic valve leaflets towards the ostia during valve prosthesis implantation. The risk of ostial obstruction is higher in patients with heavily calcified leaflets, especially in those with some degree of aortic sinus effacement, low aortic implantation of a coronary ostium, and long aortic valve leaflets. However, the low incidence rate

Table 3.8 Bleeding and vascular complications after transcatheter aortic valve replacement across various registries

	Bleeding			Vascular complications	
Registry/*N*	Life-threatening	Major	Minor	Major	Minor
FRANCE 2/3,195	1.2	4.5	7.4	4.7	5.0
Canadian/339	–	–	–	13.3	–
PARTNER-EU/130	8.5		12.3	10.8	5.4
Australia New Zealand/118	–	–	–	1.9	4.6
UK-TAVI/870	–	–	–	6.3	–
Belgian/328	–	–	–	–	–
FRANCE/244	21.3			7.3	–
SOURCE/1,038	–	–	–	10.6	10.4
European registry/646	–	–	–	5.6[a]	
German/697	19.5[b]				
Italian/663	3.2		–	3.2[c]	–

[a]Includes aortic root dissection/perforation, ventricular perforation, cardiac tamponade, and access site complications
[b]Indicated as "groin problems"
[c]Includes major access site complications and cardiac tamponade

Table 3.9 Miscellaneous complications arising after transcatheter aortic valve replacement across various registries

Registry/*N*	Coronary obstruction	Two-valve implantation	Conversion to open surgery	Valve embolization/ migration	Aortic dissection	Cardiac tamponade	Renal failure	Sepsis	Arrhythmias
FRANCE 2/3,195	–	2.3	0.4	1.3	–	–	–	–	–
Canadian/339	0.9	2.7	1.8	2.0	–	–	2.6	2.9	8.1
PARTNER-EU/130	0.8	0.8	2.3	2.3	–	–	1.5	–	–
Australia New Zealand/118	–	–	–	0	–	–	–	–	–
UK-TAVI/870	–	0.8	0.7	–	–	–	–	–	–
Belgian/328	–	1.2	–	2.7	–	–	6.0	–	–
FRANCE/244	1.2	–	–	0.8	–	2.0	1.6	2.8	–
SOURCE/1,038	0.6	2.1	2.7	0.3	–	–	4.3	–	–
European registry/646	0	2.6	0.5	–	0.6	1.4	–	–	–
German/697	0.1	–	0.7	–	0.4	1.8	–	–	–
Italian/663	–	3.6	0.8	0.6	–	1.2	–	–	2.0

of coronary obstruction has precluded a specific recommendation on the cutoff for the distance between the coronary ostia and the aortic annulus, size of the sinus of Valsalva, or the amount of leaflet calcification that should contraindicate TAVR, due to prohibitive risk of coronary ostial obstruction. Notably, although coronary obstruction is at times met with catastrophic consequences, there are numerous anecdotal descriptions in the current literature that report the feasibility and success of performing a coronary angioplasty through the struts of the transcatheter aortic valve [54–56].

Valve embolization or valve migration is another infrequent complication that may be encountered after TAVR. The incidence of this complication was observed to be 0.3–2.7 % across all registries (Table 3.9). Meticulous pre-procedure annulus measurements, optimal valve positioning, proper placement of temporary pacemaker lead during rapid pacing, full balloon inflation at the time of valve deployment, and complete balloon deflation before stopping rapid pacing are of crucial importance to prevent valve embolization.

The incidence of renal failure requiring dialysis has ranged from 1.5 to 6.0 % across various registries. Renal insufficiency has been observed to be an important predictor of adverse acute and midterm outcomes in patients undergoing TAVR [19, 36, 57–59]. The Canadian registry reported that frail patients undergoing TAVR were more likely to develop acute renal failure requiring hemodialysis compared to the rest of the study population [20].

Post-procedure Aortic Regurgitation

Moderate or severe paravalvular AR has been shown to be associated with increased risk of death at follow-up [23, 26]. Whether the degree of AR is responsible for an early mortality or is merely a marker for adverse outcomes is not presently known. Moderate to severe AR is encountered less commonly as compared to mild paravalvular AR after TAVR. The clinical significance of mild paravalvular AR is currently unclear.

Table 3.10 Post-procedure aortic regurgitation (grade 2 or higher) after transcatheter aortic valve replacement

Registry/*N*	30-day follow-up	Long-term follow-up
FRANCE 2/3,195	18.7	6 months: 18.7 1 year: 20.3
Canadian/339	6.0	–
PARTNER-EU/130	47.0	1 year: 25.0
Australia New Zealand/118	60.0	6 months: 40.4
UK-TAVI/870	13.6	–
FRANCE/244	9.5	–
SOURCE/1,038	1.9[a]	–
German/697	17.6	–
Italian/663	20.1	1 year: 17.8 2 years: 16.5 3 years: 10.1

[a]AR grade 3+ or higher

Small studies have demonstrated no adverse effects of mild AR on left ventricular function at medium-term follow-up period [60]. However, if TAVR expands to be a treatment option for lower-risk, younger individuals, there may be a lower tolerance towards mild paravalvular AR, requiring revisions in valve design to ensure flush circumferential annular apposition.

AR can occur after TAVR due to several different mechanisms, including malposition (too high or too low), undersizing, severe calcification of the annulus impairing proper sealing, valvular AR due to overstretching of the stent, and leaflet malfunction. When longer follow-up is available, it remains possible that leaflet degeneration or structural issues with the valves may be observed; however, this has not been currently observed or appreciated.

Several anatomical correlates have been associated with an increased rate of moderate to severe paravalvular AR and include heavy valvular calcification of the native aortic valve, a large aortic annulus, a small valve area, and a high angle between the ascending aorta and the left ventricular outflow tract (especially in the case of the CoreValve). Numerous studies have also suggested that echocardiography might undersize aortic annulus measurements compared to CT. This undersizing may be associated with an increased risk of significant paravalvular AR after the implantation of a smaller prosthesis. Table 3.10 demonstrates the incidence of post-procedure AR upon short-term and intermediate-term follow-up. The incidence of moderate or severe AR at 30 days after TAVR has been observed between 6.0 and 60 % across various registries. The incidence of moderate or severe AR at 1-year follow-up has been observed to be 17.8, 20.3, and 25.0 % in the Italian, FRANCE 2, and PARTNER-EU registries, respectively [23, 24, 30]. The 2- and 3-year follow-up AR rates were reported to be 16.5 and 10.1 % in the Italian CoreValve registry [36]. Severe intra-procedural AR due to an imprecise implantation of the valve may be treated with either implantation of a second valve, that is, valve-in-valve treatment [61, 62] or by catheter-based repositioning of the valve [61, 63]. Paravalvular aortic valvular leakage can also be treated by implantation of a plug device [64, 65], while misplacement of the device may be treated by retraction (if partially released) followed by reimplantation [63]. However, such rescue interventions are extremely challenging and time-consuming and impart a propensity to trigger further complications. These issues will be directly addressed by next-generation transcatheter heart valves that are capable of complete repositioning.

Edwards Valve Versus CoreValve

Most of the contemporary registry data are limited to centers that perform only balloon-expandable or self-expanding TAVR but not both; this is a significant limitation in drawing inferences about the comparison of two strategies. One potential advantage to the self-expanding CoreValve system is the smaller delivery catheter system (18 Fr) for the transfemoral access, as historically compared to the 22–24 Fr size necessary for the Edwards valve implantation. These disparities in delivery system size may be significantly mitigated given the introduction of smaller sheath delivery systems for the Edwards valve. In limited centers that implant both types of valves, valve selection has been related to annulus sizing, femoral artery access, and availability of newer delivery systems. The CoreValve is available in a 31 mm size as compared to 29 mm being the largest available Edwards valve. On the other hand, the Edwards valve has an advantage of a lower incidence of conduction abnormalities and need for permanent pacemaker implantation post-procedurally. The self-expanding nitinol frame of the CoreValve is believed to have higher radial forces and has a propensity for pacemaker with deeper implantation.

Table 3.11 demonstrates the incidence rates of death, MI, and stroke in patients undergoing TAVR stratified by the valve type. Among the Edwards valve cohorts, the 30-day incidence of death, MI, and stroke ranged between 8.5–13.8 %, 1.2–4.6 %, and 2.3–5.2 %, respectively. Among the CoreValve cohorts, the 30-day incidence of death, MI, and

Table 3.11 Incidence of death, myocardial infarction, and stroke in patients undergoing transcatheter aortic valve replacement stratified by valve type

	All-cause mortality		Myocardial infarction		Stroke	
Registry/*N*	30 days	Follow-up	30 days	Follow-up	30 days	Follow-up
Edwards valve						
FRANCE 2/2,107	9.6	6 months: 18.1 1 year: 24.0	–	1 year: 0.8	–	1 year: major (1.9) minor (1.9)
Canadian/339	10.6	8 months: 22.1	1.2	–	2.3	–
PARTNER-EU/130	13.8	6 months: 26.9 1 year: 36.9	4.6	6 months: 6.2 1 year: 6.2	2.3	6 months: 5.4 1 year: 6.9
UK-TAVI/410	8.5	1 year: 20.6 2 years: 28.3	1.5	–	4.2	–
Belgian/187	11.8	1 year: 27.2	–	–	Stroke: 5.0 TIA: 1.1	–
FRANCE/166	12.0	–	–	–	3.6	–
SOURCE/1,038	8.5	–	–	–	2.6	–
CoreValve						
FRANCE 2/1,043	9.4	6 months: 19.6 1 year: 23.7	–	1 year: 1.9	–	1 year: major (2.6), minor (1.7)
Australia New Zealand/118	5.6	10.5	–	–	1.7	–
UK-TAVI/452	5.8	1 year: 21.7 2 years: 23.9	1.1	–	4.0	–
Belgian/141	10.6	1 year: 21.3	–	–	Stroke: 3.6 TIA: 0.7	–
FRANCE/78	14.1	–	–	–	3.8	–
European registry/646	8.0	–	0.6	–	1.9	–
Italian/663	5.9	1 year: 14.9 2 years: 30.3 3 years: 34.8	0[a]	1 year: 1.2 3 years: 1.2	1.2[a]	1 year: 2.6 3 years: 3.9

[a]Only procedural rates available. 30-day event rate was not available

stroke ranged between 5.6–14.1 %, 0–1.1 %, and 1.2–4.0 %, respectively. The distribution of long-term all-cause mortality also appears to be similar between the two valve types across the available registries (Table 3.11).

Transfemoral Versus Non-transfemoral Approaches

Table 3.12 demonstrates the incidence rates of all-cause mortality and stroke in the patients undergoing transfemoral and transapical TAVR. In the transfemoral cohorts, the 30-day and 1-year mortality rates were observed to be 5.5–11.1 % and 18.0–24.7 %, respectively. In the transapical cohorts, the 30-day and 1-year mortality rates were observed to be 10.3–18.8 % and 32.3–50.7 %, respectively. Several registries have reported significantly higher all-cause mortality among patients undergoing transapical TAVR as compared to those undergoing transfemoral TAVR [21, 26, 27]. The difference is likely secondary to the higher-risk profile of the patients undergoing transapical TAVR as compared to the patients undergoing transfemoral TAVR, as well as technical procedural features. As is clearly evident in Table 3.12, the logistic EuroSCORE in the transapical TAVR is consistently higher than that in the transfemoral cohort. Although inadequate peripheral vascular access is the most common reason for transapical approach, the transapical patients are higher-risk individuals because of a systematic selection bias that has occurred with the delivery approach. The selection bias results in a significantly higher prevalence of comorbidities in the transapical cohort, thereby resulting in a higher short-term and intermediate-term mortality.

Hemodynamic Improvement Following TAVR

The favorable clinical efficacy of TAVR is likely secondary to excellent hemodynamic results obtained post-procedurally. Most studies have demonstrated mean residual transsystolic aortic valvular gradients <15 mmHg with aortic valve areas >1.5 cm^2 [19]. Importantly, these hemodynamic results are

Table 3.12 Comparison of mortality and stroke rates across various registries stratified by transapical and transfemoral approaches

	Transapical TAVR					Transfemoral TAVR				
Registry (transapical *N*/transfemoral *N*)	Mean (SD) logistic EuroSCORE	30 day mortality	30-day stroke	Long-term mortality	Long-term stroke	Mean (SD) logistic EuroSCORE	30-day mortality	30-day stroke	Long-term mortality	Long-term stroke
FRANCE 2 (567/2,361)	24.8 (14.7)	13.9	–	6 months: 22.4 1 year: 32.3	1 year: major (2.1), minor (2.3)	21.2 (14.7)		–	6 months: 17.2 1 year: 21.7	1 year: major (2.2), minor (1.5)
Canadian (177/162)	–[a]	11.3	1.7	8 months: 19.8	–	–[a]	9.5	3.0	8 months: 24.7	–
PARTNER-EU (69/61)	33.8 (14.4)	18.8	1.4	6 months: 42.0 1 year: 50.7	6 months: 5.8 1 year: 7.2	25.7 (11.5)	8.2	3.3	6 months: 9.8 1 year: 21.3	6 months: 4.9 1 year: 6.6
UK-TAVI (271[b]/599)	21.4 (14.4–33.6)[c]	10.7	4.1	1 year: 27.7 2 years: 36.7	–	17.1 (11.0–25.5)[c]	5.5	4.0	1 year: 18.5 2 years: 22.5	–
Belgian (88/99)	33.0 (17.0)	14.0	8.2	6 months: 29.0 1 year: 37.0	–	29.0 (15.0)	6.0	2.1	6 months: 9.0 1 year: 18.0	–
FRANCE (71/161)	26.8 (11.6)	16.9	2.8	–	–	25.2 (11.2)	11.1	4.3	–	–
SOURCE (575/463)	29.1 (16.3)	10.3	2.6	–	–	25.7 (14.5)	6.3	2.4	–	–

[a]Mean logistic EuroSCORE was not reported in this registry. Mean (SD) STS scores in the transapical cohort were 10.5(6.9) and 9.0 (5.8)% in the transapical and transfemoral TAVR cohorts, respectively ($p=0.034$)
[b]Transapical TAVR outcomes not reported separately. The outcomes for "other routes" were compared with those after transfemoral TAVR
[c]Median (interquartile range)

sustained at an intermediate-term follow-up. In the PARTNER trial, Smith et al. demonstrated the superior hemodynamics of transcatheter valves compared to SAVR in the high-risk cohort of severe AS patients [14]. These good hemodynamic results might be attributable to systematic oversizing of the transcatheter valve with respect to the aortic annulus, although some studies have suggested that the frame of the transcatheter valve adapts to the dimensions of the aortic annulus and that the final aortic valve area after TAVR is mainly determined by the size of aortic annulus evaluated by echocardiography [66–68]. In addition, the stent of the transcatheter valves is much thinner than the stented valve used for SAVR, resulting in minimal obstruction to blood flow. This potential improvement in valve hemodynamics achieved after TAVR has translated into significant improvement in the left ventricular ejection fraction—especially for those patients with low pre-procedural ejection fractions. Clavel et al. have demonstrated that the ventricular function in most patients with ejection fraction <50 % undergoing TAVR had normalized at 1-year follow-up period and this compared favorably with those patients with low ejection fraction undergoing surgical AVR [69]. Similarly in the REVIVAL trial, Kodali et al. demonstrated an improvement in ejection fraction from 36.2 to 50.1 % at 30 days in patients with depressed pre-procedural ventricular function undergoing TAVR [60]. Although the valve hemodynamics is excellent after TAVR, residual paravalvular AR remains an important issue, which needs to be addressed in near future.

Symptom and Quality of Life Improvement Following TAVR

Improvements in the NYHA functional class following TAVR have been consistently reported for all published registries to date. A large majority of patients described NYHA Class III or IV symptoms prior to undergoing TAVR and improve to Class I or II at midterm follow-up [19]. Exercise capacity, evaluated using the 6-min walk test, has also been shown to improve after TAVR [70, 71]. In addition, several studies have demonstrated marked improvement in quality of life parameters at 6–12 months after implantation using well-validated instruments like Short Form 36 (SF-36), Kansas City Cardiomyopathy Questionnaire (KCCQ), EuroQol-5D (EQ-5D), and Duke Activity Status Index Questionnaire [72–78]. Improvement in quality of life and activities of daily living may rank in the highest of benefits of TAVR in an elderly population of patients who prefer to add life to their years rather than years to their life.

The PARTNER-EU registry reported that 82.1 % of the patients undergoing TAVR reported an improvement in NYHA class, with 87.2 % being in Class I or II [24]. In addition, this registry reported that 73.2 % of the patients experienced a significant improvement in the KCCQ overall summary score, which is specific for assessment of quality of life in cardiac patients [24]. Limited studies have documented lack of improvement in quality of life or functional status among patients with comorbidities like severe mitral regurgitation or chronic kidney disease [74–79]. Future studies are needed to delineate specific patient populations who are unlikely to demonstrate benefit for quality or quantity of life, in order to ensure cost-effective application of this novel technology.

Long-Term Follow-Up Studies

Surgically implanted aortic bioprostheses have shown 10-year freedom from prosthetic failure in the range of 60–90 %, with younger patients predisposed towards premature deterioration [80, 81]. At 5 years, freedom from structural valve failure is generally greater than 95 %. Although premature failure requiring repeat operation or leading to adverse clinical consequences has been well described for SAVR, freedom from repeat operation at 5 years is also generally greater than 95 % [80, 81]. Whether TAVR can achieve similar outcomes remains to be seen.

Given the recent introduction of TAVR, data regarding long-term outcomes is limited. Gurvitch et al. reported a survival rate of 51 % at 3-year follow-up in a cohort of 88 patients, who had undergoing TAVR with the balloon-expandable Cribier-Edwards or Edwards SAPIEN valve between January 2005 and December 2006 [82]. After discounting patients who died within the first 30 days as a result of procedure-related complication, the survival rates were 74 and 61 % at 2- and 3-year follow-up periods, respectively [82]. Further, the incidence of MI, stroke, and pacemaker implantation at 3-year follow-up was 8.6, 8.6, and 7.1 %, respectively. In the surviving patients who were in NYHA Class III and IV at baseline, 85 and 100 % of patients had improved by at least one functional NYHA class, respectively. This study demonstrated good valve durability, with no evidence of structural deterioration or need for reoperation at the median follow-up of 3.7 years. A small reduction in the valve area with a small increase in the valve gradient was observed upon follow-up. However, the authors surmised that these changes were likely to be clinically insignificant given their small magnitude and the sustained clinical functional improvement. It was noted that the annualized aortic valve area reduction of 0.06 cm^2 and a gradient progression of 3.8 % was similar to the gradient progression reported in surgically implanted bioprostheses [83].

Long-term follow-up results of the Italian CoreValve registry demonstrated a sustained clinical and functional cardiovascular benefit among patients undergoing TAVR with 18 Fr CoreValve up to a 3-year follow-up period [36]. In this study, all-cause mortality was 30.3 and 34.8 % at 2- and 3-year follow-up, respectively. Cardiovascular-related mortality was reported to be 12.1 and 13.5 %, respectively, implying that non-cardiovascular deaths accounted for majority of deaths on follow-up. There were sustained improvements in the NYHA functional class as well as aortic valve area at 2- and 3-year follow-up periods [36]. Buellesfeld reported a 2-year survival rate of 59.7 % in the CoreValve safety and efficacy study [84]. In further analysis, the authors reported that patients who were classified as high-risk prior to undergoing TAVR had twice the risk of major adverse events at 2-year follow-up period, compared to the patients in the moderate-risk category [84].

Conclusions

TAVR has demonstrated great promise in treatment of high-risk patients with severe symptomatic AS. The efficacy of TAVR has been clearly demonstrated on early and midterm outcomes with both available devices. Although the adverse effect profile is slightly different for the Edwards valve and the CoreValve, a large number of patients derive survival and functional benefit after implantation of either device. It has been shown that with careful screening, proper training, and proctoring, short-term procedural success can be achieved in most patients. The data from the available multicenter registries indicates that proper patient selection may play a vital role to the cost-effective utilization of this revolutionary technology. The impact of comorbid conditions like frailty, respiratory failure, pulmonary hypertension, and severe mitral regurgitation on long-term outcomes following TAVR needs to be definitively established and is currently in its process through the performance of high-quality large-scale registries.

References

1. Charlson E, Legedza AT, Hamel MB. Decision-making and outcomes in severe symptomatic aortic stenosis. J Heart Valve Dis. 2006;15(3):312–21.
2. Vahanian A, Baumgartner H, Bax J, Butchart E, Dion R, Filippatos G, Flachskampf F, Hall R, Iung B, Kasprzak J, Nataf P, Tornos P, Torracca L, Wenink A, Task Force on the Management of Valvular Hearth Disease of the European Society of Cardiology; ESC Committee for Practice Guidelines. Guidelines on the management of valvular heart disease: the Task Force on the Management of Valvular Heart Disease of the European Society of Cardiology. Eur Heart J. 2007;28(2):230–68.
3. Iung B, Baron G, Butchart EG, Delahaye F, Gohlke-Ba¨rwolf C, Levang OW, Tornos P, Vanoverschelde JL, Vermeer F, Boersma E, Ravaud P, Vahanian A. A prospective survey of patients with valvular heart disease in Europe: the Euro Heart Survey on Valvular Heart Disease. Eur Heart J. 2003;13:1231–43.
4. Wendt D, Osswald BR, Kayeser K, Thielmann M, Tossios P, Massoudy P, Kamler M, Jakob H. STS score is superior to the EuroSCORE in determining mortality in high risk patients undergoing isolated aortic valve replacement. Ann Thorac Surg. 2009;2:468–74.
5. O'Brien SM, Shahian DM, Filardo G, Ferraris VA, Haan CK, Rich JB, Normand SL, DeLong ER, Shewan CM, Dokholyan RS, Peterson ED, Edwards FH, Anderson RP, for the Society of Thoracic Surgeons Quality Measurement Task Force. The Society of Thoracic Surgeons 2008 cardiac surgery risk models, part 2: isolated valve surgery. Ann Thorac Surg. 2009;1(suppl):S23–42.

6. Varadarajan P, Kapoor N, Bansal RC, Pai RG. Clinical profile and natural history of 453 nonsurgically managed patients with severe aortic stenosis. Ann Thorac Surg. 2006;82:2111–5.
7. Pai RG, Kapoor N, Bansal RC, Varadarajan P. Malignant natural history of asymptomatic severe aortic stenosis: benefit of aortic valve replacement. Ann Thorac Surg. 2006;82:2116–22.
8. Brown JM, O'Brien SM, Wu C, Sikora JA, Griffith BP, Gammie JS. Isolated aortic valve replacement in North America comprising 108,687 patients in 10 years: changes in risks, valve types, and outcomes in the Society of Thoracic Surgeons National Database. J Thorac Cardiovasc Surg. 2009;137(1):82–90.
9. Grossi EA, Schwartz CF, Yu PJ, Jorde UP, Crooke GA, Grau JB, Ribakove GH, Baumann FG, Ursumanno P, Culliford AT, Colvin SB, Galloway AC. High-risk aortic valve replacement: are the outcomes as bad as predicted? Ann Thorac Surg. 2008;85:102–7.
10. Kalavrouziotis D, Li D, Buth KJ, Le´gare´ JF. The European System for Cardiac Operative Risk Evaluation (EuroSCORE) is not appropriate for withholding surgery in high risk patients with aortic stenosis: a retrospective cohort study. J Cardiothorac Surg. 2009;4:32–40.
11. Leontyev S, Walther T, Borger MA, Lehmann S, Funkat AK, Rastan A, Kempfert J, Falk V, Mohr FW. Aortic valve replacement in octogenarians: utility of risk stratification with EuroSCORE. Ann Thorac Surg. 2009;5:1440–5.
12. Cribier A, Eltchaninoff H, Bash A, Borenstein N, Tron C, Bauer F, Derumeaux G, Anselme F, Laborde F, Lean MB. Percutaneous transcatheter implantation of an aortic valve prosthesis for calcific aortic stenosis: first human case description. Circulation. 2002;106:3006–8.
13. Piazza N, Otten A, Schultz C, Onuma Y, Garcia-Garcia HM, Boersma E, de Jaegere P, Serruys PW. Adherence to patient selection criteria in patients undergoing transcatheter aortic valve implantation with the 18F CoreValve ReValving System. Heart. 2010;96(1):19–26.
14. Smith CR, Leon MB, Mack MJ, Miller DC, Moses JW, Svensson LG, Tuzcu EM, Webb JG, Fontana GP, Makkar RR, Williams M, Dewey T, Kapadia S, Babaliaros V, Thourani VH, Corso P, Pichard AD, Bavaria JE, Herrmann HC, Akin JJ, Anderson WN, Wang D, Pocock SJ, PARTNER Trial Investigators. Transcatheter versus surgical aortic-valve replacement in high-risk patients. N Engl J Med. 2011;364(23):2187–98.
15. Thygesen K, Alpert JS, White HD, Jaffe AS, Apple FS, Galvani M, Katus HA, Newby LK, Ravkilde J, Chaitman B, Clemmensen PM, Dellborg M, Hod H, Porela P, Underwood R, Bax JJ, Beller GA, Bonow R, Van der Wall EE, Bassand JP, Wijns W, Ferguson TB, Steg PG, Uretsky BF, Williams DO, Armstrong PW, Antman EM, Fox KA, Hamm CW, Ohman EM, Simoons ML, Poole-Wilson PA, Gurfinkel EP, Lopez-Sendon JL, Pais P, Mendis S, Zhu JR, Wallentin LC, Fernandez-Aviles F, Fox KM, Parkhomenko AN, Priori SG, Tendera M, Voipio-Pulkki LM, Vahanian A, Camm AJ, De Caterina R, Dean V, Dickstein K, Filippatos G, Funck-Brentano C, Hellemans I, Kristensen SD, McGregor K, Sechtem U, Silber S, Widimsky P, Zamorano JL, Morais J, Brener S, Harrington R, Morrow D, Lim M, Martinez-Rios MA, Steinhubl S, Levine GN, Gibler WB, Goff D, Tubaro M, Dudek D, Al-Attar N. Universal definition of myocardial infarction. J Am Coll Cardiol. 2007;50:2173–95.
16. Cutlip DE, Windecker S, Mehran R, Boam A, Cohen DJ, van Es GA, Steg PG, Morel MA, Mauri L, Vranckx P, McFadden E, Lansky A, Hamon M, Krucoff MW, Serruys PW. Clinical end points in coronary stent trials: a case for standardized definitions. Circulation. 2007;115:2344–51.
17. Leon MB, Piazza N, Nikolsky E, Blackstone EH, Cutlip DE, Kappetein AP, Krucoff MW, Mack M, Mehran R, Miller C, Morel MA, Petersen J, Popma JJ, Takkenberg JJ, Vahanian A, van Es GA, Vranckx P, Webb JG, Windecker S, Serruys PW. Standardized endpoint definitions for transcatheter aortic valve implantation clinical trials: a consensus report from the Valve Academic Research Consortium. Eur Heart J. 2011;32(2):205–17.
18. Antonini-Canterin F, Leiballi E, Capanna M, Burelli C, Cassin M, Macor F, Grandis U, Nicolosi GL. Association between carotid and coronary artery disease in patients with aortic valve stenosis: an angiographic study. Angiology. 2009;60:596–600.
19. Rodés-Cabau J. Transcatheter aortic valve implantation: current and future approaches. Nat Rev Cardiol. 2011;9(1):15–29.
20. Rodés-Cabau J, Webb JG, Cheung A, Ye J, Dumont E, Feindel CM, Osten M, Natarajan MK, Velianou JL, Martucci G, DeVarennes B, Chisholm R, Peterson MD, Lichtenstein SV, Nietlispach F, Doyle D, DeLarochellière R, Teoh K, Chu V, Dancea A, Lachapelle K, Cheema A, Latter D, Horlick E. Transcatheter aortic valve implantation for the treatment of severe symptomatic aortic stenosis in patients at very high or prohibitive surgical risk: acute and late outcomes of the multicenter Canadian experience. J Am Coll Cardiol. 2010;55(11):1080–90.
21. Thomas M, Schymik G, Walther T, Himbert D, Lefèvre T, Treede H, Eggebrecht H, Rubino P, Michev I, Lange R, Anderson WN, Wendler O. Thirty-day results of the SAPIEN aortic Bioprosthesis European Outcome (SOURCE) Registry: a European registry of transcatheter aortic valve implantation using the Edwards SAPIEN valve. Circulation. 2010;122(1):62–9.
22. Piazza N, Grube E, Gerckens U, den Heijer P, Linke A, Luha O, Ramondo A, Ussia G, Wenaweser P, Windecker S, Laborde JC, de Jaegere P, Serruys PW. Procedural and 30-day outcomes following transcatheter aortic valve implantation using the third generation (18 Fr) corevalve revalving system: results from the multicentre, expanded evaluation registry 1-year following CE mark approval. EuroIntervention. 2008;4(2):242–9.
23. Gilard M, Eltchaninoff H, Iung B, Donzeau-Gouge P, Chevreul K, Fajadet J, Leprince P, Leguerrier A, Lievre M, Prat A, Teiger E, Lefevre T, Himbert D, Tchetche D, Carrié D, Albat B, Cribier A, Rioufol G, Sudre A, Blanchard D, Collet F, Dos Santos P, Meneveau N, Tirouvanziam A, Caussin C, Guyon P, Boschat J, Le Breton H, Collart F, Houel R, Delpine S, Souteyrand G, Favereau X, Ohlmann P, Doisy V, Grollier G, Gommeaux A, Claudel JP, Bourlon F, Bertrand B, Van Belle E, Laskar M, FRANCE 2 Investigators. Registry of transcatheter aortic-valve implantation in high-risk patients. N Engl J Med. 2012;366(18):1705–15.
24. Lefèvre T, Kappetein AP, Wolner E, Nataf P, Thomas M, Schächinger V, De Bruyne B, Eltchaninoff H, Thielmann M, Himbert D, Romano M, Serruys P, Wimmer-Greinecker G, PARTNER EU Investigator Group. One year follow-up of the multi-centre European PARTNER transcatheter heart valve study. Eur Heart J. 2011;32(2):148–57.
25. Meredith I. The Australia-New Zealand multicenter TAVR registry experience. 2011. http://www.tctmd.com/show.aspx?id=109728. Accessed 7 Jun 2012.
26. Moat NE, Ludman P, de Belder MA, Bridgewater B, Cunningham AD, Young CP, Thomas M, Kovac J, Spyt T, MacCarthy PA, Wendler O, Hildick-Smith D, Davies SW, Trivedi U, Blackman DJ, Levy RD, Brecker SJ, Baumbach A, Daniel T, Gray H, Mullen MJ. Long-term outcomes after transcatheter aortic valve implantation in high-risk patients with severe aortic stenosis: the U.K. TAVI (United Kingdom Transcatheter Aortic Valve Implantation) Registry. J Am Coll Cardiol. 2011;58(20):2130–8.
27. Bosmans JM, Kefer J, De Bruyne B, Herijgers P, Dubois C, Legrand V, Verheye S, Rodrigus I, Belgian TAVI Registry Participants. Procedural, 30-day and one year outcome following CoreValve or Edwards transcatheter aortic valve implantation: results of the Belgian national registry. Interact Cardiovasc Thorac Surg. 2011;12(5):762–7.

28. Eltchaninoff H, Prat A, Gilard M, Leguerrier A, Blanchard D, Fournial G, Iung B, Donzeau-Gouge P, Tribouilloy C, Debrux JL, Pavie A, Gueret P, FRANCE Registry Investigators. Transcatheter aortic valve implantation: early results of the FRANCE (FRench Aortic National CoreValve and Edwards) registry. Eur Heart J. 2011;32(2):191–7.
29. Zahn R, Gerckens U, Grube E, Linke A, Sievert H, Eggebrecht H, Hambrecht R, Sack S, Hauptmann KE, Richardt G, Figulla HR, Senges J, German Transcatheter Aortic Valve Interventions-Registry Investigators. Transcatheter aortic valve implantation: first results from a multi-centre real-world registry. Eur Heart J. 2011;32(2):198–204.
30. Tamburino C, Capodanno D, Ramondo A, Petronio AS, Ettori F, Santoro G, Klugmann S, Bedogni F, Maisano F, Marzocchi A, Poli A, Antoniucci D, Napodano M, De Carlo M, Fiorina C, Ussia GP. Incidence and predictors of early and late mortality after transcatheter aortic valve implantation in 663 patients with severe aortic stenosis. Circulation. 2011;123(3):299–308.
31. Rodés-Cabau J, Dumont E, De LaRochellière R, Doyle D, Lemieux J, Bergeron S, Clavel MA, Villeneuve J, Raby K, Bertrand OF, Pibarot P. Feasibility and initial results of percutaneous aortic valve implantation including selection of the transfemoral or transapical approach in patients with severe aortic stenosis. Am J Cardiol. 2008;102(9):1240–6.
32. Jilaihawi H, Chakravarty T, Weiss RE, Fontana GP, Forrester J, Makkar RR. Meta-analysis of complications in aortic valve replacement: comparison of Medtronic-Corevalve, Edwards-Sapien and surgical aortic valve replacement in 8,536 patients. Catheter Cardiovasc Interv. 2012;80(1):128–38.
33. de Vincentiis C, Kunkl AB, Trimarchi S, Gagliardotto P, Frigiola A, Menicanti L, Di Donato M. Aortic valve replacement in octogenarians: is biologic valve the unique solution? Ann Thorac Surg. 2008;85(4):1296–301.
34. Gulbins H, Malkoc A, Ennker J. Combined cardiac surgical procedures in octogenarians: operative outcome. Clin Res Cardiol. 2008;97(3):176–80.
35. Melby SJ, Zierer A, Kaiser SP, Guthrie TJ, Keune JD, Schuessler RB, Pasque MK, Lawton JS, Moazami N, Moon MR, Damiano Jr RJ. Aortic valve replacement in octogenarians: risk factors for early and late mortality. Ann Thorac Surg. 2007;83(5):1651–6.
36. Ussia GP, Barbanti M, Petronio AS, Tarantini G, Ettori F, Colombo A, Violini R, Ramondo A, Santoro G, Klugmann S, Bedogni F, Maisano F, Marzocchi A, Poli A, De Carlo M, Napodano M, Fiorina C, De Marco F, Antoniucci D, de Cillis E, Capodanno D, Tamburino C, CoreValve Italian Registry Investigators. Transcatheter aortic valve implantation: 3-year outcomes of self-expanding CoreValve prosthesis. Eur Heart J. 2012;33(8):969–76.
37. Vahanian A, Alfieri O, Al-Attar N, Antunes M, Bax J, Cormier B, Cribier A, De Jaegere P, Fournial G, Kappetein AP, Kovac J, Ludgate S, Maisano F, Moat N, Mohr F, Nataf P, Piérard L, Pomar JL, Schofer J, Tornos P, Tuzcu M, van Hout B, Von Segesser LK, Walther T, European Association of Cardio-Thoracic Surgery; European Society of Cardiology; European Association of Percutaneous Cardiovascular Interventions. Transcatheter valve implantation for patients with aortic stenosis: a position statement from the European Association of Cardio-Thoracic Surgery (EACTS) and the European Society of Cardiology (ESC), in collaboration with the European Association of Percutaneous Cardiovascular Interventions (EAPCI). Eur Heart J. 2008;29(11):1463–70.
38. Ranucci M, Guarracino F, Castelvecchio S, Baldassarri R, Covello RD, Landoni G, ACEF Score Research Group. Surgical and transcatheter aortic valve procedures. The limits of risk scores. Interact Cardiovasc Thorac Surg. 2010;11(2):138–41.
39. Dewey TM, Brown D, Ryan WH, Herbert MA, Prince SL, Mack MJ. Reliability of risk algorithms in predicting early and late operative outcomes in high-risk patients undergoing aortic valve replacement. J Thorac Cardiovasc Surg. 2008;135(1):180–7.
40. Rosenhek R, Iung B, Tornos P, Antunes MJ, Prendergast BD, Otto CM, Kappetein AP, Stepinska J, Kaden JJ, Naber CK, Acartürk E, Gohlke-Bärwolf C. ESC Working Group on Valvular Heart Disease Position Paper: assessing the risk of interventions in patients with valvular heart disease. Eur Heart J. 2012;33(7):822–8, 828a, 828b.
41. Kahlert P, Doettger P, Mori K, Al-Rashid F, Thielmann M, Wendt D, Jakob H, Erbel R, Eggebrecht H. Cerebral embolization during Transcatheter Aortic Valve Implantation (TAVI): a transcranial Doppler study. Circulation. 2010;122:A18122.
42. Szeto WY, Augoustides JG, Desai ND, Moeller P, McGarvey ML, Walsh E, Bannan A, Herrmann HC, Bavaria JE. Cerebral embolic exposure during transfemoral and transapical transcatheter aortic valve replacement. J Card Surg. 2011;26(4):348–54.
43. Lichtenstein SV, Cheung A, Ye J, Thompson CR, Carere RG, Pasupati S, Webb JG. Transapical transcatheter aortic valve implantation in humans: initial clinical experience. Circulation. 2006;114(6):591–6.
44. Kahlert P, Knipp SC, Schlamann M, Thielmann M, Al-Rashid F, Weber M, Johansson U, Wendt D, Jakob HG, Forsting M, Sack S, Erbel R, Eggebrecht H. Silent and apparent cerebral ischemia after percutaneous transfemoral aortic valve implantation: a diffusion-weighted magnetic resonance imaging study. Circulation. 2010;121(7):870–8.
45. Piazza N, Onuma Y, Jesserun E, Kint PP, Maugenest AM, Anderson RH, de Jaegere P, Serruys PW. Early and persistent intraventricular conduction abnormalities and requirements for pacemaking after percutaneous replacement of the aortic valve. JACC Cardiovasc Interv. 2008;1:310–6.
46. El-Khally ZTB, Staniloae C, Theroux P, Dubuc M, Roy D, Guerra P, Macle L, Talajic M. Prognostic significance of newly acquired bundle branch block after aortic valve replacement. Am J Cardiol. 2004;94:1008–11.
47. Thomas JL, Dickstein RA, Parker Jr FB, Potts JL, Poirier RA, Fruehan CT, Eich RH. Prognostic significance of the development of left bundle conduction defects following aortic valve replacement. J Thorac Cardiovasc Surg. 1982;84:382–6.
48. Sinhal A, Altwegg L, Pasupati S, Humphries KH, Allard M, Martin P, Cheung A, Ye J, Kerr C, Lichtenstein SV, Webb JG. Atrioventricular block after transcatheter balloon expandable aortic valve implantation. JACC Cardiovasc Interv. 2008;1(3):305–9.
49. Jilaihawi H, Chin D, Vasa-Nicotera M, Jeilan M, Spyt T, Ng GA, Bence J, Logtens E, Kovac J. Predictors for permanent pacemaker requirement after transcatheter aortic valve implantation with the CoreValve bioprosthesis. Am Heart J. 2009;157(5):860–6.
50. Nuis RJ, Van Mieghem NM, Schultz CJ, Tzikas A, Van der Boon RM, Maugenest AM, Cheng J, Piazza N, van Domburg RT, Serruys PW, de Jaegere PP. Timing and potential mechanisms of new conduction abnormalities during the implantation of the Medtronic CoreValve System in patients with aortic stenosis. Eur Heart J. 2011;32(16):2067–74.
51. Baan Jr J, Yong ZY, Koch KT, Henriques JP, Bouma BJ, Vis MM, Cocchieri R, Piek JJ, de Mol BA. Factors associated with cardiac conduction disorders and permanent pacemaker implantation after percutaneous aortic valve implantation with the CoreValve prosthesis. Am Heart J. 2010;159(3):497–503.
52. Fraccaro C, Buja G, Tarantini G, Gasparetto V, Leoni L, Razzolini R, Corrado D, Bonato R, Basso C, Thiene G, Gerosa G, Isabella G, Iliceto S, Napodano M. Incidence, predictors, and outcome of conduction disorders after transcatheter self-expandable aortic valve implantation. Am J Cardiol. 2011;107(5):747–54.
53. Bagur R, Manazzoni JM, Dumont É, Doyle D, Perron J, Dagenais F, Mathieu P, Baillot R, Charbonneau É, Metrás J, Mohammadi S,

Côté M, Philippon F, Voisine P, Rodés-Cabau J. Permanent pacemaker implantation following isolated aortic valve replacement in a large cohort of elderly patients with severe aortic stenosis. Heart. 2011;97(20):1687–94.

54. Kapadia SR, Svensson L, Tuzcu EM. Successful percutaneous management of left main trunk occlusion during percutaneous aortic valve replacement. Catheter Cardiovasc Interv. 2009;73(7):966–72.
55. Stabile E, Sorropago G, Cioppa A, Cota L, Agrusta M, Lucchetti V, Rubino P. Acute left main obstructions following TAVI. EuroIntervention. 2010;6(1):100–5.
56. Gogas BD, Zacharoulis AA, Antoniadis AG. Acute coronary occlusion following TAVI. Catheter Cardiovasc Interv. 2011;77(3):435–8.
57. Nuis RJ, Van Mieghem NM, Tzikas A, Piazza N, Otten AM, Cheng J, van Domburg RT, Betjes M, Serruys PW, de Jaegere PP. Frequency, determinants, and prognostic effects of acute kidney injury and red blood cell transfusion in patients undergoing transcatheter aortic valve implantation. Catheter Cardiovasc Interv. 2011;77(6):881–9.
58. Sinning JM, Ghanem A, Steinhäuser H, Adenauer V, Hammerstingl C, Nickenig G, Werner N. Renal function as predictor of mortality in patients after percutaneous transcatheter aortic valve implantation. JACC Cardiovasc Interv. 2010;3(11):1141–9.
59. Bagur R, Webb JG, Nietlispach F, Dumont E, De Larochellière R, Doyle D, Masson JB, Gutiérrez MJ, Clavel MA, Bertrand OF, Pibarot P, Rodés-Cabau J. Acute kidney injury following transcatheter aortic valve implantation: predictive factors, prognostic value, and comparison with surgical aortic valve replacement. Eur Heart J. 2010;31(7):865–74.
60. Kodali SK, O'Neill WW, Moses JW, Williams M, Smith CR, Tuzcu M, Svensson LG, Kapadia S, Hanzel G, Kirtane AJ, Leon MB. Early and late (one year) outcomes following transcatheter aortic valve implantation in patients with severe aortic stenosis (from the United States REVIVAL trial). Am J Cardiol. 2011;107(7):1058–64.
61. Grube E, Buellesfeld L, Mueller R, Sauren B, Zickmann B, Nair D, Beucher H, Felderhoff T, Iversen S, Gerckens U. Progress and current status of percutaneous aortic valve replacement: results of three device generations of the CoreValve Revalving system. Circ Cardiovasc Interv. 2008;1:167–75.
62. Piazza N, Schultz C, de Jaegere PP, Serruys PW. Implantation of two selfexpanding aortic bioprosthetic valves during the same procedure-Insights into valve-in-valve implantation ("Russian doll concept"). Catheter Cardiovasc Interv. 2009;73:530–9.
63. Vavouranakis M, Vrachatis DA, Toutouzas KP, Chrysohoou C, Stefanadis C. "Bail out" procedures for malpositioning of aortic valve prosthesis (CoreValve). Int J Cardiol. 2010;145(1):154–5.
64. Shapira Y, Hirsch R, Kornowski R, Hasdai D, Assali A, Vaturi M, Sievert H, Hein R, Battler A, Sagie A. Percutaneous closure of perivalvular leaks with Amplatzer occluders: feasibility, safety, and short-term results. J Heart Valve Dis. 2007;16:305–13.
65. Hammerstingl C, Werner N, Nickenig G. Symptomatic paravalvular leakage after mechanical aortic valve replacement in a critically ill patient: why not just "plug" the hole? Eur J Echocardiogr. 2009;10:576–8.
66. Zegdi R, Ciobotaru V, Noghin M, Sleilaty G, Lafont A, Latrémouille C, Deloche A, Fabiani JN. Is it reasonable to treat all calcified stenotic aortic valves with a valved stent? Results from a human anatomic study in adults. J Am Coll Cardiol. 2008;51(5):579–84.
67. Schultz CJ, Weustink A, Piazza N, Otten A, Mollet N, Krestin G, van Geuns RJ, de Feyter P, Serruys PW, de Jaegere P. Geometry and degree of apposition of the CoreValve ReValving system with multislice computed tomography after implantation in patients with aortic stenosis. J Am Coll Cardiol. 2009;54(10):911–8.
68. Clavel MA, Rodés-Cabau J, Dumont É, Bagur R, Bergeron S, De Larochellière R, Doyle D, Larose E, Dumesnil JG, Pibarot P. Validation and characterization of transcatheter aortic valve effective orifice area measured by Doppler echocardiography. JACC Cardiovasc Imaging. 2011;4(10):1053–62.
69. Clavel MA, Webb JG, Rodés-Cabau J, Masson JB, Dumont E, De Larochellière R, Doyle D, Bergeron S, Baumgartner H, Burwash IG, Dumesnil JG, Mundigler G, Moss R, Kempny A, Bagur R, Bergler-Klein J, Gurvitch R, Mathieu P, Pibarot P. Comparison between transcatheter and surgical prosthetic valve implantation in patients with severe aortic stenosis and reduced left ventricular ejection fraction. Circulation. 2010;122(19):1928–36.
70. Gotzmann M, Hehen T, Germing A, Lindstaedt M, Yazar A, Laczkovics A, Mumme A, Mügge A, Bojara W. Short-term effects of transcatheter aortic valve implantation on neurohormonal activation, quality of life and 6-minute walk test in severe and symptomatic aortic stenosis. Heart. 2010;96(14):1102–6.
71. Bagur R, Rodés-Cabau J, Dumont E, Larochellière RD, Doyle D, Bertrand OF, Côté M, Poirier P, Pibarot P. Exercise capacity in patients with severe symptomatic aortic stenosis before and six months after transcatheter aortic valve implantation. Am J Cardiol. 2011;108(2):258–64.
72. Ussia GP, Mulè M, Barbanti M, Cammalleri V, Scarabelli M, Immè S, Capodanno D, Ciriminna S, Tamburino C. Quality of life assessment after percutaneous aortic valve implantation. Eur Heart J. 2009;30(14):1790–6.
73. Krane M, Deutsch MA, Bleiziffer S, Schneider L, Ruge H, Mazzitelli D, Schreiber C, Brockmann G, Voss B, Bauernschmitt R, Lange R. Quality of life among patients undergoing transcatheter aortic valve implantation. Am Heart J. 2010;160(3):451–7.
74. Bagur R, Rodés-Cabau J, Dumont E, De Larochellière R, Doyle D, Pibarot P, Côté M, Clavel MA, Villeneuve J, Gutiérrez M, Poirier P, Bertrand OF. Performance-based functional assessment of patients undergoing transcatheter aortic valve implantation. Am Heart J. 2011;161(4):726–34.
75. Bekeredjian R, Krumsdorf U, Chorianopoulos E, Kallenbach K, Karck M, Katus HA, Rottbauer W. Usefulness of percutaneous aortic valve implantation to improve quality of life in patients >80 years of age. Am J Cardiol. 2010;106(12):1777–81.
76. Gonçalves A, Marcos-Alberca P, Almeria C, Feltes G, Hernández-Antolín RA, Rodríguez E, Rodrigo JL, Cobiella J, Maroto L, Cardoso JC, Macaya C, Zamorano JL. Quality of life improvement at midterm follow-up after transcatheter aortic valve implantation. Int J Cardiol. 2013;162(2):117–22.
77. Gotzmann M, Bojara W, Lindstaedt M, Ewers A, Bösche L, Germing A, Lawo T, Bechtel M, Laczkovics A, Mügge A. One-year results of transcatheter aortic valve implantation in severe symptomatic aortic valve stenosis. Am J Cardiol. 2011;107(11):1687–92.
78. Reynolds MR, Magnuson EA, Lei Y, Leon MB, Smith CR, Svensson LG, Webb JG, Babaliaros VC, Bowers BS, Fearon WF, Herrmann HC, Kapadia S, Kodali SK, Makkar RR, Pichard AD, Cohen DJ, Placement of Aortic Transcatheter Valves (PARTNER) Investigators. Health-related quality of life after transcatheter aortic valve replacement in inoperable patients with severe aortic stenosis. Circulation. 2011;124(18):1964–72.
79. Gotzmann M, Pljakic A, Bojara W, Lindstaedt M, Ewers A, Germing A, Mügge A. Transcatheter aortic valve implantation in patients with severe symptomatic aortic valve stenosis-predictors of mortality and poor treatment response. Am Heart J. 2011;162(2): 238–45.e1.
80. Jamieson WR, Rosado LJ, Munro AI, Gerein AN, Burr LH, Miyagishima RT, Janusz MT, Tyers GF. Carpentier-Edwards standard porcine bioprosthesis: primary tissue failure (structural valve deterioration) by age groups. Ann Thorac Surg. 1988;46(2): 155–62.
81. Jamieson WR, Munro AI, Miyagishima RT, Allen P, Burr LH, Tyers GF. Carpentier-Edwards standard porcine bioprosthesis:

clinical performance to seventeen years. Ann Thorac Surg. 1995;60(4):999–1006.
82. Gurvitch R, Wood DA, Tay EL, Leipsic J, Ye J, Lichtenstein SV, Thompson CR, Carere RG, Wijesinghe N, Nietlispach F, Boone RH, Lauck S, Cheung A, Webb JG. Transcatheter aortic valve implantation: durability of clinical and hemodynamic outcomes beyond 3 years in a large patient cohort. Circulation. 2010;122(13):1319–27.
83. Kulik A, Masters RG, Bédard P, Hendry PJ, Lam BK, Rubens FD, Mesana TG, Ruel M. Postoperative lipid-lowering therapy and bioprosthesis structural valve deterioration: justification for a randomised trial? Eur J Cardiothorac Surg. 2010;37(1):139–44.
84. Buellesfeld L, Gerckens U, Schuler G, Bonan R, Kovac J, Serruys PW, Labinaz M, den Heijer P, Mullen M, Tymchak W, Windecker S, Mueller R, Grube E. 2-year follow-up of patients undergoing transcatheter aortic valve implantation using a self-expanding valve prosthesis. J Am Coll Cardiol. 2011;57(16):1650–7.

4 Transcatheter Aortic Valve Replacement: An Interventionist's View

Melanie Freeman and John G. Webb

Abstract

Calcific aortic stenosis is the most common acquired valvular heart disease, and its prevalence is increasing significantly with the aging population. Once symptoms of angina, syncope, or heart failure develop, average survival is 2–3 years [1]. Traditionally, surgical aortic valve replacement (SAVR) has been the definitive treatment for severe symptomatic aortic stenosis; however, many patients do not undergo surgery as they are considered high risk or inoperable due to age and comorbidities [2].

Keywords

Transcatheter aortic valve implantation • Transcatheter aortic valve replacement • Bioprosthesis • Aortic stenosis • Valve-in-valve • Aortic valve

Introduction

Calcific aortic stenosis is the most common acquired valvular heart disease, and its prevalence is increasing significantly with the aging population. Once symptoms of angina, syncope, or heart failure develop, average survival is 2–3 years [1]. Traditionally, surgical aortic valve replacement (SAVR) has been the definitive treatment for severe symptomatic aortic stenosis; however, many patients do not undergo surgery as they are considered high risk or inoperable due to age and comorbidities [2].

Percutaneous transcatheter aortic valve replacement (TAVR) has been developed as an alternative to surgical AVR in those who are high risk or not candidates for SAVR. TAVR was first described in humans by Cribier in 2002 [3]. The transcatheter valve was delivered via an anterograde technique from the venous circulation, by subsequent transseptal puncture into the left heart and passage of the valve through the mitral and into the aortic position. Later, a transarterial retrograde approach was developed—a technique in wide use today [4]—and followed by additional approaches including transapical, transaxillary, and transaortic techniques.

Since its advent, TAVR has been performed in over 50,000 patients worldwide. TAVR has evolved into a reproducible procedure with steadily improving clinical outcomes and is now emerging as the standard of care in patients with severe aortic stenosis who are considered inoperable [5] and an accepted alternative to surgery for patients at high risk for conventional aortic valve replacement [6].

Techniques of Transcatheter Aortic Valve Replacement

TAVR is most often performed utilizing the transfemoral retrograde approach, with alternative access approaches usually reserved for patients with concomitant severe peripheral arterial disease.

M. Freeman, MBBS, FRACP (✉)
J.G. Webb, MD, FRCPC, FACC
Department of Cardiology, St Paul's Hospital,
1081 Burrard Street, Vancouver, BC V6Z 1Y6, Canada
e-mail: mfreeman@providencehealth.bc.ca;
webb@providencehealth.bc.ca

J.K. Min et al. (eds.), *Multimodality Imaging for Transcatheter Aortic Valve Replacement*,
DOI 10.1007/978-1-4471-2798-7_4, © Springer-Verlag London 2014

Transfemoral Approach

The common femoral artery, at the level of the femoral head, is the primary access site for the transfemoral approach owing to its relatively large size and compressibility. The side with the largest and least diseased, tortuous, or calcified iliofemoral artery—as assessed by a screening angiogram and/or multidetector computed tomographic (CT) angiography—is selected for placement of the sheath. The potential site of access is assessed first with fluoroscopy and/or ultrasound, and arterial access is gained by percutaneous puncture. Alternatively, a surgical cutdown is utilized to access the femoral artery. A smaller percutaneous sheath is inserted into the femoral artery on the contralateral side for placement of a pigtail catheter in the ascending aorta for root angiography.

The TAVR procedure may be performed under local or general anesthesia. Following balloon valvuloplasty, the valve prosthesis is passed across the aortic valve and positioned under fluoroscopic and transesophageal echocardiographic (TEE) guidance. Balloon-expandable valves are deployed under rapid ventricular pacing at a rate of 160–220 bpm to minimize cardiac output and therefore minimize unintentional motion of the valve during balloon dilatation. Self-expanding valves are advanced across the aortic valve within a delivery catheter and deployed by retracting the outer sheath of the delivery catheter generally without rapid pacing. Once the delivery system is retrieved, the femoral access site is closed utilizing previously inserted percutaneous sutures or repaired surgically if a surgical cutdown was used.

Transapical Approach

The transapical approach was first described in 2006 with balloon-expandable valves [7]. A sheath is placed surgically in the left ventricular apex, accessed through a small left anterolateral minithoracotomy. Following balloon valvuloplasty, the valve prosthesis and balloon catheter are passed over a wire into the left ventricle and positioned within the aortic annulus under fluoroscopic and transesophageal echocardiographic guidance.

This approach may be considered if the iliofemoral arterial system is of sufficiently small diameter, calcified, or tortuous and not technically suitable for delivery of the device. Also taken into consideration is the angulation of the aorta and arch. In particular, a transverse or extremely unfolded ascending aorta may increase the difficulty of delivery and positioning of the balloon-expandable devices. It has been suggested that with advances in device technology and a reduction in delivery system profiles for the transarterial approach, alternative access approaches will be limited to less than 30 % of TAVR procedures [8]. Contraindications to the transapical approach include previous left ventricular surgery using a patch, calcified pericardium, severe respiratory disease, and a non-reachable left ventricular apex [9].

Axillary/Subclavian Approach

The axillary/subclavian approach is an alternative access route in those excluded from the transfemoral approach; however, it has the similar limitations with respect to vessel caliber, calcification, and tortuosity. The left axillary artery is surgically isolated through a sort subclavicular incision although percutaneous access and closure are occasionally utilized. The sheath is passed through the axillary artery and into the ascending aorta, and the transcatheter heart valve (THV) is delivered in a retrograde fashion across the native aortic valve [10, 11].

Transaortic Approach

Recently, direct access through the ascending aorta has been described [12]. This involves a minimally invasive right second or third intercostal minithoracotomy or ministernotomy with introduction of the THV directly into the ascending aorta and retrograde passage across the diseased aortic valve. This approach has been utilized for patients in whom transarterial approaches are suboptimal and in those with chest wall abnormalities, severe respiratory disease, or poor left ventricular function, excluded from the transapical approach [13]. Potential advantages over the transapical approach include reduced myocardial injury and bleeding, in addition to a more familiar surgical technique to cardiac surgeons.

Transcatheter Valves

Two THV designs have been widely used in clinical practice over the last few years: the balloon-expandable Edwards SAPIEN and SAPIEN XT valves (Edwards Lifesciences Inc., Irvine, USA) and the CoreValve ReValving System.

Edwards SAPIEN and SAPIEN XT Valves

The Edwards transcatheter heart valves (Edwards Lifesciences Inc., Irvine, USA), available in SAPIEN™ and the newer-generation SAPIEN XT™, consist of bovine pericardial leaflets, mounted on a balloon-expandable frame (Fig. 4.1). The pericardium is treated with an anti-calcification

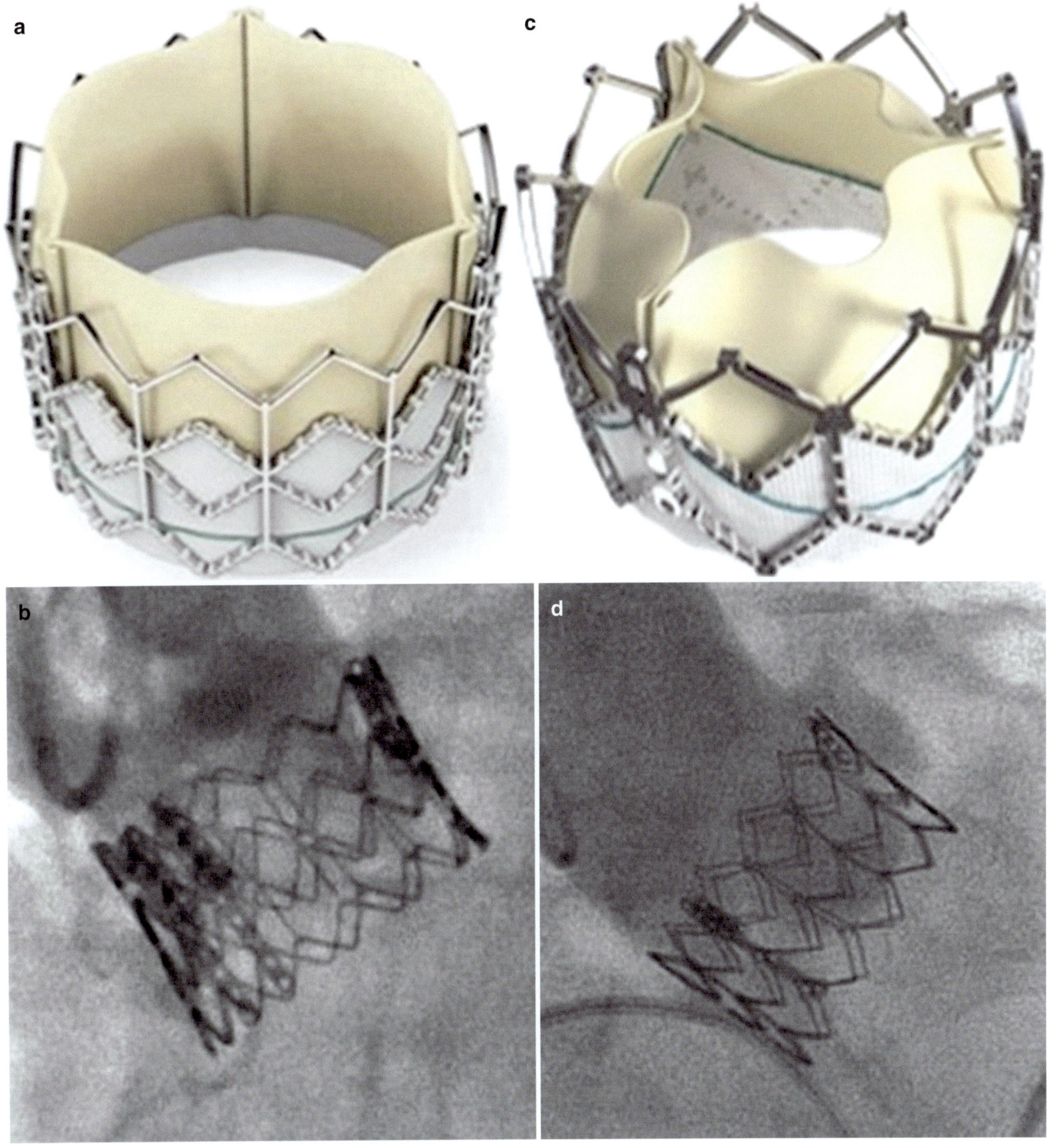

Fig. 4.1 Current balloon-expandable transcatheter heart valves: Edwards SAPIEN THV (**a**) schemata and (**b**) following deployment with aortography and Edwards SAPIEN XT THV (**c**) schemata and (**d**) following deployment with aortography

treatment used in surgical heart valves. The ventricular portion of the frame is covered with a fabric sealing cuff to provide an annular seal for minimization of post-TAVR paravalvular leak.

The SAPIEN™ THV utilizes a stainless steel frame and is available in two sizes, with external diameters of 23 and 26 mm and heights of 14.3 and 16.1 mm, respectively, once fully deployed. The newer SAPIEN XT™ THV consists of a cobalt chromium frame; the strength of the alloy is greater allowing a reduction in strut thickness with fewer stent struts and therefore a lower-profile device for delivery. As a result, radial strength may be lower. It is available in four sizes, with external diameters of 20, 23, 26, and 29 mm and heights of 13.5, 14.3, 17.2, and 19.1 mm, respectively (Fig. 4.2).

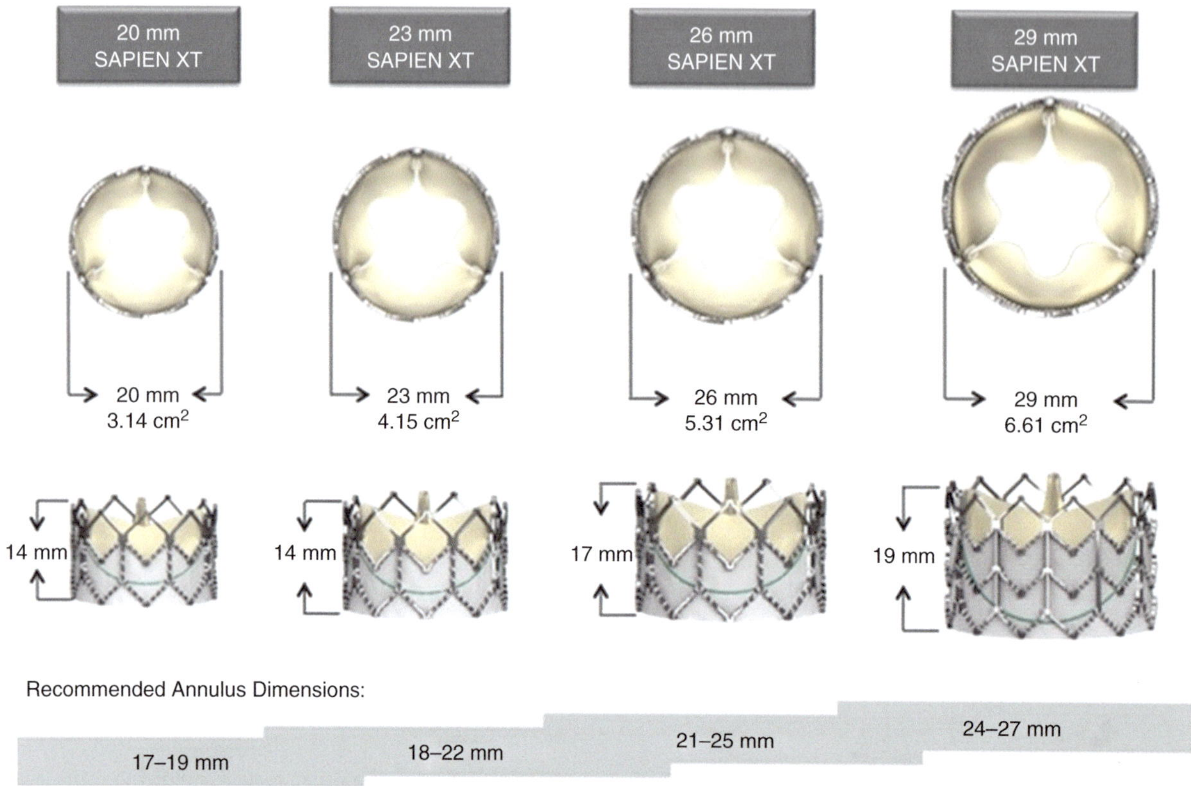

Fig. 4.2 Edwards SAPIEN XT dimensions and recommended annulus sizes

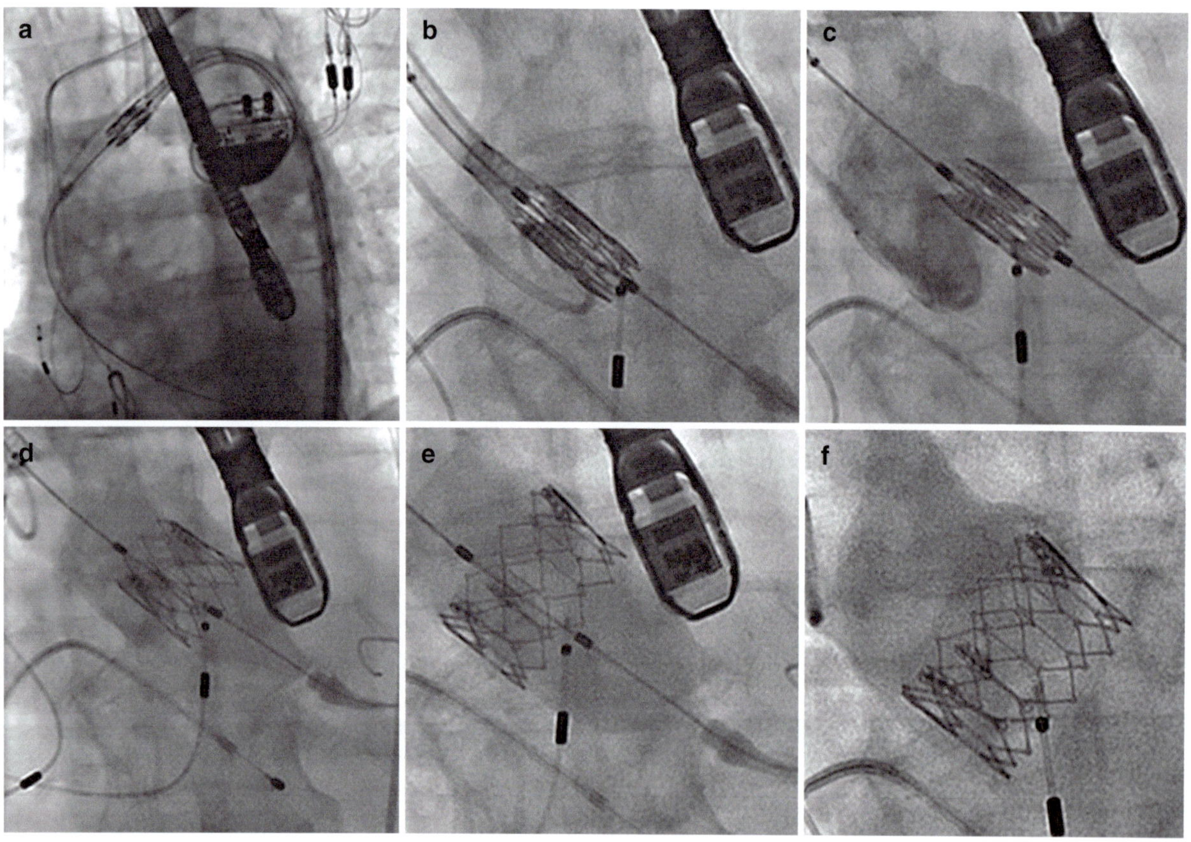

Fig. 4.3 Transfemoral delivery of Edwards balloon-expandable transcatheter heart valve. (**a**) Passage of the valve across the aortic arch. (**b**) Crossing the native aortic valve. (**c**) Positioning of the valve utilizing aortography and transesophageal echocardiography. (**d**) Partial balloon expansion of the transcatheter heart valve. (**e**) Full balloon expansion of the transcatheter heart valve. (**f**) Post implantation aortography

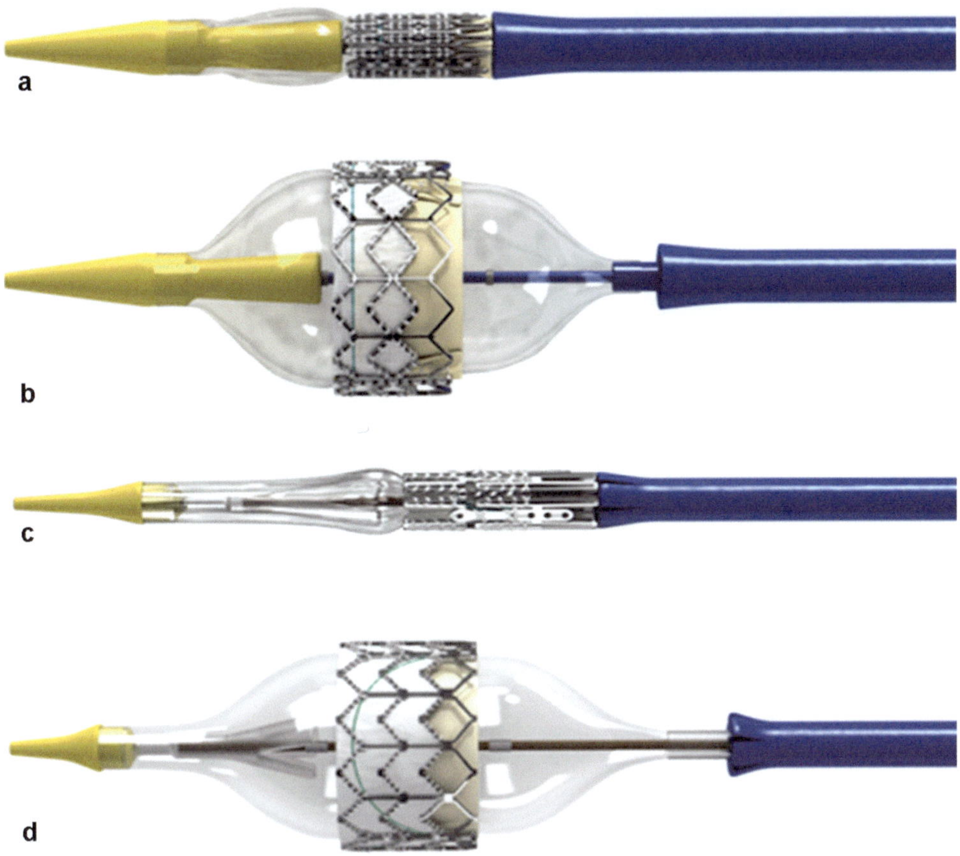

Fig. 4.4 Edwards balloon-expandable delivery systems. Retroflex 3 delivery system with (**a**) crimped valve and (**b**) balloon-expanded valve and Novaflex + delivery system with (**c**) valve crimped and (**d**) balloon-expanded valve

Table 4.1 Edward SAPIEN and SAPIEN XT sizes, sheath dimensions, and recommended minimum artery diameter

		SAPIEN		SAPIEN XT			
THV size (mm)		23	26	20	23	26	29
Sheath ID (French)		22	24	16	16	18	20
Sheath OD (mm)	Unexpanded	8.4	9.2	6.7	6.7	7.2	8
	Expanded with valve	–	–	8.9	8.9	8.9	9.9
Recommended minimum artery diameter (mm)		7	8	6	6	6.5	7

The current manufacturer's recommendations are to select device size according to two-dimensional long-axis TEE measurements of the aortic annulus, although emerging evidence by CT has challenged the accuracy of such measurements. The 23 mm valve is recommended for use in patients with annulus diameters of 18–22 mm and the 26 mm in patients with annulus diameters of 21–25 mm, while the 29 mm SAPIEN XT valve is recommended for use in patients with annulus diameters of 24–27 mm.

The Edwards THVs are generally implanted utilizing a transarterial or transapical approach. For transarterial implantation (Fig. 4.3), the SAPIEN THV is compressed onto the Retroflex 3 delivery system that is introduced into the femoral artery via a 22 or 24 F sheath for the 23 and 26 mm valves, respectively. The newer-generation SAPIEN XT is crimped onto the lower-profile Novaflex delivery system, resulting in lower sheath sizes of 16, 18, and 20 F for the 23, 26, and 29 mm valves, respectively (Fig. 4.4). This lower-profile delivery system has expanded the number of patients eligible for the transfemoral approach who would otherwise have been excluded due to small vessel diameter and has resulted in a significant reduction in vascular complications [14]. Recommended minimal luminal diameters of the iliofemoral system are demonstrated in Table 4.1 for each valve and sheath size. These recommendations, however, do not take into account vessel calcification, atheroma, and tortuosity. In the absence of severe disease, a relatively compliant artery may accommodate a slightly larger sheath size.

For the transapical approach, the THV is crimped onto the balloon and delivered using the shorter Ascendra delivery system for the SAPIEN THV and the Ascendra 2 delivery system for the SAPIEN XT.

CoreValve

The CoreValve ReValving System™ (Medtronic Inc., Irvine, USA) consists of porcine pericardial leaflets mounted within a self-expanding nitinol frame (Fig. 4.5). The current-generation device is compressed within its Accutrak™ delivery catheter and introduced through an 18 French sheath. It is manufactured in 26, 29, and 31 mm outer diameters, as measured at the ventricular part of the frame, recommended for use in patients with annulus diameters of

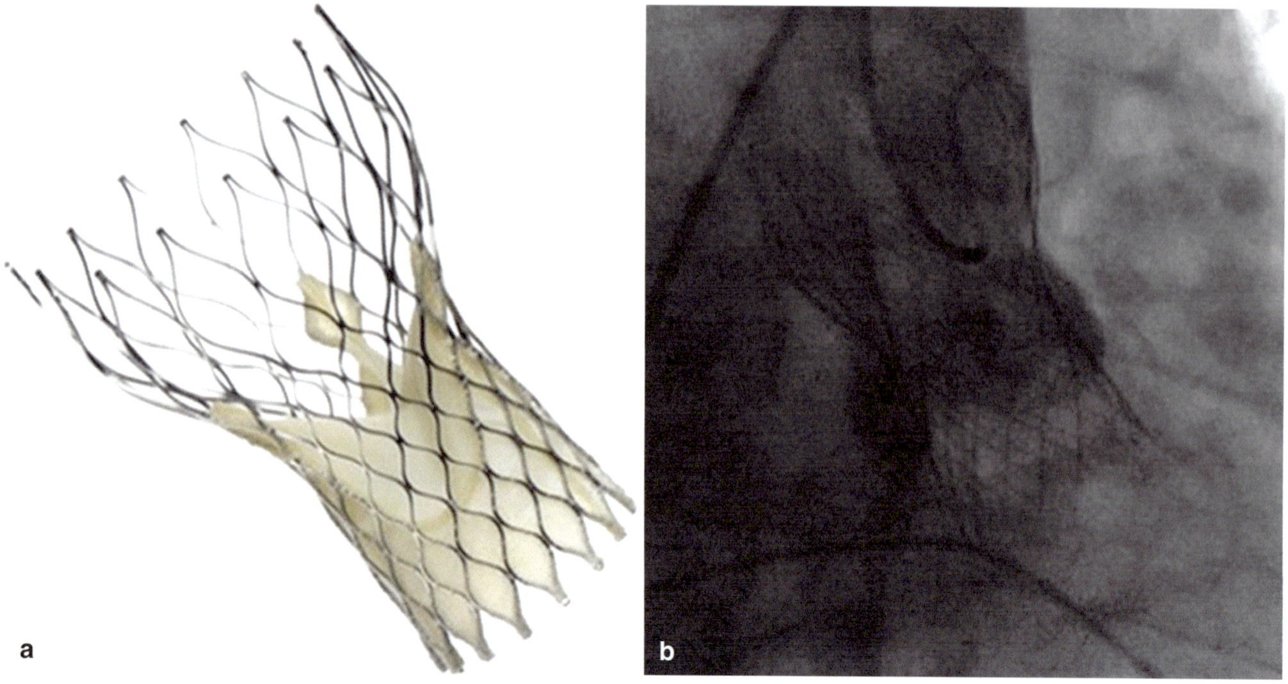

Fig. 4.5 CoreValve ReValving System (**a**) schemata and (**b**) following deployment with aortography

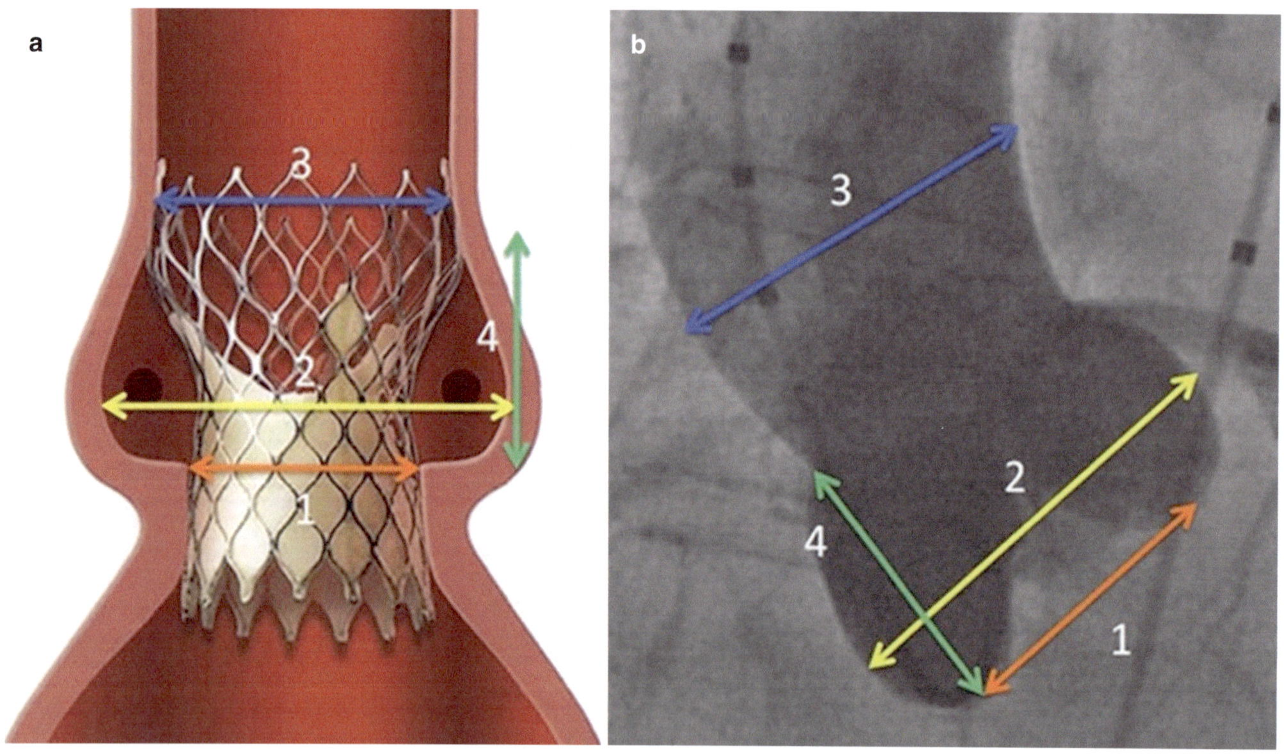

Fig. 4.6 Aortic root and annulus measurements required for CoreValve demonstrated on (**a**) schemata and (**b**) aortography. The required measurements include (*1*) aortic annulus diameter, (*2*) sinus of Valsalva width, (*3*) ascending aorta width, and (*4*) sinus of Valsalva height

20–23, 23–27, and 26–29 mm, respectively. The frame has an overall length of up to 55 mm, and in addition to anchoring at the level of the annulus and valve leaflets, the CoreValve extends superiorly to anchor in the ascending aorta.

Careful evaluation of the aortic root and ascending aorta, in addition to that of the aortic annulus, is required to avoid compromise of the coronary artery ostia and avoid valve embolization (Fig. 4.6). It is recommended that a coronary ostial height of 15 mm is required to ovoid coronary obstruction if the 12 mm skirt is deployed too aortic. Additionally, the sinus of Valsalva width needs to be greater than 27 mm for the 26 mm device and greater than 29 mm for the larger devices, to ensure a space surrounding the central waist of the device, to house the displaced native valve leaflets. The recommended maximum diameter of the ascending aorta is 40, 43, and 43 mm for the 26, 29, and 31 mm devices, respectively, to allow for satisfactory anchoring of the device at its upper portion (Table 4.2). Care must be taken in those patients with bypass grafts to ensure the device does not interfere with graft ostia.

Since the CoreValve is self-expanding, it has the potential benefit of partial retrieval if positioned incorrectly (Fig. 4.7). Disadvantages when compared with the SAPIEN valves include a higher rate of atrioventricular block, pacemaker insertion, paravalvular regurgitation, and the potential late consequences of covering the coronary ostia.

Table 4.2 CoreValve dimensions and manufacturer's recommendations

		26 mm	29 mm	31 mm
Annulus diameter (mm)		20–23	23–27	26–29
Dimensions of expanded valve (mm)	Inflow	26	29	31
	Constriction	22	23	23
	Outflow	40	44	44
	Length	55	53	52
Ascending aorta diameter (mm)		≤40	≤43	≤43
Sinus of Valsalva	Width (mm)	≥27	≥29	≥29
	Height (mm)	≥15	≥15	≥15
Sheath ID (French)		18	18	18
Recommended minimum artery diameter (mm)		≥6	≥6	≥6

Newer Valves

Several newer transcatheter heart valves are under evaluation, including the Lotus™ valve (Boston Scientific Inc., USA), Portico™ (St Jude Medical Inc., USA), Engager™ (Medtronic Inc., USA) [15], JenaClip™ (JenaValve Inc., DE) [16, 17], Acurate (Symetis Inc., CH), and Direct Flow™ valves (Direct Flow Medical Inc., USA) (Fig. 4.8) [18, 19]. Generally, these next-generation valves are self-expanding and include features that may facilitate valve positioning and improve annular sealing, with lower-profile delivery systems to accommodate smaller vessel diameters. These valves are currently under clinical evaluation and it remains unclear whether outcomes will be inferior, comparable, or superior to current-generation THVs.

Patient Selection and Evaluation

Although feasible in most patients with severe aortic stenosis, TAVR is generally utilized in patients not suitable for surgical AVR, who are likely to derive functional and survival benefit. The evaluation of potential TAVR patients is a complex process involving a multidisciplinary team approach; key members of the team include the primary cardiologist, interventional cardiologist, cardiothoracic surgeon, vascular surgeon, cardiac anesthesiologist and perfusionist, echocardiographers, and cardiac imaging specialists, as well as specialized nursing. This multidisciplinary approach is also applied during performance of the procedure and postoperative care of the patient [20].

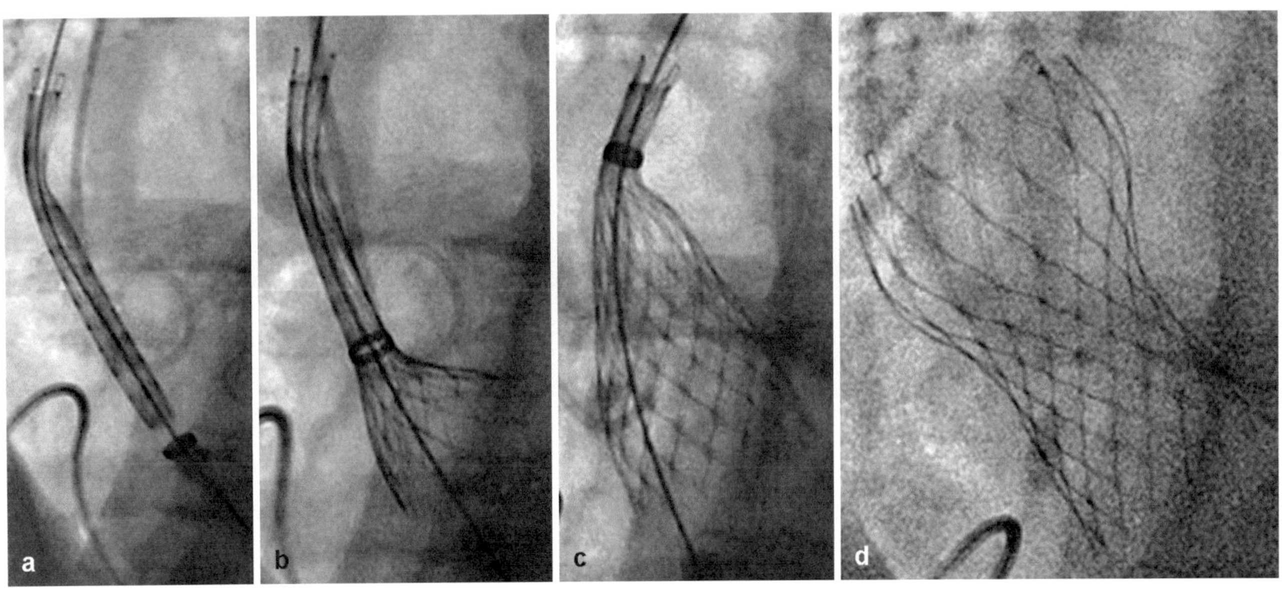

Fig. 4.7 Delivery of the CoreValve ReValving System: (**a**) Crossing the native aortic valve. (**b**) Retraction of the outer sheath. (**c**) Partial release of the transcatheter heart valve at which point it is still possible to retrieve the valve. (**d**) Full expansion of the prosthesis extending from just below the insertion of the native leaflets to the supracoronary aorta

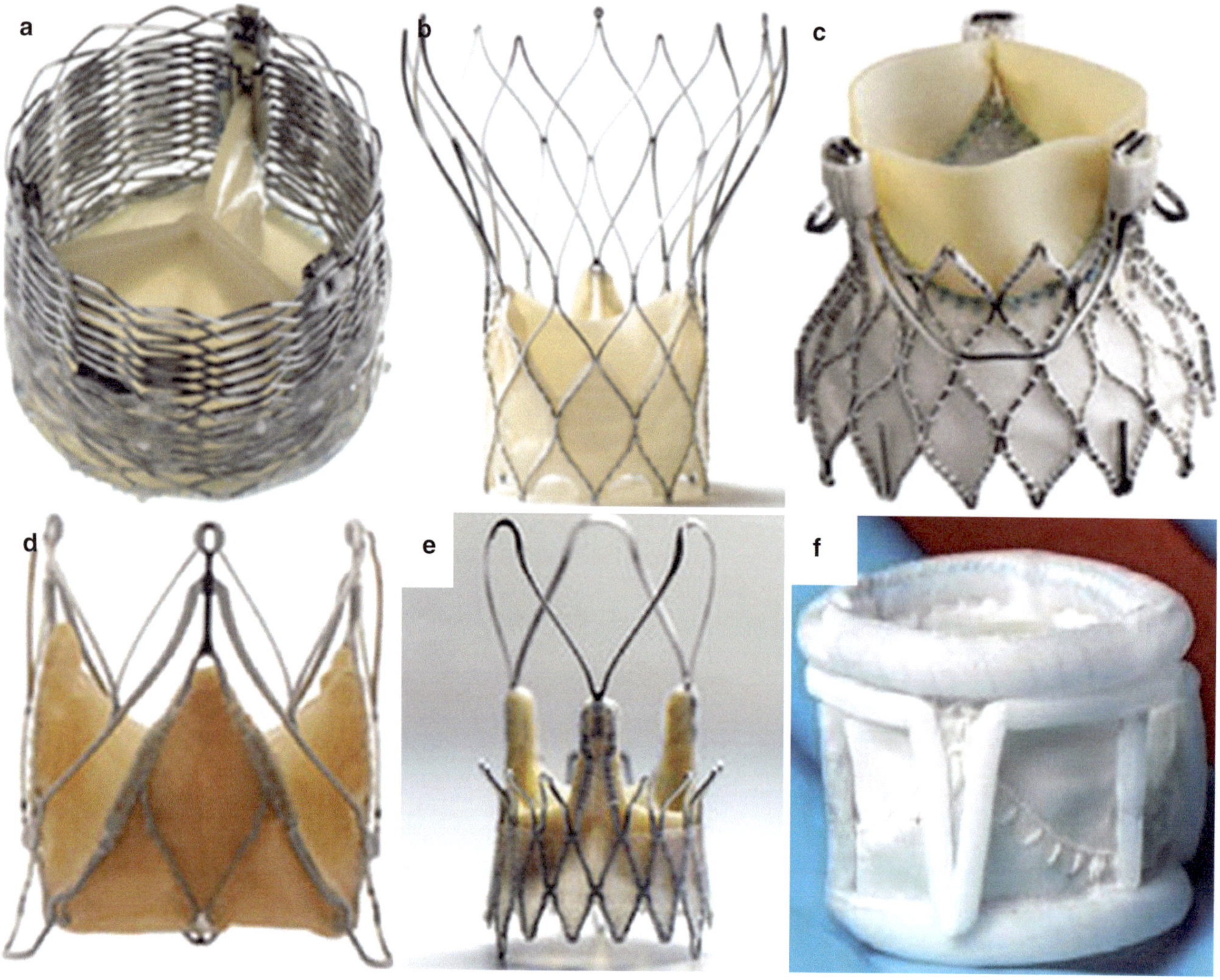

Fig. 4.8 Newer transcatheter heart valves under evaluation: (**a**) Lotus valve (Boston Scientific Inc. USA), (**b**) Portico valve(St. Jude Medical Inc. USA), (**c**) Engager valve(Medtronic Inc. USA), (**d**) JenaClip valve (JenaValve Inc. DE), (**e**) Acurate valve (Symetis Inc. Ch), and (**f**) Direct Flow valve (Direct Flow Medical Inc. USA)

"High-risk" surgical patients are often defined as having a Society of Thoracic Surgeons Predicted Risk of Mortality (STS-PROM) at 30 days of greater than 10 % or logistic EuroSCORE of greater than 20 % (Box 4.1). These risk calculators are often limited, however, and do not account for several pertinent clinical risk factors, such as previous coronary artery bypass grafting with patent grafts, porcelain aorta, previous chest radiotherapy, severe lung disease, and liver cirrhosis.

A comprehensive evaluation involving transthoracic echocardiography, coronary angiography, aortic angiography, and CT is required prior to TAVR to assess the aortic annulus dimensions and geometry, access site, and approach. Transthoracic echocardiography is used to assess valve morphology, transaortic gradient, valvular regurgitation, calcification, orifice area, and other concomitant cardiac

Box 4.1 Variable Within the Society of Thoracic Surgery (STS) and EuroSCORE

STS for Aortic Value Replacement	EuroSCORE
Age	Age
Gender	Gender
Race	Renal impairment
Weight	Extracardiac arteriopathy
Height	Poor mobility
Diabetes	Previous cardiac surgery
Renal function	Chronic lung disease
Hypertension	Active endocarditis
Endocarditis	Critical pre-operative state
Chronic lung diseases	Diabetes on insulin

STS for Aortic Value Replacement	EuroSCORE
Immunosuppresive therapy	NYHA heart failure class
Peripheral vascular disease	CCS class 4 angina
Cerebrovascular disease	LV function
Prior CABG	Recent myocardial infarction within 90 days
Prioi valve surgery	Pulmonary hypertension
Previous other cardiac – PCI	Operation urgency
Prior myocardial infarction	Surgical weight
Cardiac presentation (symptoms or ACS)	Surgery on thoracic aorta
Congestive heart failure	
Cardiogenic shock	
Resuscitation	
Arrhythmia	
Preoperative inotropes	
Number of diseased coronary vessels	
Left main disease	
Ejection fraction	
Aortic stenosis	
Mitral stenosis	
Aortic regurgitation	
Mitral regurgitation	
Tricuspid regurgitation	
First or reoperative surgery	
Status of procedure (e.g., elective versus urgent)	
Intraoperative intraaortic balloon pump	
Resection of sub-aortic stenosis	
Mitral surgery needed	
Tricuspid surgery needed	
Pulmonic surgery needed	
LVAD surgery required	
Other non-cardiac procedure required	
Unplanned procedure performed	
Other cardiac surgery performed	

pathologies. It is also used as a screening tool to evaluate aortic annulus dimensions prior to device selection. Final valve sizing, however, is usually dependant on intraoperative two-dimensional long-axis TEE measurements. Three-dimensional annular sizing with 3-D echocardiography and CT is emerging as a potentially more accurate way of sizing the aortic annulus, the latter of which is utilized by many operators including our own. Generally, the implanted valve should be slightly larger than the annulus size to minimize the risk of malapposition, paravalvular leak, and valve embolization associated with undersizing. Excessive oversizing, however, may result in incomplete stent expansion potentially affecting valve hemodynamics or aortic root injury or rupture.

Arterial access is assessed with the combination of invasive angiography and contrast-enhanced CT (Fig. 4.9). As discussed above, the evaluation of arterial dimensions and the presence or absence of atheroma, calcification, and tortuosity is fundamental in the assessment of the TAVR patient in minimizing potential major vascular complications.

The aortic root is assessed using invasive angiography and contrast MDCT to evaluate root and valvular calcification, left main height from the left coronary cusp insertion (due to risk of coronary obstruction), and technical issues related to each valve type and delivery system. Left and right heart catheterizations are also performed to assess the presence of pulmonary hypertension and coronary ischemia and the need for revascularization prior to TAVR. Percutaneous revascularization may be considered as a staged procedure in the presence of a large ischemic burden; however, in the majority of cases, this is not required. Measurement of the aortic transvalvular pressure gradient and calculation of aortic valve orifice area may be useful in cases of aortic stenosis of uncertain severity on transthoracic echocardiography.

Ideally, TAVR should be performed in regional centers of excellence with a dedicated heart valve program and high procedural volumes [20]. The procedure may be undertaken in a cardiac catheterization laboratory with modifications or in a hybrid operating room equipped with high-quality fluoroscopic imaging; the facilities need to be large enough to accommodate sophisticated X-ray imaging integrated with echocardiography, cardiopulmonary bypass and intra-aortic balloon pump machines, and anesthesia equipment, with surgical sterility standards mandatory.

Complications of TAVR

Procedural Complications

Vascular Complications

Vascular events, primarily unplanned iliofemoral repair, are not an infrequent complication of TAVR and have been reported in up to 34 % of patients [21]. These vascular events are not limited to access sites but may involve any site at which instrumentation occurs. Potential complications include aortic dissection, ventricular perforation, and access site complications including dissection, stenosis, perforation, arteriovenous fistula, pseudoaneurysm, hematoma, nerve injury, and compartment syndrome. With the transapical approach, potential access site complications include bleeding, left ventricular pseudoaneurysm formation with or without rupture, and hemodynamic instability requiring

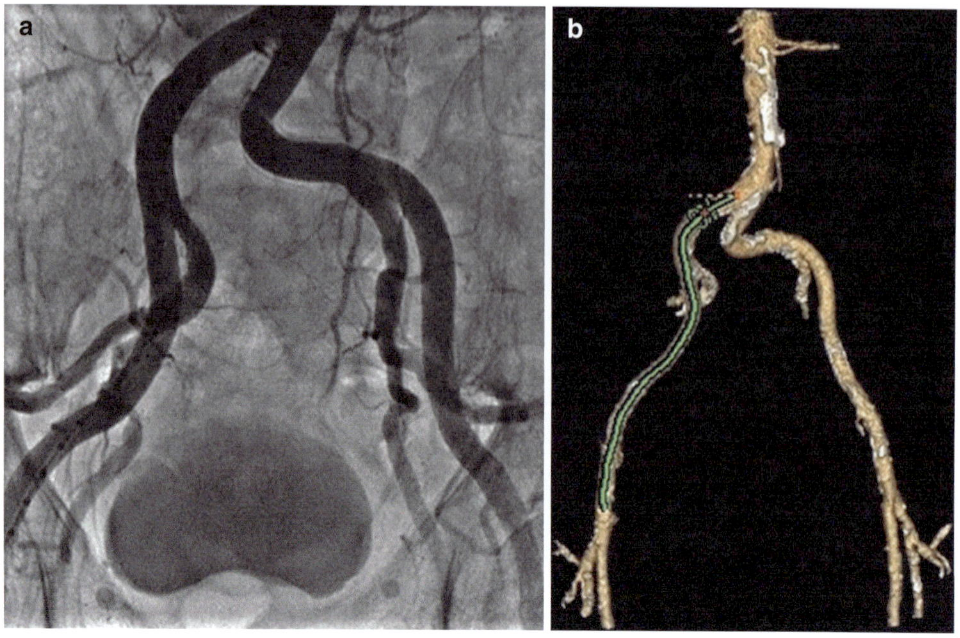

Fig. 4.9 Iliofemoral assessment with (**a**) angiography and (**b**) MDCT

urgent cardiopulmonary bypass support. Additionally, excessive balloon dilatation and oversizing of the valve may result in aortic root or annulus rupture.

More recently, a significant reduction in the incidence of vascular events has been reported, with the frequency of major vascular complications now reported as low as 1 % in experienced centers [14]. This explanation that underlies this significant improvement has been largely attributed to increased operator experience, better vascular screening, and smaller sheath sizes with improved delivery systems. As a general rule, vascular access complications are more likely to occur when the minimum artery diameter is less than the sheath external diameter, particularly in the presence of significant atheroma and calcification.

Stroke and Neurological Events

The risk of stroke due to dislodgement and subsequent embolization of atheromatous debris from the aortic arch or from the calcified valve itself has been reported to range between 2 and 11% [22–25]. Additionally, new foci of microinfarction have been reported in up to 85 % as detected by diffusion-weighted magnetic resonance imaging performed soon after TAVR [26]. Although this is reported more frequently following TAVR as compared with conventional SAVR, TAVR patients are generally older with more comorbidities. The clinical significance of these cerebral perfusion defects remains unclear with no apparent association with neurological events or clinical impairment of neurocognitive function.

Cerebral protection devices that divert debris downstream in the aorta are currently in development [27, 28]. These filter devices are delivered percutaneously, typically via the right radial or brachial artery, and positioned within the aortic arch to shield the great vessels. They allow ongoing cerebral perfusion but aim to divert emboli away from the cerebral circulation, where they are less harmful or can be treated effectively without sequelae. Results of clinical trials to address this real concern are keenly anticipated.

Coronary Occlusion

Mechanical coronary obstruction following TAVR is a rare but potentially catastrophic complication, yet occurring in less than 1 % of patients. Possible mechanisms of obstruction are numerous and include inappropriate valve positioning leading to impingement of the coronary ostia by the THV sealing cuff; displacement of bulky native valve leaflets by the THV device; embolization of calcium, thrombus, or air; and dissection of the aortic root. Patients at increased risk of coronary obstruction include those with low-lying coronary ostia (often defined as <12 mm from the basal leaflet insertion), bulky native leaflets, and a narrow aortic root with shallow sinuses of Valsalva, limiting lateral displacement of the native valve leaflets. If this is a concern, aortic root angiography performed at the time of balloon valvuloplasty will help assess the risk [29].

Early identification of ischemia following valve implantation is vital and may be identified by the presence of unexplained hypotension, electrocardiographic changes, and hypokinesis of the left ventricle as seen on echocardiography. Urgent coronary angiography and revascularization are sometimes required, either by percutaneous stent implantation or coronary artery bypass grafting.

Valve Malposition and Embolization

Valve malposition is described as being subvalvular when it is placed "too low" or supravalvular when placed "too high." If positioned subvalvularly, annular sealing may be compromised resulting in significant paravalvular regurgitation with hemodynamic compromise. If deployed lower in the left ventricular outflow tract, ventricular arrhythmias or interference with the mitral valve apparatus may result. In contrast, supravalvular malpositioning may result in aortic regurgitation, coronary occlusion, or valve embolization. Malposition has been attributed to poor visualization and imaging, poor THV positioning, ineffective rapid ventricular pacing resulting in a suboptimal reduction in transaortic flow and cardiac motion, valve undersizing, and potential displacement from other cardiac structures such as subaortic stenosis or a mitral valve prosthesis [30].

With improved operator experience, there has been a significant reduction in balloon-expandable valve malpositioning, with current rates of valve embolization at less than 0.5 % [31]. Embolization can be successfully managed by partially inflating the deployment balloon within the prosthesis and withdrawing both the balloon and prosthesis into the smaller diameter portion of the transverse or descending aorta. The prosthesis is then deployed in an area of the aorta where it will not impede normal flow in any vascular territory. If THV embolization occurs into the left ventricle, conversion to open heart surgery with removal of the device is required. Malpositioning of self-expandable valves is less likely to result in embolization; however, the relatively longer and larger-diameter prostheses may require snaring and withdrawal into the ascending or descending aorta.

Renal Impairment

Acute kidney injury has been reported in 12–28 % of patients undergoing TAVR, with up to 2 % requiring dialysis [22]. Potential causes of acute kidney injury include the administration of contrast media, transfusion, periods of severe hypotension during rapid ventricular pacing, balloon valvuloplasty, and valve deployment, and the risk of cholesterol embolization as a result of catheter manipulation within diffusely atheromatous aortas. Additionally, many TAVR patients are elderly with an element of underlying renal impairment prior to the procedure. Although many patients show an improvement in their eGFR following TAVR, the presence of acute kidney injury has been associated with a 4-fold risk in postoperative mortality [32].

Conduction Disturbance

Atrioventricular (AV) block is a well-described complication of TAVR. Since the AV conduction system passes superficially through the interventricular septum in close proximity to the aortic valve, injury may occur during valve implantation resulting in partial or complete heart block [33]. Up to 6 % of patients undergoing TAVR with the Edwards SAPIEN THV require pacemaker insertion [34, 35], and this is comparable to rates of pacemaker insertion following surgical AVR [6]. Rates of pacemaker insertion are significantly higher with CoreValve, occurring in up to one third of patients [36, 37]. Risk factors include advanced age, preexisting conduction abnormalities (particularly right bundle branch block) [38], and prosthesis oversizing. In the majority of patients requiring pacemaker insertion, this is apparent shortly following TAVR, although late heart block may occasionally occur [39].

Prosthesis-Related Complications

Prosthesis–Patient Mismatch

Prosthesis–patient mismatch (PPM) occurs when the effective orifice area (EOA) of a normally functioning prosthetic valve is too small in relation to body size, resulting in suboptimal hemodynamic performance of the valve with higher transvalvular gradients. It is often described as being present when the indexed EOA (iEOA) is less than or equal to 0.85 cm^2/m^2 (moderate PPM); severe PPM is defined as an iEOA less than or equal to 0.65 cm^2/m^2. PPM in surgical prostheses has been shown to have a negative effect on left ventricular regression and systolic function, NYHA class, and freedom from congestive heart failure. Moreover, it has been associated with increased early and late mortality [40]. Although, conceptually, PPM following TAVR should be largely avoided by appropriate sizing prior to surgery, it is frequently encountered following SVR with moderate PPM reported in 20–70 % and severe PPM in up to 28 %.

Following TAVR, severe PPM has been reported in 11–16 %, while moderate PPM has been reported in 18–32 %, with higher rates occurring following CoreValve implantation [41–44]. Although this incidence compares favorably with surgical prostheses, the effect of PPM after TAVR on clinical outcome is largely unknown.

Paravalvular and Valvular Regurgitation

Paravalvular aortic regurgitation (PAR) is common with the current THVs and is most commonly encountered as a result of incorrect positioning or due to undersizing of the valve in relation to the native annulus. Approximately 85 % of patients have some degree of PAR [45], but the majority of these have trivial or mild AR with no impact on clinical outcomes. Significant PAR, however, has been shown to be a strong predictor of in-hospital mortality [46]. If the valve is incompletely expanded, balloon valvuloplasty may reduce the leak; however, an undersized SAPIEN-type valve cannot be expanded larger than its fabric sealing cuff, and an undersized CoreValve cannot be expanded above its predetermined dimension of the nitinol frame. If severe PAR is present, implantation of a second THV overlapping the first may be useful.

Prosthetic Valve Thrombosis and Endocarditis

As with surgical prostheses, valve thrombosis and endocarditis can occur following TAVR, with isolated cases reported in the literature [47, 48]. Additionally, mitral valve injury with native valve endocarditis has been described [49]. Although a rare complication, it is likely that more cases will be reported as the procedure becomes more widely used. Criteria for diagnosis and management guidelines are similar as those used for surgical prostheses.

Transcatheter Valve-in-Valve Implantation

When surgical bioprosthetic valves fail, requiring reoperation, perioperative morbidity and mortality are high—especially in the setting of increased age, poor left ventricular ejection fraction, renal impairment, pulmonary disease, and the need for coronary artery bypass grafting in addition to valve replacement. Encouraging results have been reported with transcatheter valve-in-valve (ViV) implantation, in which a THV is inserted within the degenerated bioprosthesis.

ViV implantation has been successfully performed within the aortic, mitral, tricuspid, and pulmonary positions. Aortic bioprostheses may be accessed by the transfemoral, transaortic, transaxillary, or transapical routes. The mitral bioprosthesis is most often accessed via the transapical approach; however, the transvenous–transeptal approach has also been successfully described. Pulmonary and tricuspid bioprostheses may be accessed transvenously through the internal jugular, superior vena cava, or femoral vein; an open transatrial route with direct puncture into the right atrium may also be utilized to access the tricuspid valve.

The THV is positioned so that the stent frame anchors on the prosthetic sewing ring. Many surgical bioprostheses have radiopaque markers or rings providing fluoroscopic landmarks for transcatheter valve placement. Since these landmarks differ for each type of bioprosthesis, a good understanding of the radiographic appearance of the valvular prosthesis and the relationship between the markers and the sewing ring is required to aid with positioning. Additionally, knowledge of the internal diameter of the surgical bioprosthesis is imperative, since the THV should be sized accordingly; in most cases, the internal diameter of a surgical prosthesis is significantly smaller than the labeled valve size. As a result, those with smaller surgical bioprostheses (<21 mm) may not be eligible for THV implantation [50–53]. Although the long-term durability of ViV implants remains unknown, early experience suggests that TAVR may be a viable option and particularly desirable in those with prohibitive surgical risk.

Future Directions

SVR remains the standard of care for most patients with symptomatic severe aortic stenosis; however, excellent outcomes have been demonstrated with TAVR. TAVR has evolved as the standard of care for inoperable patients with severe aortic stenosis and is a viable alternative for selected high-risk operable patients. As device technology continues to improve, and longer-term follow-up is obtained—particularly regarding valve durability—it is possible that TAVR will become the preferred treatment option in moderate and, potentially, some low-risk patients with severe symptomatic aortic stenosis.

References

1. Bonow RO, Carabello BA, Kanu C, de Leon Jr AC, Faxon DP, Freed MD, Gaasch WH, Lytle BW, Nishimura RA, O'Gara PT, et al. ACC/AHA 2006 guidelines for the management of patients with valvular heart disease: a report of the American College of Cardiology/American Heart Association Task Force on Practice Guidelines (writing committee to revise the 1998 Guidelines for the Management of Patients With Valvular Heart Disease): developed in collaboration with the Society of Cardiovascular Anesthesiologists: endorsed by the Society for Cardiovascular Angiography and Interventions and the Society of Thoracic Surgeons. Circulation. 2006;114(5):e84–231.
2. Bouma BJ, van der Meulen JH, van den Brink RB, Arnold AE, Smidts A, Teunter LH, Lie KI, Tijssen JG. Variability in treatment advice for elderly patients with aortic stenosis: a nationwide survey in The Netherlands. Heart. 2001;85(2):196–201.
3. Cribier A, Eltchaninoff H, Bash A, Borenstein N, Tron C, Bauer F, Derumeaux G, Anselme F, Laborde F, Leon MB. Percutaneous transcatheter implantation of an aortic valve prosthesis for calcific aortic stenosis: first human case description. Circulation. 2002; 106(24):3006–8.
4. Webb JG, Chandavimol M, Thompson CR, Ricci DR, Carere RG, Munt BI, Buller CE, Pasupati S, Lichtenstein S. Percutaneous aortic valve implantation retrograde from the femoral artery. Circulation. 2006;113(6):842–50.
5. Leon MB, Smith CR, Mack M, Miller DC, Moses JW, Svensson LG, Tuzcu EM, Webb JG, Fontana GP, Makkar RR, et al. Transcatheter aortic-valve implantation for aortic stenosis in patients who cannot undergo surgery. N Engl J Med. 2010;363(17):1597–607.
6. Smith CR, Leon MB, Mack MJ, Miller DC, Moses JW, Svensson LG, Tuzcu EM, Webb JG, Fontana GP, Makkar RR, et al. Transcatheter versus surgical aortic-valve replacement in high-risk patients. N Engl J Med. 2011;364(23):2187–98.
7. Lichtenstein SV, Cheung A, Ye J, Thompson CR, Carere RG, Pasupati S, Webb JG. Transapical transcatheter aortic valve implantation in humans: initial clinical experience. Circulation. 2006;114(6):591–6.
8. Rodes-Cabau J. Progress in transcatheter aortic valve implantation. Rev Esp Cardiol. 2010;63(4):439–50.

9. Vahanian A, Alfieri O, Al-Attar N, Antunes M, Bax J, Cormier B, Cribier A, De Jaegere P, Fournial G, Kappetein AP, et al. Transcatheter valve implantation for patients with aortic stenosis: a position statement from the European Association of Cardio-Thoracic Surgery (EACTS) and the European Society of Cardiology (ESC), in collaboration with the European Association of Percutaneous Cardiovascular Interventions (EAPCI). Eur Heart J. 2008;29(11):1463–70.
10. Modine T, Obadia JF, Choukroun E, Rioufoul G, Sudre A, Laborde JC, Leprince P. Transcutaneous aortic valve implantation using the axillary/subclavian access: feasibility and early clinical outcomes. J Thorac Cardiovasc Surg. 2011;141(2):487–91, 491 e1.
11. Bruschi G, Fratto P, De Marco F, Oreglia J, Colombo P, Botta L, Cannata A, Moreo A, De Chiara B, Lullo F, et al. The trans-subclavian retrograde approach for transcatheter aortic valve replacement: single-center experience. J Thorac Cardiovasc Surg. 2010;140(4):911–5, 915 e1–2.
12. Bapat V, Thomas M, Hancock J, Wilson K. First successful trans-catheter aortic valve implantation through ascending aorta using Edwards SAPIEN THV system. Eur J Cardiothorac Surg. 2010;38(6):811–3.
13. Latsios G, Gerckens U, Grube E. Transaortic transcatheter aortic valve implantation: a novel approach for the truly "no-access option" patients. Catheter Cardiovasc Interv. 2010;75(7):1129–36.
14. Toggweiler S, Gurvitch R, Leipsic J, Wood DA, Willson AB, Binder RK, Cheung A, Ye J, Webb JG. Percutaneous aortic valve replacement vascular outcomes with a fully percutaneous procedure. J Am Coll Cardiol. 2012;59(2):113–8.
15. Falk V, Walther T, Schwammenthal E, Strauch J, Aicher D, Wahlers T, Schafers J, Linke A, Mohr FW. Transapical aortic valve implantation with a self-expanding anatomically oriented valve. Eur Heart J. 2011;32(7):878–87.
16. Lauten A, Ferrari M, Petri A, Ensminger SM, Gummert JF, Boudjemline Y, Schubert H, Schumm J, Hekmat K, Schlosser M, et al. Experimental evaluation of the JenaClip transcatheter aortic valve. Catheter Cardiovasc Interv. 2009;74(3):514–9.
17. Kempfert J, Rastan AJ, Mohr FW, Walther T. A new self-expanding transcatheter aortic valve for transapical implantation – first in man implantation of the JenaValve. Eur J Cardiothorac Surg. 2011;40(3):761–3.
18. Schofer J, Schluter M, Treede H, Franzen OW, Tubler T, Pascotto A, Low RI, Bolling SF, Meinertz T, Reichenspurner H. Retrograde transarterial implantation of a nonmetallic aortic valve prosthesis in high-surgical-risk patients with severe aortic stenosis: a first-in-man feasibility and safety study. Circ Cardiovasc Interv. 2008;1(2):126–33.
19. Treede H, Tubler T, Reichenspurner H, Grube E, Pascotto A, Franzen O, Mueller R, Low R, Bolling SF, Meinertz T, et al. Six-month results of a repositionable and retrievable pericardial valve for transcatheter aortic valve replacement: the Direct Flow Medical aortic valve. J Thorac Cardiovasc Surg. 2010;140(4):897–903.
20. Holmes Jr DR, Mack MJ. Transcatheter valve therapy a professional society overview from the american college of cardiology foundation and the society of thoracic surgeons. J Am Coll Cardiol. 2011;58(4):445–55.
21. Leon MB, Piazza N, Nikolsky E, Blackstone EH, Cutlip DE, Kappetein AP, Krucoff MW, Mack M, Mehran R, Miller C, et al. Standardized endpoint definitions for transcatheter aortic valve implantation clinical trials: a consensus report from the Valve Academic Research Consortium. J Am Coll Cardiol. 2011;57(3): 253–69.
22. Nuis RJ, Piazza N, Van Mieghem NM, Otten AM, Tzikas A, Schultz CJ, van der Boon R, van Geuns RJ, van Domburg RT, Koudstaal PJ, et al. In-hospital complications after transcatheter aortic valve implantation revisited according to the valve academic research consortium definitions. Catheter Cardiovasc Interv. 2011;78(3):457–67.
23. Grube E, Schuler G, Buellesfeld L, Gerckens U, Linke A, Wenaweser P, Sauren B, Mohr FW, Walther T, Zickmann B, et al. Percutaneous aortic valve replacement for severe aortic stenosis in high-risk patients using the second- and current third-generation self-expanding CoreValve prosthesis: device success and 30-day clinical outcome. J Am Coll Cardiol. 2007;50(1):69–76.
24. Himbert D, Descoutures F, Al-Attar N, Iung B, Ducrocq G, Detaint D, Brochet E, Messika-Zeitoun D, Francis F, Ibrahim H, et al. Results of transfemoral or transapical aortic valve implantation following a uniform assessment in high-risk patients with aortic stenosis. J Am Coll Cardiol. 2009;54(4):303–11.
25. Lefevre T, Kappetein AP, Wolner E, Nataf P, Thomas M, Schachinger V, De Bruyne B, Eltchaninoff H, Thielmann M, Himbert D, et al. One year follow-up of the multi-centre European PARTNER transcatheter heart valve study. Eur Heart J. 2011;32(2): 148–57.
26. Kahlert P, Knipp SC, Schlamann M, Thielmann M, Al-Rashid F, Weber M, Johansson U, Wendt D, Jakob HG, Forsting M, et al. Silent and apparent cerebral ischemia after percutaneous transfemoral aortic valve implantation: a diffusion-weighted magnetic resonance imaging study. Circulation. 2010;121(7):870–8.
27. Naber CK, Ghanem A, Abizaid AA, Wolf A, Sinning JM, Werner N, Nickenig G, Schmitz T, Grube E. First-in-man use of a novel embolic protection device for patients undergoing transcatheter aortic valve implantation. EuroIntervention. 2012;8(1):43–50.
28. Carpenter JP, Carpenter JT, Tellez A, Webb JG, Yi GH, Granada JF. A percutaneous aortic device for cerebral embolic protection during cardiovascular intervention. J Vasc Surg. 2011;54(1):174–181 e1.
29. Webb JG. Coronary obstruction due to transcatheter valve implantation. Catheter Cardiovasc Interv. 2009;73(7):973.
30. Al Ali AM, Altwegg L, Horlick EM, Feindel C, Thompson CR, Cheung A, Carere RG, Humphries K, Ye J, Masson JB, et al. Prevention and management of transcatheter balloon-expandable aortic valve malposition. Catheter Cardiovasc Interv. 2008;72(4): 573–8.
31. Thomas M, Schymik G, Walther T, Himbert D, Lefevre T, Treede H, Eggebrecht H, Rubino P, Michev I, Lange R, et al. Thirty-day results of the SAPIEN aortic Bioprosthesis European Outcome (SOURCE) Registry: a European registry of transcatheter aortic valve implantation using the Edwards SAPIEN valve. Circulation. 2010;122(1):62–9.
32. Bagur R, Webb JG, Nietlispach F, Dumont E, De Larochelliere R, Doyle D, Masson JB, Gutierrez MJ, Clavel MA, Bertrand OF, et al. Acute kidney injury following transcatheter aortic valve implantation: predictive factors, prognostic value, and comparison with surgical aortic valve replacement. Eur Heart J. 2010;31(7):865–74.
33. Piazza N, de Jaegere P, Schultz C, Becker AE, Serruys PW, Anderson RH. Anatomy of the aortic valvar complex and its implications for transcatheter implantation of the aortic valve. Circ Cardiovasc Interv. 2008;1(1):74–81.
34. Godin M, Eltchaninoff H, Furuta A, Tron C, Anselme F, Bejar K, Sanchez-Giron C, Bauer F, Litzler PY, Bessou JP, et al. Frequency of conduction disturbances after transcatheter implantation of an Edwards Sapien aortic valve prosthesis. Am J Cardiol. 2010;106(5): 707–12.
35. Sinhal A, Altwegg L, Pasupati S, Humphries KH, Allard M, Martin P, Cheung A, Ye J, Kerr C, Lichtenstein SV, et al. Atrioventricular block after transcatheter balloon expandable aortic valve implantation. JACC Cardiovasc Interv. 2008;1(3):305–9.
36. Eltchaninoff H, Prat A, Gilard M, Leguerrier A, Blanchard D, Fournial G, Iung B, Donzeau-Gouge P, Tribouilloy C, Debrux JL, et al. Transcatheter aortic valve implantation: early results of the FRANCE (FRench Aortic National CoreValve and Edwards) registry. Eur Heart J. 2011;32(2):191–7.

37. Bleiziffer S, Ruge H, Horer J, Hutter A, Geisbusch S, Brockmann G, Mazzitelli D, Bauernschmitt R, Lange R. Predictors for new-onset complete heart block after transcatheter aortic valve implantation. JACC Cardiovasc Interv. 2010;3(5):524–30.
38. Baan Jr J, Yong ZY, Koch KT, Henriques JP, Bouma BJ, Vis MM, Cocchieri R, Piek JJ, de Mol BA. Factors associated with cardiac conduction disorders and permanent pacemaker implantation after percutaneous aortic valve implantation with the CoreValve prosthesis. Am Heart J. 2010;159(3):497–503.
39. Piazza N, Nuis RJ, Tzikas A, Otten A, Onuma Y, Garcia-Garcia H, Schultz C, van Domburg R, van Es GA, van Geuns R, et al. Persistent conduction abnormalities and requirements for pacemaking six months after transcatheter aortic valve implantation. EuroIntervention. 2010;6(4):475–84.
40. Pibarot P, Dumesnil JG. Prosthesis-patient mismatch: definition, clinical impact, and prevention. Heart. 2006;92(8):1022–9.
41. Tzikas A, Piazza N, Geleijnse ML, Van Mieghem N, Nuis RJ, Schultz C, van Geuns RJ, Galema TW, Kappetein AP, Serruys PW, et al. Prosthesis-patient mismatch after transcatheter aortic valve implantation with the medtronic CoreValve system in patients with aortic stenosis. Am J Cardiol. 2010;106(2):255–60.
42. Jilaihawi H, Chin D, Spyt T, Jeilan M, Vasa-Nicotera M, Bence J, Logtens E, Kovac J. Prosthesis-patient mismatch after transcatheter aortic valve implantation with the Medtronic-Corevalve bioprosthesis. Eur Heart J. 2010;31(7):857–64.
43. Ewe SH, Muratori M, Delgado V, Pepi M, Tamborini G, Fusini L, Klautz RJ, Gripari P, Bax JJ, Fusari M, et al. Hemodynamic and clinical impact of prosthesis-patient mismatch after transcatheter aortic valve implantation. J Am Coll Cardiol. 2011;58(18):1910–8.
44. Clavel MA, Webb JG, Pibarot P, Altwegg L, Dumont E, Thompson C, De Larochelliere R, Doyle D, Masson JB, Bergeron S, et al. Comparison of the hemodynamic performance of percutaneous and surgical bioprostheses for the treatment of severe aortic stenosis. J Am Coll Cardiol. 2009;53(20):1883–91.
45. Rodes-Cabau J, Webb JG, Cheung A, Ye J, Dumont E, Feindel CM, Osten M, Natarajan MK, Velianou JL, Martucci G, et al. Transcatheter aortic valve implantation for the treatment of severe symptomatic aortic stenosis in patients at very high or prohibitive surgical risk: acute and late outcomes of the multicenter Canadian experience. J Am Coll Cardiol. 2010;55(11):1080–90.
46. Abdel-Wahab M, Zahn R, Horack M, Gerckens U, Schuler G, Sievert H, Eggebrecht H, Senges J, Richardt G. Aortic regurgitation after transcatheter aortic valve implantation: incidence and early outcome. Results from the German transcatheter aortic valve interventions registry. Heart. 2011;97(11):899–906.
47. Piazza N, Marra S, Webb J, D'Amico M, Rinaldi M, Boffini M, Comoglio C, Scacciatella P, Kappetein AP, de Jaegere P, et al. Two cases of aneurysm of the anterior mitral valve leaflet associated with transcatheter aortic valve endocarditis: a mere coincidence? J Thorac Cardiovasc Surg. 2010;140(3):e36–8.
48. Trepels T, Martens S, Doss M, Fichtlscherer S, Schachinger V. Images in cardiovascular medicine. Thrombotic restenosis after minimally invasive implantation of aortic valve stent. Circulation. 2009;120(4):e23–4.
49. Wong DR, Boone RH, Thompson CR, Allard MF, Altwegg L, Carere RG, Cheung A, Ye J, Lichtenstein SV, Ling H, et al. Mitral valve injury late after transcatheter aortic valve implantation. J Thorac Cardiovasc Surg. 2009;137(6):1547–9.
50. Webb JG, Wood DA, Ye J, Gurvitch R, Masson JB, Rodes-Cabau J, Osten M, Horlick E, Wendler O, Dumont E, et al. Transcatheter valve-in-valve implantation for failed bioprosthetic heart valves. Circulation. 2010;121(16):1848–57.
51. Piazza N, Bleiziffer S, Brockmann G, Hendrick R, Deutsch MA, Opitz A, Mazzitelli D, Tassani-Prell P, Schreiber C, Lange R. Transcatheter aortic valve implantation for failing surgical aortic bioprosthetic valve: from concept to clinical application and evaluation (part 2). JACC Cardiovasc Interv. 2011;4(7):733–42.
52. Piazza N, Bleiziffer S, Brockmann G, Hendrick R, Deutsch MA, Opitz A, Mazzitelli D, Tassani-Prell P, Schreiber C, Lange R. Transcatheter aortic valve implantation for failing surgical aortic bioprosthetic valve: from concept to clinical application and evaluation (part 1). JACC Cardiovasc Interv. 2011;4(7):721–32.
53. Gurvitch RCA, Ye J, Wood DA, Willson AB, Toggweiler S, Binder R, Webb JG. Transcatheter valve-in-valve implantation for failed surgical bioprosthetic valves. J Am Coll Cardiol. 2011;58: 2196–209.

Transcatheter Aortic Valve Replacement: A Surgeon's View

5

Gregory P. Fontana, Carlos E. Ruiz, and Chad Kliger

Abstract

Conventional surgical aortic valve replacement (SAVR) via a traditional sternotomy with cardiopulmonary bypass and aortic cross-clamping has been the only therapeutic option for patients with severe aortic stenosis (AS) and, hence, the gold standard for treatment. With the introduction of minimally invasive SAVR, transcatheter aortic valve replacement (TAVR), and now combined hybrid surgical-transcatheter approaches, alternative therapies for the complex AS patient are available. Furthermore, the ability to better evaluate this population and guide procedures using multimodality imaging has developed. Many challenges remain, but it is clear that with a multidisciplinary approach that includes the collaboration of cardiac surgeons, interventionalists, and imaging specialists, care to this challenging patient population will continue to evolve.

Keywords

Minimally invasive • Antegrade transapical • Retrograde transaortic • Fusion imaging

Introduction

For years, conventional surgical aortic valve replacement (SAVR) via a traditional sternotomy approach with cardiopulmonary bypass, cardiac arrest, and aortic cross-clamping was the only therapeutic option and, hence, the gold standard for treatment of severe aortic stenosis. SAVR has been shown to improve symptoms and prolong survival in patients with severe, symptomatic aortic stenosis (AS) [1]. In the absence of surgical intervention, patients develop the progressive symptoms of angina, syncope, and heart failure, with the onset of symptoms heralding a mortality rate of approximately 25 % per year [2, 3].

In low-risk patients and at experienced centers, the perioperative mortality from the Society of Thoracic Surgery (STS) database is less than 1 % for isolated SAVR [4]. However, this average increases to 2.6 % for isolated SAVR in higher-risk patients and nearly doubles with the addition of a concomitant coronary bypass surgery (CABG) procedure [5–7]. Furthermore, mortality rates continue to rise with each decade over 80 years of age [7, 8].

As life expectancy continues to lengthen and the number of elderly patients with AS grows, the proportion of AS patients at increased risk for complications from SAVR is expected to rise, particularly given their advanced age and multitude of comorbidities. In addition, patients' clinical profiles have changed over time with more AS patients possessing a greater number of adverse risk factors. Risk factors—including age >80 years, female gender, pulmonary hypertension, severe native coronary atherosclerosis, prior cardiac surgery, severely depressed left ventricular function

G.P. Fontana, MD (✉)
Department of Cardiothoracic Surgery, Lenox Hill Heart and Vascular Institute-North Shore/LIJ Health System, 130 East 77th Street, 9th Floor Black Hall, New York, NY 10021-10075, USA
e-mail: gfontana@nshs.edu

C. Kliger, MD, MS • C.E. Ruiz, MD, PhD
Department of Cardiology, Lenox Hill Heart and Vascular Institute-North Shore/LIJ Health System, 130 East 77th Street, 9th Floor Black Hall, New York, NY 10075, USA
e-mail: ckliger@nshs.edu; cruiz@nshs.edu

J.K. Min et al. (eds.), *Multimodality Imaging for Transcatheter Aortic Valve Replacement*, DOI 10.1007/978-1-4471-2798-7_5, © Springer-Verlag London 2014

≤30 %, and New York Heart Association (NYHA) class III or IV heart failure—can increase mortality to nearly 20 % [9–12].

Until now, numerous patients have been refused SAVRs in the presence of comorbidities that include severe symptoms, low ejection fraction, neurologic dysfunction, frailty, previous cardiac surgery, chronic lung disease, renal insufficiency, and associated coronary artery disease [13]. Many of these high-risk patients have not even been referred for surgical evaluation due to these factors, and treatments options were never discussed with the patients and their families. Even among those for whom careful discussion has been made, rates of refusal or denial for SAVR ranged from 30 to 60 % [14].

Since the introduction of transcatheter aortic valve replacement (TAVR), a true minimally invasive alternative for the complex aortic stenosis patient is now available. By avoiding a sternotomy, the need for extracorporeal circulation, and general anesthesia, it is possible to exclude the diseased aortic valve, implant a transcatheter valve, and correct the hemodynamic abnormality with generally robust results [15–18]. In addition, TAVR has made accessible combined hybrid surgical-transcatheter approaches and more innovative, minimally invasive SAVR for low- and intermediate-risk patients that have been excluded from clinical trials. Germane to the choice of procedure, the ability to better evaluate severe AS patients and guide procedures using multimodality imaging has evolved. Many challenges remain for the treatment of AS, but it is clear that with a multidisciplinary approach that includes the collaboration of cardiac surgeons, interventionalists, and imaging specialists, care to this complex patient population will continue to evolve.

Evolution of a Minimally Invasive Approach

Conventional surgery has been the reference therapy for AS since the 1960s. Following sternotomy and the initiation of cardiopulmonary bypass, the aorta is cross-clamped and an aortotomy is performed. The native cusps are typically excised and calcific debris removed from the aortic annulus. A mechanical or bioprosthetic valve is subsequently sutured into place within the annulus replacing the native valve. The aortotomy site is closed, the cross clamp is released, and the patient is weaned from cardiopulmonary bypass.

Since 1996, minimally invasive techniques have been used for cardiac surgery with a multitude of alternative incisions [19, 20]. These alternative incisions include the right parasternal incision through the second to fifth intercostal cartilage, a right anterior thoracotomy in the third intercostal space, and, most commonly, an upper mini-sternotomy that extends into the third or fourth intercostal space using a J or inverted T incision [21, 22]. Minimally invasive approaches are being performed in an effort to reduce postoperative complications including pain, risk of pulmonary dysfunction, infection, and sternal dehiscence. It can also be easily extended to provide additional exposure, if required.

Performing surgery without the exposure afforded by median sternotomy encouraged alternative methods for cardiopulmonary bypass access and axillary and femoral cannulation [22]. However, central aortic cannulation is preferred when safe and feasible. Similarly, cardioplegia can be administered either antegrade from an aortic cannula or retrograde from the coronary sinus via transjugular catheterization or transatrially [23]. Although the benefits of these techniques are yet to be clearly demonstrated, there is evidence of shorter ventilator dependence, intensive care stay, and transfusion requirements, especially in higher-risk patients [24–26]. Furthermore, multimodality imaging has allowed for procedural modifications and adjustments such as incision selection and cannulation strategies to address the location of bypass grafts and cardiac structures, increasing overall safety [27].

In 2002, Cribier performed the first TAVR via a transfemoral approach [28]. This approach can be performed through either standard percutaneous arterial access or now, less commonly, surgical exposure. The transfemoral approach is used for the majority of retrograde deployments and requires large-bore access of the common femoral artery for passage of a large French delivery sheath and transcatheter valve through the arterial vascular system, traversing the aortic arch. Balloon aortic valvuloplasty is first performed to facilitate implantation of the prosthesis, yet the necessity in all AS patients remains unclear. Subsequent implantation of either a balloon-expandable or self-expanding prosthesis is performed.

Alternative approaches to TAVR have emerged as a viable option for patients with significant thoracic aortic pathology such as an unfolded aorta, arch atheromata, or unsuitable iliofemoral anatomy, due either to severe peripheral vascular disease, circumferential calcification, extensive iliofemoral tortuosity, small-caliber vasculature, or prior vascular surgery. They include retrograde subclavian/transaxillary, antegrade transapical, and retrograde transaortic approaches. These approaches provide a shorter distance between the device and the valve, allowing for improved operator control and manipulation of the delivery system during valve deployment. Nonetheless, a disadvantage persists, as surgical exposure is required. Therefore, the choice of approach becomes dependent on anatomical patient-related factors and the expertise of the multidisciplinary team.

Retrograde Subclavian/Transaxillary Approach

The subclavian or transaxillary approach is typically obtained via subclavicular surgical cutdown, similar to an incision for pacemaker implantation [29, 30]. Access that may be obtained with the use of a synthetic graft attached directly to the subclavian artery or directly using the Seldinger technique

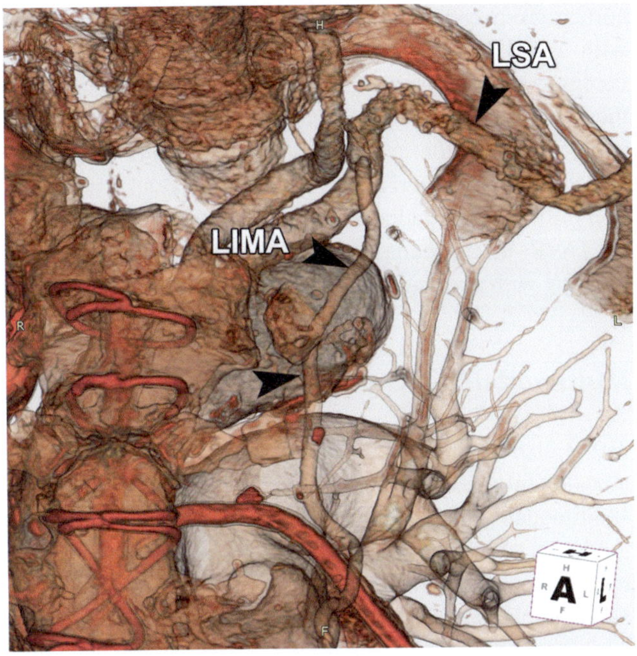

Fig. 5.1 Computed tomographic angiography reveals significant left subclavian artery (*LSA*) tortuosity as it traverses the thoracic inlet, making it more prone to injury for a retrograde subclavian/transaxillary approach. In addition, a left internal mammary artery (*LIMA*) bypass graft to the left anterior descending artery is present

has been reported. The left subclavian artery is primarily used because of its more favorable route following the natural curve of the ascending aorta and aortic arch. The right subclavian artery can be used when the heart is in a more vertical orientation.

This approach is utilized as an alternative in patients with unsuitable iliofemoral access. It provides a shorter distance to the aortic valve improving steering and control of the device. The subclavian artery, however, can be especially tortuous as it traverses the thoracic inlet, making it more prone to injury [31] (Fig. 5.1). Subclavian artery thrombosis and dissections with downstream extension involving the carotid arteries and causing subsequent neurologic deficits are a potential complication. The presence of internal mammary artery bypass graft and a dominant left vertebral artery is a relative contraindication and can risk myocardial and cerebral ischemia if flow is compromised when the delivery system is similar in caliber to the subclavian artery.

Antegrade Transapical Approach

The transapical approach to TAVR is performed via a left anterolateral mini-thoracotomy between the fifth and sixth intercostal space under general anesthesia [32]. The incision site is determined by palpation, fluoroscopy, transthoracic echocardiography, and/or multidetector computed tomography (CT). Transapical access is achieved by placing two purse-string, pledgeted sutures within the apical myocardium and introducing the delivery sheath into the left ventricle.

Apical complications are less than 1 % in experienced centers [33, 34]. The avoidance of traversing the aortic arch potentially reduces liberation of cerebral emboli. The short distance from the LV apex to aortic valve allows for improved operator maneuverability and control during valve deployment. Patients with an intended more ventricular valve positioning, such as in patients with low implanted coronary arteries, a prior mitral prosthesis, or mild septal hypertrophy that is not a contraindication for TAVR, may be easier to achieve when delivery forces can be directed toward the apex [35].

The major downsides of transapical approach are the concerns for apical bleeding, pseudoaneurysm, or apical scar, especially in patients with left ventricular dysfunction [36]. Cardiac muscle of the elderly, high-risk, frail patient can be friable, a quality not typically identifiable on CT. In addition, further pulmonary impairment with patients having underlying lung disease may be a consequence of the thoracotomy. Current data suggests faster recovery times after transapical TAVR, with early and late morbidity and mortality comparable with that of minimally invasive SAVR [37] [38].

Retrograde Transaortic TAVR Approach

The transaortic or direct aortic approach to TAVR is performed through a mini-sternotomy or right mini-thoracotomy through the second intercostal space, with dissection of the underlying tissue to expose the ascending aorta [39, 40]. For mini-sternotomy, a small supraclavicular counter incision is made with a tunnel created to the sternotomy site in order to secure sheath placement and orient the line of delivery to the aortic valve. A mini-sternotomy provides excellent exposure to all aortic orientations.

The first series of patients to undergo direct aortic approach TAVR were poor candidates for transfemoral and transapical approaches due to severe pulmonary impairment or marked chest wall deformities, suggesting a population well suited for this approach [40]. Delivery avoiding the aortic arch may also potentially reduce a source of cerebral emboli. With the avoidance of thoracic wall trauma and subsequent postoperative pain, which may occur with the transapical approach, there may be less impairment in respiratory function. Nonetheless, reported procedural outcomes between transapical and direct aortic approaches are similar [40].

The Complex Aortic Stenosis Patient

In addition to the multitude of medical comorbidities, technical difficulties arise which can make SAVR a challenge. These challenges include heavily calcified and/or atheromatous

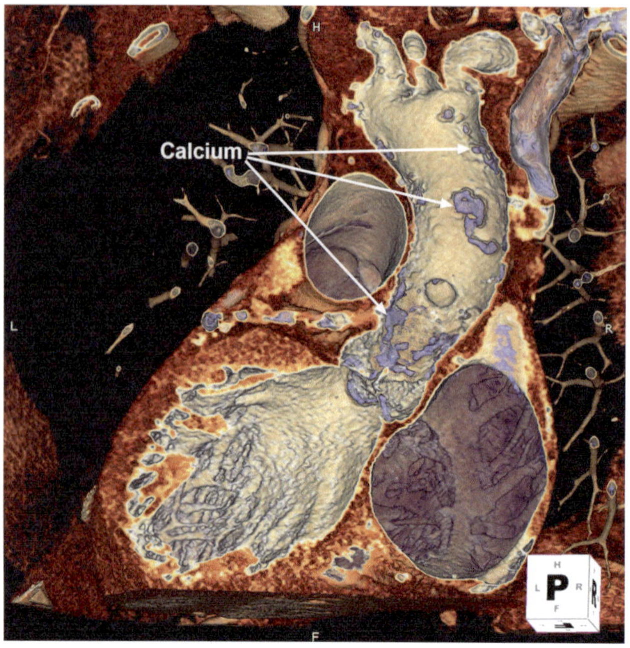

Fig. 5.2 3D volume-rendered computed tomographic images can be performed of the aorta. Using the cut-plane function, portions of the aortic root and ascending aorta are virtually removed to reveal extensive calcific atherosclerotic disease

ascending aorta such as a porcelain aorta, prior CABG surgery with patent bypass grafts that can be damaged during sternotomy or dissection, and multiple redo surgeries with extensive scar tissue or sequelae of chest and/or mediastinal radiation (Fig. 5.2). Calcification of the ascending aorta is commonly present in the elderly surgical population. Traditional options have been ascending aortic replacement and/or endarterectomy under circulatory arrest with subsequent cross-clamping and cardiopulmonary bypass and apical-descending aortic conduits, all adding significant risk to the patient.

Furthermore, similar technical difficulties arise that can make TAVR a challenge. Heavy peripheral arterial calcification, atherosclerosis, tortuosity, and smaller-caliber arterial vasculature can make access and delivery system advancement difficult and dangerous [4]. Ulcerative plaque and mobile atheroma within the aortic arch and great vessel increase the potential risk of dislodgement during catheter manipulation and subsequent embolization. Significant proximal septal bulging, particularly in patients with left ventricular outflow tract obstruction, and a prior mitral valve prosthesis may prevent adequate positioning at risk for transcatheter valve embolization into the aorta. Myomectomy during SAVR can address septal hypertrophy, but this is not the case for TAVR.

In addition, bulky aortic leaflet calcification may increase the risk of coronary occlusion and paravalvular regurgitation [41, 42]. Displacement of leaflet edge calcification into the aortic root space may obstruct the coronary ostium in patients with a low ostial height. Calcification within the device-landing zone may resist deployment of a transcatheter prosthesis, causing a gap between the prosthesis and the native valve. An Agatston calcium valve score above 3,000 may portend an increased risk for relevant paravalvular regurgitation [43]. Overall, addressing the risks and benefits of SAVR or TAVR in the complex patient requires multimodality imaging with a multidisciplinary analysis and discussion.

Multimodality Imaging in Aortic Stenosis

TAVR, like minimally invasive SAVR, lacks the direct visualization provided by a conventional open, SAVR procedure. Multimodality imaging for preprocedural assessment and for guidance within the hybrid laboratory offers an alternative means of visualization to achieve important information for valve implantation. More advanced imaging such as 3D transesophageal echocardiography (TEE), MDCT, and, more recently, CTA-fluoroscopy or rotational angiography-fluoroscopy fusion imaging is becoming essential for AS management.

In SAVR, conventional selective angiography is the standard diagnostic tool for anatomic evaluation of native coronary arteries and bypass grafts. However, it neither provides the surgeon with complete information on the proximity of the aorta, the right ventricle, coronary arteries, and grafts to the sternum nor the extent of aortic disease. CT with 3D volume rendering is able to show the relationship of these structures to one another with cut-plane able to virtually remove structures in order to visualize underlying anatomy [44] (Fig. 5.3). Median sternotomy in the setting of an adherent right ventricle, bypass grafts, or innominate vein can lead to catastrophic bleeding or myocardial injury.

Curved multiplanar reconstructions can be performed of the aorta to identify aortic calcification and atherosclerosis and the location of bypass grafts, all in relation to the aortic valve. In addition to surveying the substernal, mediastinal, and cardiac anatomy for abnormalities, CT also aids in preoperative decision analysis and cannulation strategies. It is more commonly performed prior to isolated valve procedures and has been showed to markedly reduce postoperative stroke rates, with the selection of cannulation site and clamping strategy largely influenced by CT [27, 44]. Occasionally, TEE, along with 3D full-volume mode images, can reveal advanced atherosclerosis with mobile and pedunculated atheroma (Fig. 5.4).

Regardless of the fact that conventional surgical approach allows for intraprocedural sizing of the prosthesis, an accurate preoperative assessment can improve procedure and prosthesis selection. The role of multimodality imaging in choosing the prosthesis as well as implantation technique becomes

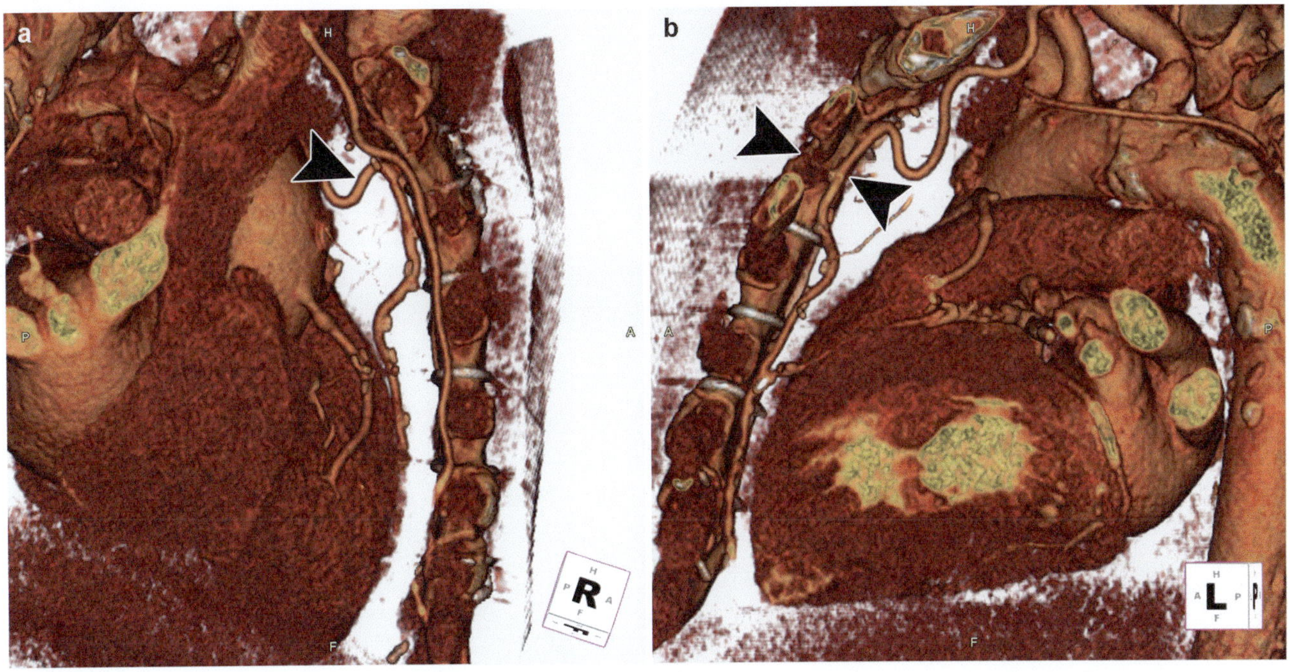

Fig. 5.3 3D cardiac reconstruction using volume-rendering techniques shows the relationship of the aorta, right ventricle, coronary arteries, and bypass grafts in relation to the sternum. In the right lateral (**a**) and left lateral (**b**) orientations, the left internal mammary artery bypass graft (*black arrowhead*) is visualized adherent to the posterior sternum

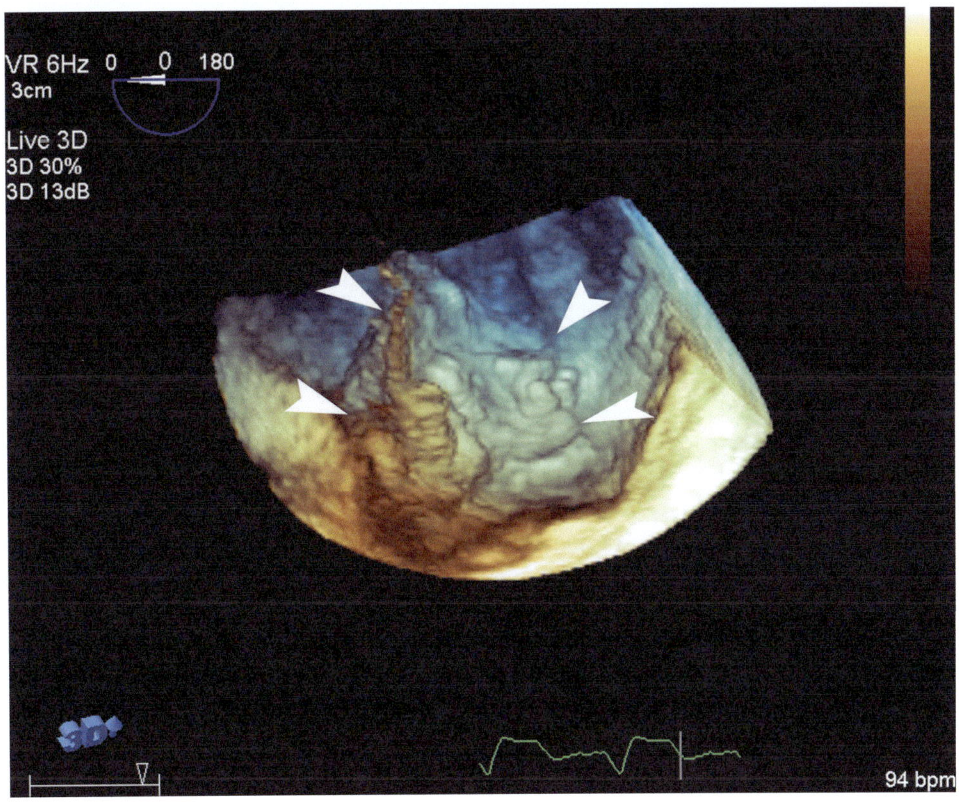

Fig. 5.4 3D transesophageal echocardiography with full-volume mode reveals advanced atherosclerosis with large, mobile atheroma with the edges identified (*white arrowheads*)

widely recognized as valuable for TAVR. Multimodality imaging, in particular CT and TEE, allows for accurate estimation of prosthesis size [45]. Accurate preoperative valve sizing may help to avoid postoperative patient-prosthesis mismatch for patients at high risk. This can also allow for optimal selection of implantation technique: supra-annular versus

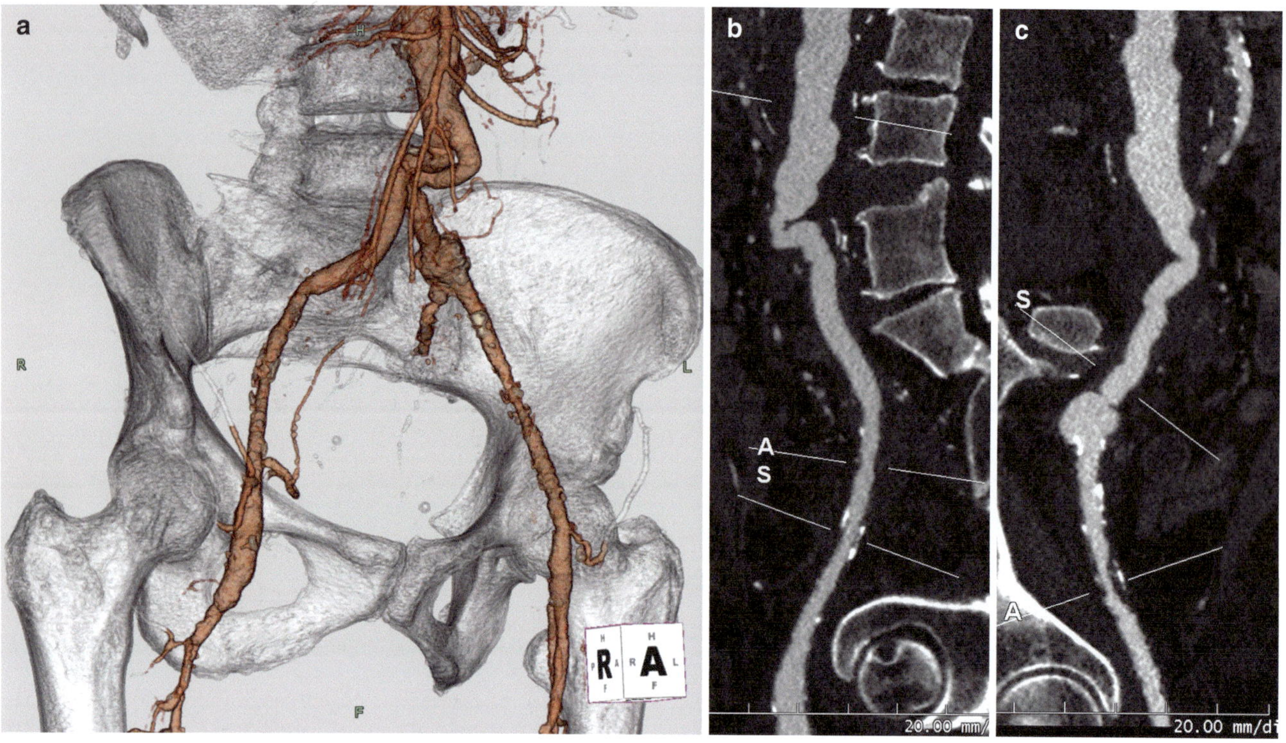

Fig. 5.5 (**a**) Computed tomographic angiography (CTA) with 3D volume rendering of the aortic bifurcation and iliofemoral system reveals tortuosity of the bilateral aortoiliac junction. Curved multiplanar reconstruction (MPR) of the right (**b**) and left (**c**) iliofemoral system shows the acute angle at the aortoiliac junction and evidence of calcific and non-calcific disease of the bilateral iliac arteries (A and S identify the axial cut-planes perpendicular to the centerline that can be moved along the vasculature, used to determine luminal dimensions)

intra-annular, the need for aortic root enlargement, and stented versus stentless or mechanical prostheses.

In TAVR, CT provides a comprehensive assessment of the iliofemoral arteries, thoracoabdominal aorta, ascending aorta, aortic root, and aortic annulus (Fig. 5.5). Atherosclerotic burden, degree of calcification, and tortuosity can be easily determined for safety of vascular access and delivery [4]. Measurements of the ascending aorta can assess the ability for successful implantation of self-expanding valves and of the aortic root to assess for the potential for coronary occlusion. Analysis and measurements of annular size and shape are crucial for appropriate prosthesis sizing. Furthermore, quantification and localization of leaflet/annular calcification is possible, but its role in conduction system abnormalities, coronary obstruction, paravalvular regurgitation, and cerebrovascular events and the ability to modify TAVR techniques to reduce complications are developing.

Real-time 3D TEE is also an important modality for preprocedural and intraprocedural assessment of TAVR. Similar to CT, precise assessment of the aortic root and annulus can be made, potentially reducing the chance of sizing error [4]. 3D visualization allows for improved positioning of transcatheter valve and determination of implantation depth during valve deployment. In addition, 3D TEE can help to evaluate the extent of and precise location of the aortic regurgitation jet following valve implantation (Fig. 5.6). In SAVR, improved localization of a paravalvular leak together with defect dimensions can assist in procedural management and need for immediate revision.

Fusion imaging is playing an increasing role in TAVR [46, 47]. It provides the ability to merge the 3D data of important cardiac and surrounding structures from either CT angiography or rotational angiography with live 2D fluoroscopy, while preserving the spatial and temporal resolution of fluoroscopy. The fundamentals of fusion imaging are described in a later chapter. There are predominately two proprietary softwares available that employ fuse CT or rotational angiography with fluoroscopy: HeartNavigator (Philips Healthcare, Best Netherlands) and syngo DynaCT (Siemens Medical, Berlin Germany). Syngo DynaCT utilizes intraprocedural rotational angiography images, reducing variables that can alter cardiac anatomy compared to a preprocedural CT angiography. Nevertheless, the primary utility of fusion imaging in TAVR includes the localization of aortic valve anatomy, determination of valve size, identification of optimal c-arm positioning, and guidance for valve deployment.

The role of fusion imaging in hybrid approaches to TAVR remains undefined but has been utilized for the retrograde transaortic and antegrade transapical approaches (Fig. 5.7). The optimal position for direct aortic cannulation

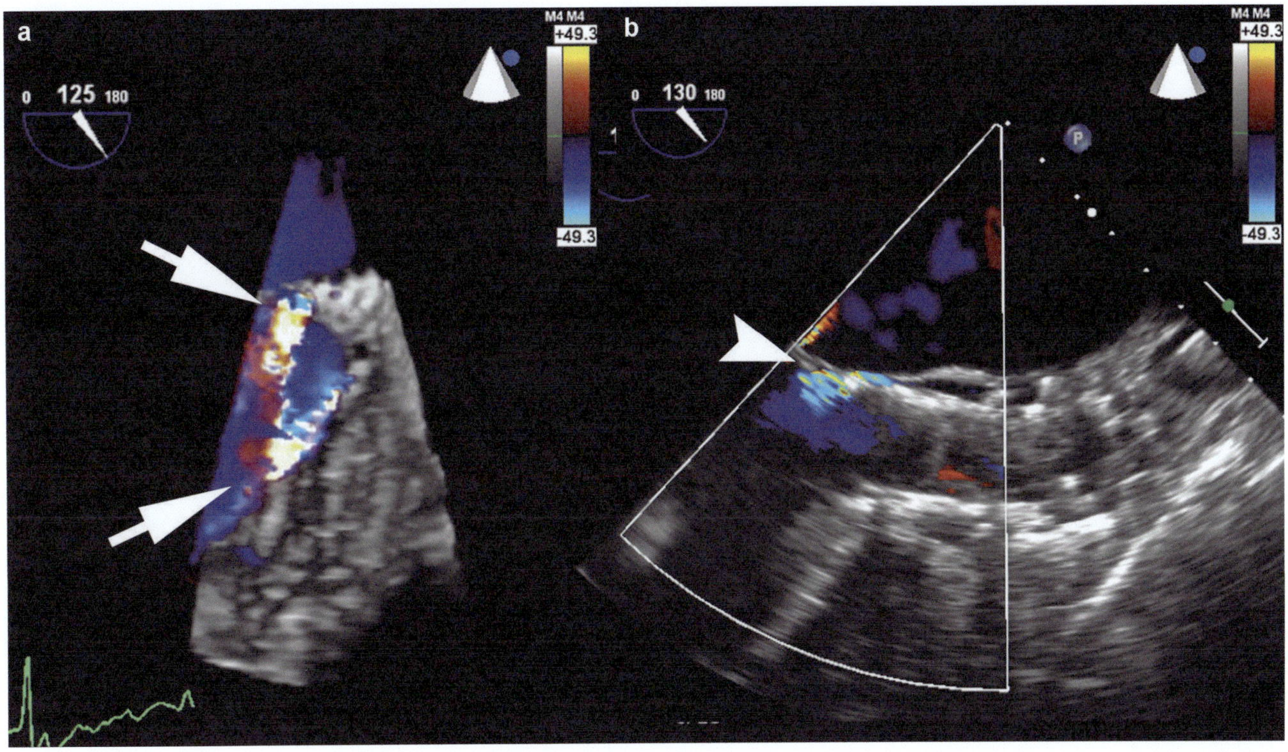

Fig. 5.6 (**a**) 3D full-volume transesophageal echocardiography with color Doppler reveals two jets of aortic paravalvular regurgitation (*white arrows*) around a self-expanding CoreValve prosthesis (Medtronic, Minneapolis MN). (**b**) 2D long-axis view of the aorta after CoreValve valve-in-valve (ViV) implantation demonstrates mild residual paravalvular regurgitation (*white arrowhead*)

can be determined based on preprocedural CT angiography images. A site is selected that is away from atherosclerotic plaque and is a sufficient distance from the aortic annulus to allow for transcatheter deployment while still maintaining sheath access. In addition, maintaining an entry site away from bypass grafts if present and providing the correct orientation for deployment is equally important.

A landmark can be placed at this site and CT angiography and fluoroscopy images co-registered such that the landmark moves with the c-arm and can guide transaortic entry. Also, an outline of the right internal mammary artery overlayed onto fluoroscopy can guide incision such that the medial edge of right anterior thoracotomy incision is 1.5–2 cm lateral to the sternal edge. For the antegrade transapical approach, preprocedural CT angiography and fusion imaging can help identify transapical access site both on the skin and on the left ventricle, determining the shortest trajectory of entry that is in direct line with the aortic valve.

The Burden of Paravalvular Regurgitation

Paravalvular leak is a serious complication associated with SAVR. Paravalvular leaks occur in 2–10 % of the surgical implants in the aortic position with 1–5 % having clinical symptoms of congestive heart failure and/or hemolysis [48, 49]. A result of incomplete seal between the sewing ring and annulus, paravalvular leaks can occur early due to technical aspects of surgery or later due to suture dehiscence or gradual resorption of incompletely debrided annular calcification.

The same problem of paravalvular regurgitation that has burdened SAVR also occurs with TAVR. It is generally caused by inadequate expansion of the prosthesis from either underinflation or calcification. It can also occur with incorrectly sized prostheses or improper positioning. Nearly one-third of patients have paravalvular regurgitation that is more than mild. Although the incidence of residual mild or moderate paravalvular regurgitation is significantly higher in TAVR compared to SAVR, moderate-severe and severe postprocedural regurgitation is rare [17]. Nonetheless, even mild paravalvular regurgitation is associated with increased late mortality [17].

Surgical correction of paravalvular leak related to surgical prosthesis involves either repair of the leak by direct suturing, patch closure, or autologous tissue incorporation or re-replacement of the valve. Transcatheter techniques have been adapted to paravalvular leak closure with reasonable success [50]. For transcatheter prostheses, acute techniques of balloon post-dilatation, valve-in-valve implantation, or valve repositioning, depending on the prosthesis type and the mechanism, can be employed. Percutaneous

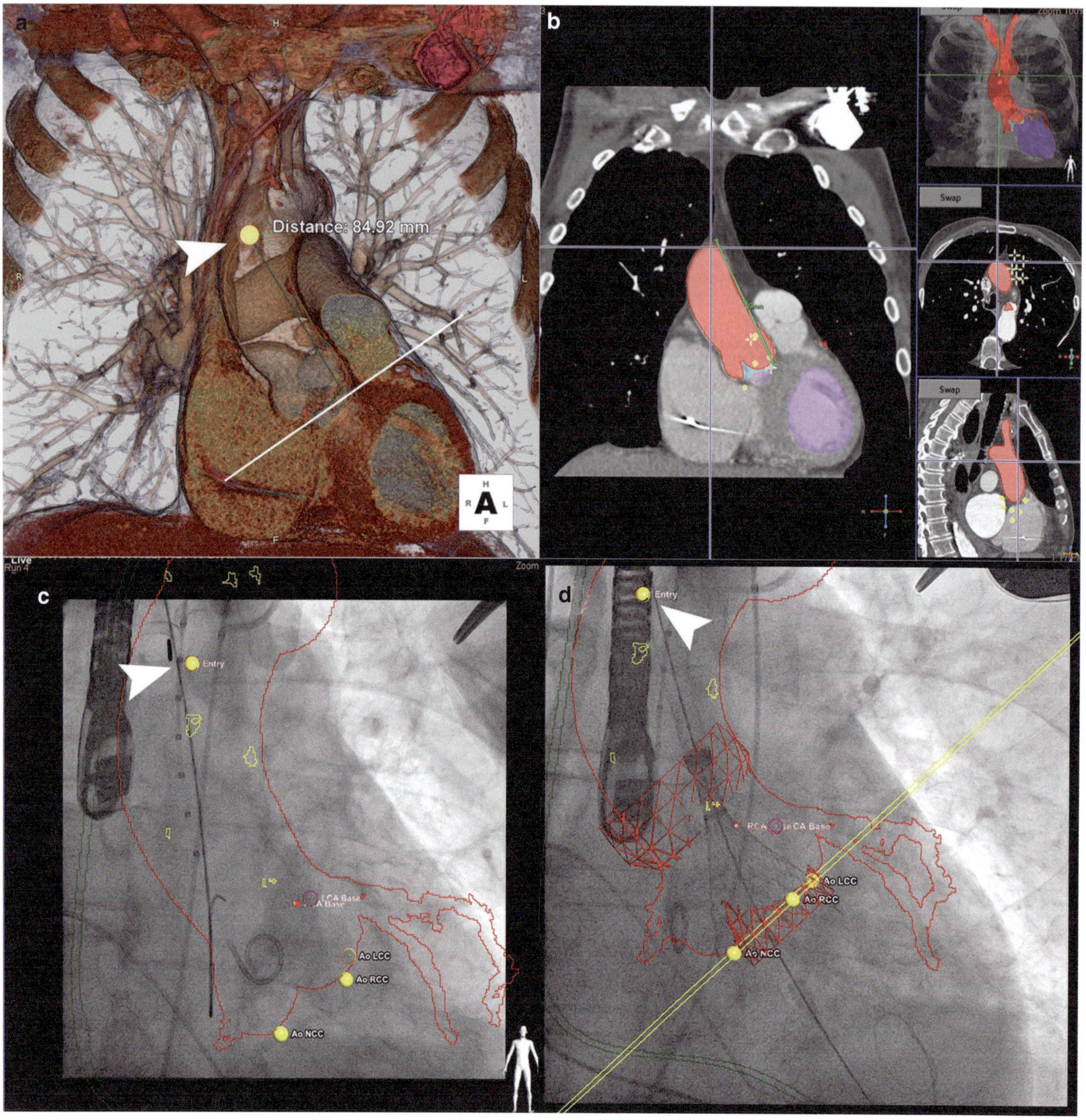

Fig. 5.7 Fusion imaging for retrograde transaortic approach. (**a**) Preprocedural computed tomographic angiography (CTA) with 3D cardiac reconstruction is used to identify an optimal position (*arrowhead, yellow dot*) for direct aortic cannulation, away from atherosclerotic plaque and with sufficient distance from the aortic annulus (>6 cm recommended for CoreValve implantation). (**b**) Segmentation of volume-rendered images identifies the aorta along with the coronary arteries and bypass grafts (*red*) and left ventricle (*purple*) on sagittal, axial, and coronal views. (**c**) Registration is performed to match the position and scale of the overlayed CTA onto fluoroscopy. The aorta and coronary arteries (*red outline*), nadir of coronary cusps and direct aortic access and tip of the delivery sheath (*arrowhead*) are visualized. (**d**) Deployment of the CoreValve is visualized at one third deployment (CoreValve Medtronic, Minneapolis MN; HeartNavigator Philips Healthcare, Best Netherlands)

paravalvular closure of a transcatheter prosthesis has been performed 3–6 months after TAVR to allow for endothelialization and stabilization, but further evaluation is warranted [51].

Multidisciplinary Team Approach

Analyzing the risk of conventional SAVR is clearly more complicated in extreme and high-risk patients. Preoperative risk stratification models such as the Society of Thoracic Surgeons and the EuroSCORE may be useful to stratify potential candidates by providing a quantitative assessment [52]. However, AS patients are a very heterogeneous group with varying life expectancies, comorbidities, and functional status. Current scores have not been designed to evaluate this population and do not capture all of the relevant variables [53].

The limitations of scoring systems underlie the importance of the multidisciplinary team approach. These scoring systems are only part of the process, and the decision whether to perform conventional SAVR, minimally invasive SAVR, or TAVR can be made jointly with a multidisciplinary team [54]. Frailty is an important consideration and remains a predominately subjective assessment. Slow gait speed and reduced grip strength have been examined and are being prospectively studied.

Future of Transcatheter Aortic Stenosis Therapy

Devices that have a lower profile and are repositionable and retrievable with improved intrinsic technological designs and size variations will have the potential to improve efficacy and reduce the rates of complications even further. A further reduction of paravalvular regurgitation is critical and will occur by increasing the size of available prostheses and/or adding sealing technology to existing stents.

Port access or an entirely percutaneous transapical approach to TAVR may be a possibility, capitalizing on the advantages of transapical approach while reducing access-related morbidities. Current TA closure methods of using the "off-label" Amplatzer family of occlusive devices (St. Jude Medical, Minneapolis MN), in particular the Amplatzer Ductal Occluder (ADO) and Vascular Plug II (AVP II), would likely be ineffective given the large diameter (>12 F) of the current TAVR delivery systems [55]. Effective transapical closure systems are being evaluated and may provide of efficacious and safe means to preclose and exit the left ventricle.

Expanding the use of transcatheter therapy to other patient populations including severe aortic regurgitation (lack of annular calcification needed to anchor a transcatheter valve), presence of existing mitral prosthesis (rigid struts may reduce transcatheter stability and valve durability), and bicuspid aortic valves (poor valve seating and paravalvular regurgitation) may be possible with iterative or novel devices.

The recent utilization of transcatheter valve-in-valve implantation for the treatment of a degenerated bioprosthesis has been performed [56]. The rigid stent of a bioprosthesis can provide an optimal landing zone for a transcatheter valve. For high-risk surgical patients, TAVR valve-in-valve implantation is an option to reduce invasiveness and avoid the potential technical difficulties of a repeat procedure. Repeat cardiac surgery may carry significant risks in this population, with a reported mortality of 6–15 % [57, 58]. Although efficacy, safety, and long-term durability are unclear, the potential to obviate the need for redo valve surgery in the high-risk patient is a possibility. In turn, knowing that transcatheter therapy may be a possibility, expanding the use of early bioprosthesis implantation instead of mechanical valves may be a future consideration for the complex cardiac patient.

Finally, TAVR trials have included the highest-risk patients, within the top tenth percentile [8]. Expanding the use of TAVR to other population would require comparable procedural 30-day mortality and other standardized clinical endpoints as defined by the Valve Academic Research Consortium (VARC) [59]. In addition, valve durability would need to be similar to that of current surgical standards. Although valve-in-valve implantation does provide a potential means to rescue failed valves, more study is required.

Conclusion

Transcatheter aortic valve replacement with its multidisciplinary team approach, intricate multimodality imaging assessment and guidance, and hybrid surgical-transcatheter approaches have bridged the disciplines of cardiac surgery, interventional cardiology, and cardiac imaging. With more innovative, minimally invasive SAVR techniques, our ability to manage a broader range of the growing complex aortic stenosis population is expanding and constantly evolving.

References

1. Pai RG, Kapoor N, Bansal RC, Varadarajan P. Malignant natural history of asymptomatic severe aortic stenosis: benefit of aortic valve replacement. Ann Thorac Surg. 2006;82(6):2116–22. Epub 2006/11/28.
2. Ross Jr J, Braunwald E. Aortic stenosis. Circulation. 1968;38(1 Suppl):61–7. Epub 1968/07/01.
3. Lester SJ, Heilbron B, Gin K, Dodek A, Jue J. The natural history and rate of progression of aortic stenosis. Chest. 1998;113(4): 1109–14. Epub 1998/04/29.
4. Holmes Jr DR, Mack MJ, Kaul S, Agnihotri A, Alexander KP, Bailey SR, et al. 2012 ACCF/AATS/SCAI/STS expert consensus document on transcatheter aortic valve replacement: developed in collaboration with the American Heart Association, American Society of Echocardiography, European Association for Cardio-Thoracic Surgery, Heart Failure Society of America, Mended Hearts, Society of Cardiovascular Anesthesiologists, Society of Cardiovascular Computed Tomography, and Society for Cardiovascular Magnetic Resonance. J Thorac Cardiovasc Surg. 2012;144(3):e29–84. Epub 2012/08/18.
5. Rankin JS, Hammill BG, Ferguson Jr TB, Glower DD, O'Brien SM, DeLong ER, et al. Determinants of operative mortality in valvular heart surgery. J Thorac Cardiovasc Surg. 2006;131(3):547–57. Epub 2006/03/07.

6. Bloomstein LZ, Gielchinsky I, Bernstein AD, Parsonnet V, Saunders C, Karanam R, et al. Aortic valve replacement in geriatric patients: determinants of in-hospital mortality. Ann Thorac Surg. 2001;71(2):597–600. Epub 2001/03/10.
7. Jamieson WR, Edwards FH, Schwartz M, Bero JW, Clark RE, Grover FL. Risk stratification for cardiac valve replacement. National Cardiac Surgery Database. Database Committee of The Society of Thoracic Surgeons. Ann Thorac Surg. 1999;67(4): 943–51. Epub 1999/05/13.
8. Mack MJ. Does transcatheter aortic valve implantation mean the end of surgical aortic valve replacement? Tex Heart Inst J. 2010;37(6):658–9. Epub 2011/01/13.
9. Kodali S, Schwartz A. Transcatheter valve repair and replacement. Annu Rev Med. 2009;60:1–11. Epub 2008/11/18.
10. Kuwaki K, Amano A, Inaba H, Yamamoto T, Matsumura T, Dohi S, et al. Predictors of early and mid-term results in contemporary aortic valve replacement for aortic stenosis. J Card Surg. 2012;27(2):139–45. Epub 2012/02/15.
11. Nowicki ER, Birkmeyer NJ, Weintraub RW, Leavitt BJ, Sanders JH, Dacey LJ, et al. Multivariable prediction of in-hospital mortality associated with aortic and mitral valve surgery in Northern New England. Ann Thorac Surg. 2004;77(6):1966–77. Epub 2004/06/03.
12. Edwards FH, Peterson ED, Coombs LP, DeLong ER, Jamieson WR, Shroyer ALW, et al. Prediction of operative mortality after valve replacement surgery. J Am Coll Cardiol. 2001;37(3):885–92. Epub 2001/11/06.
13. Iung B, Cachier A, Baron G, Messika-Zeitoun D, Delahaye F, Tornos P, et al. Decision-making in elderly patients with severe aortic stenosis: why are so many denied surgery? Eur Heart J. 2005;26(24):2714–20. Epub 2005/09/06.
14. Dua A, Dang P, Shaker R, Varadarajan P, Pai RG. Barriers to surgery in severe aortic stenosis patients with Class I indications for aortic valve replacement. J Heart Valve Dis. 2011;20(4):396–400. Epub 2011/08/26.
15. Leon MB, Smith CR, Mack M, Miller DC, Moses JW, Svensson LG, et al. Transcatheter aortic-valve implantation for aortic stenosis in patients who cannot undergo surgery. N Engl J Med. 2010;363(17):1597–607. Epub 2010/10/22.
16. Smith CR, Leon MB, Mack MJ, Miller DC, Moses JW, Svensson LG, et al. Transcatheter versus surgical aortic-valve replacement in high-risk patients. N Engl J Med. 2011;364(23):2187–98. Epub 2011/06/07.
17. Kodali SK, Williams MR, Smith CR, Svensson LG, Webb JG, Makkar RR, et al. Two-year outcomes after transcatheter or surgical aortic-valve replacement. N Engl J Med. 2012;366(18):1686–95. Epub 2012/03/27.
18. Makkar RR, Fontana GP, Jilaihawi H, Kapadia S, Pichard AD, Douglas PS, et al. Transcatheter aortic-valve replacement for inoperable severe aortic stenosis. N Engl J Med. 2012;366(18): 1696–704. Epub 2012/03/27.
19. Cosgrove 3rd DM, Sabik JF, Navia JL. Minimally invasive valve operations. Ann Thorac Surg. 1998;65(6):1535–8; discussion 8–9. Epub 1998/07/01.
20. Fontana GP. Minimally invasive cardiac surgery. Chest Surg Clin N Am. 1998;8(4):871–90. Epub 1999/01/26.
21. Jegaden O, Lapeze J, Farhart F, de Gevigney G. Aortic valve stenosis after previous coronary bypass: transcatheter valve implantation or aortic valve replacement? J Cardiothorac Surg. 2012;7:47. Epub 2012/05/31.
22. Iribarne A, Easterwood R, Chan EY, Yang J, Soni L, Russo MJ, et al. The golden age of minimally invasive cardiothoracic surgery: current and future perspectives. Future Cardiol. 2011;7(3):333–46. Epub 2011/06/02.
23. Schmitto JD, Mokashi SA, Cohn LH. Minimally-invasive valve surgery. J Am Coll Cardiol. 2010;56(6):455–62. Epub 2010/07/31.
24. Korach A, Shemin RJ, Hunter CT, Bao Y, Shapira OM. Minimally invasive versus conventional aortic valve replacement: a 10-year experience. J Cardiovasc Surg. 2010;51(3):417–21. Epub 2010/06/05.
25. Liu J, Sidiropoulos A, Konertz W. Minimally invasive aortic valve replacement (AVR) compared to standard AVR. Eur J Cardiothorac Surg. 1999;16 Suppl 2:S80–3. Epub 1999/12/29.
26. Murtuza B, Pepper JR, Stanbridge RD, Jones C, Rao C, Darzi A, et al. Minimal access aortic valve replacement: is it worth it? Ann Thorac Surg. 2008;85(3):1121–31. Epub 2008/02/23.
27. Khan NU, Yonan N. Does preoperative computed tomography reduce the risks associated with re-do cardiac surgery? Interact Cardiovasc Thorac Surg. 2009;9(1):119–23. Epub 2009/04/03.
28. Cribier A, Eltchaninoff H, Bash A, Borenstein N, Tron C, Bauer F, et al. Percutaneous transcatheter implantation of an aortic valve prosthesis for calcific aortic stenosis: first human case description. Circulation. 2002;106(24):3006–8. Epub 2002/12/11.
29. Grube E, Laborde JC, Gerckens U, Felderhoff T, Sauren B, Buellesfeld L, et al. Percutaneous implantation of the CoreValve self-expanding valve prosthesis in high-risk patients with aortic valve disease: the Siegburg first-in-man study. Circulation. 2006;114(15):1616–24. Epub 2006/10/04.
30. Asgar AW, Mullen MJ, Delahunty N, Davies SW, Dalby M, Petrou M, et al. Transcatheter aortic valve intervention through the axillary artery for the treatment of severe aortic stenosis. J Thorac Cardiovasc Surg. 2009;137(3):773–5. Epub 2009/03/05.
31. Caceres M, Braud R, Roselli EE. The axillary/subclavian artery access route for transcatheter aortic valve replacement: a systematic review of the literature. Ann Thorac Surg. 2012;93(3):1013–8. Epub 2012/01/10.
32. Blumenstein J, Van Linden A, Arsalan M, Moellmann H, Liebtrau C, Walther T, et al. Transapical access: current status and future directions. Expert Rev Med Devices. 2012;9(1):15–22. Epub 2011/12/08.
33. Wendler O, Walther T, Nataf P, Rubino P, Schroefel H, Thielmann M, et al. Trans-apical aortic valve implantation: univariate and multivariate analyses of the early results from the SOURCE registry. Eur J Cardiothorac Surg. 2010;38(2):119–27. Epub 2010/03/09.
34. Walther T, Thielmann M, Kempfert J, Schroefel H, Wimmer-Greinecker G, Treede H, et al. PREVAIL TRANSAPICAL: multicentre trial of transcatheter aortic valve implantation using the newly designed bioprosthesis (SAPIEN-XT) and delivery system (ASCENDRA-II). Eur J Cardiothorac Surg. 2012;42(2):278–83. Epub 2012/02/02.
35. Rodes-Cabau J, Dumont E, Miro S, Doyle D, De Larochelliere R, Clavel MA, et al. Apical aortic valve implantation in a patient with a mechanical valve prosthesis in mitral position. Circ Cardiovasc Interv. 2008;1(3):233. Epub 2009/12/25.
36. Al-Attar N, Ghodbane W, Himbert D, Rau C, Raffoul R, Messika-Zeitoun D, et al. Unexpected complications of transapical aortic valve implantation. Ann Thorac Surg. 2009;88(1):90–4. Epub 2009/06/30.
37. Walther T, Schuler G, Borger MA, Kempfert J, Seeburger J, Ruckert Y, et al. Transapical aortic valve implantation in 100 consecutive patients: comparison to propensity-matched conventional aortic valve replacement. Eur Heart J. 2010;31(11):1398–403. Epub 2010/03/18.
38. Zierer A, Wimmer-Greinecker G, Martens S, Moritz A, Doss M. Is transapical aortic valve implantation really less invasive than minimally invasive aortic valve replacement? J Thorac Cardiovasc Surg. 2009;138(5):1067–72. Epub 2009/09/11.
39. Bruschi G, De Marco F, Fratto P, Oreglia J, Colombo P, Paino R, et al. Direct aortic access through right minithoracotomy for implantation of self-expanding aortic bioprosthetic valves. J Thorac Cardiovasc Surg. 2010;140(3):715–7. Epub 2010/04/16.

40. Bapat V, Khawaja MZ, Attia R, Narayana A, Wilson K, Macgillivray K, et al. Transaortic transcatheter aortic valve implantation using Edwards Sapien valve: a novel approach. Catheter Cardiovasc Interv. 2012;79(5):733–40. Epub 2011/08/02.
41. Webb JG, Chandavimol M, Thompson CR, Ricci DR, Carere RG, Munt BI, et al. Percutaneous aortic valve implantation retrograde from the femoral artery. Circulation. 2006;113(6):842–50. Epub 2006/02/08.
42. John D, Buellesfeld L, Yuecel S, Mueller R, Latsios G, Beucher H, et al. Correlation of device landing zone calcification and acute procedural success in patients undergoing transcatheter aortic valve implantations with the self-expanding CoreValve prosthesis. JACC Cardiovasc Interv. 2010;3(2):233–43. Epub 2010/02/23.
43. Koos R, Mahnken AH, Dohmen G, Brehmer K, Gunther RW, Autschbach R, et al. Association of aortic valve calcification severity with the degree of aortic regurgitation after transcatheter aortic valve implantation. Int J Cardiol. 2011;150(2):142–5. Epub 2010/03/31.
44. Lapar DJ, Ailawadi G, Irvine Jr JN, Lau CL, Kron IL, Kern JA. Preoperative computed tomography is associated with lower risk of perioperative stroke in reoperative cardiac surgery. Interact Cardiovasc Thorac Surg. 2011;12(6):919–23. Epub 2011/03/11.
45. Mizia-Stec K, Pysz P, Jasinski M, Adamczyk T, Drzewiecka-Gerber A, Chmiel A, et al. Preoperative quantification of aortic valve stenosis: comparison of 64-slice computed tomography with transesophageal and transthoracic echocardiography and size of implanted prosthesis. Int J Cardiovasc Imaging. 2012;28(2):343–52. Epub 2011/02/01.
46. Schrofel HBN, van der Boomen R. Transcatheter aortic valve implantation in a hybrid operating room using HeartNavigator. Medicamundi. 2010;53:2–9.
47. Kempfert J, Falk V, Schuler G, Linke A, Merk D, Mohr FW, et al. Dyna-CT during minimally invasive off-pump transapical aortic valve implantation. Ann Thorac Surg. 2009;88(6):2041. Epub 2009/11/26.
48. Ionescu A, Fraser AG, Butchart EG. Prevalence and clinical significance of incidental paraprosthetic valvar regurgitation: a prospective study using transoesophageal echocardiography. Heart. 2003;89(11):1316–21. Epub 2003/11/05.
49. Davila-Roman VG, Waggoner AD, Kennard ED, Holubkov R, Jamieson WR, Englberger L, et al. Prevalence and severity of paravalvular regurgitation in the Artificial Valve Endocarditis Reduction Trial (AVERT) echocardiography study. J Am Coll Cardiol. 2004;44(7):1467–72. Epub 2004/10/07.
50. Ruiz CE, Jelnin V, Kronzon I, Dudiy Y, Del Valle-Fernandez R, Einhorn BN, et al. Clinical outcomes in patients undergoing percutaneous closure of periprosthetic paravalvular leaks. J Am Coll Cardiol. 2011;58(21):2210–7. Epub 2011/11/15.
51. Whisenant B, Jones K, Horton KD, Horton S. Device closure of paravalvular defects following transcatheter aortic valve replacement with the Edwards Sapien valve. Catheter Cardiovasc Interv. 2012;81:901–5. Epub 2012/05/15.
52. Dewey TM, Brown D, Ryan WH, Herbert MA, Prince SL, Mack MJ. Reliability of risk algorithms in predicting early and late operative outcomes in high-risk patients undergoing aortic valve replacement. J Thorac Cardiovasc Surg. 2008;135(1):180–7. Epub 2008/01/09.
53. Ben-Dor I, Gaglia Jr MA, Barbash IM, Maluenda G, Hauville C, Gonzalez MA, et al. Comparison between Society of Thoracic Surgeons score and logistic EuroSCORE for predicting mortality in patients referred for transcatheter aortic valve implantation. Cardiovasc Revasc Med. 2011;12(6):345–9. Epub 2011/07/12.
54. Bleiziffer S, Ruge H, Mazzitelli D, Schreiber C, Hutter A, Laborde JC, et al. Results of percutaneous and transapical transcatheter aortic valve implantation performed by a surgical team. Eur J Cardiothorac Surg. 2009;35(4):615–20; discussion 20–1. Epub 2009/02/24.
55. Jelnin V, Dudiy Y, Einhorn BN, Kronzon I, Cohen HA, Ruiz CE. Clinical experience with percutaneous left ventricular transapical access for interventions in structural heart defects a safe access and secure exit. JACC Cardiovasc Interv. 2011;4(8):868–74. Epub 2011/08/20.
56. Webb JG, Wood DA, Ye J, Gurvitch R, Masson JB, Rodes-Cabau J, et al. Transcatheter valve-in-valve implantation for failed bioprosthetic heart valves. Circulation. 2010;121(16):1848–57. Epub 2010/04/14.
57. Eitz T, Fritzsche D, Kleikamp G, Zittermann A, Horstkotte D, Korfer R. Reoperation of the aortic valve in octogenarians. Ann Thorac Surg. 2006;82(4):1385–90. Epub 2006/09/26.
58. Jamieson WR, Burr LH, Miyagishima RT, Janusz MT, Fradet GJ, Ling H, et al. Re-operation for bioprosthetic aortic structural failure – risk assessment. Eur J Cardiothorac Surg. 2003;24(6):873–8. Epub 2003/12/04.
59. Leon MB, Piazza N, Nikolsky E, Blackstone EH, Cutlip DE, Kappetein AP, et al. Standardized endpoint definitions for transcatheter aortic valve implantation clinical trials: a consensus report from the Valve Academic Research Consortium. J Am Coll Cardiol. 2011;57(3):253–69. Epub 2011/01/11.

Transcatheter Aortic Valve Replacement (TAVR): A Clinician's Perspective Aortic Stenosis: Natural and Unnatural (Treated) History

6

Blase A. Carabello

Abstract

Symptomatic aortic stenosis (AS) is a fatal illness with only one cure, aortic valve replacement. Over the past 40 years the etiology of AS has changed from congenital and rheumatic causes to that of atherosclerotic inflammatory calcific disease. As the etiology of the disease has changed so has the age of onset changed, now often occurring in seventh, eighth and ninth decades of life. With age comes age-related comorbidities that increase the risk of surgery of preclude it all together, until now relegating the patient to an AS-related death.

The advent of transcatheter AVR (TAVR) offers a game changing intervention that allows for definitive therapy for patients who otherwise would be untreatable. While the benefits are striking, this therapy is in its infancy and it will continue to evolve over the next decade. While more mature, cardiac surgery is also evolving into a safer more applicable mode of treatment. Our patients will obtain the best result when a team of physicians representing the best aspects of cardiac surgery, cardiac intervention and non-invasive cardiology work together to help the patient decide which therapeutic option is best for him or her. In this way TAVR will find its optimal place in our armamentarium for the treatment of aortic stenosis.

Keywords

Aortic valve • Aortic stenosis • Heart surgery • Transcatheter heart valve

Aortic Stenosis: Natural and Unnatural (Treated) History

Aortic stenosis (AS) is a progressive narrowing of the aortic valve, forcing the left ventricle (LV) to generate an ever-increasing pressure to overcome the obstruction. This pressure overload, initially borne by the development of hypertrophy (LVH), eventually causes LV damage, altered coronary blood flow, and both systolic and diastolic LV dysfunctions [1–7]. Once these pathologic changes result in the onset of the classic symptoms of angina, syncope, and/or heart failure, the course of the disease is radically altered so that patients begin to die at the rate of 2 % per month unless the aortic valve is replaced (Fig. 6.1) [8–10].

In many years since the publication of these classic data, some aspects of AS have remained the same, while others have changed. Constant in the natural history is the poor prognosis once symptoms develop unless durable relief of

B.A. Carabello, MD
Department of Medicine,
The W.A. "Tex" and Deborah Moncrief,
Jr., Baylor College of Medicine, Medical Care Line Executive,
Veterans Affairs Medical Center,
Houston, TX, USA

Department of Medicine,
Center for Heart Valve Disease,
St. Luke's Episcopal Hospital, Baylor College of Medicine,
Houston, TX, USA

Department of Medicine, Veterans Affairs Medical Center,
Medical Service (111), 2002 Holcombe Boulevard,
Houston, TX 77030, USA
e-mail: blaseanthony.carabello@med.va.gov

J.K. Min et al. (eds.), *Multimodality Imaging for Transcatheter Aortic Valve Replacement*,
DOI 10.1007/978-1-4471-2798-7_6, © Springer-Verlag London 2014

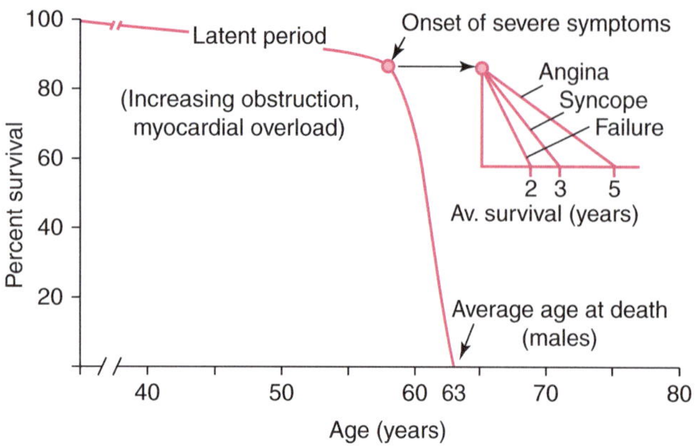

Fig. 6.1 The natural history of aortic stenosis (AS) is depicted. Following a long asymptomatic period during which survival is nearly normal, mortality rises sharply with the onset of the classic symptoms of angina, syncope, and heart failure (Taken with permission from Ross and Braunwald and modified from [8])

outflow obstruction can be achieved [11]. Relief is afforded only by aortic valve replacement. Balloon valvotomy offers palliation but does not alter mortality [11, 12]. A second constant of AS is its progressive nature. Once considered to be a "degenerative" disease, it is now clear that AS is an inflammatory process much akin to atherosclerosis [13]. Inflammation in turn leads to progressive calcification and narrowing of the valve orifice. Not surprisingly, statin therapy, so successful in the treatment of coronary artery disease, was investigated as possibly effective in retarding the progression of AS. While the concept that calcification of the aortic valve in AS can be slowed or reversed is an important therapeutic target, statins failed to achieve the goal of reducing progression of AS [14–16]. Thus, there continues to be no effective medical therapy for AS.

On the other hand two major changes in AS that have occurred over the past 40 years are its usual etiology and consequently the age at onset. The etiologies of AS of the patients comprising the data from 40 years ago were primarily rheumatic heart disease and/or congenital AS. Today calcific atherosclerotic disease is the major cause of AS in developed countries, producing severe disease and thus symptom onset in patients in their 60s, 70s, and 80s as opposed to 40s and 50s [17]. With advancing age comes a host of comorbidities that increase the risk of standard AVR therapy. In turn the older age of AS patients often presents physician and patient with a therapeutic dilemma. Symptomatic AS remains a lethal disease but the usual cure, surgical AVR, may pose too high a risk to perform safely.

Standard Indications for Surgical AVR

The AHA/ACC Guidelines for the Management of Patients with Valvular Heart Disease list only 3 class 1 (general agreement that the procedure is useful and effective) indications for AVR [18]. These are (1) symptomatic severe AS, (2) severe AS with LV dysfunction, and (3) severe AS in a patient undergoing another cardiac operation. Other less certain indications for AVR in asymptomatic patients include a 2a (most would recommend) indication for patients with moderate AS undergoing another cardiac operation [19] and several 2b (may be beneficial) indications: (1) an abnormal response to exercise [20, 21], (2) a heavily calcified valve or proof of rapid progression from frequent observations of valve area over time [22], and (3) very severe AS with an AVA of <0.6 cm [23]. In the past severe left ventricular hypertrophy has also been considered an indication for AVR in asymptomatic patients with severe AS.

These indications for AVR assume that the operation will take place in an otherwise relatively healthy individual. However, as noted above, the typical AS patient today is often aged, and with age comes multiple extra-valvular comorbidities that affect the risk of AVR. This risk can be estimated using a variety of risk calculators based upon the results of thousands of previous operations. One of the most widely used of such instruments is that sponsored by the Society of Thoracic Surgeons (STS). Figure 6.2 demonstrates how collectively adding risk factors affects total operative STS-predicted risk of mortality and morbidity [24]. Even extensive cardiac problems including repeat cardiac surgery, the additional presence of coronary artery disease, and left ventricular dysfunction do not increase the risk of surgical AVR to the point of inoperability. However, when advanced noncardiac disease is added to the mix, surgical mortality increases dramatically such that risk of surgery outweighs its benefit.

TAVR

For the practicing clinician considering a patient for AVR, the following clinical scenario may be of particular benefit through the decision-making process:

History of Present Illness: An 82-year-old woman is referred for evaluation of a heart murmur that she has known about for many years. Over the past 6 months, she has noted near syncope when she climbs the stairs to her bedroom in her two-story home. Accordingly, she has limited her activity to a bed to chair existence, living in a downstairs bedroom.

Past Medical History: She has a past history of insulin-requiring diabetes which has resulted in peripheral vascular disease, a remote stroke from which she has fully recovered, and moderately severe kidney disease (creatinine 3.5 mg/dl). She suffered a non-ST segment elevation myocardial infarction 6 years ago.

Physical Examination: Blood pressure was 112/67. Heart rate was 72.

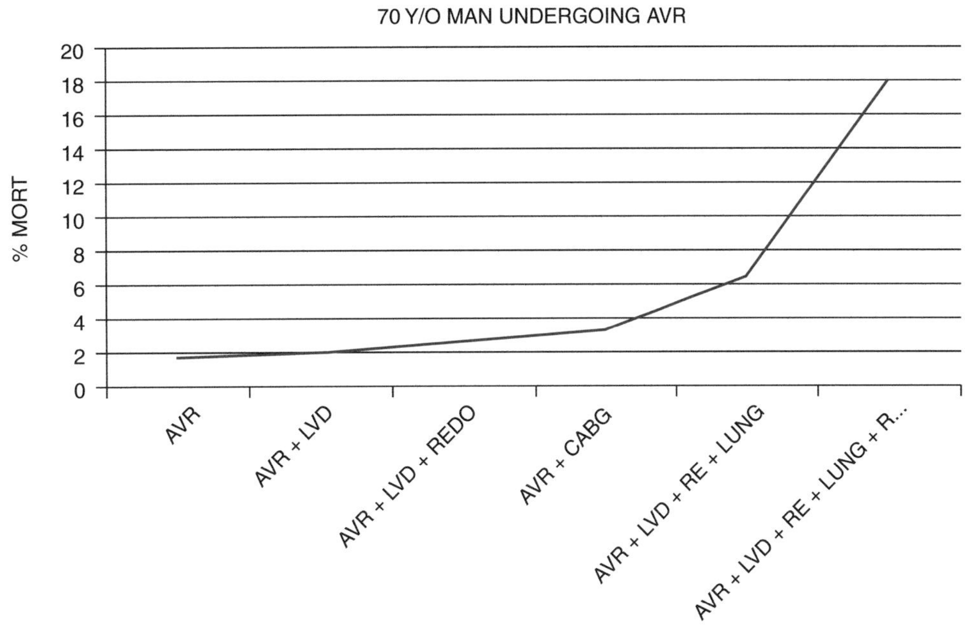

Fig. 6.2 Mortality for aortic valve replacement for AS as assessed by STS (see above) risk calculator is shown as various cardiac and noncardiac comorbidities accrue (Taken from Carabello [24])

Neck: Carotid upstrokes delayed. Estimated central venous pressure: 7 cm H_2O.

Chest: Clear.

Heart: Apical impulse forceful, 5th interspace, midclavicular line; 3/6 late-peaking SEM radiating to the neck.

Extremities: Pedal pulses absent; no edema.

Echocardiography: Severe aortic stenosis; aortic valve area 0.7 cm [2], mean gradient 55 mmHg. Ejection fraction 0.45.

Coronary Angiography: Non-obstructive disease of the left coronary artery; chronic total right coronary occlusion.

STS Mortality Risk Score: 19; risk of morbidity and mortality 41.

The patient presented above represents a common conundrum in the treatment of patients with AS. With advancing age she has also developed extra-cardiac diseases that have added substantially to the risk of a standard AVR. Further, even if she survived surgery, prolonged hospitalization due to complications or discharge to a rehabilitation center to treat her deconditioning and other medical problems might vitiate the potential benefit to surgical AVR. Indeed these negative consequences of AVR in such patients have relegated many such patients to the inevitable downward spiral of untreated AS as shown in Fig. 6.1.

The advent of the transcatheter aortic valve replacement (TAVR) now offers a less invasive approach to aortic valve replacement [11, 25, 26]. Instead of requiring open heart surgery and extracorporeal circulatory support, AVR is provided by deployment of a stented bioprosthesis via catheter manipulation from the arterial tree to the aortic annulus or transapically, through the left ventricle. The two TAVRs available in the USA are the Edwards Sapien valve (available commercially) and the Medtronic's CoreValve (in clinical trials). The Edwards valve is approved (as of this writing) in the USA for use only from the transfemoral and transapical approach in inoperable and those at very high surgical risk. The valve has also been deployed from other arterial sites in clinical trials here and commercially in Europe where general use was approved several years ago.

Approval in the USA was largely predicated upon the success of the PARTNER trial (Fig. 6.3) [11, 25, 26] that showed a large survival benefit of TAVR over medical therapy. In a second arm of the trial, TAVR proved equal in survival to standard AVR in high risk but operable patients. Initially there appeared to be an increased risk of stroke for TAVR. This risk persisted for 1 year after valve replacement, but stroke rate equalized after 2 years because of increased late risk in the surgical group [26]. Importantly TAVR not only increased survival but also relieved symptoms and enhanced the quality of life.

Thus, the clinician treating the AS patient previously thought to be inoperable now has a safer less invasive option that is truly a "game changer."

Effects of TAVR on Aortic Stenosis Therapy

The availability of TAVR obviously provides a novel effective alternative to surgical AVR for treating AS. However, the effects of TAVR go beyond the procedure itself. It has revived an interest in AS and its therapy. It has been estimated that half of patients with severe AS never receive AVR because they or their physicians think they are too ill or too old for surgery [27, 28]. TAVR has brought many of these previously untreated patients to medical attention. In many cases such patients turn out to be excellent candidates for surgical AVR despite their advanced years because age by

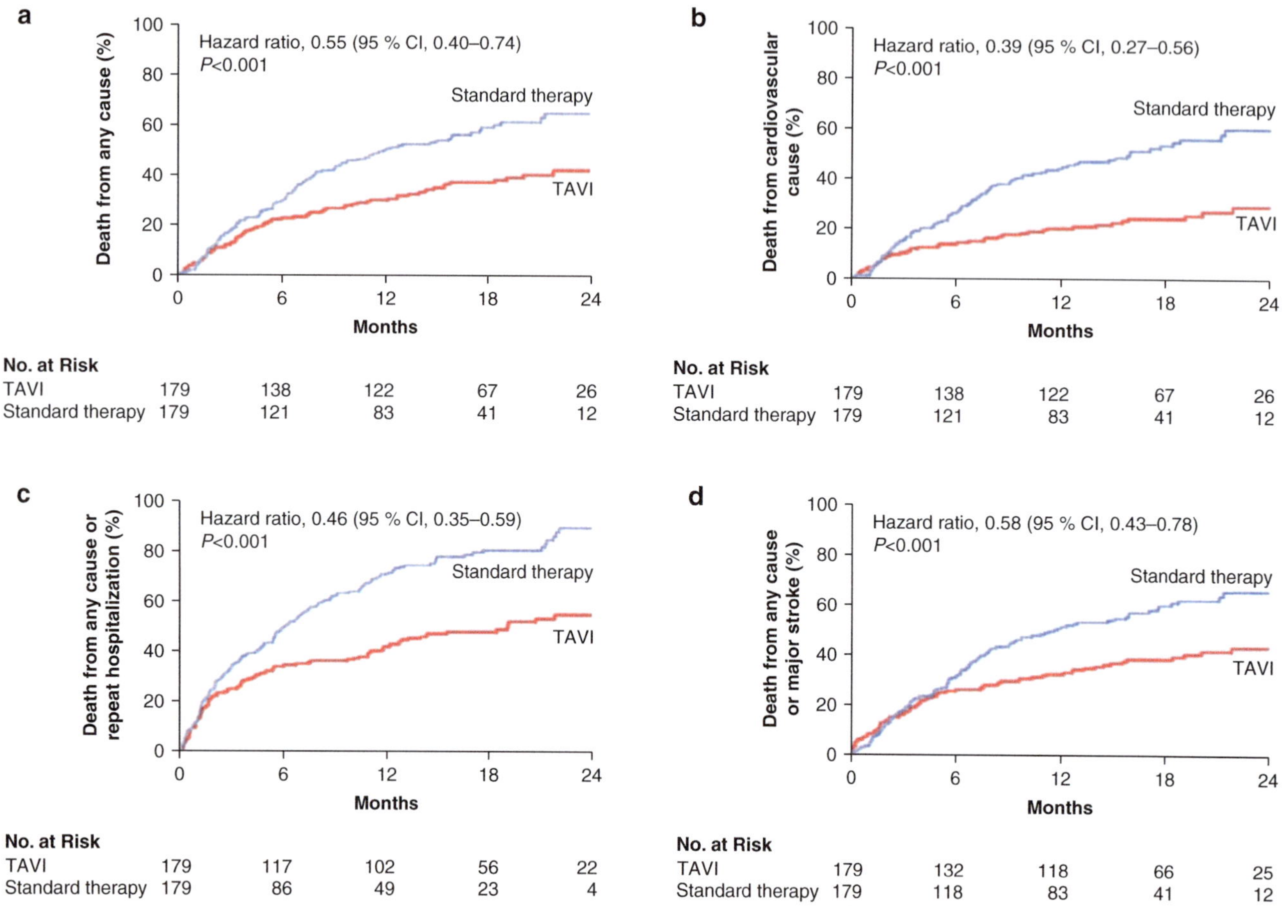

Fig. 6.3 (**a**) Death from any cause, (**b**) cardial death, (**c**) all cause mortality or hospitalization, (**d**) all cause mortality or major stroke. Data from the PARTNER trial comparing outcome with TAVR versus "medical therapy" showing striking benefit for TAVR are shown (Taken from Leon et al. [11])

itself is only a modest contributor to surgical risk (Fig. 6.2). The net effect is that between TAVR and surgical AVR, many more patients can now benefit from mechanical relief of AS.

Pitfalls to Be Overcome

Access and Delivery

Extensive use of TAVR in Europe and elsewhere gives some insight as to the immediate future of TAVR in the USA. In Europe over 60,000 valves roughly split between the CoreValve and the Edwards Sapien valve have been implanted from the femoral, transaxillary, transfemoral, and transaortic routes. While the Edwards delivery system is through a 24 or 28 F sheath in the USA, smaller delivery systems employing 18 F devices are use in Europe. Obviously the smaller the delivery device that can be used, the easier and more applicable the procedure becomes. Additionally the valve sizes available in the USA include only 23 and 26 mm diameter housings that then must fit into a given patient's aortic annulus. Larger annuli may prevent the valve from seating properly, leading either to paravalvular aortic regurgitation or valve embolization. Smaller annuli may prevent valve deployment or lead to annular rupture. The technical development of more valve sizes will also increase applicability to more patients.

Stroke

The arm of PARTNER trial that randomized high risk but operable patients to surgery versus TAVR demonstrated an increased initial risk of stroke in patients receiving TAVR versus those undergoing conventional surgery. The difference persisted at 1 year after the procedure but disappeared at 2 years owing to increased stroke in the surgical arm. It is likely that manipulating TAVR past the head vessels dislodges debris that embolizes thereby representing, initially, a cause of higher stroke rates. That the population involved is already at high risk for naturally occurring stroke probably accounts for how the surgical arm "caught up" to the TAVR arm. Stroke will always be a concern especially in this group of patients for whom independent living is often one of their greatest concerns. Smaller catheter sizes affording easier delivery and the possible use of carotid protection devices may help to reduce stroke rate in the future. Freedom from stroke will be an especially important consideration when lower-risk patients are considered for TAVR versus surgical AVR.

Paravalvular Aortic Insufficiency

Paravalvular leak is observed frequently following TAVR either because the valve does not fully occupy the native annulus or because calcified remnants of the native valve prevent proper seating of the TAVR. More than mild post-TAVR aortic insufficiency is now reported to be a leading cause of morbidity and mortality following the procedure [26, 29]. It is likely that the LV, previously adapted to the pressure overload of AS by the development of concentric LVH, responds very poorly to the volume needs of aortic insufficiency. Volume overload in this circumstance predictably would force the LV to operate at very high filling pressures resulting in pulmonary congestion and heart failure.

Liberalization of Use

Where will TAVR go from here? It is likely that Medtronic's CoreValve will also be approved for USA use in the near future. Other valves with different characteristics will almost certainly be developed adding to choices available for TAVR. There will almost undoubtedly be an interest for use of transcatheter heart valves in lower-risk patients by both practitioners and patients who by experience in many medical arenas have demonstrated a preference for less invasive procedures. The degree to which TAVR will replace surgical AVR will obviously depend on valve durability, delivery device size, ease of delivery, and overall safety. Obviously a TAVR valve that lasted a decade, that had the same or better risk profile compared to surgery, and that could be delivered through a relatively small sheath would significantly impact the penetration of TAVR into the overall therapy of AS.

Valve-in-Valve Use

There are now several instances where a TAVR has been successfully placed inside a previously surgically implanted bioprosthesis that has suffered structural deterioration [30]. It is conceivable that this could become a purposeful strategy in the treatment of AS. A bioprosthesis would be inserted surgically in relatively young patients, assuming that if it failed a TAVR could be placed valve-in-valve thus making bioprosthesis even more attractive for valve replacement. While this concept may prove to be sound, a larger body of data that includes long term follow-up thus allowing discernment that the benefits outweigh the risks of such a strategy must be available before we routinely recommend it for widespread clinical use.

The Heart Team

Currently the decision to recommend TAVR to a patient with AS is highly complex and dependent upon excellent imaging of the arterial tree and aortic annulus; a knowledge of the patient and his/her comorbidities, estimation of the risk of surgical AVR, and a general assessment that the patient will benefit from TAVR. In certain cases, patients thought too ill for surgical AVR are in fact excellent candidates for the procedure. In other cases, some patients are so ill that benefit from TAVR is highly unlikely. Both the decision about which, if any, procedure is best for the patient as well as deployment itself should not be left to a single practitioner or to members of single specialty. The decision should be made by team of experts representing all fields of cardiovascular practice so that a consensus of opinion can be reached, assuring that the patient will receive the best therapy for his/her overall condition, applied by those with the best skills to do so.

Summary

For the patient with aortic stenosis and for the healthcare provider treating AS patients, TAVR represents a significant advance, the impact of which is enormous. TAVR provides life-saving and quality-of-life improving therapy for patients that previously would have suffered sudden death or prolonged death fraught with heart failure. It is likely that we are in only the dawning of an era of transcatheter valve implantation. Future technological developments are likely to improve the outcomes and increase the ease of deployment, still further affecting the treatment for AS and other valvular heart diseases. Irrespective of these advances, it will require the input from a balanced heart team to ensure that our patients receive the therapy that best fit each patient's risks and needs.

References

1. Grossman W, Jones D, McLarin LP. Wall stress and patterns of hypertrophy in the human left ventricle. J Clin Invest. 1975;53:332–41.
2. Marcus ML, Doty DB, Hiratzka LF, Wright CB, Eastham CL. Decreased coronary reserve: a mechanism for angina pectoris in patients with aortic stenosis and normal coronary arteries. N Engl J Med. 1982;307:1362–6.

3. Hess OM, Ritter M, Schneider J, Grimm J, Turina M, Krayenbuehl HP. Diastolic stiffness and myocardial structure in aortic valve disease before and after valve replacement. Circulation. 1984;69: 855–65.
4. Levy D, Garrison RJ, Savage DD, Kannel WB, Castelli WP. Prognostic implications of echocardiographically determined left ventricular mass in the Framingham heart study. N Engl J Med. 1990;322:1561–6.
5. Kupari M, Turto H, Lommi J. Left ventricular hypertrophy in aortic valve stenosis: preventive or promotive of systolic dysfunction and heart failure. Eur Heart J. 2005;26:1790–6.
6. Huber D, Grimm J, Loch R, Krayenbuehl HP. Determinants of ejections performance in aortic stenosis. Circulation. 1981; 64:126–34.
7. Zile MR, Brutsaert DL. New concepts in diastolic dysfunction and diastolic heart failure: part II – causal mechanisms and treatment. Circulation. 2002;105:1503–8.
8. Ross Jr J, Braunwald E. Aortic stenosis. Circulation. 1968; 38:61–7.
9. Selzer A. Changing aspects of the natural history of valvular aortic stenosis. N Engl J Med. 1987;317:91–8.
10. Schwarz F, Baumann P, Manthey J, et al. The effect of aortic valve replacement on survival. Circulation. 1982;66:1105–10.
11. Leon M, Smith CR, Mack M, Miller DC, Moses JW, Svensson LG, Tuzcu EM, Webb JG, Fontana GP, Makkar RR, Brown DL, Block PC, Guyton RA, Pichard AD, Bavaria JE, Hermann HC, Douglas PS, Petersen JL, Akin JJ, Anderson WN, Wang D, Pocock S, PARTNER Trial Investigators. Transcatheter aortic-valve implantation for aortic stenosis in patients who cannot undergo surgery. N Engl J Med. 2010;363(17):1597–607.
12. Otto CM, Mickel MC, Kennedy JW, et al. Three-year outcome after balloon aortic valvuloplasty: insights into prognosis of valvular aortic stenosis. Circulation. 1994;89:642–50.
13. Otto CM, Kuusisto J, Reichenbach DD, Gown AM, O'Brien KD. Characterization of the early lesion of 'degenerative' valvular aortic stenosis: histological and immunohistochemical studies. Circulation. 1994;90:844–53.
14. Cowell SJ, Newby DE, Prescott RJ, et al. A randomized trial of intensive lipid-lowering therapy in calcific aortic stenosis. N Engl J Med. 2005;352:2389–97.
15. Rossebo AB, Pedersen TR, Boman K, et al. Intensive lipid lowering with simvastatin and ezetimibe in aortic stenosis. N Engl J Med. 2008;359:1343–56.
16. Chan KL, Teo K, Dumesnil JG, Ni A, Tam J, ASTRONOMER Investigators. Effect of lipid lowering with rosuvastatin on progression of aortic stenosis: results of the aortic stenosis progression observation: measuring effects of rosuvastatin (ASTRONOMER) trial. Circulation. 2010;121(2):306–14.
17. Roberts WC, Ko JM, Hamilton C. Comparison of valve structure, valve weights, and severity of the valve obstruction in 1849 patients having isolated aortic valve replacement for aortic valve stenosis (with or without associated aortic regurgitation) studied at 3 different medical centers in 2 different time periods. Circulation. 2005;112(25):3919–29.
18. Bonow R, Carabello BA, Chatterjee K, de Leon Jr AC, Faxon DP, Freed MD, Gaasch WH, Lytle BW, Nishimura RA, O'Gara PT, O'Rourke RA, Otto CM, Shah PM, Shanewise JS, Smith Jr SC, Jacobs AK, Adams CD, Anderson JL, Antman EM, Fuster V, Halperin JL, Hiratzka LF, Hunt SA, Lytle BW, Nishimura R, Page RL, Riegel B. ACC/AHA 2006 guidelines for the management of patients with valvular heart disease: a report of the American College of Cardiology/American Heart Association task force on practice guidelines (writing committee to revise the 1998 guidelines for the management of patients with valvular heart disease) developed in collaboration with the Society of Cardiovascular Anesthesiologist endorsed by the Society for Cardiovascular Angiography and Interventions and the Society of Thoracic Surgeons. Circulation. 2006;114(5):e84–231.
19. Pereira JJ, Balaban K, Lauer M, Lytle B, Thomas JD, Garcia MJ. Aortic valve replacement in patients with mild or moderate aortic stenosis and coronary bypass surgery. Am J Med. 2005;118(7):735–42.
20. Das P, Rimington H, Chambers J. Exercise testing to stratify risk in aortic stenosis. Eur Heart J. 2005;26(13):1309–13.
21. Amato MC, Moffa PJ, Werner KE, Ramires JA. Treatment decision in asymptomatic aortic valve stenosis: role of exercise testing. Heart. 2001;86(4):381–6.
22. Rosenhek R, Binder T, Porenta G, et al. Predictors of outcome in severe, asymptomatic aortic stenosis. N Engl J Med. 2000; 343:611–7.
23. Rosenhek R, Zilberszac R, Schemper M, Czerny M, Mundigler G, Graf S, Bergler-Klein J, Grimm M, Gabriel H, Mauerer G. Natural history of very severe aortic stenosis. Circulation. 2010; 121(1):151–6.
24. Carabello BA. The placement of aortic transcatheter valve (PARTNER) trial: the view of a cardiologist. Circulation. 2012;125(25):3240–2.
25. Smith CR, Leon MB, Mack MJ, Miller DC, Moses JW, Svensson LG, Tuzcu EM, Webb JG, Fontana GP, Makkar RR, Williams M, Dewey T, Kapadia S, Babaliaros V, Thourani VH, Corso P, Pichard AD, Bavaria JE, Herrmann HC, Akin JJ, Anderson WN, Wang D, Pocock SJ, PARTNER Trial Investigators. Transcatheter versus surgical aortic-valve replacement in high-risk patients. N Engl J Med. 2011;364(23):2187–98. Epub 2011 Jun 5.
26. Kodall SK, Williams MR, Smith CR, Svensson LG, Webb JG, Makkar RR, Fontana GP, Dewey TM, Thourani VH, Pichard AD, Fischbein M, Szeto WY, Lim S, Greason KL, Teirstein PS, Malaisrie SC, Douglas PS, Hahn RT, Whisenant B, Zajarias A, Wang D, Akin JJ, Anderson WN, Leon MB, PARTNER Trial Investigators. Two-year outcomes after transcatheter or surgical aortic-valve replacement. N Engl J Med. 2012;366(18): 1686–95. Epub 2012 Mar 26.
27. Pai RG, Kapoor N, Bansal RC, Varadarajan P. Malignant natural history of asymptomatic severe aortic stenosis: benefit of aortic valve replacement. Ann Thorac Surg. 2006;82(6):2116–22.
28. Varadarajan P, Kapoor N, Bansal RC, Pai RG. Clinical profile and natural history of 453 nonsurgically managed patients with severe aortic stenosis. Ann Thorac Surg. 2006;82(6):2111–5.
29. Tamburino C, Capodanno D, Ramondo A, Petronio AS, Ettori F, Santoro G, Klugmann S, Bedogni F, Maisano F, Marzocchi A, Poli A, Antoniucci D, Napodano M, De Carlo M, Fiorina C, Ussia GP. Incidence and predictors of early and late mortality after transcatheter aortic valve implantation in 663 patients with severe aortic stenosis. Circulation. 2011;123(3):299–308. Epub 2011 Jan 10.
30. Webb JG, Wood DA. Current status of transcatheter aortic valve replacement. J Am Coll Cardiol. 2012;60:483–92.

Transcatheter Aortic Valve Replacement: What the Near-Term Future Holds and What Evidence Is Needed?

7

Hasan Jilaihawi, Tarun Chakravarty, and Raj Makkar

Abstract

Transcatheter aortic valve replacement (TAVR) is a rapidly evolving therapy that already has a strong evidence base in both inoperable and high-risk patients with severe calcific aortic stenosis. Its ongoing growth as a treatment modality in the near future demands a rigorous approach to clinical research to provide evidence to support its long-term safety and efficacy. This evidence will come in several important areas: (1) refining the indications for TAVR, (2) improving its safety, and (3) building on the success of the first-generation devices with novel designs and concepts. The indications for this technology are being refined, and although the primary focus is on aortic stenosis, exciting new applications are emerging that will require rigorous evaluation and present new challenges. Improving the safety and efficacy of TAVR is of paramount importance, and there is a growing evidence base that concurrent advances in imaging techniques are helping to reduce complications that can arise with TAVR. Several new TAVR devices are emerging, which are each being evaluated in clinical studies.

Keywords

Evidence based • Future • TAVR • Indications • Complications • Novel TAVR devices

Transcatheter aortic valve replacement (TAVR) is a rapidly evolving therapy that already has a strong evidence base in both inoperable and high-risk patients with severe calcific aortic stenosis. Since the inception of the clinical experience of TAVR over 10 years ago by Dr Alain Cribier, its usage has increased exponentially, with over 50,000 implants worldwide so far [1]. Its ongoing growth as a treatment modality in the near future demands a rigorous approach to clinical research to provide evidence to support its long-term safety and efficacy. This evidence will come in several important areas: refining the indications for TAVR, improving its safety, and building on the success of the first-generation devices with novel designs and concepts. Multimodality imaging is fundamental to each of these concepts, and the potential impact of imaging on the evidence-based future of TAVR will be the subject of this chapter.

Refining the Indications for TAVR: Expansion and Limitation

TAVR has been shown to improve both survival and quality of life in a randomized controlled trial in patients with severe aortic stenosis (AS) who cannot have surgery [2, 3] (Fig. 7.1a). In turn, it has demonstrated similar outcomes in a randomized comparison to surgical aortic valve replacement (SAVR) in high-risk operative candidates with severe AS [4] (Fig. 7.1b), but with more rapid improvements in quality of life [5]. The next phase in the evolution of clinical indications for TAVR is gathering evidence on lower surgical

H. Jilaihawi, MD, MRCP (✉) • T. Chakravarty, MD
R. Makkar, MD, FACC
Department of Cardiology, Cedars-Sinai Heart Institute, Cedars-Sinai Medical Center, 8700 Beverly Boulevard, Los Angeles, CA 90048, USA
e-mail: hasanjilaihawi@gmail.com; tarun.chakravarty@cshs.org; raj.makkar@cshs.org

J.K. Min et al. (eds.), *Multimodality Imaging for Transcatheter Aortic Valve Replacement*, DOI 10.1007/978-1-4471-2798-7_7, © Springer-Verlag London 2014

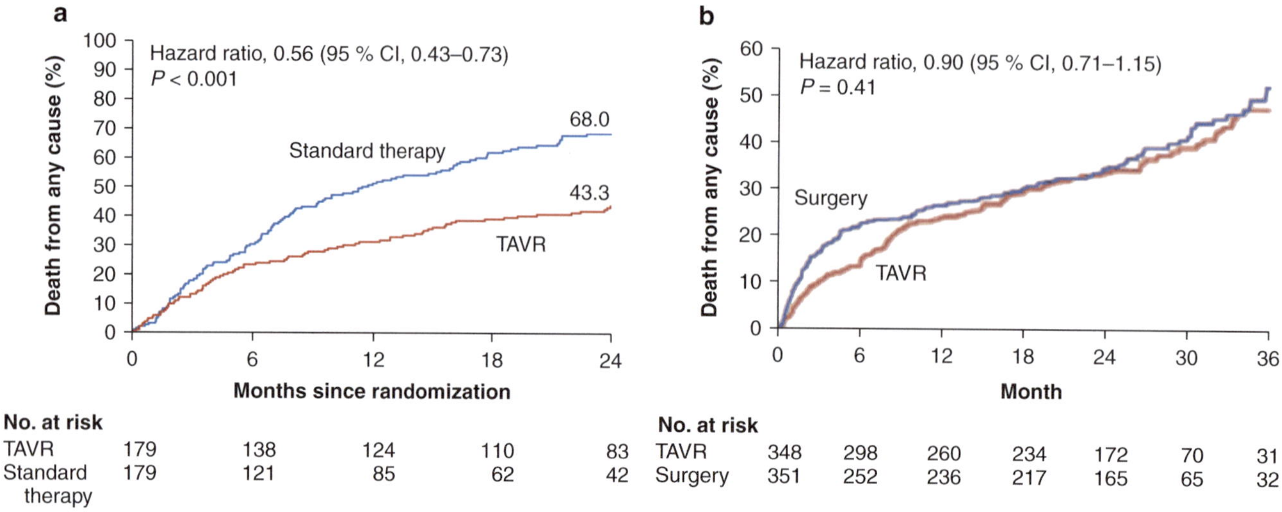

Fig. 7.1 Effect of transcatheter aortic valve replacement (TAVR) on survival in patients with severe symptomatic aortic stenosis in the randomized controlled PARTNER trial. (**a**) In inoperable patients (PARTNER trial cohort B), TAVR results in significantly improved 2-year survival, compared to standard therapy, including balloon valvuloplasty (Reprinted from Makkar et al. [3], with permission from the Massachusetts Medical Society). (**b**) In operable patients (PARTNER trial cohort A), 2-year survival is similar between TAVR and surgical aortic valve replacement (Reprinted from Kodali et al. [16], with permission from the Massachusetts Medical Society)

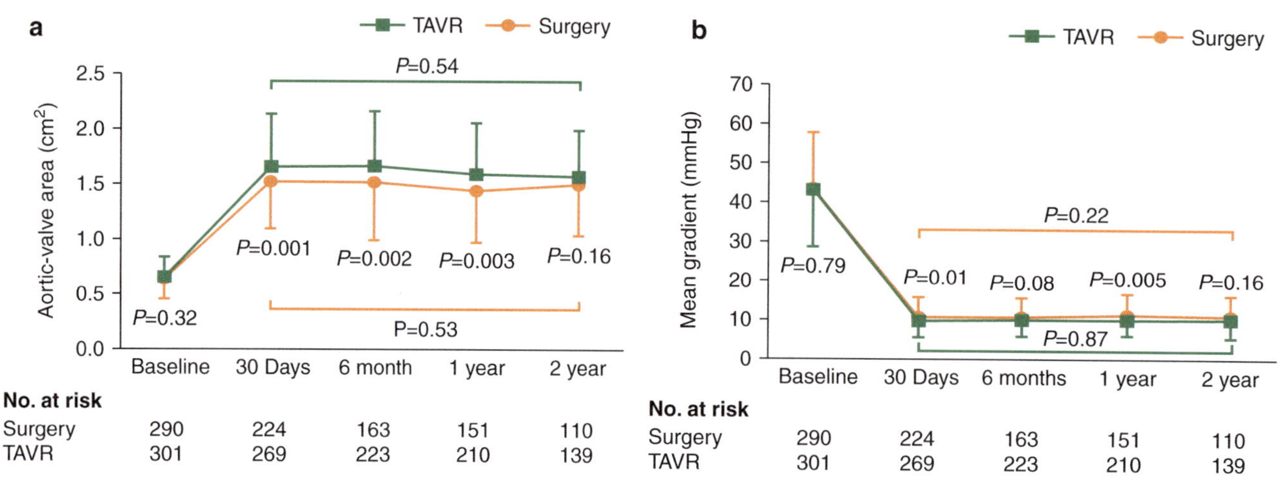

Fig. 7.2 In the randomized controlled PARTNER trial, transcatheter aortic valve replacement resulted in a sustained improvement in aortic valve area (**a**) and mean gradient (**b**), up to 2 years [2]

risk patients, to establish whether TAVR will offer benefit not only to the high-risk minority but also to the intermediate- and low-risk majority of patients with this condition. This process is already underway in a randomized controlled trial of TAVR vs SAVR in patients at intermediate surgical risk (PARTNER IIA trial).

Risk has been arbitrarily defined according to the Society of Thoracic Surgeons (STS) database scoring system, with low risk as STS <4, intermediate-risk STS 4–8, and high-risk STS >8 [6]. If TAVR offers favorable data compared to SAVR in the intermediate-risk group, the referral base for this technology will increase significantly, and its true potential will be realized. There remain important caveats to the expansion of TAVR beyond such cohorts. Low surgical risk patients are still best treated by SAVR until evidence accumulates for intermediate-risk patients. This is for several reasons. Importantly, the durability of TAVR has only been demonstrated to 3 years [3, 7] (Fig. 7.2), with the longest surviving patients with TAVR only followed to around 6 years, whereas several studies have demonstrated long-term durability of surgical bioprostheses as long as 15 years and beyond [8]. Moreover, the safety of the procedure and ongoing refinements in the technology have a growing evidence base in this regard, but it will take time to address all the shortcomings of

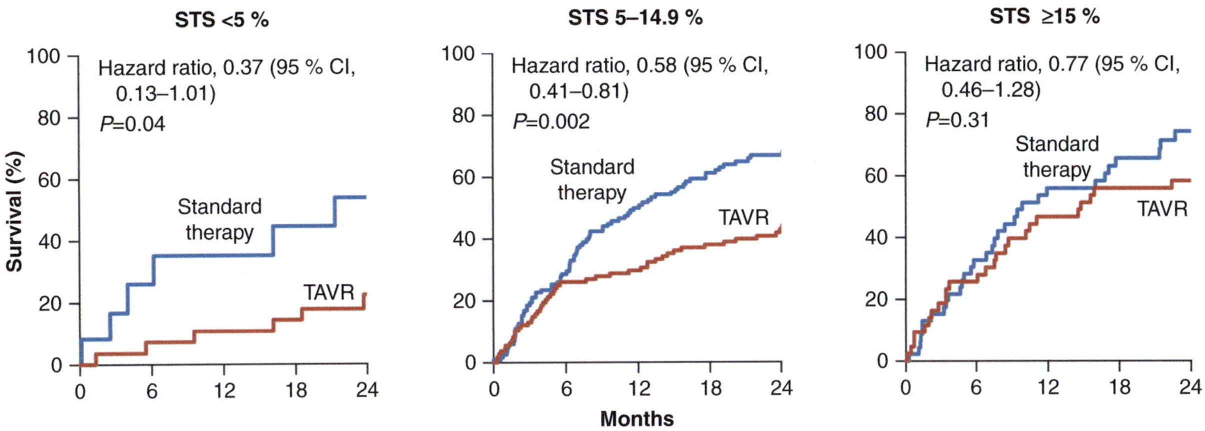

No. at risk															
TAVR	28	26	25	24	16	108	80	76	67	52	43	32	23	19	15
Standard therapy	12	8	7	6	5	119	84	59	42	29	47	29	19	14	8

Fig. 7.3 Stratification of 2-year mortality according to STS score (<5 %, 5–14.9 %, or ≥15 %) in inoperable patients with severe symptomatic aortic stenosis in the randomized, controlled PARTNER trial. The survival benefit of transcatheter aortic valve replacement, in comparison to standard therapy, diminishes with a higher STS score, with no survival benefit from TAVR in patients with STS score ≥15 % [1]

the early generation devices and procedures; these will be discussed in the next section of this chapter.

Conversely, although procedures are often technically feasible in the patients with prohibitive surgical risk, they may be clinically futile in some patients, in whom TAVR should not be performed. There will be an important focus in identifying such patients, so that an unnecessary and costly procedure may be avoided. There already exists some data in this regard. In a subset analysis cohort B of the PARTNER trial, patients at the highest surgical risk by STS score (STS ≥15) had no survival benefit with TAVR in comparison to medical therapy [3] (Fig. 7.3). Imaging may offer some insight into this group of patients; for instance, novel MRI techniques can quantify cardiac fibrosis reliably [9] and could identify patients with AS and advanced fibrosis that may not benefit from TAVR. At the other end of the spectrum, imaging may help stratify risk of cardiac structural deterioration in asymptomatic patients with severe AS, whose treatment remains controversial [10]. TAVR, with its less invasive nature than open surgery, may one day offer a viable treatment option in such patients.

Novel Indications for TAVR

TAVR also offers promise in the treatment of patients for conditions other than native aortic valve stenosis. The failing surgical bioprosthesis is an important and exciting new indication for TAVR [11, 12] (Fig. 7.4), potentially limiting the risk of redo operation. Data is currently accumulating in the form of single-center and multicentric registries, but a randomized trial is merited to provide definitive evidence supporting this strategy. There is also increasing technical data regarding how best to select a particular TAVR for a specific failing bioprosthesis, which patients and bioprostheses can be treated in a straightforward manner and which may pose increased risks, such as coronary occlusion [13].

Native aortic regurgitation is also an exciting new indication for TAVR and presents new challenges [14]. For instance, the use of a balloon expandable device is not feasible as the presence of leaflets without substantial calcification offers much less of an anchor. The vast majority of next-generation TAVR devices comprise self-expanding designs that will be more likely to address this clinical problem. Anchoring a transcatheter bioprosthesis to a native aortic valve in the absence of stenosis will also demand a more rigorous attention to multimodality imaging, ascertaining the qualitative and quantitative aspects of the aortic valvar complex. New challenges may arise; for instance, in stenotic valves leaflet mobility is restricted, with a low risk of coronary occlusion presented only by the most bulky leaflets or in cases of great proximity of the coronary ostia to the aortic annulus. In contrast, in predominant native aortic valve regurgitation, the leaflets are hypermobile and may come close to or even reach the level of the coronary ostia in systole. Indeed, advanced multimodality imaging may draw on lessons for new TAVR indications from cases already performed and provides ongoing data for the safety and efficacy of TAVR for all potential indications.

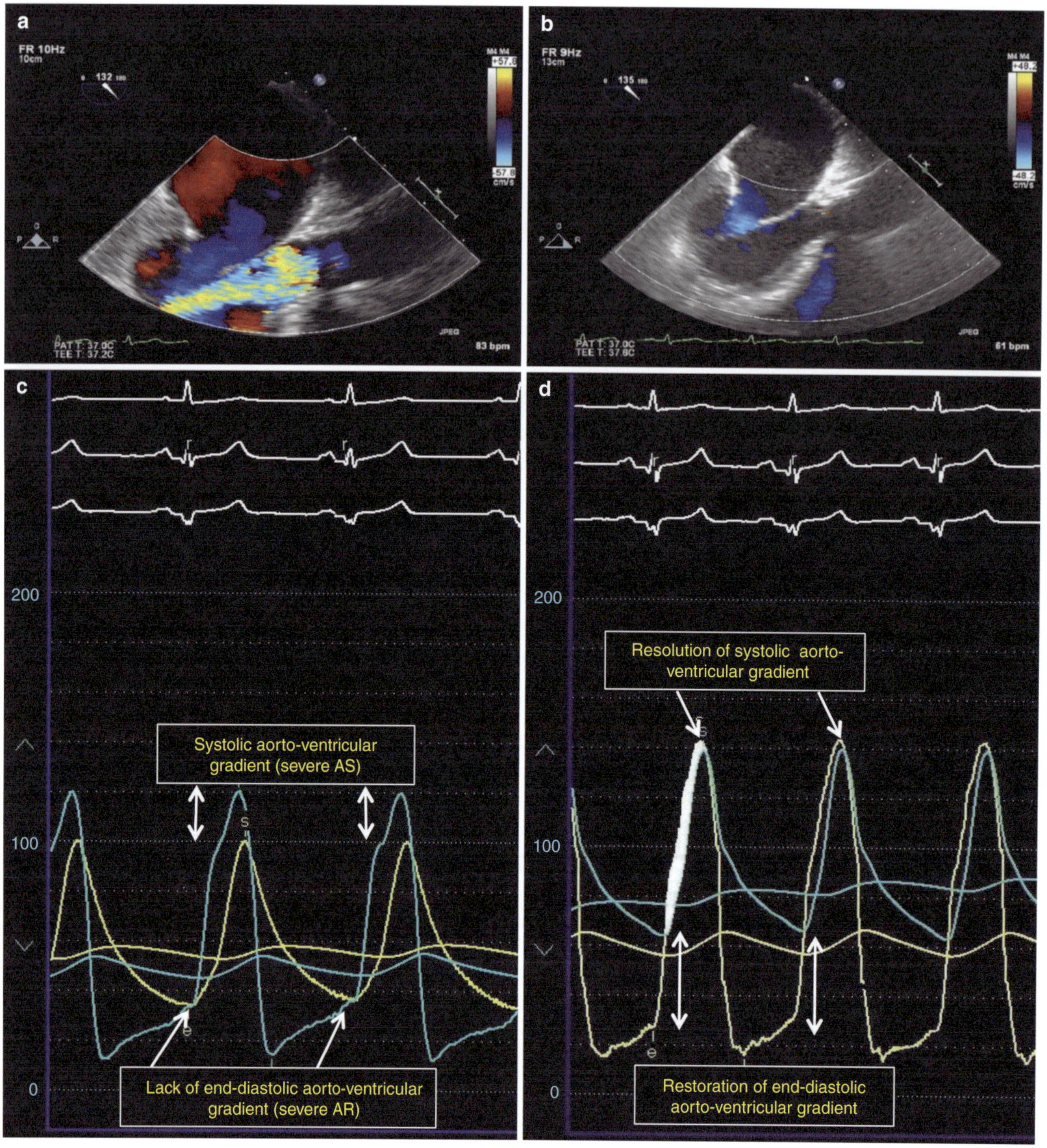

Fig. 7.4 Valve-in-valve implantation of Edwards-SAPIEN valve by transcatheter aortic valve replacement (TAVR) for degenerative bioprosthetic aortic valve stenosis (AS) with regurgitation (AR). (**a**, **b**) Echocardiographic findings: Severe bioprosthetic valve degenerative aortic stenosis and aortic regurgitation (**a**) resolved after valve-in-valve implantation (**b**). (**c**, **d**) Hemodynamic findings: resolution of systolic aorto-ventricular gradient and restoration of end-diastolic aorto-ventricular gradient after valve-in-valve implantation

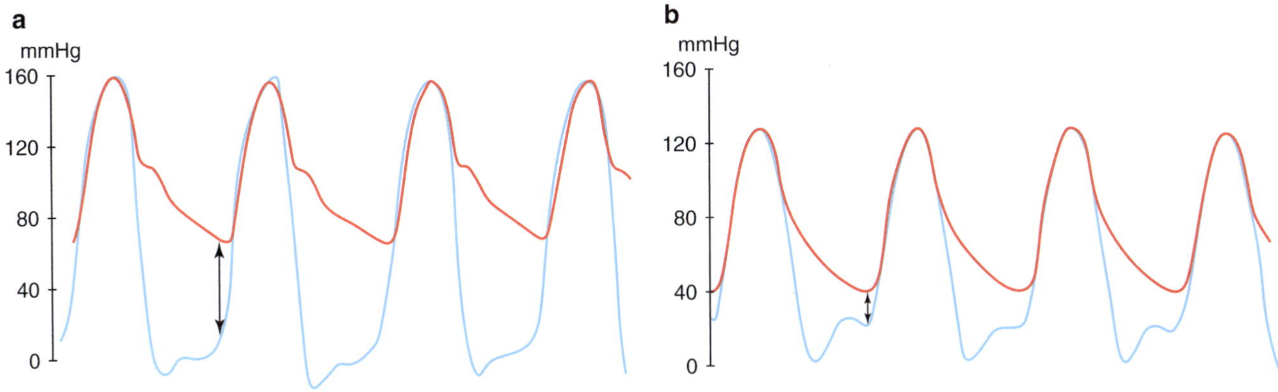

Fig. 7.5 Calculation of aortic regurgitation (AR) index. AR Index is calculated by measuring left ventricular end-diastolic pressure (LVEDP) (*blue line*) and diastolic blood pressure (DBP) in the aorta (*red line*) simultaneously. (**a**) Patient without periprosthetic AR. AR index = ([65 – 10]/160) × 100 = 34.4. (**b**) Patient with moderate periprosthetic AR. AR index = ([40 – 20]/130) × 100 = 15.4 (Reprinted from Sinning et al. [18], with permission from Elsevier Inc)

Limiting the Complications and Improving the Safety and Efficacy of TAVR

Although a lot has been learnt from the early experience of TAVR, several complications that limit the safety and efficacy of this technology are an important focus for future study. Many of these will be addressed in later chapters of this book but the near-term future evidence required for the principal issues of concern will be discussed here.

Paravalvular Regurgitation

Paravalvular AR is an important complication post-TAVR. It is more than moderate in 10 % of cases and has been shown consistently to be associated with increased mortality [15–17]. Two-year follow-up of patients in cohort A of the PARTNER study seemed to suggest that lower degrees of PV AR, even mild PV AR, are also associated with increased mortality [16]. This may be attributable to difficulties in PV AR assessment and underestimation of severity by TEE. An important study recently demonstrated that a transcatheter hemodynamic assessment of PV AR severity (Fig. 7.5) offered mortality prediction of incremental prognostic value to echocardiographic assessment [18]. Further studies are merited as to whether this should be the gold standard for the quantification of this complication. There is a fundamental need for more evidence for optimal imaging for the prevention and assessment of this complication. Recently, contrast cross-sectional CT has been shown to predict paravalvular AR much more reliably than 2D TEE [19, 20] (Fig. 7.6). However, due to renal impairment, many patients undergoing TAVR cannot receive the contrast required for accurate cross-sectional CT assessment of the aortic annulus. Although MRI and 3D TEE offer considerable potential in this regard, evidence of their reliability to the standard of contrast CT is lacking at this time.

Stroke

Stroke is an important and much feared complication of both transcatheter and surgical aortic valve replacements. The PARTNER IA study demonstrated a higher incidence of stroke after TAVR than surgery; differences were small but significant early post-procedure but not significant at 1- and 2-year follow-up [4]. Detailed and objective-specialized neurological assessment is thus an integral part of the PARTNER IIA study, mandatory before and after every TAVR and SAVR procedure. Proponents of the transapical approach initially attributed many neuroembolic events with the transfemoral approach to the requirement to negotiate an often atheromatous aortic arch [21]. Subsequent data has shown no difference in either clinical stroke [22] or imaging evidence of neuroembolic events by diffusion-weighted MRI [23]. A detailed analysis of strokes in the PARTNER IIB study showed the majority of post-TAVR embolic stroke events to be periprocedural with late stroke often attributable to hemorrhage (Fig. 7.7) and falls [3]. Important studies investigating the timing of these periprocedural events have shown them to be most marked at the time of valve deployment [24], which points to the main source being the valve leaflets. This supports the need for embolic protection devices.

There are at least three embolic protection devices customized to TAVR (Fig. 7.8). Two are CE marked and under ongoing evaluation in Europe and Canada. The first to be approved in Europe, in May 2010, was the Embrella Embolic Deflector [25], which is inserted by right radial approach, consists of

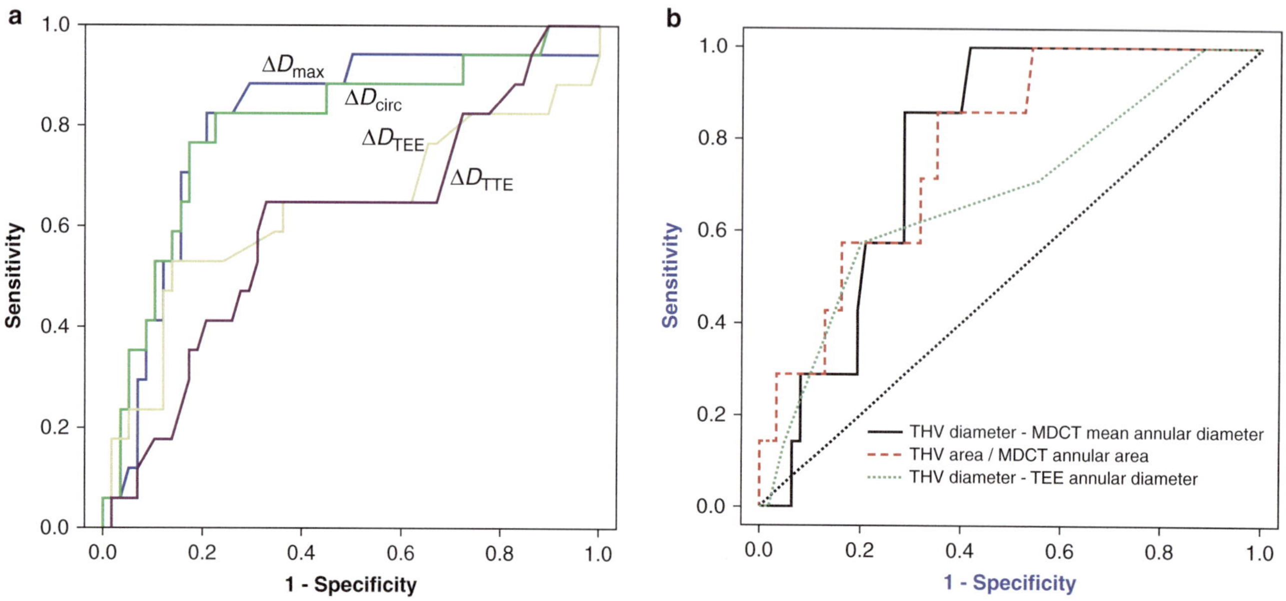

Fig. 7.6 Comparison of cross-sectional CT and transesophageal echocardiography (TEE) for predicting paravalvular aortic regurgitation (AR) after transcatheter aortic valve replacement (TAVR) using area under the receiver-operating characteristic curves method. (**a**) The cross-sectional CT-derived parameters (ΔD_{max} and ΔD_{circ}) have greater discriminatory value for predicting paravalvular AR after TAVR than TEE-derived parameters ($\Delta D_{TEE(max)}$ and $\Delta_{TEE(circ)}$) (Reprinted from Jilaihawi et al. [19], with permission from Elsevier Inc). (**b**) The MDCT-derived parameters (MDCT mean annular diameter and MDCT annular area) have greater discriminatory value for predicting paravalvular AR after TAVR than TEE-derived parameters (TEE annular diameter) (Reprinted from Willson et al. [20], with permission from Elsevier Inc.). *Abbreviations*: *THV* transcatheter heart valve. ΔD_{max}, (CT-derived non-orthogonal true maximum annular diameter) – (THV size); ΔD_{circ}, [(CT-derived perimeter of the traced polygon)/π] – (THV size); $\Delta D_{TEE(max)}$, (TEE-derived non-orthogonal true maximum annular diameter) – (THV size); $\Delta_{TEE(circ)}$, [(TEE-derived perimeter of the traced polygon)/π] – (THV size)

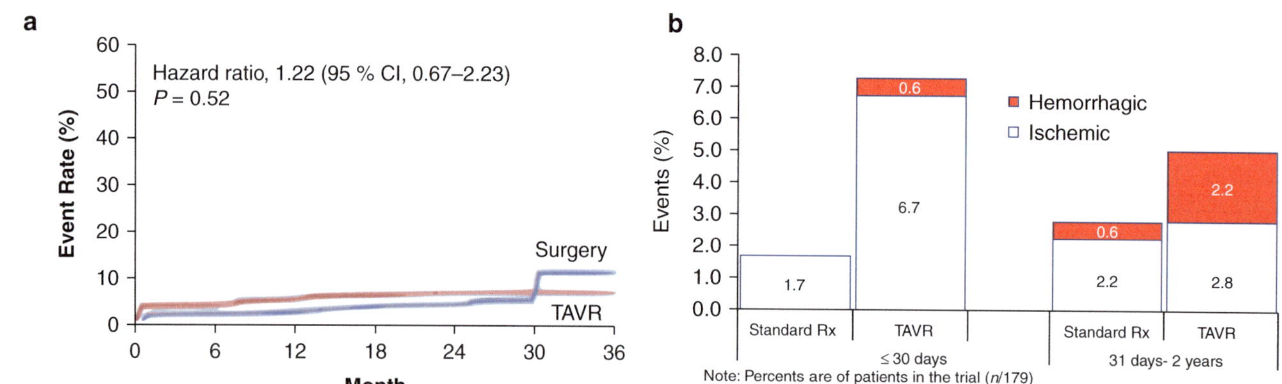

No. at risk

TAVR	348	287	249	224	162	65	28
Surgery	351	246	230	211	160	62	31

Note: Percents are of patients in the trial (*n*/179)

	≤ 30 Days	31 days - 2 years
All stroke	**p = 0.010**	**p = 0.319**
Ischemic stroke	p = 0.017	p = 0.437
Hemorrhagic stroke	p = 0.316	p = 0.160

Fig. 7.7 Comparison of transcatheter aortic valve replacement (TAVR) with surgical aortic valve replacement (SAVR) and standard therapy. (**a**) The stroke rates at 2 years were not statistically different between TAVR and SAVR in the operable cohort in the PARTNER trial [2]. (**b**) The stroke rates in the inoperable cohort in the PARTNER trial were higher with TAVR in comparison with standard therapy, both at 30 days and 2 years. The excess strokes in the TAVR group in the first 30 days were attributable to a greater number of ischemic strokes in that group. Beyond 30 days and up to 2 years, the excess of strokes was attributable to hemorrhagic events [1]

two panels that open in a clam-like configuration, and acts as a deflective shield covering the right innominate and left carotid ostia. Importantly, it does not collect debris but prevents cerebral embolization by covering the ostia of the great arch vessels. Gerckens et al. used the device in 20 TAVR patients [26]—with 18 available for final analysis—and achieved coverage of the innominate artery and the left common carotid artery in all patients; 60 % of the patients also received additional coverage of the left subclavian artery. Post-procedure MRI in 15 of the patients found new cerebral lesions in 11/15 subjects, with an average of 4.36 lesions per patient, comparing favorably with studies of patients

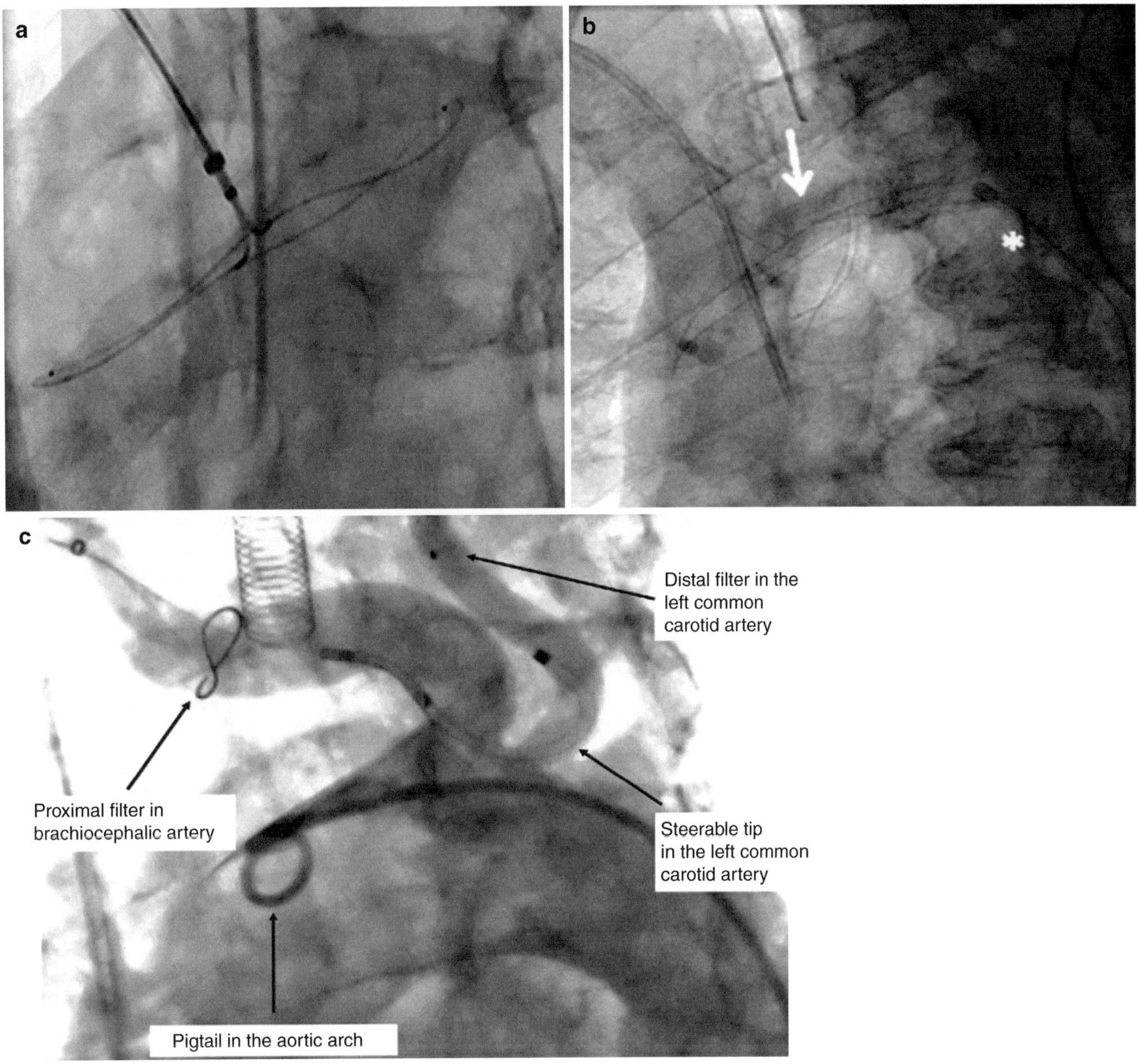

Fig. 7.8 Embolic protection devices for transcatheter aortic valve replacement (TAVR). (**a**) Embrella Embolic Deflector System (Embrella Cardiovascular, Inc., Wayne, Pennsylvania) (Reprinted from Nietlispach et al. [25], with permission from Elsevier Inc.). (**b**) SMT Embolic Deflection Device (SMT Medical Technologies, Herzliya, Israel) (Reprinted from Onsea et al. [40], with permission from Europa Digital & Publishing). (**c**) Claret Dual Filter System (Claret Medical, Santa Rosa, CA) (Reprinted from Naber et al. [41], with permission from Europa Digital & Publishing)

undergoing TAVR without embolic protection. Like Embrella, SMT is also an embolic deflector device. It has been evaluated in a small feasibility study, reported by Stella et al. [26]: 15 patients received the SMT device during TAVR. One patient suffered a transient ischemic attack (TIA) at 4 days following the procedure, and one suffered a stroke after 5 days. MRI showed a 50 % reduction in new cerebral lesions compared to 25 % in control patients. The CE mark study started in January 2012.

The Montage System is manufactured by Claret Medical and achieved CE mark approval in October 2011. It is inserted by unilateral 6 Fr radial or brachial access and facilitates insertion of a filter in both right innominate and left carotid arteries. Naber et al. reported its use in 40 TAVR patients [26]: although there were no procedural TIAs or minor or major strokes, within 30 days of the procedure, one patient suffered a minor stroke, two suffered major strokes, and six patients died (all non-device related). Although the latter device has the largest clinical experience to date, further studies are required to establish the efficacy of all of these devices, with a fundamental need for randomized studies. Given the relatively low incidence of clinical stroke,

DW-MRI will be an important surrogate outcome, although it appears to detect many clinically silent events that remain of unclear significance.

Access-Related Complications

The transfemoral approach, when feasible, is the preferred access approach for TAVR. Both improved imaging of the peripheral vasculature and careful case selection for transfemoral cases have been associated with a marked reduction in peripheral vascular complications over time [27] and will be discussed in later chapters. Technological advances have resulted in further reductions in the profile of TAVR devices, which have also been associated with a reduction in vascular complications [28]. Improved peripheral vascular techniques have facilitated a truly percutaneous approach with preclosure of the femoral access site and the avoidance of the need for cutdown in the majority of cases [29]. The contingency planning required for bail-out maneuvers in the event of vascular complication have also, most likely, improved outcomes.

However, there remain a significant proportion of patients who, due to peripheral vascular disease or small vasculature, cannot safely undergo the transfemoral approach at this time. It is in these patients that the optimal access approach is yet to be determined. Although the transapical approach was the first alternative approach [30], transaortic [31] and transaxillary [32] are now promising alternatives. Each of the 3 has relative merits. The latter two approaches demand retrograde crossing of the aortic valve but avoid disruption of the left ventricular apex. The transaortic approach cannot be performed in a true porcelain aorta. The transaxillary approach requires axillary vasculature of adequate dimension, which is often observed in larger patients with peripheral vascular disease but not smaller patients. Recently, a propensity-matched study demonstrated similar outcomes of transaxillary and transfemoral TAVR. A head-to-head randomized study of the transaortic and transapical approaches is also merited to provide further evidence required for decision making for the optimal approach in a particular patient.

Evidence for Novel TAVR Devices

The landscape of available devices for TAVR is dramatically changing. From only 2 first-generation devices, several new prostheses are emerging, some from the original companies (Edwards Lifesciences and Medtronic CoreValve) but many more from start-up companies (Fig. 7.9). Those that have entered the clinical arena, and the evidence supporting them, as well as the future evidence required will be discussed here.

The First-Generation TAVR Devices and Their Iterations

The Edwards Sapien valve is to date the only TAVR device with evidence-based data in a randomized controlled trial and, as such, is the only FDA-approved device in commercial use today. The Medtronic CoreValve device and the next-generation Edwards Sapien (XT) device are presently being evaluated in randomized controlled trials in the United States, although a large body of nonrandomized safety and efficacy data already exists for these prostheses from Europe. The principal difference between these devices is the short balloon expandable stent frame of the Edwards device, whereas a self-expanding stent frame carries the Medtronic CoreValve valve. A direct-randomized comparison has not yet been performed and is unlikely to happen. Clear differences do exist in the form of a considerably greater pacemaker requirement with the Medtronic CoreValve device which has been demonstrated in multiple-single and multicenter registries and meta-analyses [22, 33, 34]. The data from meta-analyses suggests that the incidence of other complications is broadly similar [33, 34]. There is some data to support an excess of paravalvular leak with the Medtronic CoreValve device, but this is most likely related to operators utilization of different imaging modalities to assess this complication, with fluoroscopy used by CoreValve operators, which tends to overestimate AR, relative to echocardiographic assessment favored by Edwards operators [22].

Fig. 7.9 Fluoroscopic appearance of deployed transcatheter aortic valves. (**a**) Edwards-SAPIEN trascatheter heart valve (Edwards Lifesciences Corporation, Irvine, CA). (**b**) Sapien XT transcatheter heart valve (Edwards Lifesciences Corporation, Irvine, CA). (**c**) CoreValve (Medtronic Inc., Minneapolis, MN) (Reprinted from Grube et al. [42], with permission from Elsevier Inc.). (**d**) Sadra Lotus (Boston Scientific Corporation, Natick, MA) (Reprinted from Buellesfeld et al. [36], with permission from Wiley Periodicals Inc.). (**e**) Portico valve (St. Jude Medical, Inc., St. Paul, MN) (Reprinted from Willson et al. [43], with permission from Elsevier Inc.). (**f**) Direct Flow Medical (Direct Flow Medical, Inc., Santa Rosa, CA) (Reprinted from Schofer et al. [44], with permission from Lippincott Williams & Wilkins). (**g**) Heart Leaflet Technologies (Bracco Diagnostics, Inc., Princeton, New Jersey) (Image courtesy of HLT, Inc., © 2012). (**h**) JenaValve (JenaValve Technology, Inc., Wilmington, DE) (Reprinted from Treede et al. [45], with permission from Oxford University Press). (**i**) Acurate valve (Symetis Inc., Ecublens, Switzerland) (Reprinted from Kempfert et al. [46], with permission from Oxford University Press). (**j**) Engager valve (Medtronic Inc., Minneapolis, MN) (Reprinted from Falk et al. [47] with permission from Oxford University Press)

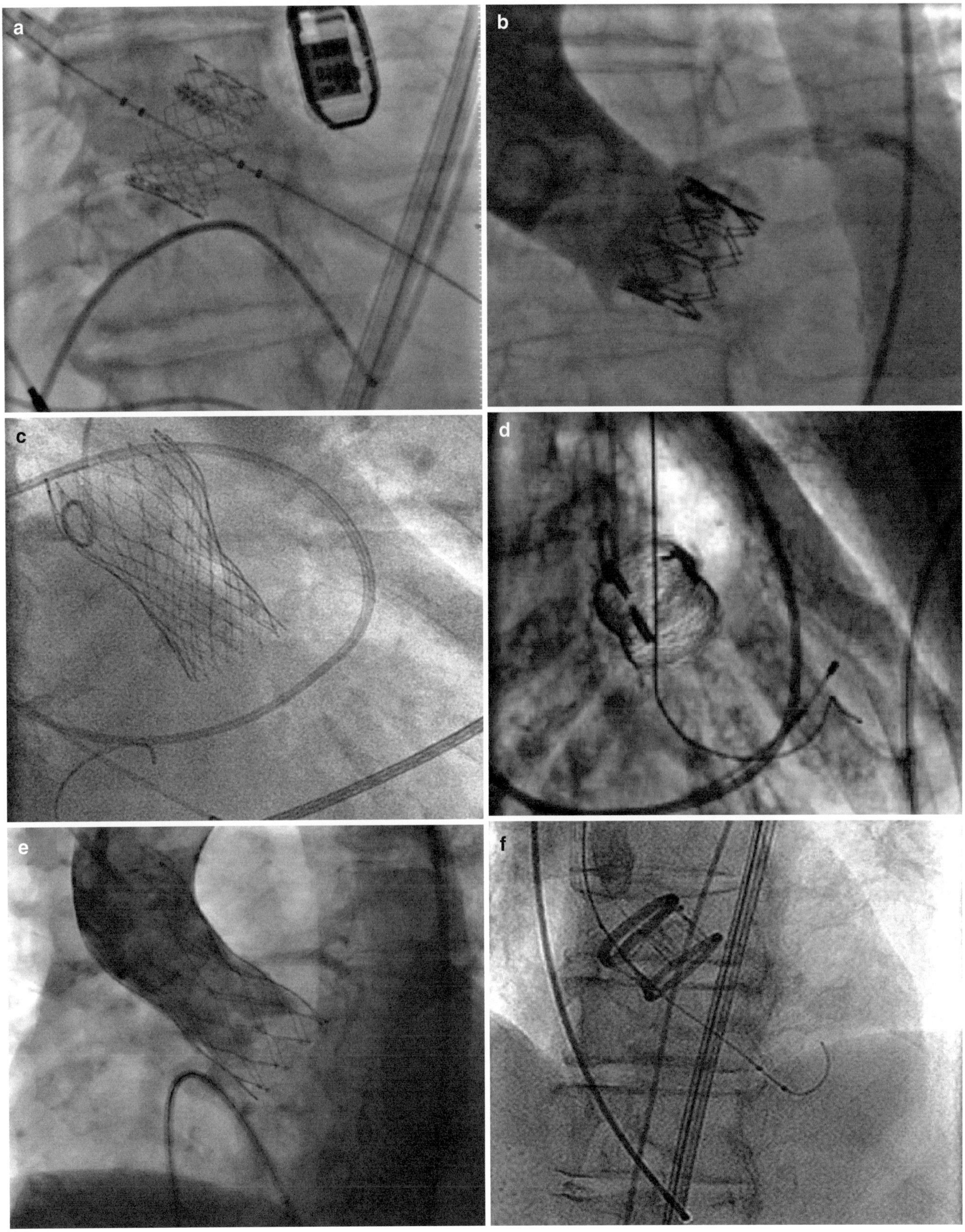
a
b
c
d
e
f

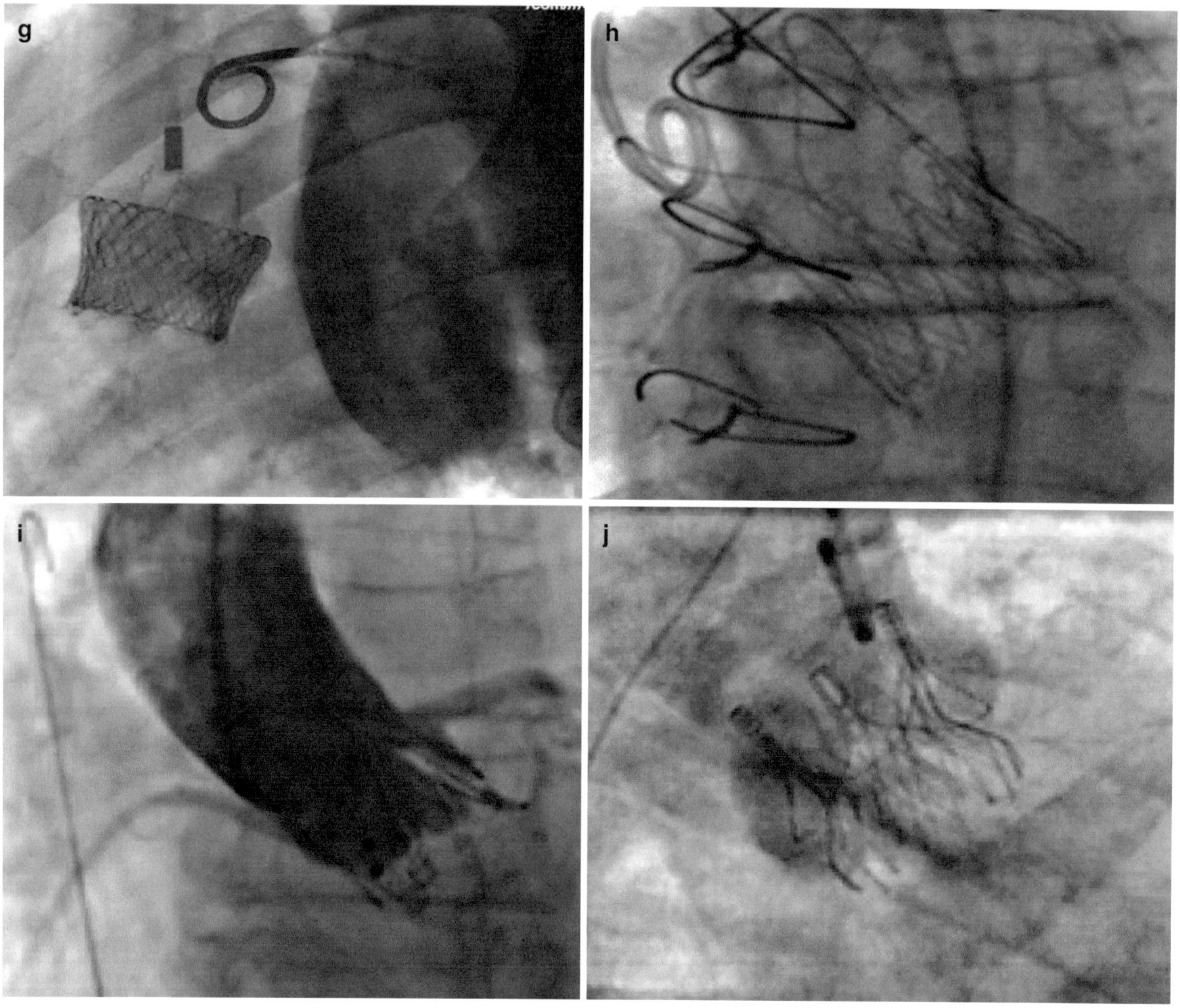

Fig. 7.9 (continued)

Important iterations have been made in both the Medtronic CoreValve and Edwards devices from their respective first-generation devices. The Edwards Sapien (stainless steel stent frame, Retroflex 3 delivery system) has now been superseded in Europe by the Sapien XT (cobalt chromium stent frame, NovaFlex delivery system), with access profile reduced to 18–19 Fr from 22 to 24 Fr [28]. This is facilitated by the NovaFlex's unique in vivo balloon mounting system; the valve is crimped on the shaft of the delivery system and has a mechanism that facilitates movement upward to the balloon after the delivery system has already been placed in the descending thoracic aorta. There is mounting evidence that this is resulting in less groin complication [28]. The comparison between Sapien and XT valves and their delivery systems has been performed in randomized fashion in the PARTNER IIB transfemoral study, data of which has not yet been presented. Further iterations in the Edwards system have included the eSheath, an introducer sheath which expands from 16 Fr to 18/19 Fr on advancement of the valve delivery system inside it and later returns to the reduced profile once the valve has passed through it; this is in clinical use outside the USA and is being used as part of the PARTNER II trial in the United States. Evidence is awaited as to whether this will further reduce groin complications. Forthcoming further developments from Edwards Lifesciences include the Sapien 3 valve, an ultra-low profile balloon expandable platform with additional features designed to further reduce PV, and a lower profile delivery system which passes through a 14 Fr eSheath; this is under evaluation in Europe and Canada. Edwards Lifesciences is also releasing another device, the Centera, a self-expanding repositionable valve with a motorized delivery system and a 14 Fr eSheath; the first-in-man experience has been completed for this device and data is awaited. Little information is available on either of these devices and is eagerly awaited.

With its self-expanding design, the Medtronic CoreValve has offered 18 Fr access from its inception but more recently has a stabilizing system (Accutrak) for device positioning, which has some evidence of benefit in the accuracy of placement [35]. The CoreValve device is being evaluated in high-risk and inoperable patients in the FDA US pivotal trial. It is being evaluated in intermediate-risk patients in the International SURTAVI trial (STS 3–8 outside the USA and 4–8 in the USA). A forthcoming iteration in the CoreValve device for small annuli is the Evolut™ 23 mm, which incorporates Trufit™ technology, said to incorporate a greater adaptability to aortic annular geometry.

Novel Retrievable Designs

A highly desirable property for TAVR is a prosthesis that is not only repositionable but also retrievable. Although this can be performed to some extent with the Medtronic CoreValve, this is associated with an excess of vascular complication and stroke. Several novel TAVR prostheses are specifically designed to be safely retrieved prior to final deployment, in the event of initial malpositioning.

The first of these repositionable prostheses was the Lotus Sadra valve [36], with a first-in-man procedure performed in 2007 and reported in 2008. Boston Scientific completed acquisition of Sadra Medical in January 2011 and completed a European clinical trial evaluating the prosthesis, the REPRISE I study, in April 2012. This comprised three sites in Australia that enrolled only 11 patients. Positive results were achieved with no mortality and no moderate or severe paravalvular regurgitation; however, there was one stroke. The REPRISE II study is an international registry that is to enroll up to 120 patients in up to 15 sites in Australia and Europe, it is expected to be completed in the first half of 2013, and its data will be used to support CE mark regulatory approval.

The Direct Flow Medical (DFM) valve is a nonmetallic repositionable and retrievable device which comprises bovine pericardial leaflets attached to an inflatable polyester fabric cuff; the cuff has independently inflatable ventricular and aortic rings which are first inflated with contrast saline, correct positioning and function confirmed, then the contrast saline exchanged under positive pressure with a solidifying inflation media that hardens to form a permanent support structure [37]. The first patient was treated in 2007, a first-in-man experience was reported in 2008, and favorable follow-up to 2 years was recently reported in 16 high-risk patients demonstrated no paravalvular regurgitation more than minimal. A larger study for CE mark approval, DISCOVER, began in 2011.

Portico is a self-expanding, fully repositionable and retrievable device from St Jude Medical. First-in-man was performed in June 2011 and a small 10-patient series was recently reported by two Canadian centers, with good clinical outcomes [38]. The European clinical trial started in late 2011 and a US trial is planned for 2013.

Heart Leaflet Technologies (HLT) valve, recently acquired by Bracco SpA, is also a self-expanding retrievable, repositionable device, with 17 Fr profile. It consists of a nitinol weave cuff with a braided polyester lining; this carries a porcine pericardial valve. After an encouraging 8-patient first-in-man experience on cardiopulmonary bypass, data with off-pump is the next phase of data awaited.

Novel Transapical Designs

Three other designs, with present iterations delivered by transapical approach, have been developed that are specifically designed to conform to aortic annular geometry: JenaValve, Symetis, and Medtronic Embracer [39]. The JenaValve is also a retrievable and repositionable device that is currently available for the TA approach. It comprises a specific anchoring mechanism that provides a "paperclip"-like active fixation mechanism with a slow pullback during deployment, with tactile feedback when the aortic aspect of the "paperclip" makes contact with the aortic leaflets. CE mark approval was granted in September 2011 after a 7-site German registry of 73 patients demonstrated favorable safety data.

Similarly, Symetis' Accurate TA system is a transapical prosthesis with 3 sizes and anchors the aortic leaflets with tactile feedback to the operator during positioning. It is not retrievable but has a stabilization arch that anchors the device gently to the proximal ascending aorta. It received a CE mark in September 2011 after FIM and pilot studies, collectively evaluating 90 patients in five German centers, demonstrated safety. Larger studies are underway, with a European post-market surveillance study, SAVI (Symetis Aortic Valve Implantation Registry) and a 150-patient, 15 center, US pivotal study planned.

The Medtronic Embracer is also a self-expanding, anatomically orientated device. Like the JenaValve, it comprises "paperclip-like" support arms that are positioned over the native leaflets but also incorporates rotational positioning, with commissures that are orientated to correspond to the native commissures. Acquired by Medtronic from a start-up company, Ventor, in 2009, a CE mark study has been completed early this year, with data awaited. There were initial problems with poor coaxiality of the support arms and uncovered commissural posts resulting in aortic dissection that prompted a redesigned flexible soft-tip over-the-wire delivery catheter that covers the entire prosthesis up to the stage of deployment. This iteration was studied in the CE mark study.

Several additional prostheses exist and are at earlier stages of study; these include the AorTx valve, the Paniagua valve, the 3 Fr valve, and the Palmaz-Bailey.

Conclusions

The near-term future of TAVR is rapidly evolving. The indications for this technology are being refined and although the primary focus is on aortic stenosis, exciting new applications are emerging that will require rigorous evaluation and present new challenges. Improving the safety and efficacy of TAVR is of paramount importance and there is a growing evidence base that concurrent advances in imaging techniques are helping to reduce complications that can arise with TAVR. Several new TAVR devices are emerging, which are each being evaluated in clinical studies. Each of these devices will require specific imaging tools for procedural planning, intraprocedural, and post-procedural imaging that will be the subject of subsequent chapters in this book.

References

1. Webb JG, Wood DA. Current status of transcatheter aortic valve replacement. J Am Coll Cardiol. 2012. doi:10.1016/j.jacc.2012.01.071. S0735-1097(12)01582-3 [pii].
2. Leon MB, Smith CR, Mack M, Miller DC, Moses JW, Svensson LG, et al. Transcatheter aortic-valve implantation for aortic stenosis in patients who cannot undergo surgery. N Engl J Med. 2011;363(17):1597–607. doi:10.1056/NEJMoa1008232.
3. Makkar RR, Fontana GP, Jilaihawi H, Kapadia S, Pichard AD, Douglas PS, et al. Transcatheter aortic-valve replacement for inoperable severe aortic stenosis. N Engl J Med. 2012;366(18):1696–704. doi:10.1056/NEJMoa1202277.
4. Smith CR, Leon MB, Mack MJ, Miller DC, Moses JW, Svensson LG, et al. Transcatheter versus surgical aortic-valve replacement in high-risk patients. N Engl J Med. 2011;364(23):2187–98. doi:10.1056/NEJMoa1103510.
5. Reynolds MR, Magnuson EA, Wang K, Thourani VH, Williams M, Zajarias A, et al. Health-related quality of life after transcatheter or surgical aortic valve replacement in high-risk patients with severe aortic stenosis: results from the PARTNER (Placement of AoRTic TraNscathetER Valve) trial (Cohort A). J Am Coll Cardiol. 2012. doi:10.1016/j.jacc.2012.03.075. S0735-1097(12)02138-9 [pii].
6. Holmes Jr DR, Mack MJ, Kaul S, Agnihotri A, Alexander KP, Bailey SR, et al. 2012 ACCF/AATS/SCAI/STS expert consensus document on transcatheter aortic valve replacement. J Am Coll Cardiol. 2012;59(13):1200–54. doi:10.1016/j.jacc.2012.01.001. S0735-1097(12)00002-2 [pii].
7. Gurvitch R, Wood DA, Tay EL, Leipsic J, Ye J, Lichtenstein SV, et al. Transcatheter aortic valve implantation: durability of clinical and hemodynamic outcomes beyond 3 years in a large patient cohort. Circulation. 2010;122(13):1319–27. doi:10.1161/CIRCULATIONAHA.110.948877. CIRCULATIONAHA.110.948877 [pii].
8. Ruggieri VG, Flecher E, Anselmi A, Lelong B, Corbineau H, Verhoye JP, et al. Long-term results of the Carpentier-Edwards supraannular aortic valve prosthesis. Ann Thorac Surg. 2012. doi:10.1016/j.athoracsur.2012.05.003. S0003-4975(12)01049-1 [pii].
9. Flett AS, Hayward MP, Ashworth MT, Hansen MS, Taylor AM, Elliott PM, et al. Equilibrium contrast cardiovascular magnetic resonance for the measurement of diffuse myocardial fibrosis: preliminary validation in humans. Circulation. 2010;122(2):138–44. doi:10.1161/CIRCULATIONAHA.109.930636. CIRCULATIONAHA.109.930636 [pii].
10. Shah PK. Severe aortic stenosis should not be operated on before symptom onset. Circulation. 2012;126(1):118–25. doi:10.1161/CIRCULATIONAHA.111.079368. 126/1/118 [pii].
11. Eggebrecht H, Schafer U, Treede H, Boekstegers P, Babin-Ebell J, Ferrari M, et al. Valve-in-valve transcatheter aortic valve implantation for degenerated bioprosthetic heart valves. JACC Cardiovasc Interv. 2011;4(11):1218–27. doi:10.1016/j.jcin.2011.07.015. S1936-8798(11)00690-X [pii].
12. Piazza N, Bleiziffer S, Brockmann G, Hendrick R, Deutsch MA, Opitz A, et al. Transcatheter aortic valve implantation for failing surgical aortic bioprosthetic valve: from concept to clinical application and evaluation (part 1). JACC Cardiovasc Interv. 2011;4(7):721–32. doi:10.1016/j.jcin.2011.03.016. S1936-8798(11)00392-X [pii].
13. Gurvitch R, Cheung A, Bedogni F, Webb JG. Coronary obstruction following transcatheter aortic valve-in-valve implantation for failed surgical bioprostheses. Catheter Cardiovasc Interv. 2011;77(3):439–44. doi:10.1002/ccd.22861.
14. Yeow WL, Roberts-Thomson P, Shetty S, Yong G. Expanding role for transcatheter aortic valve replacement: successful transfemoral implantation of a Medtronic CoreValve for severe aortic regurgitation. Heart Lung Circ. 2012. doi:10.1016/j.hlc.2012.03.010. S1443-9506(12)00095-9 [pii].
15. Moat NE, Ludman P, de Belder MA, Bridgewater B, Cunningham AD, Young CP, et al. Long-term outcomes after transcatheter aortic valve implantation in high-risk patients with severe aortic stenosis: the U.K. TAVI (United Kingdom Transcatheter Aortic Valve Implantation) Registry. J Am Coll Cardiol. 2011;58(20):2130–8. doi:10.1016/j.jacc.2011.08.050. S0735-1097(11)03339-0 [pii].
16. Kodali SK, Williams MR, Smith CR, Svensson LG, Webb JG, Makkar RR, et al. Two-year outcomes after transcatheter or surgical aortic-valve replacement. N Engl J Med. 2012;366(18):1686–95. doi:10.1056/NEJMoa1200384.
17. Tamburino C, Capodanno D, Ramondo A, Petronio AS, Ettori F, Santoro G, et al. Incidence and predictors of early and late mortality after transcatheter aortic valve implantation in 663 patients with severe aortic stenosis. Circulation. 2011;123(3):299–308. doi:10.1161/CIRCULATIONAHA.110.946533. CIRCULATIONAHA.110.946533 [pii].
18. Sinning JM, Hammerstingl C, Vasa-Nicotera M, Adenauer V, Lema Cachiguango SJ, Scheer AC, et al. Aortic regurgitation index defines severity of peri-prosthetic regurgitation and predicts outcome in patients after transcatheter aortic valve implantation. J Am Coll Cardiol. 2012;59(13):1134–41. doi:10.1016/j.jacc.2011.11.048. S0735-1097(12)00192-1 [pii].
19. Jilaihawi H, Kashif M, Fontana G, Furugen A, Shiota T, Friede G, et al. Cross-sectional computed tomographic assessment improves accuracy of aortic annular sizing for transcatheter aortic valve replacement and reduces the incidence of paravalvular aortic regurgitation. J Am Coll Cardiol. 2012;59(14):1275–86. doi:10.1016/j.jacc.2011.11.045. S0735-1097(12)00077-0 [pii].
20. Willson AB, Webb JG, Labounty TM, Achenbach S, Moss R, Wheeler M, et al. 3-dimensional aortic annular assessment by multidetector computed tomography predicts moderate or severe paravalvular regurgitation after transcatheter aortic valve replacement: a multicenter retrospective analysis. J Am Coll Cardiol. 2012;59(14):1287–94.
21. Walther T, Schuler G, Borger MA, Kempfert J, Seeburger J, Ruckert Y, et al. Transapical aortic valve implantation in 100 consecutive patients: comparison to propensity-matched conventional aortic valve replacement. Eur Heart J. 2010;31(11):1398–403. doi:10.1093/eurheartj/ehq060. ehq060 [pii].
22. Gilard M, Eltchaninoff H, Iung B, Donzeau-Gouge P, Chevreul K, Fajadet J, et al. Registry of transcatheter aortic-valve implantation in high-risk patients. N Engl J Med. 2012;366(18):1705–15. doi:10.1056/NEJMoa1114705.

23. Rodes-Cabau J, Dumont E, Boone RH, Larose E, Bagur R, Gurvitch R, et al. Cerebral embolism following transcatheter aortic valve implantation: comparison of transfemoral and transapical approaches. J Am Coll Cardiol. 2011;57(1):18–28. doi:10.1016/j.jacc.2010.07.036. S0735-1097(10)04224-5 [pii].
24. Erdoes G, Basciani R, Huber C, Stortecky S, Wenaweser P, Windecker S, et al. Transcranial Doppler-detected cerebral embolic load during transcatheter aortic valve implantation. Eur J Cardiothorac Surg. 2012;41(4):778–83. doi:10.1093/ejcts/ezr068. ezr068 [pii]; discussion 83–4.
25. Nietlispach F, Wijesinghe N, Gurvitch R, Tay E, Carpenter JP, Burns C, et al. An embolic deflection device for aortic valve interventions. JACC Cardiovasc Interv. 2010;3(11):1133–8. doi:10.1016/j.jcin.2010.05.022. S1936-8798(10)00643-6 [pii].
26. TCT. Embolic Protection Devices for TAVR Show Promise. 2011. http://www.tctmd.com/show.aspx?id=110221.
27. Lange R, Bleiziffer S, Mazzitelli D, Elhmidi Y, Opitz A, Krane M, et al. Improvements in transcatheter aortic valve implantation outcomes in lower surgical risk patients: a glimpse into the future. J Am Coll Cardiol. 2012;59(3):280–7. doi:10.1016/j.jacc.2011.10.868. S0735-1097(11)04829-7 [pii].
28. Mussardo M, Latib A, Chieffo A, Godino C, Ielasi A, Cioni M, et al. Periprocedural and short-term outcomes of transfemoral transcatheter aortic valve implantation with the Sapien XT as compared with the Edwards Sapien valve. JACC Cardiovasc Interv. 2011;4(7):743–50. doi:10.1016/j.jcin.2011.05.004. S1936-8798(11)00370-0 [pii].
29. Toggweiler S, Gurvitch R, Leipsic J, Wood DA, Willson AB, Binder RK, et al. Percutaneous aortic valve replacement: vascular outcomes with a fully percutaneous procedure. J Am Coll Cardiol. 2012;59(2):113–8. doi:10.1016/j.jacc.2011.08.069. S0735-1097(11)04616-X [pii].
30. Lichtenstein SV, Cheung A, Ye J, Thompson CR, Carere RG, Pasupati S, et al. Transapical transcatheter aortic valve implantation in humans: initial clinical experience. Circulation. 2006;114(6):591–6. doi:10.1161/CIRCULATIONAHA.106.632927. CIRCULATIONAHA.106.632927 [pii].
31. Bapat V, Khawaja MZ, Attia R, Narayana A, Wilson K, Macgillivray K, et al. Transaortic Transcatheter Aortic valve implantation using Edwards Sapien valve: a novel approach. Catheter Cardiovasc Interv. 2012;79(5):733–40. doi:10.1002/ccd.23276.
32. Petronio AS, De Carlo M, Bedogni F, Maisano F, Ettori F, Klugmann S, et al. 2-year results of CoreValve implantation through the subclavian access: a propensity-matched comparison with the femoral access. J Am Coll Cardiol. 2012. doi:10.1016/j.jacc.2012.04.014. S0735-1097(12)01498-2 [pii].
33. Genereux P, Head SJ, Van Mieghem NM, Kodali S, Kirtane AJ, Xu K, et al. Clinical outcomes after transcatheter aortic valve replacement using valve academic research consortium definitions: a weighted meta-analysis of 3,519 patients from 16 studies. J Am Coll Cardiol. 2012;59(25):2317–26. doi:10.1016/j.jacc.2012.02.022. S0735-1097(12)00927-8 [pii].
34. Jilaihawi H, Chakravarty T, Weiss RE, Fontana GP, Forrester J, Makkar RR. Meta-analysis of complications in aortic valve replacement: comparison of Medtronic-Corevalve, Edwards-Sapien and surgical aortic valve replacement in 8,536 patients. Catheter Cardiovasc Interv. 2012;80(1):128–38. doi:10.1002/ccd.23368.
35. Chorianopoulos E, Krumsdorf U, Pleger ST, Katus HA, Bekeredjian R. Improved procedural results after CoreValve implantation with the new AccuTrak delivery system. J Interv Cardiol. 2012;25(2):174–9. doi:10.1111/j.1540-8183.2011.00695.x.
36. Buellesfeld L, Gerckens U, Grube E. Percutaneous implantation of the first repositionable aortic valve prosthesis in a patient with severe aortic stenosis. Catheter Cardiovasc Interv. 2008;71(5):579–84. doi:10.1002/ccd.21470.
37. Treede H, Tubler T, Reichenspurner H, Grube E, Pascotto A, Franzen O, et al. Six-month results of a repositionable and retrievable pericardial valve for transcatheter aortic valve replacement: the Direct Flow Medical aortic valve. J Thorac Cardiovasc Surg. 2010;140(4):897–903. doi:10.1016/j.jtcvs.2010.01.017. S0022-5223(10)00050-4 [pii].
38. Willson AB, Rodes-Cabau J, Wood DA, Leipsic J, Cheung A, Toggweiler S, et al. Transcatheter aortic valve replacement with the St. Jude Medical Portico Valve: first-in-human experience. J Am Coll Cardiol.2012.doi:10.1016/j.jacc.2012.02.045.S0735-1097(12)01253-3 [pii].
39. Walther T, Mollmann H, van Linden A, Kempfert J. Transcatheter aortic valve implantation transapical: step by step. Semin Thorac Cardiovasc Surg. 2011;23(1):55–61. doi:10.1053/j.semtcvs.2011.05.006. S1043-0679(11)00064-5 [pii].
40. Onsea K, et al. First-in-man experience with a new embolic deflection device in transcatheter aortic valve interventions. EuroIntervention. 2012;8(1):51–6.
41. Naber CK, et al. First-in-man use of a novel embolic protection device for patients undergoing transcatheter aortic valve implantation. EuroIntervention. 2012;8(1):43–50.
42. Grube E, et al. Percutaneous aortic valve replacement for severe aortic stenosis in high-risk patients using the second- and current third-generation self-expanding CoreValve prosthesis: device success and 30-day clinical outcome. J Am Coll Cardiol. 2007;50(1):69 76.
43. Willson AB, et al. Transcatheter aortic valve replacement with the St. Jude Medical Portico valve: first-in-human experience. J Am Coll Cardiol. 2012;60(7):581–6.
44. Schofer J, et al. Retrograde transarterial implantation of a nonmetallic aortic valve prosthesis in high-surgical-risk patients with severe aortic stenosis: a first-in-man feasibility and safety study. Circ Cardiovasc Interv. 2008;1(2):126–33.
45. Treede H, et al. Transapical transcatheter aortic valve implantation using the JenaValve™ system: acute and 30-day results of the multicentre CE-mark study. Eur J Cardiothorac Surg. 2012;41(6):e131–8.
46. Kempfert J, et al. Trans-apical aortic valve implantation using a new self-expandable bioprosthesis: initial outcomes. Eur J Cardiothorac Surg. 2011;40(5):1114–9.
47. Falk V, et al. Transapical aortic valve implantation with a self-expanding anatomically oriented valve. Eur Heart J. 2011;32(7):878–87.

Structural Design of Transcatheter Aortic Valves: General Concepts Related to Imaging

8

Jeffrey J. Popma, Alexandra Almonacid, Diana Litmanovich, and George Gellert

Abstract

Transcatheter aortic valve replacement (TAVR) is an alternative approach in patients deemed "high risk" or "inoperable" for surgical aortic valve replacement (sAVR) [1–4]. A number of novel transcatheter heart valves (THVs) have been developed over the past decade, each with unique features that may provide potential advantages in patients undergoing TAVR. Unlike surgical valves, wherein the native aortic valve is resected, directly visualized, and a surgical valve is sewn into the aortic annulus, aortic THVs must expand and both conform to the native aortic annulus and interact with critical structures in the aortic valvar complex, including the thickened and rigid native valve leaflets and left ventricular outflow tract and membranous septum.

Keywords

Aortic stenosis • Structural design • Positioning • Novel valve designs

Introduction

Transcatheter aortic valve replacement (TAVR) is an alternative approach in patients deemed "high risk" or "inoperable" for surgical aortic valve replacement (sAVR) [1–4]. A number of novel transcatheter heart valves (THVs) have been developed over the past decade, each with unique features that may provide potential advantages in patients undergoing TAVR. Unlike surgical valves, wherein the native aortic valve is resected, directly visualized, and a surgical valve is sewn into the aortic annulus, aortic THVs must expand and both conform to the native aortic annulus and interact with critical structures in the aortic valvar complex, including the thickened and rigid native valve leaflets and left ventricular outflow tract and membranous septum.

Careful planning for TAVR is needed using an integrated assessment of noninvasive and invasive imaging studies, including coronary angiography, contrast aortography, two- (2D) and three-dimensional (3D) transthoracic (TTE) and transesophageal echocardiography (TEE), multidetector CT angiography (MDCT), and cardiac magnetic resonance imaging (CMR). Each of these imaging techniques provides complementary information related to optimal valve sizing and aortic THV selection. In contrast to echocardiography and CMR, MDCT is associated with substantial radiation

J.J. Popma, MD (✉) • A. Almonacid, MD • G. Gellert, MD
Interventional Cardiology Clinical Services, Beth Israel Deaconess Medical Center, 185 Pilgrim Road, Boston, MA 02215, USA

Departments of Internal Medicine (Cardiovascular Division) and Radiology, Beth Israel Deaconess Medical Center, Boston, MA, USA

Department of Anesthesia, Banner Good Samaritan Medical Center, Phoenix, AZ, USA
e-mail: jpopma@bidmc.harvard.edu

D. Litmanovich, MD
Department of Radiology, Beth Israel Deaconess Medical Center, Boston, MA, USA

Departments of Internal Medicine (Cardiovascular Division) and Radiology, Beth Israel Deaconess Medical Center, Boston, MA, USA

Department of Anesthesia, Banner Good Samaritan Medical Center, Phoenix, AZ, USA

Relationship with Industry: Jeffrey J. Popma: Research Grants: Medtronic Vascular, Boston Scientific, Abbott Vascular, Cordis Corporation, Medrad, Covidien. Advisory Boards: Boston Scientific, Abbott Vascular.

J.K. Min et al. (eds.), *Multimodality Imaging for Transcatheter Aortic Valve Replacement*, DOI 10.1007/978-1-4471-2798-7_8, © Springer-Verlag London 2014

Table 8.1 Ionizing radiation in cardiac imaging

	Representative effective dose valve (mSv)	Representative effective dose valve (mSv)
Chest X-ray PA and lateral	0.1	0.05–0.24
Diagnostic invasive coronary angiography	7	2–16
Coronary CT angiography		
64-slice MDCT, retrospective gating	12	9–19
64-slice MDCT, reduced tube voltage	6	3–8
64-slice MDCT, prospective triggering	3	2–4
264 or 320 MD row CT	4	2–8

Adapted from [5]

MDCT multidetector CT

doses [5] (Table 8.1). Moreover, another concern for MDCT is the administration of 80–100 cc of iodinated contrast, which can cause nephrotoxicity in the elderly population. Yet MDCT has proven invaluable for the precise characterization of the aortic valvar complex in an effort to avoid complications and improve valve sizing.

The purpose of this manuscript is to outline the specific anatomic considerations for TAVR, to describe the aortic valvar complex and its components, and to outline how these anatomic structures are influenced by the aortic THV selected.

Fatigue Testing and Long-Term Durability

Long-term durability is a critical design component for aortic THVs. The Food and Drug Administration (FDA) Draft Guidance for Industry and FDA standards for Heart Valves published in 2010 provides an overview of the preclinical requirements for durability testing of prosthetic heart valves, including aortic THVs [6]. THV regulatory submissions are required to contain a "risk analysis" for the aortic THVs in which the probability and degree of harm associated with a device due to frame or valve malfunction is estimated and an appropriate plan is outlined to mitigate these risks [6]. Required testing includes material property testing (e.g., stainless steel, cobalt chromium, nitinol), biologic safety, hemodynamic and structural performance, device durability, component fatigue testing, and device-specific testing [6].

A required component to the aortic THV and THV component durability testing is accelerated wear testing (AWT), described in ISO 5840:2005 documents [6]. AWT is performed for 600 million cycles in rigid valves and their components and 200 million cycles in flexible valves [6]. Pulsatile flow and physiologic loading conditions are tested using a variety of physiologic parameters, including radial, linear, and axial compression, bending, torsion, shear stress and fluid drag, among other physiologic stresses (Fig. 8.1, Box 8.1). Aortic THV and the load-bearing, nonbiological components of flexible replacement heart valves (e.g., stent wire) are individually fatigue tested to 600 million cycles [6]. Animal studies are also recommended to assure long-term biologic stability and human post-mortem studies may be useful to understand the tissue interactions of THVs once implanted [6].

The development of preclinical test conditions for aortic THVs is based on the estimation of the "anticipated clinical environment" (i.e., physiologic conditions) of the deformed and calcified aortic annulus in elderly patients. A description of these conditions is more challenging when the native aortic valve is not removed and remained in place [6]. MDCT reconstructions in patients treated aortic THVs have been useful in determining these boundary limits [7], but these studies are limited by their resolution to identify more subtle changes in aortoventricular compliance. A more precise characterization of aortic THVs in their physiology state may be provided by 3D TEE. Creation of an imaging database that included MDCT and TEE to determine boundary limits for the testing of aortic THVs is needed.

General Properties of Aortic Transcatheter Heart Valves (THV)

Aortic THVs have been designed to displace the native aortic valve and replace it with a bioprosthetic valve that expands and conforms to the native aortic valvar complex. This is typically performed using either a balloon-expandable or self-expanding frame or polymeric sleeve. Aortic THVs vary by the access site, sheath size, composition of the supportive frame and valve leaflets, length of the frame and valve leaflets, length and thickness of the skirt used to prevent perivalvular regurgitation (PVR), and retrievability and repositionability. Design components of contemporary aortic transfemoral THVs are found in Table 8.2, and anatomic requirements for these valves are found in Table 8.3. Each valve interacts with the underlying aortic valvar complex in unique ways due to their unique design components.

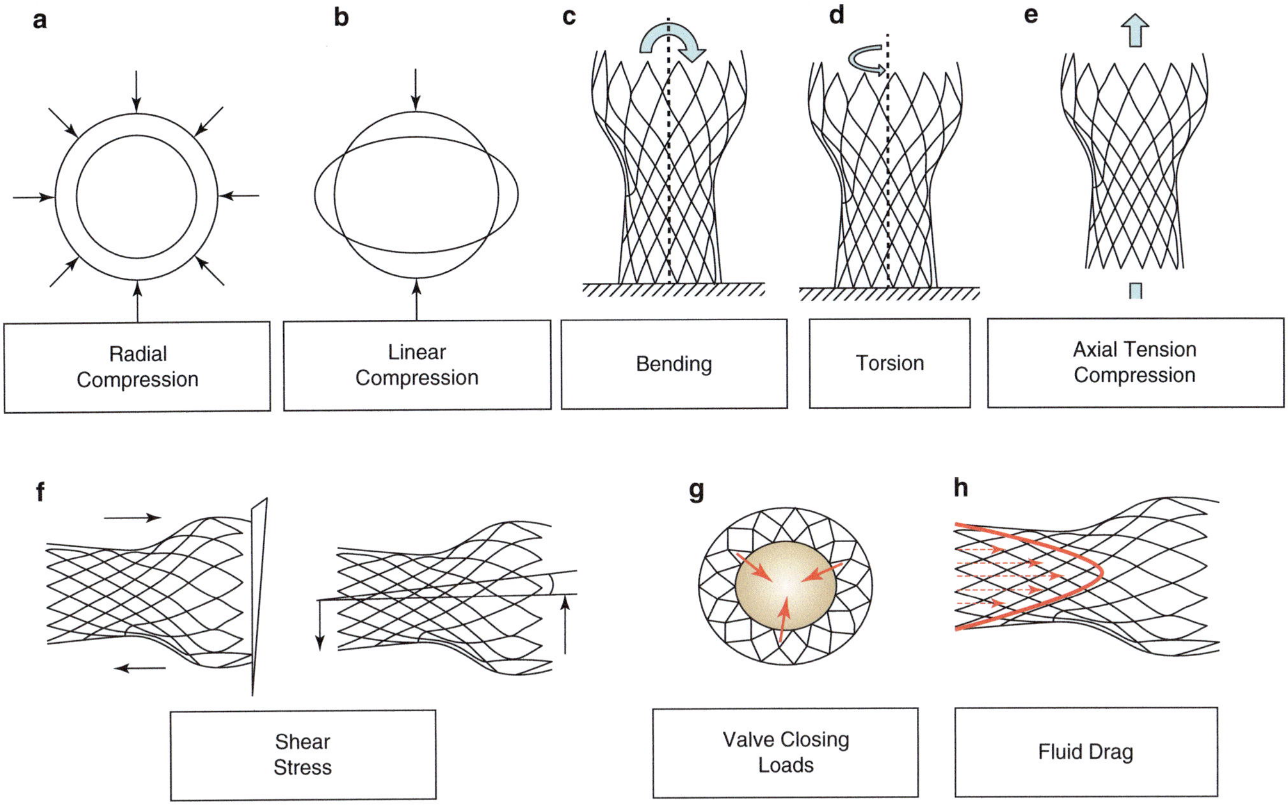

Fig. 8.1 Physical stress properties with THV. *Radial compression* (**a**) describes loading applied in a net uniform circumferential detection perpendicular to the centroidal axis of the frame resulting in a reduction of the cross-sectional diameter. *Linear compression* (**b**) applies to loading applied in a nonuniform manner predominantly from the side of the frame perpendicular to the centroidal axis resulting in a "flattened" elliptical cross-sectional profile. *Bending* (**c**) characterizes the behavior of the frame when loading is applied in a nonuniform manner resulting in a flexure (bending) of the frame that the centroidal axis post-loading is arced versus linear. *Torsion* (**d**) characterized the behavior of the frame when torque loading is applied perpendicular to the centroidal axis resulting in an angulated shear deformation of the frame that the centroidal axis is "twisted" versus linear. *Axial compression* (**e**) describes loading in a net uniform manner across the ends of the frame parallel with the centroidal axis resulting in shortening in the length of the frame. *Shear stress* (**f**) applies to directional loading in a non-normal manner predominantly from one side of the frame either parallel or tangential to the centroidal axis resulting in a canted structure about an unchanged linear centroidal axis. *Valve closing loads* (**g**) characterizes the behavior of the frame when blood pressure loading is applied across the closed valve during diastole resulting in local deformations of the frame in vicinity of the commissural attachment points. *Fluid drag* (**h**) is defined as the loading applied in a net axial direction imposed by wall shear stresses resulting from flow interactions with the inner surface of the valve (Courtesy of Medtronic, Inc)

Edwards SAPIEN Balloon-Expandable THV

The SAPIEN Valve (Edwards Lifesciences, Irvine, CA) is a trileaflet bioprosthesis made of bovine pericardium mounted on a balloon-expandable stainless steel stent. The distal half of the stent contains a fabric cuff that limits stent expansion and decreases perivalvular insufficiency. The valve is currently available as a 23 mm valve whose frame height is 14.5 mm and a 26 mm valve whose frame height is 16 mm (Fig. 8.2a). The newer generation SAPIEN XT has modified scallop-shaped leaflets that provide superior hemodynamic properties and coaptation that are mounted on a cobalt-chromium alloy stent with thinner struts, giving it a lower profile. Both valves are available in 23 and 26 mm sizes. In contrast to the RetroFlex 3 transcatheter delivery system that requires introduction of a 22 or 24 Fr sheath, respectively, the NovaFlex delivery system has reduced the sheath size to 18 Fr for the 23 mm XT valve and 19 Fr for the 26 mm valve.

Box 8.1 Physiologic Forces on TAVR Valves (see Fig. 8.1)
- Radial
- Linear
- Axial compression
- Bending, torsion
- Valve closing loads
- Fluid drag

Table 8.2 General design characterization of aortic transfemoral transcatheter heart valves

	Manufacturer	OD sheath (Fr)	Frame	Deployment	Sizes	Valve material	Skirt material	Retrievable
SAPIEN								
Ascendra	Edwards	22 24	Stainless Steel	Balloon expandable	23, 26	Bovine pericardium	Bovine pericardium	No
XT	Edwards	18	Cobalt Chromium	Balloon expandable	23, 26	Bovine pericardium	Bovine pericardium	No
CoreValve	Medtronic	18	Nitinol	Self-expanding	23, 26, 29, 31	Porcine pericardium	Porcine pericardium	Partially
Portico	St. Jude	18	Nitinol	Self-expanding	23 mm	Bovine pericardium	Porcine pericardium	Complete
Sadra Lotus	Boston Scientific	18	Nitinol	Self-expanding	23 mm, 27 mm	Bovine pericardium	Bovine pericardium	Complete
Direct Flow	Direct Flow Medical	18/22		Saline injection	23 mm	Bovine pericardium	Polymer Nylon sleeve	Partially

Fr French, *OD* outer diameter

Table 8.3 Aortic valvar requirements for aortic transfemoral transcatheter valves

	Aortic annulus								
	Diameter (mm)	Area (mm^2)	Perimeter (mm)	Annular eccentricity[a]	SOV width (mm)	Coronary height (mm)	SOV height (mm)	Tubular aorta (mm)	AV angle (°)
SAPIEN Ascendra									
23 mm	18–23	254.5–415.2	56.5–72.3	–	–	–	–	–	Any
26 mm	23–25	415.2–490.9	72.3–78.5	–	–	–	–	–	Any
CoreValve									
23 mm	18–20	254.5–314.2	56.5–62.8	–	≥25	–	≥15	≤34	<70
26 mm	20–23	314.2–415.2	62.8–72.3	–	≥27	–	≥15	≤40	< 70
29 mm	23–27	415.5–572.6	72.3–84.8	–	≥29	–	≥15	≤43	<70
31 mm	26–29	530.9–660.5	81.6–91.1	–	≥29	–	≥15	≤43	<70
Sadra Lotus									
23 mm	18–23	254.5–415.2	56.5–72.3	–	–	>14 (>11)	–	–	Any
27 mm	23–27	415.2–572.6	72.3–84.8	–	–	>14 (>11)	–	–	Any
Portico									
23 mm	19–21	283.4–346.2	59.7–65.9	≥0.7	≥27	NA	≥15 mm	≤36 (≤38)	<30 (<45)
Direct Flow									
23 mm	19–23	283.4–415.2	59.7–72.3	–	–	–	–	–	Any

AV atrioventricular angle, *SOV* sinus of Valsalva

[a]Parenthesis notes that criteria are borderline but potentially acceptable. Annular eccentricity is defined as a minor/major axis ratio

CoreValve Revalving System

The CoreValve Revalving System (Medtronic, Inc., Maple Grove, MN) is comprised of three components that include a self-expanding nitinol support frame with cells configured in a diamond cell design that anchors a trileaflet porcine pericardial tissue valve, an 18 Fr delivery catheter, and a disposable loading system. CoreValve frames are currently available in 23, 26, 29, and 31 mm sizes for an aortic diameter range of 18–20, 20–23, 24–27, and 26–29 mm, respectively (Fig. 8.2b). The nitinol frame that is approximately 50 mm in length was specifically designed for optimal functionality, stability, and durability (Fig. 8.2b) and has three levels of radial and hoop strength. The frame inflow exerts high radial expansive force to secure the frame within the aortic annular location. The strength of this portion of the frame prevents annular recoil allows the frame to partially conform to the noncircular shape of the aortic annulus. In addition, it prevents frame migration and minimizes the occurrence of perivalvular leaks. The "constrained" center portion of the frame has high hoop strength that resists size and shape deformation, which is critical as this portion of the frame contains the "supra-annular" valve leaflets. The frame is concave at this location to avoid the coronary ostium with the native valve and allows coronary cannulation after the implantation. The outflow portion of the frame exerts low radial forces and serves to orient the frame to the aorta parallel to flow through the valve. The porcine pericardium was selected due to its lower profile (compared with bovine pericardium) and durability, and the three leaflet elements are constructed with long commissures to enhance durability.

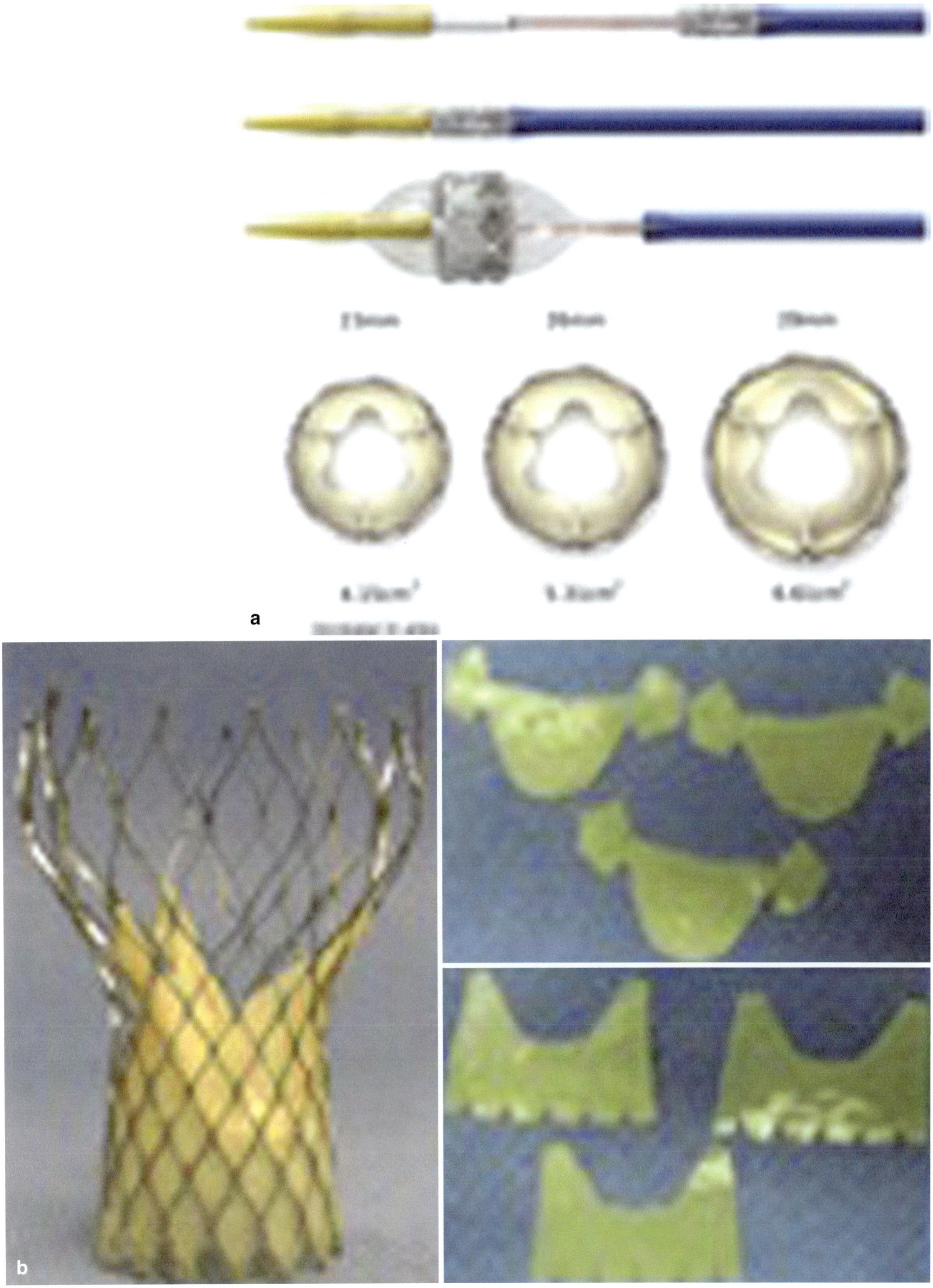

Fig. 8.2 Aortic transcatheter heart valves. Edwards SAPIEN (**a**), Medtronic CoreValve (*left panel*) and six porcine pericardial components (*right panel*) (**b**), SADRA Lotus (**c**), St. Jude Portico (**d**), Direct Flow Medical (**e**), Symetis ACURATE (**f**), Medtronic Engager (**g**), Heart Leaflet Technology (**h**), and JenaValve (**i**)

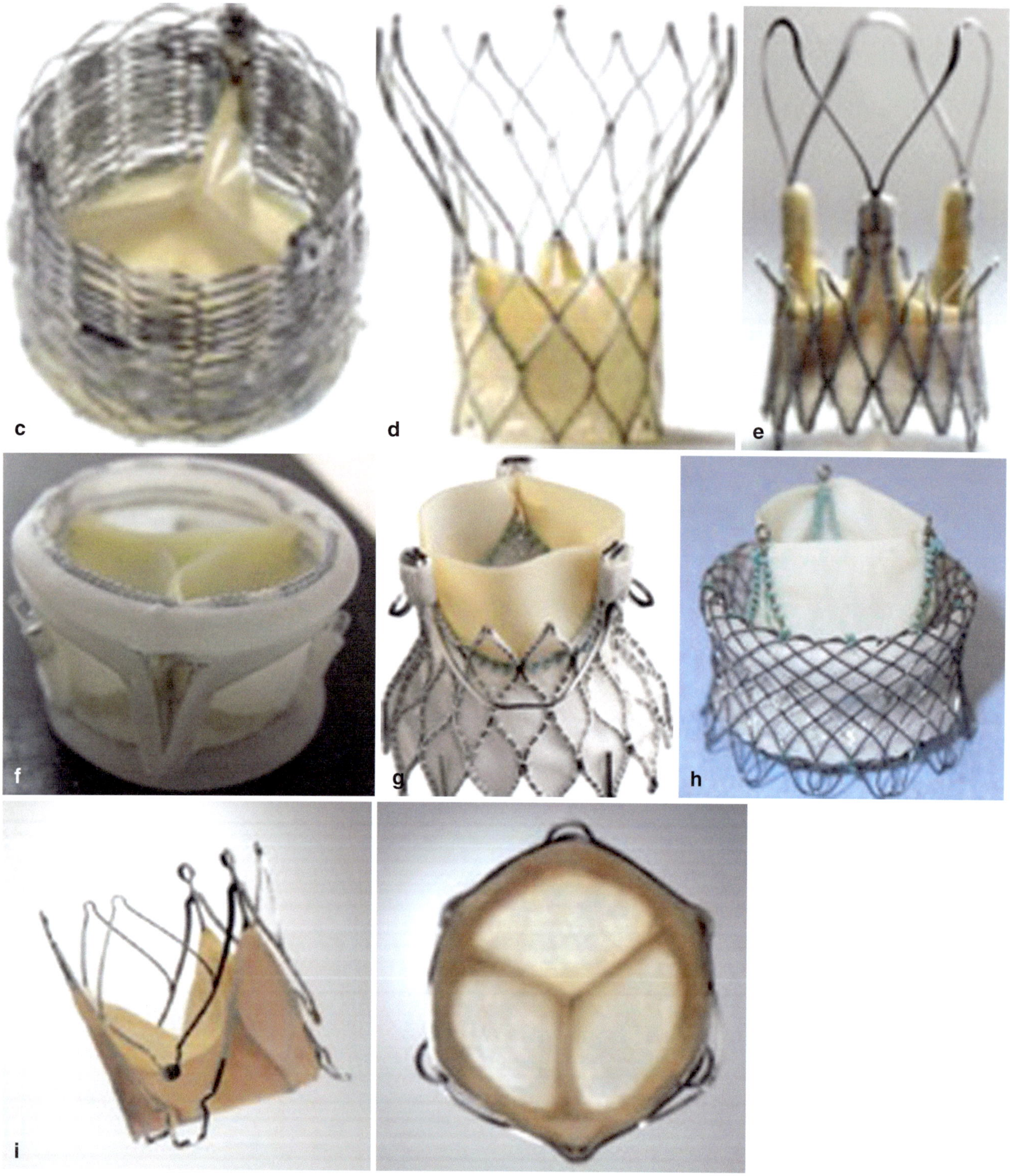

Fig. 8.2 (continued)

Portico Self-ExpandingTHV

The Portico THV (St. Jude Medical, St. Paul, MN) consists of a delivery catheter that contains a soft tapered nose cone located on an 18 Fr capsule that contains a trileaflet bovine pericardial valve that is attached to the frame using three retention tabs [8] (Fig. 8.2c). A porcine pericardial sealing cuff is used to minimize perivalvular leak. The Portico valve is sized according to the nominal external stent diameter at the valvular level and is available in a 23 mm size [8]. A desirable feature is the potential to be deployed to the point of functionality while allowing for controlled recapture, followed either by repositioning and redeployment or by removal [8].

Sadra LOTUS Self-Expanding

The Lotus Valve System (Sadra Medical, Inc., Los Gatos, California) is a trileaflet bovine pericardial valve that is attached to a self-expanding nitinol mesh by three supporting posts (Fig. 8.2d). There is an adaptive seal at the lower end of the frame that is designed to conform to the aortic annulus and prevent perivalvular leak. The Lotus valve is available in 23 and 27 mm sizes and is delivered via an 18 Fr Sheath. If the THV does not conform appropriately to the annulus due to undersizing or incomplete expansion, it can be recaptured and retrieved prior to final release. The radial expansive force of the valve renders the aortic annular more circular than ellipsoid after deployment.

Direct Flow Medical

The Direct Flow Medical THV (Direct Flow Medical, Inc., Santa Rosa, California) is designed as a trileaflet bovine pericardial tissue valve that is attached to an inflatable framework with a slightly tapered, conformable polyester fabric cuff [9] (Fig. 8.2e). The device system is comprised of a bovine, trileaflet pericardial tissue valve, a sheathed delivery and recovery system, and a Dacron fabric cuff that is inflated with saline-contrast to conform to the native annulus. Ventricular and aortic cuff rings are independently inflatable. After the saline-contrast cuff inflation ensures the position and sealing of the device with fluoroscopy, the saline-contrast mixture is exchanged for an inflation medium that solidifies and hardens to form a permanent support structure [10].

Symetis ACURATE TA

The Symetis ACURATE TA (Symetis, Ecublens Switzerland) is composed of a surgical-quality porcine tissue valve mounted on a self-expandable nitinol stent that is partially covered by a polyethylene terephthalate (PET) skirt (Fig. 8.2f) [11]. The delivery system has a flexible isodiametric shaft and ergonomic design allowing for a controlled, sheathless, atraumatic, and two-step implantation [11]. It is available primarily as a transapical device, but retrograde designs are currently under consideration.

Engager Valve

The Engager™ Aortic Valve bioprosthesis (Medtronic, Inc., Minneapolis, MN, USA) is a biological heart valve prosthesis composed of three leaflets, cut from tissue fixated bovine pericardium, sewn to a polyester sleeve, and mounted on a compressible and self-expanding nitinol frame (Fig. 8.2g) [12]. The stent assembly consists of a shaped main frame and a support frame, which are coupled together so as to form the commissural posts of the valve [12]. The bioprosthesis is available in 23 and 26 mm size with an inflated frame length of 25.5 and 27.5 mm, respectively [12]. These two sizes are designed to fit an effective aortic annulus MDCT between 21 and 26.5 mm, corresponding to a TTE annulus diameter between 19 and 26 mm [12].

JenaValve

The JenaValve™ AVR system (Jena Technologies, Munich, Germany) is designed as a trileaflet porcine root tissue valve. It is attached to a low-profile nitinol stent with flexible stent posts supporting the valve leaflets and positioning feelers for accurate placement of the prosthesis with regard to the native valve leaflets [13] (Fig. 8.2h). The valve prosthesis is available in 23, 25, and 27 mm sizes for implantation in native aortic annuli ranging from 21 to 27 mm in diameter. The transapical device is available using a sheathless 32 Fr delivery catheter [13].

Heart Leaflet Technologies

The Heart Leaflet Technologies (HLT) valve (Heart Leaflet Technologies, Inc., Maple Grove, Minnesota) is comprised of a trileaflet porcine pericardial tissue valve, a superelastic nitinol wire form that supports the valve structure, a superelastic nitinol mesh, and a braided polyester liner integrated within the support structure to prevent regurgitant flow around the valve (Fig. 8.2i).

Noninvasive Assessment of the Aortic Valvar Complex

Noninvasive characterization of the aortic valvar complex includes the aortic annulus, sinus of Valsalva (SOV), coronary arteries, tubular aorta, left ventricular outflow tract, and the aortomitral continuity which are all considered for aortic THV selection (Table 8.3). The central component of the complex is the aortic valve that is typically comprised of three semilunar leaflets that are anchored in the basal annular plane and extend to the tubular aorta (Fig. 8.3).

Aortic Annulus

Proper sizing of the aortic annulus has become a central component of TAVR. The aortic annulus generally has an elliptical shape with anchor points at the nadir of each of three aortic leaflets. The caudal valvar insertion points extend into the left ventricular outflow tract forming a virtual ring that is referred to as the basal annular ring. The true anatomic ventricular arterial juncture is located approximately 3 mm superior to basal annular ring [14–16]. While earlier clinical studies used 2D

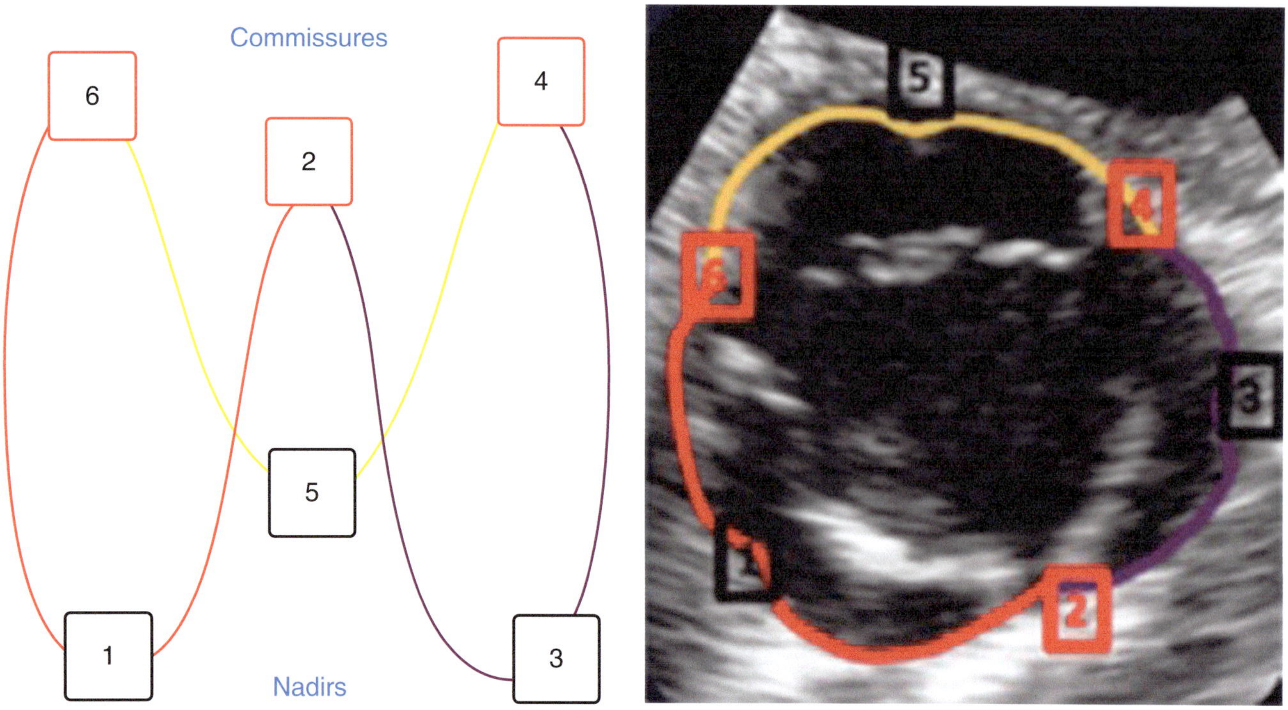

Fig. 8.3 The aortovalvular backbone. Annulus orientation as seen on two-dimensional aortic short axis view. *Red* – right coronary cusp annulus, *purple* – left coronary cusp annulus, *yellow* – noncoronary cusp annulus, 1 – 3 – 5 Nadirs, 2 – 4 – 6 commissures

TTE or TEE for annular sizing, more recent studies have demonstrated the value of MDCT for the precise determination of annular dimensions [17–19]. The most important principle of MDCT analysis is the alignment of the basal annular plane of the three sinuses. Maximal diameters, perpendicular diameters, average diameters, area, and perimeters have all been used to determine the appropriate annular diameter (Fig. 8.4).

A number of series have compared TTE, TEE, MDCT, and contrast angiography for the assessment of aortic annular dimensions [14–16, 20–25] (Table 8.3). In general, MDCT provides larger annular measurements than echocardiography. In a series of 45 consecutive patients with severe aortic stenosis referred for TAVR, correlations between TTE, TEE, and MDCT were good but the difference between MDCT and TTE (1.22 ± 1.3 mm) or TEE (1.52 ± 1.1 mm) was larger than the difference between TTE and TEE (0.6 ± 0.8 mm); $p=0.03$ and $p<0.0001$, respectively [23]. A decision based on MDCT measurements would have modified the TAVR strategy in a large number of patients (40–42 %) [23]. Cardiac MR (CMR) has also been used to estimate the annular dimensions [20]. In a series of 202 consecutive patients assessed by CMR, MDCT, and TTE for TAVR, close agreement was observed between CMR and MDCT in the dimensions of the aortic annulus and similarly for sinus of Valsalva, sinotubular junction, and ascending aortic measures [20]. Agreement between TTE-derived measures and either CMR or MDCT was less precise [20]. Intraobserver and interobserver variabilities were lowest with CMR [20].

The benefit of THV sizing based on MDCT and CMR (compared with TEE or TTE) has been shown in several studies [20]. In a series of 109 patients who underwent MDCT prior to balloon-expandable SAPIEN stent placement, appropriate sizing of the aortic annulus using mean diameters, area, and circumference correlated with the development of perivalvular regurgitation [26]. MDCT was repeated after TAVR to assess THV eccentricity (1 – (short diameter/long diameter)) and expansion (MDCT measured THV area/nominal THV area). Moderate or severe paravalvular aortic regurgitation was associated with TAVR undersizing [26]. The difference between THV size and MDCT annular size was predictive of PAR. The area under the curve (AUC) was 0.81 for the mean diameter, 0.80 for area, and 0.76 for circumference [26]. Annular eccentricity was not associated with PAR [26]. In this series, 35.3 and 45.1 % of aortic THVs were undersized relative to the MDCT mean diameter and area, respectively [26]. In another series, the presence and severity of AR after TAVR were associated with larger aortic valve annulus measurements by both CMR ($p=0.03$) and MDCT ($p=0.04$) but not TTE-derived measures ($p=0.10$) [20]. In patients undergoing imaging assessment for TAVR, the presence and severity of AR after TAVR were associated with larger aortic annulus measurements by both CMR and MDCT (but not TTE) [20].

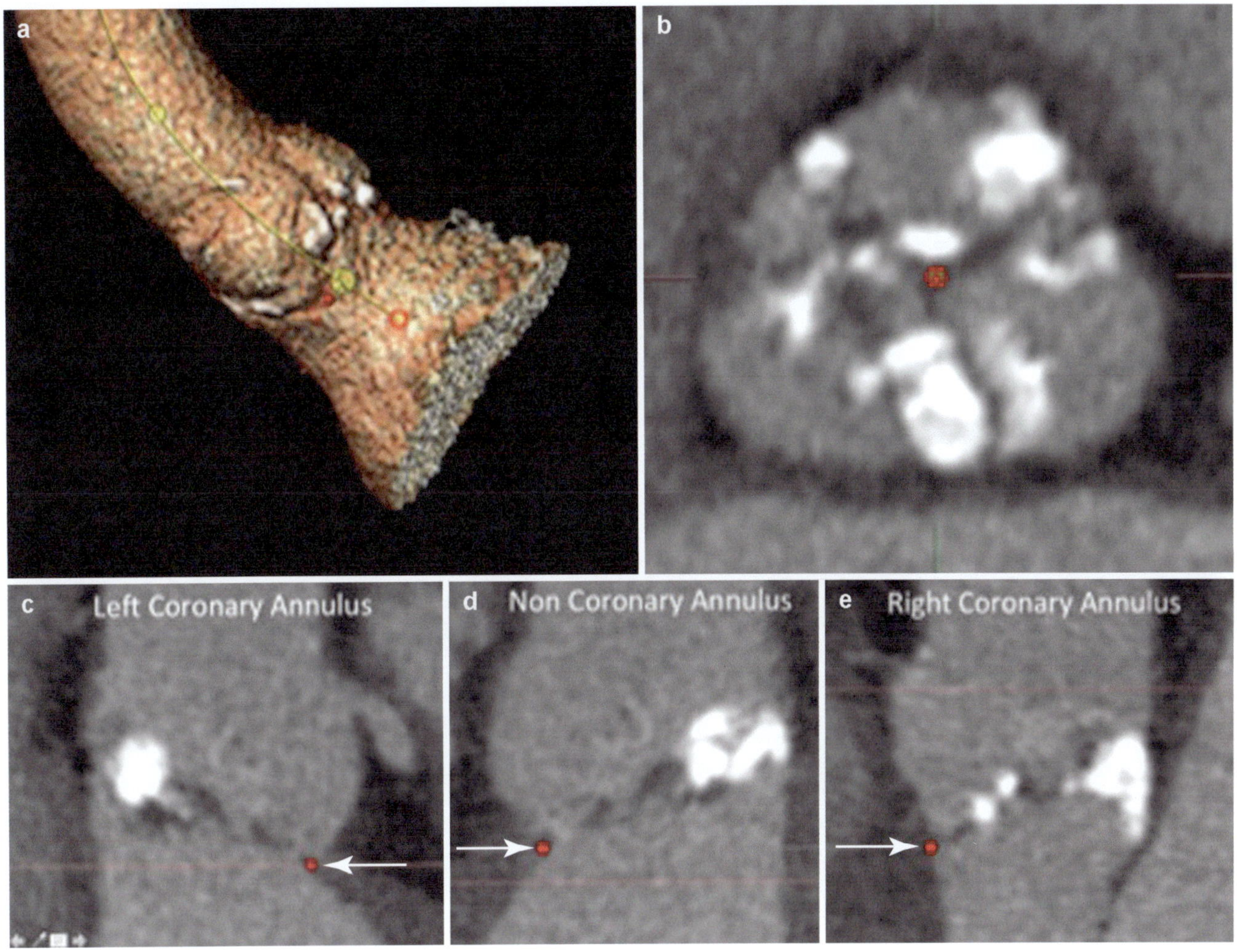

Fig. 8.4 Aortic annulus. Quantitative measure of the aortic annulus begins volume rendering of the aortovalvular complex and the creation of the aortoventricular centerline that will facilitate the creation of the double oblique (MPR) images for identification of the basal annular plane (**a**). The cross-sectional view of the double oblique (MPR) demonstrating the cross section of the sinus of Valsalva (**b**) allows identification of the basal annulus of the left coronary annulus (**c**, *arrow*), noncoronary annulus (**d**, *arrow*), and right coronary basal annulus (**e**, *arrow*). This then allows alignment of the basal annular plane of all three coronary sinuses (**f**). Measurements including the maximal diameter, perpendicular to the maximal diameter, area, and perimeter measurements (**g**)

A number of parameters can be used to estimate the annular diameter (Table 8.4). In a series of 75 patients undergoing MDCT, the minimal and maximal annular diameter differed by 6.5 mm (5.7–7.2), $p<0.001$] indicating an elliptical shape of the annulus in the majority of cases [19]. Estimation of the annular diameter using area and perimeter measurements seemed to be associated with better outcomes in these patients (Table 8.5) [19]. In another series of 136 patients, the discriminatory value of multiple CT annular measures for post-TAVR perivalvular aortic regurgitation was compared with 2D echocardiographic measures [27]. In receiver-operating characteristic models, cross-sectional MDCT parameters had the highest discriminatory value for post-TAVR perivalvular regurgitation [27]. The area under the curve was 0.82 for maximal cross-sectional diameter minus prosthesis size ($p<0.001$) and 0.81 for circumference-derived cross-sectional diameter minus prosthesis size ($p<0.001$) [27]. In contrast, traditional echocardiographic measures were nondiscriminatory in relation to post-TAVR PV aortic regurgitation [27]. In an analysis of 46 patients with MDCT, the aortic annulus plane was reconstructed at 10 % increments over the cardiac cycle [28]. In both subjects with normal and with calcified aortic valves, minimum diameter increased in systole (12.3±7.3 % and 9.8±3.4 %, respectively; $p<0.001$), and ellipticity index decreased (12.7±8.8 % and 10.3±2.7 %, respectively; $p<0.001$) [28]. The cross-sectional area (CSA) increased by 11.2±5.4 % and 6.2±4.8 %, respectively ($p<0.001$) [28]. Perimeter increase was negligible in patients with calcified valves (0.56±0.85 %; $p<0.001$) [28]. Relative percentage differences between maximum and minimum values were significantly smallest for perimeter compared with all other

Table 8.4 Comparative studies of imaging modalities for the aortovalvular complex in patients with aortic stenosis

Author	Number of patients	Modalities	Structures analyzed	Findings
Altiok et al. [14]	49	2D TTE 2D TEE 3D TEE Contrast angiography MDCT	Annulus Distance from annulus to left main	Sagittal diameters determined by angiography, TTE, 2D TEE, 3D TEE, and MDCT were smaller than coronal diameters determined by angiography, 3D TEE, and MDCT Coronal and sagittal diameters determined by 3D TEE were in high agreement with corresponding measurements by MDCT (23.60 ± 1.89 vs 23.46 ± 2.07 mm and 22.19 ± 1.96 vs 22.27 ± 2.01 mm, respectively; mean ± SD) There was a high correlation between MDCT and 3D TEE for the definition of coronal and sagittal aortic annulus diameters ($r = 0.88$, SEE = 0.89 mm and $r = 0.77$, SEE = 1.26 mm, respectively) Correlation of 3D TEE (13.47±1.67 mm) and DSCT (13.64±1.82 mm) in the analysis of the distance between aortic annulus and left main coronary artery ostium was better ($r = 0.54$, SEE = 1.55 mm) than between angiography (14.85 ± 3.84 mm) and MDCT ($r = 0.35$, SEE = 1.77 mm)
Dashkevich et al. [15]	33	2D TEE MDCT Hager Dilator	Annulus	Calculated average diameter by MDCT correlated significantly with intraoperative measurements ($r = 0.923$, $p < 0.001$) and with the size of implanted valve ($r = 0.867$, $p < 0.001$), while correlation of TEE and intraoperative measurements was weak ($r = 0.523$, $p = 0.002$) TEE tends to underestimate the dimensions of aortic annulus
Jabbour et al. [20]	202	3D TEE MDCT CMR	Annulus Sinus of Valsalva Sinotubular junction Ascending aorta diameters	Close agreement was observed between CMR and MDCT in dimensions of the aortic annulus (bias, -0.4 mm; 95 % limits of agreement: -5.7–5.0 mm), and similarly for sinus of Valsalva, sinotubular junction, and ascending aortic measures Agreement between TTE-derived measures and either CMR or MDCT was less precise. Intraobserver and interobserver variability were lowest with CMR The presence and severity of AR after TAVR were associated with larger aortic valve annulus measurements by both CMR ($p = 0.03$) and MDCT ($p = 0.04$) but not TTE-derived measures ($p = 0.10$). Neither MDCT nor CMR measures of annulus eccentricity, however, predicted AR after TAVR ($p = 0.33$ and $p = 0.78$, respectively)
Gurvich et al. [16]	50	2D TEE MDCT	Annulus	Most reproducible measurements were the area-derived diameter and basal ring average diameter (inter-reader intraclass correlation coefficient: 0.87 [95 % confidence interval: 0.81–0.92] and 0.80 [95 % confidence interval: 0.70–0.87], respectively; intrareader >0.90 for all readers) MDCT measurements were generally larger than TEE diameters (mean difference of 1.5 ± 1.6 mm and 1.1 ± 1.7 mm, respectively) When a strategy of valve sizing is undertaken using these MDCT measurements using an echocardiographic sizing scale, a different THV size would be selected in 44 and 40 % of cases, respectively When adjusting the sizing cutoffs to account for the differences in observed diameters, this was reduced to 10–12 % ($p < 0.01$ for both, respectively)
Hutter et al. [21]	187	2D TTE 2D TEE MDCT	Annulus	The mean aortic annuli were 22.6 ± 2.0 mm measured with MDCT, 22.3 ± 2.5 mm with TTE, and 22.9 ± 2.2 mm with TEE. Despite a strong correlation between the measurement techniques, relevant statistical spread occurred with differences up to 3 mm in all measurement methods Inter- and intraobserver variability was good for TEE and less satisfactory for MDCT measurements TEE measurements taken as decisive parameter for the implantation changed the implantation strategy in 15.5 % of patients and did not show an increased rate of procedural complications

Kempfert et al. [22]	26	2D TEE MDCT Intraoperative	Annulus	MDCT end-systolic echocardiographic diameters showed best agreement with intraoperative direct sizing) Mean difference for TEE versus intraoperative = 0.5 mm Mean difference for TTE versus intraoperative = 0.38 mm Mean difference for MDCT versus intraoperative = −0.56 In patients with an oval-shaped annulus, MDCT demonstrated the best agreement with intraoperative (mean difference = −0.32)
Meso Rubio et al. [59]	40	2D TTE 2D TEE Contrast angiography MDCT	Annulus	The best correlation was obtained with TTE and TEE ($r = 0.93$, $p < 0.001$) The correlation of TTE and TEE with angiography also was good ($r = 0.58$, $p < 0.001$ and $r = 0.53$, $p < 0.001$, respectively) Correlations between these techniques and computed tomography were poor (p = NS for all comparisons) The best agreement between estimated aortic annulus and implanted valve size was obtained with TTE and TEE (kappa = 0.88 and 0.76)
Messika-Zeitoun et al. [23]	45	TTE TEE MDCT	Annulus	Correlations between methods were good but the difference between MDCT and TTE (1.22 ± 1.3 mm) or TEE (1.52 ± 1.1 mm) was larger than the difference between TTE and TEE (0.6 ± 0.8 mm; $p = 0.03$ and $p < 0.0001$, respectively) Agreement between TTE and TEE overall was good (kappa = 0.68), but TAVR strategy would have been different in 8 patients (17 %) Agreement between MDCT and TTE or TEE was only modest (kappa = 0.28 and 0.27), and a decision based on MDCT measurements would have modified the TAVR strategy in a large number of patients (40–42 %). Implantation, performed in 34 patients (76 %) based on TEE measurements, was successful in all but 1 patient with grade 3/4 regurgitation
Tamborini et al. [24]	122	3D TEE MDCT	Left coronary Cusp length Distance from annulus to left main	Preoperatively, 3D TEE aortic annulus-LM ($r = 0.83$) and LCC ($r = 0.69$) significantly correlated with MDCT. Postoperatively, 3D TEE prosthesis-LM distance was 2.1 ± 1.9 mm. The prosthesis reached or exceeded LM in 6 and 10 cases, respectively. Prosthesis overlap with mitral leaflet was 4.7 ± 1.8 mm. Significant correlation between the 3D TEE computed and nominal length of the prosthesis was found ($r = 0.61$). No correlations were found between prosthesis-mitral leaflet overlap and aortic regurgitation or PPM
Tzikas et al. [25]	70	TTE Contrast angiography MDCT	Annulus	MDCT coronal view provided the largest mean annulus diameter (26.3 mm) followed by CA (24.4 mm), MDCT mean (23.7 mm), TTE (22.6 mm), and MDCT sagittal (21.8 mm) view Differences in the annulus measurements were significant: MDCT coronal view versus CA (= 2.0 mm, $r = 0.72$), CA versus MDCT mean (=0.2 mm, $r = 0.76$), MDCT mean versus TTE (=1.3 mm, $r = 0.61$), TTE versus MDCT sagittal view (=0.9 mm, $r = 0.59$), CA versus TTE (=1.5 mm, $r = 0.57$) Interobserver variability for TTE = 0.29 mm, $r = 0.57$, for CA = 0.14 mm, $r = 0.77$, and MDCT mean = 0.20 mm, $r = 0.95$

2D two dimensional, *3D* three dimensional, *CA* contrast angiography, *CMR* cardiac magnetic resonance imaging, *LM* left main, *MDCT* multidetector CT, *PPM* permanent pacemaker, *SEE* standard error of the estimate, *TEE* transesophageal echocardiography, *TTE* transthoracic echocardiography parameters [28]. The aortic annulus, generally elliptical, assumes a more round shape in systole, thus increasing CSA without substantial change in perimeter. Aortic annulus perimeter appears therefore ideally suited for accurate sizing in patients undergoing TAVR [28]. 3D TEE reconstructions of the aortic annulus may also provide better correlations with MDCT than 2D TTE or TEE alone (Fig. 8.5).

Table 8.5 Comparisons of measurement of annular dimensions

	N=75
Minimum diameter	21.4 (2.8)
Maximum diameter	26.9 (2.8)
Mean diameter	24.1 (2.6)
Mean from perimeter	24.3 (2.1)
Mean from cross-sectional area	23.6 (2.0)

Adapted from [19]

Different aortic THVs interact with the aortic annulus in different ways. These features include the frame material (e.g., stainless steel, cobalt chromium, nitinol, polymer nylon sleeve), method of frame expansion (e.g., balloon-expandable, self-expanding), frame sizes, length and thickness of frame skirt, frame eccentricity, and location of the valve leaflets (Table 8.2). In general, oversizing (10–20 %) of the CoreValve device is recommended for the range of annulus size (Fig. 8.6), whereas

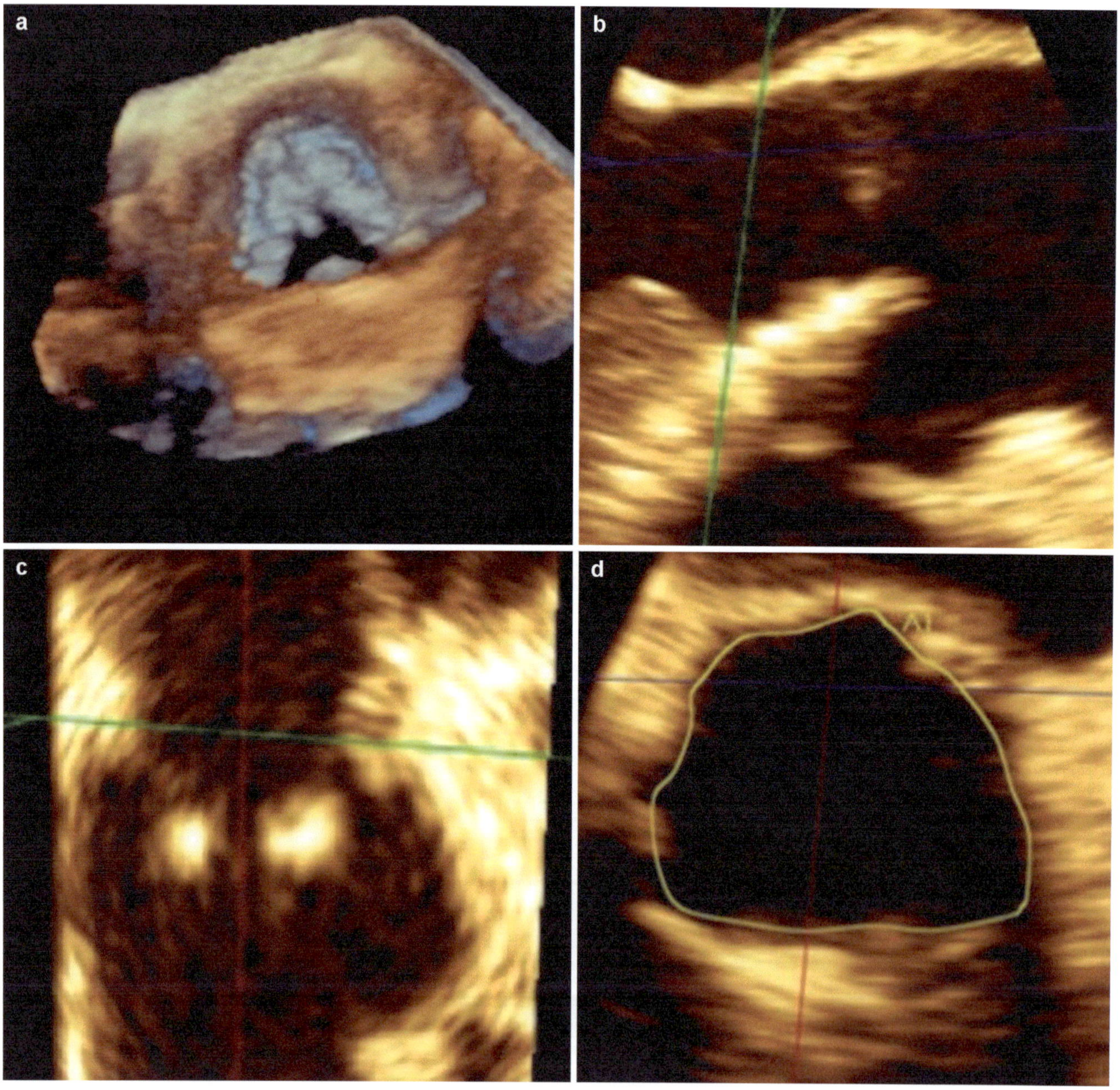

Fig. 8.5 Annular measurements using 3D transesophageal echocardiography (TEE). 3D TEE Image of a calcified aortic valve (**a**). Alignment of the three MPR planes (two shown in **b** and **c**) to obtain the annular diameter in the short axis view (**d**). *MPR* multiplanar reformat

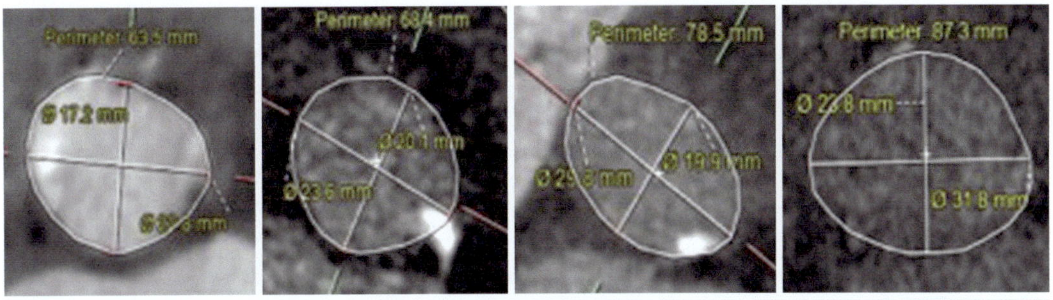

Valve size	23 (A)	26 (B)	29 (C)	31 (D)
Annular perimeter	63.5	68.4	78.5	87.3
Valve perimeter	72.2	81.6	91.1	97.3
% Oversize	12 %	16 %	14 %	10 %

Fig. 8.6 Annular measurement for aortic transcatheter heart valve selection. For THV, ranges of the CoreValve provide annular diameters from 18 to 29 for the 23, 26, 29, and 31 mm valves. Examples of perimeters are selected to provide oversizing from 10 to 20 %.

less (5–10 %) oversizing is recommended for the SAPIEN THV due to its balloon-expandable method of deployment that reshapes the eccentric annulus into more of a circle.

In contrast to self-expanding THV, wherein the annulus maintains its asymmetric shape after THV, balloon-expandable THV alters the annular shape to a more circular conformation. In a series of 53 patients undergoing balloon-expandable TAVR, MDCT assessment of the aortic valve apparatus was performed at baseline and at 1 month [29]. At baseline, MDCT demonstrated an ellipsoid shape of the aortic valve annulus with significantly larger coronal diameter when compared with sagittal diameter (25.1 ± 2.4 vs 22.9 ± 2.0 mm, $p < 0.001$) [29]. At follow-up, MDCT showed a noncircular deployment of the prosthesis in only six (14 %) patients [29]. Moderate post-procedural aortic regurgitation was observed in five (11 %) patients. These patients showed significantly larger aortic valve annulus (27.3 ± 1.6 vs 24.8 ± 2.4 mm, $p = 0.007$) and more calcified native valves (4,174 ± 1,604 vs 2,444 ± 1,237 HU, $p = 0.005$) at baseline and less favorable deployment of the prosthesis after TAVR [29].

The location of malapposition after TAVR has also been demonstrated using MDCT, and malapposition was seen predominantly at the aortomitral fibrous continuity and the aspect of the largest diameter of the aortic annulus on the inside curve of the ascending aorta [7]. Paravalvular regurgitation was less frequent in the area that contains the ventricular membranous septum and the area between the non- and right coronary sinus [7].

Sinus of Valsalva

The aortic root is the direct continuation of the left ventricular outflow tract and extends to the tubular aorta [30]. The walls of the sinuses are made of the same fibro-collagenous tissues as the aorta and support the valvar leaflets in semilunar fashion [31]. The widths of the sinuses of Valsalva (SOV) are important reservoirs for coronary perfusion with THV (Fig. 8.7).

Measurements of the SOV using MDCT provide insights into whether the THV will be accommodated within the sinus without causing coronary occlusion from displacement of the native valve leaflets (Fig. 8.8). SOV parameters for the various THVs are found in Table 8.3. 3D TEE may also provide sufficient information about the relative positioning of the aortic valve leaflets within the SOV and a useful tool for the prediction of complications after TAVR (Fig. 8.9).

Aortic Valve Leaflets

Coaptation of the native aortic valve is dependent on the integrity of the aortic valve leaflets and the sinotubular junction. Variations of leaflet length, height, width, and surface area result in differing volumes of the respective SOVs (Fig. 8.10). Variations in leaflet conformation are also found in patients with aortic stenosis, confounded by the degenerative changes and deformation imposed by progressive calcification and

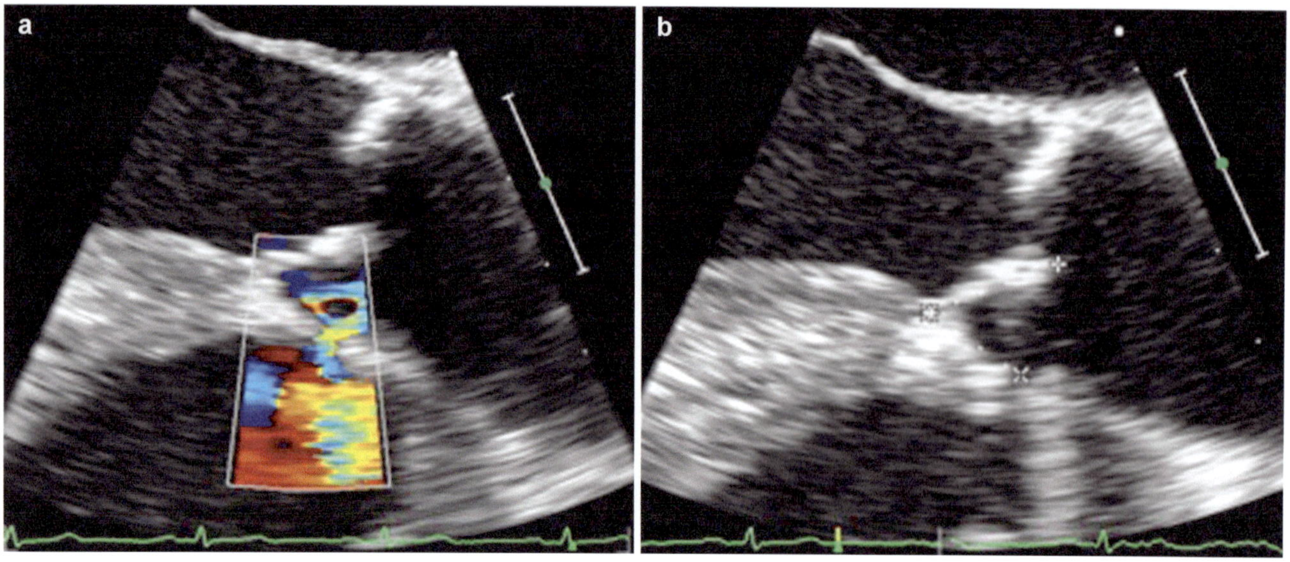

Fig. 8.7 Sinus of Valsalva and effective cusp height. Imaging plane used to define the leaflet height and effective cusp height. (**a**), Leaflet height, defined as the longest length of the cusp from the annulus to the cusp tip, was measured in diastole from the long-axis view going through the center of each cusp. Effective cusp height, defined as the vertical distance between the cusps from the annulus to the cusp tip, was measured in diastole from the same plane as the cusp height. (**b**), Schematic diagram illustrating leaflet height and effective cusp height. *STJ* sinotubular junction, *LH* leaflet height, *ECH* effective cusp height (Reproduced from [43] with permission)

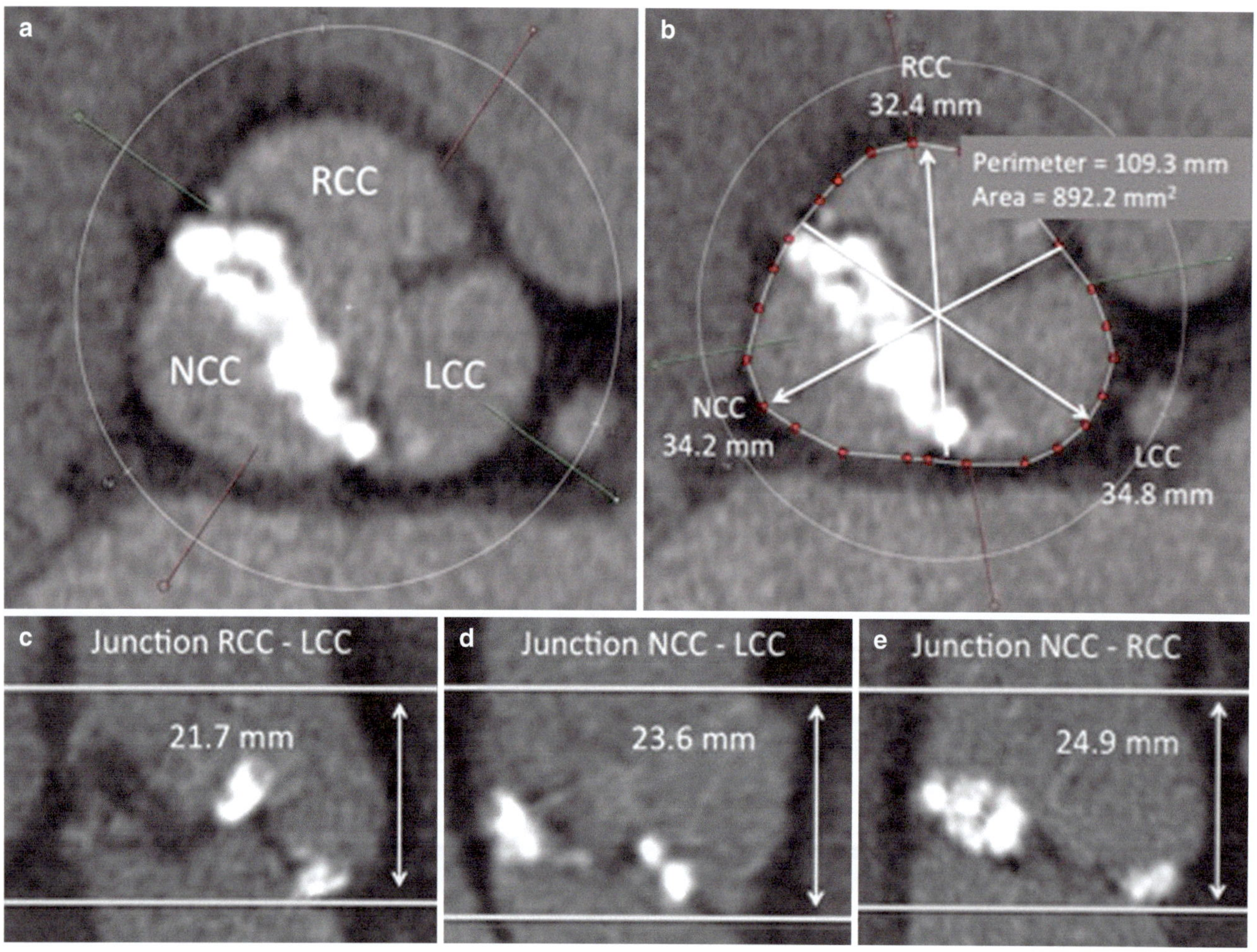

Fig. 8.8 MDCT measurements of the sinus of Valsalva (SOV). SOV measurements are obtained from the double oblique (MPR). Reconstruction of the SOV provides identification of the right coronary cusp (*RCC*), left coronary cusp (*LCC*), and noncoronary cusp (*NCC*) (**a**). The width for each SOV is obtained by measurement from the commissure to the opposite sinus. In addition, a perimeter and an area of the SOV are obtained (**b**). The height of the SOV can be obtained at the junction of the RCC and LCC (**c**), NCC and LCC (**d**), and NCC and RCC (**e**)

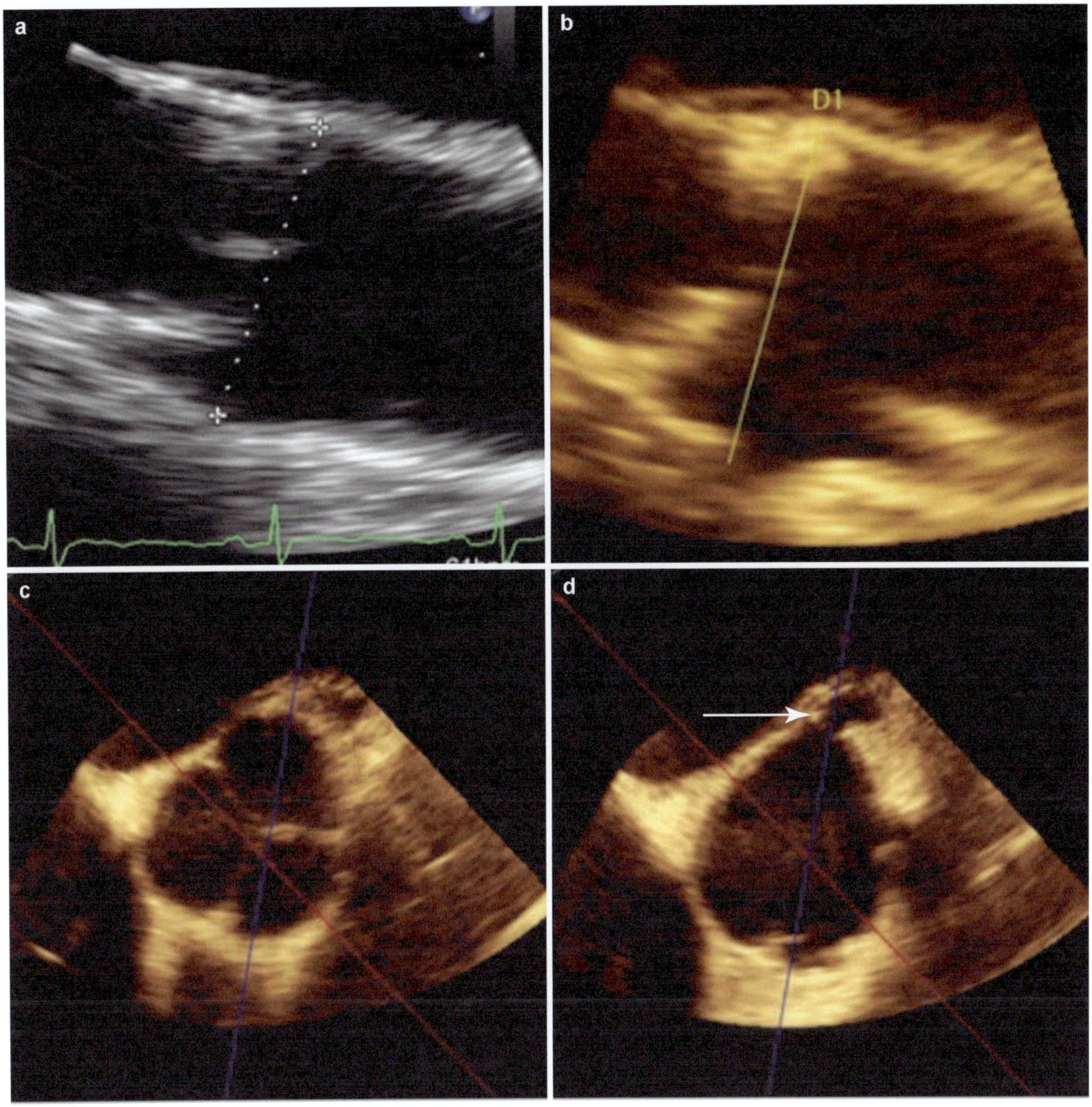

Fig. 8.9 Echocardiographic assessment of the sinus of Valsalva. TEE image of the sinus of Valsalva using 2D (**a**) and 3D (**b**) imaging. The 3D TEE short axis imaging of the SOV during diastole (**c**). The origin of the left main artery is seen during systole (**d**, *arrow*). *TEE* transesophageal echocardiography

fibrosis of the native valve. Inequalities in leaflet length imparting eccentricity of the annulus and sinus of Valsalva have led to underestimation of the annular diameters using cross-sectional echocardiography. 2D TEE may provide information about the thickness of the aortic leaflets and their relative position to the SOV and the coronary artery origin (Fig. 8.11).

Aortic valve calcification (AVC) predicts cardiovascular and coronary event risk independent of traditional risk factors and inflammatory biomarkers [32]. The degree of aortic valve calcification assessed by echocardiography has been correlated with the occurrence of paravalvular regurgitation after TAVR [32–35]. In a series of 100 patients treated with the CoreValve Revalving System, the amount and distribution of calcification was semiquantitatively assessed and graded on a 1 to 4 scale (device "landing zone" calcification score [DLZ-CS]) [36]. The Agatston score and calcification at the landing zone showed a significant correlation with the grade of perivalvular regurgitation [36]. The distribution and quantification of the aortic valve can be obtained using novel analytic methods (Fig. 8.12). In another series of patients undergoing TAVR, although there was no association between the distribution of AVC and the degree of paraval-

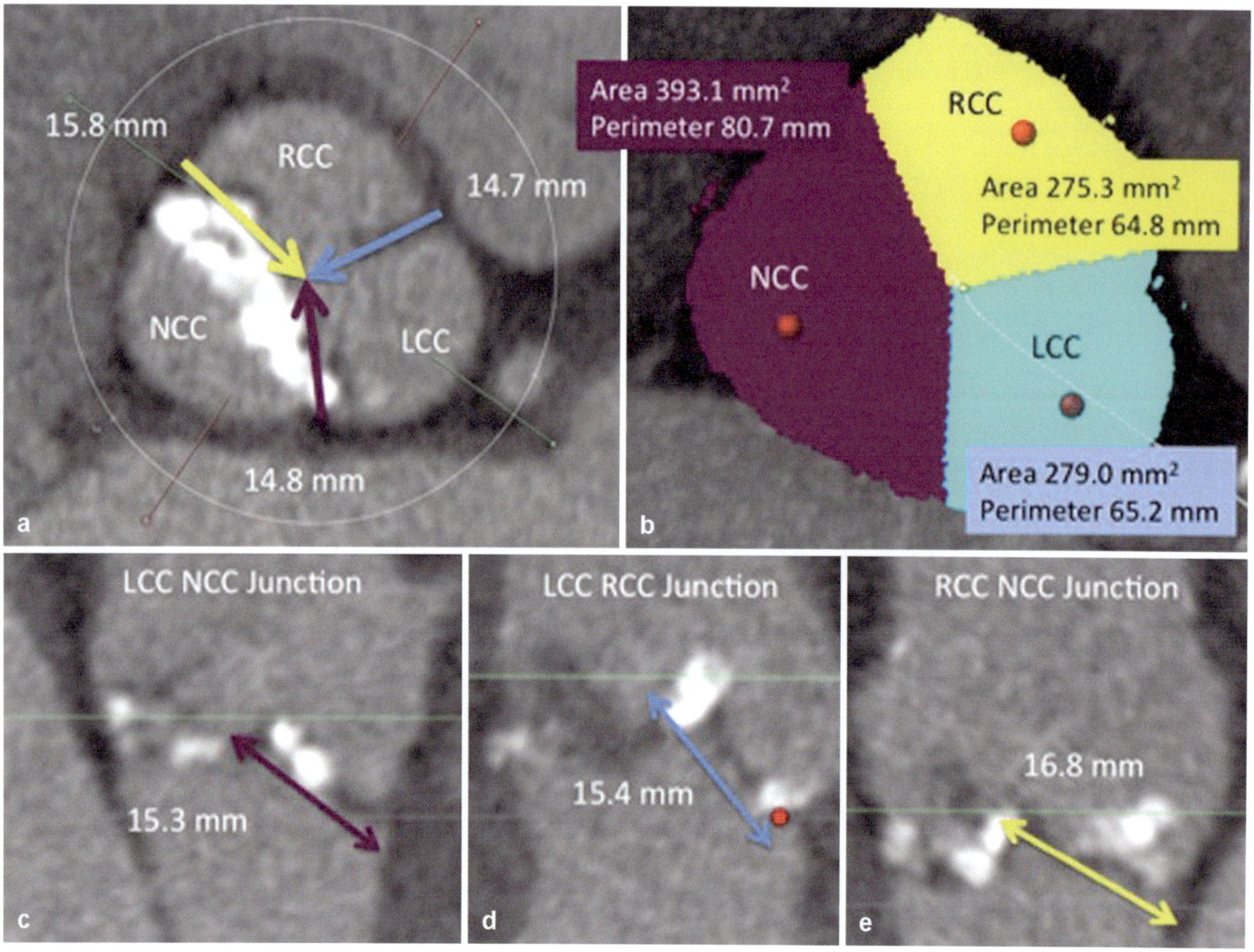

Fig. 8.10 Quantitation of leaflet lengths. The lengths of the commisures can be estimated from the cross-sectional images (**a**), and the maximal cross-sectional area and perimeters of the three sinuses can be estimated (**b**). The coaptation length between the left coronary cusp (*LCC*) and the noncoronary cusp (*NCC*) is illustrated in *purple* (**c**). The coaptation length between the LCC and the right coronary cusp (*RCC*) is shown in *blue* (**d**). The coaptation length of the RCC and NCC is shown in *yellow* (**e**)

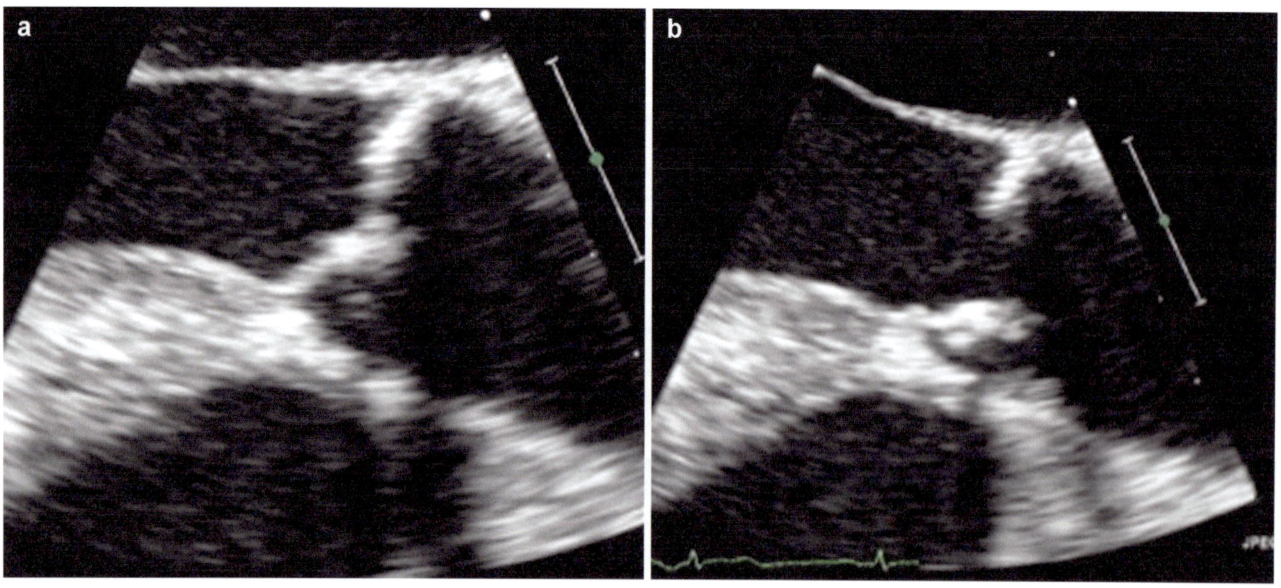

Fig. 8.11 Coronary cusp thickness and length. TEE can be used to measure the cusp length and thickness during diastole (**a**) and systole (**b**). *TEE* transesophageal echocardiography

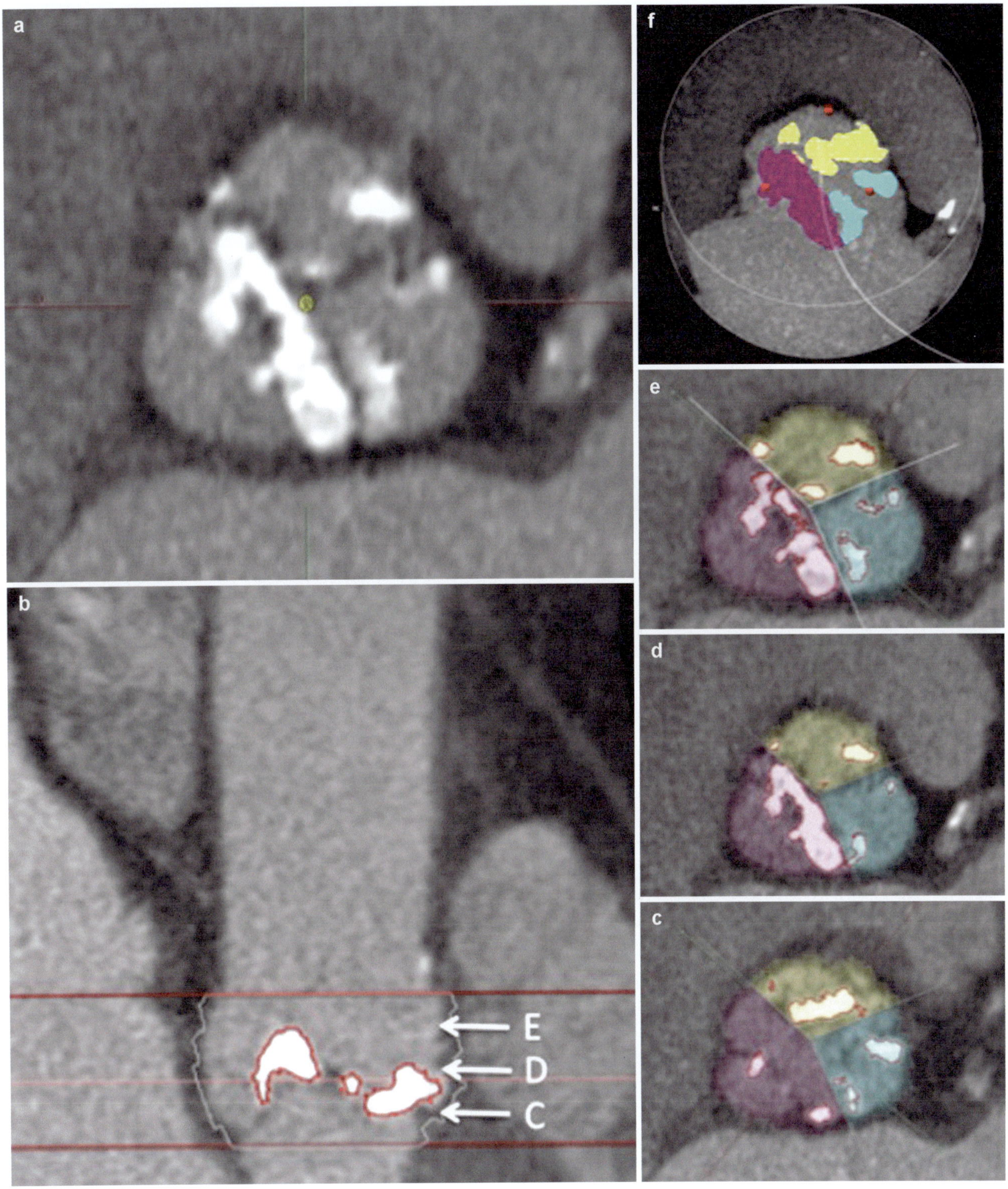

Fig. 8.12 Aortic valve calcification. The degree of calcification of the aortic valve can be qualitatively assessed in the cross-sectional view of the sinus of Valsalva (**a**). Using quantitative techniques that visualize a threshold of voxel density (usually greater than 600 HU), the stretch CMPR view can localize the calcium location within the aortic valve (**b**). Color coding of the three valve leaflets allows identification of calcium near the basal annular place (**c**), inferior portion of the sinus of Valsalva (**d**), and superior aspect of the sinus of Valsalva (**e**). These voxel densities are summed using a Hockey Puck display (**f**) that provides both the volume (in mm^3) and mass (in mg) of calcium in the aortic valve

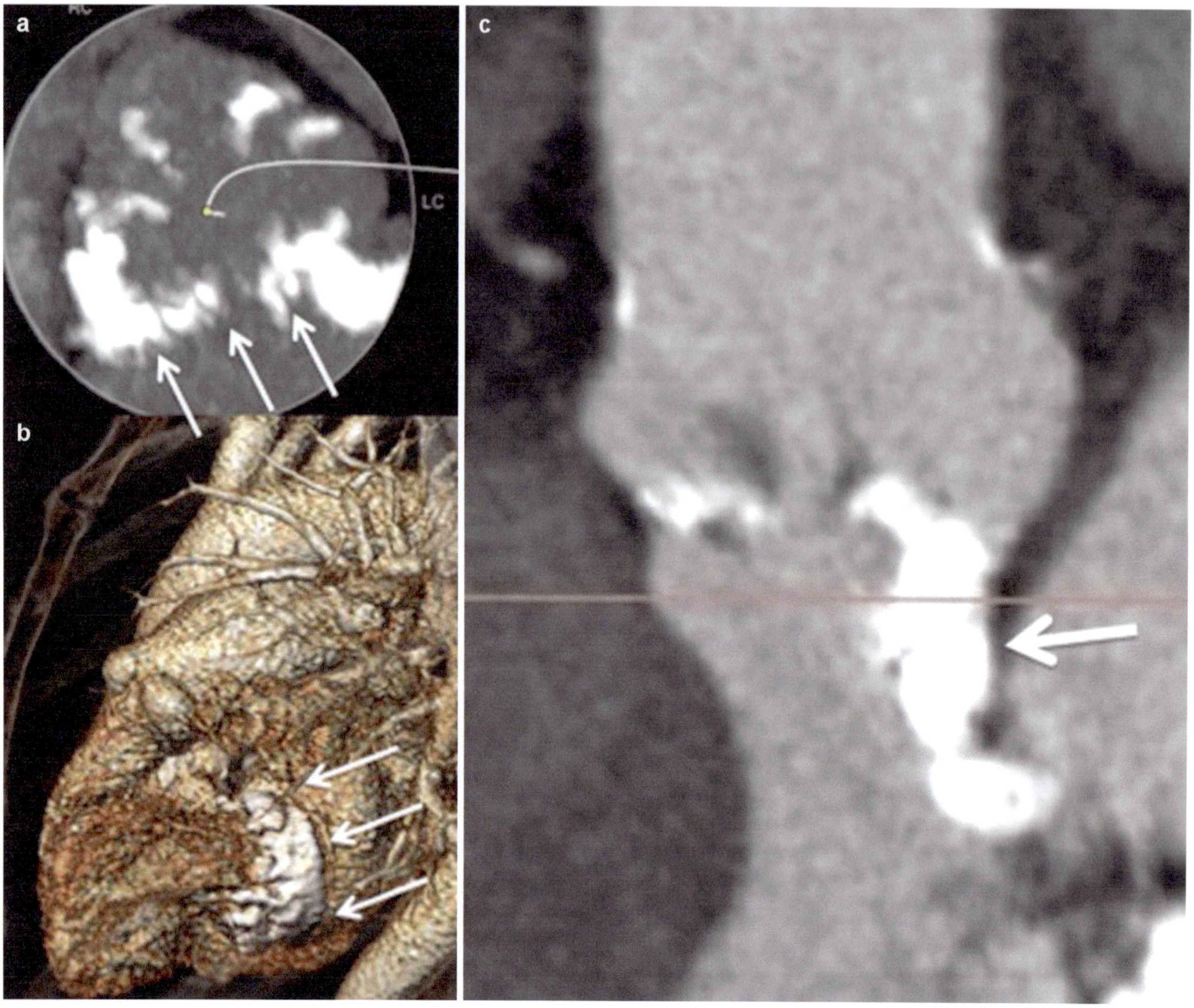

Fig. 8.13 Mitral annular calcification. The double oblique reconstruction of the aortic annulus demonstrates severe calcification in the aortomitral continuity (**a**, *arrows*). The double oblique projection with volume rendering of the mitral valve shows the posterior distribution of severe mitral annular calcification (**b**, *arrows*). There is extensive calcification of the aortomitral continuity seen in the double oblique (MPR) projection (**c**, *arrows*). *MPR* multiplanar reformat

vular aortic regurgitation after TAVR as assessed by angiography ($r=-0.02$, $p=0.88$), Agatston AVC scores were significantly higher in patients with aortic regurgitation grade ≥3 (5,055 ± 1,753, $n=3$) than in patients with aortic regurgitation grade <3 (1,723 ± 967, $p=0.03$, $n=54$) [37]. Agatston AVC scores >3,000 were associated with relevant perivalvular AR. There was a significant correlation between the severity of AVC and the degree of AR after aortic valve replacement ($r=0.50$, $p<0.001$) [37].

The need for post-deployment balloon dilatation is higher in patients with severe valvular calcification, associated with a higher rate of cerebrovascular events [38]. Calcification of the aortomitral continuity that extends to the mitral valve may also increase the risk of annular rupture with balloon dilatation (Fig. 8.13).

Coronary Arteries

The coronary arteries generally arise within the sinuses of Valsalva, usually just below the level of the sinotubular junction. A number of methods have been used to estimate the relationship of the coronary arteries to the aortic annulus [39–44] (Table 8.6). The right coronary artery generally lies higher than the left coronary arteries, although substantial inter-patient variability requires that these measures are performed in all patients prior to TAVR [42] (Fig. 8.14).

Degenerative aortic stenosis may result in longitudinal remodeling of the sinus of Valsalva [43]. One study that compared annular dimensions of 25 patients treated with severe calcific aortic stenosis and 25 elderly gender-matched controls [43] found that compared with the control group, the AS group

Table 8.6 Relationship of the coronary arteries to the aortic annulus

Author	Number Pts	Method	Annulus to RCA	Range (mm)	Annulus to LCA (mm)	Range (mm)
Jatene et al. [39]	100	Autopsy	–	–	13.3	–
McAlpine et al. [40]	100	Autopsy	18.5±2.5	–	18.5±2.5	–
Chorianopoulos et al. [41]	54	Contrast angiography	–	–	19.4+2.7	–
Knight et al. [44]	150	MDCT	17.0±3.6	10.4–28.5	15.3±3.1	9.8–29.3
	75	Autopsy	14.9±4.3	5–24	16.0±3.6	9–24
Akhtar et al. [43]	50	MDCT				
No aortic stenosis	25		15.2+2.5	–	15.6+2.7	–
Aortic stenosis	25		13.6+2.8	–	13.4+3.2	–
Tops et al. [42]	169	MDCT				
No aortic stenosis	150		17.2+3.3	–	14.4+2.8	
Aortic stenosis	19		17.3+3.6		14.0+3.3	

LCA left coronary artery, *MDCT* multidetector CT, *Pts* patients, *RCA* right coronary artery

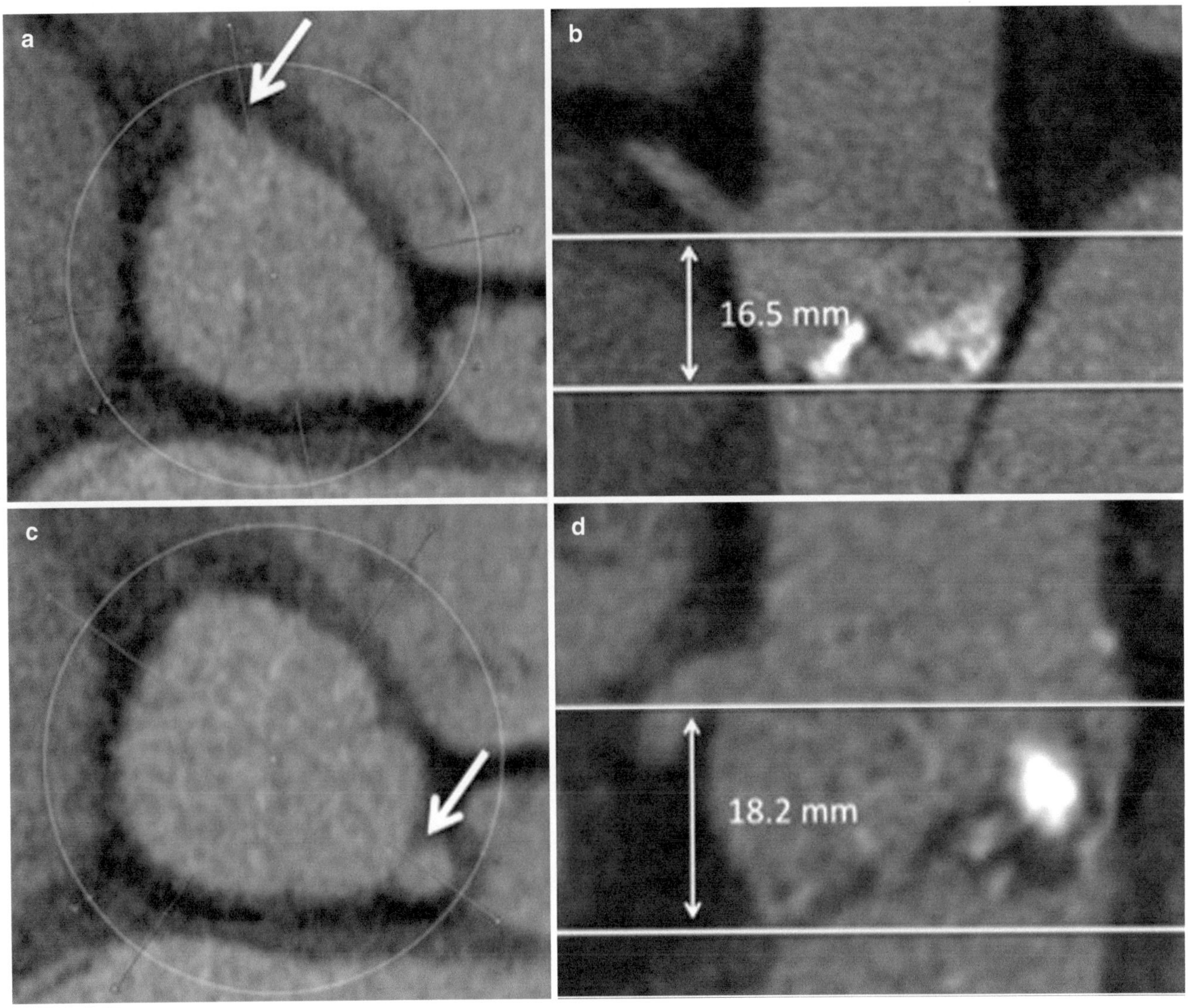

Fig. 8.14 Coronary artery height. The height of the right coronary artery is determined by identifying the origin of the right coronary artery from the cross section of MPR (**a**, *arrow*) and then measuring the height of the coronary artery above the basal annular plane (**b**). In a similar fashion, the origin of the left coronary artery is identified from the cross section of the MPR (**c**, *arrow*) and then measuring the height of the left coronary artery above the basal annular plane (**d**). In this case, the left coronary artery lies higher than the right coronary artery. *MPR* multiplanar reformat

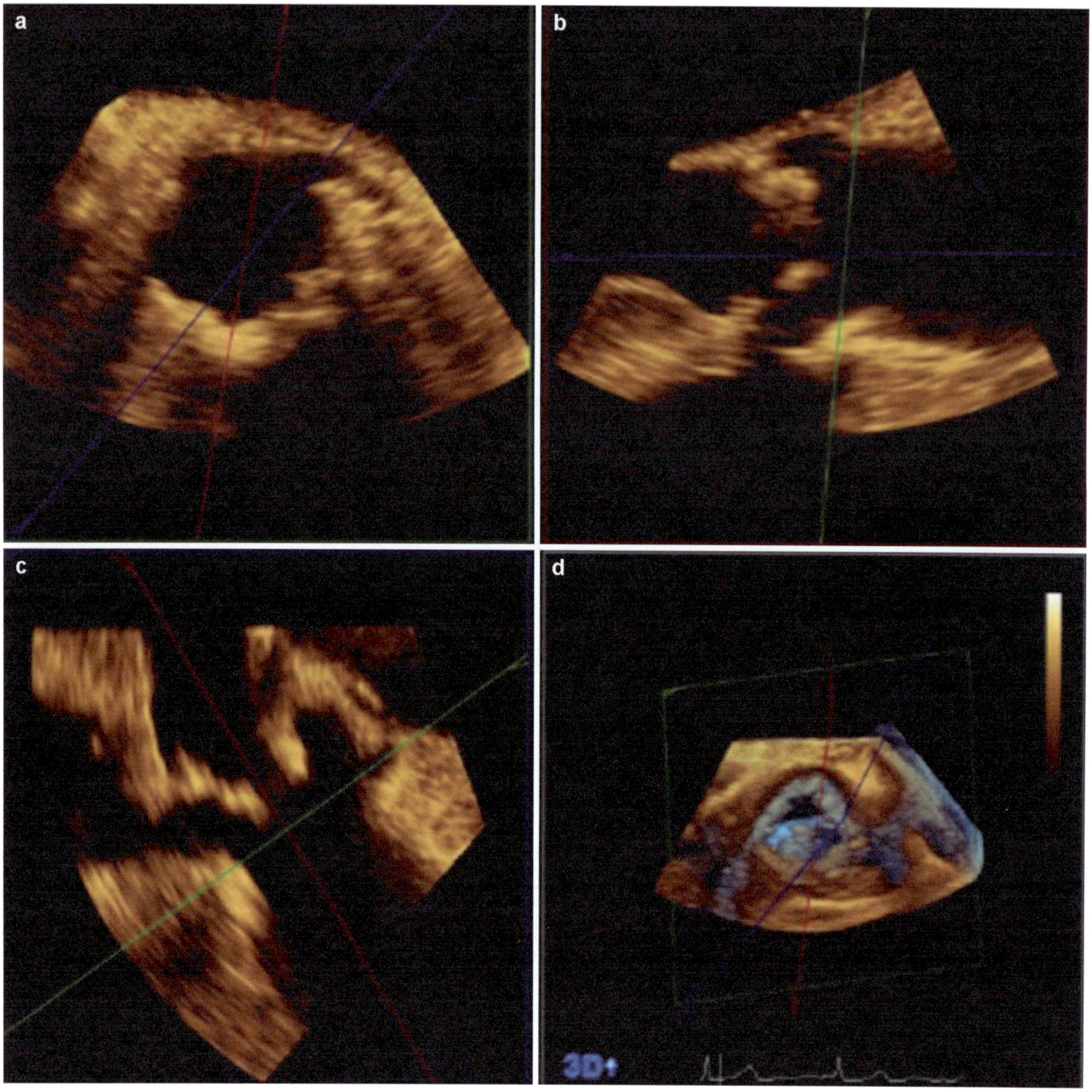

Fig. 8.15 3D Transesophageal echocardiogram. 3D TEE identification of the origin of the left coronary artery using oblique tools (**a–d**). *TEE* transesophageal echocardiography

showed a reduced distance from the aortic valve annulus to the left coronary artery ostium (13.4 ± 3.2 mm vs 15.6 ± 2.7 mm; $p = 0.01$) [43]. There was a similar reduction in the distance from the aortic valve annulus to the right coronary artery ostium in the AS group compared with the control group (13.6 ± 2.8 vs 15.2 ± 2.5 mm; $p = 0.04$) [43]. The longitudinal distance from the aortic valve annulus to the sinotubular junction was also reduced in the AS group compared with the control group (16.7 ± 2.0 vs 21.0 ± 2.3 mm; $p < 0.01$) [43]. The presence of longitudinal remodeling was not confirmed in a second study [42], although there were a smaller number of patients with aortic stenosis in the study. Although MDCT has been considered the "gold standard" for assessing the location of the coronary ostia and their relationship to the sinuses of Valsalva, TEE may also be a useful technique for identification of coronary location and patency before and after TAVR to identify the location of the left (Fig. 8.15) and right coronary arteries. In a correlative study of 122 patients undergoing TAVR, 3D TEE and MDCT measurements of the distance between the left main coronary artery and the aortic annulus

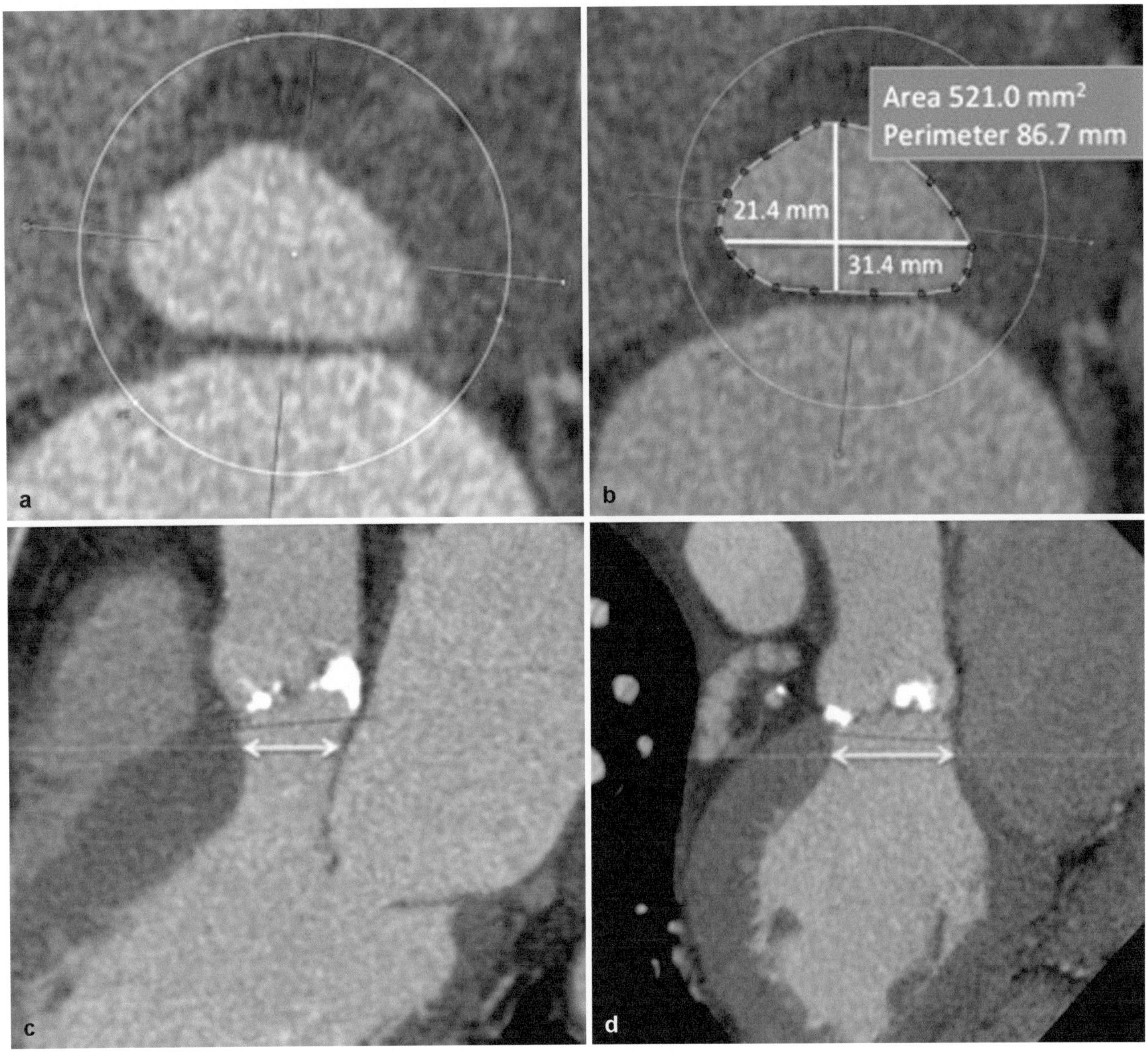

Fig. 8.16 Left ventricular outflow tract. The cross section of the left ventricular outflow tract (LVOT) can be indentified 2–4 mm inferior to the basal annular plane (**a**). Maximum and perpendicular to the maximum diameters, it is also often eccentric in appearance (**b**). The eccentricity of the LVOT can be appreciated in the orthogonal double oblique (MPR) views (**c**, **d**, *double-sided arrows*). *MPR* multiplanar reformat

($r=0.83$) and of the length of the left coronary cusp ($r=0.69$) were well correlated [24]. Using a balloon-expandable THV, the 3D TEE estimation of the distance of the THV to left main distance was 2.1 ± 1.9 mm after TAVR. The THV reached or exceeded left main height in 60 % of patient cases [24].

Coronary occlusion has been reported following TAVR [45–50]. There are several potential sources of coronary ostial obstruction, including a long native valve leaflet; inappropriately high positioning of the sealing cuff; atheroma, calcification, thrombosis, or air embolism; or dissection of the aortic root [49]. Patients at particular risk for coronary occlusion are those with a low-lying (<10–12 mm) coronary ostium, those with bulky native leaflets, and those with a narrow root with shallow sinuses of Valsalva [49]. Measurement of the height of the coronary arteries relative to their supporting valvar sinuses and dimensions of the coronary arteries is essential prior to TAVR [17].

Left Ventricular Outflow Tract

The left ventricular outflow tract between the basal annulus and the anatomic ventricular aortic junction is primarily comprised of fibrous tissue rather than muscular tissue [31] (Fig. 8.16). The triangle between the noncoronary and the left coronary aortic sinuses is in continuity with

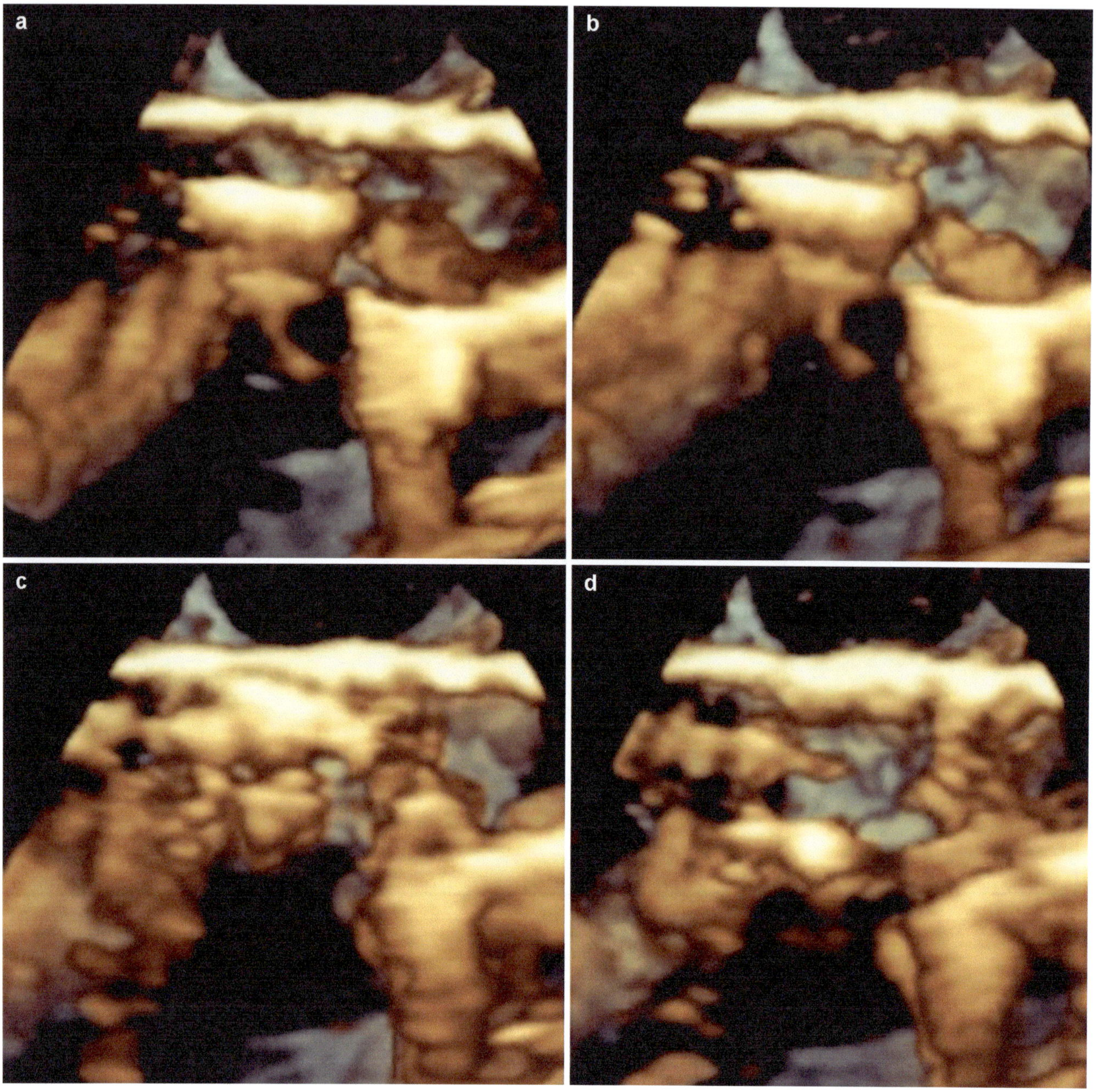

Fig. 8.17 Deployment of a balloon-expandable SAPIEN THV using 3D transesophageal echocardiography. Positioning of the unexpanded balloon-expandable frame is seen in (**a**). Partial deployment of the frame is shown in (**b**) and (**c**). Full deployment of the frame is shown in (**d**)

the anterior leaflet of the mitral valve, and the triangle between the right coronary aortic sinus and the noncoronary sinus forms the membranous septum [31]. Importantly, the atrioventricular node is located just inferior to the apex of the triangle adjacent to the membranous septum and is adjacent to the membranous septum of the left ventricular outflow tract just below the aortic valve [31]. The atrioventricular node continues as the bundle of His, then gives rise to the fascicles of the left bundle branch along the membranous septum [31]. Injury to this region predisposes to the development of conduction disturbances after TAVR.

Proper position of the aortic THV at the annulus just to the left of the LVOT and aortic annulus is critical during THV placement. Placement can be facilitated using intraoperative 3D TEE (Fig. 8.17). Deep positioning of the THV into the left ventricular outflow tract may cause injury to the interventricular septum and arteriovenous conduction system. Accordingly, the incidence of permanent pacemaker placement due high-degree atrioventricular block or symptomatic bradycardia is higher with balloon-expandable (2.5–11.5 %) and self-expanding (9.3–43 %) TAVR than with surgical aortic valve replacement (3.2–8.5 %) [51]. Any direct trauma or mechanical stress to the His bundle at the region of the membranous septum and right trigone beneath the noncoronary and right coronary cusps might explain the occurrence of new conduction abnormalities leading to complete AV Block after TAVR.

The increased requirement for PPM with TAVR likely relates to the direct trauma and mechanical stress applied by the THV directly in the region of the membranous septum and right fibrous trigone located just below the level of the right coronary and noncoronary sinuses. The higher frequency of conduction system abnormalities with the CoreValve THV is likely due to the longer length of the CoreValve frame relative to the SAPIEN device as well as the continued expansive forces of the nitinol frame onto the membranous septum after deployment. The continued pressure with self-expanding THV may also explain the later occurrence of this event after CoreValve placement. While the development of conduction system abnormalities has been associated with a worsened outcome in patients who did not receive a permanent pacemaker [52], patients who require a PPM after CoreValve TAVR have a similar outcome as those who do not receive a PPM [53]. The availability of the improved Accutrak delivery system with the CoreValve THV has allowed higher implantation depths [54] and potentially lower PPM requirements [55, 56].

Aortomitral Curtain and Mitral Anterior Leaflet

The triangle of the left coronary sinus and the noncoronary sinus is continuous with the aortic leaflet and the anterior leaflet of mitral valve [31] (Fig. 8.18). The aortomitral curtain ends in the fibrous continuity, which are thickened to form the left and right fibrous trigones. Inadvertent placement of the aortic valvar prosthesis too low within the left ventricular outflow tract, therefore, may impinge upon the anterior leaflet of the mitral valve [57, 58].

Aortoventricular Angle

The severity of the angle between the proximal aortic, the annulus, and the left ventricular outflow tract is an important consideration for aortic THVs that have a long length and require deployment perpendicular to the annular plane. For the CoreValve THV, the maximal aortoventricular angle is 70° for deployment from the iliofemoral or left subclavian approaches. Due to angulation from the right subclavian into the ascending aorta, the maximal aortoventricular angle that is recommended is 30°. With careful case planning, the aortoventricular angle is less important for the direct aortic approach, as the angulation of the delivery catheter can be better controlled by the site of aortotomy. The aortoventricular angle is best determined from the coronary (MPR) view by determining the angle of the horizontal plane at the level of the ventricle and the aortic annulus angulation (Fig. 8.19).

Aortic Root and Aortic Arch

Aortic root dimensions should be carefully evaluated in patients undergoing TAVR, particularly with those THV with a longer length. For example, orientation of the direction of the CoreValve flow occurs with the CoreValve frame contact of the inner and outer curvature of the aorta. Aortic root dilation more than 43 or 45 mm about the basal aortic annulus precluded the use of the 29 and 31 mm CoreValve THV, and dilation of the aortic root more than 40 mm precludes use of the 23 and 26 mm CoreValve device. Aortic root size is of less concern for those valves that are short in length and primarily confined to the aortic annulus and sinus of Valsalva.

The extent and distribution of AVC also determines both surgical operability as well as the ability to perform direct aortic access (Fig. 8.20). In a series of 237 patients, MDCTs scans were analyzed for the distribution of calcium within the ascending aorta. The vast majority of patients had calcification in the aortic arch (64.9 %) and aortic root (92.8 %). Only one patient had diffuse calcification in the ascending aorta precluding a transaortic or direct aortic procedure. MDCT can also be used for case planning for the median sternotomy (Fig. 8.21) or right thoracotomy (Fig. 8.22).

This chapter has reviewed a number of important components of the aortic valvar complex with specific considerations for patients undergoing transcatheter aortic valve replacement. Both short- and long-term complications can be mitigated with careful pre-procedural imaging. Appropriate annular sizing may reduce the degree of paravalvular regurgitation after TAVR, and better position may lessen the need for permanent pacemaker implantation. Characterization of the thickness and length of the degenerated leaflets, identification of the origin of the coronary arteries, and the width of the sinus of Valsalva may prevent the occurrence of coronary occlusion. Quantification of the degree of valvar calcification and its location relative to the annulus may identify those patients at risk for annular rupture. Pre-procedural imaging may also allow clinicians to select the THV best suited to the patient's specific anatomy.

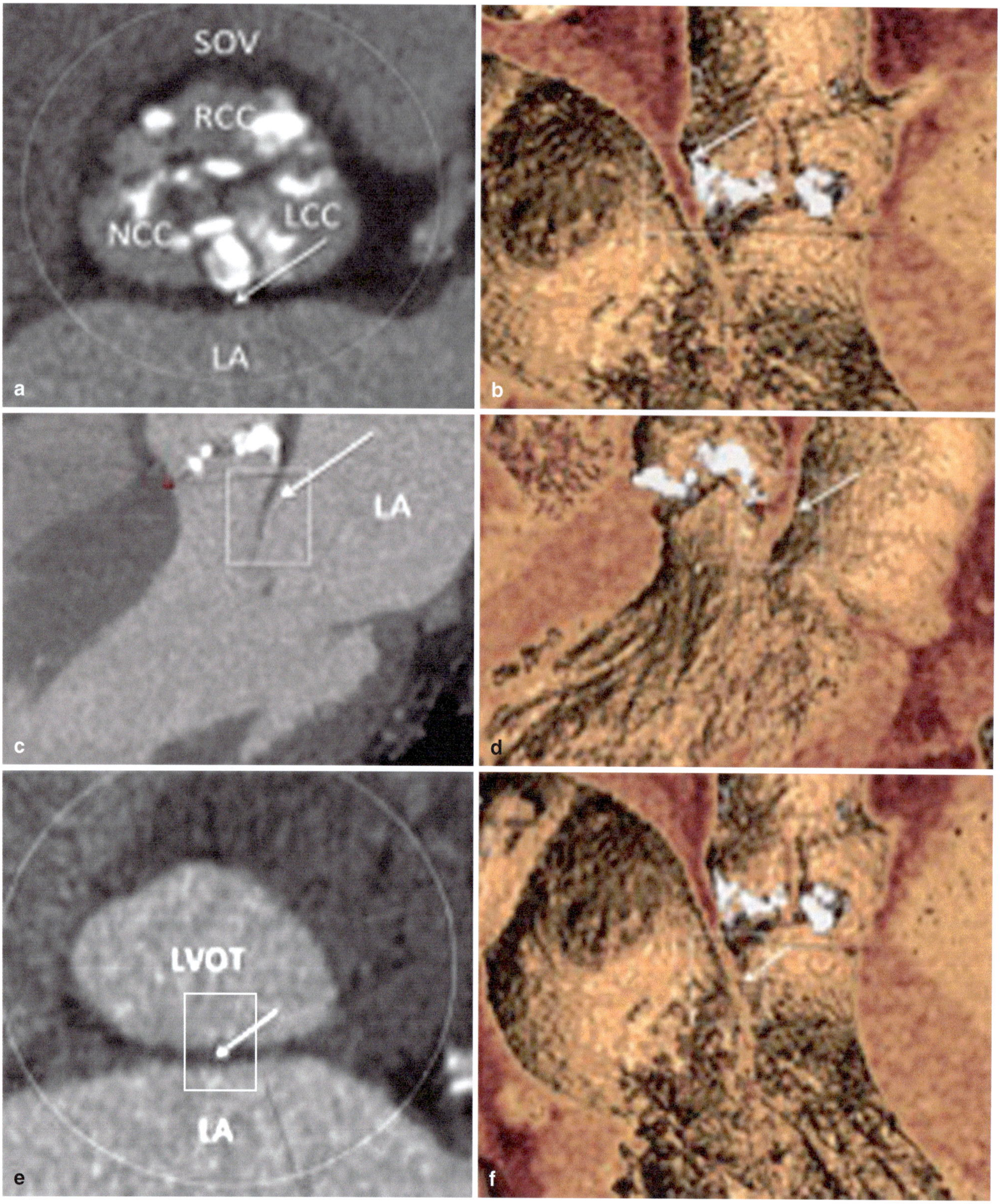

Fig. 8.18 Aortomitral continuity. The sinus of Valsalva (SOV) view can be used to identify the junction of the left coronary cusp (LCC) and the noncoronary sinus (RCC). Adjacent to this is the aortomitral continuity (*arrow*) that separates the SOV from the left atrium (LA) (**a**). The double oblique projection with volume rendering identifies the region of the aortomitral continuity (**b**, *box, with arrow*). The aortomitral continuity is visualized in the double oblique (MPR) at the level of the annulus (**c**, *box, with arrow*). The double oblique projection with volume rendering identifies the region of the aortomitral continuity at the level of the aortic annulus (**d**, *box, with arrow*). The aortomitral continuity is visualized in the double oblique (MPR) at the level of the left ventricular outflow tract (**e**, *box, with arrow*). The double oblique projection with volume rendering identifies the region of the aortomitral continuity at the level of the left ventricular outflow tract (**f**, *box, with arrow*)

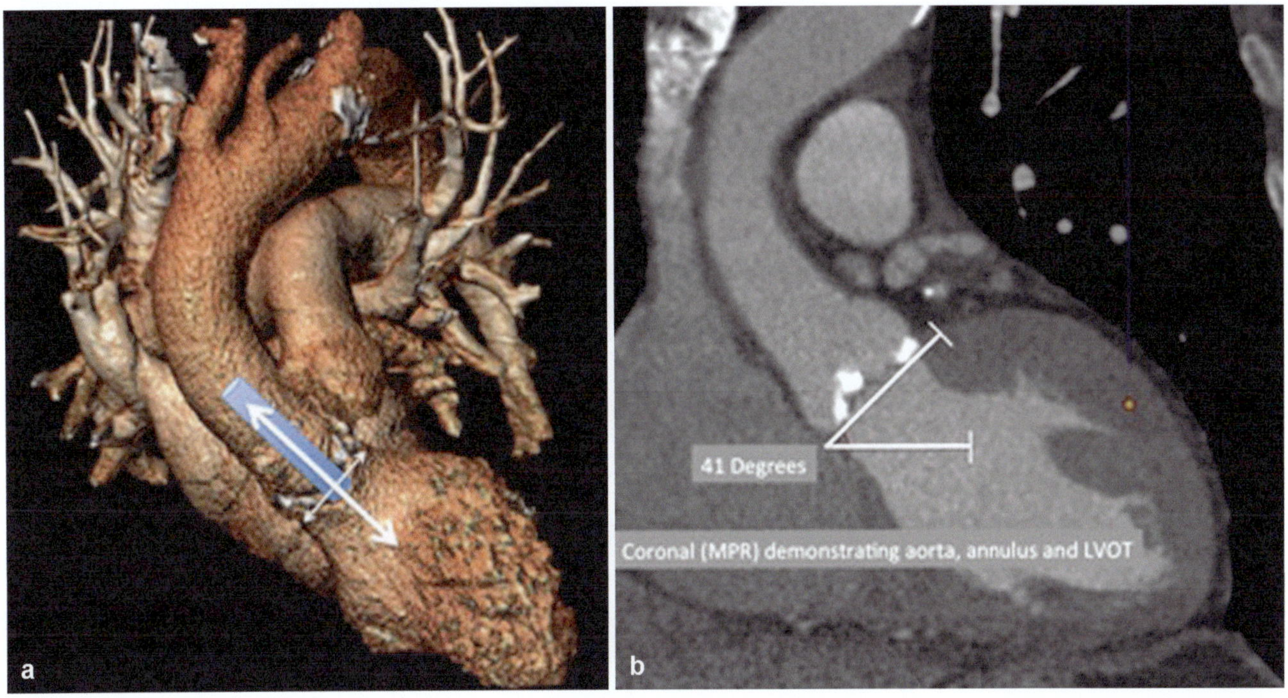

Fig. 8.19 Aortoventricular angulation. Volume rendering of the aortovalvular complex (**a**). The double-sided arrows show the central plan of the aorta (*large arrow*), aortic valve annulus (*small arrow*), and left ventricular outflow tract to guide optimal placement of the aortic THV (cylinder). Coronal MPR demonstrating aorta, annulus, and left ventricular outflow tract (LVOT) (**b**). The aortoventricular angle is determined by angle of the horizontal plane and the angle of the aortic annulus. In this case, the aortoventricular angle is 41°

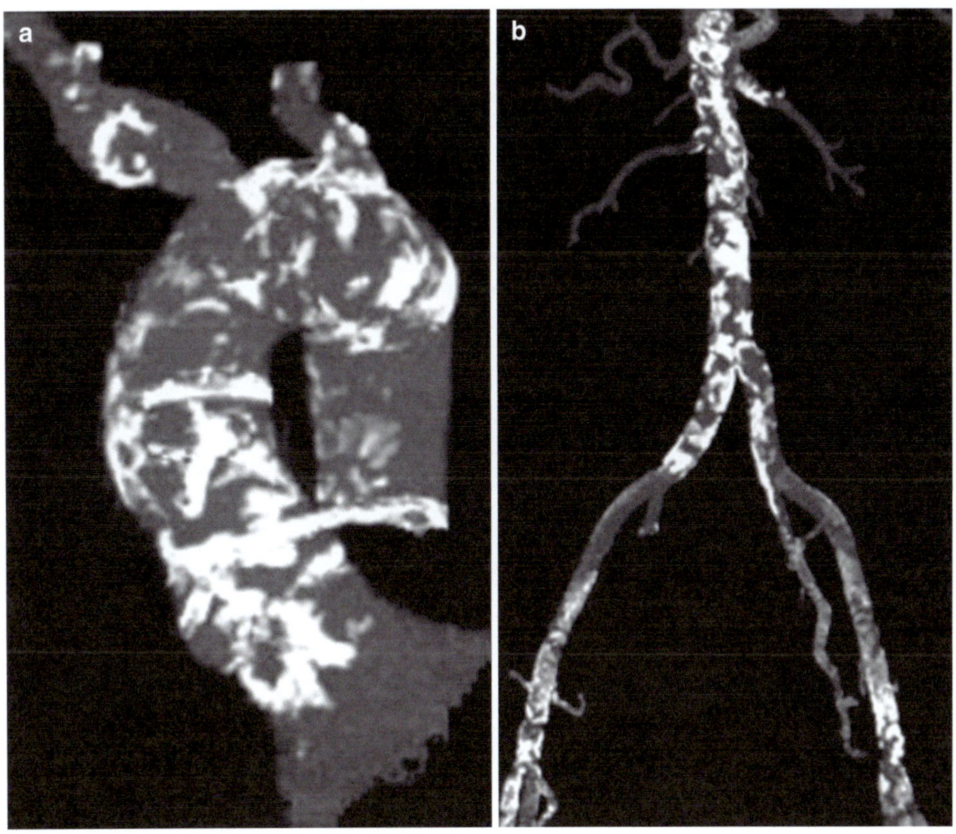

Fig. 8.20 Aortic calcification. Extensive calcification of the ascending aorta (**a**). Extensive calcification of the abdominal aorta, iliacs, and femoral arteries (**b**)

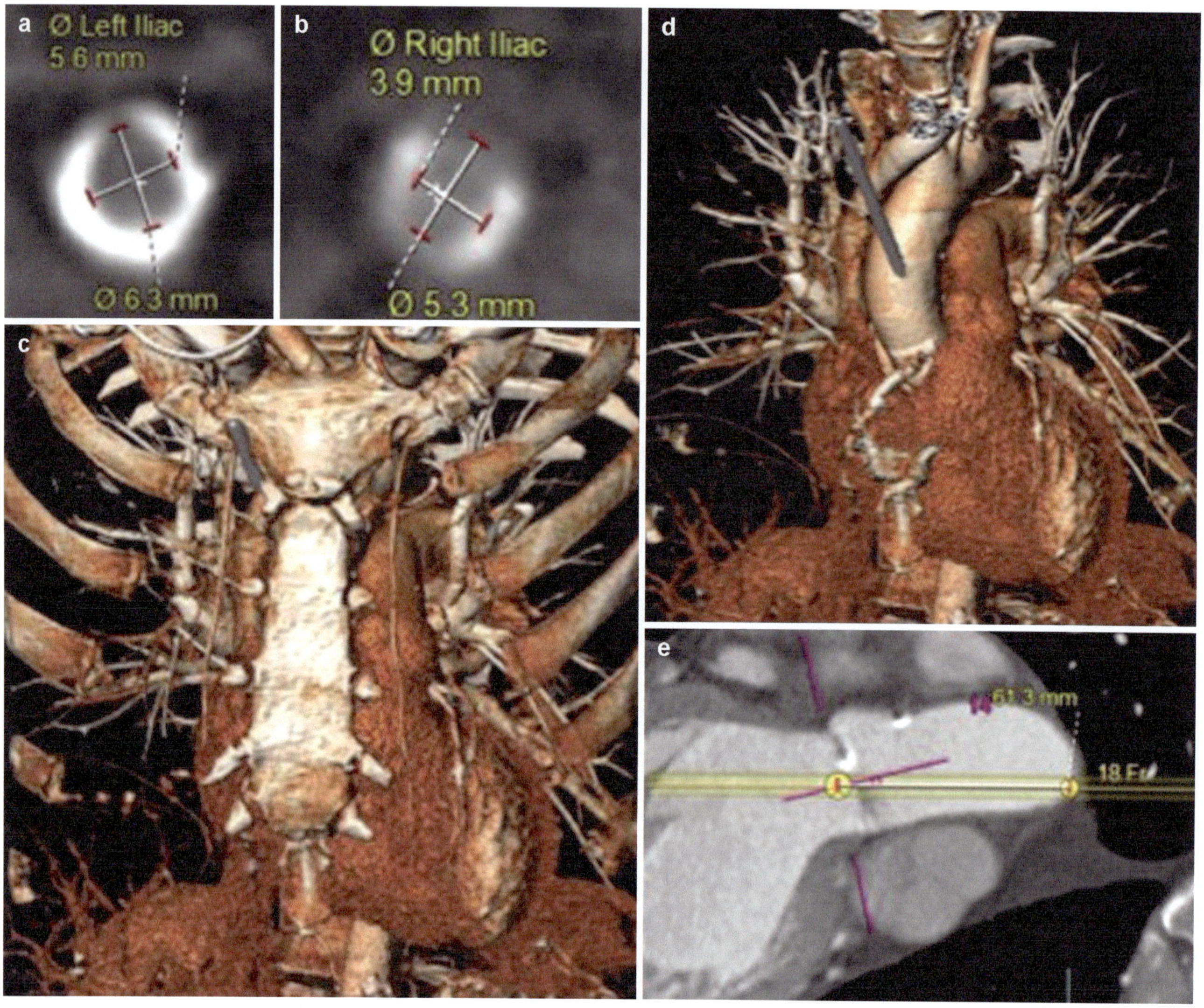

Fig. 8.21 Case planning for median hemi-sternotomy direct aortic approach. The left iliac artery (**a**) and right iliac artery (**b**) have small diameters and concentric calcification that preclude advancement of an 18 Fr sheath from the iliofemoral approach. CTA reconstruction of the chest wall and aorta shows the optimal approach for aortotomy (**c**, *cylinder*). The aortic route is visualized with the sternum removed (**d**, *cylinder*). Based on this insertion point, the angulation of implantation can be determined and the distance from the aortic annulus and the aortotomy site can be determined.

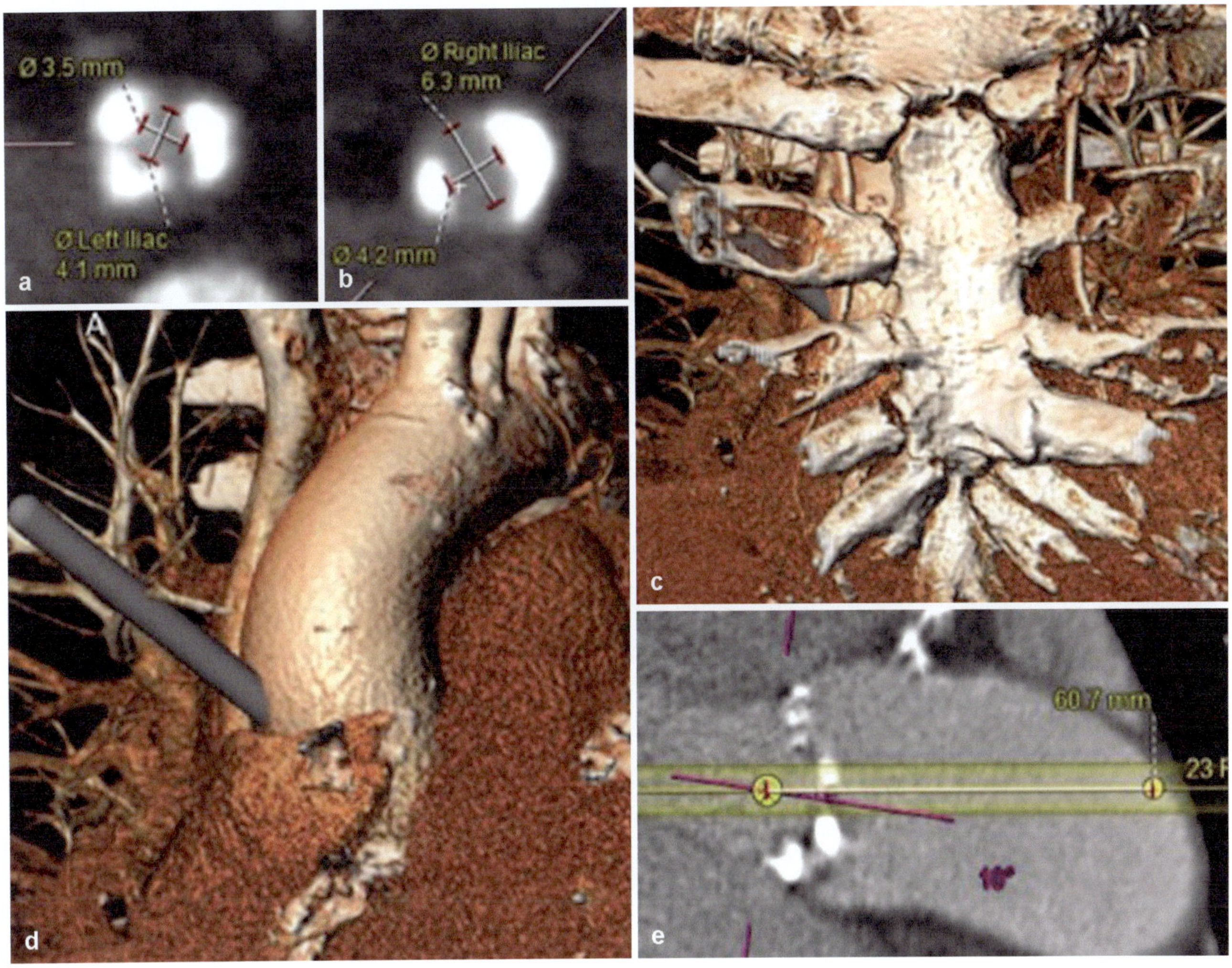

Fig. 8.22 Case planning for right thoracotomy direct aortic approach. The left iliac artery (**a**) and right iliac artery (**b**) have small diameters and concentric calcification that preclude advancement of an 18 Fr sheath from the iliofemoral approach. CTA reconstruction of the chest wall and aorta shows the optimal approach for aortotomy (**c**, *cylinder*). The aortic route is visualized with the sternum removed (**d**, *cylinder*). Based on this insertion point, the angulation of implantation can be determined and the distance from the aortic annulus and the aortotomy site can be determined. *CTA* computed tomographic angiography

References

1. Kodali SK, Williams MR, Smith CR, Svensson LG, Webb JG, Makkar RR, et al. Two-year outcomes after transcatheter or surgical aortic-valve replacement. N Engl J Med. 2012;366(18):1686–95.
2. Makkar RR, Fontana GP, Jilaihawi H, Kapadia S, Pichard AD, Douglas PS, et al. Transcatheter aortic-valve replacement for inoperable severe aortic stenosis. N Engl J Med. 2012;366(18):1696–704.
3. Reynolds MR, Magnuson EA, Lei Y, Walczak J, Vilaine K, Zajarias A, et al. Cost effectiveness of transcatheter aortic valve replacement compared with surgical aortic valve replacement in patients with severe aortic stenosis: results from the PARTNER trial. J Am Coll Cardiol. 2011;58(20):xiii.
4. Reynolds MR, Magnuson EA, Wang K, Lei Y, Vilain K, Walczak J, et al. Cost-effectiveness of transcatheter aortic valve replacement compared with standard care among inoperable patients with severe aortic stenosis: results from the placement of aortic transcatheter valves (PARTNER) trial (Cohort B). Circulation. 2012;125(9): 1102–9.
5. Paterick TE, Jan MF, Paterick ZR, Tajik AJ, Gerber TC. Cardiac imaging modalities with ionizing radiation: the role of informed consent. JACC Cardiovasc Imaging. 2012;5(6):634–40.
6. FDA. Draft Guidance for Industry and FDA Staff: Heart Valves – Investigational Device Exemption (IDE) and Premarket Approval (PMA) Applications. http://www.fda.gov/medicaldevices/deviceregulationandguidance/guidancedocuments/ucm193096.htm. 2011.
7. Schultz CJ, Tzikas A, Moelker A, Rossi A, Nuis RJ, Geleijnse MM, et al. Correlates on MDCT of paravalvular aortic regurgitation after transcatheter aortic valve implantation using the medtronic CoreValve prosthesis. Catheter Cardiovasc Interv. 2011;78(3):446–55.
8. Willson AB, Rodes-Cabau J, Wood DA, Leipsic J, Cheung A, Toggweiler S, et al. Transcatheter aortic valve replacement with the St. Jude Medical Portico valve: first-in-human experience. J Am Coll Cardiol. 2012;60(7):581–6.
9. Low RI, Bolling SF, Yeo KK, Ebner A. Direct flow medical percutaneous aortic valve: proof of concept. EuroIntervention. 2008;4(2):256–61.

10. Gada H, Kapadia SR, Tuzcu EM, Svensson LG, Marwick TH. Markov model for selection of aortic valve replacement versus transcatheter aortic valve implantation (without replacement) in high-risk patients. Am J Cardiol. 2012;109(9):1326–33.
11. Kempfert J, Treede H, Rastan AJ, Schonburg M, Thielmann M, Sorg S, et al. Transapical aortic valve implantation using a new self-expandable bioprosthesis (ACURATE TA): 6-month outcomes. Eur J Cardiothorac Surg. 2013;43(1):52–6.
12. Sundermann SH, Grunenfelder J, Corti R, Rastan AJ, Linke A, Lange R, et al. Feasibility of the Engager aortic transcatheter valve system using a flexible over-the-wire design. Eur J Cardiothorac Surg. 2012;42(4):e48–52.
13. Treede H, Mohr FW, Baldus S, Rastan A, Ensminger S, Arnold M, et al. Transapical transcatheter aortic valve implantation using the JenaValve system: acute and 30-day results of the multicentre CE-mark study. Eur J Cardiothorac Surg. 2012;41(6):e131–8.
14. Altiok E, Koos R, Schroder J, Brehmer K, Hamada S, Becker M, et al. Comparison of two-dimensional and three-dimensional imaging techniques for measurement of aortic annulus diameters before transcatheter aortic valve implantation. Heart. 2011;97(19):1578–84.
15. Dashkevich A, Blanke P, Siepe M, Pache G, Langer M, Schlensak C, et al. Preoperative assessment of aortic annulus dimensions: comparison of noninvasive and intraoperative measurement. Ann Thorac Surg. 2011;91(3):709–14.
16. Gurvitch R, Webb JG, Yuan R, Johnson M, Hague C, Willson AB, et al. Aortic annulus diameter determination by multidetector computed tomography: reproducibility, applicability, and implications for transcatheter aortic valve implantation. JACC Cardiovasc Interv. 2011;4(11):1235–45.
17. Leipsic J, Gurvitch R, Labounty TM, Min JK, Wood D, Johnson M, et al. Multidetector computed tomography in transcatheter aortic valve implantation. JACC Cardiovasc Imaging. 2011;4(4):416–29.
18. Schoenhagen P, Tuzcu EM, Kapadia SR, Desai MY, Svensson LG. Three-dimensional imaging of the aortic valve and aortic root with computed tomography: new standards in an era of transcatheter valve repair/implantation. Eur Heart J. 2009;30(17):2079–86.
19. Schultz CJ, Moelker A, Piazza N, Tzikas A, Otten A, Nuis RJ, et al. Three dimensional evaluation of the aortic annulus using multislice computer tomography: are manufacturer's guidelines for sizing for percutaneous aortic valve replacement helpful? Eur Heart J. 2010;31(7):849–56.
20. Jabbour A, Ismail TF, Moat N, Gulati A, Roussin I, Alpendurada F, et al. Multimodality imaging in transcatheter aortic valve implantation and post-procedural aortic regurgitation: comparison among cardiovascular magnetic resonance, cardiac computed tomography, and echocardiography. J Am Coll Cardiol. 2011;58(21):2165–73.
21. Hutter A, Opitz A, Bleiziffer S, Ruge H, Hettich I, Mazzitelli D, et al. Aortic annulus evaluation in transcatheter aortic valve implantation. Catheter Cardiovasc Interv. 2010;76(7):1009–19.
22. Kempfert J, Van Linden A, Lehmkuhl L, Rastan AJ, Holzhey D, Blumenstein J, et al. Aortic annulus sizing: echocardiographic vs. computed tomography derived measurements in comparison with direct surgical sizing. Eur J Cardiothorac Surg. 2012;42(4):627–33.
23. Messika-Zeitoun D, Serfaty JM, Brochet E, Ducrocq G, Lepage L, Detaint D, et al. Multimodal assessment of the aortic annulus diameter: implications for transcatheter aortic valve implantation. J Am Coll Cardiol. 2010;55(3):186–94.
24. Tamborini G, Fusini L, Gripari P, Muratori M, Cefalu C, Maffessanti F, et al. Feasibility and accuracy of 3DTEE versus CT for the evaluation of aortic valve annulus to left main ostium distance before transcatheter aortic valve implantation. JACC Cardiovasc Imaging. 2012;5(6):579–88.
25. Tzikas A, Schultz CJ, Piazza N, Moelker A, Van Mieghem NM, Nuis RJ, et al. Assessment of the aortic annulus by multislice computed tomography, contrast aortography, and trans-thoracic echocardiography in patients referred for transcatheter aortic valve implantation. Catheter Cardiovasc Interv. 2011;77(6):868–75.
26. Willson AB, Webb JG, Labounty TM, Achenbach S, Moss R, Wheeler M, et al. 3-dimensional aortic annular assessment by multidetector computed tomography predicts moderate or severe paravalvular regurgitation after transcatheter aortic valve replacement: a multicenter retrospective analysis. J Am Coll Cardiol. 2012;59(14):1287–94.
27. Jilaihawi H, Kashif M, Fontana G, Furugen A, Shiota T, Friede G, et al. Cross-sectional computed tomographic assessment improves accuracy of aortic annular sizing for transcatheter aortic valve replacement and reduces the incidence of paravalvular aortic regurgitation. J Am Coll Cardiol. 2012;59(14):1275–86.
28. Hamdan A, Guetta V, Konen E, Goitein O, Segev A, Raanani E, et al. Deformation dynamics and mechanical properties of the aortic annulus by 4-dimensional computed tomography insights into the functional anatomy of the aortic valve complex and implications for transcatheter aortic valve therapy. J Am Coll Cardiol. 2012;59(2):119–27.
29. Delgado V, Ng AC, van de Veire NR, van der Kley F, Schuijf JD, Tops LF, et al. Transcatheter aortic valve implantation: role of multi-detector row computed tomography to evaluate prosthesis positioning and deployment in relation to valve function. Eur Heart J. 2010;31(9):1114–23.
30. Anderson RH. Clinical anatomy of the aortic root. Heart. 2000;84(6):670–3.
31. Anderson R, Becker A, Piazza N. The anatomy of the aortic valvar complex. In: Serruys P, Piazza N, Cribier A, Webb J, Laborde J-C, de Jaegere P, editors. Transcatheter aortic valve implantation: tips and tricks to avoid failure. New York/London: Informa Healthcare; 2010. p. 1–17.
32. Owens DS, Budoff MJ, Katz R, Takasu J, Shavelle DM, Carr JJ, et al. Aortic valve calcium independently predicts coronary and cardiovascular events in a primary prevention population. JACC Cardiovasc Imaging. 2012;5(6):619–25.
33. Yared K, Garcia-Camarero T, Fernandez-Friera L, Llano M, Durst R, Reddy AA, et al. Impact of aortic regurgitation after transcatheter aortic valve implantation: results from the REVIVAL trial. JACC Cardiovasc Imaging. 2012;5(5):469–77.
34. Haensig M, Lehmkuh L, Holzhey D, Mukherjee C, Kempfert J, Walther T, et al. Aortic valve calcium scoring (AVCS) is a predictor of significant paravalvular aortic insufficiency in transapical aortic valve implantation. J Am Coll Cardiol. 2011;58(20):B203.
35. Haensig M, Lehmkuhl L, Rastan AJ, Kempfert J, Mukherjee C, Gutberlet M, et al. Aortic valve calcium scoring is a predictor of significant paravalvular aortic insufficiency in transapical-aortic valve implantation. Eur J Cardiothorac Surg. 2012;41(6):1234–40.
36. John D, Buellesfeld L, Yuecel S, Mueller R, Latsios G, Beucher H, et al. Correlation of Device landing zone calcification and acute procedural success in patients undergoing transcatheter aortic valve implantations with the self-expanding CoreValve prosthesis. JACC Cardiovasc Interv. 2010;3(2):233–43.
37. Koos R, Mahnken AH, Dohmen G, Brehmer K, Gunther RW, Autschbach R, et al. Association of aortic valve calcification severity with the degree of aortic regurgitation after transcatheter aortic valve implantation. Int J Cardiol. 2011;150(2):142–5.
38. Nombela-Franco L, Rodes-Cabau J, DeLarochelliere R, Larose E, Doyle D, Villeneuve J, et al. Predictive factors, efficacy, and safety of balloon post-dilation after transcatheter aortic valve implantation with a balloon-expandable valve. JACC Cardiovasc Interv. 2012;5(5):499–512.
39. Jatene MB, Monteiro R, Guimaraes MH, Veronezi SC, Koike MK, Jatene FB, et al. Aortic valve assessment. Anatomical study of 100 healthy human hearts. Arq Bras Cardiol. 1999;73(1):75–86.

40. McAlpine W. An introduction to the aortoventricular unit. In: McAlpine W, editor. An anatomical atlas for clinical diagnosis, radiological investigation, and surgical treatment. Berlin: Springer; 1975. p. 9–27.
41. Abedin Z, Goldberg J. Origin and length of left main coronary artery: its relation to height, weight, sex, age, pattern of coronary distribution, and presence or absence of coronary artery disease. Cathet Cardiovasc Diagn. 1978;4(3):335–40.
42. Tops LF, Wood DA, Delgado V, Schuijf JD, Mayo JR, Pasupati S, et al. Noninvasive evaluation of the aortic root with multislice computed tomography implications for transcatheter aortic valve replacement. JACC Cardiovasc Imaging. 2008;1(3):321–30.
43. Akhtar M, Tuzcu EM, Kapadia SR, Svensson LG, Greenberg RK, Roselli EE, et al. Aortic root morphology in patients undergoing percutaneous aortic valve replacement: evidence of aortic root remodeling. J Thorac Cardiovasc Surg. 2009;137(4):950–6.
44. Knight J, Kurtcuoglu V, Muffly K, Marshall Jr W, Stolzmann P, Desbiolles L, et al. Ex vivo and in vivo coronary ostial locations in humans. Surg Radiol Anat. 2009;31(8):597–604.
45. Gogas BD, Zacharoulis AA, Antoniadis AG. Acute coronary occlusion following TAVR. Catheter Cardiovasc Interv. 2011;77(3):435–8.
46. Kapadia SR, Svensson L, Tuzcu EM. Successful percutaneous management of left main trunk occlusion during percutaneous aortic valve replacement. Catheter Cardiovasc Interv. 2009;73(7):966–72.
47. Tuzcu EM, Kapadia SR. Left main occlusion with transcatheter aortic valve replacement. Catheter Cardiovasc Interv. 2011;78(4):660–1.
48. Seipelt RG, Hanekop GG, Schoendube FA, Schillinger W. Heart team approach for transcatheter aortic valve implantation procedures complicated by coronary artery occlusion. Interact Cardiovasc Thorac Surg. 2012;14(4):431–3.
49. Webb JG. Coronary obstruction due to transcatheter valve implantation. Catheter Cardiovasc Interv. 2009;73(7):973.
50. Gurvitch R, Cheung A, Bedogni F, Webb JG. Coronary obstruction following transcatheter aortic valve-in-valve implantation for failed surgical bioprostheses. Catheter Cardiovasc Interv. 2011;77(3):439–44.
51. Bagur R, Rodes-Cabau J, Gurvitch R, Dumont E, Velianou JL, Manazzoni J, et al. Need for permanent pacemaker as a complication of transcatheter aortic valve implantation and surgical aortic valve replacement in elderly patients with severe aortic stenosis and similar baseline electrocardiographic findings. JACC Cardiovasc Interv. 2012;5(5):540–51.
52. Houthuizen P, Van Garsse LA, Poels TT, de Jaegere P, van der Boon RM, Swinkels BM, et al. Left bundle-branch block induced by transcatheter aortic valve implantation increases risk of death. Circulation. 2012;126(6):720–8.
53. Buellesfeld L, Stortecky S, Heg D, Hausen S, Mueller R, Wenaweser P, et al. Impact of permanent pacemaker implantation on clinical outcome among patients undergoing transcatheter aortic valve implantation. J Am Coll Cardiol. 2012;60(6):493–501.
54. Chorianopoulos E, Krumsdorf U, Pleger ST, Katus HA, Bekeredjian R. Improved procedural results after CoreValve implantation with the new AccuTrak delivery system. J Interv Cardiol. 2012;25(2):174–9.
55. Munoz-Garcia A, Garcia JMH, Briales JHA, Navarro MFJ, Franco A, Mora MJM, et al. Impact of the need for permanent pacemaker requirement after coreValve prosthesis implantation with the new Accutrak delivery Catheter System. J Am Coll Cardiol. 2011;58(20):B202.
56. Tchetche D, Modine T, Farah B, Vahdat O, Sudre A, Koussa M, et al. Update on the need for a permanent pacemaker after transcatheter aortic valve implantation using the CoreValve(R) Accutrak system. EuroIntervention. 2012;8(5):556–62.
57. Piazza N, Marra S, Webb J, D'Amico M, Rinaldi M, Boffini M, et al. Two cases of aneurysm of the anterior mitral valve leaflet associated with transcatheter aortic valve endocarditis: a mere coincidence? J Thorac Cardiovasc Surg. 2010;140(3):e36–8.
58. Wong DR, Boone RH, Thompson CR, Allard MF, Altwegg L, Carere RG, et al. Mitral valve injury late after transcatheter aortic valve implantation. J Thorac Cardiovasc Surg. 2009;137(6):1547–9.
59. Mesa Rubio D, Suarez de Lezo Cruz Conde J, Alvarez-Osorio MP, Ruiz Ortiz M, Delgado Ortega M, Leon del Pino Mdel C, et al. Measurement of aortic valve annulus using different cardiac imaging techniques in transcatheter aortic valve implantation: agreement with finally implanted prosthesis size. Echocardiography. 2011;28(4):388–96.
60. Schultz CJ, Weustink A, Piazza N, Otten A, Mollet N, Krestin G, et al. Geometry and degree of apposition of the CoreValve ReValving system with multislice computed tomography after implantation in patients with aortic stenosis. J Am Coll Cardiol. 2009;54(10):911–8.

Native and Prosthetic Valve Stenosis

9

Pei-Hsiu Huang and David P. Faxon

Abstract

Aortic stenosis (AS) is the most common valvular heart disease in adults. Left untreated, AS inevitably worsens and leads to significant morbidity and mortality. Replacing the aortic valve, whether by surgical means or, more recently, transcatheter procedures, remains the only definitive therapy for treating AS. The increasing interest in AS has driven the need for a more sophisticated understanding of the pathophysiology and national history of AS. This chapter focuses primarily on discussion of AS, including etiology, pathophysiology, clinical presentation, hemodynamics, natural history, and medical and surgical therapy.

Keywords

Aortic stenosis • Prosthetic valve • Epidemiology • Pathophysiology • Natural history • Transcatheter aortic valve replacement • Surgical aortic valve replacement • Balloon aortic valvuloplasty • Medical treatment

Introduction

Aortic stenosis (AS) is the most common valvular heart disease in adults and, if left untreated, leads to significant morbidity and mortality. Calcification of a normal trileaflet (Fig. 9.1a) or congenital bicuspid aortic valve (Fig. 9.1b) comprises the principal etiologies of aortic valve stenosis in adults. The incidence of rheumatic AS, where adhesions and commissural fusion cause leaflet thickening and restricted motion (Fig. 9.1c), has declined as the frequency of rheumatic fever has decreased in developed nations [1]. The only effective therapy in the past for severe AS has been surgical valve replacement. With the development of transcatheter aortic valve replacement (TAVR), a significant number of patients who are high risk for surgery are now being considered for TAVR. The increasing interest in AS has driven the need for a more sophisticated understanding of the pathophysiology and national history of AS. This chapter focuses primarily on discussion of AS, including etiology, pathophysiology, clinical presentation, hemodynamics, natural history, and medical and surgical therapy.

Historical Perspective

The pathologist Lazare Rivière first described aortic valve stenosis in 1663 [2]. A few years later in 1672, Carolus Rayger reported a case of sudden death due to AS [3]. Pathological evaluations in both of these cases demonstrated heavy calcifications of the aortic valve, but the young age of these patients caused physicians to relate their stenotic valves to congenital causes. It was not until 1812 that Napoleon's physician Jean Corvisart described the clinical manifestations of AS [4] with William Stokes describing the characteristic murmur decades later in 1854 [5]. Following the introduction of cardiac catheterization in 1955, Schnabel characterized the

P.-H. Huang, MD
Cardiovascular Division, Department of Medicine, Brigham and Women's Hospital, Harvard Medical School, 75 Francis Street, Boston, MA 02115, USA
e-mail: phuang@alum.emory.edu

D.P. Faxon, MD (✉)
Cardiovascular Division, Department of Medicine, Brigham and Women's Hospital, Harvard Medical School, 1620 Tremont Street, OBC-3-12J, Boston, MA 02115, USA
e-mail: dfaxon@partners.org

J.K. Min et al. (eds.), *Multimodality Imaging for Transcatheter Aortic Valve Replacement*, DOI 10.1007/978-1-4471-2798-7_9, © Springer-Verlag London 2014

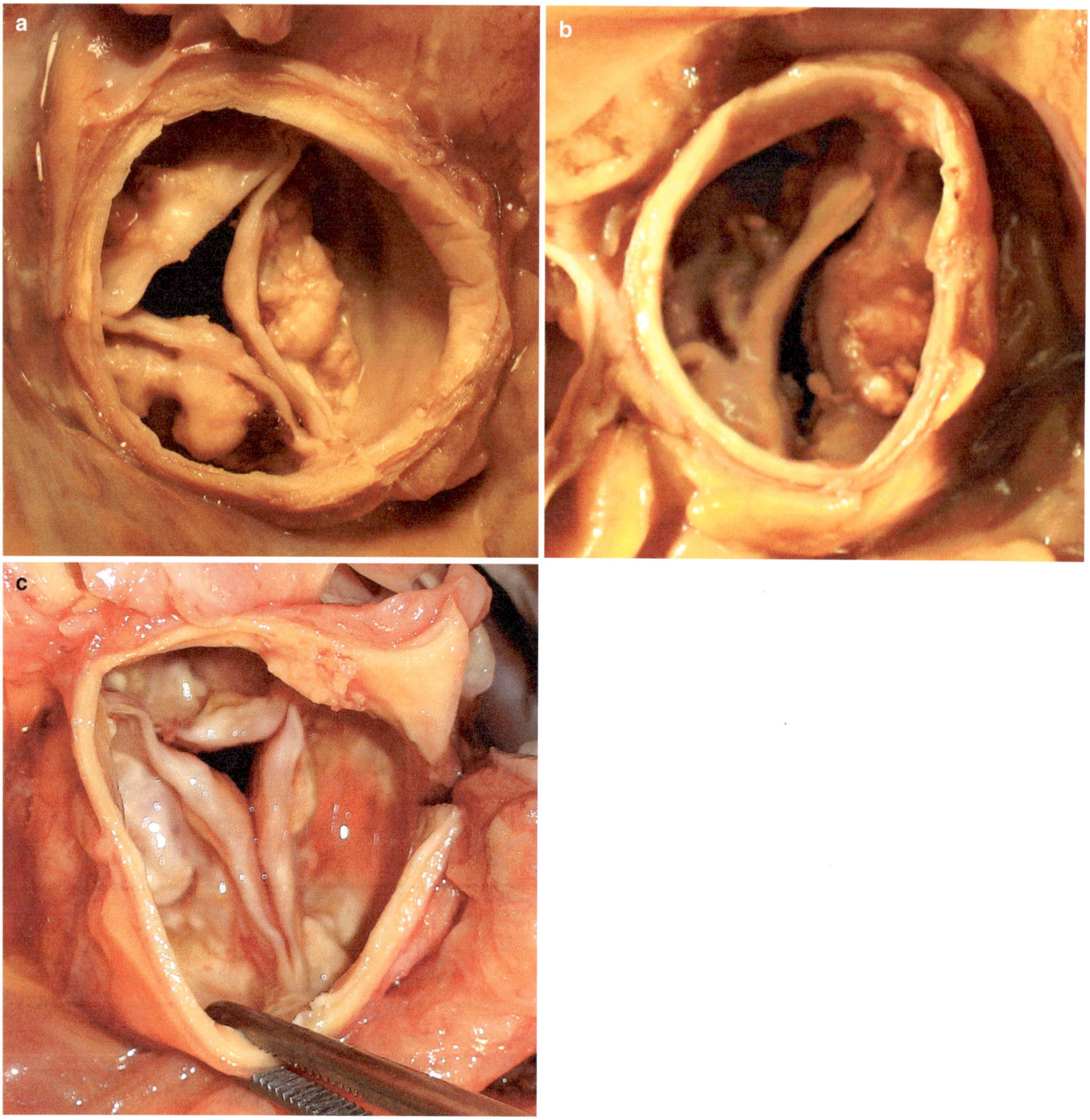

Fig. 9.1 Etiologies of valvular stenosis: (**a**) Calcific aortic valve stenosis. (**b**) Congenital bicuspid aortic valve stenosis. (**c**) Rheumatic aortic valve stenosis (Images courtesy of Michael A. Seidman, M.D., Ph.D., Cardiovascular Pathology Fellow, Department of Pathology, Brigham & Women's Hospital and Harvard Medical School, Boston, MA)

hemodynamic basis of assessing the severity of AS by simultaneous measurement of aortic and left ventricular pressures [6]. Using these pressure measurements, Gorlin developed a formula to calculate the orifice area of the stenotic aortic valve [7], and this became the gold standard technique to quantitate the degree of AS until the development of accurate noninvasive echocardiographic methods.

The early surgical treatments for AS were fraught with high rates of morbidity and mortality. In 1913, Tuffier performed the first operation for AS, a digital commissurotomy, which was of limited success. The era of aortic valve replacement (AVR) started with the implantation of the first prosthetic aortic valve in 1952 by Hufnagel. Introduction of cardiopulmonary bypass in the mid-1950s helped transform AVR into the standard of care for severe AS where the volume has grown to more than 300,000 surgical valve replacements worldwide each year [8]. Transcatheter aortic valve replacement (TAVR) was approved in Europe in 2007, and it

Table 9.1 Prevalence of valvular heart diseases in population-based studies

	Age (years)					*p* value for trend	Frequency adjusted to 2000 US adult population
	18–44	45–54	55–64	65–74	≥75		
Participants (*n*)	4,351	696	1,240	3,879	1,745		202,128,094
Male, *n* (%)	1,959 (45 %)	258 (37 %)	415 (33 %)	1,586 (41 %)	826 (47 %)		100,994,367 (48 %)
Mitral regurgitation (*n*=449)	23, 0.5 % (0.3–0.8)	1, 0.1 % (0–0.8)	12, 1.0 %(0.5–1.8)	250, 6.4 % (5.7–7.3)	163, 9.3 % (8.1–10.9)	<0.0001	1.7 % (1.5–1.9)
Mitral stenosis (*n*=15)	0, 0 % (0–0.1)	1, 0.1 % (0–0.8)	3, 0.2 % (0.1–0.7)	7, 0.2 % (0.1–0.4)	4, 0.2 % (0.1–0.6)	0.006	0.1 % (0.02–0.2)
Aortic regurgitation (*n*=90)	10, 0.2 % (0.1–0.4)	1, 0.1 % (0–0.8)	8, 0.7 % (0.3–1.3)	37, 1.0 % (0.7–1.3)	34, 2.0 % (1.4–2.7)	<0.0001	0.5 % (0.3–0.6)
Aortic stenosis (*n*=102)	1, 0.02 % (0–0.1)	1, 0.1 % (0–0.8)	2, 0.2 % (0.6–1.9)	50, 1.3 % (1.0–1.7)	48, 2.8 % (2.1–3.7)	<0.0001	0.4 % (0.3–0.5)
Any valve disease							
Overall (*n*=615)	31, 0.7 % (0.5–1.0)	3, 0.4 % (0.1–1.3)	23, 1.9 %(1.2–2.8)	328, 8.5 % (7.6–9.4)	230, 13.2 % (11.7–15.0)	<0.0001	2.5 % (2.2–2.7)
Women (*n*=365)	19, 0.8 % (0.5–1.3)	1, 0.2 % (0.01–1.3)	13, 1.6 % (0.9–2.7)	208, 9.1 % (8.0–10.4)	115, 12.6 % (10.6–15.0)	<0.0001	2.4 % (2.1–2.8)
Men (*n*=259)	12, 0.6 % (0.3–1.1)	2, 0.8 % (0.1–2.8)	10, 2.4 % (1.2–4.4)	120, 7.6 % (6.3–9.0)	115, 14.0 % (11.7–16.6)	<0.0001	2.5 % (2.1–2.9)

From Nkomo et al. [10]
Data presented as *n*, % (95 % confidence interval)

is estimated that 60,000 have since been placed worldwide. The Edwards Sapien valve was approved in the USA in 2011 and significant growth in the use of TAVR is anticipated.

Epidemiology

The prevalence of AS steadily increased in the nineteenth century as a result of the rise in the incidence of rheumatic heart disease. Recognition of the association of rheumatic fever with cardiac disease is largely attributable to J. B. Boullaud in 1835. At its peak in 1,900, an estimated 1 in 1,000 people in the USA had the disease, but the incidence subsequently declined dramatically to less than 3,000 cases each year and a mortality of <1 % [9].

The current prevalence of valvular heart disease is not well defined. The difficulty of determining the true prevalence of valvular heart disease stems from the long asymptomatic latent phase of the disease, a factor likely contributing to the significant underdiagnosis in the elderly. Additionally, many studies are affected by a selection bias of patients referred for screening echocardiography and, thus, likely do not capture the true prevalence. Pooled analysis from three large epidemiologic studies provides the best estimates, reporting a 2.5 % prevalence of valvular heart disease in the general population (Table 9.1) [10]. The prevalence of valvular heart disease increases with age. In those above the age of 75 years, the prevalence of valvular heart disease rises to nearly 12 % (Fig. 9.2).

Currently in the USA, degenerative calcific AS comprises the most common cause of AS, largely the result of the

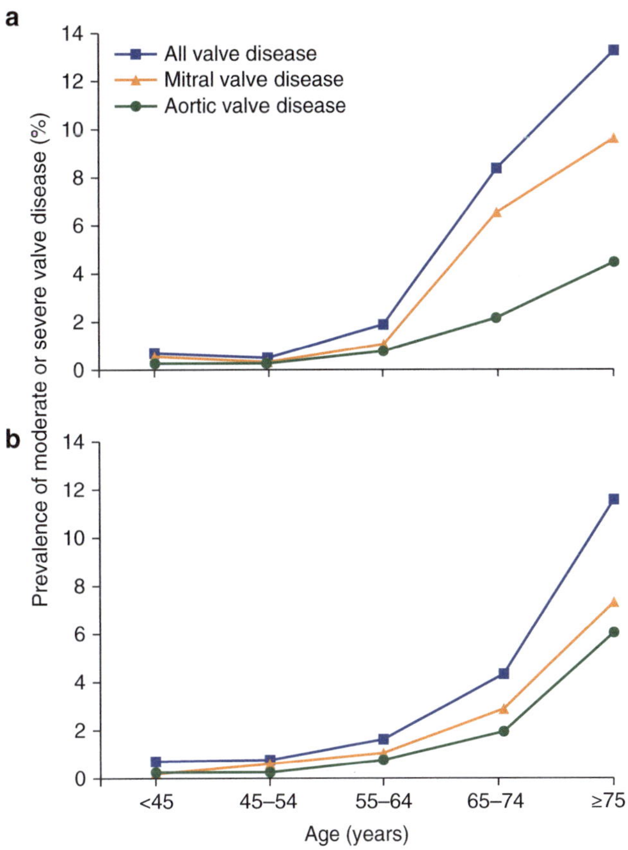

Fig. 9.2 Prevalence of valvular heart disease by age from (**a**) pooled population-based studies and (**b**) an Olmsted County community study (From Nkomo et al. [10])

Table 9.2 Etiology of native left-sided single valve disease

	Aortic stenosis $n=1,197$	Aortic regurgitation $n=369$	Mitral stenosis $n=336$	Mitral regurgitation $n=877$
Degenerative (%)	81.9	50.3	12.5	61.3
Rheumatic (%)	11.2	15.2	85.4	14.2
Endocarditis (%)	0.8	7.5	0.6	3.5
Inflammatory (%)	0.1	4.1	0	0.8
Congenital (%)	5.4	15.2	0.6	4.8
Ischemic (%)	0	0	0	7.3
Other (%)	0.6	7.7	0.9	8.1

From Iung et al. [11]

aging population. The Euro Heart Survey in 2003 found that among those with AS, 82 % were due to degenerative disease, 11 % from rheumatic causes, and 5 % from congenital causes (Table 9.2) [11]. In underdeveloped countries, however, rheumatic heart disease continues as the major cause of valvular heart disease.

Pathophysiology

The understanding of the pathophysiology of degenerative AS has significantly advanced with improved understanding of the cellular mechanisms and the process of calcification [12, 13]. Leaflet thickening and calcification, which progress to calcified nodules, form the hallmark of calcific AS (Fig. 9.3). These calcium deposits eventually compromise valve leaflet mobility, in effect narrowing the effective valve orifice. The pathological findings are well described and reviewed in a separate section of this text.

Current evidence suggests that oxidative stress initiates early valve sclerosis. The combination of lipid deposition, neuroendocrine, and hemodynamic factors may propagate these changes. In susceptible patients, valvular interstitial and endothelial cells develop an osteoblastic phenotype and begin producing pro-calcific mediators, collagen, and osteopontin to ultimately promote bone formation. The progression of disease is due to both oxidant stress and inflammation causing an increase in extracellular matrix deposition and calcification. Despite the known role of the renin-angiotensin system and lipids, clinical trials have not demonstrated the effectiveness ACE inhibitors or statins in slowing the progression of AS [14–20]. Recent evidence suggests that genetic factors, particularly inflammatory and lipid markers such as IL-10 and Apo B, may be important predictors of calcific aortic disease [21].

Progression to severe AS occurs gradually over a period of several decades. As obstruction of the left ventricular outflow worsens, the left ventricle (LV) remodels to compensate for the significant systolic pressure overload. This remodeling leads to development of concentric left ventricular hypertrophy where the ventricular chamber remains a normal size despite an increase in the wall thickness [22, 23]. The resulting increase in wall thickness allows LV to maintain normal wall stress (i.e., afterload) in the setting of elevated chamber pressures and a normal ejection fraction [24]. However, a normal ejection fraction does not necessarily indicate normal contractility, as the former may be the augmented by preload reserve. When the ventricular hypertrophy cannot adequately compensate for the degree of pressure overload due to severe outflow obstruction, the ejection fraction begins to decline [24, 25]. At this point, decreased myocardial contractility potentially contributes to the depressed ejection fraction as well [26].

As a consequence of left ventricular hypertrophy and interstitial fibrosis of the cardiac myocytes, the left ventricular chamber compliance decreases causing diastolic dysfunction [27, 28]. The increased stiffness of the LV creates higher pressures at all volumes requiring elevation in diastolic filling pressures. In this setting, a prominent *a*-wave is seen on the pressure tracing due to its more forceful contraction and the decreased compliance of the LV. Indeed, left atrial contraction contributes a great deal to left ventricular filling in these situations [29]. This becomes important in situations where left atrial contraction is lost and can lead to a significant decline in left ventricular performance. After AVR to relieve the left ventricular outflow obstruction, the hypertrophic LV may regress though the concentric stiffness from residual interstitial fibrosis still results in diastolic dysfunction [27].

In the absence of significant volume overload, patients with AS typically experience the classic symptoms on exertion. The mechanisms for development of systolic and diastolic heart failure are discussed above. Syncope probably occurs as a result of a combination of mechanisms [30]. The most direct mechanism relates to the inability to augment cardiac output adequately in the presence of a fixed outflow obstruction. During exercise, the deficit of cardiac output in the setting of a drop in systemic arterial resistance causes a fall in blood pressure and syncope. Various arrhythmias including atrial flutter, atrial fibrillation, and ventricular tachycardia have been observed in patients with AS during episodes of syncope. Additional postulated mechanisms include a vasodepressor effect from left ventricular baroreceptor activation as a response to highly elevated LV pressures during exercise [31].

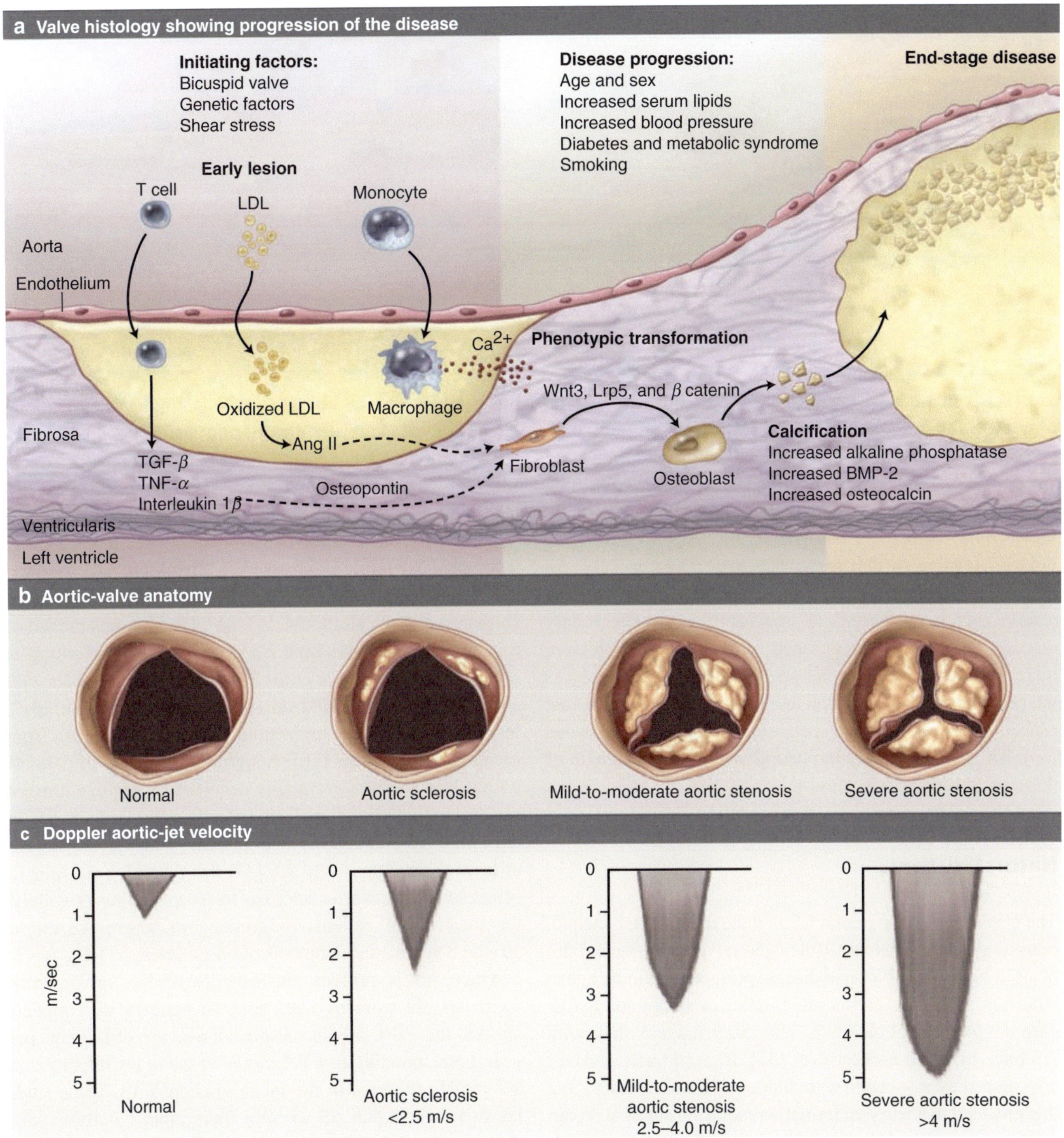

Fig. 9.3 Pathophysiology of calcific aortic stenosis. (**a**) The histology of the early lesion is characterized by a subendothelial accumulation of oxidized low-density lipoprotein (*LDL*), production of angiotensin (*Ang*) II, and inflammation with T lymphocytes and macrophages. Disease progression occurs by several mechanisms including local production of proteins, such as osteopontin, osteocalcin, and bone morphogenetic protein 2 (*BMP-2*), which mediate tissue calcification; activation of inflammatory signaling pathways including tumor necrosis factor-*α* (*TNF-α*), tumor growth factor-*β* (*TGF-β*), the complement system, C-reactive protein, and interleukin-1*β*; and changes in tissue matrix including the accumulation of tenascin C, and upregulation of matrix metalloproteinase-2 and alkaline phosphatase activity. In addition, leaflet fibroblasts undergo phenotypic transformation into osteoblasts, regulated by the Wnt3-Lrp5-*β* catenin signaling pathway. Microscopic accumulations of extracellular calcification (Ca^{2+}) are present early in the disease process, with progressive calcification as the disease progresses and areas of frank bone formation in end-stage disease. The corresponding changes in the aortic valve anatomy are viewed from the aortic side with the valve open in systole (**b**) and the corresponding Doppler aortic jet velocity (**c**) (From Otto [142])

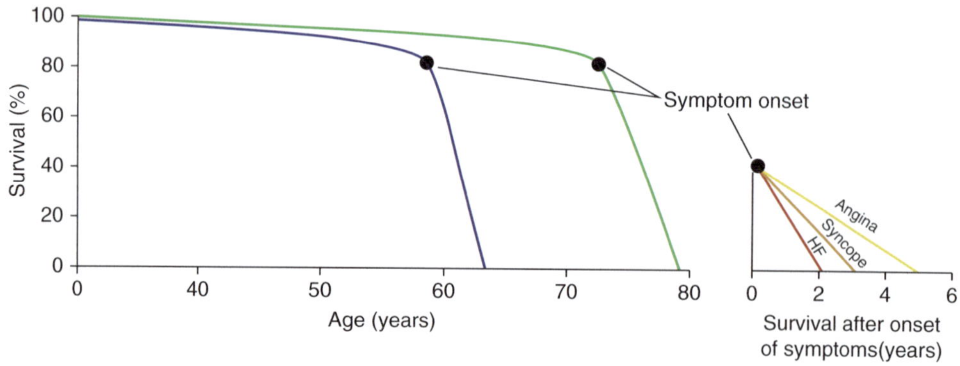

Fig. 9.4 Natural history of aortic stenosis. The *blue line* represents the disease course as described by Ross and Braunwald. In contemporary times, the disease course may more closely represent the *green line*. The average survival after development of heart failure (*HF*), syncope, or angina is shown in the *inset* (Figure derived from Ross et al. [38])

A suggested mechanism for angina in AS focuses on the oxygen supply/demand mismatch that is accentuated during exercise or periods of tachycardia to cause subendocardial ischemia. The hypertrophied LV in AS consumes more oxygen due to the increased myocardial muscle mass, increased work from systolic pressure overload, and prolonged ejection period due to LV outflow obstruction. At rest, coronary blood flow, while elevated in absolute terms, may be normal or reduced relative to the myocardial mass. Additionally, the hypertrophied ventricle also has a limited coronary flow reserve even in the absence of significant epicardial coronary disease [32, 33]. The elevated intraventricular pressure increases the transmyocardial pressure, which can compress the coronary microcirculation and affect coronary perfusion, especially when coronary perfusion pressure is exceeded [34]. The prolonged ejection period also limits the length of diastole and coronary perfusion.

Natural History

The etiologies of congenital AS include unicuspid, bicuspid, or tricuspid valve anatomy. Unicuspid valves cause severe stenosis at birth while bicuspid disease presents in middle age to elderly. Despite this earlier presentation of symptomatic disease, up to 20 % of elderly patients 80 years and older with AS have bicuspid aortic valves [35]. Bicuspid aortic valves are commonly associated with dilation of the ascending aorta that can lead to aneurysm formation requiring surgical repair. Additionally, bicuspid aortic valves may cluster within families, exhibiting an autosomal dominant with incomplete penetrance pattern of heredity [36]. Tricuspid congenital aortic valve disease is less common and difficult to distinguish from acquired disease. Of the acquired causes, rheumatic disease typically presents in the fifth and sixth decade, with younger presentation in underdeveloped countries [37]. Degenerative calcific aortic valve disease is a disease of the elderly increasing significantly with age above 65 years.

Patients with AS progress through the various stages of disease over a period of many decades. The spectrum of disease includes aortic sclerosis (thickened and calcified valve leaflets without obstruction) at the mild end and moves through worsening degrees of obstruction to severe AS at its most severe. Progression of disease is highlighted by a long latent phase lasting decades during which patients remain asymptomatic and have a low risk of cardiac or sudden death [38, 39]. However, the rate of survival rapidly declines following the onset of symptoms (Fig. 9.4).

An estimated 26 % of the population over the age of 65 years old have aortic sclerosis [40]. Histologic data suggests that aortic sclerosis occurs through a degenerative process similar to that of calcific AS [41–45]. Despite the absence of a significant hemodynamic effect on cardiac performance, aortic sclerosis is not an entirely benign lesion. Patients with aortic sclerosis identified on echocardiogram have a 50 % increase in the risk of myocardial infarction and death from cardiovascular causes [46]. A significant portion of patients with aortic sclerosis eventually develop AS. Up to a third of patients with aortic sclerosis eventually progress to having at least mild AS and that 2.5 % of patients with aortic sclerosis ultimately develop severe AS [47–49]. Although the time to progressing from aortic sclerosis to severe AS varies widely, the majority of patients progressing to severe AS do so around 8 years after diagnosis of aortic sclerosis [47].

Once AS is present, the severity of the valve stenosis invariably worsens with time. In patients with moderate AS, the valve area decreases an average of 0.1 cm^2 per year, corresponding to a 0.3 m/s increase in jet velocity and a 7 mmHg increase in the mean gradient [50]. Some studies also suggest that AS worsens more rapidly in those with degenerative calcific AS compared with those having congenital or rheumatic aortic valve stenosis [51].

At the onset of symptoms, survival of patients with AS decreases precipitously. Braunwald and Ross reported that in patients with severe AS, death occurs approximately 2 years after the onset of heart failure, 3 years after syncope related to valve stenosis, and 5 years after developing angina (Fig. 9.4) [38]. Subsequent studies have consistently demonstrated similarly poor prognosis of patients with symptomatic severe AS who do not undergo AVR [39, 52–61]. In the PARTNER trial, death occurred in nearly 70 % of patients randomized to contemporary medical therapy over

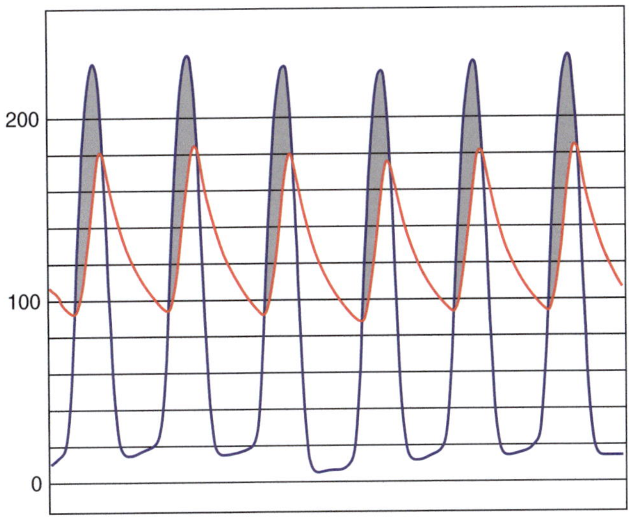

Fig. 9.5 Simultaneous left ventricular (*blue*) and aortic (*red*) pressures as measured by cardiac catheterization. The shaded region (*gray*) highlights the transaortic valve gradient

2 years, which included the use of balloon aortic valvuloplasty [60, 61].

Hemodynamic Assessment

When the physical examination raises suspicion for AS, the next step of the evaluation involves hemodynamic measurements to determine the severity of the valve stenosis. Historically, cardiac catheterization represented the diagnostic standard in hemodynamic assessment because of its ability to obtain direct, real-time pressure measurements of both the LV and aorta (Fig. 9.5). Obtaining a mean transvalvular gradient and cardiac output allows for calculation of the aortic valve orifice area [7]. Noninvasive hemodynamic assessment by echocardiography has largely replaced invasive catheterization and offers several potential advantages [62]. The transaortic valve gradient can be determined by Doppler data and the aortic valve orifice area determined through the concept of flow conservation via the continuity equation. Table 9.3 details the criteria for classifying the severity of AS [62]. Both measures correlate well to catheterization data and have been validated in multiple studies. Echocardiography also allows for direct visualization of the aortic valve anatomy, assessment of LV function, and evaluation for coexisting valvular lesions. Certain situations such as severe hypertension, pressure recovery in small aortas, and low-flow, low-gradient states may affect the accuracy of the echocardiographic assessment of AS. In these cases and in those where noninvasive studies either do not provide adequate assessment or do not correlate with clinical findings, hemodynamics by cardiac catheterization may be helpful in characterizing the severity of the valve stenosis.

Table 9.3 Classification of aortic stenosis severity

	Mild	Moderate	Severe
Aortic jet velocity (m/s)	2.6–2.9	3.0–4.0	>4.0
Mean gradient (mmHg)	<20[a] (<30)	20–40[a] (30–50[b])	>40[a] (>50[b])
AVA (cm^2)	>1.5	1.0–1.5	<1.0
Indexed AVA (cm^2/m^2)	>0.85	0.6–0.85	<0.6
Velocity ratio	>0.50	0.25–0.50	<0.25

Adapted from Baumgartner et al. [62]
AVA aortic valve area
[a]American Heart Association/American College of Cardiology Guidelines
[b]European Society of Cardiology Guidelines

Asymptomatic Patients

The gradual progression of the severity of outflow tract obstruction occurs over a long period, perhaps 10–15 years. During this latent period, clinical outcomes of patients with mild to moderate stenosis remain favorable [63]. The prognosis of patients with moderate to severe stenosis also remains favorable as long as they remain asymptomatic [63]. The risk of sudden death in asymptomatic patients is less than 1 % per year [64]. However, close follow-up is mandatory, as the disease will inevitably progress. The degree of stenosis at which patients develop symptoms is variable with symptomatic patients generally having more severe stenosis [65]. The rate of progression to symptomatic AS has been studied extensively. The strongest predictor of symptom development is the Doppler velocity of the antegrade aortic valve jet [64, 66, 67]. Those with moderate to severe aortic valve calcification or a rapidly increasing aortic valve velocity also have poor clinical outcomes [63]. Furthermore, in asymptomatic patients with very severe AS (peak antegrade aortic jet velocity of ≥5.0 m/s by echocardiography), AVR or cardiac death occurred in 36 % at 1 year and 64 % at 2 years [59]. In that study, the subgroup of patients with a Doppler velocity of ≥5.5 m/s had the worst outcomes, with the rate of AVR or death occurring in 56 % at 1 year and 75 % at 2 years.

Patients with asymptomatic AS may underestimate the degree of their symptoms, making evaluation and management difficult for the physician. As symptoms develop over a long period of time, patients may slowly self-limit and not perceive the development of symptoms or simply attribute progressive deconditioning to natural aging. In evaluating patients with asymptomatic severe AS, exercise stress testing and stress echocardiography may help with assessment of exercise capacity and functional valve hemodynamics to guide decision-making [68]. Risk scores may also help with assessment of asymptomatic patients. Female sex, peak aortic velocity, and B-type natriuretic peptide independently predict need for AVR or death within 24 months, suggesting that valve interventions could also benefit select asymptomatic patients with severe AS [69].

Symptomatic Patients

When AS becomes moderate to severe, patients may present with the classic symptoms of angina, exertional dyspnea or congestive heart failure, and syncope. At this stage, patients have a poor long-term prognosis if the LV outflow obstruction is not treated. In addition to angina due to the effects of ventricular hypertrophy from AS, patients often have angina from concomitant coronary atherosclerosis. Up to half of patients with severe AS also have significant coronary artery disease [70, 71]. Accordingly the ACC/AHA valvular heart disease guidelines suggest coronary angiography in patients over the age of 35 with risk factors for coronary disease being considered for AVR (Box 9.1) [72]. While patients commonly experience dyspnea with exertion, frank congestive heart failure typically occurs during later stages of the disease when ventricular function deteriorates and cardiac output declines from chronic LV outflow obstruction. In situations where poor LV function and decreased cardiac output result in low aortic valve gradients—termed low-flow, low-gradient AS—estimating the degree of AS becomes challenging. The characteristic late peaking systolic murmur of aortic valve stenosis becomes subtle and easy to overlook. In the elderly patients, other typical physical findings such as *parvis* and *tardis* pulse, single second heart sound, and a precordial thrill may be absent. On echocardiography, motion of a calcified aortic valve may appear restricted due to the low cardiac output of a poorly functioning ventricle alone. Using dobutamine to augment cardiac output aids in differentiating this "pseudo AS" from true severe AS [68]. Patients displaying contractile reserve with dobutamine also have more favorable outcomes, including improvement in LV function, after AVR [73–76]. Invasive hemodynamic assessment by cardiac catheterization can also help in assessment in these patients.

Box 9.1 ACC/AHA Guideline Indications for Aortic Valve Replacement [72]

Class I	AVR is indicated for symptomatic patients with severe AS. (*Level of Evidence: B*)
	AVR is indicated for symptomatic patients with severe AS undergoing coronary artery bypass graft surgery. (*Level of Evidence: C*)
	AVR is indicated for symptomatic patients with severe AS undergoing surgery on the aorta or other heart valves. (*Level of Evidence: C*)
	AVR is recommended for patients with severe AS and LV systolic dysfunction (ejection fraction less than 0.50). (*Level of Evidence: C*)
Class IIa	AVR is reasonable for patients with moderate AS undergoing CABG or surgery on the aorta or other heart valves. (*Level of Evidence: B*)
Class IIb	AVR may be considered for asymptomatic patients with severe AS and abnormal response to exercise (e.g., development of symptoms or asymptomatic hypotension). (*Level of Evidence: C*)
	AVR may be considered for adults with severe asymptomatic if there is a high likelihood of rapid progression (age, calcification, and CAD) or if surgery might be delayed at the time of symptom onset. (*Level of Evidence: C*)
	AVR may be considered in patients undergoing CABG who have mild AS when there is evidence, such as moderate to severe valve calcification, that progression may be rapid. AVR may be considered for asymptomatic patients with severe AS and abnormal response to exercise (e.g., development of symptoms or asymptomatic hypotension). (*Level of Evidence: C*)
	AVR may be considered for asymptomatic patients with extremely severe AS (aortic valve area less than 0.6 cm^2, mean gradient greater than 60 mmHg, and jet velocity greater than 5.0 m/s) when the patient's expected operative mortality is 1.0 % or less. AVR may be considered for asymptomatic patients with severe AS and abnormal response to exercise (e.g., development of symptoms or asymptomatic hypotension). (*Level of Evidence: C*)
Class III	AVR is not useful for the prevention of sudden death in asymptomatic patients with AS who have none of the findings listed under the Class IIa/IIb recommendations. (*Level of Evidence: B*)

AVR aortic valve replacement, *AS* aortic stenosis, *LV* left ventricle, *CAD* coronary artery disease, *CABG* coronary artery bypass surgery

Medical Treatment

Medical treatment of symptomatic AS offers limited benefit as no current therapy has demonstrated the ability to alter the disease course. The contemporary understanding of calcific AS attributes valve calcification to an active process rather than a passive degenerative one. Several studies have demonstrated the association of calcific AS with the traditional risk factors and cellular mechanisms of atherosclerosis [15, 40, 43, 45, 77–81]. Despite the suggestion that these risk factors may represent targets of therapy [82, 83], none have yet effectively delayed or prevented progression of aortic valve stenosis. While reports had showed the potential benefit of statins and angiotensin-converting enzyme inhibitors in preventing disease progression [14–19], the large-scale, prospective, randomized trial failed to demonstrate a benefit of using atorvastatin to slow the progression of AS over 3 years of follow-up [20].

In spite of the lack of benefit in affecting disease progression, medical therapy plays a definite role in symptomatic management of heart failure from AS, particularly in patients whose comorbidities preclude them from undergoing an AVR operation. Some precautions need to be considered in patients with severe AS. Beta-adrenergic antagonists may depress left ventricular contractility and worsen heart failure. Diuretics help manage fluid accumulation in those with heart failure but as in the case of other antihypertensive agents, excessive diuresis will decrease preload excessively and impact LV filling and thus cardiac output, which can lead to orthostatic symptoms or syncope.

The use of vasodilators has been thought to improve hemodynamics in AS. Vasodilators should be used cautiously as hypotension could cause detrimental hemodynamic effects in patients with severe AS. However, multiple studies have demonstrated that vasodilator agents may be well tolerated when used judiciously. Sodium nitroprusside [84, 85] and angiotensin-converting enzyme inhibitor [86–88] administration may result in hemodynamic and symptomatic improvement at the cost of hypotension in some cases. More recently, a small pilot study suggested that phosphodiesterase type 5 inhibition with sildenafil also improves hemodynamics in patients with severe AS [89].

Atrial arrhythmias are uncommon in isolated aortic valve disease, likely because left atrial enlargement occurs late in the disease process. In the hypertrophied LV of AS, the atrial contraction can contribute a significant portion of LV filling, and these patients may quickly deteriorate to developing heart failure. Patients with severe AS may also have significant hypotension due the sudden fall of cardiac output when these episodes develop so treatment should be administered promptly.

Aortic Valve Replacement

Currently, AVR is the only definitive treatment for relieving the left ventricular outflow tract obstruction in AS. The timing of surgery should correspond to the onset of symptoms as patients have a poor long-term prognosis after this point (Box 9.1). Replacement of the stenotic valve immediately improves hemodynamics, improves symptoms, and ultimately improves survival [54, 90, 91]. Patients with LV dysfunction also have a similar survival benefit, but they may not have a pronounced improvement in symptoms or LV function if the initial LV dysfunction did not occur as a direct consequence of the LV outflow obstruction [74, 76, 92–94]. Presence of LV contractile reserve on dobutamine stress echocardiography appears to positively affect postoperative outcomes [73–76]. However, even in the absence of LV contractile reserve, patients had better outcomes with aortic valve replacement compared with medical therapy [76].

Operative mortality in patients without significant comorbidities such as LV dysfunction ranges between 2 and 5 % at most centers in North America, having decreased over the period between 1997 and 2006 [95]. In patients younger than 70 years old, the operative mortality for isolated AVR is as low as 1 %. The 2008 report from the Society of Thoracic Surgeons National Database Committee found that the overall operative mortality for those undergoing isolated AVR is 3.2 % and for those having AVR and concomitant CABG is 5.6 % [96, 97]. Factors that increase the perioperative risk of mortality include older age, presence of LV dysfunction, higher New York Heart Association (NYHA) functional class, presence of CAD, renal dysfunction, and chronic pulmonary disease. Notably, the increasing life expectancy will lead to a growing population of elderly patients with AS. As centers gain more experience in performing AVR in elderly patients, perioperative mortality has improved, with contemporary risks ranging from 4 to 6 % [98–100]. Age alone should no longer preclude these patients from undergoing surgery. However, elderly patients often have multiple additional comorbidities that increase surgical risk [101]. Risk estimation can be performed using the commonly used, well-validated risk scores from the Society of Thoracic Surgeons [96, 97, 102] and the European System for Cardiac Operative Risk Evaluation [103].

Despite the potential benefits gained through AVR, a large portion of patients with symptomatic severe AS do not undergo the operation. Several series have reported that between 40 and 60 % of potential surgical candidates with severe AS underwent AVR [58, 104–106]. Common reasons for foregoing aortic valve surgery include increased surgical risk due to comorbidities and age as well as patient refusal. In some cases, patients had not undergone evaluation by a cardiac surgeon [58]. One series demonstrated a racial disparity among patients undergoing AVR due to the difference in the rates of patient refusal [106].

In recent years, development of transcatheter aortic valve replacement (TAVR) has introduced an alternative to the traditional aortic valve surgery for treatment of patients with severe AS. The landmark first human implantation was performed by Cribier and his team on April 16, 2002, in a patient with significant comorbidities that made him ineligible for surgical intervention [107]. Since then, around 50,000 patients worldwide have undergone TAVR through 2011 [108]. Two transcatheter valve systems are currently in widespread use: the CoreValve self-expandable valve (Medtronic Inc., Minneapolis, Minnesota) and the Edwards Sapien balloon-expandable valve (Edwards Lifesciences LLC, Irvine, California). A variety of other investigational devices may see their way into clinical trials soon.

The current indications for TAVR include use in patients at high operative risk for undergoing a traditional surgical AVR. The US pivotal PARTNER trial randomized two subsets of patients to standard-of-care therapy or TAVR. In the first subset of patients considered unsuitable candidates for surgical AVR, TAVR resulted in an absolute reduction in death of 31 % through 2 years of follow-up compared with standard medical therapy, which included the use of balloon aortic valvuloplasty in 84 % of patients [61]. The other subset of patients included high-risk surgical candidates (STS score ≥10 %), and TAVR resulted in similar rates of death and symptomatic improvement through the 2-year follow-up [109]. Numerous registries including the German Transcatheter Aortic Valve Interventions Registry [110], SOURCE Registry [111], UK TAVI Registry [112], ADVANCE study [113], CoreValve Italian Registry [114], and FRANCE 2 [115] have provided additional data on outcomes with TAVR and experience with additional indications.

Balloon Aortic Valvuloplasty

Percutaneous balloon dilation of a stenotic aortic valve in patients with calcific AS was initially developed as a potential alternative to surgical AVR. Cribier first reported the use of balloon aortic valvuloplasty (BAV) in three adult patients with severe AS [116]. The procedure has since moved through many roles in the treatment of calcific AS. Balloon dilation of a calcified aortic valve primarily causes fracture of the leaflet calcium deposits and less commonly separation of fused commissures [117, 118]. While this may result in an immediate, though modest, increase in valve area and hemodynamic improvements, the gains are short-lived [119–122]. Restenosis and recurrence of symptoms occurred in most patients within 6–12 months and patients continued to have a poor prognosis despite the initial procedural success. With post-procedure survival rates of 52–84 % at 1 year and 23–37 % at 3 years, BAV does not appear to significantly alter the natural history of the disease [120–122]. However, in patients who subsequently underwent AVR after BAV, 95 % survived after 1 year, making this a potential therapeutic "bridge" to more definitive treatment [122]. BAV has also been used as a palliative treatment in some settings. The use of BAV steadily declined in the late 1980s and 1990s but has met renewed interest in the era of TAVR as a preliminary treatment for patients in whom the benefits of AVR remain uncertain [123–125].

Prosthetic Valve Stenosis

Patients undergoing AVR typically end up with either a mechanical aortic valve prosthesis or a biological aortic valve prosthesis (bioprosthetic valve). Mechanical valve prostheses carry the advantage of longer durability at the cost of requiring treatment with systemic anticoagulation. On the other hand, bioprosthetic valves allow patients to avoid long-term anticoagulation but lack the longevity due to degeneration compared with their mechanical counterparts. As such, bioprosthetic valves have traditionally been reserved for use in patients over the age of 65 years, in whom studies have demonstrated excellent survival and freedom from reoperation [126–128]. Contemporary surgical practice has seen increasing use of bioprotheses in patients younger than 65 years undergoing surgery for left heart valve replacement [95, 129, 130]. The issue of bioprosthetic valve degeneration (Fig. 9.6) will become more common as more patients survive longer than the expected durability of these devices (Fig. 9.7).

The mechanisms responsible for bioprosthetic valve failure include leaflet degeneration, calcification, and destruction or structural compromise due to thrombus, pannus, or paravalvular leaks. Younger age at implant, mitral valve position, and renal failure comprise some of the common risk factors for bioprosthetic valve failure [131–134]. The typical risk factors for atherosclerosis such as hypercholesterolemia, metabolic syndrome, and diabetes have also been implicated in the degeneration of bioprosthetic valves [135–137]. In the current bioprosthetic heart valves, freedom from failure at 10 years is 70–90 % and at 15 years is 40 and 70 % [128, 131, 132, 134]. Unfortunately, patients undergoing reoperation do so at an elevated risk because of older age and comorbidities [138–140]. This patient population represents another potential use for TAVR as an alternative to reoperation [141].

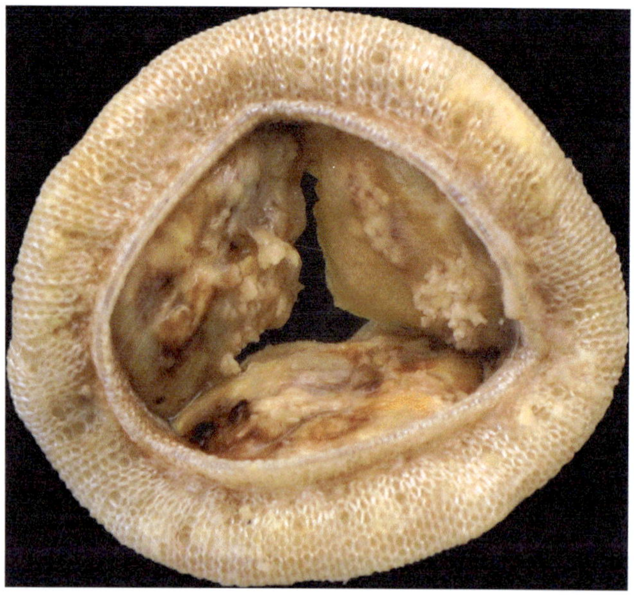

Fig. 9.6 Bioprosthetic valve degeneration (Image courtesy of Michael A. Seidman, M.D., Ph.D., Cardiovascular Pathology Fellow, Department of Pathology, Brigham & Women's Hospital and Harvard Medical School, Boston, MA)

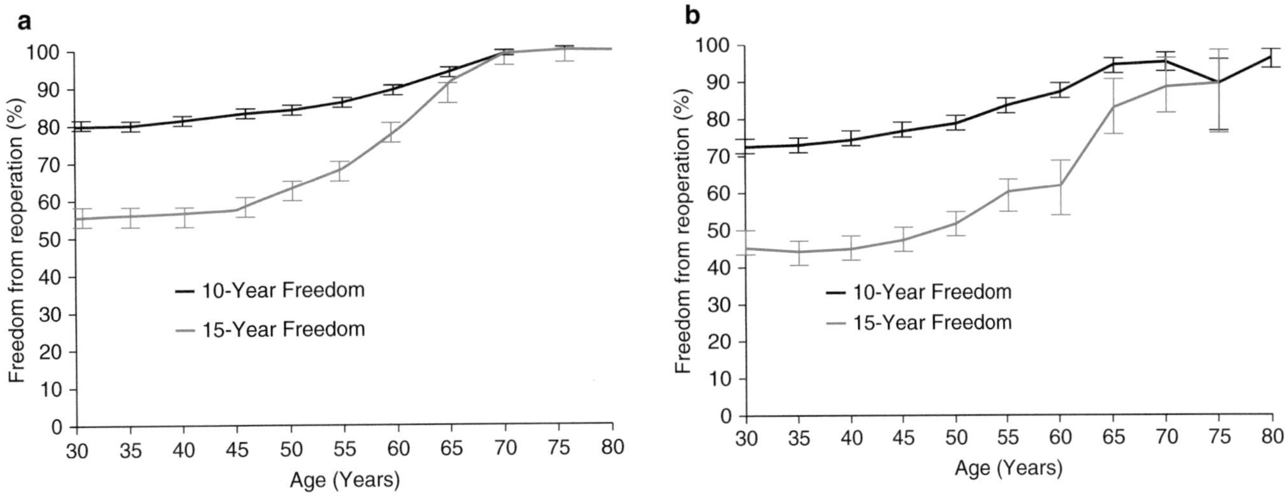

Fig. 9.7 Freedom from reoperation at 10 and 15 years (95 % confidence interval) according to age at operation for aortic valve replacement (**a**) and mitral valve replacement (**b**) (From Chan et al. [128])

Conclusion

Calcific AS commonly affects the elderly population and the prevalence is increasing as the population ages. Left untreated, the chronic obstruction of the LV outflow results in the slow deterioration of LV performance, eventually leading to heart failure and death. While the current understanding of the mechanisms responsible for development of AS is limited, newer concepts may lead to innovative preventive therapy. The only effective treatment is either surgical AVR or TAVR as medical therapy has a limited role and balloon valvuloplasty does not appear to confer long-term benefit. Earlier diagnosis should allow for consideration for valve replacement at an optimal time to prevent the serious consequences of untreated disease.

References

1. Selzer A. Changing aspects of the natural history of valvular aortic stenosis. N Engl J Med. 1987;317(2):91–8.
2. Rivière L. Opera Medica Universa. Observationum medicarum, centuria IV, observatio XXI, Cordis palpitatio pulses inaequalitas. Sumptibus Antoni, Cellier: Lugduni; 1663. p. 83.
3. Bonet T. Sepulchretum; sive, anatomia practica, ex cadaveribos morbo denatis, proponens historias et observationes omnium humani corporis affectuum. Genevae: Sumptibus Leonardi Chouet; 1679. p. 702.
4. Corvisart JN. Essai sur les maladies et les lésions organiques du coeur. Paris, 1806. Translated by J. Gates, 1812. In: Willius FA, Keys TE, editors. Cardiac classics. St. Louis: CV Mosby; 1941. p. 285.
5. Stokes W. The diseases of the heart and aorta. Extreme ossific disease of the aortic orifice. Dublin: Hodges and Smith; 1854. p. 139–58.
6. Schnabel Jr T, Blakemore W, Kuo P, Langfield S. Left heart catheterization in aortic and mitral disease. J Clin Invest. 1955;34:915–23.
7. Gorlin R, Gorlin SG. Hydraulic formula for calculation of the area of the stenotic mitral valve, other cardiac valves, and central circulatory shunts. I. Am Heart J. 1951;41(1):1–29.
8. Weinberg EJ, Schoen FJ, Mofrad MRK. A computational model of aging and calcification in the aortic heart valve. PLoS One. 2009;4(6):e5960.
9. Roger VL, Go AS, Lloyd-Jones DM, et al. Heart disease and stroke statistics – 2011 update: a report from the American Heart Association. Circulation. 2011;123(4):e18–209.
10. Nkomo VT, Gardin JM, Skelton TN, Gottdiener JS, Scott CG, Enriquez-Sarano M. Burden of valvular heart diseases: a population-based study. Lancet. 2006;368(9540):1005–11.
11. Iung B, Baron G, Butchart EG, et al. A prospective survey of patients with valvular heart disease in Europe: The Euro Heart Survey on Valvular Heart Disease. Eur Heart J. 2003;24(13):1231–43.
12. Leopold JA. Cellular mechanisms of aortic valve calcification. Circ Cardiovasc Interv. 2012;5(4):605–14.
13. Rajamannan NM, Evans FJ, Aikawa E, et al. Calcific aortic valve disease: not simply a degenerative process: a review and agenda for research from the National Heart and Lung and Blood Institute Aortic Stenosis Working Group. Executive summary: calcific aortic valve disease-2011 update. Circulation. 2011;124(16):1783–91.
14. Aronow WS, Ahn C, Kronzon I, Goldman ME. Association of coronary risk factors and use of statins with progression of mild valvular aortic stenosis in older persons. Am J Cardiol. 2001;88(6):693–5.
15. Pohle K, Mäffert R, Ropers D, et al. Progression of aortic valve calcification: association with coronary atherosclerosis and cardiovascular risk factors. Circulation. 2001;104(16):1927–32.
16. Shavelle DM, Takasu J, Budoff MJ, Mao S, Zhao XQ, O'Brien KD. HMG CoA reductase inhibitor (statin) and aortic valve calcium. Lancet. 2002;359(9312):1125–6.
17. O'Brien KD, Probstfield JL, Caulfield MT, et al. Angiotensin-converting enzyme inhibitors and change in aortic valve calcium. Arch Intern Med. 2005;165(8):858–62.
18. Bellamy MF, Pellikka PA, Klarich KW, Tajik AJ, Enriquez-Sarano M. Association of cholesterol levels, hydroxymethylglutaryl coenzyme-A reductase inhibitor treatment, and progression of aortic stenosis in the community. J Am Coll Cardiol. 2002;40(10):1723–30.
19. Rosenhek R, Rader F, Loho N, et al. Statins but not angiotensin-converting enzyme inhibitors delay progression of aortic stenosis. Circulation. 2004;110(10):1291–5.
20. Cowell SJ, Newby DE, Prescott RJ, et al. A randomized trial of intensive lipid-lowering therapy in calcific aortic stenosis. N Engl J Med. 2005;352(23):2389–97.

21. Bosse Y, Mathieu P, Pibarot P. Genomics: the next step to elucidate the etiology of calcific aortic valve stenosis. J Am Coll Cardiol. 2008;51(14):1327–36.
22. Sasayama S, Ross J, Franklin D, Bloor CM, Bishop S, Dilley RB. Adaptations of the left ventricle to chronic pressure overload. Circ Res. 1976;38(3):172–8.
23. Spann JF, Bove AA, Natarajan G, Kreulen T. Ventricular performance, pump function and compensatory mechanisms in patients with aortic stenosis. Circulation. 1980;62(3):576–82.
24. Krayenbuehl HP, Hess OM, Ritter M, Monrad ES, Hoppeler H. Left ventricular systolic function in aortic stenosis. Eur Heart J. 1988;9(Suppl E):19–23.
25. Gunther S, Grossman W. Determinants of ventricular function in pressure-overload hypertrophy in man. Circulation. 1979; 59(4):679–88.
26. Huber D, Grimm J, Koch R, Krayenbuehl HP. Determinants of ejection performance in aortic stenosis. Circulation. 1981;64(1): 126–34.
27. Hess OM, Ritter M, Schneider J, Grimm J, Turina M, Krayenbuehl HP. Diastolic stiffness and myocardial structure in aortic valve disease before and after valve replacement. Circulation. 1984;69(5):855–65.
28. Murakami T, Hess OM, Gage JE, Grimm J, Krayenbuehl HP. Diastolic filling dynamics in patients with aortic stenosis. Circulation. 1986;73(6):1162–74.
29. Stott DK, Marpole DG, Bristow JD, Kloster FE, Griswold HE. The role of left atrial transport in aortic and mitral stenosis. Circulation. 1970;41(6):1031–41.
30. Schwartz LS, Goldfischer J, Sprague GJ, Schwartz SP. Syncope and sudden death in aortic stenosis. Am J Cardiol. 1969;23(5):647–58.
31. Richards AM, Nicholls MG, Ikram H, Hamilton EJ, Richards RD. Syncope in aortic valvular stenosis. Lancet. 1984;2(8412):1113–6.
32. Marcus ML, Doty DB, Hiratzka LF, Wright CB, Eastham CL. Decreased coronary reserve: a mechanism for angina pectoris in patients with aortic stenosis and normal coronary arteries. N Engl J Med. 1982;307(22):1362–6.
33. Rajappan K, Rimoldi OE, Dutka DP, et al. Mechanisms of coronary microcirculatory dysfunction in patients with aortic stenosis and angiographically normal coronary arteries. Circulation. 2002;105(4):470–6.
34. Hittinger L, Mirsky I, Shen YT, Patrick TA, Bishop SP, Vatner SF. Hemodynamic mechanisms responsible for reduced subendocardial coronary reserve in dogs with severe left ventricular hypertrophy. Circulation. 1995;92(4):978–86.
35. Roberts WC, Janning KG, Ko JM, Filardo G, Matter GJ. Frequency of congenitally bicuspid aortic valves in patients ≥80 years of age undergoing aortic valve replacement for aortic stenosis (with or without aortic regurgitation) and implications for transcatheter aortic valve implantation. Am J Cardiol. 2012;109(11):1632–6.
36. Braverman AC, Güven H, Beardslee MA, Makan M, Kates AM, Moon MR. The bicuspid aortic valve. Curr Probl Cardiol. 2005;30(9):470–522.
37. Marijon E, Mirabel M, Celermajer DS, Jouven X. Rheumatic heart disease. Lancet. 2012;379(9819):953–64.
38. Ross JJ, Braunwald E. Aortic stenosis. Circulation. 1968;38(1 Suppl):61–7.
39. Kelly TA, Rothbart RM, Cooper CM, Kaiser DL, Smucker ML, Gibson RS. Comparison of outcome of asymptomatic to symptomatic patients older than 20 years of age with valvular aortic stenosis. Am J Cardiol. 1988;61(1):123–30.
40. Stewart BF, Siscovick D, Lind BK, et al. Clinical factors associated with calcific aortic valve disease. Cardiovascular Health Study. J Am Coll Cardiol. 1997;29(3):630–4.
41. Olsson M, Dalsgaard CJ, Haegerstrand A, Rosenqvist M, Rydén L, Nilsson J. Accumulation of T lymphocytes and expression of interleukin-2 receptors in nonrheumatic stenotic aortic valves. J Am Coll Cardiol. 1994;23(5):1162–70.
42. Olsson M, Rosenqvist M, Nilsson J. Expression of HLA-DR antigen and smooth muscle cell differentiation markers by valvular fibroblasts in degenerative aortic stenosis. J Am Coll Cardiol. 1994;24(7):1664–71.
43. Otto CM, Kuusisto J, Reichenbach DD, Gown AM, O'Brien KD. Characterization of the early lesion of "degenerative" valvular aortic stenosis. Histological and immunohistochemical studies. Circulation. 1994;90(2):844–53.
44. O'Brien KD, Kuusisto J, Reichenbach DD, et al. Osteopontin is expressed in human aortic valvular lesions. Circulation. 1995;92(8): 2163–8.
45. O'Brien KD, Reichenbach DD, Marcovina SM, Kuusisto J, Alpers CE, Otto CM. Apolipoproteins B, (a), and E accumulate in the morphologically early lesion of "degenerative" valvular aortic stenosis. Arterioscler Thromb Vasc Biol. 1996;16(4):523–32.
46. Otto CM, Lind BK, Kitzman DW, Gersh BJ, Siscovick DS. Association of aortic-valve sclerosis with cardiovascular mortality and morbidity in the elderly. N Engl J Med. 1999;341(3):142–7.
47. Cosmi JE, Kort S, Tunick PA, et al. The risk of the development of aortic stenosis in patients with "benign" aortic valve thickening. Arch Intern Med. 2002;162(20):2345–7.
48. Faggiano P, Antonini-Canterin F, Erlicher A, et al. Progression of aortic valve sclerosis to aortic stenosis. Am J Cardiol. 2003; 91(1):99–101.
49. Novaro GM, Katz R, Aviles RJ, et al. Clinical factors, but not C-reactive protein, predict progression of calcific aortic-valve disease: the Cardiovascular Health Study. J Am Coll Cardiol. 2007; 50(20):1992–8.
50. Bonow RO, Carabello BA, Chatterjee K, et al. 2008 Focused Update Incorporated Into the ACC/AHA 2006 Guidelines for the Management of Patients With Valvular Heart Disease. J Am Coll Cardiol. 2008;52(13):e1–142.
51. Wagner S, Selzer A. Patterns of progression of aortic stenosis: a longitudinal hemodynamic study. Circulation. 1982;65(4):709–12.
52. Frank S, Johnson A, Ross J. Natural history of valvular aortic stenosis. Br Heart J. 1973;35(1):41–6.
53. Chizner MA, Pearle DL, deLeon AC. The natural history of aortic stenosis in adults. Am Heart J. 1980;99(4):419–24.
54. Schwarz F, Baumann P, Manthey J, et al. The effect of aortic valve replacement on survival. Circulation. 1982;66(5):1105–10.
55. Turina J, Hess O, Sepulcri F, Krayenbuehl HP. Spontaneous course of aortic valve disease. Eur Heart J. 1987;8(5):471–83.
56. Horstkotte D, Loogen F. The natural history of aortic valve stenosis. Eur Heart J. 1988;9(Suppl E):57–64.
57. Lindroos M, Kupari M, Heikkilä J, Tilvis R. Prevalence of aortic valve abnormalities in the elderly: an echocardiographic study of a random population sample. J Am Coll Cardiol. 1993;21(5): 1220–5.
58. Bach DS, Siao D, Girard SE, Duvernoy C, McCallister BD, Gualano SK. Evaluation of patients with severe symptomatic aortic stenosis who do not undergo aortic valve replacement: the potential role of subjectively overestimated operative risk. Circ Cardiovasc Qual Outcomes. 2009;2(6):533–9.
59. Rosenhek R, Zilberszac R, Schemper M, et al. Natural history of very severe aortic stenosis. Circulation. 2010;121(1):151–6.
60. Leon MB, Smith CR, Mack M, et al. Transcatheter aortic-valve implantation for aortic stenosis in patients who cannot undergo surgery. N Engl J Med. 2010;363(17):1597–607.
61. Makkar RR, Fontana GP, Jilaihawi H, et al. Transcatheter aortic-valve replacement for inoperable severe aortic stenosis. N Engl J Med. 2012;366(18):1696–704.
62. Baumgartner H, Hung J, Bermejo J, et al. Echocardiographic assessment of valve stenosis: EAE/ASE recommendations for clinical practice. J Am Soc Echocardiogr. 2009;22(1):1–23.
63. Rosenhek R, Binder T, Porenta G, et al. Predictors of outcome in severe, asymptomatic aortic stenosis. N Engl J Med. 2000;343(9):611–7.

64. Pellikka PA, Sarano ME, Nishimura RA, et al. Outcome of 622 adults with asymptomatic, hemodynamically significant aortic stenosis during prolonged follow-up. Circulation. 2005;111(24):3290–5.
65. Varadarajan P, Kapoor N, Bansal RC, Pai RG. Clinical profile and natural history of 453 nonsurgically managed patients with severe aortic stenosis. Ann Thorac Surg. 2006;82(6):2111–5.
66. Otto CM, Burwash IG, Legget ME, et al. Prospective study of asymptomatic valvular aortic stenosis. Clinical, echocardiographic, and exercise predictors of outcome. Circulation. 1997;95(9):2262–70.
67. Rosenhek R, Klaar U, Schemper M, et al. Mild and moderate aortic stenosis. Natural history and risk stratification by echocardiography. Eur Heart J. 2004;25(3):199–205.
68. Picano E, Pibarot P, Lancellotti P, Monin JL, Bonow RO. The emerging role of exercise testing and stress echocardiography in valvular heart disease. J Am Coll Cardiol. 2009;54(24):2251–60.
69. Monin JL, Lancellotti P, Monchi M, et al. Risk score for predicting outcome in patients with asymptomatic aortic stenosis. Circulation. 2009;120(1):69–75.
70. Ramsdale DR, Bennett DH, Bray CL, Ward C, Beton DC, Faragher EB. Angina, coronary risk factors and coronary artery disease in patients with valvular disease. A prospective study. Eur Heart J. 1984;5(9):716–26.
71. Vandeplas A, Willems JL, Piessens J, De Geest H. Frequency of angina pectoris and coronary artery disease in severe isolated valvular aortic stenosis. Am J Cardiol. 1988;62(1):117–20.
72. Bonow RO, Carabello BA, Chatterjee K, et al. 2008 Focused update incorporated into the ACC/AHA 2006 guidelines for the management of patients with valvular heart disease: a report of the American College of Cardiology/American Heart Association Task Force on Practice Guidelines (Writing Committee to Revise the 1998 Guidelines for the Management of Patients With Valvular Heart Disease): endorsed by the Society of Cardiovascular Anesthesiologists, Society for Cardiovascular Angiography and Interventions, and Society of Thoracic Surgeons. Circulation. 2008;118(15):e523–661.
73. Quéré J-P, Monin JL, Lévy F, et al. Influence of preoperative left ventricular contractile reserve on postoperative ejection fraction in low-gradient aortic stenosis. Circulation. 2006;113(14):1738–44.
74. Lévy F, Laurent M, Monin JL, et al. Aortic valve replacement for low-flow/low-gradient aortic stenosis operative risk stratification and long-term outcome: a European multicenter study. J Am Coll Cardiol. 2008;51(15):1466–72.
75. Clavel MA, Fuchs C, Burwash IG, et al. Predictors of outcomes in low-flow, low-gradient aortic stenosis: results of the multicenter TOPAS Study. Circulation. 2008;118(14 Suppl):S234–42.
76. Tribouilloy C, Lévy F, Rusinaru D, et al. Outcome after aortic valve replacement for low-flow/low-gradient aortic stenosis without contractile reserve on dobutamine stress echocardiography. J Am Coll Cardiol. 2009;53(20):1865–73.
77. Olsson M, Thyberg J, Nilsson J. Presence of oxidized low density lipoprotein in nonrheumatic stenotic aortic valves. Arterioscler Thromb Vasc Biol. 1999;19(5):1218–22.
78. O'Brien KD, Shavelle DM, Caulfield MT, et al. Association of angiotensin-converting enzyme with low-density lipoprotein in aortic valvular lesions and in human plasma. Circulation. 2002;106(17):2224–30.
79. Wilmshurst PT, Stevenson RN, Griffiths H, Lord JR. A case-control investigation of the relation between hyperlipidaemia and calcific aortic valve stenosis. Heart. 1997;78(5):475–9.
80. Ngo MV, Gottdiener JS, Fletcher RD, Fernicola DJ, Gersh BJ. Smoking and obesity are associated with the progression of aortic stenosis. Am J Geriatr Cardiol. 2001;10(2):86–90.
81. Taylor HA, Clark BL, Garrison RJ, et al. Relation of aortic valve sclerosis to risk of coronary heart disease in African-Americans. Am J Cardiol. 2005;95(3):401–4.
82. Palta S, Pai AM, Gill KS, Pai RG. New insights into the progression of aortic stenosis: implications for secondary prevention. Circulation. 2000;101(21):2497–502.
83. Rajamannan NM, Otto CM. Targeted therapy to prevent progression of calcific aortic stenosis. Circulation. 2004;110(10):1180–2.
84. Ikram H, Low CJ, Crozier IG, Shirlaw T. Hemodynamic effects of nitroprusside on valvular aortic stenosis. Am J Cardiol. 1992;69(4):361–6.
85. Khot UN, Novaro GM, Popović ZB, et al. Nitroprusside in critically ill patients with left ventricular dysfunction and aortic stenosis. N Engl J Med. 2003;348(18):1756–63.
86. Martínez Sánchez C, Henne O, Arceo A, et al. [Hemodynamic effects of oral captopril in patients with critical aortic stenosis]. Arch Inst Cardiol Mex. 1996;66(4):322–30.
87. Chockalingam A, Venkatesan S, Subramaniam T, et al. Safety and efficacy of angiotensin-converting enzyme inhibitors in symptomatic severe aortic stenosis: Symptomatic Cardiac Obstruction-Pilot Study of Enalapril in Aortic Stenosis (SCOPE-AS). Am Heart J. 2004;147(4):E19.
88. O'Brien KD, Zhao XQ, Shavelle DM, et al. Hemodynamic effects of the angiotensin-converting enzyme inhibitor, ramipril, in patients with mild to moderate aortic stenosis and preserved left ventricular function. J Investig Med. 2004;52(3):185–91.
89. Lindman BR, Zajarias A, Madrazo JA, et al. Effects of phosphodiesterase type 5 inhibition on systemic and pulmonary hemodynamics and ventricular function in patients with severe symptomatic aortic stenosis. Circulation. 2012;125(19):2353–62.
90. Murphy ES, Lawson RM, Starr A, Rahimtoola SH. Severe aortic stenosis in patients 60 years of age or older: left ventricular function and 10-year survival after valve replacement. Circulation. 1981;64(2 Pt 2):II184–8.
91. Kvidal P, Bergström R, Hörte LG, Stahle E. Observed and relative survival after aortic valve replacement. J Am Coll Cardiol. 2000;35(3):747–56.
92. Smith N, McAnulty JH, Rahimtoola SH. Severe aortic stenosis with impaired left ventricular function and clinical heart failure: results of valve replacement. Circulation. 1978;58(2):255–64.
93. Connolly HM, Oh JK, Orszulak TA, et al. Aortic valve replacement for aortic stenosis with severe left ventricular dysfunction. Prognostic indicators. Circulation. 1997;95(10):2395–400.
94. Pereira JJ, Lauer MS, Bashir M, et al. Survival after aortic valve replacement for severe aortic stenosis with low transvalvular gradients and severe left ventricular dysfunction. J Am Coll Cardiol. 2002;39(8):1356–63.
95. Brown JM, O'Brien SM, Wu C, Sikora JAH, Griffith BP, Gammie JS. Isolated aortic valve replacement in North America comprising 108,687 patients in 10 years: changes in risks, valve types, and outcomes in the Society of Thoracic Surgeons National Database. J Thorac Cardiovasc Surg. 2009;137(1):82–90.
96. O'Brien SM, Shahian DM, Filardo G, et al. The Society of Thoracic Surgeons 2008 cardiac surgery risk models: part 2–isolated valve surgery. Ann Thorac Surg. 2009;88(1 Suppl):S23–42.
97. Shahian DM, O'Brien SM, Filardo G, et al. The Society of Thoracic Surgeons 2008 cardiac surgery risk models: part 3–valve plus coronary artery bypass grafting surgery. Ann Thorac Surg. 2009;88(1 Suppl):S43–62.
98. Vasques F, Messori A, Lucenteforte E, Biancari F. Immediate and late outcome of patients aged 80 years and older undergoing isolated aortic valve replacement: a systematic review and meta-analysis of 48 studies. Am Heart J. 2012;163(3):477–85.
99. Mølstad P, Veel T, Rynning S. Long-term survival after aortic valve replacement in octogenarians and high-risk subgroups. Eur J Cardiothorac Surg. 2012;42:934–40.
100. Di Eusanio M, Fortuna D, Cristell D, et al. Contemporary outcomes of conventional aortic valve replacement in 638 octogenarians: insights from an Italian Regional Cardiac Surgery Registry (RERIC). Eur J Cardiothorac Surg. 2012;41(6):1247–52; discussion 1252–3.

101. Iung B. Management of the elderly patient with aortic stenosis. Heart. 2008;94(4):519–24.
102. Shahian DM, O'Brien SM, Filardo G, et al. The Society of Thoracic Surgeons 2008 cardiac surgery risk models: part 1–coronary artery bypass grafting surgery. Ann Thorac Surg. 2009;88(1 Suppl):S2–22.
103. Nashef SA, Roques F, Michel P, Gauducheau E, Lemeshow S, Salamon R. European system for cardiac operative risk evaluation (EuroSCORE). Eur J Cardiothorac Surg. 1999;16(1):9–13.
104. Bouma BJ, van Den Brink RB, van Der Meulen JH, et al. To operate or not on elderly patients with aortic stenosis: the decision and its consequences. Heart. 1999;82(2):143–8.
105. Charlson E, Legedza ATR, Hamel MB. Decision-making and outcomes in severe symptomatic aortic stenosis. J Heart Valve Dis. 2006;15(3):312–21.
106. Yeung M, Kerrigan J, Sodhi S, et al. Racial Differences in Rates of Aortic Valve Replacement in Patients With Severe Aortic Stenosis. Am J Cardiol. 2013 [Epub ahead of print].
107. Cribier A, Eltchaninoff H, Bash A, et al. Percutaneous transcatheter implantation of an aortic valve prosthesis for calcific aortic stenosis: first human case description. Circulation. 2002;106(24):3006–8.
108. Leon MB. TAVR – The year in review (2011 and 2012 so far)… and a 10-year anniversary. Transcath Valve Ther. Seattle, WA; 2012.
109. Kodali SK, Williams MR, Smith CR, et al. Two-year outcomes after transcatheter or surgical aortic-valve replacement. N Engl J Med. 2012;366(18):1686–95.
110. Zahn R, Gerckens U, Grube E, et al. Transcatheter aortic valve implantation: first results from a multi-centre real-world registry. Eur Heart J. 2011;32(2):198–204.
111. Thomas M, Schymik G, Walther T, et al. One-year outcomes of cohort 1 in the Edwards SAPIEN Aortic Bioprosthesis European Outcome (SOURCE) registry: the European registry of transcatheter aortic valve implantation using the Edwards SAPIEN valve. Circulation. 2011;124(4):425–33.
112. Moat NE, Ludman P, de Belder MA, et al. Long-term outcomes after transcatheter aortic valve implantation in high-risk patients with severe aortic stenosis: the U.K. TAVI (United Kingdom Transcatheter Aortic Valve Implantation) Registry. J Am Coll Cardiol. 2011;58(20):2130–8.
113. Linke A, Gerckens U, Wenaweser P, et al. Treatment of high risk aortic stenosis patients with transcatheter Medtronic CoreValve implantation: results from the international multi-center ADVANCE study. J Am Coll Cardiol. 2012;59(13s1):E8.
114. Ussia GP, Barbanti M, Petronio AS, et al. Transcatheter aortic valve implantation: 3-year outcomes of self-expanding CoreValve prosthesis. Eur Heart J. 2012;33(8):969–76.
115. Gilard M, Eltchaninoff H, Iung B, et al. Registry of transcatheter aortic-valve implantation in high-risk patients. N Engl J Med. 2012;366(18):1705–15.
116. Cribier A, Savin T, Saoudi N, Rocha P, Berland J, Letac B. Percutaneous transluminal valvuloplasty of acquired aortic stenosis in elderly patients: an alternative to valve replacement? Lancet. 1986;1(8472):63–7.
117. McKay RG, Lock JE, Safian RD, et al. Balloon dilation of mitral stenosis in adult patients: postmortem and percutaneous mitral valvuloplasty studies. J Am Coll Cardiol. 1987;9(4):723–31.
118. Isner JM, Samuels DA, Slovenkai GA, et al. Mechanism of aortic balloon valvuloplasty: fracture of valvular calcific deposits. Ann Intern Med. 1988;108(3):377–80.
119. Block PC, Palacios IF. Clinical and hemodynamic follow-up after percutaneous aortic valvuloplasty in the elderly. Am J Cardiol. 1988;62(10 Pt 1):760–3.
120. Ferguson JJ, Riuli EP, Massumi A, et al. Balloon aortic valvuloplasty: the Texas Heart Institute experience. Tex Heart Inst J. 1990;17(1):23–30.
121. Otto CM, Mickel MC, Kennedy JW, et al. Three-year outcome after balloon aortic valvuloplasty. Insights into prognosis of valvular aortic stenosis. Circulation. 1994;89(2):642–50.
122. Lieberman EB, Bashore TM, Hermiller JB, et al. Balloon aortic valvuloplasty in adults: failure of procedure to improve long-term survival. J Am Coll Cardiol. 1995;26(6):1522–8.
123. Ussia GP, Capodanno D, Barbanti M, et al. Balloon aortic valvuloplasty for severe aortic stenosis as a bridge to high-risk transcatheter aortic valve implantation. J Invasive Cardiol. 2010;22(4):161–6.
124. Tissot C-M, Attias D, Himbert D, et al. Reappraisal of percutaneous aortic balloon valvuloplasty as a preliminary treatment strategy in the transcatheter aortic valve implantation era. EuroIntervention. 2011;7(1):49–56.
125. Malkin CJ, Judd J, Chew DP, Sinhal A. Balloon aortic valvuloplasty to bridge and triage patients in the era of trans-catheter aortic valve implantation. Catheter Cardiovasc Interv. 2012;81(2):358–63.
126. Khan SS, Trento A, DeRobertis M, et al. Twenty-year comparison of tissue and mechanical valve replacement. J Thorac Cardiovasc Surg. 2001;122(2):257–69.
127. Ruel M, Chan V, Bédard P, et al. Very long-term survival implications of heart valve replacement with tissue versus mechanical prostheses in adults. Circulation. 2007;116(11 Suppl):I294–300.
128. Chan V, Malas T, Lapierre H, et al. Reoperation of left heart valve bioprostheses according to age at implantation. Circulation. 2011;124(11 Suppl):S75–80.
129. Gammie JS, Sheng S, Griffith BP, et al. Trends in mitral valve surgery in the United States: results from the Society of Thoracic Surgeons Adult Cardiac Surgery Database. Ann Thorac Surg. 2009;87(5):1431–7; discussion 1437–9.
130. Barnett SD, Ad N. Surgery for aortic and mitral valve disease in the United States: a trend of change in surgical practice between 1998 and 2005. J Thorac Cardiovasc Surg. 2009;137(6):1422–9.
131. Jamieson WR, Rosado LJ, Munro AI, et al. Carpentier-Edwards standard porcine bioprosthesis: primary tissue failure (structural valve deterioration) by age groups. Ann Thorac Surg. 1988;46(2):155–62.
132. Jamieson WR, Munro AI, Miyagishima RT, Allen P, Burr LH, Tyers GF. Carpentier-Edwards standard porcine bioprosthesis: clinical performance to seventeen years. Ann Thorac Surg. 1995;60(4):999–1006; discussion 1007.
133. Fann JI, Miller DC, Moore KA, et al. Twenty-year clinical experience with porcine bioprostheses. Ann Thorac Surg. 1996;62(5):1301–11; discussion 1311–2.
134. Ruel M, Kulik A, Rubens FD, et al. Late incidence and determinants of reoperation in patients with prosthetic heart valves. Eur J Cardiothorac Surg. 2004;25(3):364–70.
135. Briand M, Pibarot P, Després J-P, et al. Metabolic syndrome is associated with faster degeneration of bioprosthetic valves. Circulation. 2006;114(1 Suppl):I512–7.
136. Shetty R, Pibarot P, Audet A, et al. Lipid-mediated inflammation and degeneration of bioprosthetic heart valves. Eur J Clin Invest. 2009;39(6):471–80.
137. Lorusso R, Gelsomino S, Lucà F, et al. Type 2 diabetes mellitus is associated with faster degeneration of bioprosthetic valve: results from a propensity score-matched Italian multicenter study. Circulation. 2012;125(4):604–14.
138. Jones JM, O'kane H, Gladstone DJ, et al. Repeat heart valve surgery: risk factors for operative mortality. J Thorac Cardiovasc Surg. 2001;122(5):913–8.
139. Maganti M, Rao V, Armstrong S, Feindel CM, Scully HE, David TE. Redo valvular surgery in elderly patients. Ann Thorac Surg. 2009;87(2):521–5.
140. Leontyev S, Borger MA, Davierwala P, et al. Redo aortic valve surgery: early and late outcomes. Ann Thorac Surg. 2011;91(4):1120–6.
141. Gurvitch R, Cheung A, Ye J, et al. Transcatheter valve-in-valve implantation for failed surgical bioprosthetic valves. J Am Coll Cardiol. 2011;58(21):2196–209.
142. Otto CM. Calcific aortic stenosis – time to look more closely at the valve. N Engl J Med. 2008;359(13):1395–8.

Low-Flow and Low-Gradient Aortic Stenosis Consideration in the Context of TAVR

10

Alper Ozkan and Paul Schoenhagen

Abstract

Aortic valve replacement (AVR) is the definitive treatment for patients with symptomatic, severe AS, typically defined as aortic valve area <1 cm^2 and mean transvalvular gradient >40 mmHg. Surgical AVR is associated with substantial improvement in symptomatic status and increased survival for patient with normal and decreased LV function. In contrast, patients with low-gradient severe AS have considerable increased operative risk and less potential benefit from AVR. Low-gradient AS is generally seen in patients with low EF; however, a significant percentage of patients with severe AS may present with low-gradient despite preserved LVEF ("paradoxical" low-flow and low-gradient stenosis). In patients with low-gradient AS, clarification of disease severity and prediction of outcome are clinically challenging. Dobutamine stress echocardiography can help to distinguish true from pseudo AS, and assessment of LV contractile reserve provides important prognostic data regarding outcome. Patients with low-flow and low-gradient severe AS are characterized by a poor natural prognosis, and therefore AVR should not be withheld. The experience with TAVR in patients with low-flow and low-gradient AS is limited, in particular as a high gradient is typically required for inclusion in clinical trials. However, because TAVR is associated with considerably lower operative risk in comparison to standard surgery, it is intuitive that TAVR may be a promising treatment option for patients with low-flow and low-gradient severe AS.

Keywords

Low-flow and low-gradient aortic stenosis • Low LVEF • Preserved LVEF • TAVR

Abbreviations

AS	Aortic stenosis
AVA	Aortic valve area
CR	Contractile reserve
DI	Dimensionless index
DSE	Dobutamine stress echocardiography
EF	Ejection fraction
LF	Low flow
LG	Low gradient
LV	Left ventricle/ventricular
LVOT	Left ventricular outflow tract
SAVR	Surgical aortic valve replacement
SV	Stroke volume
TAVR	Transcatheter aortic valve replacement

A. Ozkan, MD
Department of Cardiovascular Medicine, Cleveland Clinic, 9500 Euclid Avenue/JJ5-208A, Cleveland, OH 44195, USA
e-mail: ozkana@ccf.org

P. Schoenhagen, MD (✉)
Department of Cardiology, Imaging Institute and Heart and Vascular Institute, Cleveland Clinic, J1-4, Cleveland, OH 44195, USA
e-mail: schoenp1@ccf.org

J.K. Min et al. (eds.), *Multimodality Imaging for Transcatheter Aortic Valve Replacement*, DOI 10.1007/978-1-4471-2798-7_10, © Springer-Verlag London 2014

Introduction

Aortic stenosis (AS) is the most common valvular pathology and a common reason for valve replacement in industrialized countries [1]. Although degenerative AS has a long asymptomatic period, once symptoms develop, prognosis is poor if left untreated. Surgical aortic valve replacement (SAVR) is the recommended therapeutic approach for the symptomatic severe AS patients [2]. Following AVR, symptomatic recovery and improved survival have been well established in patients with normal preoperative LV function [3] but also in patients with LV dysfunction. A subgroup of patients with low-flow and low-gradient (LF-LG) severe AS also derive benefit from valve replacement, but surgery is associated with increased perioperative mortality. Therefore, management decisions in this population are challenging and risk-benefit ratio of AVR in comparison to medical treatment is still a controversial issue. This chapter reviews the pathophysiology of low-gradient AS, describes diagnostic challenges, and discusses the potential role of TAVR.

Definition of Low-Gradient AS

Severe AS is defined as aortic valve area <1 cm^2 and mean transvalvular gradient >40 mmHg. Although there is no universal definition of low-gradient AS, it can be defined as aortic valve area (AVA) less than 1 cm^2 with a mean gradient less than 30–40 mmHg [2].

The pressure gradient across a stenotic valve is a dynamic measurement that depends upon not only the valve orifice area but also transvalvular flow. While largely dependent on transvalvular flow, aortic valvular systolic gradients are also affected by heart rate, blood pressure, and inotropic state. Therefore, a relatively low transvalvular gradient can be measured in a patient with severe AS and decreased cardiac output secondary to reduced LV systolic performance. LF-LG AS is most commonly seen in patients with LV systolic dysfunction (5–10 % of AS population), but most patients with low EF have normal or high transvalvular gradients. Importantly, recent studies demonstrate that LG severe AS can be encountered in patients with normal LVEF, and this clinical entity is called "paradoxical low-flow and low-gradient severe AS" [4]. These data demonstrate that LF-LG AS describes a heterogeneous patient population. The clinical impact of low-gradient AS is incompletely understood and there is in particular limited data evaluating the relative impact of low gradient and LVEF.

Low-Gradient Aortic Stenosis with Reduced LVEF

Pathophysiology

Due to chronic pressure overload associated with significant AS, LV hypertrophy develops in order to normalize increased LV wall stress and maintain forward stroke volume. Increased wall stress causes diminished subendocardial blood flow, which results in subendocardial ischemia and fibrosis over time. Increased LV mass complicated by myocardial fibrosis initially leads to LV diastolic dysfunction and later to decreasing LV systolic performance and eventually LV dilatation. Due to failing LV performance, this phenomenon of "afterload mismatch" results in inability of the LV to generate a normal systolic pressure and/or gradient across the severely stenotic valve [5]. On the other hand, LV failure can coexist in patient with AS secondary to ischemic or nonischemic cardiomyopathy. In this subset of patients, as the primary problem is "intrinsic LV dysfunction," low gradients can be found across mildly or moderately stenotic valve. Whether the problem is afterload mismatch or intrinsic LV dysfunction, traditional cutoff values (mean gradient >40 mmHg or peak transvalvular aortic velocity >4 m/s) cannot be used for the definition of severity of AS. Therefore, understanding of disease severity along with distinguishing true AS from pseudo AS is challenging.

Distinguishing True from Pseudo AS

In order to predict potential reversibility of LV failure and the benefit from possible aortic valve replacement, assessment of LV contractile reserve is useful (Box 10.1). Measurement of the aortic valvular hemodynamics during dobutamine infusion can help to distinguish true AS—or severe AS with LV dysfunction due to afterload mismatch—from pseudo AS (defined as LV dysfunction with mild to moderate AS) [6, 7]. Augmentation of LV systolic ejection performance with dobutamine provides transiently increased stroke volume and flow across the valve. In the subset of pseudo AS, increased flow produces an increase in AVA (i.e., increase >0.3 cm^2), whereas in the setting of true stenosis AVA does not significantly change but transvalvular gradients increase considerably (Fig. 10.1). For patients with afterload mismatch, improvement in LV ejection performance can be expected following successful AVR (Fig. 10.1).

Box 10.1 Distinguising True from Psuedo AS During Dobutamine Infusion

True	AVA does not change but transvalvular gradients increase
Pseudo	Increased flow results in increased AVA (i.e., increase >0.3 cm^2)

AS aortic stenosis, *AVA* aortic valve area

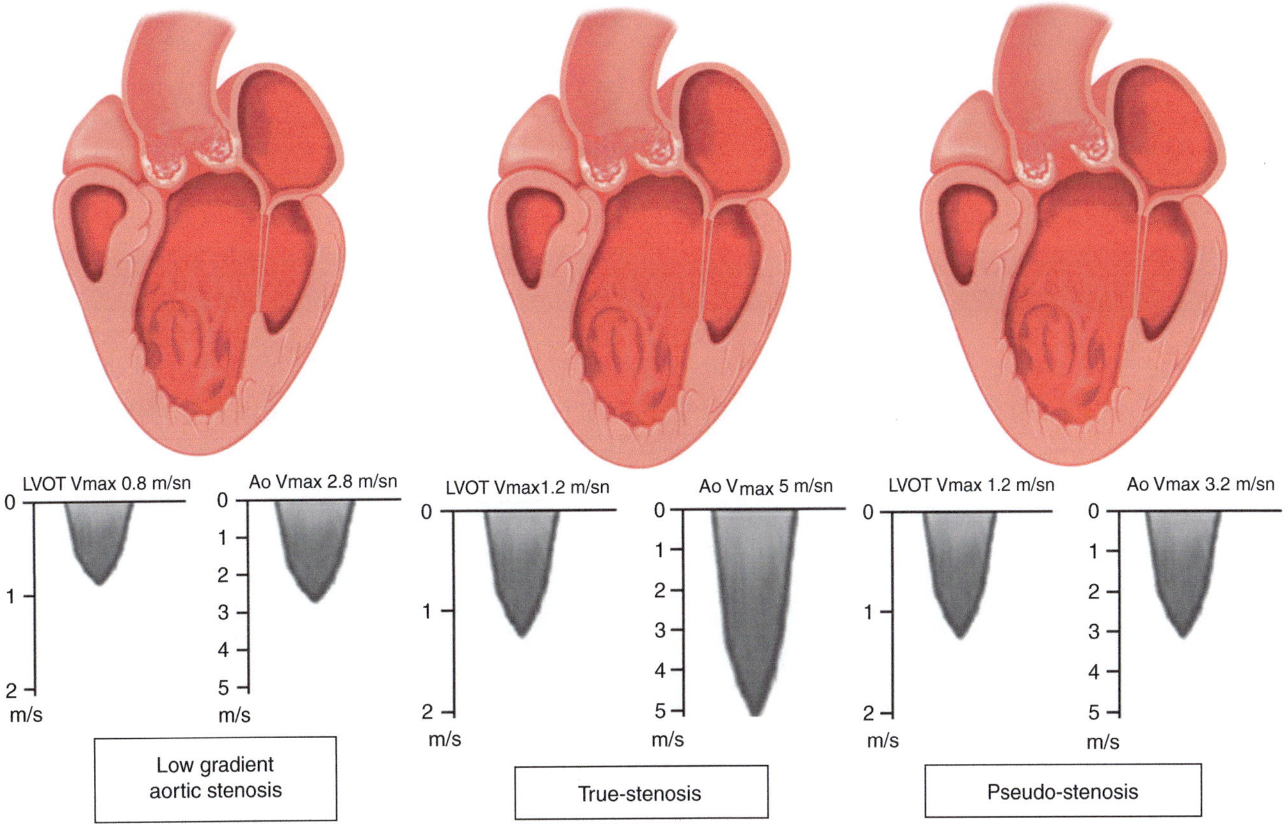

Fig. 10.1 (**a–c**) Distinguishing true AS from pseudo AS. In patients with LF-LG AS, as the continuity equation is less accurate and is known to underestimate the valve area, distinguishing the patient with severe AS causing LV dysfunction secondary to afterload mismatch (true AS) from the one who has LV dysfunction and coexisting mild to moderate AS (pseudo AS) is clinically essential. DSE can help to discriminate the two distinct pathologies; at peak stress valve area can slightly increase while gradients are dramatically increased in true AS, whereas in pseudo AS, valve area increases>0.3 cm^2 and gradients slightly increase due to moderate AS

Surgical Aortic Valve Replacement: Predictors of Outcome

In 1980, Carabello et al. demonstrated that outcomes of patients with LG and low EF AS were poor and risk of surgery was high [8]. Subsequently, in a study of 52 patients with impaired LVEF (≤35 %) and LG (<30 mmHg) AS, Connoly et al. confirmed high operative risk. Perioperative mortality was 21 %, and overall survival at 3 and 5 years was 62 and 39 %, respectively [9]. Significant improvement in symptomatic status following AVR was reported in particular younger patient age group and larger prosthesis size. However, it is still incompletely understood whether AVR in these patients improves long-term survival compared to medical therapy. Pereira et al. compared LG (<30 mmHg) severe AS patients with LV dysfunction (LVEF ≤35 %) who did and did not receive surgical valve replacement and demonstrated that there is not only symptomatic benefit but also a mortality benefit following AVR in the LG AS group. In patients who underwent AVR, 4-year survival rate was found markedly improved (79 %), as compared to medically treated patients. Together with age and serum creatinine level, AVR was found to be a main predictor of improved survival [10]. In order to better understand which patients would have more benefits from AVR, further studies tested clinical utility and prognostic importance of LV contractile reserve with dobutamine stress echocardiography (DSE).

Impact of LV Contractile Reserve (CR)

In patients with true AS, determination of LV CR with a DSE test is an essential step in clinical decision making and furthermore provides important prognostic data regarding perioperative mortality and postoperative survival. LV contractile reserve is defined as an increase in stroke volume >20 % during DSE [11] (Fig. 10.2).

Assessment of LV CR is important, because presence of LV CR indicates better survival in patients with LF-LG severe AS and reduced LVEF. In a study of 136 patients with LG (<40 mmHg) symptomatic severe AS, who underwent DSE, perioperative mortality was found 5 % in patients with LV CR versus 33 % in those without CR [12]. However, lack of LV CR should not be considered an absolute contraindication for valve replacement. In a subsequent report of 66 patients from the above study, symptomatic recovery and improvement of functional capacity after AVR were similar in those with and without LV CR [13]. Based on these data, risk stratification in patients with LF-LG AS is difficult, because symptomatic recovery and improvement of LVEF after surgery are not associated with higher operative mortality rate and decreased survival (Fig. 10.3a–f) [14].

Impact of Plasma BNP Levels

Increased plasma BNP levels have been correlated with onset of symptoms and prognosis in asymptomatic AS patients [15, 16]. In one study, 69 patients with LG (<40 mmHg) and low LVEF (40 %) were investigated with DSE to distinguish true from pseudo AS. Simultaneously, plasma BNP was analyzed in order to understand its

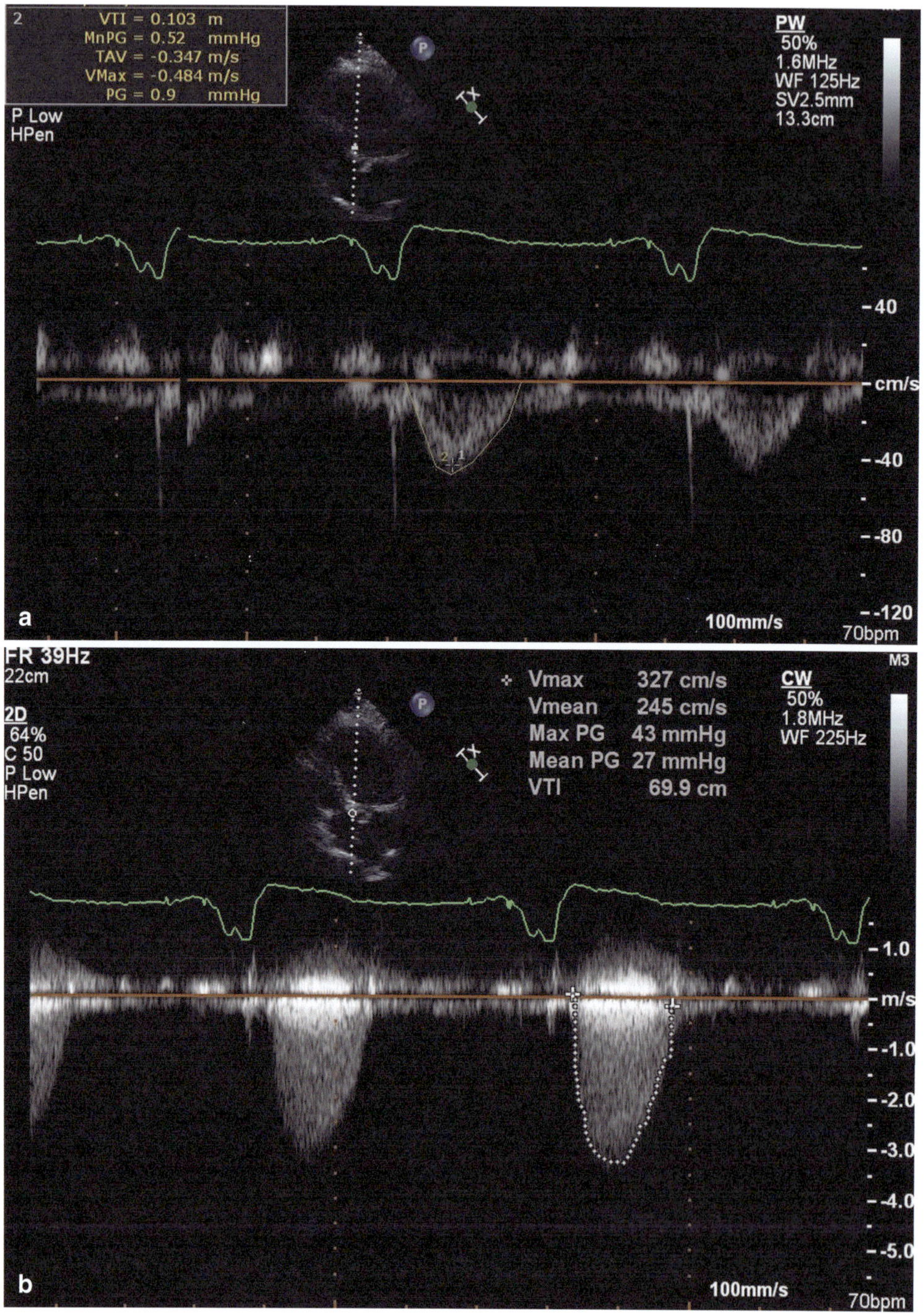

Fig. 10.2 Assessment of low-gradient AS by dobutamine stress echocardiography and LV contractile reserve. A 71-year-old man presented with shortness of breath (NYHA class III). Baseline LVEF was 20 %, calculated AVA was 0.45 cm^2, and max/mean gradients were 43/27 mmHg. DSE was performed (1) to distinguish true AS from pseudo AS and (2) to assess whether he had LV CR. (**a**) Baseline stroke volume was calculated 32 cc; (**b**) after low-dose dobutamine stroke volume and gradients were increased to 43 cc and 55/36 mmHg, respectively. (**c**) At peak DSE, stroke volume was calculated 46 cc and gradients were increased to 70/43 mmHg. LVCR was calculated as 43 %. DSE results in this patient with LF-LG AS are consistent with true AS with LV CR. This case was considered high risk for conventional SAVR due to his comorbidities, and 26 mm Edwards Sapien valve was inserted via transfemoral route

Fig. 10.2 (continued)

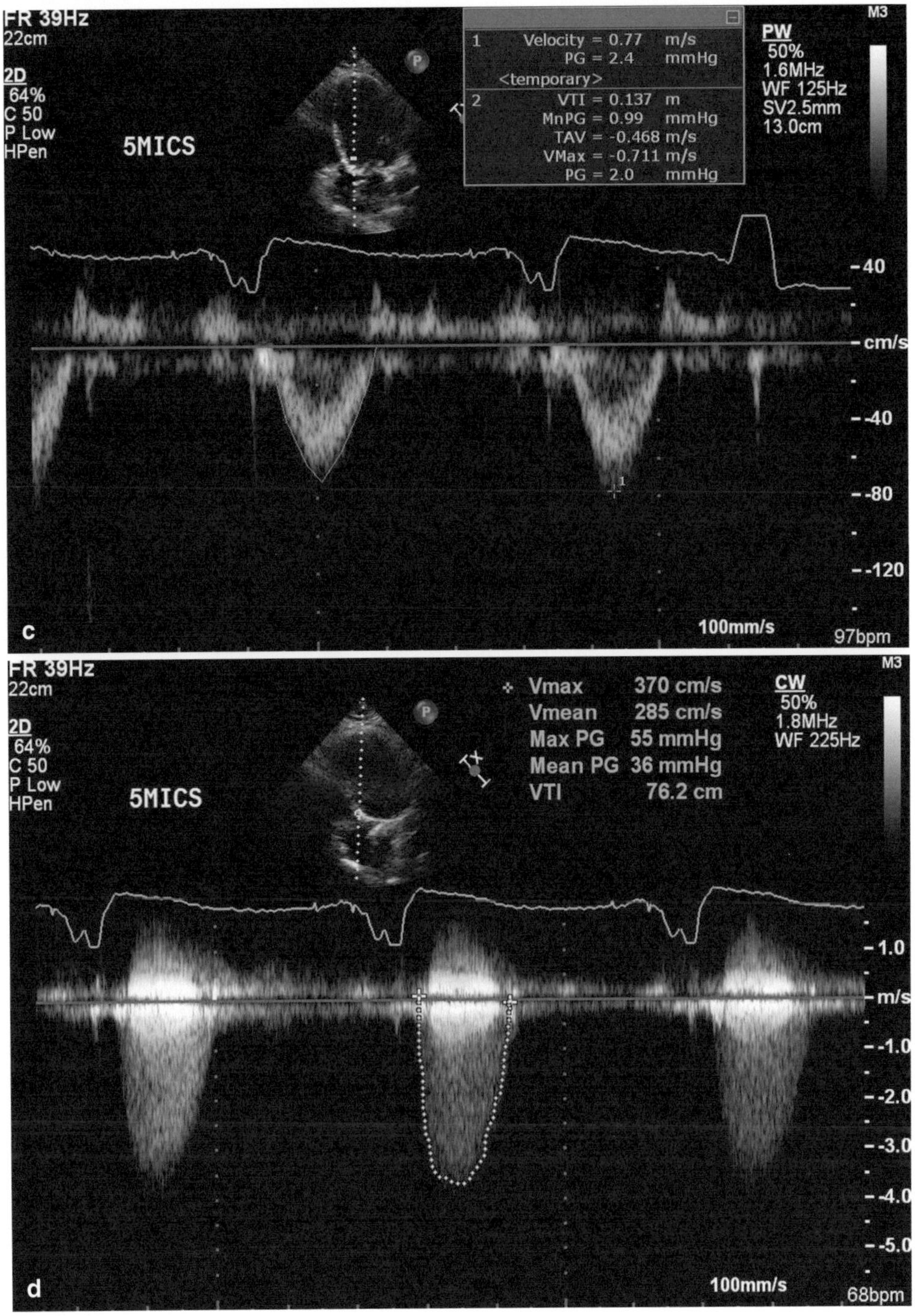

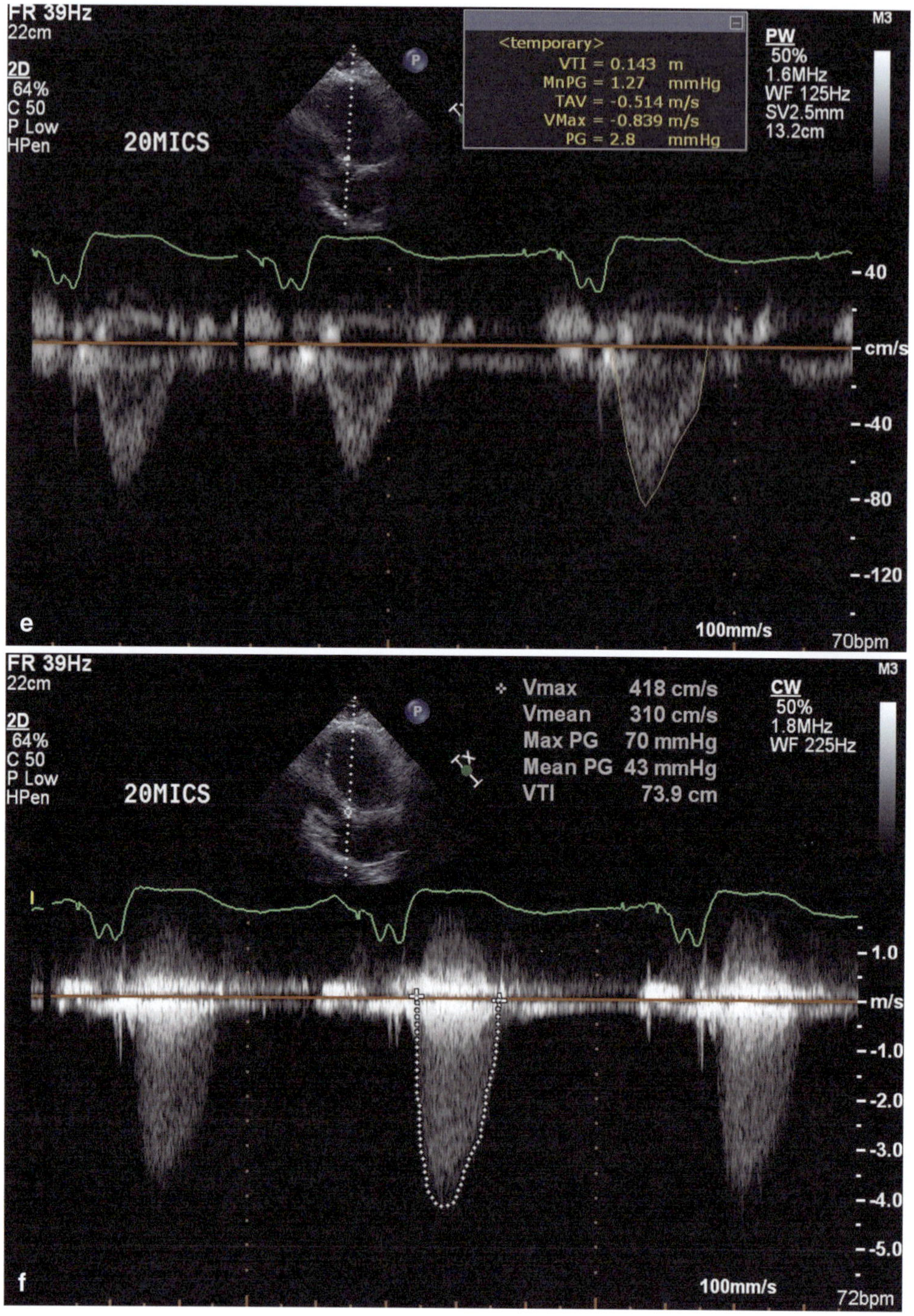

Fig. 10.2 (continued)

diagnostic and prognostic value in LF-LG AS. Patients with true AS had significantly higher BNP levels than patients with pseudo AS. However, large overlaps of BNP levels were observed between patient with pseudo and true AS. Furthermore, high plasma BNP was associated with poor outcome in the entire study cohort with a cutoff value of 550 pg/mL independent of LV CR [17]. These data suggest that increased BNP levels cannot reliably distinguish true from pseudo AS.

Low-Gradient AS in the Era of TAVR

TAVR is a promising alternative therapeutic approach for patients, who are at high risk for conventional SAVR. The Placement of Aortic Transcatheter Valves (PARTNER) trial demonstrated that in high-risk patients, TAVR is associated with significantly better outcome in comparison to standard medical therapy in non-operable patients [18] and equivalent outcomes compared to SAVR [19]. However, reflecting the fact that a gradient >40 is a specific inclusion criteria, a dedicated subgroup analysis of outcome in patient with LF-LG AS is not available. There is currently no randomized data investigating outcomes of LF-LG AS patients after TAVR. In non-randomized studies, Clavel et al. compared outcome of patients with low LVEF who received SAVR versus TAVR using propensity-matched analysis. The authors found that TAVR is associated with better LVEF recovery compared to SAVR. Recovery of LVEF was not significantly different in patients with low versus high gradients. In this study, among the 283 patients, only 71 patients underwent DSE. In this subset, the presence of LV CR was not found to be a predictor of LVEF recovery [20].

In another recent study, 38 patient with low gradients (<40 mmHg) and low LVEF (<40 %), who underwent TAVR, were compared to a group of surgically treated patient ($n = 33$). Both groups had significant improvement in LVEF with presence of high preoperative gradient being a predictor for an improvement of LVEF [21]. Gotzmann et al. studied 167 consecutive patients who underwent TAVR, of whom 15 (8 %) had LF-LG (<40 mmHg) and decreased LVEF (<40 %) [22]. While all patients showed symptomatic benefit, significant improvement of LVEF, and exercise capacity, all cause mortality at 6 months following TAVR was found considerably higher in the LF-LG group.

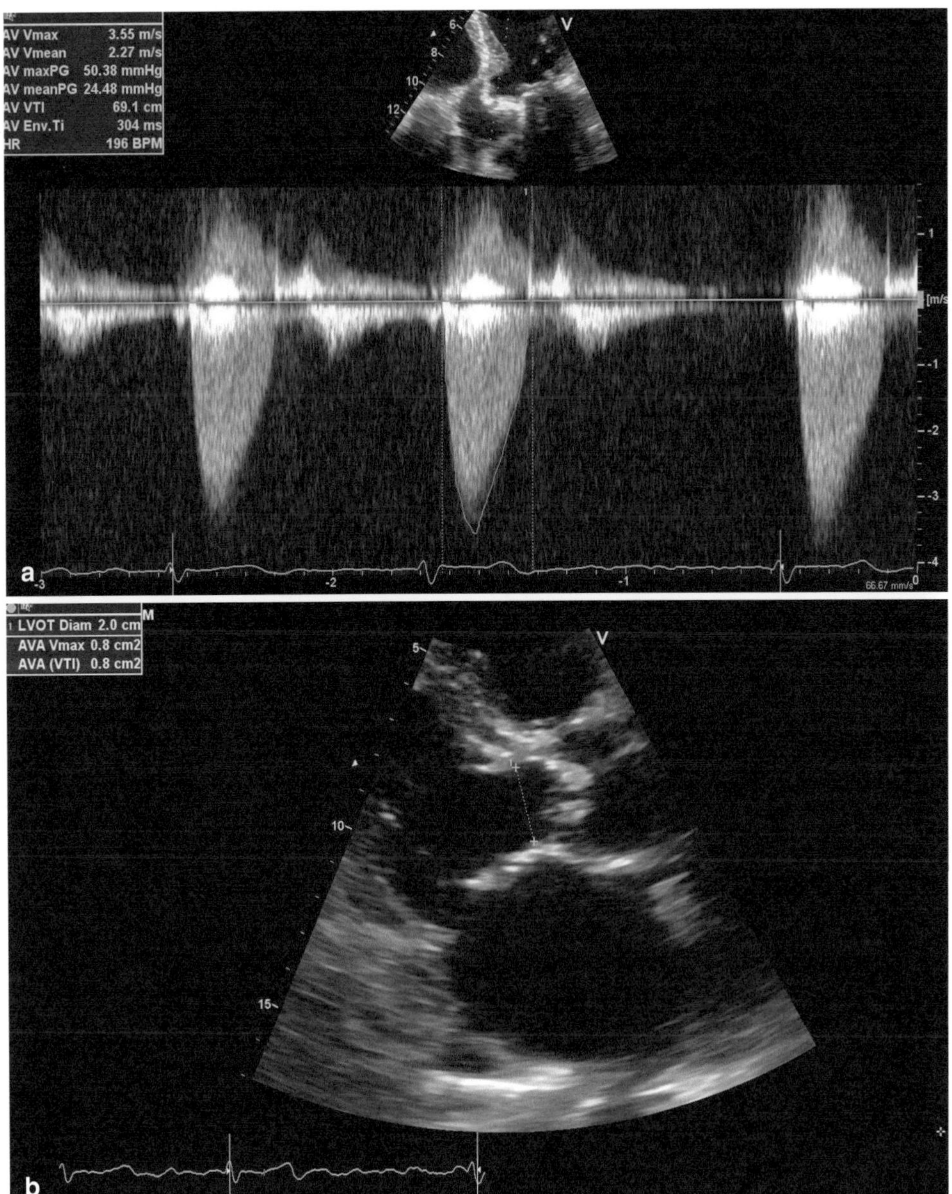

Fig. 10.3 (**a–d**) Paradoxically low-flow and low-gradient severe AS. A 78-year-old man who was diagnosed with severe AS presented with dyspnea on exertion. Calculated AVA was 0.88 cm^2 (iAVA was 0.44 cm^2/m^2 with a BSA of 2 m^2) but gradients were measured as 50/24 mmHg despite LVEF of 61 %. SVi was calculated 30.6 mL/m^2. The patient was considered as low-flow and low-gradient severe AS despite preserved LV EF. (**e–g**) Assessment of segmental and global strain by 2D STE. Global longitudinal strain was found to be 13.3 % indicating mildly decreased LV function. Decreased global strain indicates possible subtle impaired LV dysfunction. Since the patient was not a good candidate for surgical AVR due to multiple comorbidities, transcatheter aortic valve replacement (TAVi) was performed via transfemoral approach (From Ozkan [37]; with permission from AME publishing)

Fig. 10.3 (continued)

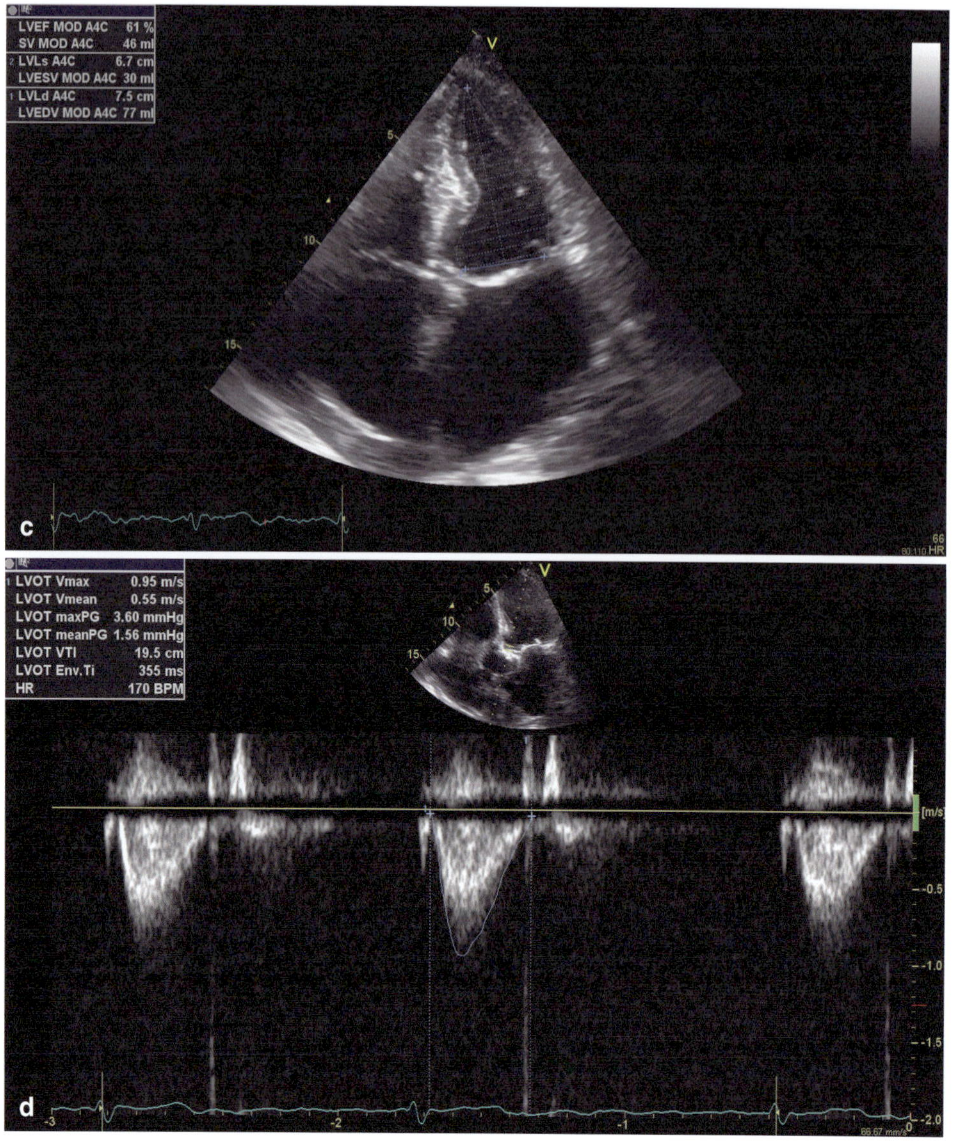

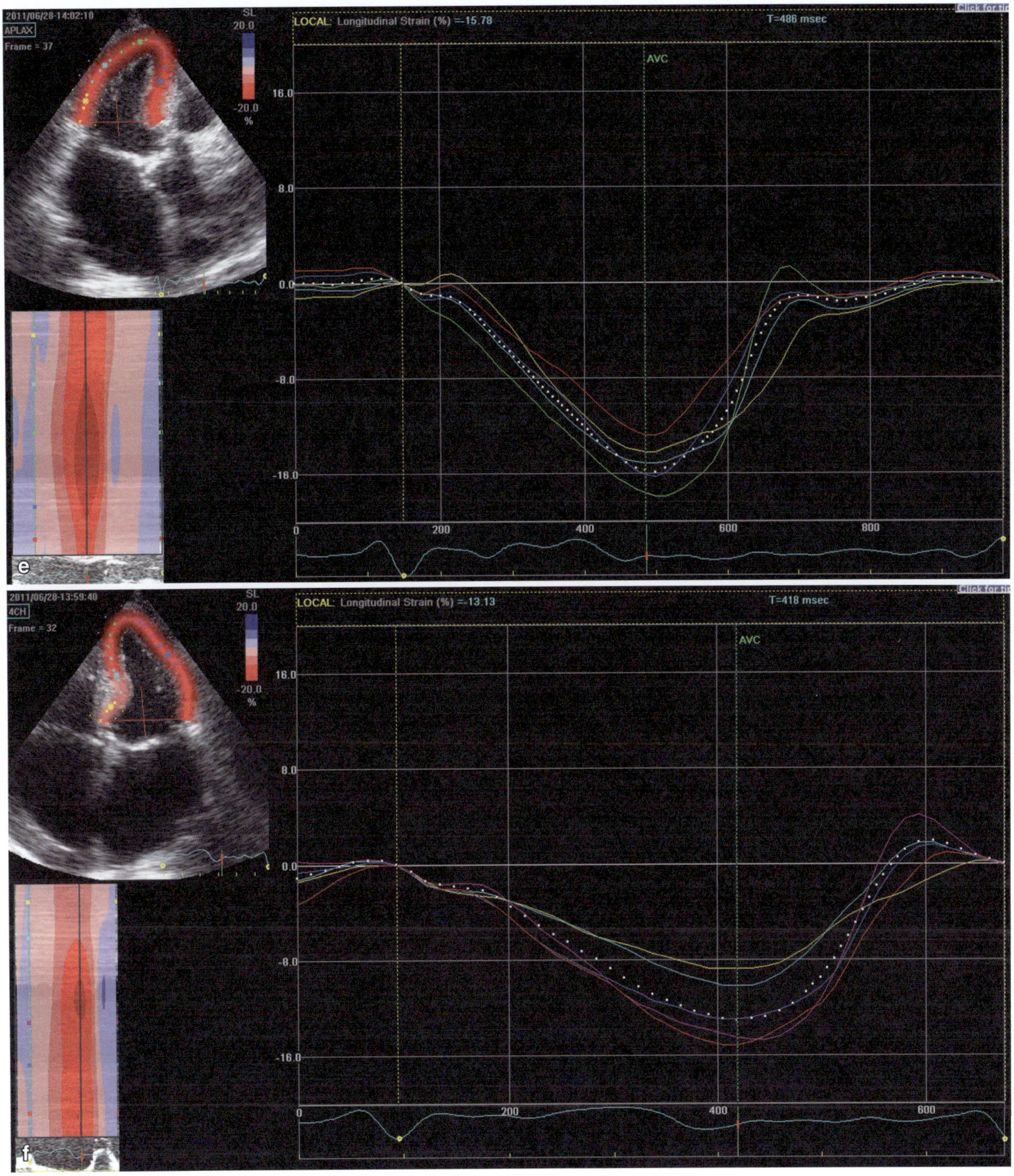

Fig. 10.3 (continued)

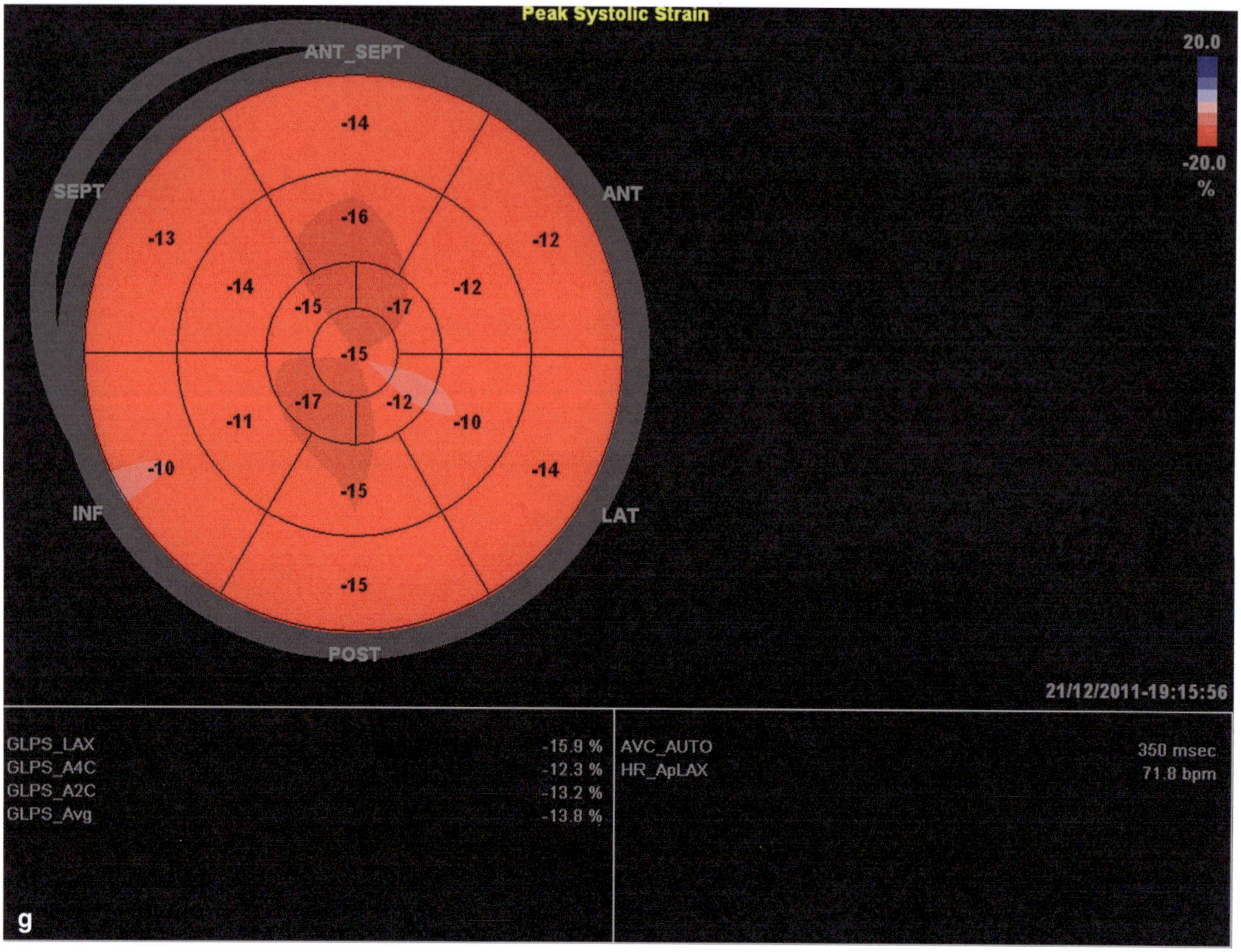

Fig. 10.3 (continued)

A recent study analyzed 126 patients after TAVR—35 patients with low-gradient AS and 91 patients with high-gradient (≥40 mmHg) AS—and confirmed that low-gradient patients are at increased risk. Although procedural success was reported as 98 %, major adverse cardiovascular events (MACE) and cardiovascular death were reported 29 and 10 %, respectively. In multivariate analysis, presence of low preoperative transvalvular gradient was found to be associated with two- to fourfold increase in hazards for MACE and cardiovascular death [23].

Mitral regurgitation has been found more common in patients undergoing TAVR. Mitral regurgitation can be responsible for both the LF-LG itself and increased surgical operative mortality in this cohort [24]. Significant regression of MR has been shown in AS patients following TAVR, a finding which may contribute to maintained forward stroke volume and associated symptomatic improvement and better outcome [25].

Low-Gradient Aortic Stenosis Despite Preserved LVEF

As described above, low-gradient severe AS is most commonly seen in patients with LV systolic dysfunction, where low cardiac output is secondary to systolic dysfunction. However, recent studies demonstrated that severe LG AS can be encountered in patients with normal LVEF. This clinical entity of "paradoxical low flow and low gradient" is consistent with more advanced stages of disease with poor prognosis [4]. However, other studies demonstrate that assessing the true frequency of this entity is confounded by inconsistent grading of aortic valve stenosis, with both echocardiography and invasive measurements [26]. The discrepancy between aortic valve area (AVA) and mean gradient (MG) can potentially cause an underestimation of stenosis and thus lead inappropriate delay of AVR [27]. In fact, previous studies show that compared to high-gradient patients, patients with LG severe AS were less frequently referred to AVR. Since AVR has been found to be associated with significant improvement in long-term survival despite low-gradient, clarification of disease severity is critical in the subgroup of LF-LG AS [28, 29].

Prevalence and Significance of Paradoxically Low-Flow and Low-Gradient AS

In a study of 512 patients with severe aortic stenosis, indexed AVA ≤0.6 cm^2/m^2, and preserved LVEF >50 %, 181 (35 %) patients had paradoxically low flow (stroke volume index ≤35 mL/m^2) [4]. When compared with normal flow patients, low-flow patients were more frequently female, had a higher prevalence of lower transvalvular gradient (32 ± 17 versus 40 ± 15 mmHg; $p < 0.001$), a lower LV diastolic volume index (52 ± 12 versus 59 ± 13 mL/m^2; $p < 0.001$), lower LVEF (62 ± 8 % versus 68 ± 7 %; $p < 0.001$), and a higher level of LV global afterload reflected by a higher valvuloarterial impedance (5.3 ± 1.3 versus 4.1 ± 0.7 $mmHg \cdot mL^{-1} \cdot m^{-2}$; $p < 0.001$). Importantly, compared with normal flow patients, low-flow patients had a lower overall 3-year survival (76 % versus 86 %; $p < 0.006$). These data suggest that this pattern of the disease represents more advanced stage of the disease, which are in turn associated with poorer outcomes.

Other studies suggest that the current focus on transvalvular gradients, when grading AS clinically, is associated with underestimation of AS severity and misdiagnosis of LG severe AS. This delay to diagnosis is also associated with a significant, and inappropriate, delay to AVR. An almost 50 % lower referral rate for AVR and twofold increase in mortality exists for patients with low-gradient AS as compared to high-gradient patients [28].

Pathophysiology

Current data suggest that LG severe AS (i.e., paradoxically low-flow and low-gradient AS) can be explained by decreased cardiac output. Postulated mechanisms include severe concentric LV hypertrophy with small LV cavity, restrictive filling pattern, and increased global afterload with decreased arterial compliance. Subtle LV myocardial dysfunction has been demonstrated by 2D Speckle Tracking Echocardiography (2D-STE) [30, 31], with increased myocardial fibrosis and decreased longitudinal mechanics also shown in previous MRI studies [32]. Increased fibrosis and subendocardial ischemia result in subtle LV systolic dysfunction with apparently normal LVEF.

Differential Diagnosis and Possible Pitfalls

It is important to differentiate patient with severe AS and low flow and low gradient ("paradoxically" LF-LG AS) from conditions of low flow and low gradient without significant AS. The latter are most commonly encountered secondary to measurement errors, including lack of correction for body size and inconsistent grading cutoff values for AS.

Measurements Errors

Discrepancies between AVA and transvalvular gradient are often secondary to errors in the measurement of transvalvular Doppler and LVOT area. Estimation of the AVA with transthoracic echocardiography is based on the continuity equation and assumes a circular LVOT. However, 3D analysis of the annulus has demonstrated a typically eccentric, oval shape in the majority of patients. Therefore, the LVOT area, measured with 3D echo or MDCT, is typically significantly higher than the LVOT area calculated from a single diameter measurement. This difference translates into a higher AVA when 3D LVOT data is used in the continuity equation [33]. These data show that congruence of measurements for severe AS significantly increases with the use of 3D LVOT measurements (Fig. 10.4).

Therefore, integration of 3D data (CT, MRI, and 3D TEE) provides a more complete understanding of the aortic root structures, resulting in more accurate calculation of LVOT and AVA area [34]. Other data suggest that indirect findings in CT can be used to clarify stenosis severity in selected patients with discrepant findings. Specifically, an aortic valve calcium score >1,651 units has been described to be associated with true severe stenosis [35].

Correction for Body Size

Patients with small body surface area can be incorrectly classified as having severe AS, if the AVA is not indexed for BSA. Likewise, a large body size may lead to an overestimation of AVA in terms of disease severity unless it is indexed. Therefore, AVA should be indexed for the body size, in particular in the context of discrepant measurement. In current guidelines, an indexed AVA cutoff value of 0.6 cm^2/m^2 is recommended as the criterion for severe AS [2].

Inconsistent Grading Cutoff Values for AS

Current guidelines define severe AS by a valve area less than 1 cm² calculated by the continuity equation and/or a mean transvalvular systolic gradient >40 mmHg, suggesting that these cutoff values correlate with each other. However, in a single-center study, evaluating 2,427 patients with AS and preserved left ventricular systolic function [3], a substantial proportion of patients (30 %) had a valve area calculated by the continuity equation less than 1 cm² but a mean gradient less than 40 mmHg [36]. According to echocardiographic results, AVA of 1 cm² was found to be correlated with a mean gradient of 22 mmHg. Conversely, a mean gradient of 40 mmHg was correlated to an in vivo AVA of 0.74 cm², while a maximum velocity of 4 cm/s corresponded to an in vivo AVA of 0.82 cm².

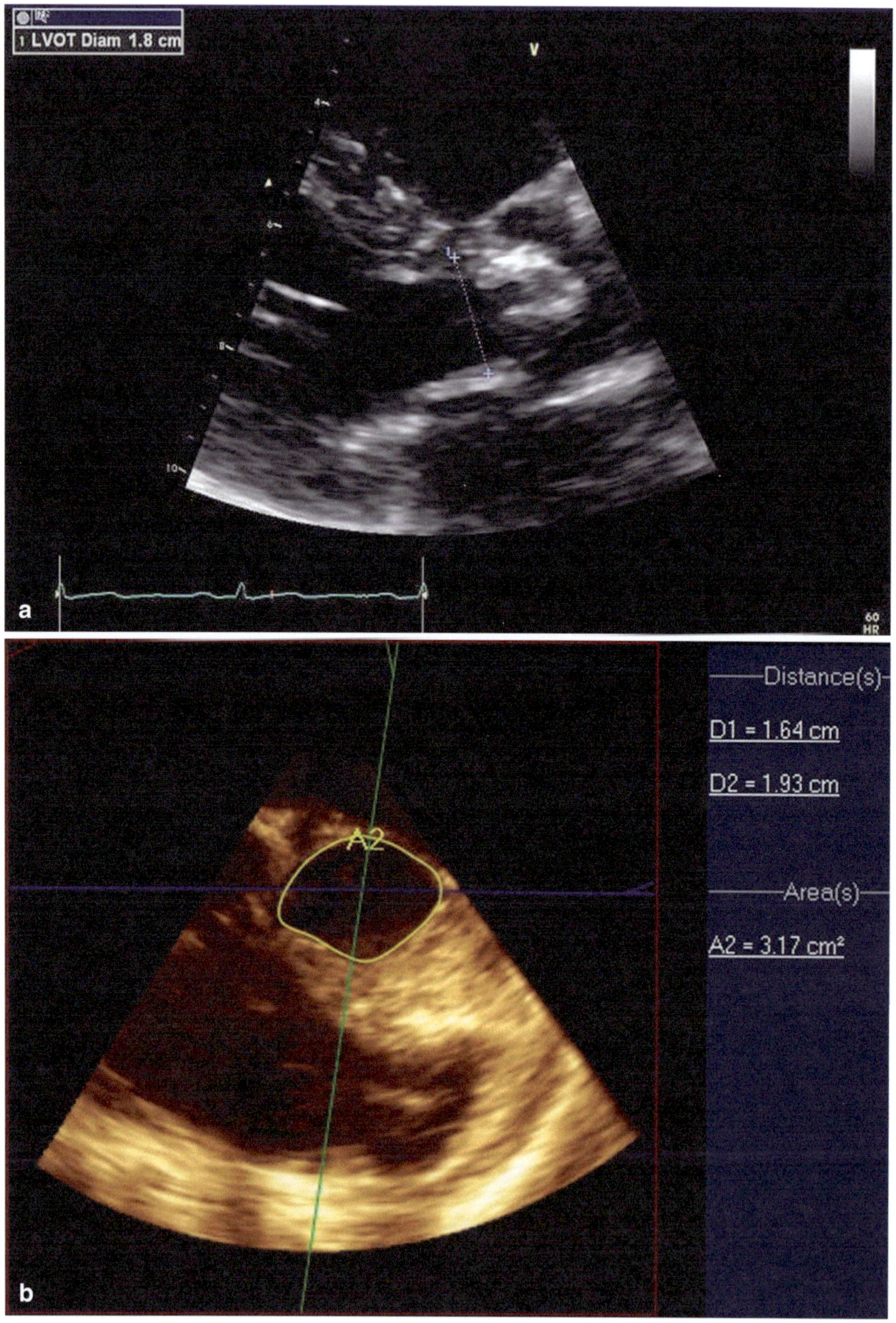

Fig. 10.4 (**a**–**c**) Importance of LVOT measurements. It is important to note that LVOT measurements play an essential role in calculating both AVA and stroke volume. Although transthoracic Doppler echocardiography provides practical approach by using continuity equation in daily practice, it may cause significant underestimation of LVOT area which leads to underestimation of AVA and low stroke volume (flow). (**a**) In this case, LVOT area was calculated 2.54 cm² by TTE; however, LVOT area was measured 3.17 cm² by 3D TEE (**b**) and 3.38 cm² by CT (**c**)

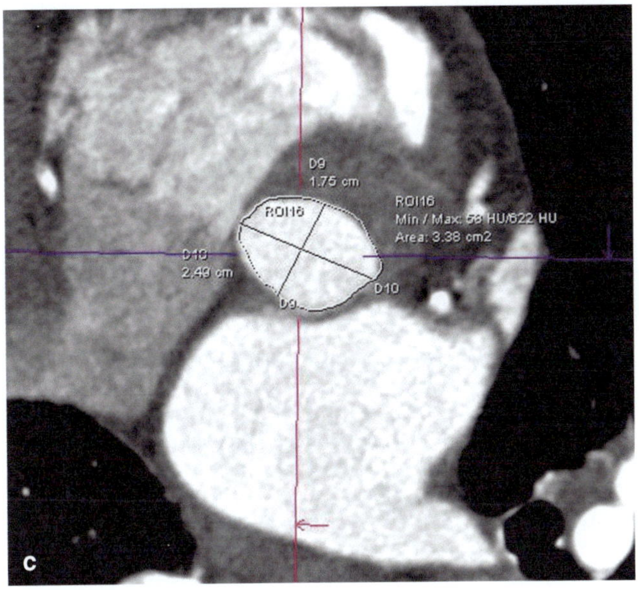

Fig. 10.4 (continued)

Conclusion

The above-described data has identified subgroups of patients with severe AS but low transvalvular gradient. While this pattern is better known in patients with LV dysfunction, recent data identified this pattern also in patients with normal LV function or milder forms of LV dysfunction. These patients experience poor outcome with medical management but also higher surgical risk than patients with normal gradient normal flow AS. The experience with TAVR in these patients is limited, in particular as high transsystolic aortic valvular gradients are typically required for inclusion in clinical trials. However, as TAVR is associated with considerably lower operative risk compared to standard surgery, it seems intuitive that TAVR may be a promising treatment option for patient with low-flow and low-gradient severe AS. In fact, recent studies confirmed that AVR is associated with significant improvement in long-term survival and with a low operative mortality in both low EF [14] and preserved LVEF [29]. A practical clinical algorithm based on current literature is proposed in Fig. 10.5. However, larger and more definitive trials are necessary in these challenging patient populations.

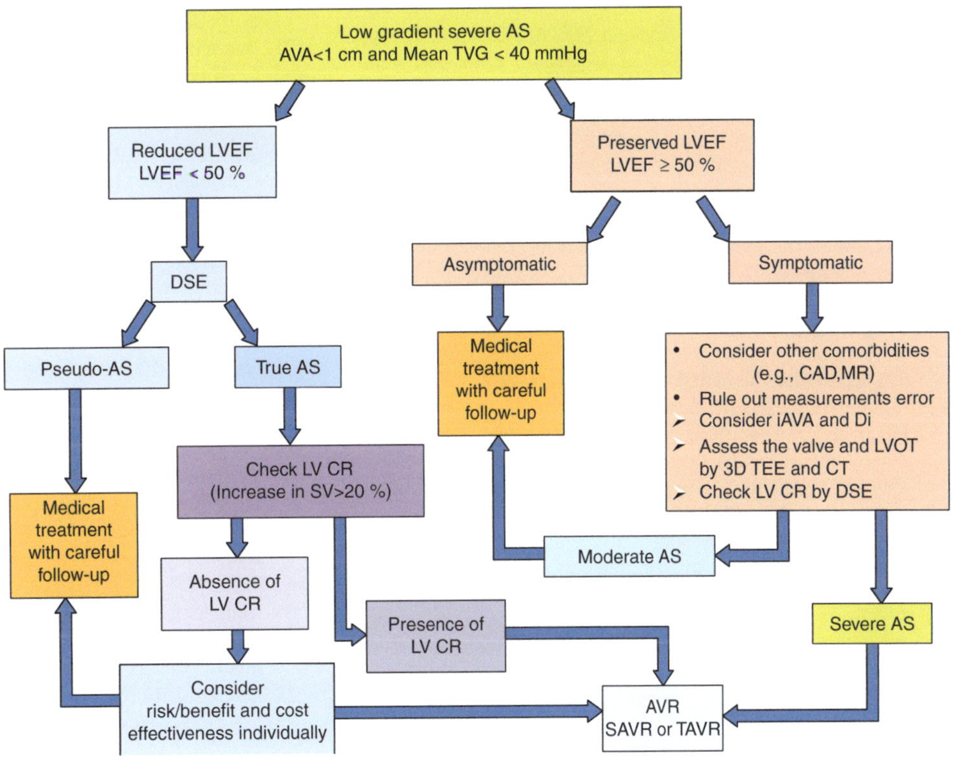

Fig. 10.5 A proposed clinical algorithm for low-gradient severe AS patients

References

1. Iung B, Baron G, Butchart EG, Delahaye F, Gohlke-Barwolf C, Levang OW, et al. A prospective survey of patients with valvular heart disease in Europe: The Euro Heart Survey on Valvular Heart Disease. Eur Heart J. 2003;24(13):1231–43.
2. American College of Cardiology/American Heart Association Task Force on Practice Guidelines, Society of Cardiovascular Anesthesiologists, Society for Cardiovascular Angiography and Interventions, Society of Thoracic Surgeons, Bonow RO, Carabello BA, et al. ACC/AHA 2006 guidelines for the management of patients with valvular heart disease: a report of the American College of Cardiology/American Heart Association Task Force on Practice Guidelines (writing committee to revise the 1998 Guidelines for the Management of Patients With Valvular Heart Disease): developed in collaboration with the Society of Cardiovascular Anesthesiologists: endorsed by the Society for Cardiovascular Angiography and Interventions and the Society of Thoracic Surgeons. Circulation. 2006;114(5):e84–231.
3. Lindblom D, Lindblom U, Qvist J, Lundstrom H. Long-term relative survival rates after heart valve replacement. J Am Coll Cardiol. 1990;15(3):566–73.
4. Hachicha Z, Dumesnil JG, Bogaty P, Pibarot P. Paradoxical low-flow, low-gradient severe aortic stenosis despite preserved ejection fraction is associated with higher afterload and reduced survival. Circulation. 2007;115(22):2856–64.
5. Ross Jr J. Afterload mismatch and preload reserve: a conceptual framework for the analysis of ventricular function. Prog Cardiovasc Dis. 1976;18(4):255–64.
6. deFilippi CR, Willett DL, Brickner ME, Appleton CP, Yancy CW, Eichhorn EJ, et al. Usefulness of dobutamine echocardiography in distinguishing severe from nonsevere valvular aortic stenosis in patients with depressed left ventricular function and low transvalvular gradients. Am J Cardiol. 1995;75(2):191–4.
7. Nishimura RA, Grantham JA, Connolly HM, Schaff HV, Higano ST, Holmes Jr DR. Low-output, low-gradient aortic stenosis in patients with depressed left ventricular systolic function: the clinical utility of the dobutamine challenge in the catheterization laboratory. Circulation. 2002;106(7):809–13.
8. Carabello BA, Green LH, Grossman W, Cohn LH, Koster JK, Collins Jr JJ. Hemodynamic determinants of prognosis of aortic valve replacement in critical aortic stenosis and advanced congestive heart failure. Circulation. 1980;62(1):42–8.
9. Connolly HM, Oh JK, Schaff HV, Roger VL, Osborn SL, Hodge DO, et al. Severe aortic stenosis with low transvalvular gradient and severe left ventricular dysfunction: result of aortic valve replacement in 52 patients. Circulation. 2000;101(16):1940–6.
10. Pereira JJ, Lauer MS, Bashir M, Afridi I, Blackstone EH, Stewart WJ, et al. Survival after aortic valve replacement for severe aortic stenosis with low transvalvular gradients and severe left ventricular dysfunction. J Am Coll Cardiol. 2002;39(8):1356–63.
11. Monin JL, Monchi M, Gest V, Duval-Moulin AM, Dubois-Rande JL, Gueret P. Aortic stenosis with severe left ventricular dysfunction and low transvalvular pressure gradients: risk stratification by low-dose dobutamine echocardiography. J Am Coll Cardiol. 2001;37(8):2101–7.
12. Monin JL, Quere JP, Monchi M, Petit H, Baleynaud S, Chauvel C, et al. Low-gradient aortic stenosis: operative risk stratification and predictors for long-term outcome: a multicenter study using dobutamine stress hemodynamics. Circulation. 2003;108(3):319–24.
13. Quere JP, Monin JL, Levy F, Petit H, Baleynaud S, Chauvel C, et al. Influence of preoperative left ventricular contractile reserve on postoperative ejection fraction in low-gradient aortic stenosis. Circulation. 2006;113(14):1738–44.
14. Tribouilloy C, Levy F, Rusinaru D, Gueret P, Petit-Eisenmann H, Baleynaud S, et al. Outcome after aortic valve replacement for low-flow/low-gradient aortic stenosis without contractile reserve on dobutamine stress echocardiography. J Am Coll Cardiol. 2009;53(20):1865–73.
15. Gerber IL, Legget ME, West TM, Richards AM, Stewart RA. Usefulness of serial measurement of N-terminal pro-brain natriuretic peptide plasma levels in asymptomatic patients with aortic stenosis to predict symptomatic deterioration. Am J Cardiol. 2005;95(7):898–901.
16. Bergler-Klein J, Klaar U, Heger M, Rosenhek R, Mundigler G, Gabriel H, et al. Natriuretic peptides predict symptom-free survival and postoperative outcome in severe aortic stenosis. Circulation. 2004;109(19):2302–8.
17. Bergler-Klein J, Mundigler G, Pibarot P, Burwash IG, Dumesnil JG, Blais C, et al. B-type natriuretic peptide in low-flow, low-gradient aortic stenosis: relationship to hemodynamics and clinical outcome: results from the Multicenter Truly or Pseudo-Severe Aortic Stenosis (TOPAS) study. Circulation. 2007;115(22):2848–55.
18. Leon MB, Smith CR, Mack M, Miller DC, Moses JW, Svensson LG, et al. Transcatheter aortic-valve implantation for aortic stenosis in patients who cannot undergo surgery. N Engl J Med. 2010;363(17):1597–607.
19. Smith CR, Leon MB, Mack MJ, Miller DC, Moses JW, Svensson LG, et al. Transcatheter versus surgical aortic-valve replacement in high-risk patients. N Engl J Med. 2011;364(23):2187–98.
20. Clavel MA, Webb JG, Rodes-Cabau J, Masson JB, Dumont E, De Larochelliere R, et al. Comparison between transcatheter and surgical prosthetic valve implantation in patients with severe aortic stenosis and reduced left ventricular ejection fraction. Circulation. 2010;122(19):1928–36.
21. Ben-Dor I, Maluenda G, Iyasu GD, Laynez-Carnicero A, Hauville C, Torguson R, et al. Comparison of outcome of higher versus lower transvalvular gradients in patients with severe aortic stenosis and low (<40%) left ventricular ejection fraction. Am J Cardiol. 2012;109(7):1031–7.
22. Gotzmann M, Lindstaedt M, Bojara W, Ewers A, Mugge A. Clinical outcome of transcatheter aortic valve implantation in patients with low-flow, low gradient aortic stenosis. Catheter Cardiovasc Interv. 2012;79:693–701.
23. Amabile N, Ramadan R, Ghostine S, Cheng S, Azmoun A, Raoux F, et al. Early and mid-term cardiovascular outcomes following TAVI: impact of pre-procedural transvalvular gradient. Int J Cardiol. 2012 (Epub ahead of print).
24. D'Onofrio A, Gasparetto V, Napodano M, Bianco R, Tarantini G, Renier V, et al. Impact of preoperative mitral valve regurgitation on outcomes after transcatheter aortic valve implantation. Eur J Cardiothorac Surg. 2012;41:1271–7.
25. Durst R, Avelar E, McCarty D, Poh KK, Friera LF, Llano MF, et al. Outcome and improvement predictors of mitral regurgitation after transcatheter aortic valve implantation. J Heart Valve Dis. 2011; 20(3):272–81.
26. Minners J, Allgeier M, Gohlke-Baerwolf C, Kienzle RP, Neumann FJ, Jander N. Inconsistencies of echocardiographic criteria for the grading of aortic valve stenosis. Eur Heart J. 2008;29(8):1043–8.
27. Dumesnil JG, Pibarot P, Carabello B. Paradoxical low flow and/or low gradient severe aortic stenosis despite preserved left ventricular ejection fraction: implications for diagnosis and treatment. Eur Heart J. 2010;31(3):281–9.
28. Barasch E, Fan D, Chukwu EO, Han J, Passick M, Petillo F, et al. Severe isolated aortic stenosis with normal left ventricular systolic function and low transvalvular gradients: pathophysiologic and prognostic insights. J Heart Valve Dis. 2008;17(1):81–8.
29. Tarantini G, Covolo E, Razzolini R, Bilato C, Frigo AC, Napodano M, et al. Valve replacement for severe aortic stenosis with low transvalvular gradient and left ventricular ejection fraction exceeding 0.50. Ann Thorac Surg. 2011;91(6):1808–15.

30. Lee SP, Kim YJ, Kim JH, Park K, Kim KH, Kim HK, et al. Deterioration of myocardial function in paradoxical low-flow severe aortic stenosis: two-dimensional strain analysis. J Am Soc Echocardiogr. 2011;24(9):976–83.
31. Ozkan A, Kapadia S, Tuzcu M, Marwick TH. Assessment of left ventricular function in aortic stenosis. Nat Rev Cardiol. 2011;8:494–501.
32. Herrmann S, Stork S, Niemann M, Lange V, Strotmann JM, Frantz S, et al. Low-gradient aortic valve stenosis myocardial fibrosis and its influence on function and outcome. J Am Coll Cardiol. 2011;58(4):402–12.
33. O'Brien B, Schoenhagen P, Kapadia SR, Svensson LG, Rodriguez L, Griffin BP, et al. Integration of 3D imaging data in the assessment of aortic stenosis: impact on classification of disease severity. Circ Cardiovasc Imaging. 2011;4(5):566–73.
34. Ng AC, Delgado V, van der Kley F, Shanks M, van de Veire NR, Bertini M, et al. Comparison of aortic root dimensions and geometries before and after transcatheter aortic valve implantation by 2- and 3-dimensional transesophageal echocardiography and multislice computed tomography. Circ Cardiovasc Imaging. 2010;3(1):94–102.
35. Cueff C, Serfaty JM, Cimadevilla C, Laissy JP, Himbert D, Tubach F, et al. Measurement of aortic valve calcification using multislice computed tomography: correlation with haemodynamic severity of aortic stenosis and clinical implication for patients with low ejection fraction. Heart. 2011;97(9):721–6.
36. Minners J, Allgeier M, Gohlke-Baerwolf C, Kienzle RP, Neumann FJ, Jander N. Inconsistent grading of aortic valve stenosis by current guidelines: haemodynamic studies in patients with apparently normal left ventricular function. Heart. 2010;96(18):1463–8.
37. Ozkan A. Low gradient "severe" aortic stenosis with preserved left ventricular ejection fraction. Cardiovasc Diagn Ther. 2012;2:19–27. doi:10.3978/j.issn.2223-3652.2012.01.01.

Pathologic Findings in Aortic Stenosis

11

Elena Ladich, Mastataka Nakano, and Renu Virmani

Abstract

With the aging of the general population in the developing world, calcific aortic stenosis (CAS) is becoming an increasingly common condition in the elderly and is associated with significant morbidity and mortality. The most common etiology in industrialized nations is tricuspid CAS, historically referred to as senile or degenerative aortic stenosis, followed by bicuspid CAS. Calcific aortic stenosis is a progressive disease exhibiting a spectrum of pathologic findings ranging from mild fibrocalcific changes in early disease, or aortic sclerosis, to end-stage stenotic lesions characterized by severe nodular calcification of valve cusps. Various atherosclerotic risk factors have been linked to CAS, leading some researchers to postulate an active cellular process similar to atherosclerosis in the development of valvular calcification. Mechanical determinants have also been emphasized, supported by pathologic observations that calcification develops at sites of maximal cuspal stress and is accelerated in congenitally abnormal valves. In addition, genetic studies are demonstrating that genetic defects may predispose patients to the development of CAS. Further insights into pathologic mechanisms underlying the initiation and progression of CAS are under investigation and may ultimately translate into novel therapeutic strategies.

Keywords

Calcific aortic stenosis • Pathology • Bicuspid aortic valve • Calcification • Risk factors • Genetics

Introduction

Calcific aortic stenosis (CAS) is the most common heart valve disease in Western society and is now the leading indication for aortic valve replacement [1]. With dramatic improvements in diagnostic imaging techniques available to clinical cardiologists, many morphologic and physiologic aspects of aortic valve disease can now be appreciated premortem. However, detailed histologic characteristics cannot be assessed by current imaging tools, particularly prior to the onset of symptomatology; therefore, pathologic examination of surgical or autopsy material remains the most definitive and direct method of assessing diseased valves. CAS is a progressive disease with precursor lesions that may remain asymptomatic for years. Precursor lesions are characterized by mild fibrocalcific thickening of the valve cusp without left ventricular outflow obstruction. With progression of disease, the cusps become increasingly fibrotic and calcified, eventually forming irregular calcific nodules on the aortic aspect of the cusp thereby interfering with the opening of the cusps. Severe CAS is responsible for the classic triad of clinical symptoms including chest pain, dyspnea, and syncope.

Recent epidemiological studies have shown that the risk factors for developing coronary atherosclerosis are similar to those for CAS. This has led to the hypothesis that there may be a similar cellular basis responsible for the development of

E. Ladich, MD • M. Nakano, MD • R. Virmani, MD (✉)
Department of Cardiovascular Pathology, CVPath Institute, Inc, 19 Firstfield Road, Gaithersburg, MD 20878, USA
e-mail: eladich@cvpath.org; mnakano@cvpath.org; rvirmani@cvpath.org

J.K. Min et al. (eds.), *Multimodality Imaging for Transcatheter Aortic Valve Replacement*, DOI 10.1007/978-1-4471-2798-7_11, © Springer-Verlag London 2014

vascular atherosclerosis and CAS. Whereas in the past CAS was considered to be a passive degenerative process related to aging, research has shown that active cellular mechanisms, some of which share common pathogenic features with coronary atherosclerosis, are responsible for CAS.

Epidemiology and Natural History

Aortic valve lesions that cause stenosis may be classified as tricuspid calcific aortic stenosis, congenital abnormalities such as unicuspid or bicuspid valves, and postinflammatory scarring (usually post-rheumatic). Over the last 50 years, pathologists have studied the etiologies of excised stenotic aortic valves examined at their institutes. In the most recent of these studies, performed at a Canadian medical center, over 1,000 consecutively excised aortic valves were analyzed: Tricuspid aortic valve was found to be the most common valve pathology (64.5 %) followed by bicuspid valve (31.9 %) and unicuspid aortic valve (3.0 %) [2] (Table 11.1).

In general, the age at presentation is quite predictive of the underlying pathologic lesion [3]. Unicuspid aortic valve occurs in 0.02 % of the population and presents in childhood, adolescence, or early adulthood and overall accounts for only 4–6 % of CAS. In contrast, bicuspid aortic valve has a prevalence of 1–2 % in the general population, a male preponderance ratio of 2:1, and is responsible for 30–50 % of surgically removed calcified aortic valves. Patients with bicuspid CAS present at an earlier age (45–55 years of age) than patients with tricuspid CAS (65–75 years) [4]. Tricuspid CAS is present in approximately 1–2 % of patients older than 65 years and 4 % of patients >85 years with men affected more commonly than women (male to female ratio = 1.6:1). With the aging of the general population in the USA, tricuspid CAS is responsible for nearly 60 % of surgical valve replacements with most patients being close to 70 years of age [2, 5].

Aortic sclerosis and stenosis are considered to represent a spectrum of the same disease process with calcification as the final common pathway leading to stenosis. While the rate of progression from mild to severe stenosis tends to be highly variable among individual patients [6], a 7-year echocardiography study observed a rate of progression to AS of any degree of approximately 16 % in elderly patients (age 70.8 ± 7.8 years) with aortic sclerosis [7]. Early sclerotic changes are characterized by fibrotic thickening and early calcification of the valve cusps without left ventricular outflow obstruction. Such changes are common in elderly patients (20–30 % in those >65 years and 48 % >85 years) and are not usually associated with a significant gradient across the valve. Aortic sclerosis however has important clinical implications beyond its identification as a precursor lesion to CAS; namely, it is associated with a 50 % increased risk of death from cardiovascular disease and myocardial infarction even in the absence of hemodynamically significant aortic valve obstruction. Whether aortic sclerosis is a marker for increased risk of cardiovascular events or has a direct effect on clinical outcomes is not known. Interestingly, in patients with mitral annular calcification, aortic valve sclerosis is observed in nearly 50 % of cases, however, CAS is only observed in 17 % [8].

A recent echocardiographic study has found that hemodynamic progression of aortic stenosis in elderly patients is dependent on underlying baseline AS severity [9]. Mean aortic valve gradients increased an average of 4, 6, and 10 mmHg/year in elderly patients with mild, moderate, and severe AS, respectively. Overall, 74 % of patients with moderate AS and 35 % of patients with mild AS progressed to severe AS. Other predictors of rapid hemodynamic progression included advanced aortic valve calcification, severe chronic renal failure, and anemia.

Severe aortic stenosis results in a pressure overloaded left ventricle with concentric left ventricular hypertrophy and normal left ventricular chamber size. Once symptomatic, aortic valve replacement with either a mechanical or bioprosthetic valve is the only definitive treatment and is usually curative. The average survival without treatment is only 2–3 years with an increased risk of sudden death.

Table 11.1 Etiology of surgically removed aortic valves

Etiology	Mayo Clinic (1965)[a] (%)	University of Minnesota (1979–1983)[b] (%)	London (1976–1979)[c] (%)	Mayo (1990)[d] (%)	AFIP (1990–1997) (%)	Toronto (2008)[e] (%)
Bicuspid	49	49	56	36	30	32
Post-rheumatic	33	23	24	9	13	11
Tricuspid degenerative	0	28	12	51	49	64
Unicuspid	10	1	0	0	6	3
Other	7	0	8	2	2	1

[a]Subramanian et al. [15]
[b]Peterson et al. [44]
[c]Davis [45]
[d]Dare et al. [46]
[e]Collins et al. [2]

Pathology of Calcific Aortic Stenosis

Calcific Aortic Stenosis (Tricuspid)

The normal aortic valve is composed of three semicircular cusps (left, right, and posterior (noncoronary)) attached to the aorta at three commissures. The cusps are thin and translucent with a thickness of less than 1 mm and two surfaces lined by endothelial cells including the ventricular surface facing the left ventricle (inflow surface) and the aortic surface (outflow surface). The aortic valve cusp has three distinct histologic layers each of which is adapted to a specific function. These layers are defined as (1) the ventricularis, a loose connective tissue layer rich in elastic fibers on the ventricular side of the cusp; (2) the spongiosa, in the middle of the cusp, composed predominantly of proteoglycans and glycosaminoglycans; (3) the fibrosa, a dense collagen layer that extends on the aortic surface. Finally, valvular interstitial cells (VICs) constitute the majority of the cells in all layers of the valve and maintain the matrix of the normal valve tissue.

We and others have described the gross and histologic features of aortic valves at autopsy as well as valve cusps removed surgically. Grossly, tricuspid CAS demonstrates calcified masses and nodules involving the aortic surface of the valve cusps in an aortic valve that was previously anatomically normal. The earliest calcification occurs at cusp attachment sites (base of cusps) and extends along the line of closure or coaptation zone. Pathologic changes may range from mild cuspal thickening in early disease (aortic sclerosis) to end-stage stenotic lesions with calcific nodules filling the involved sinuses of Valsalva (Fig. 11.1). It has been shown that the distribution of calcium in stenotic cusps is not uniform and may differ considerably between individual cusps. In one study, surgically excised cusps showed differences in weights with one cusp differing from the other two (by >0.1 g) in 61 % of valves, whereas 26 % of valves demonstrated weight differences between all three cusps. Weight differences appeared to be caused by differing quantities of calcium [10]. Interestingly, calcification is typically more pronounced in the noncoronary cusp compared with the coronary cusps. One explanation for this finding may relate to the relatively reduced diastolic pressure loads around the coronary cusps due to the presence of the coronary ostia.

Histologically, early calcification—highlighted by von Kossa staining—appears as fine stippled calcifications or small nodular concretions typically located in the fibrosa layer on the aortic aspect of the valve cusp, especially in areas of early atherosclerotic change. The ventricular surface of the valve is mostly smooth exhibiting varying degrees of fibrosis. The "hinge" area of the aortic cusps near the attachment to the aortic root at an area just below the line of valve closure are regions where early calcific deposits are found and may be related to the higher mechanical forces in these regions (Fig. 11.2) [11]. Such site-specific vulnerability to calcification has also been partially attributed to differential endothelial gene expression on the aortic versus ventricular side of aortic valve cusps. It has been shown that the fibrosa on the aortic side of the cusp displays a "calcification permissive" transcriptional profile characterized by overexpression of genes related to skeletal development, vascular calcification, and bone formation such as bone morphogenetic protein 4 (BMP4) along with decreased expression of multiple inhibitors of cardiovascular calcification [12].

As calcification progresses, there is coalescence of microcalcifications into larger complex plates and nodules, sometimes associated with surface ulceration. In a pathologic study of 247 surgically excised aortic valves (age range 17–86 years, mean 64.1 ± 13.4 years), morphologic features of aortic stenosis were present in almost 70 % of valves. Ulceration of calcific nodules was present in approximately 40 % of valves showing severe calcification [13]. In later stages, the calcification is often superimposed on a thickened and fibrotic cusp and there may be histologic evidence of bone matrix formation, osteocytes, and marrow elements.

Congenital Bicuspid and Unicuspid Valve

A congenital bicuspid aortic valve is a common congenital cardiac anomaly present in 1–2 % of the general population. Valvular stenosis is the most frequent physiologic complication affecting approximately 80 % of such valves studied at autopsy or post-valve replacement. Fifteen percent of congenital bicuspid aortic valves are surgically excised for insufficiency and only 5 % for combined aortic stenosis and aortic insufficiency [2].

Recently, macroscopic and microscopic findings have been reported in a large series of tricuspid, bicuspid, and unicuspid aortic valves removed at surgery [2]. Overall, pathologic features became progressively more severe with valves exhibiting fewer cusps (unicuspid and bicuspid) and presented at an earlier age. For example, a decreasing number of cusps were associated with an increasing frequency of cusp calcification, calcification occurring at the raphe and the base of the cusp in the presence of ossification, cartilaginous metaplasia, and ulceration. It has also been shown that bicuspid aortic valves are more likely than tricuspid valves to show high grade (grade 4) calcification [13]. The increased severity of changes in congenital valves may result from abnormal blood flow and stress distribution across the abnormal valve causing accelerated calcification and earlier failures.

An association between congenitally malformed aortic valves and aortic dissection is well known. In one series, replacement of the ascending aorta was more common in

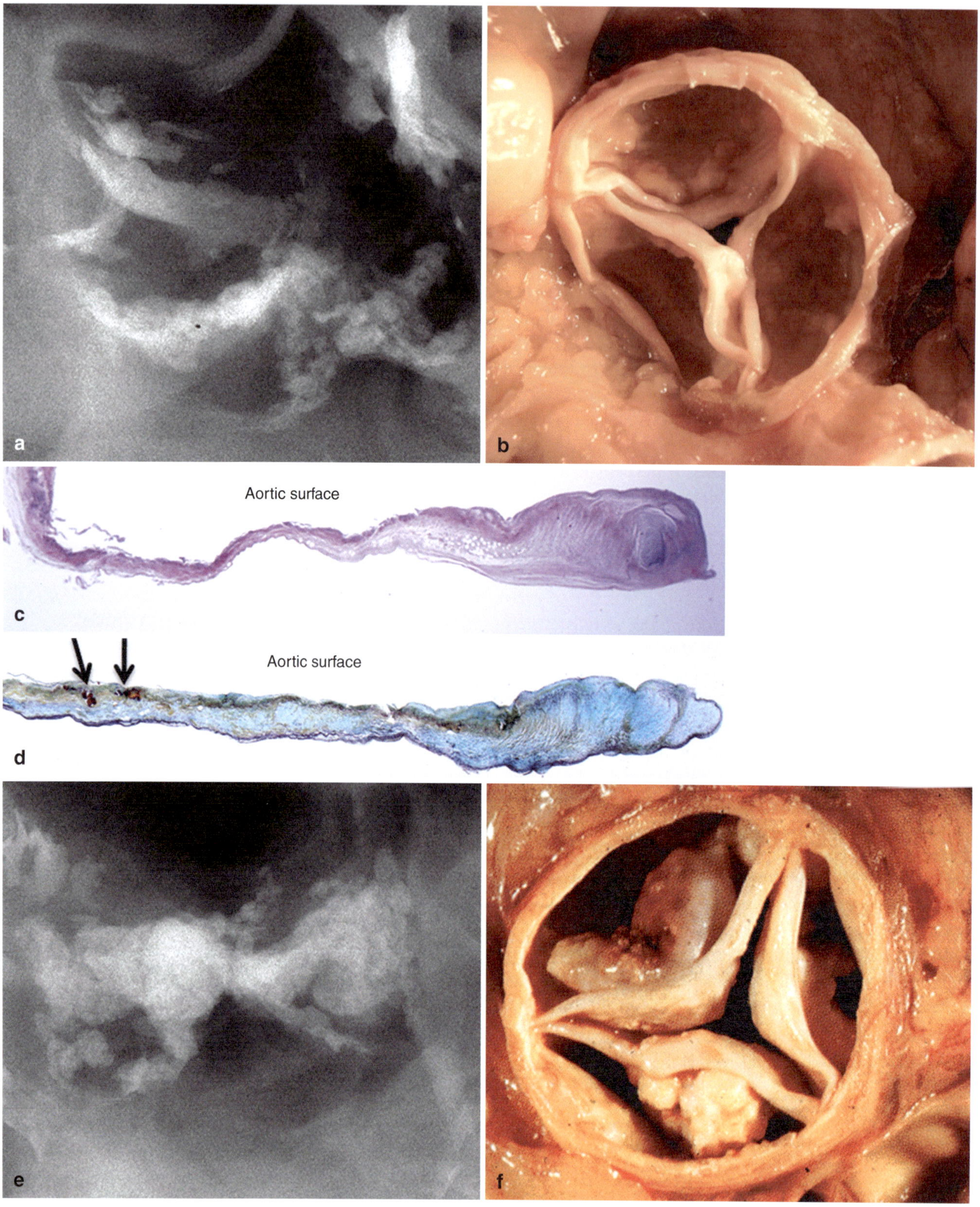

Fig. 11.1 Two aortic valves seen at autopsy showing progression of calcific aortic stenosis. (**a**, **b**) Radiograph and gross image of aortic valve from an 83-year-old female. This valve shows mild calcification with small calcific deposits on aortic surface of cusps and sparing of the free edge. (**c**, **d**) Histologic sections of cusps showing fibrotic thickening and microscopic calcific deposits in the zona fibrosa (*arrows*). (**e**, **f**). Radiograph and gross image of stenotic aortic valve from an 82-year-old female. There is marked nodular calcification of the cusps with bulky deposits on the aortic surface. (**g**, **h**) Histologic sections of the cusps show calcific nodules superimposed on a fibrotic cusp with ulceration of the aortic surface (*arrow*). Note fibrotic thickening of the ventricular surface

Fig. 11.1 (continued)

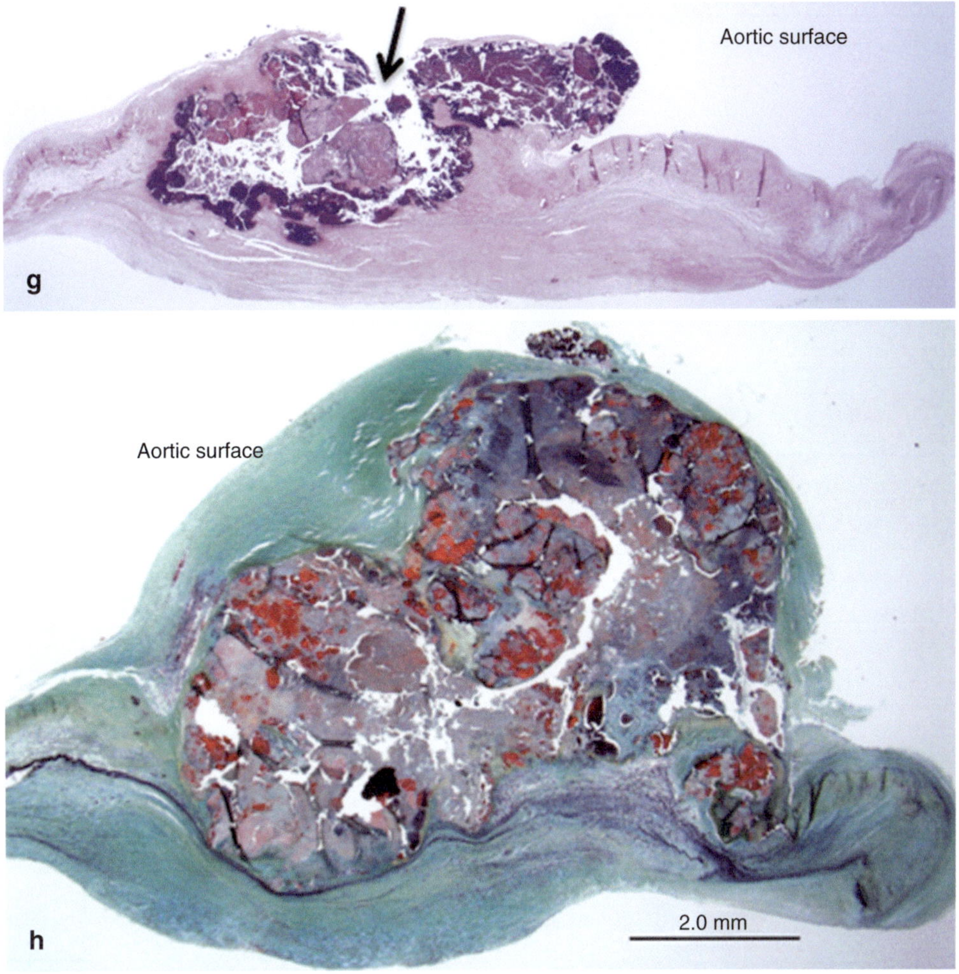

patients with congenital valves occurring in 38.8 and 54.8 % of bicuspid and unicuspid valves, respectively, compared to 16.6 % of patients with tricuspid aortic valves [2]. Of aortic dissections reported from autopsy series, a bicuspid valve was present in 10 %, five times more than the rate of bicuspid valve in the general population. The mechanism seems to be independent of hemodynamic alterations secondary to aortic stenosis and is supported by observations that aortas associated with bicuspid aortic valves have reduced fibrillin-1 content as compared to tricuspid valves. Reduction of fibrillin-1 has been associated with release of matrix metalloproteinases that may weaken the vessel wall by degrading the elastic matrix [14].

In the most common morphology of congenital bicuspid valve (about 75 % of cases), there are two cusps of unequal size with the larger conjoint cusp located anteriorly within the aortic root; the smaller cusp is typically found posteriorly. In this morphologic variant, the right and left cusps are conjoined and both coronary arteries arise from the sinus of Valsalva from the anterior conjoint cusp. The size of the conjoint cusp is typically less than two times the size of the non-conjoint cusp and contains a median raphe (aborted third commissure). The raphe may extend a variable distance from the aortic sinus toward the cusp but usually does not reach the free edge of the conjoint cusp. Less commonly, the right and noncoronary cusps are conjoint. The rarest morphology is a conjoint left and noncoronary cusp [15].

In congenital bicuspid valves, calcification begins in the raphe (if present) and develops in a linear fashion as noted on computed tomographic examination and extends into the cusp tissue, often in a radial pattern, largely sparing the true commissures (Fig. 11.3) [11]. In contrast, in rheumatic aortic stenosis, calcification is variably present and starts in the fused commissures and extends into the body of the cusp. The bicuspid aortic valve has an uneven cusp surface that is often dysplastic in appearance. When young individuals present with symptoms of stenotic congenital bicuspid valves, the cusps are typically thickened and dysplastic. The complex anatomic features of bicuspid aortic valve including cuspal thickening and raphal ridge make the valve more susceptible to higher mechanical stress compared to the tricuspid valve. In thickened dysplastic valves, the fibrotic

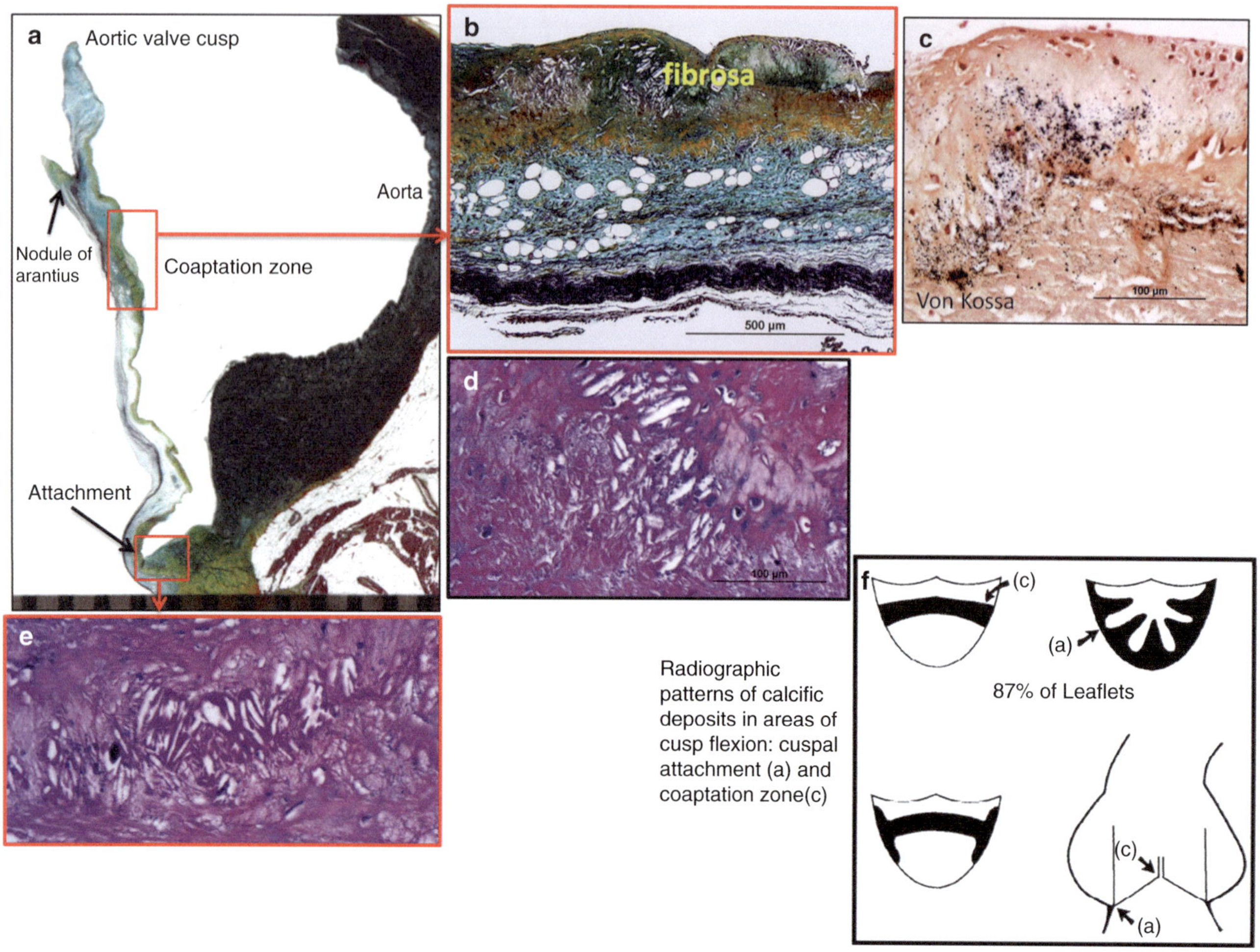

Fig. 11.2 Pattern of calcification in aortic valve cusps. (**a**) Longitudinal section of intact aortic valve cusp and aorta. The *red boxes* highlight areas of early atheromatous change with microscopic calcification in two regions: (1) the *upper box* shows an early lesion on the aortic surface at the coaptation zone and (2) an early lesion at the cuspal attachment site (*lower box*). Higher magnifications show fibrosa layer of cusp with atheromatous changes characterized by cholesterol clefts, lipid pools, and rare chronic inflammation (**b**, **d**, **e**). (**c**) Von Kossa staining highlights microscopic calcifications (*calcium stains black*). The diagram in (**f**) highlights radiographic patterns of calcific deposits in areas of cusp flexion. (*c*) Area of coaptation and (*a*) cusp attachment site. These radiographic areas mirror histologic regions of calcification (The diagram F was reproduced with permission from Thubrikar et al.[11])

thickening may be diffuse or more often is most pronounced near the line of valve closure. Histologically, calcification has been reported to occur diffusely within the cusp spongiosa in congenital bicuspid valve stenosis.

Unicuspid valves can be categorized as one of two morphologic subtypes: (1) a domed-shaped acommissural valve containing three aborted commissures (or raphe) or (2) a unicommissural valve with slit-like opening that reaches the aortic wall at its single intact commissure. Unicommissural unicuspid aortic valves account for 60 % of aortic stenosis cases in patients <15 years old [16]. Leaflet dysplasia is common and the severity of leaflet calcification is variable however dysplasia of unicuspid has been reported to be more severe compared to bicuspid valve and is dependent on patient age [2].

Risk Factors (Box 11.1)

Several epidemiological studies have identified risk factors for calcific aortic stenosis similar to those of coronary atherosclerosis including age, male gender, smoking, elevated cholesterol levels, diabetes, metabolic syndrome, hypertension, and increased lipoprotein (a) levels. CAS has also been associated with renal dysfunction and abnormalities of calcium and phosphate metabolism such as Paget's disease, hyperparathyroidism, and chronic renal failure [17, 18]. A recent prospective epidemiological study of 1,323 young adult participants with >25-year follow-up evaluated cardiovascular risk factors and valve calcium [19]. Of the modifiable risk factors, cigarette smoking and total cholesterol were strongly associated with valve calcium. In addition, important associations for HDL-C and BMI with valvular calcification were noted. Overall, this study provides new evidence that long-term exposure to adverse risk factors is associated with increased valve calcium [19].

Pathogenesis

Calcification occurs in a wide variety of clinically important cardiovascular disease such as atherosclerosis, aortic valve stenosis, ischemic myocardial calcification, and the calcification associated with bioprosthetic cardiac valves. The view that valvular calcification is primarily a consequence of age-related degeneration has been challenged by studies demonstrating that aortic valve calcification is an active cellular process with identifiable clinical and genetic risk factors with specific cellular and molecular pathways. Studies in animal models of calcific aortic stenosis and surgically excised valves have demonstrated histologic similarities to atherosclerosis lending support to the hypothesis that there is a link between atherosclerosis and CAS.

Early aortic valve sclerosis lesions have been demonstrated in hypercholesterolemic rabbits characterized by thickening of the valve leaflets with lipid deposition, endothelial cell disruption, connective tissue changes, and the presence of

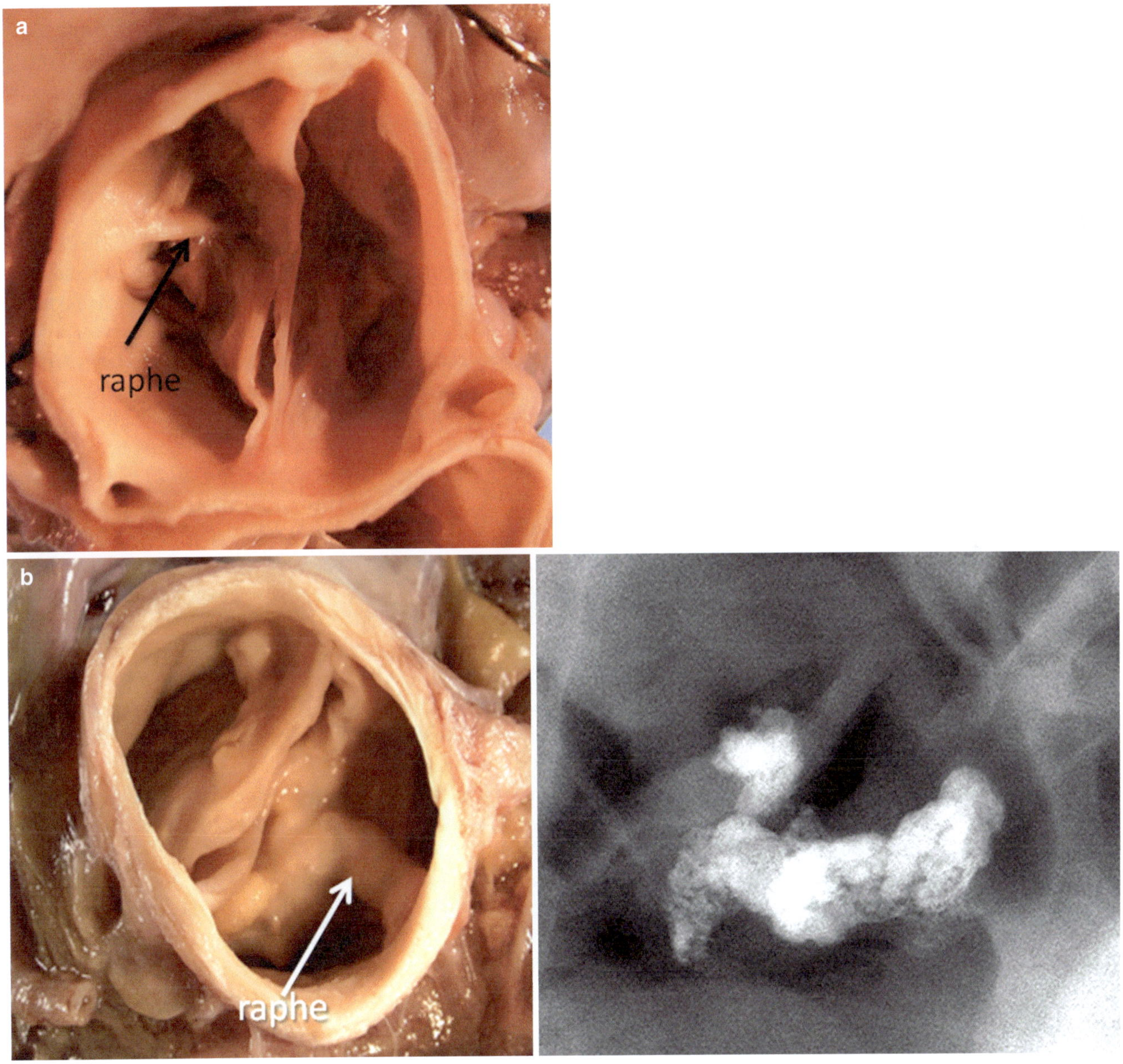

Fig. 11.3 Progression of bicuspid aortic valve calcification. (**a**) Bicuspid aortic valve viewed from the aortic surface (early lesion); calcification was limited to the raphe. (**b**) A stenotic bicuspid aortic valve obtained at autopsy from a 49-year-old male who died suddenly (late lesion). (**c**) Severe nodular calcification arising in a bicuspid valve. Note multiple nodules with ulceration through the aortic surface

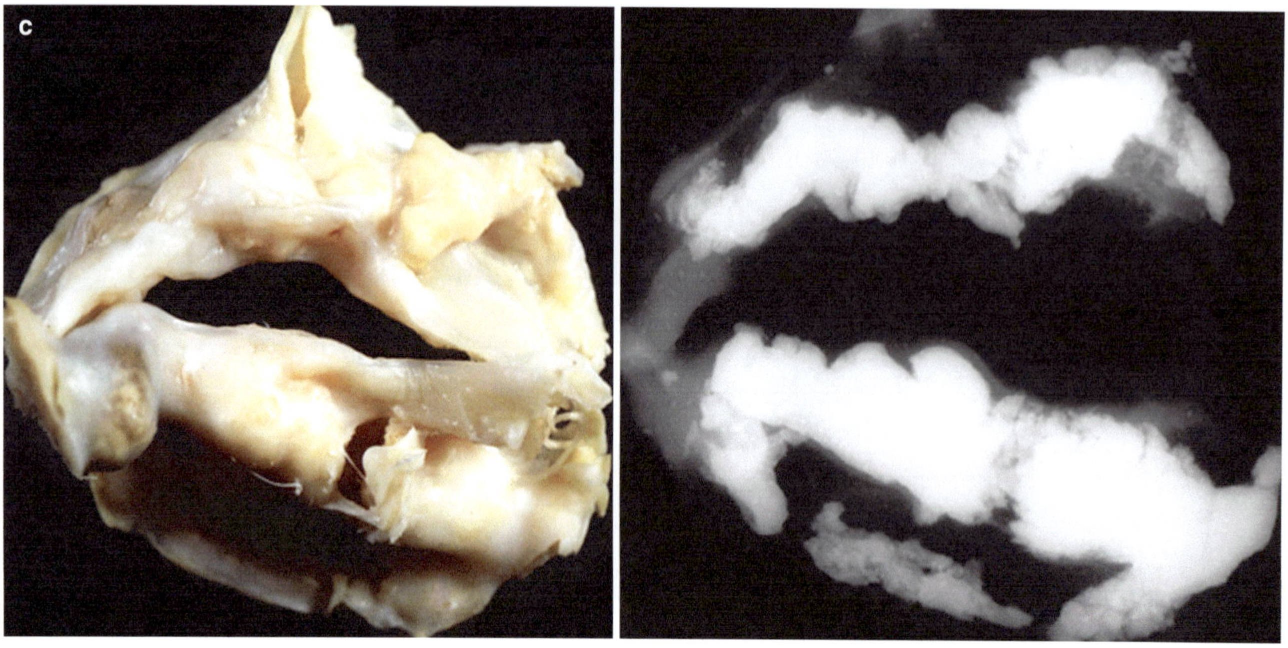

Fig. 11.3 (continued)

Box 11.1 Risk Factors for Calcific Aortic Stenosis

- Age
- Calcium and phosphate metabolism disorders
- Chronic kidney disease
- Diabetes mellitus
- Dyslipidemia
- Hypertension
- Lipoprotein (a) elevation
- Male gender
- Metabolic syndrome
- Smoking

macrophages and osteopontin [20]. In addition, studies have shown an increase in macrophages and cellular proliferation (PCNA +) associated with transformation to an osteoblast-like phenotype with calcification and bone differentiation [21]. In other studies, hypercholesterolemic rabbits demonstrated complex bone formation in calcified aortic valves associated with upregulation of the Wnt/LDL receptor-related protein 5 (Lrp5), osteopontin, and p42/44 expression [22].

Human histology studies have also demonstrated features of early aortic valve calcification that share histologic similarities with coronary atherosclerosis such as presence of lipid and inflammation. Otto et al. demonstrated intracellular and extracellular lipid in early valve lesions associated with fine stippled mineralization localized along the aortic aspect of the cusp. A cellular infiltrate composed predominantly of macrophages and T lymphocytes with few actin positive smooth muscle cells was also identified within these lesions [23].

Neovascularization and lymphohistiocytic inflammation in surgically removed stenotic calcific valves have also been consistently described. These histologic features were similar between tricuspid and bicuspid valves; however, the degree of calcification was more severe in bicuspid aortic valves compared to tricuspid valves. The results suggest a similar pathologic process leading to stenosis between BAV and TAV that becomes accelerated in BAV [13]. Other investigators have also noted neovascularization located in regions of inflammation. Cusp thickening and subsequent hypoxia have been shown to trigger the release of vascular endothelial growth factors and other proangiogenic factors [24].

Histologic similarities between CAS and atherosclerosis, however, do not prove whether atherosclerosis is responsible for the pathogenesis of CAS. In support of the view that mechanical determinants also play a role in the development of valvular calcification, it has been shown (as described above) that calcification occurs in regions of increased mechanical stress as the earliest deposits are found at the cusp attachments and near points of coaptation. Mild asymmetry of valve cusps has also been suggested as a potential precipitant of the calcification process; however, minor differences in cusp size is observed in greater than 50 % of individuals rendering it unlikely that cusp asymmetry is sufficient to account for severe stenosis in most cases [3, 25]. Nevertheless, a role for cusp asymmetry is suggested because deformed valves, such as bicuspid valves, have an abnormal distribution of stress across the cusps and calcify earlier than normal tricuspid valves.

Calcification of valve cusps may also occur as a result of mechanical "wear and tear" through the formation of nucleation sites. For example, fragmented collagen and elastin fibers resulting from mechanical disruption can serve as nucleation

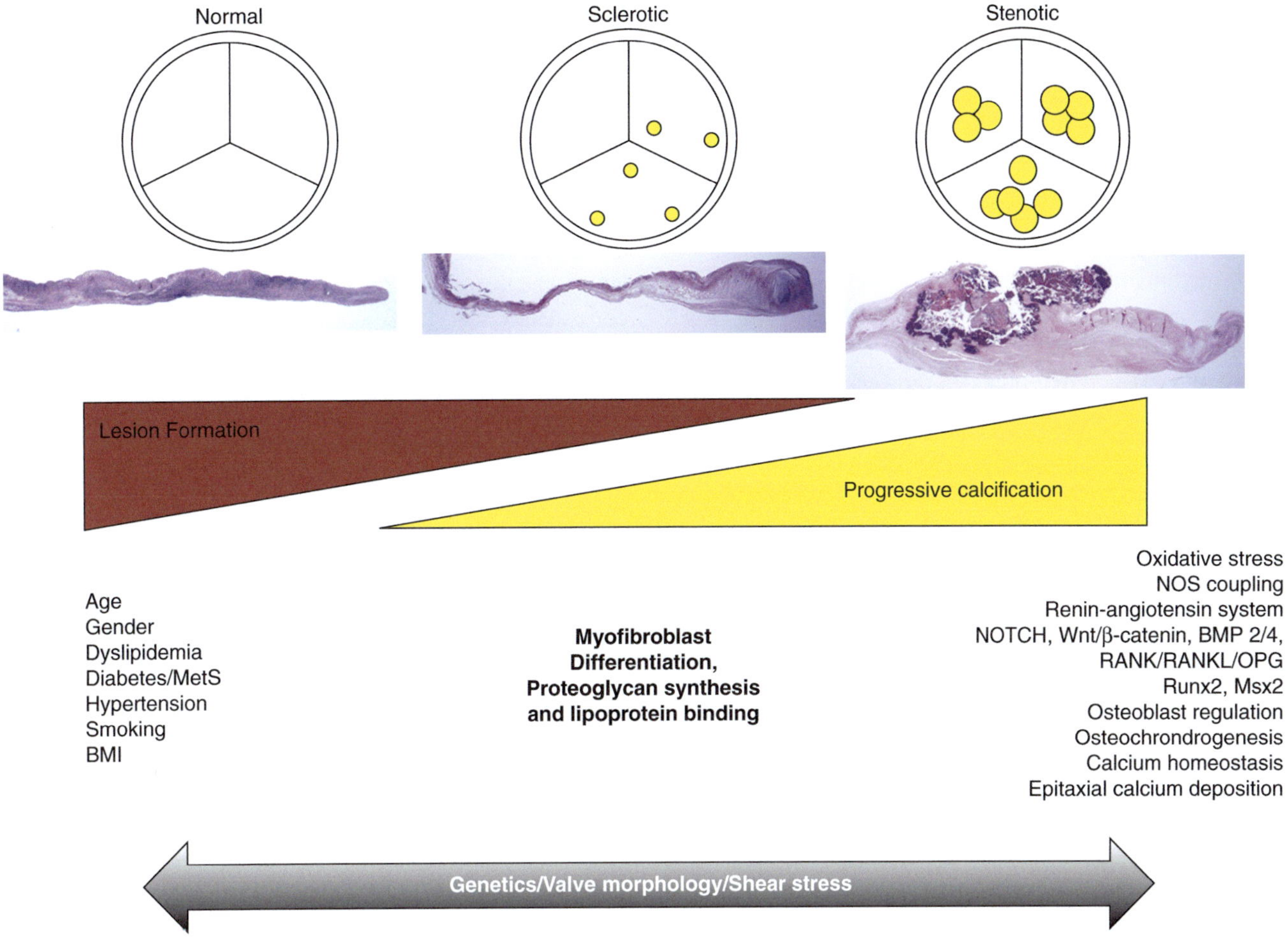

Fig. 11.4 Diagram illustrating the potential paradigm for the understanding of CAS, traditional cardiovascular risk factors promote valvular calcification via atherosclerosis. Myoblast differentiation and proteoglycan synthesis and lipoprotein binding may enhance calcification. Alternatively, transdifferentiation into osteogenic phenotypes through the upregulation of Wnt/β-catenin, RANK/RANKL/OPG, Runx2/Cbfa1, and Msx2 pathways may occur. Systemic and paracrine regulators of osteoblast function, calcium hemostasis, and dystrophic epitaxial calcification play an increasing role as calcification progresses. Genetic factors, valve morphology (e.g., unicuspid and bicuspid valves), and shear stress likely contribute to disease progression across the full spectrum of disease. *Abbreviations*: *MetS* metabolic syndrome, *NOS* nitric oxide synthase, *BMP* bone morphogenetic protein, *RANK* receptor activator of nuclear factor kappa-B (NF-κB), *RANKL* receptor activator of NFκB ligand, *OPG* osteoprotegerin, *Runx-2* Runt-related transcription factor (RUNX) family of genes which are also called core binding factor-α (Cbfα) that are involved in osteoblast differentiation, and *Msx2* Msh homeobox 2 (Modified from Owens and Otto [47])

sites for calcification [26]. In addition, it has been proposed that extracellular lipid may also serve as nucleation sites for calcification because calcific deposits and lipid droplets have been shown to localize to similar regions in the valve cusp [27].

Comparison of CAS to Atherosclerosis Lesions

Atherosclerosis, regardless of the arterial location, shares common features of intimal smooth muscle cells, foamy macrophages T cells, lipid deposition, neovascularization, and calcification. The smooth muscle cell is historically considered to be the source of atherosclerotic plaque calcification by an active process involving calcification of portions of the cell organelles called matrix vesicles. In contrast to arterial atherosclerosis, the lesions of early aortic valve disease have demonstrated few actin positive smooth muscle cells. The biology of intimal calcification within atherosclerotic regions suggests a putative role for apoptotic bodies, bone associated proteins, lipids, and inflammation in the formation of extracellular intimal calcifications [28]. In addition, immunohistochemical studies have demonstrated the co-localization of osteopontin and other calcium-binding proteins in areas of microcalcifications [29–31]. Similar to observations reported in human coronary arteries, osteopontin and other calcium-binding proteins have been identified in calcified aortic valves obtained at autopsy and surgery. Studies have shown that aortic valve calcification is composed of hydroxyapatite deposited on a bone-like matrix of collagen, osteopontin, and other minor bone matrix proteins [32, 33]. In addition, an osteoblast-like cellular phenotype was identified in calcified valves removed at the time of surgical valve replacement as shown by increased gene expression of osteopontin, bone sialoprotein, osteocalcin, and CBfa1 (the osteoblast-specific transcription factor for bone formation). These findings support the hypothesis that the cells residing in the aortic valve have the potential to differentiate into bone forming cells, which over time mineralize and express an ossification phenotype [34].

Growth factors have also been implicated in the pathogenesis of both coronary atherosclerosis and CAS. A "response to injury" hypothesis has been postulated based on evidence that injury to the valve surface initiates a cascade of events involving inflammatory mediators such as transforming growth factor beta (TGF-ß) [35]. TGF-ß has been identified in the extracellular matrix in calcified valve cusps where it was found to promote CAS through formation of calcified apoptotic alkaline phosphatase-enriched nodules. Furthermore, TGF-ß showed effects on differentiation of valvular interstitial cells increasing expression of alpha SMA, smooth muscle myosin, calponin, as well as matrix metalloproteinases suggesting that TGF-ß may induce the connective tissue alterations associated with CAS.

Genetics

A growing number of studies are providing further evidence for a genetic basis for aortic valve disease (Box 11.2). For example, genetic lipoprotein abnormalities have been identified in some patients predisposed to the development of calcific aortic stenosis. A higher prevalence of the apolipoprotein B and E2 polymorphisms was identified in patients with severe AS. In addition, a significant association of vitamin D receptor polymorphisms with calcific aortic valve stenosis has been identified in which the B allele of the vitamin D receptor is more common in these patients [36, 37]. Other genetic abnormalities include loss of function of the NOTCH 1 receptor as well as familial clustering for calcific aortic disease in western France where operated calcific aortic disease was significantly higher compared to the general population [38].

Box 11.2 Examples of Genetic Disorders Associated with Aortic Stenosis

- Apoliprotein B polymorphism
- E2 polymorphism
- Loss of function of the NOTCH 1 receptor
- Vitamin D receptor polymorphisms (B allele of the vitamin D receptor)

Statin Therapy for CAS

Given the clinical evidence that valvular lesions occur in the setting of hypercholesterolemia and elevated serum lipoprotein, there has been much clinical interest in assessing the effectiveness of statins in treating CAS. While earlier retrospective studies demonstrated an association between statin use and decreased risk of progression of aortic valve calcification, the results from prospective studies have not shown a consistent effect [39]. The RAAVE study (Rosuvastatin Affecting Aortic Valve Endothelium to Slow the Progression of Aortic Stenosis) was the first prospective study to demonstrate a positive effect of statin therapy in the treatment of AS patients with moderate to severe aortic stenosis as measured by echocardiography [40]. However, other prospective lipid-lowering trials such as SALTIRE study (Scottish Aortic Stenosis and Lipid Lowering Trial) and SEAS trial (Simvastatin and Ezetamibe in Aortic Stenosis Study) failed to show a benefit of lipid lowering on calcific aortic stenosis [41]. The recently published ASTRONOMER trial (Aortic Stenosis Progression Observation: Measuring Effects of Rosuvastatin), which randomized patients with less severe aortic valve disease, also failed to demonstrate the efficacy of statins in slowing aortic valve disease [42].

There are several possible explanations for the contradictory results between studies. It is possible that these studies involved patients with advanced disease no longer amenable to treatment. However, a study in patients with only mild to moderate disease (SEAS) also showed no benefit from statins. It is also feasible that, while atherosclerosis and CAS share some clinical and pathologic features, CAS is more complex and there may be overlapping non-atherosclerotic mechanisms involved such as shear forces and genetic factors. A recent study by Ngo et al. demonstrated nitric oxide resistance as another potential mechanism underlying aortic valve calcification [43]. Finally, the histologic features and clinical implications of calcification observed in atherosclerosis are distinct from those in calcific aortic stenosis and may explain the differing responses to statin treatment.

Conclusions

With the aging of the general population, calcific aortic stenosis is becoming an increasingly common condition in the elderly and is associated with significant morbidity and mortality. Various atherosclerotic risk factors have been linked to aortic stenosis and there are pathologic and mechanistic similarities between atherosclerosis and CAS. Other mechanisms potentially explaining the pathogenesis of CAS have also been observed, including direct mechanical force and genetic susceptibility. Yet, to date, no effective medical therapies have been identified to halt or slow progression of disease. In the near future, it will be vital to understand the differences in mild, moderate, and severe aortic valve calcification, especially the distribution of valvular calcification, and how noninvasive technologies may help identify individuals who are candidates for new techniques such as percutaneous valve replacement for treatment of aortic stenosis.

References

1. Vaishnava P, Fuster V, Goldman M, Bonow RO. Surgery for asymptomatic degenerative aortic and mitral valve disease. Nat Rev Cardiol. 2011;8(3):173–7. Epub 2011/01/19.
2. Collins MJ, Butany J, Borger MA, Strauss BH, David TE. Implications of a congenitally abnormal valve: a study of 1025 consecutively excised aortic valves. J Clin Pathol. 2008;61(4):530–6.
3. Roberts WC. The structure of the aortic valve in clinically isolated aortic stenosis: an autopsy study of 162 patients over 15 years of age. Circulation. 1970;42(1):91–7.
4. Roberts WC, Ko JM. Frequency by decades of unicuspid, bicuspid, and tricuspid aortic valves in adults having isolated aortic valve replacement for aortic stenosis, with or without associated aortic regurgitation. Circulation. 2005;111(7):920–5. Epub 2005/02/16.
5. Passik CS, Ackermann DM, Pluth JR, Edwards WD. Temporal changes in the causes of aortic stenosis: a surgical pathologic study of 646 cases. Mayo Clin Proc. 1987;62(2):119–23.
6. Faggiano P, Aurigemma GP, Rusconi C, Gaasch WH. Progression of valvular aortic stenosis in adults: literature review and clinical implications. Am Heart J. 1996;132(2 Pt 1):408–17.
7. Cosmi JE, Kort S, Tunick PA, Rosenzweig BP, Freedberg RS, Katz ES, et al. The risk of the development of aortic stenosis in patients with "benign" aortic valve thickening. Arch Intern Med. 2002;162(20):2345–7.
8. Boon A, Cheriex E, Lodder J, Kessels F. Cardiac valve calcification: characteristics of patients with calcification of the mitral annulus or aortic valve. Heart. 1997;78(5):472–4. Epub 1998/01/01.
9. Kearney LG, Ord M, Buxton BF, Matalanis G, Patel SK, Burrell LM, et al. Progression of aortic stenosis in elderly patients over long-term follow up. Int J Cardiol. 2012 (in press). doi:10.1016/j.ijcard.2012.03.139.
10. Roberts WC, Ko JM. Weights of individual cusps in operatively-excised stenotic three-cuspid aortic valves. Am J Cardiol. 2004;94(5):681–4. Epub 2004/09/03.
11. Thubrikar MJ, Aouad J, Nolan SP. Patterns of calcific deposits in operatively excised stenotic or purely regurgitant aortic valves and their relation to mechanical stress. Am J Cardiol. 1986;58(3):304–8. Epub 1986/08/01.
12. Yip CY, Simmons CA. The aortic valve microenvironment and its role in calcific aortic valve disease. Cardiovasc pathol. 2011;20(3):177–82.
13. Butany J, Collins MJ, Demellawy DE, Nair V, Israel N, Leong SW, et al. Morphological and clinical findings in 247 surgically excised native aortic valves. Can J Cardiol. 2005;21(9):747–55.
14. Fedak PW, de Sa MP, Verma S, Nili N, Kazemian P, Butany J, et al. Vascular matrix remodeling in patients with bicuspid aortic valve malformations: implications for aortic dilatation. J Thorac Cardiovasc Surg. 2003;126(3):797–806.
15. Subramanian R, Olson LJ, Edwards WD. Surgical pathology of pure aortic stenosis: a study of 374 cases. Mayo Clin Proc. 1984;59(10):683–90.
16. Roberts WC. Morphologic aspects of cardiac valve dysfunction. Am Heart J. 1992;123(6):1610–32.
17. Stewart BF, Siscovick D, Lind BK, Gardin JM, Gottdiener JS, Smith VE, et al. Clinical factors associated with calcific aortic valve disease. Cardiovascular Health Study. J Am Coll Cardiol. 1997;29(3):630–4.
18. Gotoh T, Kuroda T, Yamasawa M, Nishinaga M, Mitsuhashi T, Seino Y, et al. Correlation between lipoprotein(a) and aortic valve sclerosis assessed by echocardiography (the JMS Cardiac Echo and Cohort Study). Am J Cardiol. 1995;76(12):928–32.
19. Thanassoulis G, Massaro JM, Cury R, Manders E, Benjamin EJ, Vasan RS, et al. Associations of long-term and early adult atherosclerosis risk factors with aortic and mitral valve calcium. J Am Coll Cardiol. 2010;55(22):2491–8.
20. Cimini M, Boughner DR, Ronald JA, Aldington L, Rogers KA. Development of aortic valve sclerosis in a rabbit model of atherosclerosis: an immunohistochemical and histological study. J Heart Valve Dis. 2005;14(3):365–75.
21. Rajamannan NM, Subramaniam M, Springett M, Sebo TC, Niekrasz M, McConnell JP, et al. Atorvastatin inhibits hypercholesterolemia-induced cellular proliferation and bone matrix production in the rabbit aortic valve. Circulation. 2002;105(22):2660–5.
22. Rajamannan NM. Calcific aortic stenosis: lessons learned from experimental and clinical studies. Arterioscler Thromb Vasc Biol. 2009;29(2):162–8.
23. Otto CM, Kuusisto J, Reichenbach DD, Gown AM, O'Brien KD. Characterization of the early lesion of 'degenerative' valvular aortic stenosis. Histological and immunohistochemical studies. Circulation. 1994;90(2):844–53.
24. Mazzone A, Epistolato MC, De Caterina R, Storti S, Vittorini S, Sbrana S, et al. Neoangiogenesis, T-lymphocyte infiltration, and heat shock protein-60 are biological hallmarks of an immunomediated inflammatory process in end-stage calcified aortic valve stenosis. J Am Coll Cardiol. 2004;43(9):1670–6.
25. Vollebergh FE, Becker AE. Minor congenital variations of cusp size in tricuspid aortic valves. Possible link with isolated aortic stenosis. Br Heart J. 1977;39(9):1006–11.
26. Bailey MT, Pillarisetti S, Xiao H, Vyavahare NR. Role of elastin in pathologic calcification of xenograft heart valves. J Biomed Mater Res A. 2003;66(1):93–102.
27. Dunmore-Buyze J, Boughner DR, Macris N, Vesely I. A comparison of macroscopic lipid content within porcine pulmonary and aortic valves. Implications for bioprosthetic valves. J Thorac Cardiovasc Surg. 1995;110(6):1756–61.
28. Proudfoot D, Shanahan CM. Biology of calcification in vascular cells: intima versus media. Herz. 2001;26(4):245–51.
29. Fitzpatrick LA, Severson A, Edwards WD, Ingram RT. Diffuse calcification in human coronary arteries. Association of osteopontin with atherosclerosis. J Clin Invest. 1994;94(4):1597–604.
30. Kwon HM, Hong BK, Kang TS, Kwon K, Kim HK, Jang Y, et al. Expression of osteopontin in calcified coronary atherosclerotic plaques. J Korean Med Sci. 2000;15(5):485–93.
31. O'Brien ER, Garvin MR, Stewart DK, Hinohara T, Simpson JB, Schwartz SM, et al. Osteopontin is synthesized by macrophage, smooth muscle, and endothelial cells in primary and restenotic human coronary atherosclerotic plaques. Arterioscler Thromb. 1994;14(10):1648–56.
32. O'Brien KD, Kuusisto J, Reichenbach DD, Ferguson M, Giachelli C, Alpers CE, et al. Osteopontin is expressed in human aortic valvular lesions. Circulation. 1995;92(8):2163–8.
33. Mohler 3rd ER, Gannon F, Reynolds C, Zimmerman R, Keane MG, Kaplan FS. Bone formation and inflammation in cardiac valves. Circulation. 2001;103(11):1522–8.
34. Rajamannan NM, Subramaniam M, Rickard D, Stock SR, Donovan J, Springett M, et al. Human aortic valve calcification is associated with an osteoblast phenotype. Circulation. 2003;107(17):2181–4.
35. Li C, Xu S, Gotlieb AI. The response to valve injury. A paradigm to understand the pathogenesis of heart valve disease. Cardiovasc pathol. 2011;20(3):183–90. Epub 2010/11/16.

36. Novaro GM, Sachar R, Pearce GL, Sprecher DL, Griffin BP. Association between apolipoprotein E alleles and calcific valvular heart disease. Circulation. 2003;108(15):1804–8.
37. Ortlepp JR, Hoffmann R, Ohme F, Lauscher J, Bleckmann F, Hanrath P. The vitamin D receptor genotype predisposes to the development of calcific aortic valve stenosis. Heart. 2001;85(6):635–8.
38. Garg V, Muth AN, Ransom JF, Schluterman MK, Barnes R, King IN, et al. Mutations in NOTCH1 cause aortic valve disease. Nature. 2005;437(7056):270–4.
39. Shavelle DM, Takasu J, Budoff MJ, Mao S, Zhao XQ, O'Brien KD. HMG CoA reductase inhibitor (statin) and aortic valve calcium. Lancet. 2002;359(9312):1125–6.
40. Moura LM, Ramos SF, Zamorano JL, Barros IM, Azevedo LF, Rocha-Goncalves F, et al. Rosuvastatin affecting aortic valve endothelium to slow the progression of aortic stenosis. J Am Coll Cardiol. 2007;49(5):554–61.
41. Cowell SJ, Newby DE, Prescott RJ, Bloomfield P, Reid J, Northridge DB, et al. A randomized trial of intensive lipid-lowering therapy in calcific aortic stenosis. N Engl J Med. 2005;352(23):2389–97.
42. Chan KL, Teo K, Dumesnil JG, Ni A, Tam J. Effect of Lipid lowering with rosuvastatin on progression of aortic stenosis: results of the aortic stenosis progression observation: measuring effects of rosuvastatin (ASTRONOMER) trial. Circulation. 2010; 121(2):306–14.
43. Ngo DT, Sverdlov AL, Willoughby SR, Nightingale AK, Chirkov YY, McNeil JJ, et al. Determinants of occurrence of aortic sclerosis in an aging population. JACC Cardiovasc Imaging. 2009;2(8):919–27.
44. Peterson MD, Roach RM, Edwards JE. Types of aortic stenosis in surgically removed valves. Arch Pathol Lab Med. 1985;109:829–32.
45. Davis MJ. Pathology of cardiac valves. London: Butterworths; 1980. p. 18–58.
46. Dare AJ, Veinot JP, Edwards WD, Tazelaar HD, Schaff HV. New observations on the etiology of aortic valve disease: a surgical pathologic study of 236 cases from 1990. Hum Pathol. 1993;24:1330–8.
47. Owens DS, Otto CM. Is it time for a new paradigm in calcific aortic valve disease? JACC Cardiovasc Imaging. 2009;2(8): 928–30.

Echocardiographic Evaluation of Aortic Stenosis

12

Robert R. Moss

Abstract

Echocardiography is a definitive tool for the assessment of aortic stenosis (AS). Echocardiographic assessment should include morphology of the aortic valve and related structures as well as a functional assessment of aortic stenosis severity. Functional assessment includes peak velocity of the AS jet, mean pressure gradient, and aortic valve area. Accurate assessment and reporting of aortic stenosis require a commitment to technical excellence as well as a sophisticated understanding of the limitations of functional parameters and potential for measurement errors. Echocardiograhers should provide an overall determination of aortic stenosis severity, determine suitability for treatment with transcatheter heart valve techniques, and resolve discrepant measurements whenever possible. Three-dimensional (3D) echo has an increasing role, especially in the transcutaneous heart valve context. Finally, AS needs to be viewed in the context of the function of the heart as a whole taking into account systolic and diastolic function, cardiac remodeling, non-aortic valvular heart disease, and the influence of associated cardiac conditions.

Keywords

Aortic valve • Stenosis • Echocardiography • Transcatheter heart valve • 3D echo

Abbreviations

AF	Atrial fibrillation
AR	Aortic regurgitation
AS	Aortic stenosis
AVA	Aortic valve area
BSA	Body surface area
CW	Continuous wave
EOA	Effective orifice area
LVOT	Left ventricular outflow tract
MR	Mitral regurgitation
PSAS	Pseudosevere aortic stenosis
PW	Pulse wave
3D	Three dimensional
TEE	Transesophageal echo
THV	Transcatheter heart valve
TSAS	Truly severe aortic stenosis
VTI	Velocity-time integral

Introduction

Echocardiography is the primary imaging tool for evaluation and decision making in aortic stenosis (AS) [1] as it almost invariably offers rapid and accurate assessment of aortic valve structure and function in the context of a comprehensive cardiac evaluation. Ventricular size, systolic and diastolic function, chamber hypertrophy, and mitral and tricuspid valve disease are assessed in addition to evaluating the aortic valve. In general, echocardiography offers superior temporal resolution, and functional assessment compared to

R.R. Moss, MB, BS
Department of Cardiology,
St. Paul's Hospital, Room 474 Burrard Building,
1081 Burrard St, Vancouver, BC V6Z1Y6, Canada
e-mail: rmoss@providencehealth.bc.ca

J.K. Min et al. (eds.), *Multimodality Imaging for Transcatheter Aortic Valve Replacement*,
DOI 10.1007/978-1-4471-2798-7_12, © Springer-Verlag London 2014

other imaging modalities, but is limited in the certain patients with difficult acoustic windows and may deliver inferior spatial resolution to MRI and CT. Echocardiography has the advantage of safety, portability, availability, and cost [2].

Aortic Valve Morphology

A clear understanding of aortic valve morphology has always been an integral component in the echocardiographic assessment of aortic stenosis, but has assumed an even greater importance in the era of transcatheter heart valve (THV) implantation. AS may be categorized as subvalvular, supravalvular, or valvular. At present, as only valvular aortic stenosis is amenable to present transcatheter techniques, only valvular aortic stenosis will be discussed here.

The advent of THV techniques has provided additional insights into the subtleties and complexities of the aortic valve complex [3], as discussed in earlier chapters. The aortic valve is usually tricuspid; congenitally abnormal valves may be unicuspid, bicuspid, or rarely quadricuspid. Congenitally abnormal valves pose additional challenges for THV techniques and were considered a contraindication in the PARTNER randomized trial [4]. Congenitally abnormal valves may have larger annulus size and eccentric calcium distribution, increasing the risk of device migration or paravalvular aortic regurgitation [5]. It is thought that up to 54 % of adult calcific aortic stenosis actually represents the end stage of congenitally abnormal valves [6]. In addition, the bicuspid aortic valve may be associated with aortopathy and coarctation which have the potential to impact on decision making in THV assessment [7]. Important pathologic differences also exist between rheumatic and calcific aortic stenosis, especially in so far as calcium distribution occurs with rheumatic disease favoring the commissures, as opposed to the body of the leaflets [8, 9]. The echocardiographic report geared towards THV assessment should include a description of annulus size and LVOT dimension in the parasternal long-axis view (Fig. 12.1), leaflet morphology, and calcium distribution. Attention should also be paid to anatomic variants in the subvalvular region such as discrete upper septal thickening, (especially if associated with any degree of dynamic left ventricular outflow obstruction) and abnormalities of the aortic root including significant calcification and narrowing of the sinotubular junction. All of these factors have the potential to impact upon the safety, feasibility, and outcome associated with THV implantation. Finally, assessment of aortic valve mobility, calcium burden, and geometric orifice area by planimetry (where technically feasible) provides an important means to corroborate hemodynamic information that can be subject to various forms of error.

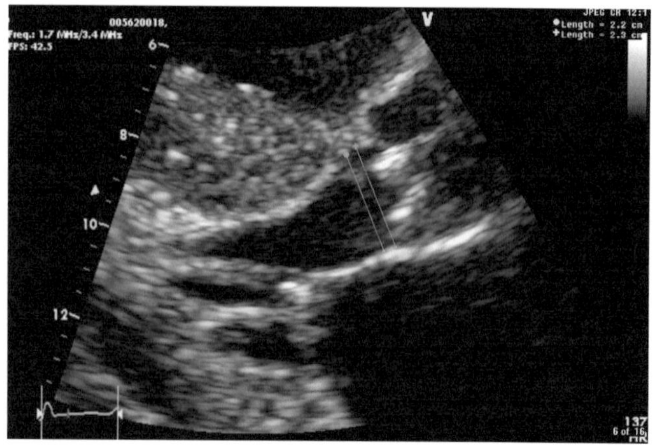

Fig. 12.1 A zoomed-up, optimized image in the parasternal long-axis view is used to measure the aortic annulus size and LVOT dimensions. The aortic annulus dimension is measured edge-to-edge at the ventricular aspect of cusp insertion. The LVOT is usually measured a little more ventricular, corresponding to the location of the PW sample volume and avoiding the zone of flow acceleration

Hemodynamic Assessment of Aortic Stenosis

The principal echocardiographic measurements used to determine aortic stenosis severity are (1) transaortic flow velocity, (2) mean pressure gradient, and (3) aortic valve area (Box 12.1).

Box 12.1 Core Echocardiographic Measurements Suggesting Severe Aortic Stenosis

- Peak transaortic flow velocity (V_{max}) >4.0 m/sec
- Mean transaortic pressure gradient >40 mmHg
- Aortic valve area (by continuity equation) of <1.0 cm^2

Supplementary Measurements

- Geometric aortic valve area (by short axis planimetry) <1.0 cm^2
- Dimensionless velocity index <0.25

Measurement of Velocity and Gradients

Echocardiography uses Doppler physics to determine blood flow velocities in the heart. Using the modified Bernoulli equation (Fig. 12.2), flow velocities are converted to pressure gradients partially because the conventional understanding of aortic valve hemodynamics was formulated in the pre-echocardiographic era. The accurate acquisition of velocity data is technically demanding and requires expertise and commitment to quality. Given that flow velocities as determined by Doppler techniques are angle dependent, alignment of the angle of the ultrasound beam as close as possible (<15°) to the direction of blood flow of the aortic jet is critical in

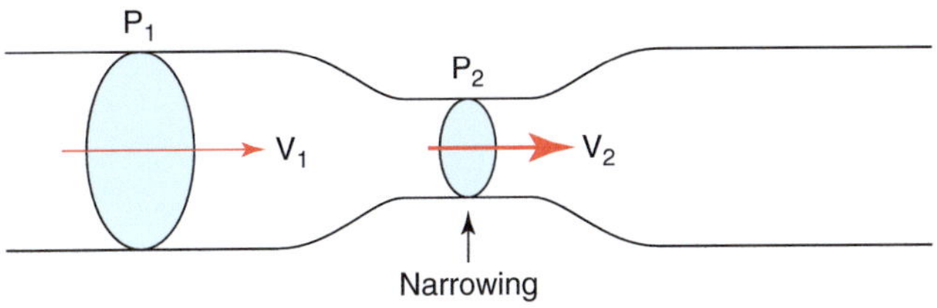

Convective element | **Inertial element** | **Viscous element**

$$\Delta P = \frac{1}{2}\rho\,(V_2^2 - V_1^2) \; + \; \rho \int_1^2 \frac{d\vec{v}}{dt} \times d\vec{s} \; + \; R(\vec{\eta})$$

where
- ΔP = The pressure difference between 2 points
- V_1 = Velocity at proximal location
- V_2 = Peak velocity downstream from stenosis
- ρ = Density of blood
- dv/dt = Change in velocity over the change in time
- ds = Distance over which pressure decreases
- R = Viscous resistance in the vessel
- η = Viscosity

Fig. 12.2 The Bernoulli equation is used to derive the pressure gradient across a stenosis from proximal and distal flow velocities. The full Bernoulli equation includes convective acceleration, intentional, and frictional elements. In practice the frictional and inertial components are ignored, and the convective element is simplified by ignoring the proximal velocity to yield the more familiar $\Delta P = 4V_2$, where ΔP is the pressure gradient and V is the maximal blood flow velocity across a stenosis, obtained using CW Doppler. When proximal velocities (V_1) are taken into account, a slightly fuller version of the simplified formula is rendered: $\Delta P = 4(V_1^2 - V_2^2)$. (From Anderson [10, p 195]. Reproducced with permission from MGA Graphics)

minimizing the error intrinsic in the Doppler equation [10]. In practice this is gained by interrogating the aortic stenosis jet from multiple windows with a continuous wave (CW) Doppler probe (Fig. 12.3). The highest obtained velocity is reported, unless atrial fibrillation is present. Where moderate or greater aortic stenosis is present, a non-imaging probe should be used, which offers the smallest footprint and optimal signal-to-noise ratio. Careful attention is paid to signal optimization especially gain settings [11]. Severe aortic stenosis usually results in a flow velocity of >4 m/s [12]. The shape of the CW ejection signal also contains additional information. In mild or moderate aortic stenosis, the signal is triangular and peaks in the early part of systole, while in severe AS it is rounded and peaks in mid-systole[13] (Fig. 12.4).

Mean Pressure Gradient

Mean pressure gradient is one of the core measurements used to gauge aortic stenosis severity. Because mean pressure gradients reflect flow velocities at all time points during systole (in contrast to peak gradient), they may contain information incremental to the measurement of peak velocity. Like flow velocity, this measurement is flow dependent and can be misleading high in states of abnormally high or low flow (see below).

Aortic Valve Area (AVA)

Determination of AVA by the continuity equation provides a useful index of aortic stenosis severity in low- and high-flow states, although this measurement is also flow dependent to a degree. It relies on the principle of conservation of mass and is given by the formula AVA × VTIAV = CSALVOT × VTILVOT (Figs. 12.4 and 12.5). When the equation is rearranged for AVA, the numerator of the equation is stroke volume across the valve. This is usually determined from an estimate of left ventricular outflow tract (LVOT) area which, when multiplied by the mean of flow velocities throughout systole in the LVOT (VTI or velocity time integral), yields stroke volume. Calculation of the LVOT area relies, in turn, upon and accurate linear assessment of the LVOT, which is obtained from a zoomed up, optimized view in the parasternal long-axis window (Fig. 12.1). The LVOT area is then calculated based on the assumption of a circular LVOT. The VTI in the LVOT is obtained using the pulse wave (PW) mode, with the sample volume positioned just proximal to the zone of flow acceleration, usually 5–10 mm ventricular to the aortic valve. An important principle is that the flow velocity should be sampled at the same point in space at which the LVOT dimension is measured. A detailed description of the technical requirements required to obtain these measurements is beyond the scope of this chapter but is well covered elsewhere [11]. Other measurements of stroke volume derived from volumetric assessment of the left ventricle by two- or three-dimensional techniques, or flow across other non-regurgitant valves (the right ventricular outflow tract for example), can occasionally be used. Once an estimate of stroke volume is obtained, the VTI of the highest-velocity transaortic signal obtained using CW mode is used to determine valve area. The continuity equation contains many assumptions and potential sources of error (see below) but works surprisingly well in clinical practice [14–17]. As with all hemodynamic measurements in aortic stenosis, accurate and reproducible results can only be obtained with superior sonographer training, a good understanding on the part of the echocardiographer of the errors and limitations intrinsic in the measurement and an overarching commitment to quality on the part of the echo lab.

Velocity Ratio

If an accurate assessment of the LVOT dimension is not obtained, the LVOT area cannot be calculated; hence, stroke volume across the LVOT cannot be determined. In

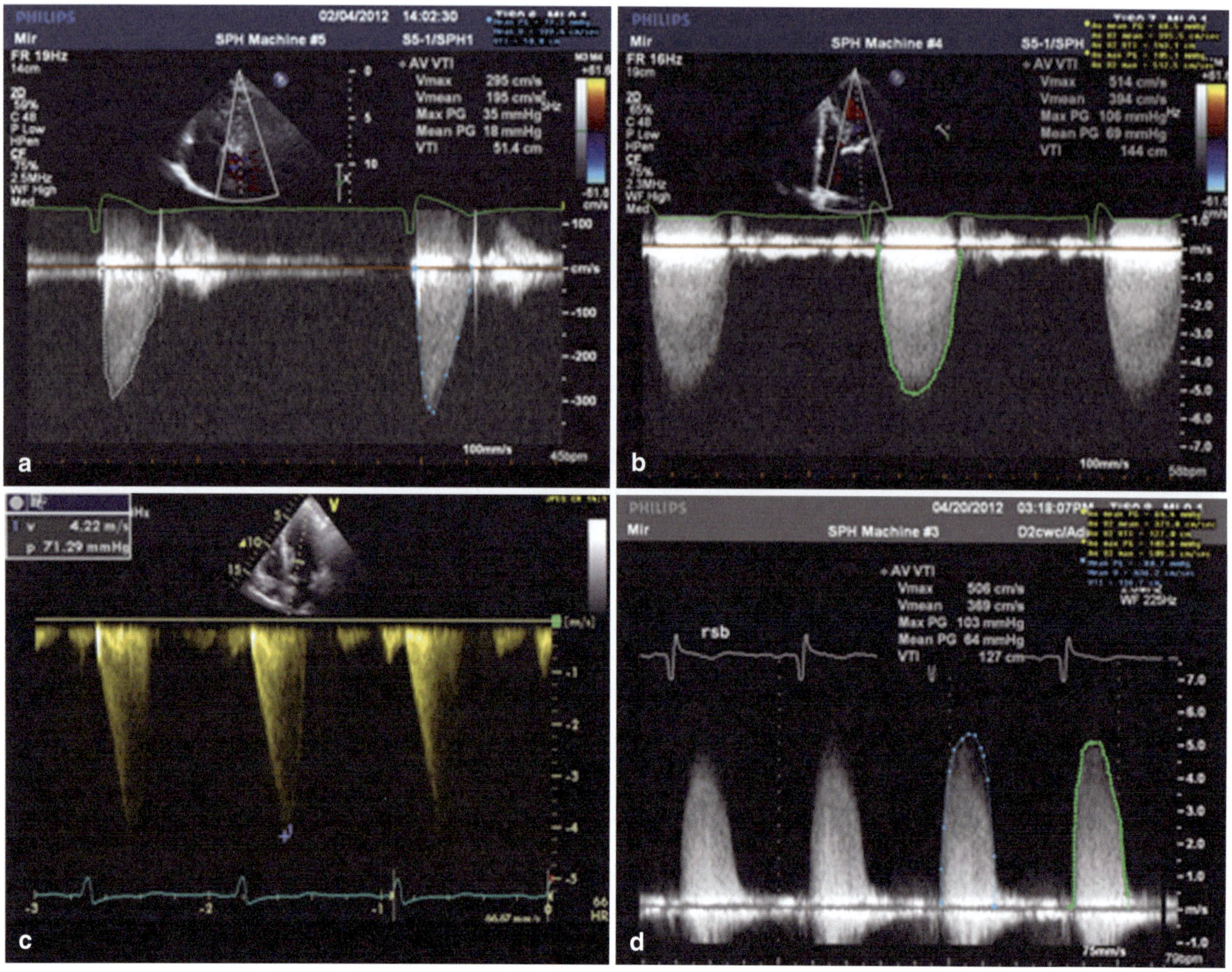

Fig. 12.3 Contrast this with the signal in Panel (**a**) where the patient has severe aortic stenosis with a peak velocity of 5.1 m/s, and a strong, rounded signal which peaks in mid-systole. Panel (**b**) shows a CW signal recorded from a patient with moderate aortic stenosis. The peak velocity is around 3.3 m/s, but importantly the signal shows peaking in the early part of systole. In panel (**c**), the patient has hypertrophic cardiomyopathy with dynamic sub-aortic obstruction. The signal is characteristically late peaking. Panel (**d**) shows a Doppler signal obtained from the right sternal border. The signal velocity from this window was highest than that obtained from the apex, resulting in a higher reported mean gradient and smaller calculated AVA

this instance, the ratio of the flow velocity in the LVOT to the flow velocity of the aortic jet may be a useful alternative to the continuity equation. Aortic stenosis is considered severe when the ratio is 0.25 or less [16]. The velocity ratio ignores natural variation of LVOT area with body size and lacks extensive outcome data supporting its use as a decision-making tool.

Experimental Measurements

A variety of experimental measurements have been proposed as alternative indices of AS severity [18–20]. In general, these measurements have been designed to more accurately determine the hemodynamic burden of aortic stenosis or to be useful in low-flow states. Because these measurements lack sufficient outcome data and may be cumbersome in a working lab, they are generally used in a niche or research setting and not presently endorsed as primary clinical working tools.

Sources of Measurement Variability, Error, and Discrepancies

Gradients and Velocities

As indicated, the major potential source of error is the misalignment of the ultrasound beam to the aortic stenotic jet. Careful attention to appropriate gain settings to avoid spectral broadening and tracing the crisp outer border when measuring the CW velocity signal are important technical

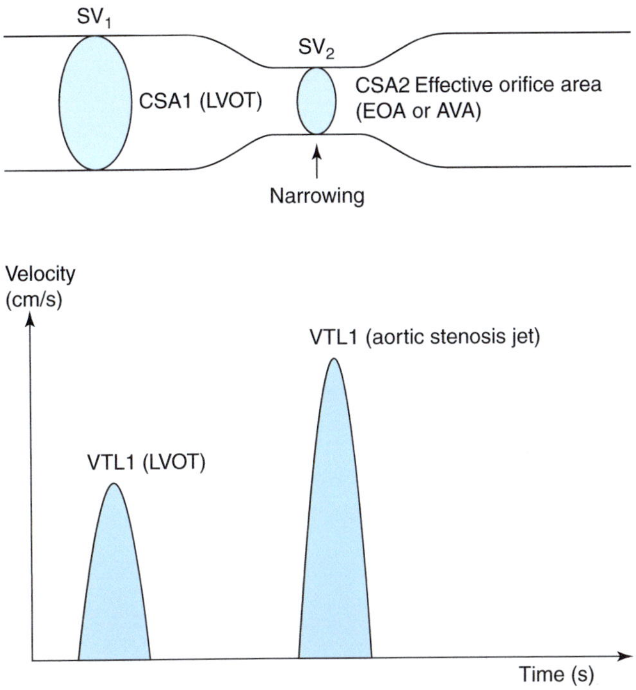

Fig. 12.4 Continuity equation. The continuity equation relies on the principle of conservation of mass. This means that flow in the LVOT must equal flow in the proximal aorta, distal to the aortic stenosis, i.e., $SV_1 = SV_2$. Given that flow is given by cross-sectional area (CSA) × velocity: CSA1 × VTI1 = CSA2 × VTI2. Solving for EOA aortic valve (or aortic valve area) yields the continuity equation. *CSA1* cross-sectional area LVOT, *VTI1* velocity time integral of LVOT, *CSA2* effective orifice area of the aortic valve (EOA or AVA), *VTI2* velocity time integral aortic stenosis jet (From Anderson [10, p 188]. Reproduced with permission from MGA Graphics)

considerations. The anticipated coefficient of variation in an tertiary echo lab with repeated measurements of the same patient is of the order of 3 % for determining the maximum velocity of the aortic and LVOT signals and somewhat greater for the determination of the VTI [15]. The simplified Bernoulli equation represents an abbreviation of the full formula in that it ignores proximal velocity as well as other hydraulic variables (see Fig. 12.2). This means that if there is significant flow acceleration in the LVOT, the pressure gradients will be overestimated if the simplified version of the Bernoulli is used. This is easily accounted for mathematically by using the more complete formula when flow velocities in the LVOT are >1.5 m/s, at least in so far as peak gradients are concerned (Fig. 12.2).

Because peak LV and peak aortic pressure do not occur at the same point in time, the peak-to-peak gradient familiar to catheterizing cardiologists is a non-physiological measurement and is invariably less than the maximum instantaneous pressure difference which is reflected in the aortic jet velocity (Fig. 12.6). This can cause a discrepancy between the catheter-derived and echo-derived peak gradient in aortic stenosis. The mean gradients are typically comparable however.

Pressure Recovery

Pressure recovery is a phenomenon that reflects the dynamic interplay between kinetic and potential energy across the aortic valve. During blood flow across the aortic valve, potential energy is converted into kinetic as flow velocity accelerates. Downstream from the stenosis, this is converted back into potential energy and pressure increases downstream [21]. The greatest pressure drop occurs at the level of the vena contracta of the stenotic jet where flow velocity is greatest; usually catheters are positioned downstream where recovery of pressure has occurred (Fig. 12.7). It is therefore not surprising that catheter-derived pressure gradients may be lower and Gorlin formula-derived valve areas higher than their echo-derived counterparts under certain circumstances [22]. Rapid pressure recovery is favored in patients with mild stenosis and small aortas [21] and is unlikely to be clinically important when the diameter of the aorta is >30 mm. Indices have been developed to account for the effects of pressure recovery; yet these are seldom used in clinical practice [18]. Notwithstanding, an awareness of the phenomenon is sometimes useful in resolving inconsistent or disparate results.

Valve Area: Planimetry

The planimetered aortic valve area is derived by tracing a short-axis view of the aortic valve (Fig. 12.8). It represents peak geometric orifice area and will be greater than the continuity valve area or effective orifice area (EOA). The EOA represents the average vena contracta area throughout the cardiac cycle and more accurately represents hemodynamic load and outcome. Imaging difficulties caused by acoustic shadowing and reverberation artifacts can compromise accuracy, and this measurement is usually considered more accurate with TEE. Identifying the plane that incorporates the minimal orifice area can be problematic especially in bicuspid valves. 3D imaging is likely to prove useful in this setting [23].

Valve Area: Continuity Equation

The continuity equation depends on the ability to accurately calculate flow across the LVOT. The measurement subject to the highest variability is that of the LVOT dimension [15]. Given that this measurement is squared, the potential for measurement error and variability is high. In addition the assumptions that underpin the continuity equation are its "Achilles heel." Specifically it assumes a circular LVOT geometry, which is untrue in some and, perhaps, most cases [24–26]. In particular, the LVOT shape can be distorted by abnormal basal septal hypertrophy or protruding mitral annular calcium. Another assumption is that of uniform velocity distribution of flow in the LVOT. It is known that the

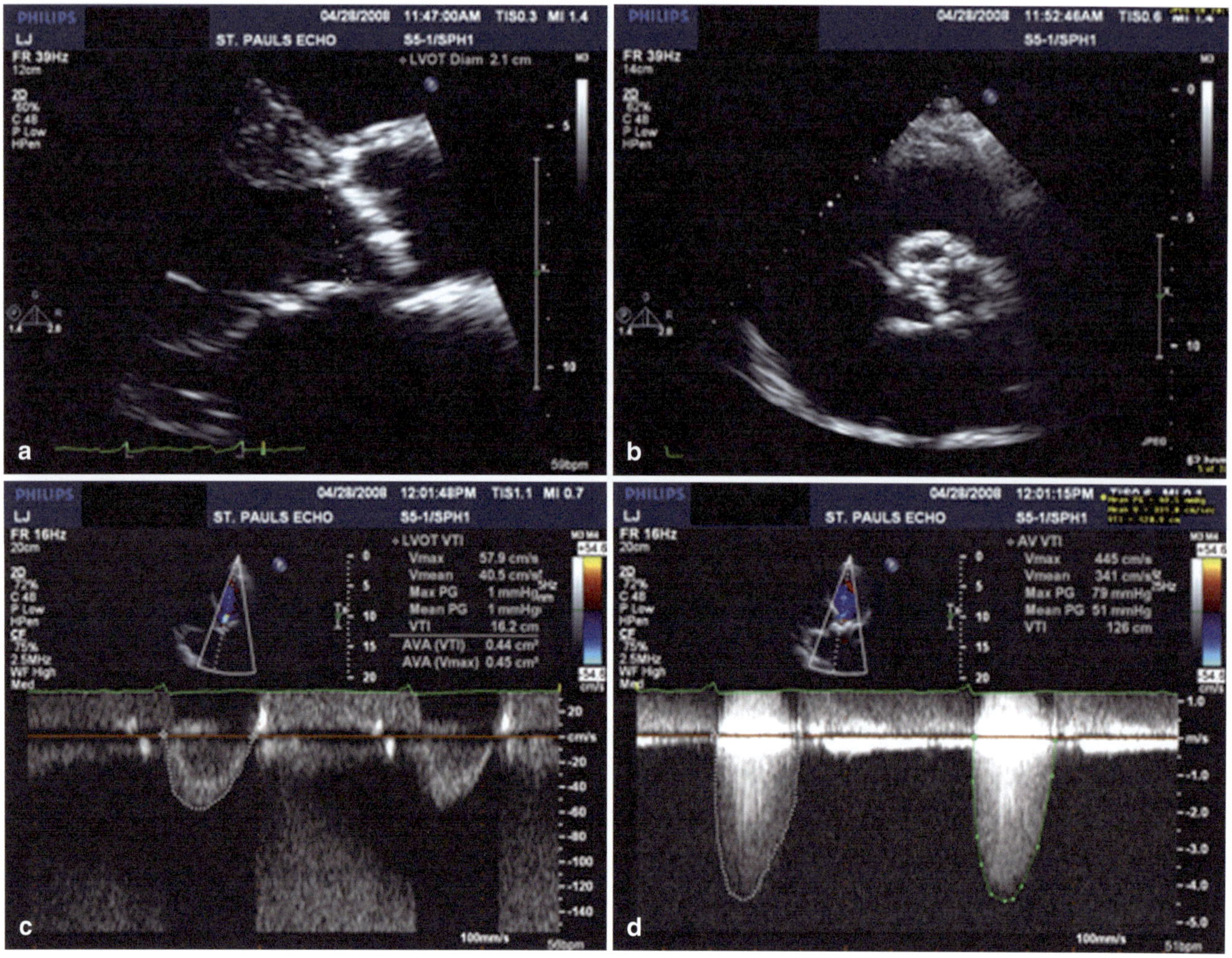

Fig. 12.5 The core elements required for AS assessment by echo are illustrated here. Panel (**a**) is a zoomed in long-axis view which shows markedly thickened cusps. A measurement of the LVOT dimension has been made. Panel (**b**) shows the VTI of flow in the LVOT, obtained with PW Doppler. This measurement is required for calculation of aortic valve area using the continuity equation. Panel (**c**) shows the aortic valve in short-axis orientation. This shows severe anatomic aortic stenosis and provides a useful confirmation of the hemodynamic measurements. Panel (**d**) shows the typical CW spectral Doppler signal of severe AS, obtained from the apical window. The measurements in this instance indicate critical AS with a valve area of 0.4 cm^2

velocity profile in the LVOT may be distorted and skewed in conditions of high subvalvular flow such as aortic regurgitation (AR). It is likely that emerging 3D techniques will allow for more accurate estimation of LVOT flow velocities and geometry, hence reducing potential for variability error in AS assessment [25].

Classification and Reporting of Aortic Stenosis

The stenotic aortic valve represents one aspect of cardiac pathology and requires understanding in the context of other parameters of structure and function—including LV ejection fraction, diastology, LV mass, aortic and mitral regurgitation, and pulmonary artery pressure. As well as, describing the morphologic appearance of the aortic valve, the three core hemodynamic measurements—peak velocity, mean pressure, and aortic valve area—are reported. In addition, a sense of the correlation between the morphologic appearance and hemodynamic measurements, and an estimate of the reliability of the hemodynamic measurements, is often useful. To minimize measurement variability the same LVOT dimension should be used in valve area calculations in serial studies. Both aortic annulus and LVOT dimensions are reported in our lab. Similarly the window where the highest aortic jet velocity was obtained should be noted.

The traditional cut points for severe AS do not take account of body size, although it seems intuitive that a 1 cm^2 valve area might be adequate for a small female with a body

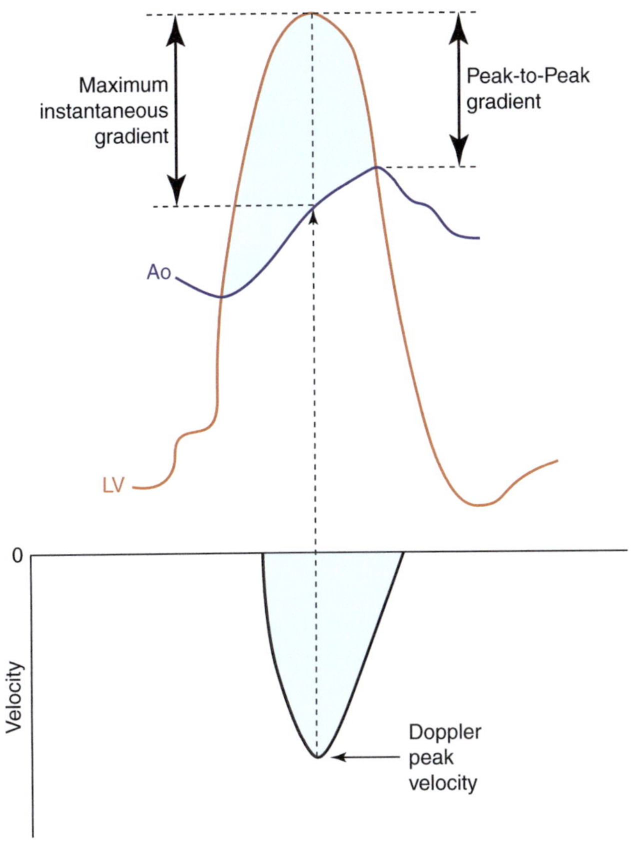

Fig. 12.6 The catheter-derived peak-to-peak gradient is compared to the Doppler-derived maximum instantaneous gradient in a patient with mild to moderate aortic stenosis. The Doppler measurement measures the gradient at the same time point in systole while the catheter gradient is a non-physiological measurement (From Anderson [10, p 198]. Reproduced with permission from MGA Graphics)

surface area of 1.4 cm^2, but represent severe or critical aortic stenosis for a much larger individual with say a BSA of 2.5 m^2 with higher cardiac output requirements. Most experts consider that it is appropriate to consider indexed valve areas in decision making in small individuals; the value is less established for larger persons. Indexed valve area cut points for mild, moderate, and severe AS have been published [11].

As the principal hemodynamic indices are at times discordant, a full echocardiographic report should contain an integrated assessment of the severity of the aortic stenosis and a statement regarding the anatomic suitability for THV, where relevant. Finally serial results obtained through time should be tabulated in matrix form for assessment of disease progression.

Resolving Discordant Measurements

Accurate echocardiographic determination of AS severity requires a combination of accurately acquired data, paired with an acute understanding of the errors and limitations of the measurement techniques—as well as the interaction between aortic stenosis and other cardiac disease states, as discussed below. While echocardiography is the primary tool for assessing AS, catheterization is occasionally acquired in borderline or equivocal cases. It should be remembered that catheter techniques and calculations based on the Gorlin formula carry their own set of inherent limitations and assumptions [27, 28].

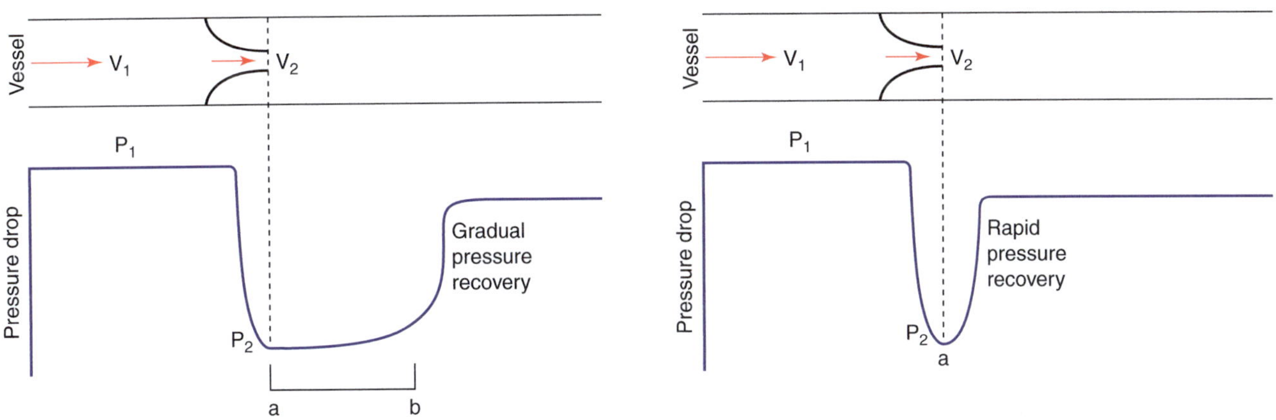

Fig. 12.7 The *left hand panel* indicates a situation where "normal" pressure recovery. The *right hand panel* indicates "rapid pressure recovery," a situation favored by small aortas and small mechanical prosthetic valves. The gradient as measured by Doppler is derived from the maximum velocity (V_2) and will reflect the "unrecovered" or maximal pressure gradient. In the *left hand panel*, the hemodynamic catheter may be positioned in the zone between *a* and *b*, i.e., the "unrecovered zone" and hence significant disparity between echo and catheter gradients is unlikely to occur. In the *right hand panel*, the hemodynamic catheter may be positioned upstream, in the zone of recovered pressure, a scenario that may lead to a discrepancy in the gradient estimate between the two techniques (From Anderson [10, p 198]. Reproduced with permission from MGA Graphics)

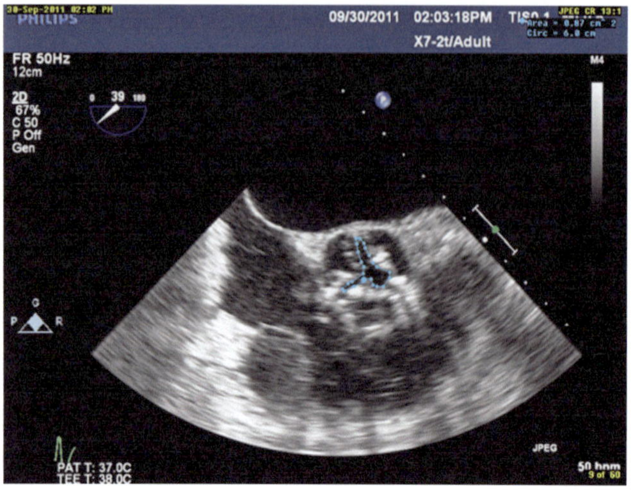

Fig. 12.8 Planimetry of the aortic valve may be useful when Doppler data is unreliable or cannot be obtained. Geometric orifice area is obtained with this technique, as opposed to effective orifice area determined with the continuity equation. In this instance, a value of 0.9 cm^2 for AVA is obtained. Effective orifice area represents the area of the vena contracta of the AS jet and is smaller than the geometric (or anatomic) orifice area. Planimetry measurements may be limited by acoustic artifacts, and care must be taken that the cut plane incorporates the smallest orifice area, a situation where 3-D imaging may be useful

Aortic Stenosis Associated with other Cardiac Conditions

AS in High-Flow States

High-flow states such as anemia or AV fistula will result in a higher gradients for a given aortic valve area. If the maximum velocity or mean gradient is taken at face value aortic stenosis, severity will be underestimated. This is avoided by careful determination of aortic valve area. In doubtful cases, morphologic appearance and planimetry of the aortic valve and the shape of the aortic ejection signal may be useful.

Coexisting LVOT Obstruction

Occasionally, the entities of dynamic LVOT obstruction and calcific aortic stenosis can coexist leading to a "stenosis-in-series" situation. This is sometimes seen where there is substantial thickening of the basal septum and mitral anatomy that favors systolic anterior motion of the mitral valve. In most cases, conventional surgical valve replacement, which allows for ventricular septal myectomy, may be indicated. Where there is significant flow acceleration in the LVOT due to outflow obstruction, the pulsed wave Doppler signal will be spectrally broadened, distorted or not even measurable due to signal aliasing. A common sonographer error is to "back up" the PW sample volume into the LV until a lower and less turbulent signal is obtained. Also, conventional assumptions in relation to LVOT circularity are unlikely to apply. The continuity equation cannot be used in this setting and planimetry is the only viable means of evaluating valvular aortic stenosis severity. The shape of the ejection signal will give a clue as to which of the two causes is the more hemodynamically important. Alternative imaging modalities may be useful in this context.

Aortic Stenosis in Low-Flow States

When left ventricular dysfunction coexists with severe aortic stenosis, a situation termed low-flow, low-gradient AS can occur. Gradients across the valve are low because cardiac output and, hence, flow across the valve are reduced. Although this group constitutes only 5–10 % of the AS population, their effective evaluation and management constitute a significant challenge. The usual definition requires the presence of AVA <1.0 cm^2, mean gradient of <30 mmHg, and LV ejection fraction <40 % [1, 29]. It is important for the echocardiographer to distinguish the two clinical scenarios in which this may arise. In the first instance the reduced LV ejection fraction is secondary to an appropriate LV response to excessive afterload imposed by severe AS; this implies the potential for recovery of the ventricular function following correction of the AS. This is sometimes referred to as truly severe AS (TSAS). In the second scenario, the LV dysfunction is present because of coexistent LV disease (such as myocardial infarction or cardiomyopathy) independent of the aortic valve disease. The ventricle may be unable to generate sufficient flow to open the valve; hence, valve area may be severely reduced in the presence of only moderate aortic stenosis. This is sometimes referred to as pseudosevere AS (PSAS). Correction of the aortic valve disease will not necessarily result in improvement of LV function in this case, although, strictly speaking, randomized outcome data comparing a conservative and interventional strategy is lacking. The most useful approach to distinguish between these two entities is to artificially augment flow across the aortic valve with dobutamine (discussed below). More recently a variant of low-flow, low-gradient aortic stenosis has been described in which LV ejection fraction is preserved. This is usually in patients with extensively remodeled, small, hypertrophic ventricles with marked diastolic dysfunction and high vascular impedance [30].

Aortic Stenosis in Atrial Fibrillation (AF)

In AF, stroke volume and therefore transaortic gradients may vary significantly with the R-R interval of the cardiac cycle. To overcome this, a minimum of five cardiac cycles for velocity and pressure measurements should be averaged. The issue gains more importance when stroke volume estimates are paired with transaortic flow velocities based on different and discordant cardiac cycles. This limitation is somewhat mitigated by averaging, with an alternative strategy being to pair two measurements with concordant R-R intervals.

AS in Prosthetic Valves

Degeneration of bioprosthetic valves is an important problem and seems likely to increase with increasing identification and treatment of aortic stenosis in the elderly. The advent of valve-in-valve THV techniques opens up the possibility of intervention to a wider population that includes those deemed too old or too sick for conventional redo surgery. Valve dysfunction should be suspected in a patient with new onset of heart failure in the context of a new or changing murmur. In general the principles for evaluation of AS are quite similar in native and prosthetic valves. The phenomenon of pressure recovery as described for native valves has also been identified as occurring *within the valve* of small bileaflet mechanical and ball-cage prostheses [31–33]. The type and size of the valve is critical in comparing obtained to referenced hemodynamic values and should be annotated on all requisitions. Knowledge of serial valve hemodynamics in patients is also critical and can be especially helpful in distinguishing patient-prosthesis mismatch from valve dysfunction. Because the major source of variance in determination of valve area is LVOT dimension, the same value (where correct) should be used in serial studies. It is important to note that smaller prostheses, especially mechanical ones that have potential for pressure recovery, can have relatively high gradients and relatively low valve areas but still be functioning normally. Severe prosthesis dysfunction is likely with a dimensionless velocity index of <0.25, a rounded velocity contour, an acceleration time of 100 ms, and an EOA of <0.8 cm^2 [32].

Mixed Aortic Stenosis and Mitral Valve Disease

Mitral regurgitation (MR) can exert significant impact on evaluation of AS in two settings. If severe MR is present, a significant proportion of stroke volume will be ejected as regurgitant flow. Hence, forward flow across the LVOT, opening forces and, therefore, transvalvular gradient and EOA of the aortic valve area can be lower than anticipated. Secondly when a non-imaging probe is used, the MR jet can be mistaken for the AS jet. This issue can be readily resolved by considering the timing of the signal and the orientation of the probe.

MR should be quantitated wherever possible, as the presence of significant mitral or aortic regurgitation may modify the clinical expression of AS and its impact on decision making. Traditional echocardiographic cut points of AS severity that assist in decision making do not take into account mixed valve disease. A patient with moderate AS and MR as assessed by echocardiography, for example, might continue to experience symptoms requiring intervention.

A not uncommon finding in AS is the presence of severe mitral annular calcium (MAC) which can cause either stenosis or regurgitation. When the MAC is exuberant and located at the anterior mitral leaflet, it can potentially involve the landing zone of the TH, V and, therefore, should be noted in the report. Finally, a complete echocardiographic report should include a statement describing the mechanism of the MR. In general, structural mitral valve disease is unlikely to improve post THV [34].

Aortic Stenosis and Hypertension

Severe concomitant hypertension in experimental models of AS has the potential to affect hemodynamic values [35]. High afterload presents with both hypertension and AS and may impact on LV ejection fraction, flow, and therefore determination of velocities gradients and valve area. For this reason, it is recommended that severe hypertension be controlled at the time of echocardiographic evaluation [11].

Mixed Aortic Stenosis and Aortic regurgitation (AR)

High flow across the valve with severe AR can increase peak velocity and mean gradient for a given valve area. In contrast, aortic valve EOA determined by the continuity equation should accurately reflect stenosis severity in this setting.

Stress Echocardiography in the Evaluation of Aortic Stenosis

Dobutamine echocardiography is used primarily in the setting of low-flow, low-gradient AS. The principle is that dobutamine augments contractility, increasing stroke volume and, hence, flow across the aortic valve. This, in theory, should help to distinguish TSAS from PSAS. In PSAS, augmented flow will result in increased opening of a relatively pliable aortic valve, and valve area will increase [20]. In TSAS, valve area will not change despite an increase in flow across the valve, and gradient should increase. In practice, dobutamine dose is augmented in staged fashion, with valve area and gradients being recorded at each increment in dobutamine dosage. Once flow is augmented towards more physiological values, the presence of PSAS can be characterized by an increase in AVA of ≥0.3 with a final AVA >1.0 cm^2 [36]. Similarly, an increase in gradient to 30–40 mmHg or a peak velocity to >4 m/s implies the presence of TSAS [11, 37]. More recently, a projected indexed AVA at the "normal" transvalvular flow rate of 250 ml/s seemed to separate TSAS from PSAS better than conventional parameters [20]. Dobutamine echo is useful, but is limited when significant augmentation of aortic flow cannot be achieved with dobutamine, a situation that can occur up to a third of cases [38]. This is termed a lack of contractile reserve and is generally defined by a failure to increase flow with dobutamine by <20 % [36]. This is typically associated with advanced myocardial disease or concomitant beta-blocker use. The finding is of prognostic importance [38] but limits the ability of echocardiography to unmask PSAS. In that situation, alternate imaging strategies, such as CT determination of calcium content of the aortic valve, can be explored [39].

Exercise echocardiography has potential role in prognostic determination and decision making in moderate to severe asymptomatic aortic stenosis. Increasing gradient with exercise, and possibly abnormal left ventricular response to exercise, has been identified as independent prognostic determinants [40].

Transesophageal Echo (TEE) in Aortic Stenosis Evaluation

While transthoracic echocardiography is the established tool for assessment of AS hemodynamics, TEE can provide incremental information in certain situations. Specifically, planimetry of the aortic valve can be useful where the continuity equation cannot be used to determine valve area. It should also be recalled that TEE assessment of the LVOT dimension (when available) can be substituted into the continuity equation where this measurement is unavailable or technically inadequate from the TTE. In the setting of THV, TEE is occasionally called upon for accurate determination of annulus dimension in patients with limited windows, and where more accurate assessment of aortic valve and root morphology is required for decision making. The accurate assessment of aortic annulus dimension is especially important when annulus dimensions are at the upper and lower limits of suitability for the available device. Very heavy or eccentric calcification of the aortic leaflets, aortic annulus and small aortic root dimensions are all factors which have the potential to impact upon decision making insofar as suitability for THV or device selection and sizing are concerned.

3D Echo in Aortic Stenosis Evaluation

Some trade-offs occur in terms of spatial and temporal resolution with 3D techniques. Temporal resolution can be augmented by reducing image volume but this reduces the field of view unless multiple volumes are 'stitched' together from sequential cardiac cycles. As this technology evolves however, the use of 3D techniques in the assessment of aortic stenosis seems likely to increase. 3D TEE imaging has already proven useful in underscoring the elliptical nature of the LVOT and annulus in many patients (Fig. 12.9) and

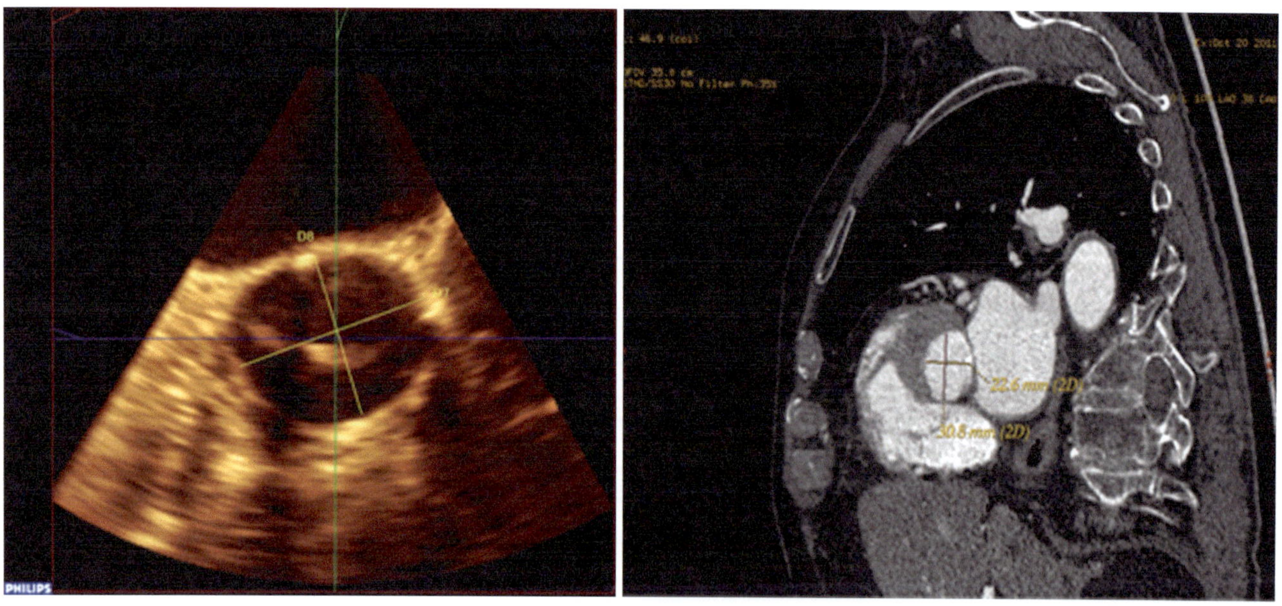

Fig. 12.9 In the *left hand panel*, a short-axis view of the aortic annulus is shown, using 3D TEE imaging in the multi-planar reconstruction (MPR) mode. The *right hand panel* shows a CT image from the same patient. Careful adjustment of the annular plane is necessary to obtain reproducible measurements. The elliptical nature of the annulus in this patient is well illustrated. In this instance the major and minor annular dimensions are measured at 23 mm by 29 mm. This compares with a CT image from the same patient where annular dimensions of 23 mm by 31 mm are obtained. Annular areas determined by planimetry using the two techniques were highly comparable

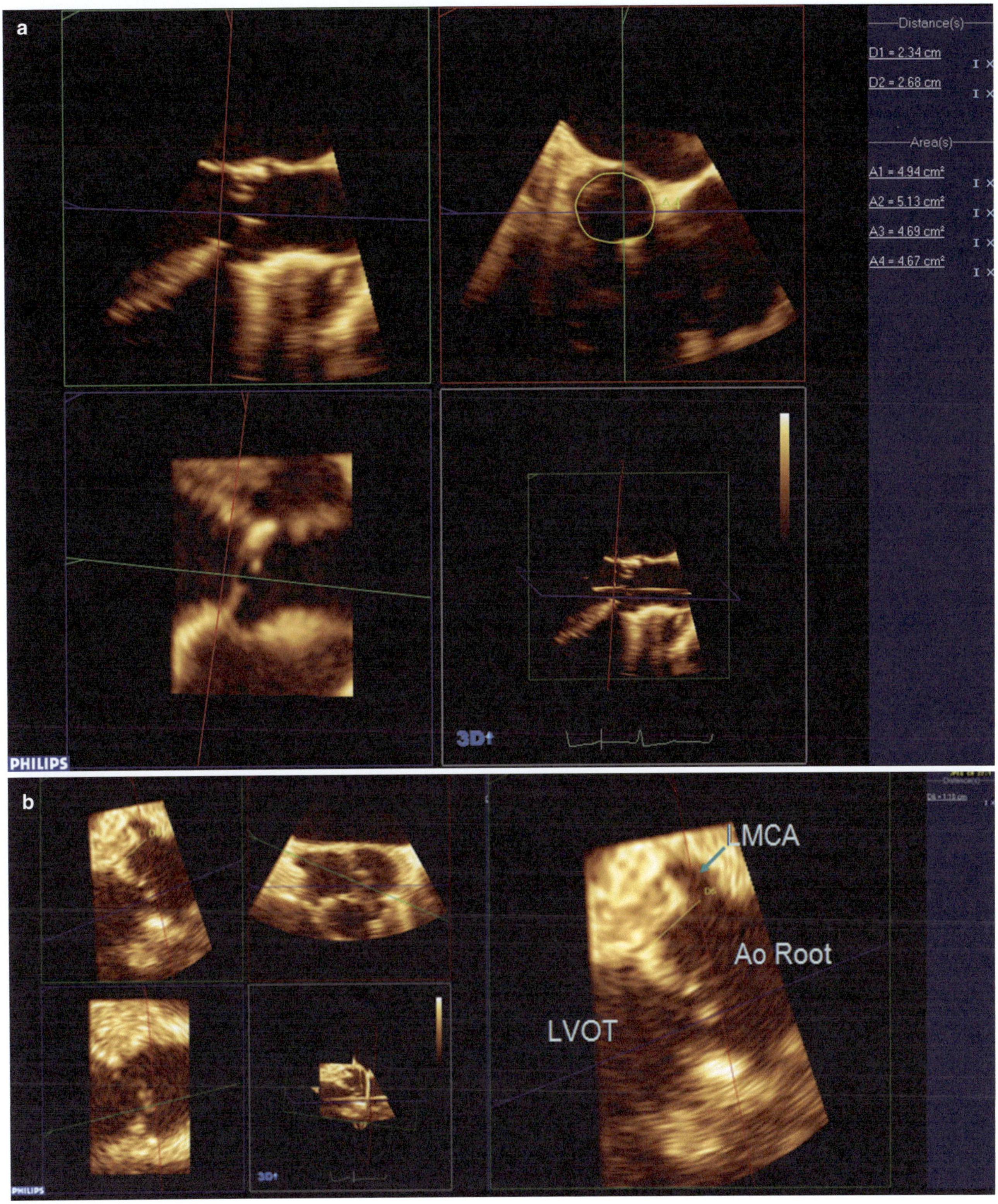

Fig. 12.10 Panel (**a**) shows the area of the aortic annulus measured from a 3-D data set using the multiplanar acquisition mode (Philips IE 33). The sagittal and coronal imaging planes are adjusted to the plane just below leaflet insertion, or until leaflet calcium just disappears. The frame is chosen for maximal aortic valve opening, usually mid-systole. The annular area is then planimetered in the short axis plane. A similar method can be used to determine the LVOT area. In Panel (**b**) The height of the left coronary above the aortic annulus is measured using 3D TEE in the MPR mode. This information can only be obtained from 3D imaging. In this instance, the measurement is 11 mm. The height of the coronary arteries above the annulus is part of the comprehensive TEE assessment prior to THV implantation, however this information is usually better obtained with CT or coronary angiography

allowing more useful and clinically appropriate measurements of these structures [41]. As focus shifts from linear measurements of the annulus towards aortic annular area as a the primary sizing paradigm, 3-D measurements of aortic annular area will become an integral part of assessment for THV device selection and sizing, especially if CT measurements are not obtainable. The 3D visualization of the aortic valve complex not only impacts on device selection in the THV setting but has the potential to improve accuracy of both planimetry and the continuity equation in the determination of valve area [25]. 3D TEE imaging can accurately determine calcium bulk and distribution and aortic root anatomy, as well as height of the left main coronary artery (Fig. 12.10). In our lab, 3D echo is principally used in the procedural setting of the THV deployment to assess aortic valve anatomy and annular size (and specifically aortic annular area) and to guide deployment of the transcatheter valve, especially if fluoroscopic views are inadequate. 3D color imaging is especially important in the post-deployment context for assessing AR mechanism, extent, and severity.

References

1. Bonow RO, Carabello BA, Chatterjee K, De Leon Jr AC, Faxon DP, Freed MD, et al. ACC/AHA 2006 guidelines for the management of patients with valvular heart disease: a report of the American College of Cardiology/American Heart Association Task Force on Practice Guidelines (writing Committee to Revise the 1998 guidelines for the management of patients with valvular heart disease) developed in collaboration with the Society of Cardiovascular Anesthesiologists endorsed by the Society for Cardiovascular Angiography and Interventions and the Society of Thoracic Surgeons. J Am Coll Cardiol. 2006;48(3):e1–148.
2. Gillam L, Otto C. Advanced approaches in echocardiography. Philadelphia: Elsevier; 2012.
3. Piazza N, de Jaegere P, Schultz C, Becker AE, Serruys PW, Anderson RH. Anatomy of the aortic valvar complex and its implications for transcatheter implantation of the aortic valve. Circ Cardiovasc Interv. 2008;1(1):74–81.
4. Leon MB, Smith CR, Mack M, Miller DC, Moses JW, Svensson LG, et al. Transcatheter aortic-valve implantation for aortic stenosis in patients who cannot undergo surgery. N Engl J Med. 2010;363(17):1597–607.
5. Zamorano JL, Badano LP, Bruce C, Chan KL, Goncalves A, Hahn RT, et al. EAE/ASE recommendations for the use of echocardiography in new transcatheter interventions for valvular heart disease. J Am Soc Echocardiogr. 2011;24(9):937–65.
6. Roberts WC, Ko JM. Frequency by decades of unicuspid, bicuspid, and tricuspid aortic valves in adults having isolated aortic valve replacement for aortic stenosis, with or without associated aortic regurgitation. Circulation. 2005;111(7):920–5.
7. Braverman AC, Guven H, Beardslee MA, Makan M, Kates AM, Moon MR. The bicuspid aortic valve. Curr Probl Cardiol. 2005;30(9):470–522.
8. Baumgartner H, Hung J, Bermejo J, Chambers JB, Evangelista A, Griffin BP, et al. Echocardiographic assessment of valve stenosis: EAE/ASE recommendations for clinical practice. Eur J Echocardiogr. 2009;10(1):1–25.
9. Otto Catherine M. Textbook of clinical echocardiography. 4th ed. Elsevier: Saunders; 2009.
10. Anderson B. Echocardiography: the normal examination and echocardiographic measurements. 2nd ed. Sydney: MGA Graphics; 2007.
11. Baumgartner H, Hung J, Bermejo J, Chambers JB, Evangelista A, Griffin BP, et al. Echocardiographic assessment of valve stenosis: EAE/ASE recommendations for clinical practice. J Am Soc Echocardiogr. 2009;22(1):1–23. quiz 101–2.
12. Otto CM. Valvular aortic stenosis: disease severity and timing of intervention. J Am Coll Cardiol. 2006;47(11):2141–51.
13. Chambers J, Rajani R, Hankins M, Cook R. The peak to mean pressure decrease ratio: a new method of assessing aortic stenosis. J Am Soc Echocardiogr. 2005;18(6):674–8.
14. Otto CM, Pearlman AS, Gardner CL, Enomoto DM, Togo T, Tsuboi H, et al. Experimental validation of Doppler echocardiographic measurement of volume flow through the stenotic aortic valve. Circulation. 1988;78(2):435–41.
15. Otto CM, Pearlman AS, Comess KA, Reamer RP, Janko CL, Huntsman LL. Determination of the stenotic aortic valve area in adults using Doppler echocardiography. J Am Coll Cardiol. 1986;7(3):509–17.
16. Oh JK, Taliercio CP, Holmes Jr DR, Reeder GS, Bailey KR, Seward JB, et al. Prediction of the severity of aortic stenosis by Doppler aortic valve area determination: prospective Doppler-catheterization correlation in 100 patients. J Am Coll Cardiol. 1988;11(6):1227–34.
17. Zoghbi WA, Farmer KL, Soto JG, Nelson JG, Quinones MA. Accurate noninvasive quantification of stenotic aortic valve area by Doppler echocardiography. Circulation. 1986;73(3):452–9.
18. Garcia D, Pibarot P, Dumesnil JG, Sakr F, Durand LG. Assessment of aortic valve stenosis severity: a new index based on the energy loss concept. Circulation. 2000;101(7):765–71.
19. Briand M, Dumesnil JG, Kadem L, Tongue AG, Rieu R, Garcia D, et al. Reduced systemic arterial compliance impacts significantly on left ventricular afterload and function in aortic stenosis: implications for diagnosis and treatment. J Am Coll Cardiol. 2005;46(2):291–8.
20. Blais C, Burwash IG, Mundigler G, Dumesnil JG, Loho N, Rader F, et al. Projected valve area at normal flow rate improves the assessment of stenosis severity in patients with low-flow, low-gradient aortic stenosis: the multicenter TOPAS (Truly or Pseudo-Severe Aortic Stenosis) study. Circulation. 2006;113(5):711–21.
21. Baumgartner H, Stefenelli T, Niederberger J, Schima H, Maurer G. "Overestimation" of catheter gradients by Doppler ultrasound in patients with aortic stenosis: a predictable manifestation of pressure recovery. J Am Coll Cardiol. 1999;33(6):1655–61.
22. Garcia D, Dumesnil JG, Durand LG, Kadem L, Pibarot P. Discrepancies between catheter and Doppler estimates of valve effective orifice area can be predicted from the pressure recovery phenomenon: practical implications with regard to quantification of aortic stenosis severity. J Am Coll Cardiol. 2003;41(3):435–42.
23. Goland S, Trento A, Iida K, Czer LS, De Robertis M, Naqvi TZ, et al. Assessment of aortic stenosis by three-dimensional echocardiography: an accurate and novel approach. Heart. 2007;93(7): 801–7.
24. Doddamani S, Grushko MJ, Makaryus AN, Jain VR, Bello R, Friedman MA, et al. Demonstration of left ventricular outflow tract eccentricity by 64-slice multi-detector CT. Int J Cardiovasc Imaging. 2009;25(2):175–81.
25. Poh KK, Levine RA, Solis J, Shen L, Flaherty M, Kang YJ, et al. Assessing aortic valve area in aortic stenosis by continuity equation: a novel approach using real-time three-dimensional echocardiography. Eur Heart J. 2008;29(20):2526–35.
26. Burgstahler C, Kunze M, Loffler C, Gawaz MP, Hombach V, Merkle N. Assessment of left ventricular outflow tract geometry in non-stenotic and stenotic aortic valves by cardiovascular magnetic resonance. J Cardiovasc Magn Reson. 2006;8(6):825–9.
27. Bermejo J, Rojo-Alvarez JL, Antoranz JC, Abel M, Burwash IG, Yotti R, et al. Estimation of the end of ejection in aortic stenosis: an

unreported source of error in the invasive assessment of severity. Circulation. 2004;110(9):1114–20.
28. Segal J, Lerner DJ, Miller DC, Mitchell RS, Alderman EA, Popp RL. When should Doppler-determined valve area be better than the Gorlin formula? Variation in hydraulic constants in low flow states. J Am Coll Cardiol. 1987;9(6):1294–305.
29. deFilippi CR, Willett DL, Brickner ME, Appleton CP, Yancy CW, Eichhorn EJ, et al. Usefulness of dobutamine echocardiography in distinguishing severe from nonsevere valvular aortic stenosis in patients with depressed left ventricular function and low transvalvular gradients. Am J Cardiol. 1995;75(2):191–4.
30. Hachicha Z, Dumesnil JG, Bogaty P, Pibarot P. Paradoxical low-flow, low-gradient severe aortic stenosis despite preserved ejection fraction is associated with higher afterload and reduced survival. Circulation. 2007;115:2856–64.
31. Chambers JB, Sprigings DC, Cochrane T, Allen J, Morris R, Black MM, et al. Continuity equation and Gorlin formula compared with directly observed orifice area in native and prosthetic aortic valves. Br Heart J. 1992;67(2):193–9.
32. Zoghbi WA, Chambers JB, Dumesnil JG, Foster E, Gottdiener JS, Grayburn PA, et al. Recommendations for evaluation of prosthetic valves with echocardiography and doppler ultrasound: a report From the American Society of Echocardiography's Guidelines and Standards Committee and the Task Force on Prosthetic Valves, developed in conjunction with the American College of Cardiology Cardiovascular Imaging Committee, Cardiac Imaging Committee of the American Heart Association, the European Association of Echocardiography, a registered branch of the European Society of Cardiology, the Japanese Society of Echocardiography and the Canadian Society of Echocardiography, endorsed by the American College of Cardiology Foundation, American Heart Association, European Association of Echocardiography, a registered branch of the European Society of Cardiology, the Japanese Society of Echocardiography, and Canadian Society of Echocardiography. J Am Soc Echocardiogr. 2009;22(9):975–1014. quiz 82–4.
33. Baumgartner H, Khan S, DeRobertis M, Czer L, Maurer G. Discrepancies between Doppler and catheter gradients in aortic prosthetic valves in vitro. A manifestation of localized gradients and pressure recovery. Circulation. 1990;82(4):1467–75.
34. Durst R, Avelar E, McCarty D, Poh KK, Friera LF, Llano MF, et al. Outcome and improvement predictors of mitral regurgitation after transcatheter aortic valve implantation. J Heart Valve Dis. 2011; 20(3):272–81.
35. Kadem L, Dumesnil JG, Rieu R, Durand LG, Garcia D, Pibarot P. Impact of systemic hypertension on the assessment of aortic stenosis. Heart. 2005;91(3):354–61.
36. Schwammenthal E, Vered Z, Moshkowitz Y, Rabinowitz B, Ziskind Z, Smolinski AK, et al. Dobutamine echocardiography in patients with aortic stenosis and left ventricular dysfunction: predicting outcome as a function of management strategy. Chest. 2001;119(6): 1766–77.
37. Nishimura RA, Grantham JA, Connolly HM, Schaff HV, Higano ST, Holmes Jr DR. Low-output, low-gradient aortic stenosis in patients with depressed left ventricular systolic function: the clinical utility of the dobutamine challenge in the catheterization laboratory. Circulation. 2002;106(7):809–13.
38. Monin JL, Quere JP, Monchi M, Petit H, Baleynaud S, Chauvel C, et al. Low-gradient aortic stenosis: operative risk stratification and predictors for long-term outcome: a multicenter study using dobutamine stress hemodynamics. Circulation. 2003;108(3):319–24.
39. Cueff C, Serfaty JM, Cimadevilla C, Laissy JP, Himbert D, Tubach F, et al. Measurement of aortic valve calcification using multislice computed tomography: correlation with haemodynamic severity of aortic stenosis and clinical implication for patients with low ejection fraction. Heart. 2011;97(9):721–6.
40. Marechaux S, Hachicha Z, Bellouin A, Dumesnil JG, Meimoun P, Pasquet A, et al. Usefulness of exercise-stress echocardiography for risk stratification of true asymptomatic patients with aortic valve stenosis. Eur Heart J. 2010;31(11):1390–7.
41. Binder RK, Webb JG, Willson AB, Urena M, Hansson NC, Norgaard BL, Pibarot P, Barbanti M, Larose E, Freeman M, Dumont E, Thompson C, Wheeler M, Moss RR, Yang TH, Pasian S, Hague C, Nguyen G, Raju R, Toggweiler S, Min JK, Wood DA, Rodés-Cabau J, Leipsic J. The impact of integration of a multidetector computed tomography annulus area sizing algorithm on outcomes of transcatheter aortic valve replacement: a prospective, multicenter, controlled trial. J Am Coll Cardiol. 2013. doi:10.1016/j.jacc.2013.04.036, pii: S0735-1097(13)01878-0.

CT Evaluation of Aortic Stenosis

13

Gudrun Feuchtner, Fabian Plank, and Hatem Alkadhi

Abstract

Multidetector row computed tomography (CT), with its capability of 4D dynamic evaluation of cardiac valves, allows for functional and morphological assessment of the aortic valve. This chapter describes the background and techniques for evaluation of the aortic valve by CT, with an emphasis on implications for use of CT for transcatheter aortic valve replacement (TAVR).

Keywords

CT (computed tomography) • Aortic stenosis • Aortic valve • Calcification

Introduction

Aortic stenosis (AS) is a common valvular disease in the aging population and carries a poor prognosis with a 1- and 5-year survival of 60 and 32 %, respectively [1]. Aortic valve replacement has, historically, been the only effective treatment in severe AS. However, elderly patients with multiple comorbidities are often not suitable for conventional open-heart surgery, with up to 40 % being declined for operation [2]. Transcatheter aortic valve replacement (TAVR) is a promising new treatment for high-risk and inoperable patients [1–3]. Multidetector row computed tomography (CT) angiography has emerged as a central imaging modality to define an individual's suitability for TAVR [3–7].

With the advent of 16-detector row CT, sufficient temporal and spatial resolution permitted, for the first time, evaluation of aortic valve morphology and function. In the ensuing years, continuous improvements in CT technology with each scanner generation, paramount benefits in image quality were achieved, allowing for reliable four-dimensional imaging—or volumetric imaging over time—of the aortic valve. This chapter describes the technique for evaluation of the aortic valve with CT, the morphology of a stenotic aortic valve, and the approach for diagnosing AS by CT. Further, we review the scientific evidence base evaluating the diagnostic performance of CT for this indication and discuss the clinical applications of CT, with a special focus on evaluation in the context of TAVR.

Basic Principles of CT

Through advances in CT technology over the past decade, four-dimensional cine imaging of aortic valve function by CT across the entire cardiac cycle has been proven feasible, largely due to advances in volume coverage, as well as temporal and spatial resolution. Current standard CT by 64-detector rows enables reliable assessment of the aortic valve, with even 16-detector row CT scanners sufficient for use. Limitations to CT should be considered for aortic valve evaluation, particularly in relation to high and irregular heart rates.

G. Feuchtner, MD (✉) • F. Plank, MD
Department of Radiology, Innsbruck Medical University, Anichstr 35, Innsbruck, 6020, Austria
e-mail: gudrun.feuchtner@gmail.com, gudrun.feuchtner@i-med.ac.at; magolin@gmail.com

H. Alkadhi, MD, MPH
Insitute of Diagnostic and Interventional Radiology, University Hospital Zurich, Raemistrasse 100, Zurich 8091, Switzerland
e-mail: hatem.alkadhi@usz.ch

J.K. Min et al. (eds.), *Multimodality Imaging for Transcatheter Aortic Valve Replacement*,
DOI 10.1007/978-1-4471-2798-7_13, © Springer-Verlag London 2014

The main benefit of cardiac CT is the possibility to evaluate cardiac valves from the same CT datasets [7] acquired for coronary arteries or aortoiliofemoral assessment, as is the case for patients being evaluated for TAVR [5–8]. If retrospective ECG gating is applied, CT also permits the simultaneous evaluation of left ventricular function and aortic valve areas.

CT Reconstruction

Retrospective ECG-gated helical CT enables image acquisition throughout the entire cardiac cycle. A dataset with axial images is typically reconstructed at 5 % steps through the entirety of the R-wave to R-wave (R-R) interval. The image quality of the aortic valve during cardiac cycle, particularly during systole, varies individually. It is necessary therefore to select the "best phase" for optimal image quality and for the measurement of the aortic valve orifice area (AVA). This "best phase" is the % of the cardiac cycle during systole when maximal aortic valve opening is present by short-axis planimetry.

When applying low radiation dose CT techniques—such as single-padded prospective ECG-triggering [9] or high-pitch coronary CTA [10]—only the diastolic phase is acquired. Thus, the aortic valve can be evaluated for morphology; 4D cine imaging quantification of the AVA is not possible. Certain CT scanners allow for a "dual-step" prospective ECG-triggered sequence, in which a second "pulsing" window is added to cover both systole and diastole with low radiation, that is, by covering the cardiac cycle from 10 to 90 % of R-R interval at a reduced tube current of 20 % mA [9]. As a result, a 4D cine imaging of the aortic valve opening and closing can be generated. This tool, while reducing radiation dose to mean 3.8 mSv requires a regular heart rate [9]. Also, imaging within the systolic phase of the cardiac cycle is limited by higher image noise, allowing a generally sufficient evaluation of the valve in primarily non-obese patients with normal body mass index.

Managing Arrhythmias and High Heart Rate

Cardiac arrhythmia such as atrial fibrillation and extrasystoles is a frequent phenomenon in patients with severe aortic stenosis being evaluated for TAVR. Arrhythmia may result in deterioration of CT image quality in that inconsistent R-R intervals may result in significant "misregistration," such as stair-step artifacts or "blurred" portions of imagery within a single selected axial slice. "ECG editing" is a tool offered by selected CT scanners and serves as an effective approach to remove those artifacts. In detail, "outlier" heartbeats—for example, an extrasystolic beat—can be "disabled" by removal from the final slices used in the reconstruction for the image dataset. Importantly, however, if the interval between heartbeats becomes too long after removing the extrasystolic heartbeat, a transverse "data loss strip" (i.e., blurred strip) appears within the image therein masking potential important anatomical structures. To resolve this artifact and to ensure diagnostic image quality, an additional second image reconstruction window can be added into the prolonged diastolic phase, so that no loss in image data coverage occurs.

While single "runaway" heartbeats can be successfully managed with "ECG editing", more complex arrhythmias such as atrial fibrillation represent a greater challenge for CT imaging. It is generally not advised to examine patients with atrial fibrillation using 16- or 64-slice CT, because diagnostic quality is not achieved in these patients. In contrast, CT scanners with higher temporal—such as dual-source CT—may allow for sufficient image quality in patients with atrial fibrillation without rapid ventricular rates [11] or in patients in sinus rhythm with slightly high heart rates.

For coronary CT imaging, beta-blockers are a mainstay to lower heart rates <65 beats/min; this allows for compensation of the limited temporal resolution of CT. In the imaging for the TAVR patient, however, beta-blockers are not recommended as the potential hypotension induced by the beta-blockade may lead to untoward hemodynamic effects.

Contrast Injection Protocols

Iodinated contrast-enhanced CT is required to morphological and functional analysis of the aortic valve (Fig. 13.1). For optimal timing of the contrast injection, it is appropriate to apply a monophasic bolus injection triggered to the arterial phase in a manner analogous to that performed for coronary CT. However, a biphasic contrast injection protocol [12] may be favorable in patients undergoing evaluation for TAVR to obtain right ventricular enhancement, which allows for comprehensive evaluation of all cardiac structures, as well as for global and regional ventricular function.

Reconstructing the Aortic Valve by CT

Given the volumetric acquisition of the aortic valve by a single CT examination, it becomes possible to review the valve morphology and function by several different methods. These include multiplanar reformations (MPR), maximal intensity projections (MIP), minimum intensity projections (MinIP), and volume rendering techniques (VRT) (Box 13.1). Each of these has benefits and limitations and is herein discussed.

Box 13.1 CT Post-processing Methods for Evaluation of Aortic Stenosis

- *4D cine loop imaging*: allows for short axis planimetry of aortic valve and assessment of mobile components of valve calcification
- *Maximal intensity projection*: not recommended as first-line technique due to partial volume artifacts
- *Minimum intensity projection*: projection of minimally dense structures reduces calcification artifact
- *Multiplanar reformat*: enables visualization review on thin slices in true long- and short-axis planes
- *Volume rendered techniques*: demonstrates location, severity and shape of valvular calcification in one view; enables easy differentiation between bicuspid and tricuspid aortic valve

Table 13.1 Standardized imaging planes for aortic valve assessment using multiplanar reformat images

Left coronal oblique
Left sagittal oblique (similar to echocardiographic three-chamber view)
Short axis (cross-sectional left ventricular outflow tract) requires multiple views from tip of leaflet to annulus

Abbreviation: *LVOT* left ventricular outflow tract

MPR visualization of the aortic valve on advanced 3D post-processing workstations or thin-client server-based solutions are a prerequisite for aortic valve assessment. The aortic valve should be reviewed on thin-slices MPR (0.5–1 mm slice width) and reconstructed in three different views shown as listed below in Table 13.1 and shown at Figure 13.1. This technique enables visualization of the valve in true long- and short-axis reformats, thereby generating accurate assessments of the aortic valve areas (AVA) over the cardiac cycle.

MIP views project the maximally dense structures within a voxel (typically calcium) and are not recommended as first-line post-processing technique for evaluation of the aortic valve morphology or sizing the AVA. MIP views are less reliable than MPR, because the thin valve leaflets may appear smaller or falsely interrupted caused by surrounding hyperattenuation due to artifactual enlargement afforded by "blooming" or partial volume artifacts. In contrast, for delineation of AVA, MinIP views, which project the minimally dense structures (and thereby reduce the calcium blooming), may be more accurate for measuring AVA although this method has not been tested against MPR or MIP in large-scale studies.

VRT methods of evaluation are useful to demonstrate the location, severity, and shape of valvular calcification at one glance (Fig. 13.2). Such 3D VRT visualization of aortic valve calcium can be useful for presentation to the TAVR team during interdisciplinary review. Protruding and/or excessive calcification—particularly at the aortic annulus or left ventricular outflow tract—may lead to complications during TAVR, such as aortic rupture or hematoma. Four-dimensional cine loop imaging of the valve in this view may also allow for assessment of mobile components of valve calcium, which may predispose an individual to embolization. Finally, VRT methods are also particularly well suited to illustrate the valve leaflets and allow for differentiation between tricuspid and bicuspid valves (Figs. 13.2 and 13.3).

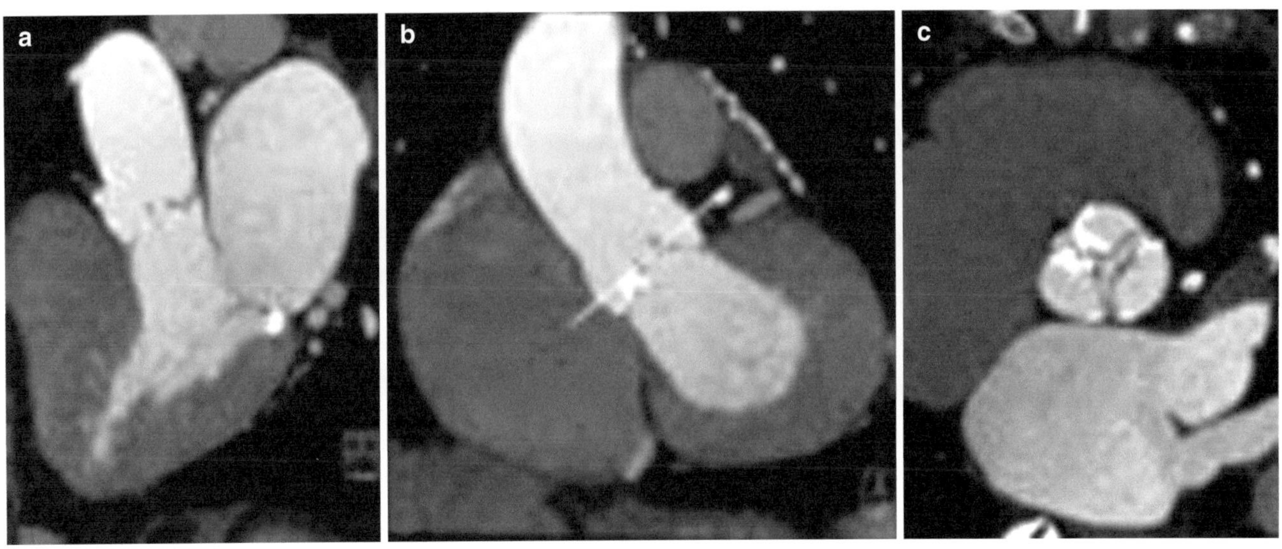

Fig. 13.1 3D standardized views of the aortic valve using multiplanar reformation (MPR). Panel (**a**) Left sagittal oblique (3-chamber view); (**b**): left coronal oblique; (**c**): short-axis view of the aortic valve during systole enabling sizing of the aortic valve orifice area (AVA). The displayed short-axis plane of panel (**c**) is indicated as *white line* in panel (**b**). The smallest AVA must be selected

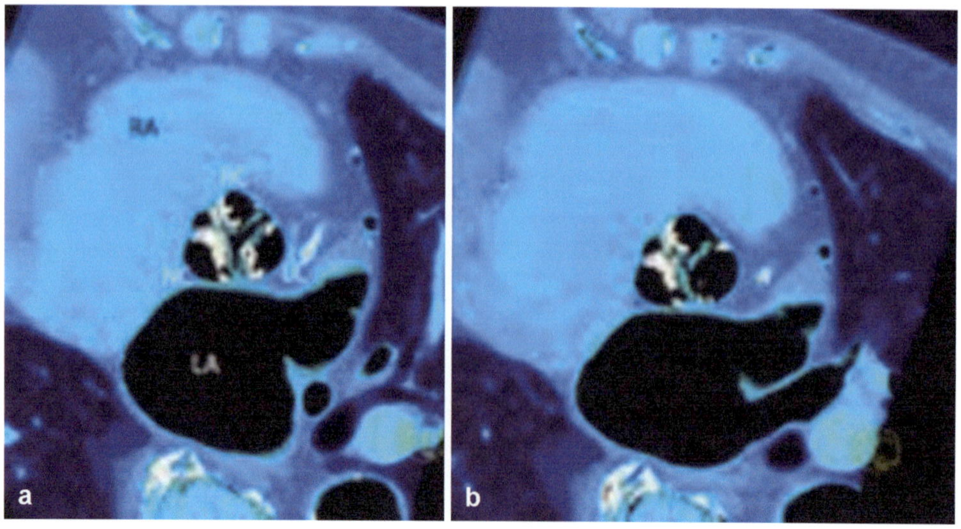

Fig. 13.2 Tricuspid aortic valve, systole versus diastole using 3D VRT. Three-dimensional VRT reconstruction shows severe aortic valve calcification in aortic stenosis during systole (Panel **a**) with open valve orifice. During end diastole (Panel **b**), the "Mercedes star" feature of tricuspid valve is shown (note a small central leakage indicating aortic valve regurgitation was found). *RC* Right coronary sinus, *LC* left coronary sinus, *NC* noncoronary sinus of Valsalva, *LA* left atrium, *RA* right atrium, axial oblique view

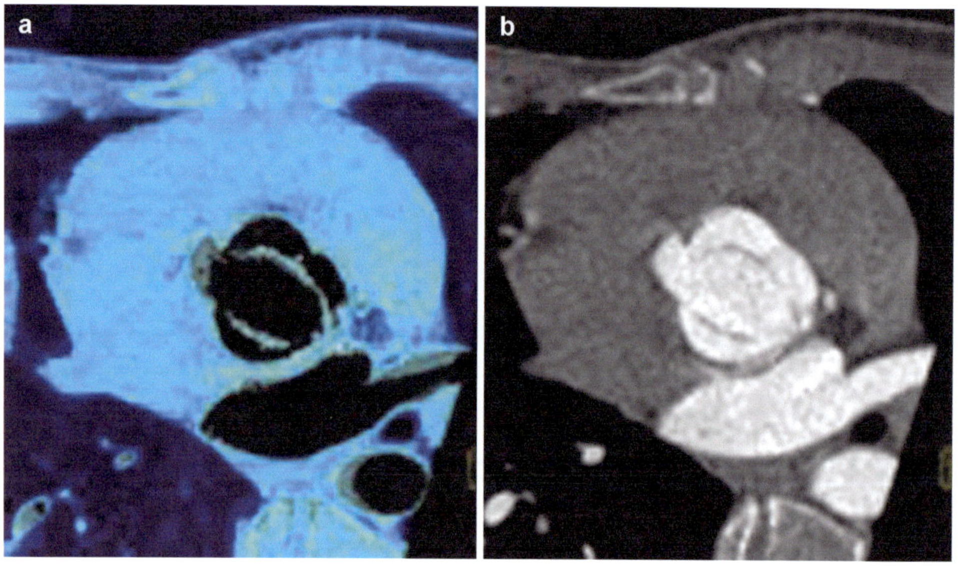

Fig. 13.3 Congenital bicuspid valve. Characteristic "fish-mouth" opening during systole illustrated on a 3D VRT (Panel **a**) and short-axis multiplanar reformation (Panel **b**). Note congenital bicuspid valve with fused left and right coronary cusp

CT for Assessment of Valve Morphology: Bicuspid Versus Tricuspid

CT has a high accuracy [13, 14] for identification of bicuspid valves, with a sensitivity of 94 % and specificity of 100 % [13]. The presence or absence of a raphe (85 and 15 %, respectively [13].) can be directly identified on CT images. The characteristic diagnostic criterion for a bicuspid valve is the "fish-mouth"-like orifice widening during systole (Fig. 13.3). Importantly, congenital primary bicuspid valves with or without raphe must be differentiated from secondary degenerative bicuspid valves. The latter arise from an originally tricuspid valve, with fusion of leaflets that can occur in the context of degenerative, rheumatic, and/or inflammatory aortic valve disease. In extremely rare cases, a quadricuspid aortic valve [15], consisting of four leaflets with an estimated incidence of 0.003–0.043 % of all congenital heart disease, may be found. For patients being considered for TAVR, a definite exclusion of bicuspid valve morphology is required as this valve type is currently considered a relative contraindication for TAVR owing to its distinct geometry.

Diagnosis of Aortic Stenosis by CT

The systolic anatomic aortic valve orifice area (AVA) is the key parameter to establish the diagnosis of aortic stenosis severity (Table 13.2), apart from a transvalvular pressure gradient. The dedicated CT reconstruction path for AVA sizing is illustrated in Fig. 13.1. A "best phase" with optimal image quality showing the phase with the maximal orifice area should be choosen [16]. Usually, the mid-systolic phases

(15–35 % of R-R interval) are the most suitable; however, dependent upon a given patient's individual heart rate, all systolic phases of the R-R interval should be reviewed. The "best phase" for sizing should entail a careful review of all of the information available—including a combination of the best image quality (with no or minimal artifacts) and the largest AVA during systole. Most importantly, all short-axis views of the aortic valve from the tip of the leaflets caudally towards the annulus should be reviewed, in order to select the smallest AVA during this maximal opening.

Numerous studies [16–28] published over the past years have shown high diagnostic accuracy of CT for measuring the AVA in comparison to other modalities. These comparisons of CT to other clinical modalities—such as transesophageal echocardiograph (TEE), transthoracic echocardiography (TTE), magnetic resonance tomography (MRT), and invasive catheterization—are summarized in Table 13.3. One meta-analysis pooling 9 studies [18] with 175 women and 262 men revealed a good agreement for determining the AVA by TTE and CT (mean Pearson correlation coefficient, $r=0.89$), mean difference of +0.03 cm^2, and an even higher agreement of CT with TEE ($r=0.99$) in 95 subjects. Similarly, another meta-analysis [19] of 14 studies with 470 subjects revealed a mean variance of +0.08 cm^2 AVA overestimation by CT, indicating a generally high intermodality agreement.

Overall, there is a tendency towards a slight systematic "overestimation" of the short-axis planimetered anatomic orifice area by CT compared to the effective orifice area by TTE, likely explained by the site of measurement and physiologic basis of Doppler flow measurement by TTE. Potential limitations associated with the use of the TTE Doppler flow velocity calculation of AVA using the continuity equation include difficulties in accurately measuring the mostly eccentric LVOT diameter and estimations of the maximal velocity of the left ventricular outflow tract (LVOT). Nevertheless, the overestimation of AVA by CT is rather small, ranging between +0.04 and +0.18 cm^2 [16–29] depending on the CT technology and the individual center's experience. In a recent study comparing dual-source CT (with higher temporal resolution) to TEE and invasive calculations using the Gorlin formula in 50 patients [27], a high correlation was observed for TEE ($r=0.93$) and for invasive methods ($r=0.97$), with a slight overestimation of the AVA by CT of +0.12 and +0.10 cm^2, respectively.

Table 13.2 Aortic stenosis severity by CT

	AVA (cm^2)
Mild	>1.5
Moderate	1.0–1.5
Severe	<1.0
Severe, critical	<0.7

Abbreviation: *AVA* aortic valve orifice area

Table 13.3 Studies comparing AVA sizing by CT compared to other imaging modalities

	N	Reference modality	CT scanner detector rows	*R* value (sensitivity, specificity)
Alkadhi (2005) [17]	20	TTE	16	0.95
Feuchtner (2005) [16]	46	TTE	16	0.89
Bouvier et al. (2006) [25]	103	TTE	16	n/a, good agreement
Pouleur (2007) [21]	48	TTE, TEE, MRI	40	0.92
Habis et al. (2007) [26]	52	TTE	64	0.76
Laissy et al. (2007) [30]	50	TTE	16	0.77
Leborgne et al. (2009) [23]	33	TTE	16	0.89
Feuchtner et al. (2007) [22]	36	TTE	64	0.88
		TEE		0.99
Tanaka et al. (2007) [24]	29	TTE	n/a	0.96
Lembcke (2008) [20]	32	TTE	40	0.86
		CATH		0.90
La Bounty et al. (2009) [27]	56[a]	TEE	64	(sensitivity 100 %, specificity 96 %)
Ropers et al. (2009) [28]	50	TEE	DSCT	0.93
		CATH		0.97
Lembcke (2009) [44]	36	TTE	64	0.91
		TEE		0.82
		CATH		0.91
Li et al. (2009) [29]	40	TTE	DSCT	0.79 (sensitivity 91 %, specificity 100 %)
Total	*647*			*0.89*

Abbreviations: *CATH* cardiac catheterization, *DSCT* dual-source CT, *TTE* transthoracic echocardiography, *TEE* transesophageal echocardiography

[a]Mixed aortic stenosis disease – non-diseased valves

Subvalvular Aortic Stenosis

Notably, CT allows for differentiation of degenerative valvular aortic stenosis from subvalvular stenosis within the LVOT caused by a hypertrophic proximal septum and/or subaortic membrane. Related specifically to TAVR, CT examination also permits a precise measurement of septal bulging, which may preclude a TAVR [16] procedure and potentially necessitate an open-heart surgery including septal myectomy.

Clinical Application of CT in Aortic Stenosis

Transthoracic echocardiography remains the mainstay for evaluation of aortic stenosis based on transvalvular pressure gradients and calculated AVA. However, Doppler flow assessment by echocardiography has some limitations: For instance, in patients with reduced left ventricular ejection fraction, low-flow, low-gradient aortic stenosis [30] has been observed, wherein low valvular flow velocity and pressure gradients are identified even while the anatomic stenosis of the valve may be severe. Alternatively, low-dose dobutamine studies may allow for differentiation of this pseudo-aortic stenosis from true aortic stenosis.

Even among patients without suspected aortic stenosis, an evaluation of the aortic valve is recommended [8] to avoid missing underlying valve disease in patients undergoing CT for other indications. Germane to this, the prevalence of aortic valve calcification is 13.3 % in patients with an intermediate pretest likelihood of CAD—who represent the majority of patients referred for CT for coronary imaging—and 7 % have an AVA less than 2 cm^2 [31]. Coronary CTA may also be performed in patients prior to conventional surgery [32] to reliably rule out significant coronary artery stenosis (sens 90 %, spec 92 % per vessel in 452 patients) and can also permit evaluation of the AVA if retrospective ECG gating was applied.

Quantification of Aortic Valve Calcification

Non-enhanced coronary artery CT calcium scoring can also provide a complementary information related to the aortic valve, specifically with regard to location, extent, and severity of aortic valve calcium (AVC) score. These non-enhanced CT scans are typically acquired at 1.5–3 mm slice thicknesses using prospective or retrospective ECG gating and at lower tube current than contrast-enhanced CT studies, thus resulting in a low radiation dose of approximal 1 mSv [33]. Similar to coronary arteries, AVC can be measured by numerous methods, including Agatston, mass, and volumetric scores. Among these, the Agatston method is more frequently employed.

The severity of AVC is known as strong prognostic parameter for outcome in asymptomatic patients with severe AS [34, 35], as shown in electron-beam and multidetector row CT studies. Asymptomatic patients with severe aortic stenosis and high calcium scores experience a significantly worse outcome than patients with low scores [34] and may be more likely scheduled for surgical valve replacement. In another study, AVC scores were a stronger predictor of major adverse clinical outcome compared to clinical parameters such as the effective orifice area, brain natriuretic peptide (BNP), or left ventricular systolic function [35].

Whether patients with more severe or differentially located AVC experience a higher risk of TAVR-associated complications—such as paravalvular leak—is currently a topic of research [36–38] Limited data have accrued to address these important topics. Koos et al. [36] report no association between the distribution of AVC, defined as the percentage of the calcium load of the most severely calcified cusp, and paravalvular leak in 59 patients. However, these investigators observed that the severity of AVC, expressed by Agatston scores >3,000, was associated with paravalvular AR, with moderate correlation to increasing AVC score ($r=0.5$). Similarly, Haensig et al. [37] recently demonstrated that higher AVC scores in patients with mild and moderate paravalvular leaks possessed higher AVC scores (3,804 and 7,387, respectively),as compared to those having no paravalvular leaks after TAVR (AVC 2,704).

In contrast, a recent study by Ewe [38] using contrast-enhanced CT for quantification of calcium (thereby precluding quantification of AVC by the Agatston method) found that calcific lesions located at the aortic annulus, rather than commissural and leaflet calcification, can predict the development of paravalvular leaks with regurgitation >grade 1. Using contrast-enhanced CT instead of calcium scores is certainly more accurate to quantify and characterize aortic valve and annular calcification, due to higher spatial resolution and minimized artifacts (e.g., motion artifacts), when selecting the best phase. In contrast, AVC scoring on non-enhanced CT calcium scores demonstrated high variability (36.2 % [39], with the lowest amount of AVC observed during diastolic phase).

These findings are of significant import as annular calcium may portend incomplete stent adaption with the aortic annulus, wherein leaflet calcium is pushed laterally into the wall (more cranially in the sinus of Valsalva) during stent deployment. John et al. [40] reported a positive but weak correlation between total calcium leaflet severity at the device landing zone and the grade of paravalvular leak after deployment ($r=0.33$, $p=0.001$) and suggested that the calcium lesion location might be of greater importance than the total amount.

There is a moderate correlation of the AVC severity by CT to aortic stenosis severity ($r=0.7$ [40], $r=0.63$ [42]). Thus, the total AVC score may be used to estimate the likelihood of definite aortic stenosis on non-enhanced coronary calcium scores. A cutoff of AVC score ≥1,100 AU provided 93 % sensitivity and 82 % specificity for severe AS diagnosis (AVA <1 cm^2), with a receiver operating characteristics (ROC) area under the curve of 0.8 [42].

Thus, the AVC score enables quantification of the severity of calcium deposits of the aortic valve and represents a prognostic marker for adverse outcome that might influence the management of patients with asymptomatic but severe aortic stenosis. A moderate relationship exists between the severity of calcification at the annulus (rather than leaflets) for complications after TAVR, including paravalvular aortic regurgitation due to incomplete prosthesis adaption. As such, an increased likelihood of intra-procedural balloon dilatation may be needed with increasing severity of aortic valvular or annular calcium [43].

Conclusion

Sizing of the anatomic aortic valve orifice area (AVA) by cardiac CT is an accurate evaluation tool for grading the severity of aortic stenosis. CT provides an alternative diagnostic modality for evaluation of aortic stenosis in selected patients, particularly in case of discordance between other modalities. For patients undergoing pre-procedural assessment for TAVR, one added advantage of CT is the opportunity to evaluate the aortic valve morphology and function and the aortoiliofemoral vascular bed from the same CT exam. Thus, a routine evaluation of cardiac valves in each CT study is routine in our institution [8]. Quantification of the severity of AVC similarly provides useful prognostic information and appears to be useful for identifying individuals who may be at increased risk of complications during and after TAVR.

References

1. Zajarias A, Cribier AG. Outcomes and safety of percutaneous aortic valve replacement. J Am Coll Cardiol. 2009;53:1829–36.
2. Holmes Jr DR, Mack MJ. Transcatheter valve therapy: a professional society overview from the American College of Cardiology Foundation and the Society of Thoracic Surgeons. Ann Thorac Surg. 2011;92:380–9.
3. Holmes D, et al. 2012 ACCF/AATS/SCAI/STS expert consensus document on transcatheter aortic valve replacement. J Am Coll Cardiol. 2012;59:1200–54.
4. Tops LF, Wood DA, Delgado V, Schuijf JD, Mayo JR, Pasupati S, Lamers FP, van der Wall EE, Schalij MJ, Webb JG, Bax JJ. Noninvasive evaluation of the aortic root with multislice computed tomography implications for transcatheter aortic valve replacement. JACC Cardiovasc Imaging. 2008;1:321–30.
5. Wuest W, Anders K, Schuhbaeck A, May MS, Gauss S, Marwan M, Arnold M, Ensminger S, Muschiol G, Daniel WG, Uder M, Achenbach S. Dual source multidetector CT-angiography before Transcatheter Aortic Valve Implantation (TAVR) using a high-pitch spiral acquisition mode. Eur Radiol. 2012;22:51–8.
6. Wood DA, Tops LF, Mayo JR, Pasupati S, Schalij MJ, Humphries K, Lee M, Al Ali A, Munt B, Moss R, Thompson CR, Bax JJ, Webb JG. Role of multislice computed tomography in transcatheter aortic valve replacement. Am J Cardiol. 2009;103:1295–301.
7. Feuchtner GM. The utility of computed tomography in the context of aortic valve disease. Int J Cardiovasc Imaging. 2009;25(6):611–4.
8. de Heer LM, Habets J, Chamuleau SA, Mali WP, van Herwerden LA, Kluin J, Budde RP. Multidetector row computed tomography assessment of the native aortic and mitral valve: a call for routine assessment of left-sided heart valves during coronary computed tomography. Cardiol Rev. 2012;20(5):222–9.
9. Feuchtner G, Goetti R, Plass A, Baumueller S, Stolzmann P, Scheffel H, Wieser M, Marincek B, Alkadhi H, Leschka S. Dual-step prospective ECG-triggered 128-slice dual-source CT for evaluation of coronary arteries and cardiac function without heart rate control: a technical note. Eur Radiol. 2010;20(9):2092–9.
10. Alkadhi H, Stolzmann P, Desbiolles L, Baumueller S, Goetti R, Plass A, Scheffel H, Feuchtner G, Falk V, Marincek B, Leschka S. Low-dose, 128-slice, dual-source CT coronary angiography: accuracy and radiation dose of the high-pitch and the step-and-shoot mode. Heart. 2010;96(12):933–8.
11. Marwan M, Pflederer T, Schepis T, Lang A, Muschiol G, Ropers D, Daniel WG, Achenbach S. Accuracy of dual-source computed tomography to identify significant coronary artery disease in patients with atrial fibrillation: comparison with coronary angiography. Eur Heart J. 2010;31(18):2230–7.
12. Vrachliotis TG, Bis KG, Haidary A, Kosuri R, Balasubramaniam M, Gallagher M, Raff G, Ross M, O'neil B, O'neill W. Atypical chest pain: coronary, aortic, and pulmonary vasculature enhancement at biphasic single-injection 64-section CT angiography. Radiology. 2007;243(2):368–76.
13. Alkadhi H, Leschka S, Trindade PT, Feuchtner G, Stolzmann P, Plass A, Baumueller S. Cardiac CT for the differentiation of bicuspid and tricuspid aortic valves: comparison with echocardiography and surgery. AJR Am J Roentgenol. 2010;195(4):900–8.
14. Tanaka R, Yoshioka K, Niinuma H, Ohsawa S, Okabayashi H, Ehara S. Diagnostic value of cardiac CT in the evaluation of bicuspid aortic stenosis: comparison with echocardiography and operative findings. AJR Am J Roentgenol. 2010;195(4):895–9.
15. Gouveia S, Martins JD, Costa G, Paramés F, Freitas I, Rebelo M, Trigo C, Pinto FF. Quadricuspid aortic valve – 10-year case series and literature review. Rev Port Cardiol. 2011;30(11):849–54.
16. Feuchtner GM, Dichtl W, Friedrich GJ, et al. Multislice computed tomography for detection of patients with aortic valve stenosis and quantification of severity. J Am Coll Cardiol. 2006;47(7):1410–7.
17. Alkadhi H, Wildermuth S, Plass A, et al. Aortic stenosis: comparative evaluation of 16-detector row CT and echocardiography. Radiology. 2006;240(1):47–55.
18. Shah RG, Novaro GM, Blandon RJ, Whiteman MS, Asher CR, Kirsch J. Aortic valve area: meta-analysis of diagnostic performance of multi-detector computed tomography for aortic valve area measurements as compared to transthoracic echocardiography. Int J Cardiovasc Imaging. 2009;25(6):601–9.
19. Abdulla J, Sivertsen J, Kofoed KF, Alkadhi H, LaBounty T, Abildstrom SZ, Kober L, Christensen E, Torp-Pedersen C. Evaluation of aortic valve stenosis by cardiac multislice computed tomography compared with echocardiography: a systematic review and meta-analysis. J Heart Valve Dis. 2009;18(6):634–43.
20. Lembcke A, Thiele H, Lachnitt A, et al. Precision of forty slice spiral computed tomography for quantifying aortic valve stenosis: comparison with echocardiography and validation against cardiac catheterization. Invest Radiol. 2008;43:719–28.

21. Pouleur AC, de Waroux JB, Pasquet A, Vanoverschelde JL, Gerber BL. Aortic valve area assessment: multidetector CT compared with cine MR imaging and transthoracic and transesophageal echocardiography. Radiology. 2007;244(3):745–54.
22. Feuchtner GM, Muller S, Bonatti J, et al. Sixty-four slice CT evaluation of aortic stenosis using planimetry of the aortic valve area. AJR Am J Roentgenol. 2007;189(1):197–203.
23. Leborgne L, Choplin Y, Renard C, et al. Quantification of aortic valve area with ECG-gated multi-detector spiral computed tomography in patients with aortic steno- sis and comparison of two image analysis methods. Int J Cardiol. 2009;135(2):266–9.
24. Tanaka H, Shimada K, Yoshida K, et al. The simultaneous assessment of aortic valve area and coronary artery stenosis using 16-slice multidetector-row computed tomography in patients with aortic stenosis comparison with echocardiography. Circ J. 2007;71: 1593–8.
25. Bouvier E, Logeart D, Sablayrolles JL, et al. Diagnosis of aortic valvular stenosis by multislice cardiac computed tomography. Eur Heart J. 2006;27:3033–8.
26. Habis M, Daoud B, Roger VL, et al. Comparison of 64-slice computed tomography planimetry and Doppler echocardiography in the assessment of aortic valve steno- sis. J Heart Valve Dis. 2007;16: 216–24.
27. LaBounty TM, Glasofer S, Devereux RB, Lin FY, Weinsaft JW, Min JK. Comparison of cardiac computed tomographic angiography to transesophageal echocardiography for evaluation of patients with native valvular heart disease. Am J Cardiol. 2009;104(10): 1421–8.
28. Ropers D, Ropers U, Marwan M, Schepis T, Pflederer T, Wechsel M, Klinghammer L, Flachskampf FA, Daniel WG, Achenbach S. Comparison of dual-source computed tomography for the quantification of the aortic valve area in patients with aortic stenosis versus transthoracic echocardiography and invasive hemodynamic assessment. Am J Cardiol. 2009;104(11):1561–7.
29. Li X, Tang L, Zhou L, Duan Y, Yanhui S, Yang R, Wu Y, Kong X. Aortic valves stenosis and regurgitation: assessment with dual source computed tomography. Int J Cardiovasc Imaging. 2009;25(6):591–600.
30. Laissy JP, Messika-Zeitoun D, Serfaty JM, et al. Comprehensive evaluation of preoperative patients with aortic valve stenosis: usefulness of cardiac multidetector computed tomography. Heart 2007;93:1121–5.
31. Aglan I, Jodocy D, Hiehs S, Soegner P, Frank R, Haberfellner B, Klauser A, Jaschke W, Feuchtner GM. Clinical relevance and scope of accidental extracoronary findings in coronary computed tomography angiography: a cardiac versus thoracic FOV study. Eur J Radiol. 2010;74(1):166–74.
32. Bettencourt N, Rocha J, Carvalho M, Leite D, Toschke AM, Melica B, Santos L, Rodrigues A, Gonçalves M, Braga P, Teixeira M, Simões L, Rajagopalan S, Gama V. Multislice computed tomography in the exclusion of coronary artery disease in patients with presurgical valve disease. Circ Cardiovasc Imaging. 2009;2(4):306–13.
33. Newton TD, Mehrez H, Wong K, Menezes R, Wintersperger BJ, Crean A, Nguyen E, Paul N. Radiation dose threshold for coronary artery calcium score with MDCT: how low can you go? Eur Radiol. 2011;21(10):2121–9.
34. Rosenhek R, Binder T, Porenta G, et al. Predictors of outcome in severe, asymptomatic aortic stenosis. N Engl J Med. 2000;343: 611–61.
35. Feuchtner GM, Müller S, Grander W, Alber HF, Bartel T, Friedrich GJ, Reinthaler M. Pachinger O, zur Nedden D, Dichtl W Aortic valve calcification as quantified with multislice computed tomography predicts short-term clinical outcome in patients with asymptomatic aortic stenosis. J Heart Valve Dis. 2006;15(4): 494–8.
36. Koos R, Mahnken AH, Dohmen G, Brehmer K, Günther RW, Autschbach R, Marx N, Hoffmann R. Association of aortic valve calcification severity with the degree of aortic regurgitation after transcatheter aortic valve implantation. Int J Cardiol. 2011;150(2):142–5.
37. Haensig M, Lehmkuhl L, Rastan AJ, Kempfert J, Mukherjee C, Gutberlet M, Holzhey DM, Mohr FW. Aortic valve calcium scoring is a predictor of significant paravalvular aortic insufficiency in transapical-aortic valve implantation. Eur J Cardiothorac Surg. 2012;41(6):1234–41.
38. Ewe SH, Ng AC, Schuijf JD, van der Kley F, Colli A, Palmen M, de Weger A, Marsan NA, Holman ER, de Roos A, Schalij MJ, Bax JJ, Delgado V. Location and severity of aortic valve calcium and implications for aortic regurgitation after transcatheter aortic valve implantation. Am J Cardiol. 2011;108(10):1470–7.
39. Ruhl KM, Das M, Koos R, Mühlenbruch G, Flohr TG, Wildberger JE, Günther RW, Mahnken AH. Variability of aortic valve calcification measurement with multislice spiral computed tomography. Invest Radiol. 2006;41(4):370–3.
40. John D, Buellesfeld L, Yuecel S, Mueller R, Latsios G, Beucher H, Gerckens U, Grube E. Correlation of device landing zone calcification and acute procedural success in patients undergoing transcatheter aortic valve implantations with the self-expanding CoreValve prosthesis. JACC Cardiovasc Interv. 2010;3:233–43.
41. Koos R, Mahnken AH, Sinha AM, Wildberger JE, Hoffmann R, Kühl HP. Aortic valve calcification as a marker for aortic stenosis severity: assessment on 16-MDCT. AJR Am J Roentgenol. 2004;183(6):1813–8.
42. Messika-Zeitoun D, Aubry MC, Detaint D, Bielak LF, Peyser PA, Sheedy PF, Turner ST, Breen JF, Scott C, Tajik AJ, Enriquez-Sarano M. Evaluation and clinical implications of aortic valve calcification measured by electron-beam computed tomography. Circulation. 2004;110(3):356–62.
43. Schultz C, Rossi A, van Mieghem N, van der Boon R, Papadopoulou SL, van Domburg R, Moelker A, Mollet N, Krestin G, van Geuns RJ, Nieman K, de Feyter P, Serruys PW, de Jaegere P. Aortic annulus dimensions and leaflet calcification from contrast MSCT predict the need for balloon post-dilatation after TAVR with the Medtronic CoreValve prosthesis. EuroIntervention. 2011;7(5):564–72.
44. Lembcke A, Kivelitz DE, Borges AC, Lachnitt A, Hein PA, Dohmen PM, Thiele H. Quantification of Aortic Valve Stenosis: Head to Head comparison of 64-slice Spiral Computed Tomography with transesophageal and transthoracic echocardiography and cardiac catheterization. Invest Radiol. 2009;44(1):7–14

MRI Evaluation of Aortic Stenosis

14

Eric Larose

Abstract

Aortic valve stenosis is a complex condition that requires the integration of both clinical and imaging data for optimal patient management. Accurate characterization of valve morphology and physiology is essential for the determination of disease severity and the planning of surgical or percutaneous intervention. Cardiovascular magnetic resonance (CMR) allows for the complete assessment of aortic valve morphology and function, along with the evaluation of important hemodynamic data points including cardiac volumes and systolic and diastolic function without the need for ionizing radiation or intravenous contrast medium. With delayed gadolinium enhancement imaging, tissue characterization is possible allowing for the identification of patients considered to be at increased risk.

Keywords

Aortic stenosis • Cardiovascular imaging • Cardiovascular magnetic resonance • Cardiac morphology and function • Velocity-encoding magnetic resonance • Myocardial tissue characterization

Introduction to Magnetic Resonance Physics Relevant to Aortic Stenosis

Magnetic resonance imaging is based on the detection of signals from hydrogen nuclei that are prevalent in the human body [1]. When a patient enters the MRI scanner, hydrogen nuclei align with and rotate about the axis of the field of the magnet. The precession, or spinning of these hydrogen nuclei, can be disturbed through the application of additional smaller magnetic field pulses. Then by applying these radiofrequency pulses in a controlled manner through "pulse sequences," images can be produced via the feedback of signals received based on the spatial distribution of the spins within the body. While most scanners currently in use for cardiovascular imaging are based on a magnetic field of 1.5 T, greater field strengths are becoming increasingly available with the potential for improved image signal, resolution, and speed.

The function of the main magnetic field is to impose a known alignment to the protons found in the body. Pulsed radiofrequency (RF) signals are then applied to temporarily disrupt the protons. The behavior of protons released from the influence of the RF signals that return to the axis imposed by the magnetic field is characteristic for the various tissue types. Longitudinal relaxation time (T1) and transverse relaxation time (T2)—in addition to proton density (PD)—provide unique tissue signatures that generate contrast in magnetic resonance (MR) imaging. The aim of sequence design is to adjust the RF pulse and readout of the signal emitted by the protons and captured by the receiver coils in

E. Larose, DVM, MD, FRCPC, FAHA
Department of Cardiology, Institut universitaire de cardiologie et de pneumologie de Québec (IUCPQ), 2725 chemin Ste-Foy, Québec, QC G1V4G5, Canada

Faculté de médecine, Université Laval, Québec City, QC, Canada
e-mail: eric.larose@criucpq.ulaval.ca

The online version of this chapter (doi:10.1007/978-1-4471-2798-7_14) contains supplementary material, which is available to authorized users.

J.K. Min et al. (eds.), *Multimodality Imaging for Transcatheter Aortic Valve Replacement*,
DOI 10.1007/978-1-4471-2798-7_14, © Springer-Verlag London 2014

order to maximize the contrast between the structures or tissues of interest. The adjustment of the RF pulse is mainly achieved by modification of the repetition time (TR) (or the time between consecutive 90° RF pulses) and of the echo time (TE) (or the time between the initial 90° RF pulse and its echo).

Among the different imaging sequences commonly used in cardiovascular magnetic resonance (CMR), black blood spin-echo sequences are typically used for general morphological imaging and basic tissue characterization, while steady-state free precession (SSFP) imaging generating 20–30 cine frames per cardiac cycle is used for general morphology as well as functional imaging. Spin-echo sequences are typically named after the dominant design characteristic, for instance, a T1-weighted sequence in which subcutaneous and pericardial fat will appear bright white or a T2-weighted sequence with short tau inversion recovery (T2 STIR) in which myocardial water content or edema associated with acute injury will appear brighter than normal myocardium. One of the strengths of CMR is the ability to perform tissue characterization through myocardial delayed enhancement imaging with gadolinium. Gadolinium is a blood-pool agent that passively redistributes and becomes highly visible in T1-weighted sequences. In the equilibrium phase of imaging at 10–15 min following the injection of gadolinium, the contrast medium has washed out of normal myocardium, but in the setting of scar or infiltrative disease, there is an increase in the distribution volume of the contrast agents within the expanded extracellular space [1]. The resulting differences in contrast distribution between normal and injured myocardium can be delineated with T1-sensitive inversion-recovery CMR methods. Beyond the proton characteristics described above, flowing blood has an important impact on the signal in the MR field. While different techniques exist, phase-contrast velocity mapping is the most widely used approach, acquiring two images with different gradient waveforms in the direction of flow measurement. The difference between both waveforms determines the pixel-by-pixel velocity map for blood flow. Measurement of blood velocity and flow is now an important component in CMR imaging of valvular disease.

The key clinical features of CMR for assessment of valvular heart disease are the ability to accurately measure morphology, function, flow, and tissue characteristics in an integrative approach to provide the full scope of information regarding the nature of disease, its severity, and the impact of the valvular process on cardiac chamber morphology and function (Box 14.1). Furthermore, CMR provides this information without the added risk of ionizing radiation or a semi-invasive approach, such as with computed tomography (CT) or transesophageal echocardiography, respectively. Finally, most of this information derived from CMR—with the exception of myocardial fibrosis—may be obtained without the use of a contrast agent, thus rendering CMR an ideal alternative for up to 52 % of patients undergoing transcatheter aortic valve replacement (TAVR) with concomitant significant chronic kidney disease [2].

Box 14.1 General MRI Evaluation Techniques Pertinent to Aortic Stenosis Evaluation

Sequence	Brief description
SSFP (Steady-state free precession)	Excellent tissue contrast between cardiac structures and blood pool in a time-resolved cine imaging sequence Useful for measuring chamber volumes, function and mass. Accurate measurement of aortic valve annulus for TAVR sizing
T2 STIR	T2-weighted sequence with short tau inversion recovery Myocardial water content or edema associated with acute injury will appear brighter than normal myocardium
MOLLI T1 mapping (modified look-locker inversion recovery)	Novel pulse sequence to evaluate for diffuse fibrosis as a predictor of recovery and/or prognosis
T1-sensitive inversion recovery (Late gadolinium enhancement)	Detection of focal myocardial scar for risk statisfication of patients with aortic stenosis Detection of myocardial infarction to assess patients pre-transapical TAVR
Phase-contrast velocity mapping	Flow imaging and quantification Measurement of valvular and vascular mean and peak velocities and regurgitant flow

Cardiovascular Magnetic Resonance Imaging for Aortic Stenosis

Imaging plays a central role in establishing the diagnosis of aortic stenosis and also helping to define the etiology of the valvular pathology. The three primary causes of valvular aortic stenosis are calcific disease of a trileaflet valve, abnormal bicuspid (or unicuspid valve) complicated by calcification, and rheumatic valve disease. Beyond establishing the precise etiology, noninvasive imaging is essential for determining disease severity, impact on cardiac morphology and function, and planning of medical or interventional therapies.

While echocardiography has been the stalwart of noninvasive assessment of aortic stenosis, the most recent appropriate use criteria proposed by the American College of Cardiology Foundation consider the performance CMR to characterize native and prosthetic cardiac valves—including short-axis planimetry of stenotic disease and quantification of regurgitant disease—as appropriate in patients with technically limited echocardiographic images [3, 4]. In addition, CMR is considered appropriate to evaluate morphology and function when information from other testing is discordant and to evaluate the contribution of a non-valvular etiology—typically with gadolinium-based tissue characterization—when mixed disease is suspected.

In our experience at Institut universitaire de cardiologie et de pneumologie de Québec of 2,500 CMR studies performed yearly, the proportion of clinical indications for assessment of valvular disease is approximately 10 %. Contraindications to CMR rarely prevent a study (<2 %) and usually consist of a non-MR compatible pacemaker or defibrillator or ferromagnetic material in or near to the central nervous system, eyes, or inner ears. Importantly, other ferromagnetic material—including sternotomy wires and most implanted heart valves and device—is not contraindicated for MR imaging (refer to www.MRIsafety.com for complete list).

While standard CMR assessment of valvular heart disease is typically performed with contrast, a robust CMR examination may be performed without gadolinium contrast if contraindications exist, such as is the case in severe kidney failure (creatinine clearance <30 cc/min). As previously stated, one important strength of CMR is its ability to perform 3D cine imaging (morphology and function) and flow measurement noninvasively and without contrast agents. In our own institutional experience, approximately 25 % of individuals undergoing TAVR have severe kidney failure. For these patients, contrast-free CMR provides all the necessary information regarding etiology and severity of valvular aortic stenosis, its consequences and concomitant disease, and morphology necessary for the planning of TAVR.

Cardiac Morphology and Function

The usefulness of CMR for cardiac morphology and function has been well described elsewhere [5]. For patients with aortic valve stenosis, an accurate measurement of left ventricular (LV) volumes, mass, and function using full 3D coverage is important to help guide therapeutic intervention and provide important prognostic information (Fig. 14.1). 3D techniques are particularly useful for the accurate measurement of ventricular volume, function, and mass when there is regional remodeling where geometrical assumptions from 2D imaging are less accurate and reliable [6]. Beyond measuring these parameters at a single time point, serial assessment of cardiac structure, morphology, and function is highly reproducible by CMR and plays a vital role in determining whether valvular disease is manifesting with progressive deterioration. The excellent spatial and contrast resolution afforded by modern bright blood sequences allows for reproducible and accurate functional analysis that has been shown to be superior to echocardiography [7, 8]. CMR has also proven helpful in accurately assessing reverse remodeling following aortic valve replacement for aortic stenosis [8–10].

Valvular Morphology and Function

Cine SSFP imaging allows the dynamic visualization of the aortic valve throughout the cardiac cycle without the need for contrast or ionizing radiation. Importantly, the aortic valve can be reformatted in any desired plane. Typically, the valve is imaged in two orthogonal long-axis views displaying the left ventricular outflow tract and aortic root and in a short-axis view following the plane of the aortic annulus and left ventricular outflow tract. Despite respiratory standstill, cardiac motion leads the aortic valve plane to temporarily migrate out of the imaging plane during the cardiac cycle. Motion correction software is required to remain in the annular plane throughout the cycle.

Dynamic imaging in short axis is also useful to first confirm the tricuspid or bicuspid nature of the aortic valve. Following that, the aortic valve area is planimetered to assess the severity of aortic stenosis (Fig. 14.2). Planimetered measurements of the aortic valve by CMR have been shown to correlate highly with measurements of AVA by transesophageal echocardiography (TEE) and retrospective ECG-gated multidetector CT [11–13]. Correlation with TEE is strongest with cine SSFP, as compared to gradient-echo sequences by CMR [14]. These same pulse sequences and image planes can be used to assess the aortic root dimensions to provide additional important information to guide surgical or percutaneous intervention [15].

Historically, morphological imaging of valvular function has proven very useful in establishing the underlying mechanism of disease but has been a poor substitute for the hemodynamic measurement of the severity of stenosis and regurgitation. While a true planimetered valve area provides excellent anatomical analysis of the aortic valve, it has been previously shown that the physiological effects, as measured by effective orifice area (EOA), outweigh the anatomical assessment—calculated as an anatomic aortic valve area (AVA)—in determining disease severity and its impact [16]. To overcome the limitations of anatomical valvular imaging with bright blood cine sequences, phase-contrast velocity mapping (PC-CMR) measures the velocity of blood flow in any given plane, allowing the precise measurement of mean and maximum velocities of the entire blood pool flowing through the vessel of interest and avoiding the dependence on interrogation angles and beam position seen with Doppler echocardiography. This method has been validated against the clinical standard Doppler echocardiography for measurement of flow velocities [17, 18] and the physiological EOA in mild to severe AS [19]. Calculating AVA by the continuity equation provides similar results whether using CMR or TTE [20]. Ongoing research aims to further refine PC-CMR in high-velocity turbulent jets of severe AS where PC-CMR has been known to underestimate peak gradients [21]. By imaging the short-axis plane immediately above the plane of the aortic valve annulus, forward and regurgitant flow is measured completely in order to determine precise regurgitant fraction, which may be underestimated by echocardiography following TAVR (Fig. 14.3) [22].

Myocardial Tissue Characterization

Severe aortic valve disease is associated with alterations in myocyte structure that can result in progressive myocardial fibrosis. Preliminary data has suggested that greater myocardial fibrosis measured by CMR may impede the improvement in LV ejection fraction following surgical valve replacement [23]. The measurement of myocardial fibrosis by CMR relies on proton relaxation characteristics. The T1 or spin–lattice relaxation time corresponds to the specific time decay constant when the proton recovers approximately 63 % of its longitudinal magnetization equilibrium value. The T1 relaxation time depends on the molecular environment of the water molecules in the tissue and therefore characterizes each tissue very specifically. T1 relaxation times vary significantly from one type of tissue to another, but also within the same tissue depending on its physiopathological status (inflammation, edema, or fibrosis). While focal fibrosis such as that incurred by ischemic cardiomyopathy may be measured by LGE as described above, diffuse fibrosis may be measured by a variety of other CMR techniques, including contrast-enhanced T1 mapping, modified look-locker inversion-recovery (MOLLI) T1 mapping, and equilibrium-contrast CMR [24]. Each method carries strengths and limitations with respect to feasibility in the clinical setting.

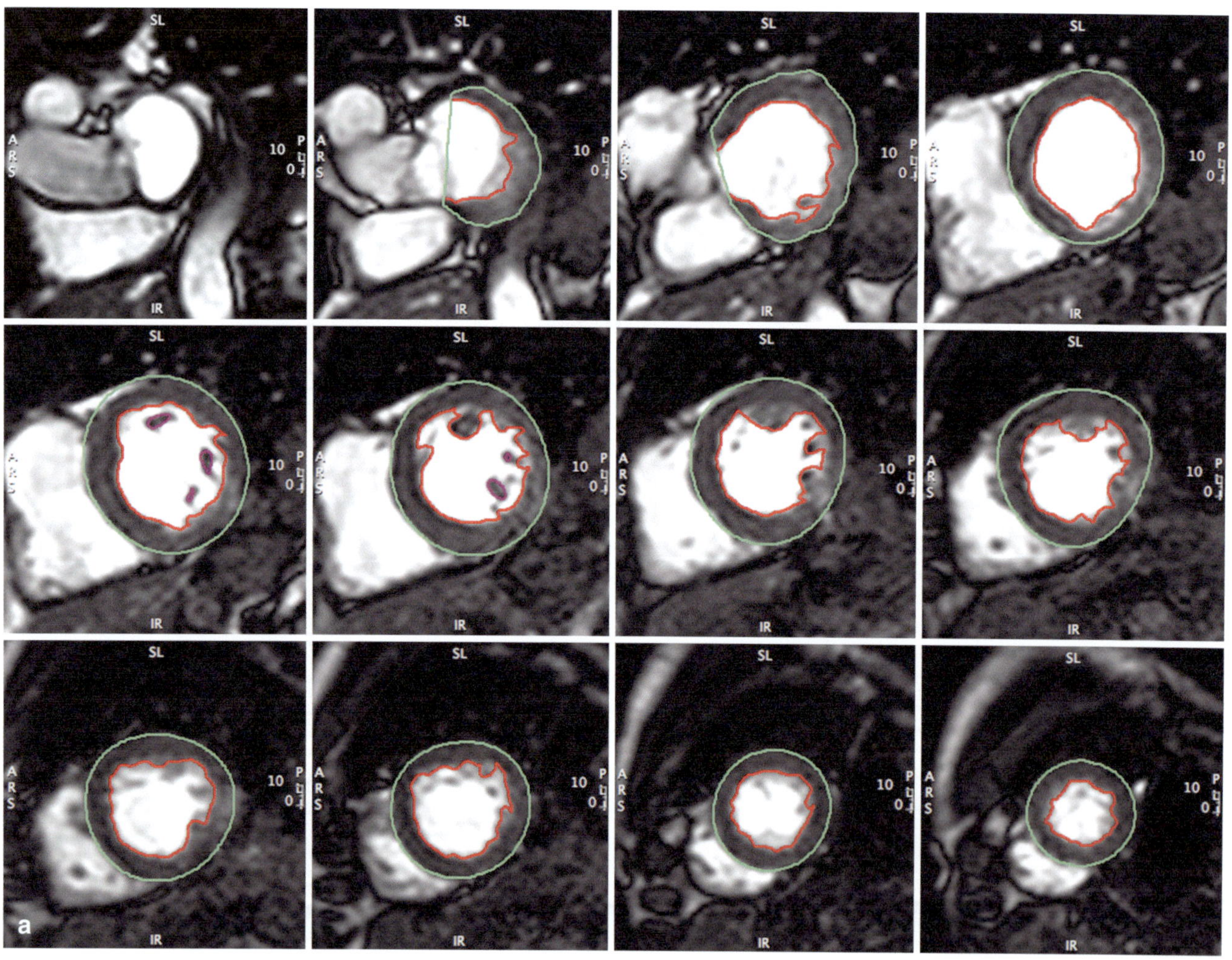

Fig. 14.1 (**a**, **b**) Full coverage of left ventricle in short axis by standard steady-state free precession (SSFP) CMR. This approach is typically used at 20–30 phases per cardiac cycle for accurate and reproducible measurement of left ventricular end-diastolic (Panel **a**) and end-systolic (Panel **b**) volumes, ejection fraction, and left ventricular mass (LVEDV, LVESV, LV mass, LVEF). Cardiac morphology and function may thus be followed serially to detect disease progression/regression without ionizing radiation

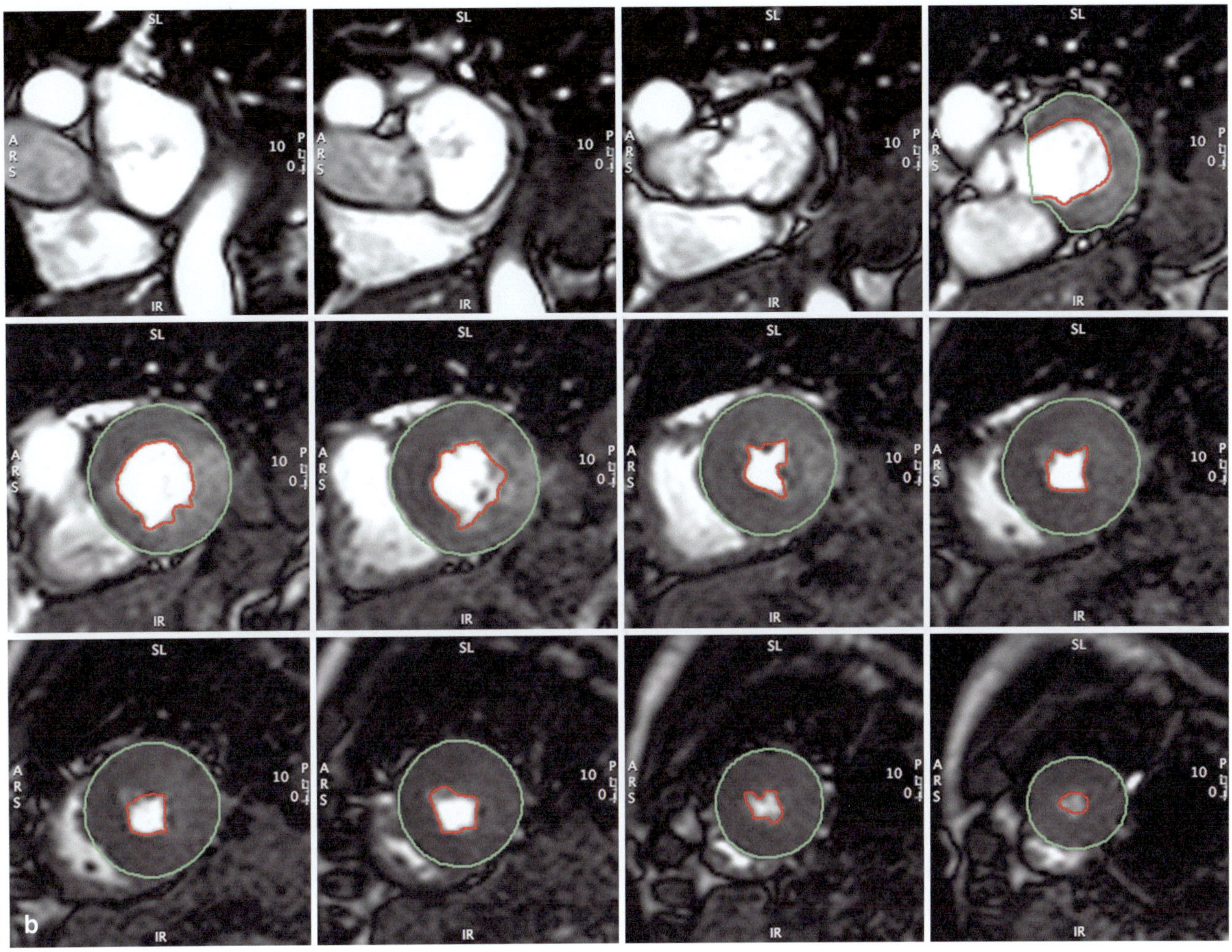

Fig. 14.1 (continued)

Focal fibrosis measured by LGE appears to be common in the setting of significant myocardial hypertrophy with wall thickness in excess of 18 mm [25, 26]. When identified, this appears to be a truly limited process commonly involving less than 5 % of the total myocardial mass. While limited in scope, the presence of LGE has important prognostic significance with a fivefold increased hazard for all-cause mortality as compared to those without delayed enhancement with comparable severity of aortic stenosis [27]. Greater fibrosis on CMR is also known to be present in low-flow severe AS, a subpopulation of AS with poorer prognosis [28]. It has also been shown that focal fibrosis on LGE CMR is an irreversible finding that does not resolve with aortic valve replacement and elimination of the afterload disturbance [29].

Magnetic resonance spectroscopy has proven useful to study myocardial high-energy phosphate (HEP) metabolism in patients. Similar to that observed with dilated cardiomyopathy, significant AS may be associated with altered myocardial HEP metabolism, which may improve following corrective surgery [30–32]. This metabolic improvement appears to occur even in the presence of patient-prosthesis mismatch [33].

Myocardial Ischemia

Inducible myocardial ischemia indicative of obstructive coronary artery disease (CAD) can be identified using CMR by adenosine-stress perfusion or dobutamine-stress functional studies [34] with high diagnostic accuracy (83 % positive predictive value and 100 % negative predictive value) for the diagnosis of obstructive coronary artery disease on invasive coronary angiography in patients with severe aortic stenosis [35].

Extra-Cardiac Magnetic Resonance for Aortic Stenosis

Magnetic resonance imaging is also useful to detect ischemic cerebral insults after correction of AS, whether by traditional or percutaneous methods [36]. Evidence of new presumably embolic cerebrovascular events has been identified in up to 68 % undergoing TAVR without a significant difference between transfemoral or transapical approaches [37] with the Sapien platform and 77 % of CoreValve TAVR procedures [38]. Brain

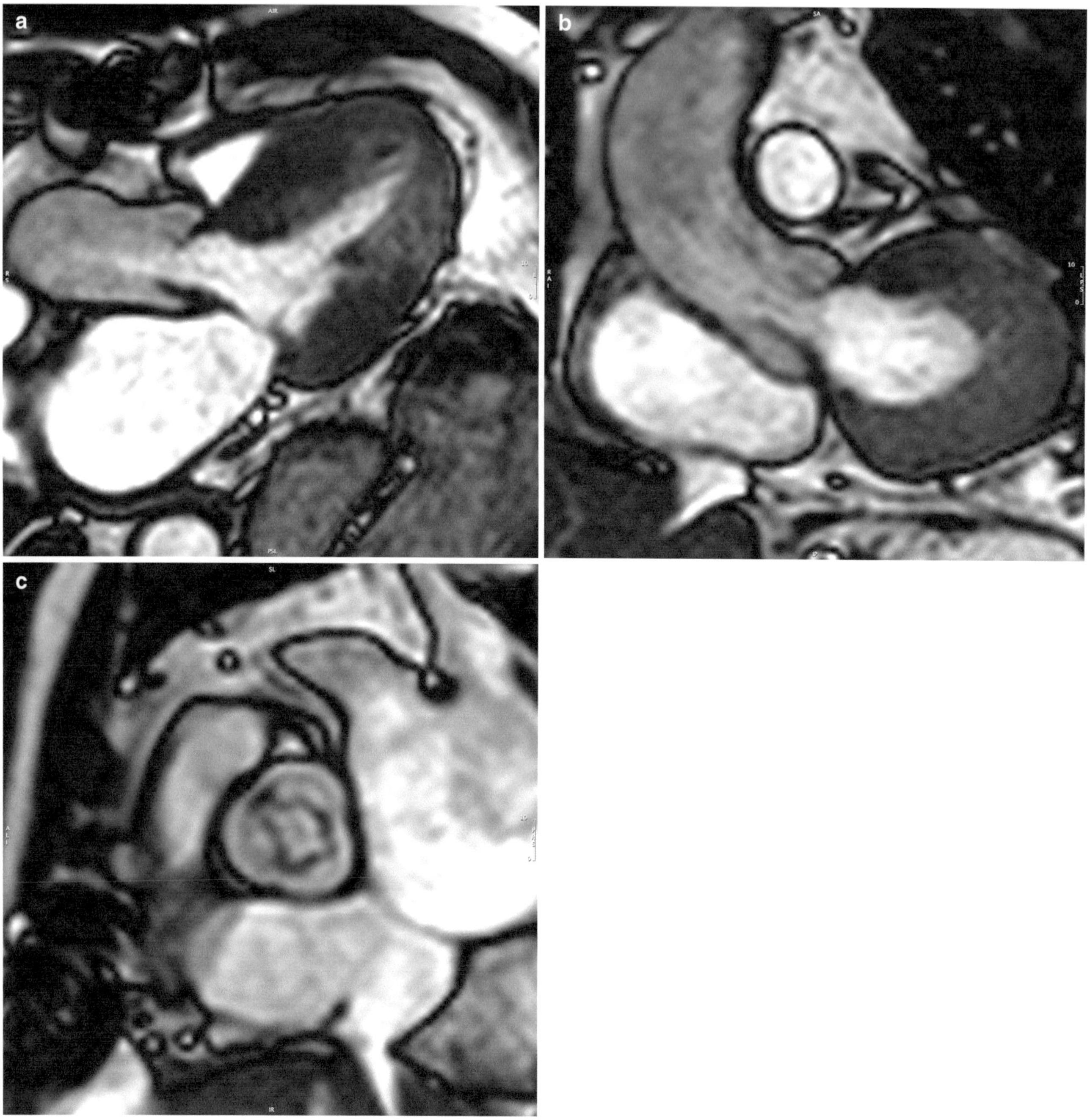

Fig. 14.2 (**a**–**c**) Cine SSFP CMR of the aortic valve, left ventricular outflow tract, and aortic root in two orthogonal long-axis planes (Panels **a** and **b**) and the short-axis plane (Panel **c**). Dynamic 3D imaging allows radiation-free and contrast-free measurement of the aortic valve opening and annulus surfaces by planimetry, as well as the annulus diameters in any given plane

MRI has also been proposed as the imaging end point for the evaluation of new embolic protection devices in TAVR [39].

Cardiovascular Magnetic Resonance in TAVR Evaluation

Planimetry of AVA by CMR has been shown to correlate well with the planimetry of the AVA by CT, transesophageal echocardiography (TEE), and transthoracic echocardiography (TTE) [15]. However, in a pilot study of 39 patients undergoing TAVR, measurements of aortic valve annulus diameter by CMR were on average 2.3 mm (11 %) larger than measurements by TTE [40]. A different study of 24 patients undergoing TAVR for severe AS supported the observation that TTE underestimates annulus size compared to TEE and CMR [41]. It would appear that a systematic difference between the 2D diameter measurements performed by TTE and CMR exists and needs to be accounted for when using CMR for annular sizing (Fig. 14.4).

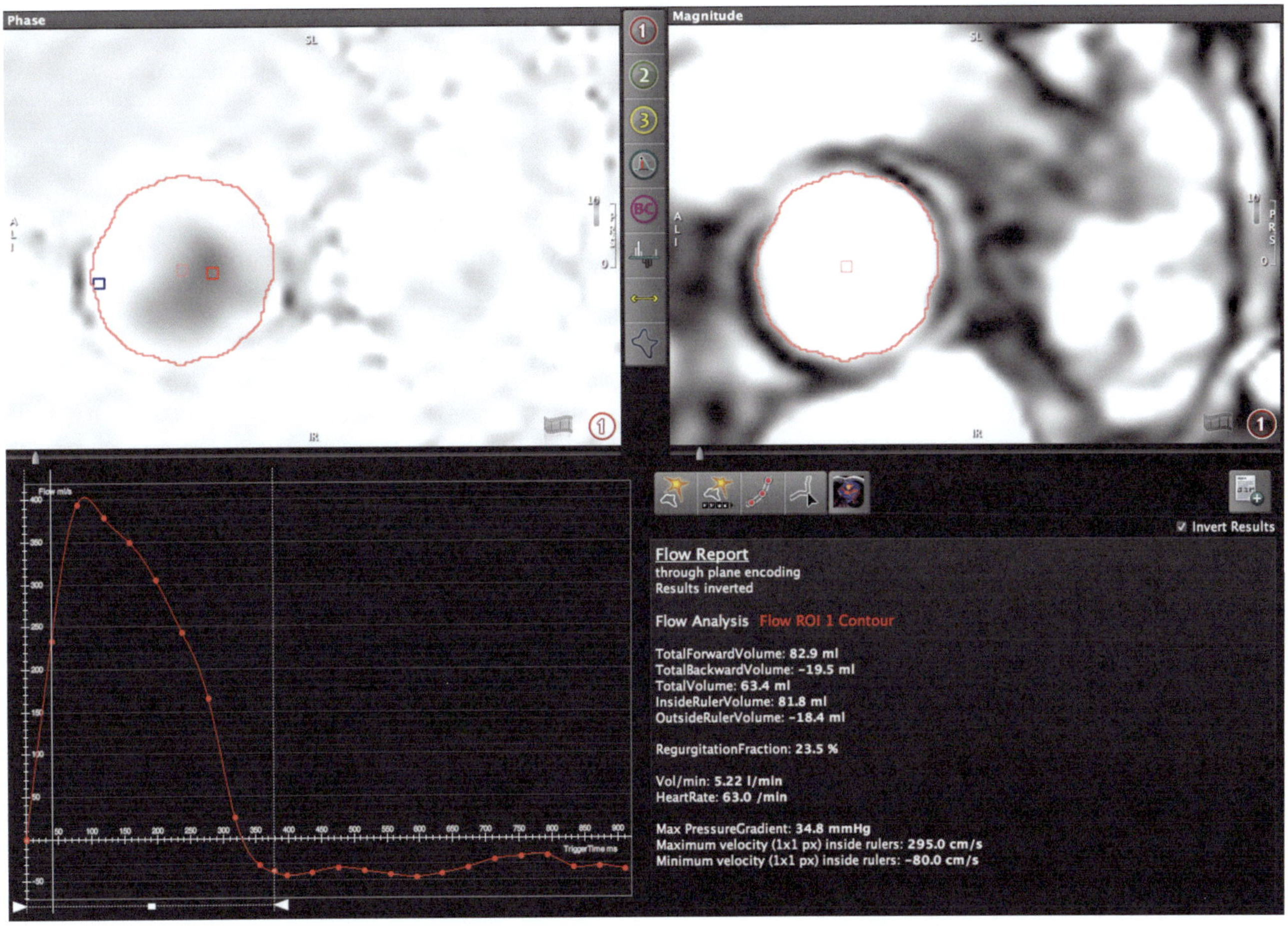

Fig. 14.3 Phase-contrast (PC-CMR) performed in the aortic root above the valve in the plane of the annulus (Fig. 14.4). Through-plane encoding measurements include a maximum velocity of 295 cm/s (maximum pressure gradient of 34.8 mmHg), total forward volume of 82.9 ml, and backward volume of 19.5 ml for a regurgitant fraction of 23.5 %. Such PC-CMR measurements do not suffer from Doppler beam angle dependency or errors brought on by multiple jets

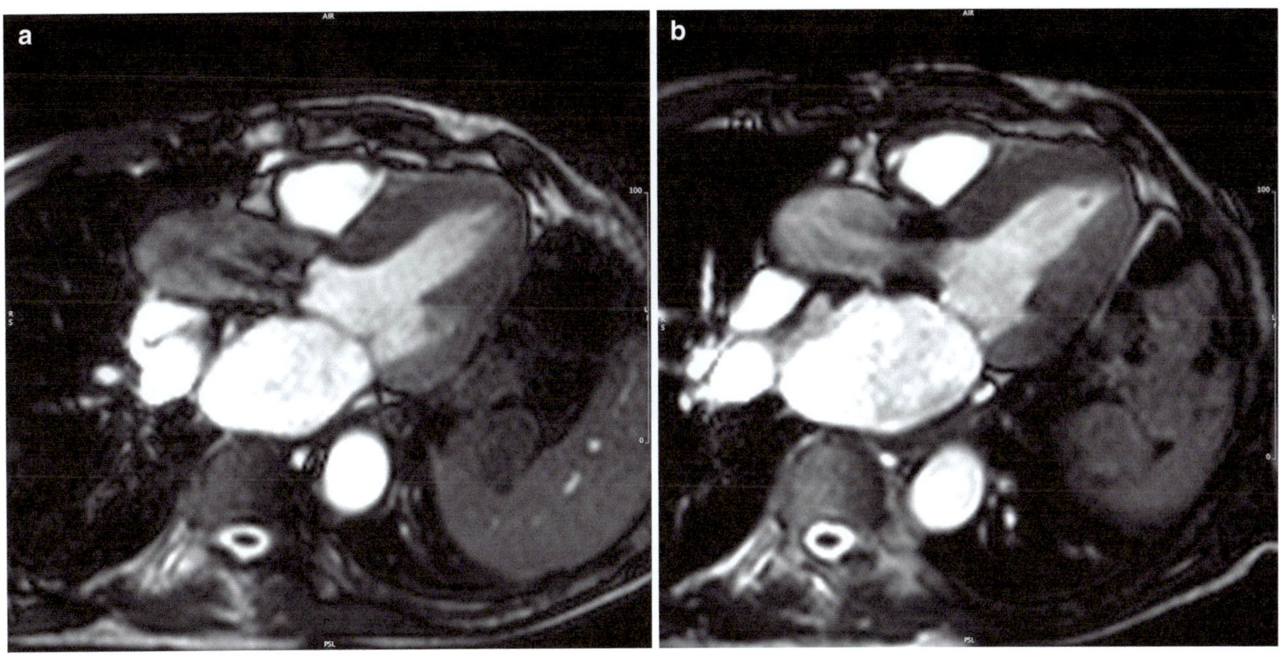

Fig. 14.4 (**a**, **b**) (Movies 14.4a and b). Long-axis cine SSFP CMR of a severely stenotic aortic valve at end systole before (Panel **a**) and after (Panel **b**) TAVR

Conclusion

Cardiovascular MR allows for the complete assessment of a patient undergoing evaluation for TAVR. CMR allows for the accurate characterization of aortic valve morphology and stenosis severity as well as left ventricular function and tissue characterization without ionizing radiation. For individuals with underlying chronic kidney disease who cannot undergo MDCT, MR appears to be a reasonable option for characterization of patients prior to TAVR.

References

1. Lockie T, Nagel E, Redwood S, et al. Use of Cardiovascular Magnetic Resonance Imaging in Acute Coronary Syndromes. Circulation. 2009;119:1671–81.
2. Leon MB, Smith CR, Mack M, et al. Transcatheter aortic-valve implantation for aortic stenosis in patients who cannot undergo surgery. N Engl J Med. 2010; 363(17):1597–607.
3. Bonow RO, Carabello BA, Chatterjee K, et al. 2008 Focused update incorporated into the ACC/AHA 2006 guidelines for the management of patients with valvular heart disease: a report of the American College of Cardiology/American Heart Association Task Force on Practice Guidelines (Writing Committee to Revise the 1998 Guidelines for the Management of Patients With Valvular Heart Disease): endorsed by the Society of Cardiovascular Anesthesiologists, Society for Cardiovascular Angiography and Interventions, and Society of Thoracic Surgeons. Circulation. 2008;118:e523–661.
4. Hendel RC, Patel MR, Kramer CM, et al. ACCF/ACR/SCCT/SCMR/ASNC/NASCI/SCAI/SIR 2006 appropriateness criteria for cardiac computed tomography and cardiac magnetic resonance imaging: a report of the American College of Cardiology Foundation Quality Strategic Directions Committee Appropriateness Criteria Working Group, American College of Radiology, Society of Cardiovascular Computed Tomography, Society for Cardiovascular Magnetic Resonance, American Society of Nuclear Cardiology, North American Society for Cardiac Imaging, Society for Cardiovascular Angiography and Interventions, and Society of Interventional Radiology. J Am Coll Cardiol. 2006;48:1475–97.
5. Pennell DJ. Cardiovascular magnetic resonance. Circulation. 2010;121:692–705.
6. Maceira AM, Prasad SK, Khan M, Pennell DJ. Normalized left ventricular systolic and diastolic function by steady state free precession cardiovascular magnetic resonance. J Cardiovasc Magn Reson. 2006;8:417–26.
7. Thiele H, Paetsch I, Schnackenburg B, et al. Improved accuracy of quantitative assessment of left ventricular volume and ejection fraction by geometric models with steady-state free precession. J Cardiovasc Magn Reson. 2002;4:327–39.
8. Biederman RW, Magovern JA, Grant SB, et al. LV reverse remodeling imparted by aortic valve replacement for severe aortic stenosis; is it durable? A cardiovascular MRI study sponsored by the American Heart Association. J Cardiothorac Surg. 2011;6:53.
9. Biederman RW, Doyle M, Yamrozik J, et al. Physiologic compensation is supranormal in compensated aortic stenosis: does it return to normal after aortic valve replacement or is it blunted by coexistent coronary artery disease? An intramyocardial magnetic resonance imaging study. Circulation. 2005;112:I429–36.
10. Breitenbach I, Harringer W, Tsui S, et al. Magnetic resonance imaging versus echocardiography to ascertain the regression of left ventricular hypertrophy after bioprosthetic aortic valve replacement: results of the REST study. J Thorac Cardiovasc Surg. 2012;144(3):640–5.
11. Bruder O, Jochims M, Hunold P, et al. Comparison of aortic valve area measured by magnetic resonance imaging and dual-source computed tomography. Acta Radiol. 2009;50:645–51.
12. Pouleur AC, le Polain de Waroux JB, Pasquet A, Vanoverschelde JL, Gerber BL. Aortic valve area assessment: multidetector CT compared with cine MR imaging and transthoracic and transesophageal echocardiography. Radiology. 2007;244:745–54.
13. Westermann Y, Geigenmuller A, Elgeti T, et al. Planimetry of the aortic valve orifice area: comparison of multislice spiral computed tomography and magnetic resonance imaging. Eur J Radiol. 2011;77:426–35.
14. Schlosser T, Malyar N, Jochims M, et al. Quantification of aortic valve stenosis in MRI-comparison of steady-state free precession and fast low-angle shot sequences. Eur Radiol. 2007;17: 1284–90.
15. Link KM, Lesko NM. The role of MR imaging in the evaluation of acquired diseases of the thoracic aorta. AJR Am J Roentgenol. 1992;158:1115–25.
16. Pibarot P, Larose E. What our eyes see is not necessarily what our heart feels. Cardiology. 2008;109:122–5.
17. Caruthers SD, Lin SJ, Brown P, et al. Practical value of cardiac magnetic resonance imaging for clinical quantification of aortic valve stenosis: comparison with echocardiography. Circulation. 2003;108:2236–43.
18. Eichenberger AC, Jenni R, von Schulthess GK. Aortic valve pressure gradients in patients with aortic valve stenosis: quantification with velocity-encoded cine MR imaging. AJR Am J Roentgenol. 1993;160:971–7.
19. Garcia J, Kadem L, Larose E, Clavel MA, Pibarot P. Comparison between cardiovascular magnetic resonance and transthoracic Doppler echocardiography for the estimation of effective orifice area in aortic stenosis. J Cardiovasc Magn Reson. 2011; 13:25.
20. Yap SC, van Geuns RJ, Meijboom FJ, et al. A simplified continuity equation approach to the quantification of stenotic bicuspid aortic valves using velocity-encoded cardiovascular magnetic resonance. J Cardiovasc Magn Reson. 2007;9:899–906.
21. O'Brien KR, Myerson SG, Cowan BR, Young AA, Robson MD. Phase contrast ultrashort TE: a more reliable technique for measurement of high-velocity turbulent stenotic jets. Magn Reson Med. 2009;62:626–36.
22. Sherif MA, Abdel-Wahab M, Beurich HW, et al. Haemodynamic evaluation of aortic regurgitation after transcatheter aortic valve implantation using cardiovascular magnetic resonance. EuroIntervention. 2011;7:57–63.
23. Azevedo CF, Nigri M, Higuchi ML, et al. Prognostic significance of myocardial fibrosis quantification by histopathology and magnetic resonance imaging in patients with severe aortic valve disease. J Am Coll Cardiol. 2010;56:278–87.
24. Flett AS, Hayward MP, Ashworth MT, et al. Equilibrium contrast cardiovascular magnetic resonance for the measurement of diffuse myocardial fibrosis: preliminary validation in humans. Circulation. 2010;122:138–44.
25. Debl K, Djavidani B, Buchner S, et al. Delayed hyperenhancement in magnetic resonance imaging of left ventricular hypertrophy caused by aortic stenosis and hypertrophic cardiomyopathy: visualisation of focal fibrosis. Heart. 2006;92:1447–51.
26. Rudolph A, Abdel-Aty H, Bohl S, et al. Noninvasive detection of fibrosis applying contrast-enhanced cardiac magnetic resonance in

different forms of left ventricular hypertrophy relation to remodeling. J Am Coll Cardiol. 2009;53:284–91.
27. Dweck MR, Joshi S, Murigu T, et al. Midwall fibrosis is an independent predictor of mortality in patients with aortic stenosis. J Am Coll Cardiol. 2011;58:1271–9.
28. Herrmann S, Stork S, Niemann M, et al. Low-gradient aortic valve stenosis myocardial fibrosis and its influence on function and outcome. J Am Coll Cardiol. 2011;58:402–12.
29. Weidemann F, Herrmann S, Stork S, et al. Impact of myocardial fibrosis in patients with symptomatic severe aortic stenosis. Circulation. 2009;120:577–84.
30. Beyerbacht HP, Lamb HJ, van Der Laarse A, et al. Aortic valve replacement in patients with aortic valve stenosis improves myocardial metabolism and diastolic function. Radiology. 2001;219:637–43.
31. Neubauer S, Horn M, Cramer M, et al. Myocardial phosphocreatine-to-ATP ratio is a predictor of mortality in patients with dilated cardiomyopathy. Circulation. 1997;96:2190–6.
32. Neubauer S, Horn M, Pabst T, et al. Cardiac high-energy phosphate metabolism in patients with aortic valve disease assessed by 31P-magnetic resonance spectroscopy. J Investig Med. 1997;45:453–62.
33. Mannacio V, Di Tommaso L, Stassano P, De Amicis V, Vosa C. Myocardial metabolism and diastolic function after aortic valve replacement for aortic stenosis: influence of patient-prosthesis mismatch. Eur J Cardiothorac Surg. 2012;41:316–21.
34. Nabi F, Malaty A, Shah DJ. Stress cardiac magnetic resonance. Curr Opin Cardiol. 2011;26:385–91.
35. Burgstahler C, Kunze M, Gawaz MP, et al. Adenosine stress first pass perfusion for the detection of coronary artery disease in patients with aortic stenosis: a feasibility study. Int J Cardiovasc Imaging. 2008;24:195–200.
36. Arnold M, Schulz-Heise S, Achenbach S, et al. Embolic cerebral insults after transapical aortic valve implantation detected by magnetic resonance imaging. JACC Cardiovasc Interv. 2010;3:1126–32.
37. Rodes-Cabau J, Dumont E, Boone RH, et al. Cerebral embolism following transcatheter aortic valve implantation: comparison of transfemoral and transapical approaches. J Am Coll Cardiol. 2011;57:18–28.
38. Fairbairn TA, Mather AN, Bijsterveld P, et al. Diffusion-weighted MRI determined cerebral embolic infarction following transcatheter aortic valve implantation: assessment of predictive risk factors and the relationship to subsequent health status. Heart. 2012;98:18–23.
39. Nietlispach F, Wijesinghe N, Gurvitch R, et al. An embolic deflection device for aortic valve interventions. JACC Cardiovasc Interv. 2010;3:1133–8.
40. La Manna A, Sanfilippo A, Capodanno D, et al. Cardiovascular magnetic resonance for the assessment of patients undergoing transcatheter aortic valve implantation: a pilot study. J Cardiovasc Magn Reson. 2011;13:82.
41. Paelinck BP, Van Herck PL, Rodrigus I, et al. Comparison of magnetic resonance imaging of aortic valve stenosis and aortic root to multimodality imaging for selection of transcatheter aortic valve implantation candidates. Am J Cardiol. 2011;108:92–8.

Positron Emission Tomography Evaluation of Aortic Stenosis

15

Mark R. Dweck, James H.F. Rudd, and David E. Newby

Abstract

Positron Emission Tomography is an emerging non-invasive imaging techniques which allows the activity of specific biochemical processes to be studied within even small structures in the body. PET has recently been applied to patients with aortic stenosis providing some key insights to the pathological processes underlying this condition. In the chapter we will review the principles of PET and how this imaging modality can be applied to heart and specifically the aortic valve.

Keywords

Aortic stenosis • Positron emission tomography • Inflammation • Calcification

Introduction

Calcific aortic stenosis (AS) is a common and increasing health-care burden. Over the last decade, the number of aortic valve replacements performed in the USA has doubled, and as the population ages, the prevalence of AS is predicted to double again by 2020 [1]. However, the underlying pathophysiology of AS remains incompletely defined, and there are currently no effective medical treatments capable of altering its course. Furthermore, reliable markers that can predict disease progression, future need for surgery, or mortality are lacking. There is therefore a pressing need to reevaluate the underlying pathophysiological processes involved [2].

With advances in technology, modern noninvasive imaging techniques such as cardiovascular computed tomography (CT) and positron emission tomography (PET) have become applicable to the heart. This has afforded the opportunity to improve our understanding of the pathogenesis underlying aortic stenosis in a noninvasive manner. Specifically combined PET and computed tomography (PET/CT) has allowed us to examine the relative contributions of two key processes: inflammation and calcification.

In this chapter, we will first examine the basic principles of PET/CT scanning and then describe how this technology has been applied to aortic stenosis. We conclude with a discussion of the work that is still required for its validation and how PET/CT might contribute to the investigation of aortic stenosis in the future.

M.R. Dweck, MD, PhD (✉) • D.E. Newby, MD, PhD
Centre for Cardiovascular Science, University of Edinburgh, Chancellor's Building, Little France Crescent, Edinburgh EH16 4SB, UK
e-mail: mdweck@staffmail.ed.ac.uk; d.e.newby@ed.ac.uk

J.H.F. Rudd, MD, PhD
Division of Cardiovascular Medicine, University of Cambridge, Addenbrooke's Hospital, Box 110, ACCI, Hills Road, Cambridge CB2 2QQ, UK
e-mail: jhfr2@cam.ac.uk

J.K. Min et al. (eds.), *Multimodality Imaging for Transcatheter Aortic Valve Replacement*,
DOI 10.1007/978-1-4471-2798-7_15, © Springer-Verlag London 2014

Positron Emission Tomography

Physics

PET is a noninvasive imaging technique, which provides information regarding the activity of specific biochemical processes within the body. The positron or antielectron is the antiparticle of the electron, having the same mass but a positive electric charge. PET tracers consist of a positron emitter, such as 18F-fluoride, 15O-oxygen, or 11C-carbon, that is attached to a molecular vehicle targeting the biochemical process of interest [3]. In the nuclei of these molecules, protons decay to neutrons (beta decay) resulting in emission of a positron and a neutrino. After a time, collision between the positron and an electron results in annihilation of both particles and the release of two photons, with a specific energy (511 keV), at 180° to one another. Detection of these photons provides the basis for PET scanning (Fig. 15.1).

PET imaging uses a dedicated camera system that involves multiple circumferential rings of detectors completely surrounding the patient. These detectors are made up of scintillation crystals, which release light when hit by a photon and convert this light into an electrical signal. PET imaging utilizes the concept that two 511 keV photons detected in close temporal proximity (within 6–12 ns) by two opposed detectors in the ring are likely to have originated from a single annihilation event in the body somewhere in a line between them or the line of response. Such simultaneous detections are termed coincidences, and these events are used to build a PET image that maps the site of tracer accumulation [3].

The resultant images provide detailed functional data regarding the biochemical process being studied; however, PET scans are limited by a lack of spatial resolution. Recently this issue has been addressed combining low resolution functional PET data with high resolution anatomical data provided by CT. PET/CT scanners incorporating both PET and CT within the same gantry have become the standard equipment of clinical PET practice. Patients lie in the same position for both scans, which allows the PET and CT scans to be superimposed upon one another. This serves two purposes: firstly, the CT can be used to perform accurate attenuation correction of the PET image; and secondly, co-registration allows precise localization of tracer uptake within small structures such as the aortic valve (Fig. 15.2).

To date, PET/CT in aortic stenosis has focused on 18F-fluorodeoxyglucose (18F-FDG) and 18F-sodium fluoride (18F-NaF) as markers of inflammation and calcification, respectively. Tracer development has largely been driven by oncology studies (Box 15.1). While both of the above tracers are used commonly to identify malignant lesions and bone metastases, their role in imaging the vasculature has only recently been investigated.

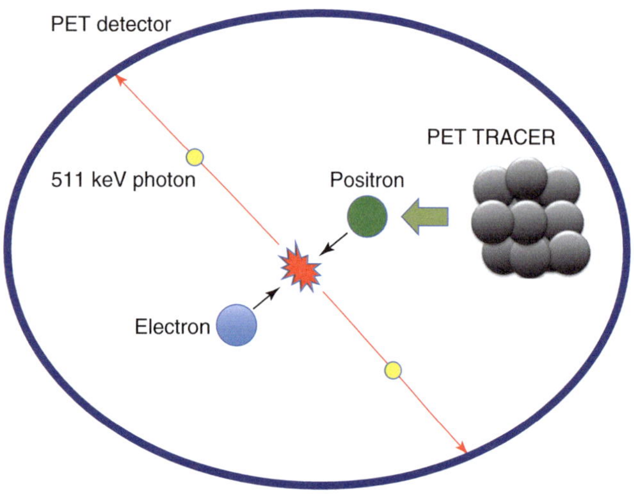

Fig. 15.1 Basic principles of positron emission tomography. PET tracers release protons which quickly collide with bystander electrons and annihilate resulting in the release of two 511 keV photons at 180° to one another. The simultaneous detection of these photons by the detector rings allows the origin of the annihilation to be pinpointed along the line or response

Box 15.1 PET Tracers for Evaluation of Aortic Stenosis

18F-flurodeoxyglucose	Glucose analogue taken up by cells via glucose transport proteins and enters the glycolytic metabolic pathway
	Following initial hexokinase step. 18F-FDG-6-phosphate cannot be metabolized further and becomes trapped, concentrating in cells with high metabolic requirements
	Thought to incorporate into inflammatory areas such as the calcifications of aortic stenosis
18F-sodium fluoride	Tracer directly produced in cyclotrons and does not require further labeling for use as IV injected PET imaging agent
	Incorporates into bone crystals via an exchange with hydroxyl groups ([hydroxyapatite crystal of bone, $(Ca_{10}(PO4)_6OH_2] \rightarrow$ [fluoroapatite $(Ca_{10}(PO_4)_6F_2)$])
	Hydroxyapatite key component of calcification in aortic stenosis

FDG flurodeoxyglucose, *PET* positron emission tomography

18F-Fluorodeoxyglucose

18F-fluorodeoxyglucose (18F-FDG) is a glucose analogue that is taken up into cells by glucose transport proteins and enters the glycolytic metabolic pathway. Following the initial hexokinase step, 18F-FDG-6-phosphate cannot be metabolized further and becomes trapped, concentrating in cells with high metabolic requirements. Increased uptake is therefore observed in malignant cells but also in arterial macrophages, which have

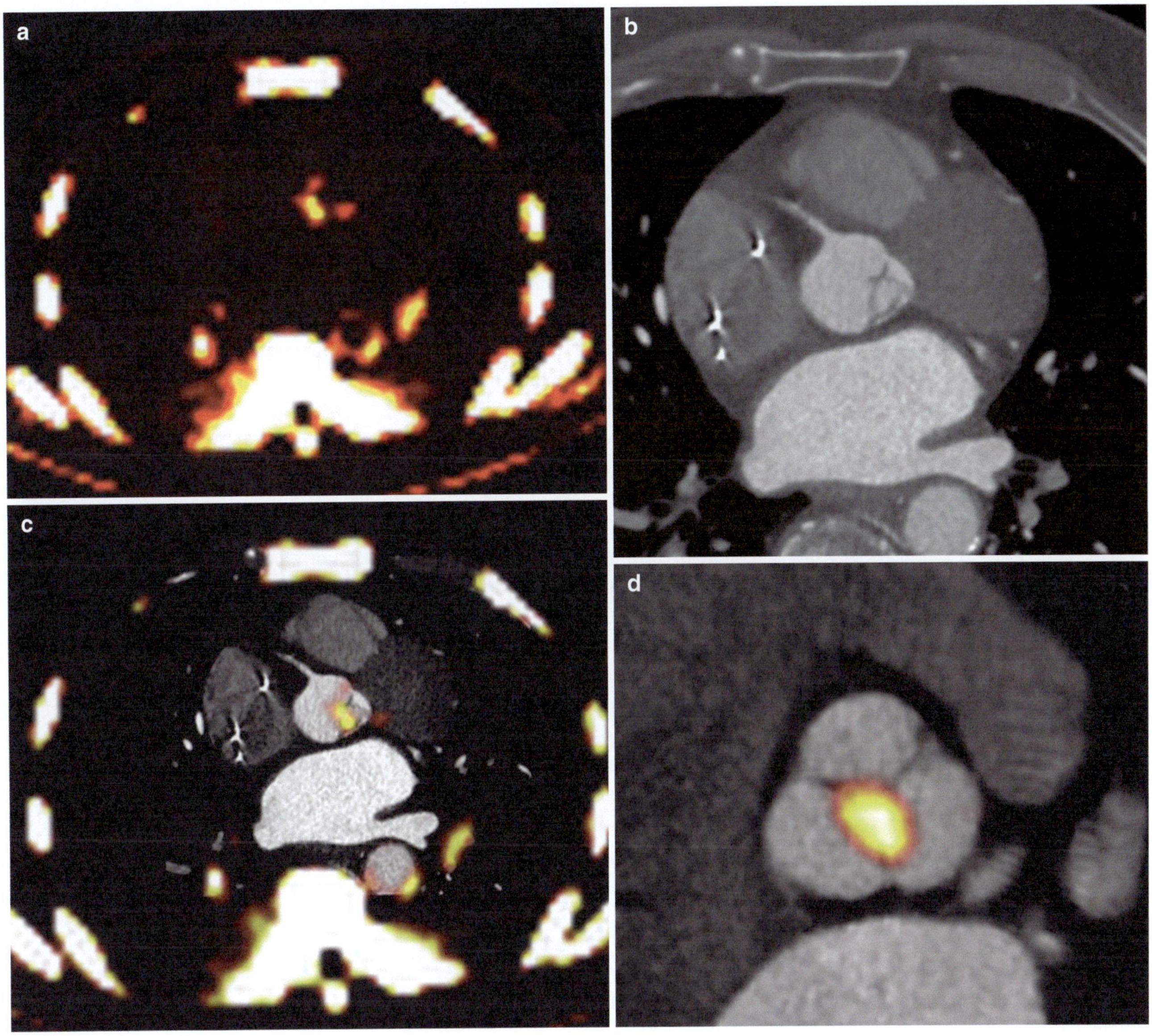

Fig. 15.2 Fusion of PET/CT scans for the assessment of aortic valve activity. (**a**) PET scan (axial view) showing activity of 18F-NaF in the thorax. (**b**) CT scan acquired at the same level during the same scan. (**c**) Fusion of the PET and CT scans identifies increased uptake in the valve. (**d**) The PET/CT image has been reorientated to provide short-axis views of the valve in a patient with aortic sclerosis. Note increased uptake in the non-coronary cusp

increased metabolic requirements compared to other cells in the vasculature. This has been the basis for vascular PET imaging using 18F-FDG, which has become an established means of quantifying vascular inflammation in both the aorta and carotid arteries [4, 5]. Rudd and colleagues first established that 18F-FDG uptake was increased in symptomatic carotid plaque following transient ischemic attack compared to contralateral lesions [5]. Subsequently the level of 18F-FDG activity has been shown to correlate with plaque macrophage burden [6] and hypoxia [7]. Arterial uptake of 18F-FDG has now been extended to the aorta, femoral, and iliac vessels displaying excellent reproducibility [8, 9] and has demonstrated considerable promise as a means of assessing novel anti-inflammatory atherosclerotic agents. Tahara and colleagues demonstrated that simvastatin significantly reduced carotid 18F-FDG uptake after 3 months of treatment. More recently 18F-FDG has been used to study a novel cholesteryl ester transfer protein (CETP) inhibitor, dalcetrapib, that appeared to result in a reduction in the carotid plaque signal [10].

18F-Sodium Fluoride (18F-NaF)

18F-sodium fluoride (18F-NaF) is a tracer that is directly produced in medical cyclotrons and does not require further labeling to an additional molecule for its use as an intravenous PET imaging tracer. It was first introduced as a bone scanning agent approximately 40 years ago. 18F-NaF directly incorporates into bone crystals via an exchange with hydroxyl groups in the hydroxyapatite crystal of bone ($Ca_{10}(PO4)_6OH_2$) to form fluorapatite ($Ca_{10}(PO_4)_6F_2$). This process can be divided into four stages as originally described by Blau and colleagues [11]. In steps 1 and 2, fluoride moves from the blood through the extracellular space to the shell of bound water around exposed crystals, a process which occurs within minutes of exposure. Step 3 is movement of the tracer on to the crystal surface and probably occurs in hours, while in step 4, 18F-NaF is incorporated into the bone crystal, which takes days or weeks. Uptake in bone is therefore thought to reflect two processes, firstly increased blood flow and secondly osteoblast and osteoclast activity [11–13], which increase the surface area of exposed hydroxyapatite to which 18F-NaF can bind [14]. Given that hydroxyapatite is also a key component of the calcification observed in aortic stenosis, the mechanism of 18F-NaF uptake in the valve is likely to be similar and predominantly reflect calcification activity since blood flow should be constant.

18F-NaF is used clinically for the detection of primary osteoblastic tumors, bone metastases, and conditions associated with high bone turnover such as Paget's disease [15, 16]. More recently, studies have described 18F-NaF uptake as a marker of calcification within carotid and aortic atheroma [17, 18] and demonstrated an association between activity and cardiovascular risk factors [18]. Our group has also extended this to the coronary arteries, in which increased activity could be localized to discrete regions of coronary plaque and identified patients who had higher rates of prior adverse cardiovascular events and increased Framingham risk scores [19].

Aortic Stenosis

Two studies have now examined uptake of 18F-FDG in aortic stenosis [20, 21] and two have examined 18F-NaF [20, 22]. However, our study was the only one to date to prospectively compare the uptake of both tracers within the same patient population and will be the initial focus of this review. We performed a prospective study of 121 patients, including 81 patients with aortic stenosis (25 mild, 33 moderate, 21 severe), 20 patients with aortic sclerosis, and 20 control patients with normal valves [20]. Patients underwent a full baseline clinical assessment, which included an echocardiographic assessment of valve severity. Subjects then underwent two PET/CT scans: the first 90 min following administration of 200 MBq of 18F-FDG and the second 60 min after injection with 125 MBq of 18F-NaF. Finally, a CT calcium score of the valve and coronary arteries was performed.

Method of Quantification

Quantification of PET activity in the aortic valve presents many challenges. In other tissue, tracer uptake is measured on axial, coronal, or sagittal images. However, the axis of the aortic valve does not lie in any of these standard imaging planes, so that quantification of tracer uptake is not straightforward using traditional methods. In order to overcome this problem, the field of view can be reorientated to provide coaxial, short-axis views of the valve (Fig. 15.2) [20]. Regions of interest can then be placed around its perimeter with greater accuracy and used to measure the mean and maximum standard uptake values (SUV) (Fig. 15.1). The SUV is the decay-corrected tissue uptake divided by the injected dose per body weight. In vascular tissue, it is influenced by tracer blood-pool activity. Therefore, the arterial SUV signal is often normalized to a venous blood SUV (measured in the SVC, which has no atheroma) to provide the tissue-to-background ratio (TBR). Tawakol and colleagues showed that TBR was related more closely to the underlying macrophage content of carotid artery plaque than the uncorrected SUV [6].

Using this technique, we demonstrated excellent measures of inter- and intra-observer reproducibility for quantification of 18F-NaF (intra-class correlation coefficients [ICC] 0.99). However, measurement of 18F-FDG was more challenging still. Glucose is the predominant energy source for the myocardium so that intense uptake of 18F-FDG is frequently observed that can spill into the plane of the aortic valve and contaminate its signal. We therefore employed stringent dietary restrictions (patients were asked to avoid ingestion of all carbohydrate for 24 h prior to the scan) in an attempt to shift the myocardium towards a fatty acid metabolism and reduce its 18F-FDG uptake. However, even despite these precautions, measures of reproducibility were poor using whole valve methods with regions of interest placed around the perimeter of the valve. We therefore adopted a second approach in which these regions were restricted to the center of the valve and well away from the myocardial signal. This resulted in a significant improvement in measures of reproducibility (ICC >0.90) without appearing to underestimate valve activity. Interestingly, Marincheva-Savcheva and colleagues independently settled on a similar center-valve technique when they approached the same problem (see below) [21].

Tracer Uptake at Different Stages of Aortic Stenosis Severity

We have observed that there is a relationship between tracer uptake and severity of aortic stenosis with both 18F-FDG and 18F-NaF. 18F-FDG was observed in a diffuse pattern across the valve. Uptake was increased in patients with both aortic sclerosis (max TBR: median 1.47 [IQR 1.31–1.61], $p<0.001$) and aortic stenosis (1.57 [1.44–1.68]; $p<0.001$) compared to control subjects (1.27 [1.21–1.40]). However, in our study, 18F-FDG activity rose progressively in patients with mild (1.44 [1.37–1.63]), moderate (1.58 [1.41–1.65]), and severe aortic stenosis (1.65 [1.55–1.85]) consistent with a modest yet sustained increase in inflammation with disease severity, even among those with advanced disease ($r^2=0.218$, $p<0.001$).

With respect to 18F-NaF, focal areas of uptake were observed in the valve in two distinct patterns (Fig. 15.2). First, activity could be observed in the absence of underlying calcium on the CT scan, suggestive of new calcification or microcalcification. Second, uptake could be observed overlying existing CT calcium. This was thought to represent regions of calcium that were remodeling towards the end-stage bone phenotype. Activity of 18F-NaF was again higher in patients with aortic sclerosis (1.96 [1.63–2.11]) and aortic stenosis (2.73 [2.30–3.22]) compared to control subjects (1.56 [1.41–1.64; both $p<0.001$) and displayed a progressive rise with increasing aortic stenosis severity ($r^2=0.540$; $p<0.001$) (Fig. 15.3). However, the rate of rise was much steeper than for 18-FDG such that there was only a modest correlation between the activity of the 2 tracers and so that in all stages of disease severity 18F-NaF uptake exceeded 18F-FDG (Fig. 15.4).

Comparisons between tracer activity in the valve and in nearby aortic atheroma provided some additional interesting

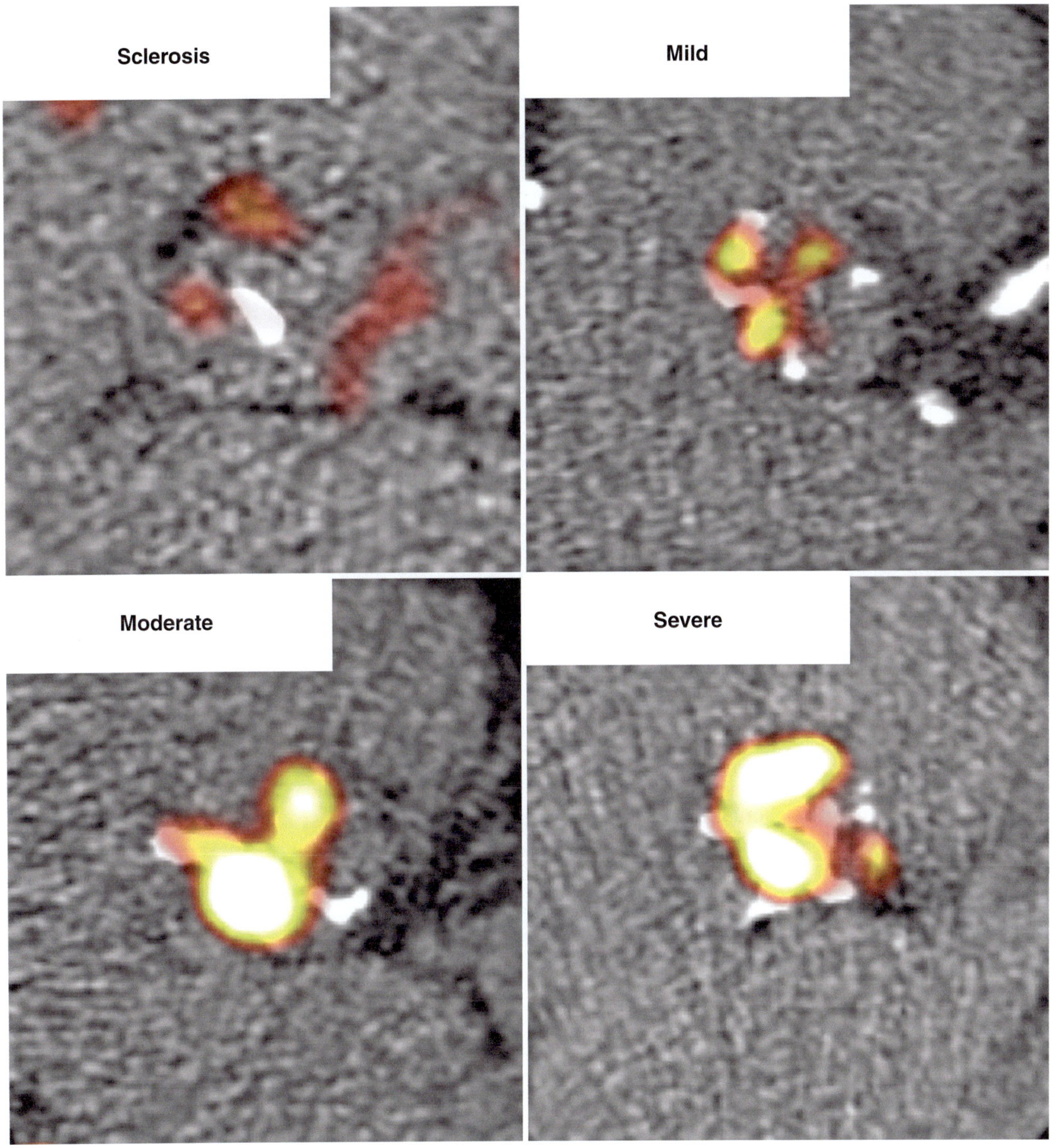

Fig. 15.3 18F-NaF activity in aortic stenosis. Fused PET/CT scans identify increased 18F-NaF activity in the valve. Increased PET uptake can be identified both overlying and remote from existing calcification. The intensity of activity increases with increasing aortic stenosis severity

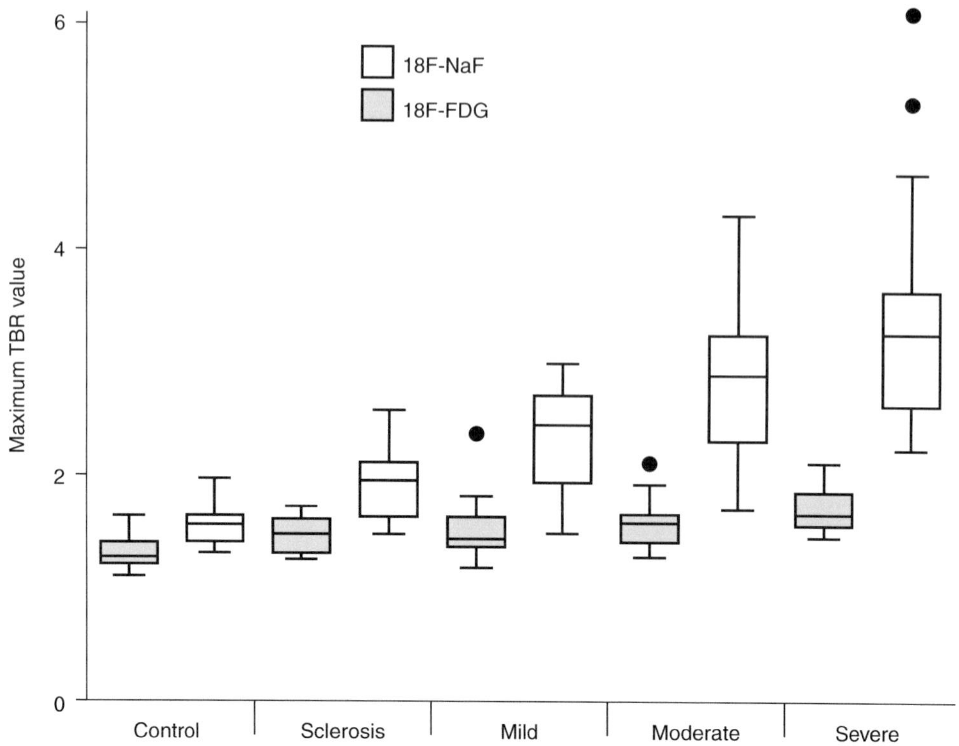

Fig. 15.4 Uptake of 18F-fluorodeoxyglucose (18F-FDG) and 18F-sodium fluoride (18F-NaF) according to the severity of aortic stenosis. Box plots showing the median and interquartile ranges of the tissue-to-background ratios (TBR) for 18F-NaF (*white boxes*) and 18F-FDG (*gray boxes*) with whiskers to 1.5× interquartile range (Reproduced with permission from the American Heart Association [20])

observations. In particular, while 18F-NaF was almost a third higher in the valve than the aorta, the reverse was true for 18F-FDG being increased in regions of atheroma [23]. Thus, calcification would appear to be accelerated in the valve compared to other vascular territories and out of proportion to the degree of inflammation. It would therefore seem to be the predominant pathological process in aortic stenosis and a better target for future therapies than inflammation.

Observational Studies of PET in Aortic Stenosis

Valvular 18F-FDG uptake was in fact first described in a study performed by Marincheva-Savcheva and colleagues [21]. They retrospectively examined aortic valve uptake in oncology patients who had a scan as part of their work up for cancer. In total, 42 patients with aortic stenosis were identified alongside 42 control patients with normal aortic valves. As discussed above, quantification was performed using a similar center-valve technique to ours, which also demonstrated increased 18F-FDG activity in the valves of patients with aortic stenosis compared to controls (TBR 1.53 [IQR: 1.42–1.76] vs. 1.34 [1.20–1.55]; $p<0.001$), with a stepwise increase in activity between patients with mild (1.50 [1.36–1.75]; $n=18$) and moderate aortic stenosis (1.70 [1.52–1.94]; $n=16$). However, in contrast to our results, they observed a reduction in 18-FDG activity among patients with severe aortic stenosis (1.51 [1.38–1.54]; $n=8$). This discrepancy aside, 18F-FDG values in the two studies were very similar and together indicate that 18F-FDG is likely to prove a useful tool in the quantification of inflammation in aortic stenosis.

18F-NaF uptake in aortic stenosis has been described in one other small study. Hyafil and colleagues examined activity in the valves of five patients with aortic stenosis who had a PET/CT scan again for oncology or rheumatic purposes [22]. Activity was higher than in 10 matched patients with normal aortic valves (TBR 2.2 [2.0–2.7] vs. 1.5 [1.5–1.7]; $p=0.008$ for both). This group did not reorient the field of view in to the plane of the valve but instead quantified activity on axial images. Nevertheless, they too achieved excellent measures of inter- and intra-observer reproducibility for the quantification of aortic valve 18F-NaF activity (ICC 0.99 and 0.98 respectively), and their results were therefore largely supportive of our own.

Future Directions

Histological Studies

In bone, 18F-NaF is known to localize to areas of exposed hydroxyapatite; however, while the same crystal is present in aortic stenosis, the exact mechanism of its uptake needs to be confirmed [11]. Ideally, this would be performed with both histological validation and kinetic modeling of 18F-NaF to establish the time course with which this tracer moves in to the valve. Early data have suggested a strong correlation between 18F-NaF activity in the valve and alkaline phosphatase staining on immunohistochemistry (performed on valves removed after aortic valve replacement) [24]; however, this was based upon only a small number ($n = 5$) of valves, and further data are required to establish that 18F-NaF truly provides a measure of calcification activity in aortic stenosis. Validation of the 18F-FDG signal in the valve is also required although this is perhaps less pressing given that uptake is very likely to be similar to that in the aorta and carotids.

Longitudinal Studies

Having established the feasibility and reproducibility of quantifying 18F-NaF and 18F-FDG uptake in the aortic valve, the key question is whether this technique can truly provide a measure of disease activity. In order to answer this issue, longitudinal studies will need to address whether tracer activity predicts the progression of aortic valve calcium scores and indeed valve narrowing. At present, the baseline calcium score provides perhaps the best prediction [25], offering hope that a more advanced approach of measuring current calcification activity may prove to be of clinical use to predict progression.

ECG and Respiratory Gating

The aortic valve moves significantly during systole and the entire structure of heart alters position in response to the changes in intrathoracic pressure that accompany respiration. While attenuation correction CT and PET scans will be affected equally by these processes, motion artifact is likely to limit our ability to localize PET uptake to specific regions of the valve. In this regard, ECG and respiratory gating techniques for both the PET and CT are available that might overcome this problem in future studies [26]. The basis for this approach is to only include diastolic PET data (when the valve is still), which can then be refined by adjusting for respiratory motion. This should allow the more accurate localization of activity to the valve, perhaps to individual cusps, although ultimately the spatial resolution of PET is limited to 3 or 4 mm by the sensitivity of the detectors.

Randomized Control Trial of Anti-calcific Medication in Aortic Stenosis

To date, there are no effective medical treatments for aortic stenosis. These are urgently required as they might avoid the need for invasive cardiac surgery in patients that are often elderly and not ideally suited to a major operation. Treatment strategies to date, such as statin therapy, have focused upon targeting lipid deposition and inflammation without success. The data from these PET studies suggest that calcification may in fact represent a better target for intervention. In principle and if the valve 18F-NaF signal can be appropriately validated, novel anti-calcific therapies could be investigated to assess whether they reduce 18F-NaF uptake. This would provide an early assessment of whether such therapies are capable of reducing calcification activity and indeed of slowing aortic valve narrowing.

Limitations of PET in Assessment of Aortic Stenosis

There are multiple limitations regarding the use of PET for assessment of aortic stenosis. Primarily these relate to its cost (often approximately $2,000 per scan) and it's relative lack of availability; although with the growing role of PET in the assessment of oncology patients, the latter is becoming less of an issue. Furthermore, there are few clinically approved radiotracers that might be used for this purpose, so that only a limited number of pathological processes can be studied at this time. While inflammation and calcification are key process in aortic stenosis, only with further tracer development will the true potential of PET to elucidate the pathophysiological mechanisms of aortic stenosis be reached. Finally, PET/CT scans are associated with radiation. Exposure to the patient is about 5 mSv per PET/CT scan, which is similar to most nuclear medicine examinations and indeed other imaging techniques using ionizing radiation. However, this issue will affect the feasibility of longitudinal PET studies and needs to take in to careful consideration especially in young patients and in those likely to undergo multiple cardiac investigations.

Conclusions

PET/CT holds promise as a research tool for the investigation of inflammation and calcification in aortic stenosis. Initial studies have demonstrated its feasibility and have suggested that calcification predominates as a mechanism underlying the disease process. Further work is required to validate the signal histologically and to investigate whether this may prove a clinically useful technique in predicting disease progression.

References

1. Nkomo VT, Gardin JM, Skelton TN, Gottdiener JS, Scott CG, Enriquez-Sarano M. Burden of valvular heart diseases: a population-based study. Lancet. 2006;368:1005–11.
2. Otto CM. Calcific aortic stenosis – time to look more closely at the valve. N Engl J Med. 2008;359:1395–8.
3. Lin EC, Abass A. PET and PET/CT. A clinical guide. New York/Stuttgart: Thieme; 2005.

4. Rudd JH, Narula J, Strauss HW, Virmani R, Machac J, Klimas M, Tahara N, Fuster V, Warburton EA, Fayad ZA, Tawakol AA. Imaging atherosclerotic plaque inflammation by fluorodeoxyglucose with positron emission tomography: ready for prime time? J Am Coll Cardiol. 2010;55:2527–35.
5. Rudd JH, Warburton EA, Fryer TD, Jones HA, Clark JC, Antoun N, Johnstrom P, Davenport AP, Kirkpatrick PJ, Arch BN, Pickard JD, Weissberg PL. Imaging atherosclerotic plaque inflammation with [18f]-fluorodeoxyglucose positron emission tomography. Circulation. 2002;105:2708–11.
6. Tawakol A, Migrino RQ, Bashian GG, Bedri S, Vermylen D, Cury RC, Yates D, LaMuraglia GM, Furie K, Houser S, Gewirtz H, Muller JE, Brady TJ, Fischman AJ. In vivo 18f-fluorodeoxyglucose positron emission tomography imaging provides a noninvasive measure of carotid plaque inflammation in patients. J Am Coll Cardiol. 2006;48:1818–24.
7. Folco EJSY, Rocha VZ, Christen T, Shvartz E, Sukhova GK, Di Carli MF, Libby P. Hypoxia but not inflammation augments glucose uptake in human macrophages. J Am Coll Cardiol. 2011; 58:603–14.
8. Rudd JH, Myers KS, Bansilal S, Machac J, Rafique A, Farkouh M, Fuster V, Fayad ZA. (18)fluorodeoxyglucose positron emission tomography imaging of atherosclerotic plaque inflammation is highly reproducible: Implications for atherosclerosis therapy trials. J Am Coll Cardiol. 2007;50:892–6.
9. Rudd JH, Myers KS, Bansilal S, Machac J, Pinto CA, Tong C, Rafique A, Hargeaves R, Farkouh M, Fuster V, Fayad ZA. Atherosclerosis inflammation imaging with 18f-fdg pet: carotid, iliac, and femoral uptake reproducibility, quantification methods, and recommendations. J Nucl Med. 2008;49:871–8.
10. Fayad ZA, Mani V, Woodward M, Kallend D, Abt M, Burgess T, Fuster V, Ballantyne CM, Stein EA, Tardif JC, Rudd JH, Farkouh ME, Tawakol A. Safety and efficacy of dalcetrapib on atherosclerotic disease using novel non-invasive multimodality imaging (dal-plaque): a randomised clinical trial. Lancet. 2011;378: 1547–59.
11. Blau M, Ganatra R, Bender MA. 18 f-fluoride for bone imaging. Semin Nucl Med. 1972;2:31–7.
12. Foldager CB, Bendtsen M, Bunger C. Pet scanning for evaluation of bone metabolism. Acta Orthop. 2009;80:737–8; author reply 738–9.
13. Hawkins RA, Choi Y, Huang SC, Hoh CK, Dahlbom M, Schiepers C, Satyamurthy N, Barrio JR, Phelps ME. Evaluation of the skeletal kinetics of fluorine-18-fluoride ion with pet. J Nucl Med. 1992;33:633–42.
14. Toegel S, Hoffmann O, Wadsak W, Ettlinger D, Mien LK, Wiesner K, Nguemo J, Viernstein H, Kletter K, Dudczak R, Mitterhauser M. Uptake of bone-seekers is solely associated with mineralisation! A study with 99mtc-mdp, 153sm-edtmp and 18f-fluoride on osteoblasts. Eur J Nucl Med Mol Imaging. 2006;33:491–4.
15. Installe J, Nzeusseu A, Bol A, Depresseux G, Devogelaer JP, Lonneux M. (18)f-fluoride pet for monitoring therapeutic response in paget's disease of bone. J Nucl Med. 2005;46:1650–8.
16. Grant FD, Fahey FH, Packard AB, Davis RT, Alavi A, Treves ST. Skeletal pet with 18f-fluoride: applying new technology to an old tracer. J Nucl Med. 2008;49:68–78.
17. Derlin T, Richter U, Bannas P, Begemann P, Buchert R, Mester J, Klutmann S. Feasibility of 18f-sodium fluoride pet/ct for imaging of atherosclerotic plaque. J Nucl Med. 2010;51:862–5.
18. Derlin T, Wisotzki C, Richter U, Apostolova I, Bannas P, Weber C, Mester J, Klutmann S. In vivo imaging of mineral deposition in carotid plaque using 18f-sodium fluoride pet/ct: Correlation with atherogenic risk factors. J Nucl Med. 2011;52:362–8.
19. Dweck MR, Chow MW, Joshi NV, Williams MC, Jones C, Fletcher AM, Richardson H, White A, McKillop G, van Beek EJ, Boon NA, Rudd JH, Newby DE. Coronary arterial 18f-sodium fluoride uptake: a novel marker of plaque biology. J Am Coll Cardiol. 2012;59:1539–48.
20. Dweck MR, Jones C, Joshi NV, Fletcher AM, Richardson H, White A, Marsden M, Pessotto R, Clark JC, Wallace WA, Salter DM, McKillop G, van Beek EJ, Boon NA, Rudd JH, Newby DE. Assessment of valvular calcification and inflammation by positron emission tomography in patients with aortic stenosis. Circulation. 2012;125:76–86.
21. Marincheva-Savcheva G, Subramanian S, Qadir S, Figueroa A, Truong Q, Vijayakumar J, Brady TJ, Hoffmann U, Tawakol A. Imaging of the aortic valve using fluorodeoxyglucose positron emission tomography increased valvular fluorodeoxyglucose uptake in aortic stenosis. J Am Coll Cardiol. 2011;57:2507–15.
22. Hyafil F, Messika-Zeitoun D, Burg S, Rouzet F, Benali K, Iung B, Vahanian A, Le Guludec D. Detection of 18fluoride sodium accumulation by positron emission tomography in calcified stenotic aortic valves. Am J Cardiol. 2012;109:1194–6.
23. Dweck MR, Khaw HJ, Sng GK, Luo EL, Baird A, Williams MC, Makiello P, Mirsadraee S, Joshi NV, van Beek EJ, Boon NA, Rudd JH, Newby DE. Aortic stenosis, atherosclerosis, and skeletal bone: Is there a common link with calcification and inflammation? Eur Heart J. 2013;34(21):1567–74.
24. Dweck MR, Richardson H, Malley TS, Cowie W, Fletcher AM, Rudd JH, Boon NA, Newby DE. Valvular 18f-naf activity in aortic stenosis. Eur Soc Cardiol Abstr. 2012.
25. Rosenhek R, Klaar U, Schemper M, Scholten C, Heger M, Gabriel H, Binder T, Maurer G, Baumgartner H. Mild and moderate aortic stenosis. Natural history and risk stratification by echocardiography. Eur Heart J. 2004;25:199–205.
26. Nakazato R, Dey D, Alexanderson E, Meave A, Jimenez M, Romero E, Jacome R, Pena M, Berman DS, Slomka PJ. Automatic alignment of myocardial perfusion pet and 64-slice coronary ct angiography on hybrid pet/ct. J Nucl Cardiol. 2012;19:482–91.

Coronary Artery Disease and Aortic Stenosis

16

Jean-Michel Paradis and Susheel K. Kodali

Abstract

Aortic stenosis (AS) is a common valve disease affecting mainly the elderly population. Risk factors for AS have been shown to be similar to those for atherosclerosis and coronary artery disease (CAD). Over the last decades, the standard treatment option for patients with AS and CAD has been surgical aortic valve replacement and coronary artery bypass grafting. However, the arrival of transcatheter aortic valve replacement has created a paradigm shift in the management of patients with AS. In the setting of this less invasive approach, the management of coexistent significant CAD remains unclear. This book chapter summarizes the actual knowledge on the topic of AS and concomitant CAD, but also identifies some unanswered questions.

Keywords

Coronary artery disease • Aortic stenosis • Aortic valve calcification • Percutaneous coronary intervention • Transcatheter aortic valve replacement • Surgical aortic valve replacement

Aortic Stenosis and Atherosclerosis

Aortic valve disease is the most common valve disease in the aging population and often occurs with CAD [1, 2]. There are compelling epidemiological and histopathological data suggesting that degenerative calcific aortic stenosis (AS) is an active and multifaceted disease that involves atherosclerotic-like and elastocalcinosis-like processes [3]. Risk factors for AS have been found to be similar to those for atherosclerosis and CAD [4]. Therefore, significant CAD is often found in patients with severe AS, and its incidence increases with age. CAD has been reported in >50 % of patients with AS who are ≥70 years of age and in >65 % of patients who are ≥80 years of age [5].

J.-M. Paradis, MD (✉) • S.K. Kodali, MD
Department of Interventional Cardiology, Columbia University Medical Center, 177 Fort Washington Avenue, 5th Floor, Room 501, New York, NY 10032, USA
e-mail: jp3153@columbia.edu; sk2427@columbia.edu

Aortic Valve Calcification and Prevalence of CAD

The prevalence of CAD in patients undergoing surgical aortic valve replacement (SAVR) increases not only with age but also with the presence of valve calcification [6]. The presence of aortic valve calcification probably indicates a systemic vascular atherosclerotic process. Roberts [7], in a necropsy study of persons aged >65 years, showed that 100 % of those with aortic valve calcification or MAC had calcific deposits in one or more coronary arteries. These findings are supported by pathological studies [8] showing that collections of foam cells, which represent early atherosclerotic lesions, may be observed on the endothelium of the epicardial coronary arteries, on the ventricular surface of the mitral valve, and on each of the aortic cusps as early as adolescence.

A study by Adler et al. demonstrated an association between aortic valve calcification and significant coronary artery disease. Thus, aortic valve calcification can serve as a window to atherosclerosis of the coronary arteries [6].

J.K. Min et al. (eds.), *Multimodality Imaging for Transcatheter Aortic Valve Replacement*, DOI 10.1007/978-1-4471-2798-7_16, © Springer-Verlag London 2014

This association is supported in a study by Otto et al. [9] showing an ~50 % increase in the risk of death from cardiovascular causes as well as myocardial infarction in patients with aortic sclerosis. This finding held true even in the absence of hemodynamically significant obstruction of the left ventricular outflow.

Coronary Flow in Aortic Stenosis

The coronary flow reserve (CFR) is defined as the maximal increase in myocardial blood flow above its resting level for a given perfusion pressure when coronary vasculature is maximally dilated. This is an integrated measure of flow through both the large epicardial coronary arteries and the microcirculation. Narrowing of the epicardial coronaries or microvascular dysfunction can cause an abnormal CFR.

Despite normal coronary arteries, patients with AS have a decreased CFR, which limits the capacity of the coronary circulation to increase flow to match myocardial oxygen demand. This impairment of CFR is certainly one of the key elements responsible for myocardial ischemia in AS patients, and this may contribute to the development of symptoms, LV dysfunction, and adverse outcomes [10]. The mechanisms underlying the reduction of CFR in AS patients remain uncertain. Initially, concentric LV hypertrophy was believed to play a central role. However, recent data have shown that the abnormally high LV workload induced by the aortic stenosis itself may really be one of the key factors explaining the impaired CFR and myocardial ischemia in these patients. In fact, reduced CFR correlates better with the hemodynamic indexes of AS severity (valve effective orifice area and transvalvular pressure gradient) than with LV mass [11].

Symptoms and CAD in Patients with AS

The presence of symptoms is typically not helpful in identifying patients with CAD in the setting of AS. The incidence of CAD is similar in patients with (43 %) and without (29 %) angina pectoris. The sensitivity of angina pectoris in identifying coronary disease was 68 %, and the specificity is 46 %. The positive predictive value was 43 % and the negative predictive value was 71 %. Several previously published studies have consistently reported that about half the patients with aortic stenosis and angina pectoris have CAD. In the other half (those with AS and angina but without CAD), a myocardial oxygen supply to demand imbalance is believed to be caused, as previously explained, by diminished coronary flow reserve. Based on these data, it is impossible to predict the presence or absence of CAD in patients with AS based on symptoms. As a result, it is recommended that all patients with AS undergo coronary angiography in preparation for valve replacement [12].

Impact of CAD on the Outcomes of Surgical Aortic Valve Replacement

The presence of CAD has been demonstrated to increase procedural risk with conventional aortic valve replacement [13, 14], and revascularization is generally recommended at the time of surgery. The ESC guidelines on valvular heart disease recommend performing complete revascularization in patients with severe AS undergoing SAVR [15]. However, interventions combining AVR and coronary artery bypass grafting are associated with an increase in postoperative mortality, compared to AVR alone [16]. Data from >10,000 patients undergoing heart surgery from the New York Cardiac Surgery Reporting System showed that mortality for isolated valve surgery was 4.4 % compared with 8.9 % for valve surgery and concomitant CABG [17]. As combined valve and coronary surgery may be associated with excessively high mortality rates and because additional medical conditions such as congestive heart failure, pulmonary disease, and renal insufficiency may further raise the risk of surgical intervention, as many as a third of all potential surgical AVR candidates are denied surgery according to the recent Euro Heart Survey [18].

Outcomes of PCI in Patients with Severe AS

Surgical AVR with CABG has been considered the main and sometimes the only treatment option, and percutaneous coronary intervention (PCI) has been performed infrequently in patients with severe AS and CAD. Therefore, the outcomes of PCI in patients with severe AS and severe CAD are largely unknown.

A group of authors has recently analyzed the short-term outcomes of 254 patients with severe AS who underwent PCI at Cleveland Clinic over a 10-year period [19]. Between 1998 and 2008, PCI was performed in patients with severe AS for one or more of the following reasons: (1) clinical presentation of ACS (UA, NSTEMI, STEMI); (2) stable angina, the symptoms of which were thought to be attributable to significant CAD rather than AS; and (3) palliation of symptoms in patients deemed inoperable for surgical AVR. The outcomes of these patients were compared to those of 508 similar risk patients derived by propensity matching. The two groups were well matched (mean age 75 years old, 62 % male, EF 45 %, stable angina 26 %, UA 39 %, NSTEMI 18 %, STEMI 5 %). The 30-day mortality was 4.3 % in patients with AS and 4.7 % in the control group (HR 0.51–1.69, $p=0.2$). In subgroup analysis of the severe AS group, patients with low EF (≤30 %) had a higher 30-day post-PCI mortality of 15.4 % compared with 1.2 % among patients with AS and an EF >30 %. Also, patients with AS and a high STS score (≥10) had a higher 30-day post-PCI mortality of 10.4 % compared with no mortality in those with AS and STS score <10. Other short-term complications of PCI such as contrast nephropathy, death, hemodynamic compromise during PCI, periprocedural MI, coronary dissection, coronary perforation, cardiac tamponade, access site hematoma, and retroperitoneal bleed were not significantly different in the two groups. At a mean follow-up of 3.7 years, 73 of 254 patients (29 %) with severe AS had undergone SAVR, with a mean duration of 15.5 months between PCI and SAVR. CABG was carried out with SAVR in 52 patients (71 %). Long-term mortality was 42.5 % in AS patients who could undergo SAVR, 68 % in AS individuals who could not undergo SAVR, and 46.7 % in the non-AS control group.

Despite the fact that this is the largest study to date comparing patients with and without severe AS undergoing PCI, a few limitations are worth mentioning. Most importantly, it was an observational, single-center study which was consequently prone to bias. As well, approximately 22 % of patients in each group underwent PCI with DES, making this largely a BMS study.

Transcatheter Aortic Valve Replacement

In the last few years, transcatheter aortic valve replacement (TAVR) has emerged as an attractive therapeutic option in patients with severe symptomatic AS and high risk for, or contraindications to, conventional AVR. Therefore, treatment paradigms will certainly change in the setting of TAVR. Coronary angiography is still strongly recommended in the assessment of eligibility to TAVR. Nevertheless, the management of CAD in the context of TAVR is not yet established [20].

Impact of CAD on the Outcomes of Transcatheter Aortic Valve Replacement

Currently published US randomized trials of TAVR systematically excluded patients with the "need for revascularization" (though antecedent PCI was occasionally performed to qualify for eligibility) and did not demonstrate any interaction between prior CAD and mortality. However, several registries have reported on the impact of CAD on outcomes after TAVR [14, 21–23].

In a study by Dewey et al. [14], the impact of previous CABG or PCI on procedural outcomes and overall survival in 201 high-risk patients undergoing TAVR (161 attempted TF and 40 attempted TA) was analyzed. In this article, patients with CAD had significantly greater rates of hyperlipidemia, chronic kidney disease, hypertension, chronic obstructive lung disease (COPD), peripheral vascular disease (PVD), previous myocardial infarction (MI), and symptoms of angina. The pooled patients with CAD also had significantly higher EuroSCORE (35.8 vs. 26.1), decreased ejection fraction (EF) (48 % vs. 54 %), larger body surface area (BSA), larger left ventricular end-diastolic volumes, and more significant mitral regurgitation. There were also a significantly greater number of patients having TA-TAVR in the pooled CAD cohort. Overall mortality after TAVR was significantly higher among the CAD group (35.7 %) in contrast with the non-CAD group (18.4 %). Logistic regression analysis found that patients who had CAD were 10.1 times more likely to die (95 % CI 2.1–174.8) within 30 days of the TAVR procedure than those who did not. There was no indication in the analysis that either CABG or PCI, individually, demonstrated more significance than the other in regard to procedural mortality. However, several limitations of this study are noteworthy. This study represents the earliest experience with TAVR in both the USA and Europe. Also, CAD was defined simply as prior revascularization (CABG or PCI), and there was no information about the degree of ischemic burden in each patient. Finally, completeness of revascularization was not reported.

In contrast to these results, a study published in 2010 [21] of 136 TAVR patients showed a similar survival rate, with no statistically significant difference between five groups stratified according to the extend of CAD assessed with the Duke myocardial jeopardy score (DMJS). Therefore, the authors concluded that in their initial Canadian cohort of patients who underwent TAVR between 2005 and 2007, the presence of CAD or nonrevascularized myocardium was not associated with an increased risk of adverse events. However, even though the 30-day mortality was not significantly different between patients with and without CAD (11.5 vs. 6.3 %), the sample size of this study was small and 15 patients had undergone PCI before TAVR, which might have impacted the results.

More recently, the Italian registry studying 663 consecutive patients who underwent TAVR with the 18 Fr CoreValve ReValving system (Medtronic) demonstrated that at a mean follow-up of 19 months, patients with concomitant CAD, as defined by previous PCI or CABG, were no more likely to develop major adverse cerebrovascular and cardiac events (MACCE) (adjusted HR 0.76; 95 % confidence interval 0.42–1.36; $p=0.353$) or all-cause mortality (adjusted HR 0.74; 95 % CI 0.40–1.36; $p=0.331$) than those without CAD [24]. Nevertheless, a higher incidence of myocardial infarction (4.8 %) was found in the group not undergoing revascularization compared with the groups where revascularization was achieved completely (0.0 %) or incompletely (1.8 %). Major limitations of this nonrandomized study were the lack of specific tools such as fractional flow reserve, intravascular ultrasound, quantitative coronary analysis or myocardial jeopardy score to assess significance of coronary stenosis, the differences in TAVR experience among the participating centers, and the use of nonstandardized outcomes definitions.

Currently, there is no clear evidence as to the importance of complete revascularization in patients prior to TAVR. Consequently, the proper approach to CAD in patients referred for TAVR should be individualized in each patient based on their clinical condition and coronary anatomy. Two important questions must be answered for each patient: (1) Will coronary anatomy impact safety of TAVR procedure and (2) will long-term survival and symptoms be impacted by CAD? For example, a patient with normal LV function and focal RCA disease is unlikely to have significant ischemic complications with TAVR and should not be revascularized in the absence of angina. A patient with multivessel disease and depressed LV function, however, may benefit from revascularization prior to valvular intervention. These answers to these clinical questions are, however, not always straightforward. In the latter patient, if LV function was normal, it would be reasonable to defer revascularization prior to TAVR.

Timing of PCI

Before TAVR

PCI in patients with significant CAD before TAVR can potentially reduce the procedural risk of TAVR and may reduce the need for revascularization after TAVR [19]. In 2012, Gasparetto et al. [25] assessed the safety and effectiveness of a selective percutaneous revascularization strategy before TAVR in a single-center prospective registry (PUREVALVE registry) including 191 consecutive patients with severe AS referred for TAVR. The presence of CAD was defined as previous percutaneous or surgical coronary revascularization and/or presence of any coronary stenosis of at least 50 %. PCI was scheduled for lesions involving proximal-to-midcoronary segments of major coronary branches. CTO and lesions in small vessels (reference diameters <2.5 mm) were not considered for revascularization. The decision to perform PCI pre-TAVR was driven first of all by symptoms, additionally by evaluation of extent of myocardium at risk and/or proven ischemia by means of invasive or noninvasive tests, and finally by technical feasibility of PCI. Thus, only the lesions associated with clinical relevance were scheduled for PCI. Use of DES or BMS was left to operator's judgement. Out of 191 patients who underwent TAVR, CAD occurred in 113 patients (59.2 %) and PCI was performed before TAVR in 20.4 % (39/113) of them. A total of 78 stents were implanted in 66 lesions. BMS were used in 56.4 % of cases. In this observational analysis with a limited number of patients, estimated survival rates at 1 month (97.4 % vs. 94.5 %) and 12 months (88.2 % vs. 81.9 %) were similar in the no CAD group compared to the CAD group. Myocardial infarction (4.4 % vs. 0 %, $p=0.08$) and major stroke (2.7 % vs. 0 %) seemed to be numerically more frequent in the CAD population, but the differences were not statistically significant. A selective clinical-based, coronary revascularization before TAVR appeared to be safe and was associated with an outcome similar to those observed in no CAD-TAVR patients.

Concomitant to TAVR

In the BERN TAVI registry [23], 256 patients undergoing TAVR were prospectively included. CAD was defined as a stenosis of >50 % in at least one coronary artery as assessed during coronary angiography or previous PCI/CABG. In patients with CAD, myocardium at risk was assessed using the DUKE myocardial jeopardy score. Of the 165 patients with CAD, 59 underwent TAVR and staged ($n=23$) or concomitant ($n=36$) PCI. Of the remaining 108 patients with CAD but no revascularization procedure, 53 patients had been completely revascularized prior to TAVR, and 55 patients had an incomplete revascularization status (DUKE myocardial jeopardy score ≥1). In this trial, chronic total occlusion (CTO) and distal segments or side branches with a small area at risk were left untreated. Clinical outcome at 30 days was similar for patients undergoing isolated TAVI as compared with TAVI combined with PCI in terms of death (5.6 vs. 10.2 %, $p=0.24$), major stroke (4.1 % vs. 3.4 %, $p=1.00$), and VARC combined safety end point (31.0 % vs. 23.7 %, $p=0.33$). Moreover, after a direct comparison between patients undergoing TAVR with concomitant PCI and those undergoing isolated TAVR, similar results were obtained with respect to these three end points. Despite the observational nature of this study, the limited number of patients, and the possibility of a selection bias (treatment strategy was left to the discretion of the operator), it seems that revascularization by means of PCI can be safely performed in addition to TAVR either as staged or a concomitant intervention.

After TAVR

The strategy of PCI after TAVR is not without risks. Valve struts may indeed interfere with cannulation of coronaries, and catheter manipulation may potentially dislodge the valve [19]. The impact of PCI done immediately after TAVR was analyzed in the study by Pasic et al. [26]. Between April 2008 and July 2011, a total of 419 subjects underwent transapical TAVR. PCI was performed in 46 (11 %) of them. Only the most significant lesions amenable to straightforward PCI were treated. Coronary artery stenosis was deemed significant only if the diseased artery supplied a large myocardial territory and the stenosis put a large myocardial area at risk. Technical procedural success was achieved in 100 % of patients, without any need for conversion to open-heart surgery. In the TA-TAVR and PCI group, survival at 12, 24 and 36 months was 87.1, 69.7, and 69.7 %, respectively. These results demonstrated that this single-stage approach seems feasible and safe.

Remaining Questions

In the era of TAVR, a number of questions about CAD and AS remain unanswered. Will the extent of CAD impact the patient's symptoms as well as long-term survival? Can TAVR be performed safely in the setting of a certain threshold of CAD? Moreover, the optimal timing to proceed with the PCI remains unclear. Also, are patients with AS and a high SYNTAX score better suited for CABG/AVR than TAVR/PCI provided that they are reasonable surgical candidates? Will the use of antiplatelet agents impact bleeding complications after TAVR, especially via the trans-apical approach? Will this concern of bleeding impact the decision of BMS vs. DES during PCI? Should we perform balloon aortic valvuloplasty before each PCI to mitigate the risk of PCI in the setting of AS, especially in patients with depressed LV function [27]? What is the ideal interval between PCI and TAVR? If TAVR precedes PCI, does PCI become even more difficult to perform (there are concerns that the prosthesis might impact the ability to engage the coronaries adequately with a guiding catheter)? Finally, as TAVR is performed in lower risk patients with better long-term prognosis independent of the AS, will the threshold for treating CAD become lower because the potential impact of the CAD on long-term mortality and quality of life will become greater?

Upcoming Studies

Currently published US randomized trials systematically excluded patients with the need of revascularization and did not demonstrate any interaction between CAD and mortality [28]. Two ongoing trials will help answer some of these questions. PARTNER 2A and SURTAVI will include patients with CAD in need of revascularization and compare outcomes following AVR with or without CABG versus TAVR with and without PCI.

PARTNER 2A Trial

The Placement of AoRTic TraNscathetER Valve Trial (PARTNER) 2A is a prospective multicenter randomized trial comparing safety and effectiveness of the Edwards SAPIEN XT THV with the NovaFlex delivery system in patients deemed to be surgical candidates with certain risk profiles versus surgical SAVR. Enrollment will consist of up to 2,000 patients with STS score ≥4 %. Study patients will undergo clinical follow-up at discharge, 30 days, 6 months, 1 year, and then annually for a minimum of 5 years. Patients with complex coronary disease, either an unprotected left main lesion or a SYNTAX score >32, are excluded from the study. However, if the patient has CAD that needs revascularization, the PARTNER 2A trial will allow the comparison between the following two arms: TAVR+PCI or SAVR+CABG.

SURTAVI Trial

The Medtronic CoreValve® SUrgical Replacement and Transcatheter Aortic Valve Implantation (SURTAVI) trial is designed to evaluate the safety and efficacy of the Medtronic CoreValve system in the treatment of symptomatic severe AS in subjects who are at intermediate risk for aortic valve surgery (STS score ≥3 and ≤8 % in Europe and STS score ≥4 and ≤8 % in the USA). Up to 2,500 patients at up to 75 global sites will be included in the trial. The SURTAVI trial will assess whether the CoreValve system is non-inferior to SAVR based on data on all-cause mortality and major stroke at 24 months. Clinical end points will be reported and adjudicated according to Valve Academic Research Consortium (VARC) standard end point definitions. All patients will be followed through 5 years. The enrollment flowchart of the SURTAVI trial is explained in the below.

Hopefully, from these studies, the best PCI strategy for different clinical scenarios will emerge. Until then, clinical judgement, good knowledge of the available limited data, and a case-by-case approach should guide the management of these complex AS patients with CAD (Box 16.1).

Box 16.1 Coronary Revascularization and TAVR

Before TAVR	Limited evidence to date
	30 days and 12 months mortality similar in revascularized versus non-revascularized patients
	Myocardial infarction and major stroke higher in individuals undergoing revascularization and/or presence of any stenosis >50 %, but not statistically different
At the time of TAVR	Limited evidence to date
	30 days mortality similar to those undergoing percutaneous revascularization versus no revascularization
After TAVR	May be technically difficult due to value struts that may interfere with percutaneous intervention
	Limited evidence to date
	Observational data for percutaneous revascularization reveals no increased need for coronary artery bypass surgery with generally high survival

TAVR transcatheter aortic valve replacement

References

1. Vandeplas A, Willems JL, Piessens J, De Geest H. Frequency of angina pectoris and coronary artery disease in severe isolated valvular aortic stenosis. Am J Cardiol. 1988;62:117–20.
2. Rapp AH, Hillis LD, Lange RA, Cigarroa JE. Prevalence of coronary artery disease in patients with aortic stenosis with and without angina pectoris. Am J Cardiol. 2001;87:1216–7, A1217.
3. Pibarot P, Dumesnil JG. Improving assessment of aortic stenosis. J Am Coll Cardiol. 2012;60:169–80.
4. Stewart BF, Siscovick D, Lind BK, Gardin JM, Gottdiener JS, Smith VE, Kitzman DW, Otto CM. Clinical factors associated with calcific aortic valve disease. Cardiovascular Health Study. J Am Coll Cardiol. 1997;29:630–4.
5. Iung B. Interface between valve disease and ischaemic heart disease. Heart. 2000;84:347–52.
6. Adler Y, Vaturi M, Herz I, Iakobishvili Z, Toaf J, Fink N, Battler A, Sagie A. Nonobstructive aortic valve calcification: a window to significant coronary artery disease. Atherosclerosis. 2002;161: 193–7.
7. Roberts WC. Morphologic features of the normal and abnormal mitral valve. Am J Cardiol. 1983;51:1005–28.
8. Thubrikar MJ, Deck JD, Aouad J, Chen JM. Intramural stress as a causative factor in atherosclerotic lesions of the aortic valve. Atherosclerosis. 1985;55:299–311.
9. Otto CM, Lind BK, Kitzman DW, Gersh BJ, Siscovick DS. Association of aortic-valve sclerosis with cardiovascular mortality and morbidity in the elderly. N Engl J Med. 1999;341: 142–7.
10. Garcia D, Camici PG, Durand LG, Rajappan K, Gaillard E, Rimoldi OE, Pibarot P. Impairment of coronary flow reserve in aortic stenosis. J Appl Physiol. 2009;106:113–21.
11. Rajappan K, Rimoldi OE, Dutka DP, Ariff B, Pennell DJ, Sheridan DJ, Camici PG. Mechanisms of coronary microcirculatory dysfunction in patients with aortic stenosis and angiographically normal coronary arteries. Circulation. 2002;105:470–6.
12. Smith Jr SC, Jacobs AK, Adams CD, Anderson JL, Antman EM, Fuster V, Halperin JL, Hiratzka LF, Hunt SA, Nishimura R, Page RL, Riegel B. ACC/AHA 2006 guidelines for the management of patients with valvular heart disease: a report of the American College of Cardiology/American Heart Association Task Force on Practice Guidelines (writing Committee to Revise the 1998 guidelines for the management of patients with valvular heart disease): developed in collaboration with the Society of Cardiovascular Anesthesiologists: Endorsed by the Society for Cardiovascular Angiography and Interventions and the Society of Thoracic Surgeons. Circulation. 2006;114:e84–231.
13. Aranki SF, Rizzo RJ, Couper GS, Adams DH, Collins Jr JJ, Gildea JS, Kinchla NM, Cohn LH. Aortic valve replacement in the elderly. Effect of gender and coronary artery disease on operative mortality. Circulation. 1993;88:II17–23.
14. Dewey TM, Brown DL, Herbert MA, Culica D, Smith CR, Leon MB, Svensson LG, Tuzcu M, Webb JG, Cribier A, Mack MJ. Effect of concomitant coronary artery disease on procedural and late outcomes of transcatheter aortic valve implantation. Ann Thorac Surg. 2010;89:758–67; discussion 767.
15. Vahanian A, Baumgartner H, Bax J, Butchart E, Dion R, Filippatos G, Flachskampf F, Hall R, Iung B, Kasprzak J, Nataf P, Tornos P, Torracca L, Wenink A. Guidelines on the management of valvular heart disease: the task force on the management of valvular heart disease of the European Society of Cardiology. Eur Heart J. 2007;28:230–68.
16. Tjang YS, van Hees Y, Korfer R, Grobbee DE, van der Heijden GJ. Predictors of mortality after aortic valve replacement. Eur J Cardiothorac Surg. 2007;32:469–74.
17. Hannan EL, Wu C, Bennett EV, Carlson RE, Culliford AT, Gold JP, Higgins RS, Smith CR, Jones RH. Risk index for predicting in-hospital mortality for cardiac valve surgery. Ann Thorac Surg. 2007;83:921–9.
18. Iung B, Baron G, Butchart EG, Delahaye F, Gohlke-Barwolf C, Levang OW, Tornos P, Vanoverschelde JL, Vermeer F, Boersma E, Ravaud P, Vahanian A. A prospective survey of patients with valvular heart disease in Europe: the euro heart survey on valvular heart disease. Eur Heart J. 2003;24:1231–43.
19. Goel SS, Agarwal S, Tuzcu EM, Ellis SG, Svensson LG, Zaman T, Bajaj N, Joseph L, Patel NS, Aksoy O, Stewart WJ, Griffin BP, Kapadia SR. Percutaneous coronary intervention in patients with severe aortic stenosis: implications for transcatheter aortic valve replacement. Circulation. 2012;125:1005–13.
20. Vahanian A, Alfieri O, Al-Attar N, Antunes M, Bax J, Cormier B, Cribier A, De Jaegere P, Fournial G, Kappetein AP, Kovac J, Ludgate S, Maisano F, Moat N, Mohr F, Nataf P, Pierard L, Pomar JL, Schofer J, Tornos P, Tuzcu M, van Hout B, Von Segesser LK, Walther T. Transcatheter valve implantation for patients with aortic stenosis: a position statement from the European Association of Cardio-Thoracic Surgery (EACTS) and the European Society of Cardiology (ESC), in collaboration with the European Association of Percutaneous Cardiovascular Interventions (EAPCI). Eur Heart J. 2008;29:1463–70.
21. Masson JB, Lee M, Boone RH, Al Ali A, Al Bugami S, Hamburger J, John Mancini GB, Ye J, Cheung A, Humphries KH, Wood D, Nietlispach F, Webb JG. Impact of coronary artery disease on outcomes after transcatheter aortic valve implantation. Catheter Cardiovasc Interv. 2010;76:165–73.
22. Gautier M, Pepin M, Himbert D, Ducrocq G, Iung B, Dilly MP, Attias D, Nataf P, Vahanian A. Impact of coronary artery disease on indications for transcatheter aortic valve implantation and on procedural outcomes. EuroIntervention. 2011;7:549–55.
23. Wenaweser P, Pilgrim T, Guerios E, Stortecky S, Huber C, Khattab AA, Kadner A, Buellesfeld L, Gloekler S, Meier B, Carrel T, Windecker S. Impact of coronary artery disease and percutaneous coronary intervention on outcomes in patients with severe aortic stenosis undergoing transcatheter aortic valve implantation. EuroIntervention. 2011;7:541–8.
24. Ussia GP, Barbanti M, Colombo A, Tarantini G, Petronio AS, Ettori F, Ramondo A, Santoro G, Klugmann S, Bedogni F, Antoniucci D, Maisano F, Marzocchi A, Poli A, De Carlo M, Fiorina C, De Marco F, Napodano M, Violini R, Bortone AS, Tamburino C. Impact of coronary artery disease in elderly patients undergoing transcatheter aortic valve implantation: insight from the italian corevalve registry. Int J Cardiol. 2012. March 27, Epub ahead of print
25. Gasparetto V, Fraccaro C, Tarantini G, Buja P, D'Onofrio A, Yzeiraj E, Pittarello D, Isabella G, Gerosa G, Iliceto S, Napodano M. Safety and effectiveness of a selective strategy for coronary artery revascularization before transcatheter aortic valve implantation. Catheter Cardiovasc Interv. 2013;81(2):376–83.
26. Pasic M, Dreysse S, Unbehaun A, Buz S, Drews T, Klein C, D'Ancona G, Hetzer R. Combined elective percutaneous coronary intervention and transapical transcatheter aortic valve implantation. Interact Cardiovasc Thorac Surg. 2012;14:463–8.
27. McKay RG, Safian RD, Berman AD, Diver DJ, Weinstein JS, Wyman RM, Cunningham MJ, McKay LL, Baim DS, Grossman W. Combined percutaneous aortic valvuloplasty and transluminal coronary angioplasty in adult patients with calcific aortic stenosis and coronary artery disease. Circulation. 1987;76:1298–306.
28. Leon MB, Smith CR, Mack M, Miller DC, Moses JW, Svensson LG, Tuzcu EM, Webb JG, Fontana GP, Makkar RR, Brown DL, Block PC, Guyton RA, Pichard AD, Bavaria JE, Herrmann HC, Douglas PS, Petersen JL, Akin JJ, Anderson WN, Wang D, Pocock S. Transcatheter aortic-valve implantation for aortic stenosis in patients who cannot undergo surgery. N Engl J Med. 2010;363: 1597–607.

17

Common Cardiac Pathologies Associated with Aortic Stenosis

Yasmin Siddiqui, Sean Moore, Subha Ghosh, and Subha V. Raman

Abstract

Given the inoperability of many patients undergoing transcatheter aortic valve replacement (TAVR), numerous other cardiac pathologies are often present. These can be represented a myriad of conditions that may alter the planned approach to TAVR. The evaluation of these conditions include traditional techniques such as echocardiography but often require advanced imaging methods including multidetector computed tomography and magnetic resonance imaging. This chapter delineates the diagnostic approach to three commonly encountered pathologies in patients with critical aortic stenosis, including mitral regurgitation, prior myocardial infarction, asymmetric septal hypertrophy. Further we describe the current practice and highlight the needs for specific research pertaining to this concomitant cardiac pathologies in patients undergoing TAVR.

Keywords

Aortic stenosis • Left ventricular hypertrophy • Mitral regurgitation • Myocardial infarction • Transcatheter valve replacement

Y. Siddiqui, BA, DO, MPH, MD (✉)
Department of Internal Medicine,
Wexner Medical Center at the Ohio State University,
395 West 12th Ave, Columbus, OH 43210, USA
e-mail: yamin.siddiqui@gmail.com

S. Moore, BS
Department of Internal Medicine,
Wexner Medical Center at the Ohio State University,
473 W. 12th Ave, Suite 200, Columbus, OH 43210, USA
e-mail: moore.1802@osu.edu

S. Ghosh, MD
Department of Radiology, Wexner Medical Center,
Ohio State University, 395 W 12TH AVENUE,
Columbus, OH 43210, USA
e-mail: subha.ghosh@osumc.edu

S.V. Raman, MD, MSEE
Department of Cardiovascular Medicine,
Ohio State University, 473 W. 12th Ave, Suite 200,
Columbus, OH 43210, USA
e-mail: raman.1@osu.edu

Introduction

Patients undergoing transcatheter aortic valve replacement (TAVR) for aortic valve stenosis are older and are often affected by comorbid conditions that impart higher procedural risk (Box 17.1). These disorders include, but are not limited to, congestive heart failure, coronary artery disease, chronic kidney disease, and pulmonary disease [1, 2]. Coexistence of other forms of left heart disease may also influence decision-making and outcomes associated with TAVR. This chapter will review common comorbid conditions in patients undergoing TAVR, focusing on mitral regurgitation, coronary artery disease, and asymmetric septal hypertrophy. Available evidence evaluating their impact on patient selection and procedural aspects of TAVR are summarized.

J.K. Min et al. (eds.), *Multimodality Imaging for Transcatheter Aortic Valve Replacement*,
DOI 10.1007/978-1-4471-2798-7_17, © Springer-Verlag London 2014

Box 17.1 Common Pathologies Associated with AS

Mitral regurgitation	Occurs in 60–90 % of patients with aortic stenosis
	Generally reduced after aortic valve replacement
	Early data indicate no increased mortality in patients with versus without mitral regurgitation after TAVR
	TAVR may potentially worsen mitral regurgitation by restriction of anterior leaflet mobility
Coronary artery disease s/p myocardial infarction	No excess risk factor association with prevalence of aortic stenosis when comparing AS patients with controls
	Discordant data as to prognosis in patients with versus without coronary artery disease following TAVR
Asymmetric septal hypertrophy	Severe asymmetric hypertrophy may onsider septal myomectomy
	Cotraindication to TAVR

TAVR transcatheter aortic valve replacement

Mitral Regurgitation

Mitral regurgitation (MR) can result from structural abnormalities of the mitral valve apparatus—including leaflets, annulus, chordae, and papillary muscles—or it may ensue from mechanisms such as dyssynchronous contraction. Ischemic heart disease may cause MR via annular dilatation, papillary muscle infarction or ischemia, or systolic tenting of the valve leaflet due to adverse LV remodeling following infarction (Figs. 17.1, 17.2, and 17.3). Often, multiple mechanisms coexist, just as nonischemic cardiomyopathy may be superimposed on ischemic heart disease and explain LV enlargement or dysfunction out of proportion to the extent of coronary artery disease.

Some degree of mitral regurgitation coexists in 60–90 % of patients with AS [3–5]. When overlaid on a condition that fundamentally limits cardiac output, MR further detracts from forward stroke volume necessary for perfusion, exacerbates left atrial and pulmonary venous hypertension, and increases the likelihood of atrial fibrillation. Increased LV pressures in AS, in turn, may exacerbate MR. "Functional" MR is defined as MR in the absence of structural abnormalities of the mitral apparatus and contributes to excess mortality post-AVR. Jeong et al. observed a hazard for late cardiac death of more than fivefold in patients with mild to moderate functional MR in patients undergoing AVR when compared to patient with no to trivial MR ($p=0.016$) [4]. In a retrospective study of elderly patients who had undergone surgical AVR, moderate MR was also shown to be an independent predictor of late mortality [6].

The underlying processes associated with the progression of calcific aortic stenosis commonly affects the mitral valve as well; prior rheumatic injury may further contribute to structural alterations of the mitral apparatus. In advanced disease, it may be difficult (and unnecessary) to ascertain the

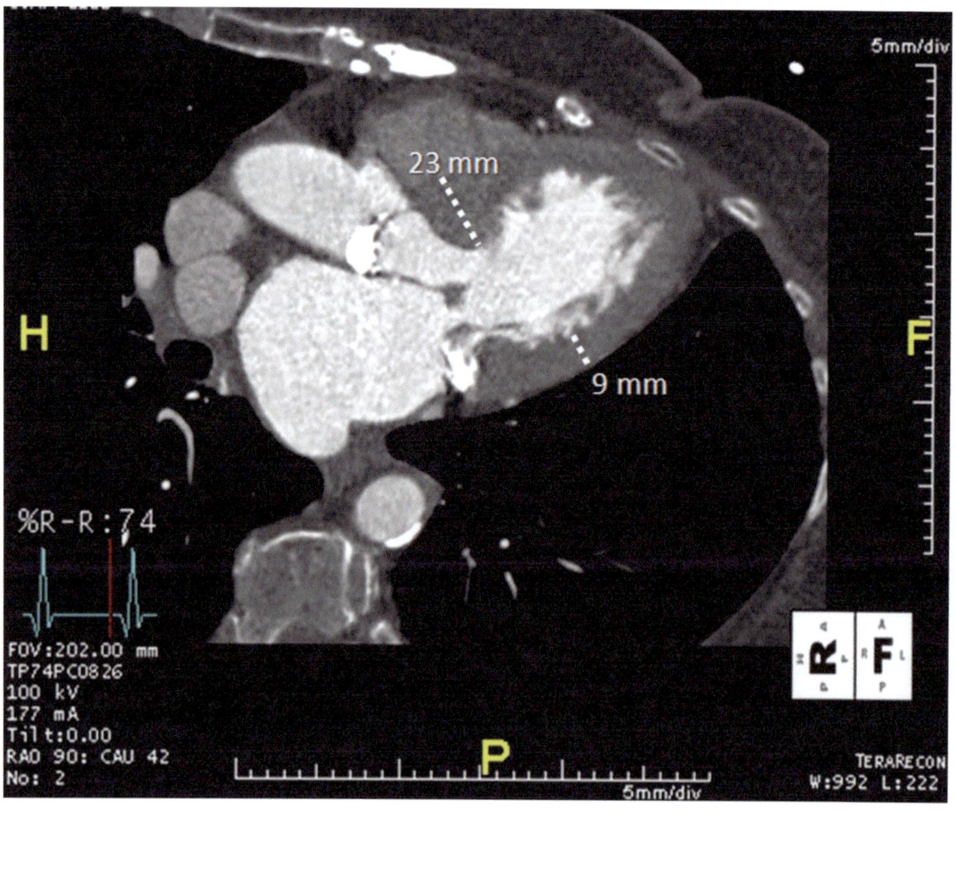

Fig. 17.1 Asymmetric septal hypertrophy is evident in this ECG-gated, multiplanar reformatted CTA that has been reconstructed in the three-chamber or LV outflow tract plane. This end-diastolic reconstruction allows measurement of the anteroseptum (23 mm) and inferolateral (9 mm) LV myocardial segments, with marked asymmetric thickening of the septum

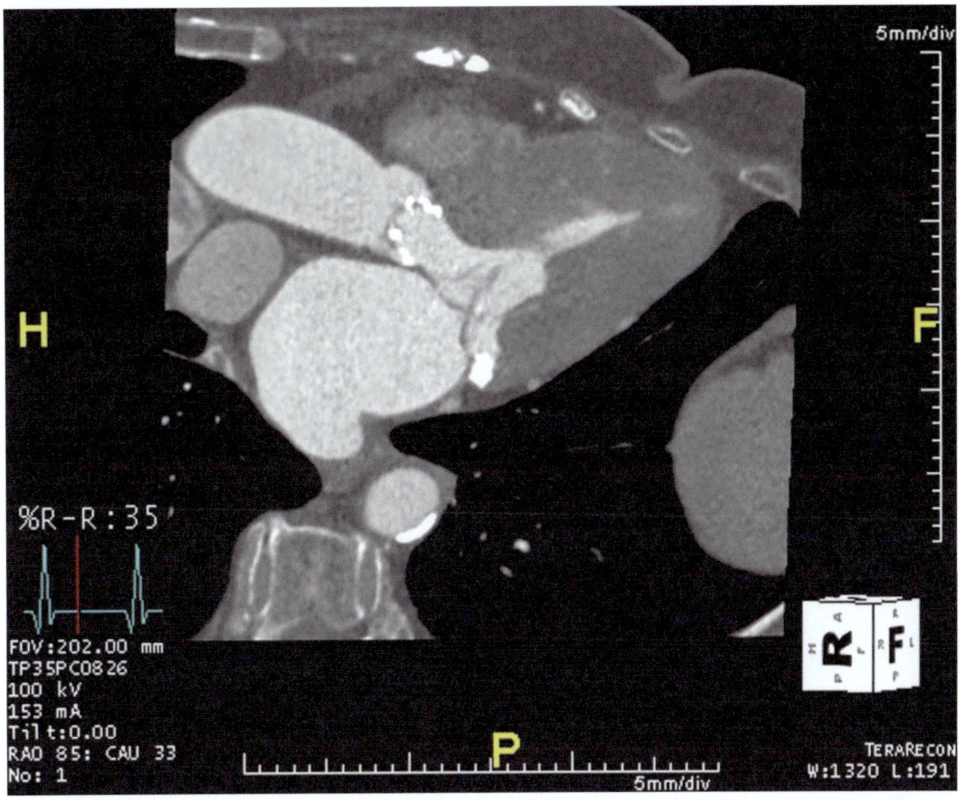

Fig. 17.2 The same CTA data acquired for Fig. 17.1 is now reconstructed at an end-systolic phase, revealing systolic encroachment into the left ventricular outflow tract by the asymmetrically thickened septum

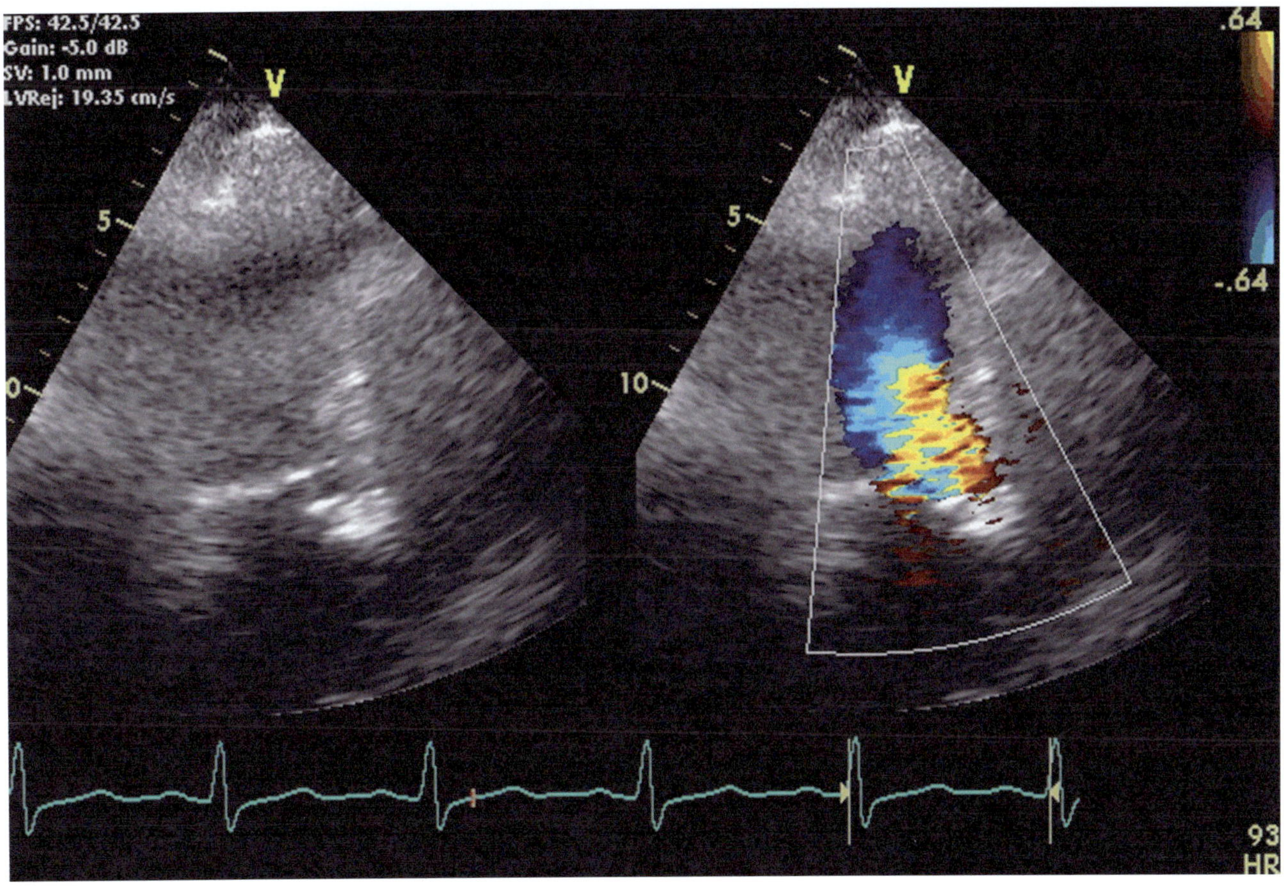

Fig. 17.3 In the same patient with evident ASH by CTA shown in Figs. 17.1 and 17.2, echocardiography acquired during systole (*left*) and with superimposed Doppler recordings (*right*) is shown from the apical 3-chamber view, indicating flow acceleration and mosaic colors with aliased velocities consistent with some degree of left ventricular outflow tract obstruction

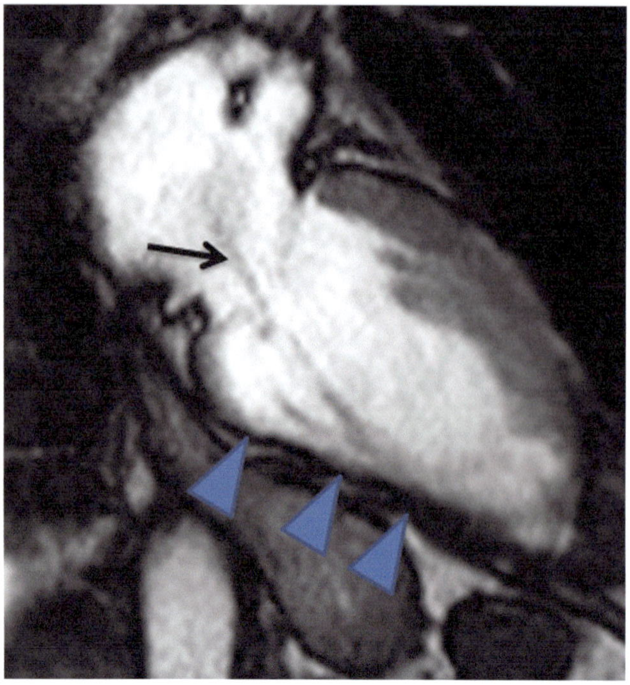

Fig. 17.4 Systolic frame from a vertical long-axis cine cardiac magnetic resonance acquisition shows a thinned inferior wall (*arrowheads*) due to prior myocardial infarction as well as a jet of turbulent mitral regurgitation flow (*arrow*)

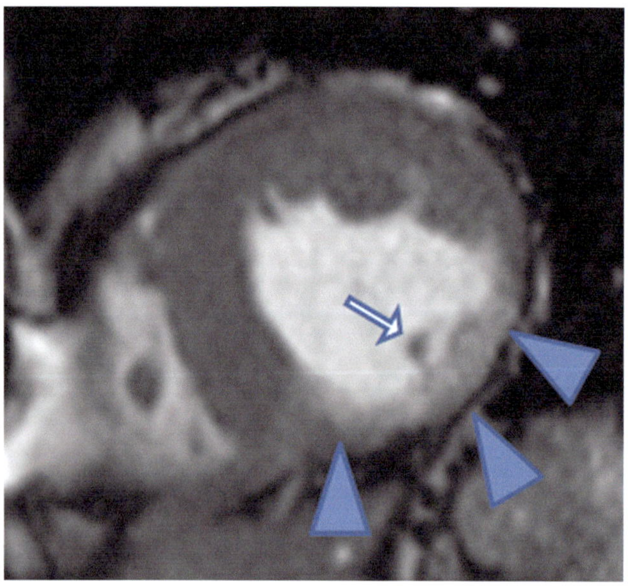

Fig. 17.5 Inferior wall thinning and contrast enhancement (*arrowheads*) are evident on this end-diastolic frame from a mid-level short-axis cine cardiac magnetic resonance acquired after contrast injection. Also note the relatively reduced mass of the posteromedial papillary muscle (*arrow*) compared to the anterolateral papillary muscle

underlying cause of MR; nonetheless, its presence and severity are generally evident by routinely transthoracic echocardiography (Figs. 17.4 and 17.5).

When severe MR is present in patients with severe AS requiring surgery, addressing both valves (e.g., AVR plus mitral valve repair) is advocated. However, for moderate MR, concomitant mitral valve repair (MVR) with AVR is a subject of debate [4]. Surgical replacement of both valves results in a higher operative risk [7, 8], and some studies suggest that moderate functional MR may regress after isolated AVR through reverse LV remodeling [9, 10]. Tassan et al. found that MR severity decreased early after AVR in a cohort of patients with normal LVEF, moderate MR, and severe aortic stenosis [11]. Lower pulmonary artery pressure and reduction in mitral annular dimension and LV mass predicted regression of MR in this echocardiography-guided investigation [11]. However, moderate to severe MR may not improve and may even increase post-AVR [10, 12, 13]. Thus, some argue for an aggressive approach for concomitant MR and AS. Vanden Eynden et al. found improved postoperative MR predicted better 10-year survival post-AVR, noting little improvement in those whose MR was a result of rheumatic disease or myxomatous degeneration [14]. While data suggest that patients with uncorrected MR after AVR have higher morbidity and mortality, ongoing evidence must accrue to ensure that correcting mild to moderate MR with aortic valve replacement consistently confers additional postoperative improvements over AVR alone [4].

In the TAVR era, studies are appropriately focused on the outcomes of patients with MR who undergo transcatheter heart valve implantations. A prospective, single-center study by D'Onofrio et al. performed echocardiography in 176 patients undergoing TAVR prior to and at discharge, 1, 3, 6, and 12 months post-procedure [15]. Despite a trend toward higher in-hospital mortality after TAVR in patients with MR as compared to patients with no MR, 20-month survival was identical in those with moderate or more severe MR compared to those with mild or less MR. In addition, MR severity fell and LV remodeling improved after TAVR.

Other studies support variable improvement of functional MR after TAVR. Durst et al. reviewed echocardiograms before and at 1-day, 3-month, and 6-month post-TAVR in 35 patients enrolled in the REVIVAL II trial (tRanscatheter EndoVascular Implantation of VALves) [16]. Those with at least 30 % reduction in vena contracta-based MR severity comprised approximately one-third of the group—so-called good responders—while the rest were deemed "poor responders." Poor responders were distinguished from good responders by the presence of mitral annular calcification causing restriction of mitral leaflet motion. Hekimian et al. studied MR in a prospective study of 119 patients that included baseline, 7-day, and 1-month post-TAVR echocardiograms [5]. Improvement in both organic and structural MR was seen at 7 days, was not influenced by the overlap of the anterior mitral leaflet and the device, and was associated with improvement in LV ejection fraction. Others have concluded that even if there is no improvement in the degree of MR after TAVR, the correction in aortic valve pathology is sufficient to improve patient outcomes by reducing left ventricular dimensions [15]. These results call for more studies with longer-term follow-up to evaluate outcomes and survival after TAVR in patients with MR.

Technical aspects of TAVR in patients with coexistent MR have been considered. Cilingiroglu and Hakeem have commented on the variable results from studies evaluating the impact of TAVR with CoreValve or Edwards Sapien valve on mitral valve function [17]. The CoreValve prosthesis can potentially worsen mitral regurgitation due to mitral annular calcification because it is usually placed 8 mm below the base of the aortic root and can potentially restrict anterior leaflet mobility [17–19]. Reproducible measurements are necessary to quantify MR as part of the careful pre-TAVR evaluation, and this information should aid in the selection of patients likely to benefit from TAVR and to guide approach, type of valve, and device position.

As with patient selection for TAVR, transcatheter mitral valve repair may be a consideration for the poor surgical candidate with significant MR. Rudolph et al. reported findings in 11 patients who underwent MitraClip placement as well as TAVR [20]. Despite technical feasibility, clinical benefit was limited, underscoring the need for further investigations as to the implications of MR on TAVR and additional interventions in the setting of significant AS.

Prior Myocardial Infarction

Aortic stenosis and coronary artery disease (CAD) often coexist. Age-related calcified aortic sclerosis has been associated with a 50 % increased risk of cardiovascular mortality and myocardial infarction in a longitudinal study of over 5,000 patients [21]. The Cardiovascular Health Study studied clinical factors associated with aortic sclerosis and stenosis in a population-based evaluation that included echocardiography [22]. Independent predictors of degenerative aortic valve disease included age, male gender, smoking, and hypertension—all risk factors for atherosclerosis. Furthermore, high lipoprotein(A) and low-density lipoprotein cholesterol levels contributed to degenerative aortic valve disease risk [22]. In contrast, Ortlepp et al. observed no excess risk factor association with prevalence of aortic stenosis when comparing AS patients with controls matched for age, sex, and angiographically defined coronary artery disease [23]. Indirectly supportive of these findings, a recent meta-analysis of statin therapy trials for aortic valve disease confirmed that treating hyperlipidemia, an established approach to attenuate atherosclerosis, does not halt progression of AS [24]. These data suggest that AS and CAD, while potentially occurring amidst a backdrop of similar

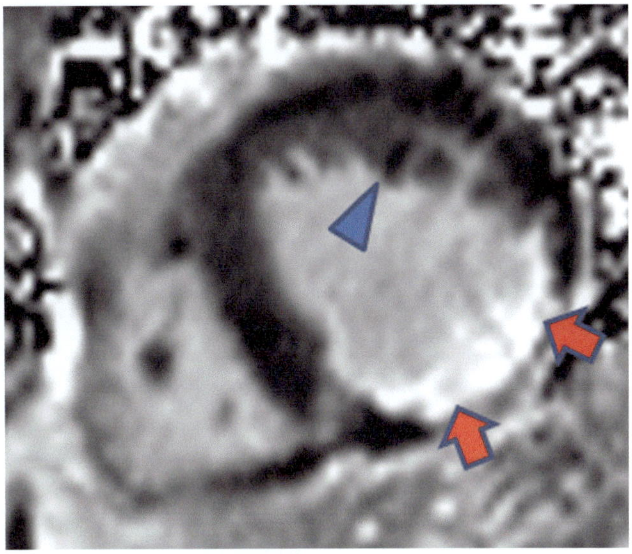

Fig. 17.6 Late post-gadolinium enhancement cardiac magnetic resonance imaging obtained 10 min after contrast shows extensive inferior wall infarct scar (*arrows*). Not seen is the posteromedial papillary muscle, which should be dark like the anterolateral papillary muscle (*arrowhead*)

risk factors, may develop via distinct mechanistic pathways. Given the excess prevalence of coronary atherosclerosis in patients referred for TAVR (Figs. 17.6, 17.7 and 17.8), thorough evaluation of CAD in this population should and is nevertheless the standard of care.

Previous studies have demonstrated that for surgical AVR, history of CAD and/or previous CABG is an independent risk factor for increased mortality [25–27]. Dewey et al. showed that CAD, as defined by previous percutaneous intervention (PCI) or coronary artery bypass graft (CABG), is a significant risk factor for mortality in patients undergoing TAVR [28]. In that study, data on operational and long-term survival was collected on 201 patients undergoing TAVR. Concomitant CAD was identified by previous cardiovascular intervention. Patients who had CAD were tenfold more likely to die within 30 days of the procedures than those without CAD. However, it is unrealistic to exclude CAD or prior MI from TAVR candidacy.

Webb et al. study reported functional improvement after TAVR in a population where 73 % had a history of previous myocardial infarction, a finding that was not associated with increased mortality at up to 2 years [29]. Drews et al. reported technical success and subsequent survival post-TAVR were similar in patients with versus without a history of previous heart surgery [30]. Ducrocq et al. also evaluated the procedural impact of previous coronary bypass surgery [31]. The study found similar 30-day mortality post-TAVR in patients with versus those without a history of CABG. Collectively, these data further position TAVR as an attractive option to repeat sternotomy or thoracotomy in patients with CAD that previously required cardiac surgery.

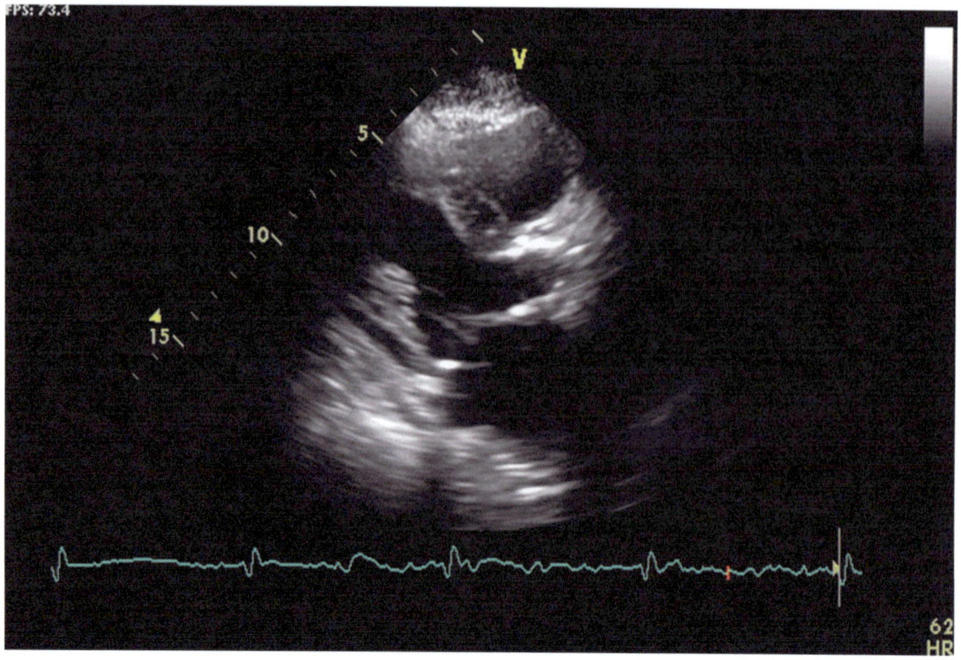

Fig. 17.7 Still frame from a transthoracic echocardiogram, parasternal view shows mitral annular calcification in a pre-TAVR patient

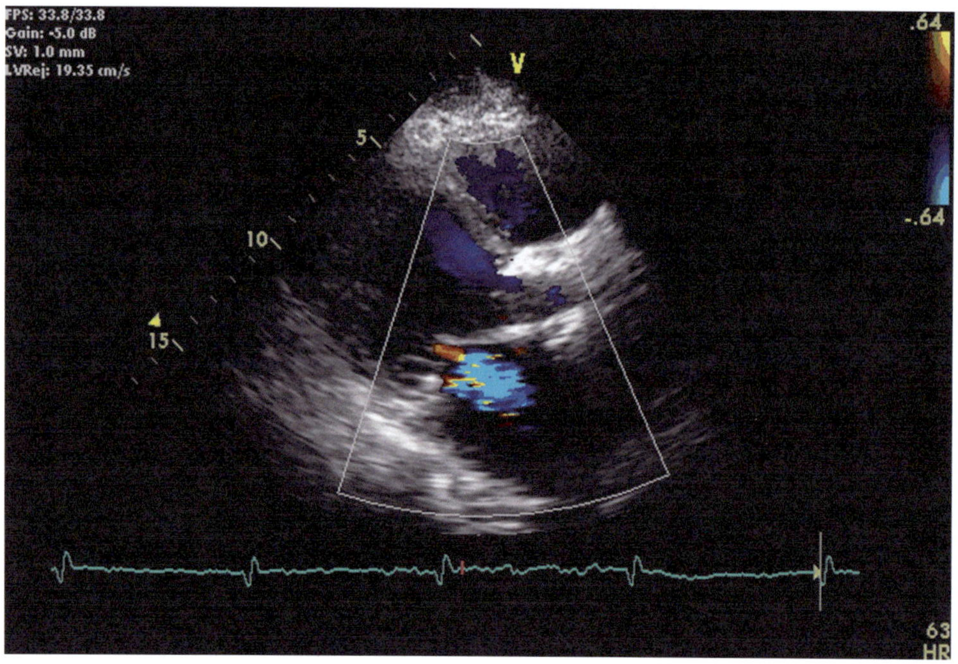

Fig. 17.8 Still frame from the same parasternal view shown in Fig. 17.7 with superimposed color Doppler demonstrates a jet of mitral regurgitation

Elective TAVR may be deferred in the setting of recent myocardial infarction (MI) (Fig. 17.9). With high prevalence of anatomic CAD detected by angiography in patients with symptomatic AS, patients who are considered too high risk for valve surgery may require catheter-based approaches to treat both CAD and AS. Pasic et al. reported initial results of combining percutaneous coronary intervention with transapical TAVR [32]. They reported technical feasibility in 46 patients undergoing both procedures simultaneously and 30-day mortality similar to what has been reported with TAVR alone. Larger randomized trials are needed to know if elective PCI combined with TAVR delivers the posited benefit of reducing post-TAVR myocardial infarction without increasing procedural complication rates. Such data may help formulate guidelines regarding when and how obstructive CAD should be treated in patients referred for TAVR.

Asymmetric Septal Hypertrophy

Asymmetric septal hypertrophy (ASH) implies nonuniform thickening of the interventricular septum in relation to the remaining myocardial segments [33, 34]. Left ventricular hypertrophy (LVH) is most commonly a compensatory

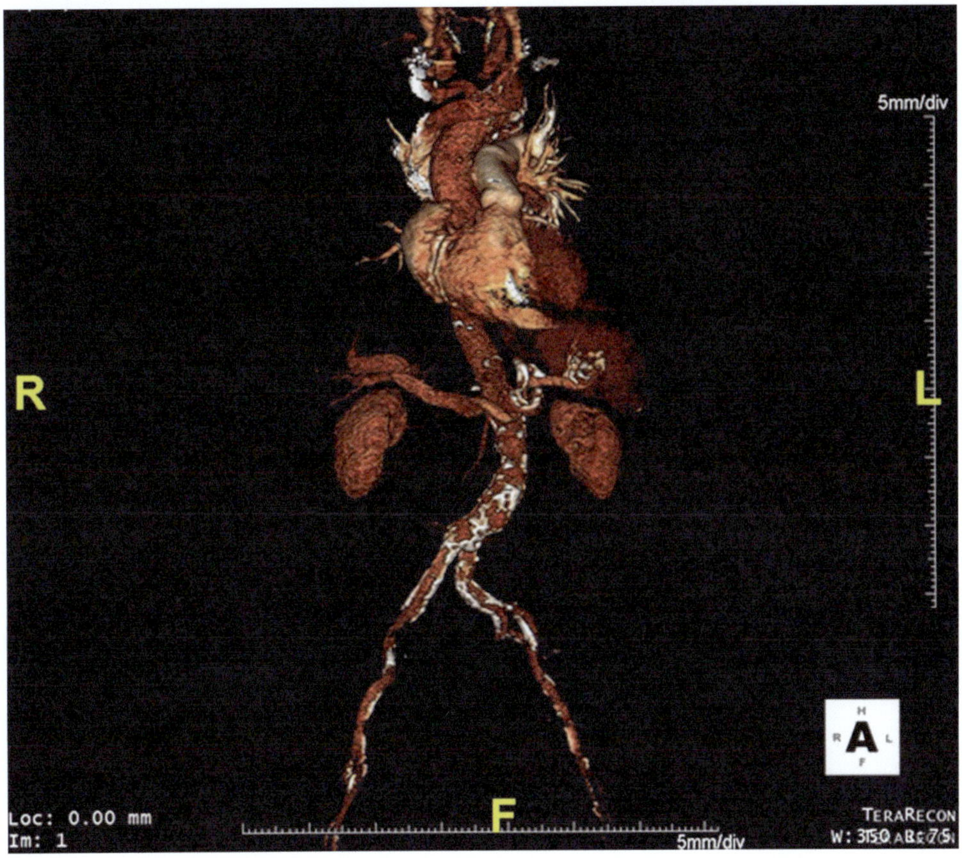

Fig. 17.9 Extensive abdominal aortic atherosclerosis is seen in this anteroposterior volume rendering of CTA data obtained during pre-TAVR evaluation

mechanism for ventricular pressure overload, either due to a rise in circulatory pressure or by a mechanical obstruction to outflow [35]. As significant aortic valve stenosis is the sine qua non prompting TAVR consideration, some degree of LVH or concentric thickening relative to a small LV cavity size is almost uniformly present in patients being evaluated for TAVR (Figs. 17.10 and 17.11).

The histopathology of LVH that develops in response to aortic stenosis involves muscle fiber hypertrophy and abnormalities of the collagen network [33, 36, 37]. Hypertrophy can be uniform and symmetric or it is most pronounced in the ventricular septum leading to ASH. ASH may lead to forward motion of the anterior leaflet of the mitral valve during systole (SAM), resulting in mitral insufficiency. ASH may also be associated with dynamic left ventricular outflow tract obstruction (LVOTO, Fig. 17.12). While ASH may conjure a possible diagnosis of hypertrophic cardiomyopathy (HCM), it should be noted that patients with HCM can coincidentally develop intrinsic disease of the aortic valve [38]. Asymmetric thickening may commonly be present in hypertension that is, in turn, a common comorbid condition in the pre-TAVR patient [39, 40]. Its presence in hypertensive patients has been shown to confer increased cardiovascular risk [40, 41].

Using M-mode echocardiography, Raj et al. reported that the prevalence of ASH in patients was 2.5 % among 119 patients with severe aortic stenosis referred for surgical aortic valve replacement (AVR) [42]. A more recent prevalence assessment, notably in asymptomatic patients with mild to moderate AS, found ASH in 22 % of the 1,719 patients enrolled in the simvastatin and ezetimibe in aortic stenosis (SEAS) trial [39]. This population was older and had a higher prevalence of hypertension as compared to the preoperative patients studied by Raj et al., and hypertension emerged as a more powerful predictor of ASH compared to AS severity.

The presence of LVH in patients with aortic stenosis increases the likelihood of developing symptoms in patients with AS. Pellikka et al. studied 622 patients with isolated, asymptomatic AS and peak velocity of at least 4 m/s and performed longitudinal assessment [43]. The likelihood of developing cardiac symptoms over the subsequent 5.4 ± 4.0 years was predicted by LVH and severity of AS. It is not known from these data, however, what degree of ASH was present.

The presence of ASH may influence the surgical approach for AVR and contribute to excess operative morbidity [39, 44]. Persistently high gradients after AVR warrant consideration of ASH along with prosthesis-patient mismatch as potential underlying mechanisms [38]. The surgical literature has described the immediate post-AVR hemodynamic changes associated with unmasked residual LVOTO leading to hemodynamic collapse as "suicide left ventricle" [45, 46]. ASH and increased LV mass overall is associated with high perioperative morbidity, and patients with multiple comorbidities and severe symptomatic aortic stenosis with ASH may be denied surgical AVR because of excessively

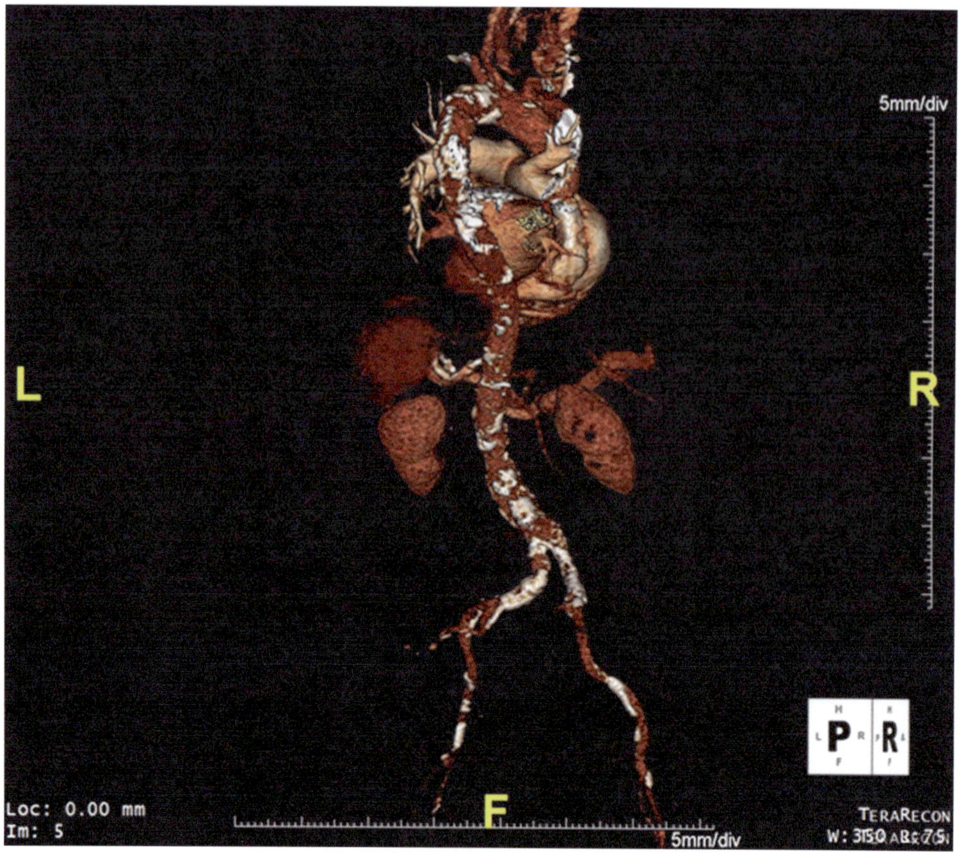

Fig. 17.10 This posteroanterior volume rendering of CTA data obtained during pre-TAVR evaluation shows atherosclerosis in the thoracic and abdominal aorta

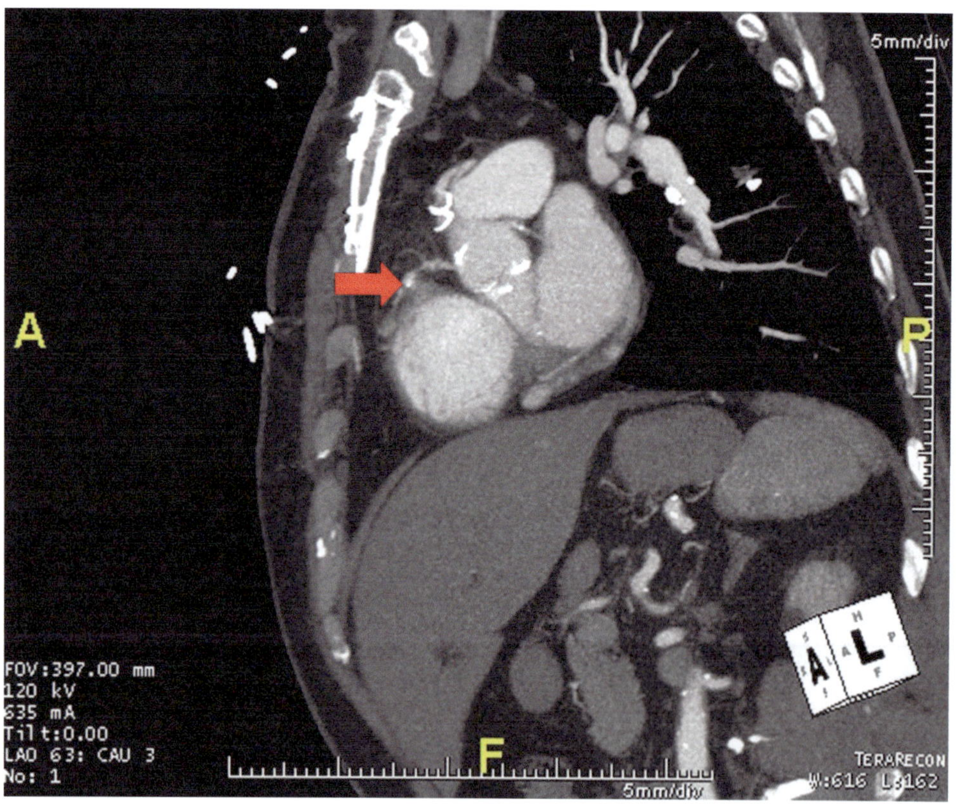

Fig. 17.11 CTA obtained prior to TAVR is shown in an oblique sagittal maximum intensity projection in a patient with prior myocardial infarction due to right coronary artery occlusion (*arrow*)

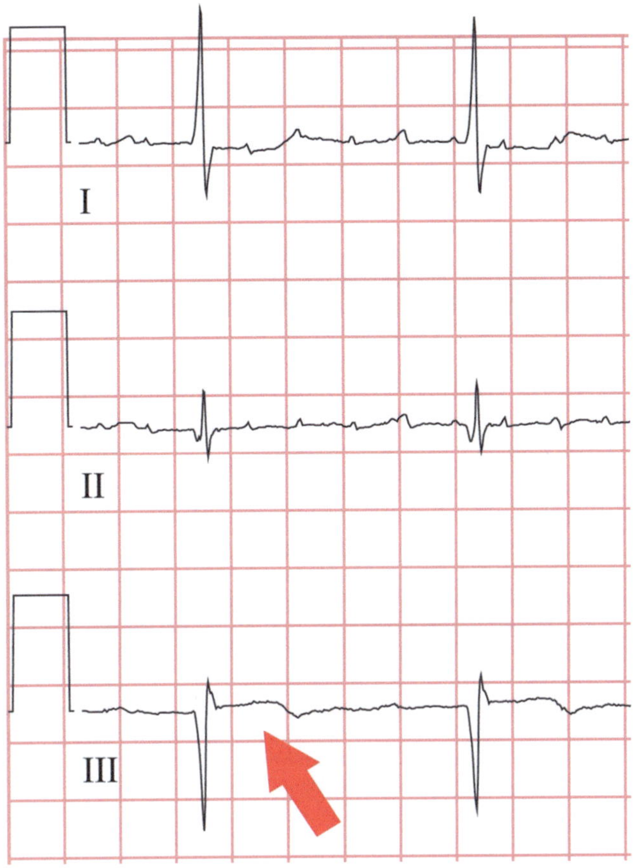

Fig. 17.12 Inferior ST-segment elevation (*arrow*) myocardial infarction is evident by electrocardiography obtained in a patient with multiple comorbidities and chest pain. Invasive pressure measurements obtained during cardiac catheterization revealed an 80 mmHg mean gradient across the aortic valve. TAVR was performed 6 months after percutaneous coronary intervention

high estimated operative risk. Mehta et al. reported echocardiographic measures of LV geometry and outcomes in 473 patients undergoing elective AVR [44]. Patients with increased left ventricular mass index experienced higher rates of post-procedural complications including respiratory failure, renal insufficiency, congestive heart failure, and atrial and ventricular arrhythmias; increased lengths of stay in the ICU; and higher in-hospital mortality. Again, the extent of asymmetric hypertrophy and the degree to which this modifies the negative impact of LVH on AVR outcomes remain to be precisely defined.

In light of potentially worse outcomes associated with ASH in the setting of significant AS, several groups have evaluated the potential benefit versus risks of doing septal myomectomy at the time of AVR. Kayalar et al. retrospectively reviewed the outcomes of 47 patients over a 10-year period who underwent AVR for severe aortic stenosis and concomitant septal myomectomy [47]. Over a mean follow-up period of 43 months, there was one death due to multisystem organ failure, complete heart block in two patients, and no iatrogenic ventricular septal defect. It would seem that operative risk is not increased with myomectomy, although randomized studies are necessary to understand the benefit compared to withholding myomectomy. Di Tommaso et al. retrospectively evaluated outcomes in 34 AVR-only versus 52 AVR plus myomectomy patients with AS [34]. They concluded that concomitant myomectomy at AVR is a safe and effective procedure that improves mass regression and LV diastolic function [34]. It is not known if percutaneous approaches such as alcohol septal ablation could be combined with TAVR in AS patients with significant ASH and LVOTO or if such an approach is necessary to improve outcomes post-TAVR.

With the development of TAVR, different technical approaches that may address ASH are being evaluated. Initially, one of the contraindications to TAVR was severe intraventricular septal hypertrophy because of the risk, among other concerns, of prosthesis displacement and migration during implantation. In 2010, Finkelstein et al. reported the first case of severe valvular AS, discrete subvalvular subaortic stenosis, and septal hypertrophy successfully treated with TAVR (CoreValve), by intentionally implanting the bioprosthetic valve in a lower position within the LV outflow tract [48]. This lower position allowed the valve struts to cover the subaortic membrane and part of the thickened septum, thus eliminating the valvular and subvalvular gradients and SAM. With regard to the Edwards Sapien prosthetic valve, Moreno et al. reported a modification of the technique leading to successful implantation of the prosthesis in two patients with septal hypertrophy and severe AS [49]. The technique modification involved minimizing the contact between the balloon and interventricular septum by repositioning the prosthetic valve asymmetrically and more distally. Dworakowski and Wendler suggest that the transapical approach rather than the retroaortic approach may be better suited for the TAVR patient with ASH [50]. The authors state that the transapical approach with antegrade passage of the device minimizes risk of prosthetic displacement due to ASH.

As described above, successful TAVR in patients with ASH can be affected by the approach, access, and position of the valve. In essentially all such patients, a transthoracic echocardiogram is available for review of LV anatomy and any LVOT obstruction before TAVR. Given the increased utility demonstrated with cardiac magnetic resonance (CMR) in robust demonstration of LV geometry along with myocardial tissue characterization in hypertension [51], hypertrophic cardiomyopathy [52], and aortic stenosis [53], CMR warrants consideration in the pre-TAVR population as well, particularly when poor acoustic windows limit precise LVOT visualization. La Manna et al. compared LV and LVOT measurements by both TTE and CMR in 49 high-risk elderly patients referred for TAVR [54]. CMR provided diagnostic information and adequate sizing in all patients, and CMR provided comparable measurements of annulus size, LVOT, and aortic valve area. Regardless of the modality chosen, the information provided by appropriate imaging regarding structure and function of the left ventricle—and the impact of ASH on LV and LVOT geometry—are an integral part of TAVR care, with implications regarding technical approach and outcomes to improve the likelihood of a successful procedure.

Conclusion

In the recent past, TAVR has emerged as a disruptive technology that demonstrates great success for aortic valve replacement in inoperable and high-risk patients. While studies to date have reported very good outcomes associated with TAVR, the presence of comorbid conditions in patients undergoing TAVR influences the risk of the procedure. Careful consideration of these comorbidities—as well as determination of the need for modification of TAVR procedures, or enhanced pre- or post-TAVR evaluation of these conditions—is an area necessary of future study.

References

1. Gurvitch R, Tay EL, Wijesinghe N, Ye J, Nietlispach F, Wood DA, Lichtenstein S, Cheung A, Webb JG. Transcatheter aortic valve implantation: lessons from the learning curve of the first 270 high-risk patients. Catheter Cardiovasc Interv. 2011;78:977–84.
2. Kodali SK, O'Neill WW, Moses JW, Williams M, Smith CR, Tuzcu M, Svensson LG, Kapadia S, Hanzel G, Kirtane AJ, Leon MB. Early and late (one year) outcomes following transcatheter aortic valve implantation in patients with severe aortic stenosis (from the United States REVIVAL trial). Am J Cardiol. 2011;107:1058–64.
3. Come PC, Riley MF, Ferguson JF, Morgan JP, McKay RG. Prediction of severity of aortic stenosis: accuracy of multiple non-invasive parameters. Am J Med. 1988;85:29–37.
4. Unger P, Dedobbeleer C, Van Camp G, Plein D, Cosyns B, Lancellotti P. Mitral regurgitation in patients with aortic stenosis undergoing valve replacement. Heart. 2010;96:9–14.
5. Hekimian G, Detaint D, Messika-Zeitoun D, Attias D, Iung B, Himbert D, Brochet E, Vahanian A. Mitral regurgitation in patients referred for transcatheter aortic valve implantation using the Edwards Sapien prosthesis: mechanisms and early postprocedural changes. J Am Soc Echocardiogr. 2012;25:160–5.
6. Barreiro CJ, Patel ND, Fitton TP, Williams JA, Bonde PN, Chan V, Alejo DE, Gott VL, Baumgartner WA. Aortic valve replacement and concomitant mitral valve regurgitation in the elderly: impact on survival and functional outcome. Circulation. 2005;112:I443–7.
7. Arom KV, Nicoloff DM, Kersten TE, Northrup 3rd WF, Lindsay WG, Emery RW. Ten-year follow-up study of patients who had double valve replacement with the St. Jude Medical prosthesis. J Thorac Cardiovasc Surg. 1989;98:1008–15; discussion 1015–16.
8. Mueller XM, Tevaearai HT, Stumpe F, Fischer AP, Hurni M, Ruchat P, von Segesser LK. Long-term results of mitral-aortic valve operations. J Thorac Cardiovasc Surg. 1998;115:1298–309.
9. Sutton M, Plappert T, Spiegel A, Raichlen J, Douglas P, Reichek N, Edmunds L. Early postoperative changes in left ventricular chamber size, architecture, and function in aortic stenosis and aortic regurgitation and their relation to intraoperative changes in afterload: a prospective two-dimensional echocardiographic study. Circulation. 1987;76:77–89.
10. Moazami N, Diodato MD, Moon MR, Lawton JS, Pasque MK, Herren RL, Guthrie TJ, Damiano RJ. Does functional mitral regurgitation improve with isolated aortic valve replacement? J Card Surg. 2004;19:444–8.
11. Tassan-Mangina S, Metz D, Nazeyllas P, Torossian F, Pop C, Bertrand J, Baehrel B, Elaerts J. Factors determining early improvement in mitral regurgitation after aortic valve replacement for aortic valve stenosis: a transthoracic and transesophageal prospective study. Clin Cardiol. 2003;26:127–31.
12. Adams PB, Otto CM. Lack of improvement in coexisting mitral regurgitation after relief of valvular aortic stenosis. Am J Cardiol. 1990;66:105–7.
13. Brasch AV, Khan SS, DeRobertis MA, Kong JH, Chiu J, Siegel RJ. Change in mitral regurgitation severity after aortic valve replacement for aortic stenosis. Am J Cardiol. 2000;85:1271–4.
14. Vanden Eynden F, Bouchard D, El-Hamamsy I, Butnaru A, Demers P, Carrier M, Perrault LP, Tardif JC, Pellerin M. Effect of aortic valve replacement for aortic stenosis on severity of mitral regurgitation. Ann Thorac Surg. 2007;83:1279–84.
15. D'Onofrio A, Gasparetto V, Napodano M, Bianco R, Tarantini G, Renier V, Isabella G, Gerosa G. Impact of preoperative mitral valve regurgitation on outcomes after transcatheter aortic valve implantation. Eur J Cardiothorac Surg. 2012;41:1271–6.
16. Durst R, Avelar E, McCarty D, Poh KK, Friera LF, Llano MF, Chu J, Anumandla AK, Rodriguez LL, Mack MJ, et al. Outcome and improvement predictors of mitral regurgitation after transcatheter aortic valve implantation. J Heart Valve Dis. 2011;20:272–81.
17. Cilingiroglu M, Hakeem A. Fate of mitral regurgitation following transcatheter aortic valve implantation: the achilles heel of core valve? Catheter Cardiovasc Interv. 2011;78:645–6.
18. Chin D. Echocardiography for transcatheter aortic valve implantation. Eur J Echocardiogr. 2009;10:i21–9.
19. Yong Z, Van Dijk K, Koch K, Vis M, et al. Effect of transcatheter aortic valve implantation with the Medtronic-CoreValve bioprosthesis on mitral valve area and pressure gradient. Eur J Echocardiogr. 2010;11 Suppl 2:ii9–11.
20. Rudolph V, Schirmer J, Franzen O, Schluter M, Seiffert M, Treede H, Reichenspurner H, Blankenberg S, Baldus S. Bivalvular transcatheter treatment of high-surgical-risk patients with coexisting severe aortic stenosis and significant mitral regurgitation. Int J Cardiol. 2013;167(3):716–20.
21. Otto CM, Lind BK, Kitzman DW, Gersh BJ, Siscovick DS. Association of aortic-valve sclerosis with cardiovascular mortality and morbidity in the elderly. N Engl J Med. 1999;341:142–7.
22. Stewart BF, Siscovick D, Lind BK, Gardin JM, Gottdiener JS, Smith VE, Kitzman DW, Otto CM. Clinical factors associated with calcific aortic valve disease. Cardiovascular Health Study. J Am Coll Cardiol. 1997;29:630–4.
23. Ortlepp JR, Schmitz F, Bozoglu T, Hanrath P, Hoffmann R. Cardiovascular risk factors in patients with aortic stenosis predict prevalence of coronary artery disease but not of aortic stenosis: an angiographic pair matched case-control study. Heart. 2003;89:1019–22.
24. Teo KK, Corsi DJ, Tam JW, Dumesnil JG, Chan KL. Lipid lowering on progression of mild to moderate aortic stenosis: meta-analysis of the randomized placebo-controlled clinical trials on 2344 patients. Can J Cardiol. 2011;27:800–8.
25. Nowicki ER, Birkmeyer NJ, Weintraub RW, Leavitt BJ, Sanders JH, Dacey LJ, Clough RA, Quinn RD, Charlesworth DC, Sisto DA, et al. Multivariable prediction of in-hospital mortality associated with aortic and mitral valve surgery in Northern New England. Ann Thorac Surg. 2004;77:1966–77.
26. Tjang YS, van Hees Y, Korfer R, Grobbee DE, van der Heijden GJ. Predictors of mortality after aortic valve replacement. Eur J Cardiothorac Surg. 2007;32:469–74.

27. Florath I, Rosendahl UP, Mortasawi A, Bauer SF, Dalladaku F, Ennker IC, Ennker JC. Current determinants of operative mortality in 1400 patients requiring aortic valve replacement. Ann Thorac Surg. 2003;76:75–83.
28. Dewey TM, Brown DL, Herbert MA, Culica D, Smith CR, Leon MB, Svensson LG, Tuzcu M, Webb JG, Cribier A, Mack MJ. Effect of concomitant coronary artery disease on procedural and late outcomes of transcatheter aortic valve implantation. Ann Thorac Surg. 2010;89:758–67; discussion 767.
29. Webb JG, Altwegg L, Boone RH, Cheung A, Ye J, Lichtenstein S, Lee M, Masson JB, Thompson C, Moss R, et al. Transcatheter aortic valve implantation: impact on clinical and valve-related outcomes. Circulation. 2009;119:3009–16.
30. Drews T, Pasic M, Buz S, Unbehaun A, Dreysse S, Kukucka M, Mladenow A, Hetzer R. Transapical aortic valve implantation after previous heart surgery. Eur J Cardiothorac Surg. 2011;39:625–30.
31. Ducrocq G, Al-Attar N, Himbert D, Messika-Zeitoun D, Iung B, Descoutures F, Nataf P, Vahanian A. Early and mid-term outcomes in patients undergoing transcatheter aortic valve implantation after previous coronary artery bypass grafting. Eur J Cardiothorac Surg. 2012;41:499–504.
32. Pasic M, Dreysse S, Unbehaun A, Buz S, Drews T, Klein C, D'Ancona G, Hetzer R. Combined elective percutaneous coronary intervention and transapical transcatheter aortic valve implantation. Interact Cardiovasc Thorac Surg. 2012;14:463–8.
33. Hess OM, Ritter M, Schneider J, Grimm J, Turina M, Krayenbuehl HP. Diastolic stiffness and myocardial structure in aortic valve disease before and after valve replacement. Circulation. 1984;69:855–65.
34. Di Tommaso L, Stassano P, Mannacio V, Russolillo V, Monaco M, Pinna G, Vosa C. Asymmetric septal hypertrophy in patients with severe aortic stenosis: the usefulness of associated septal myomectomy. J Thorac Cardiovasc Surg. 2012;145:171–5.
35. Siegenthaler W. Differential diagnosis in internal medicine: from symptom to diagnosis. Stuttgart: Georg Thieme Verlag; 2007.
36. Villari B, Campbell SE, Hess OM, Mall G, Vassalli G, Weber KT, Krayenbuehl HP. Influence of collagen network on left ventricular systolic and diastolic function in aortic valve disease. J Am Coll Cardiol. 1993;22:1477–84.
37. Krayenbuehl HP, Hess OM, Monrad ES, Schneider J, Mall G, Turina M. Left ventricular myocardial structure in aortic valve disease before, intermediate, and late after aortic valve replacement. Circulation. 1989;79:744–55.
38. Bach DS. Subvalvular left ventricular outflow obstruction for patients undergoing aortic valve replacement for aortic stenosis: echocardiographic recognition and identification of patients at risk. J Am Soc Echocardiogr. 2005;18:1155–62.
39. Tuseth N, Cramariuc D, Rieck AE, Wachtell K, Gerdts E. Asymmetric septal hypertrophy – a marker of hypertension in aortic stenosis (a SEAS substudy). Blood Press. 2010;19:140–4.
40. Verdecchia P, Porcellati C, Zampi I, Schillaci G, Gatteschi C, Battistelli M, Bartoccini C, Borgioni C, Ciucci A. Asymmetric left ventricular remodeling due to isolated septal thickening in patients with systemic hypertension and normal left ventricular masses. Am J Cardiol. 1994;73:247–52.
41. Devereux RB, Wachtell K, Gerdts E, Boman K, Nieminen MS, Papademetriou V, Rokkedal J, Harris K, Aurup P, Dahlof B. Prognostic significance of left ventricular mass change during treatment of hypertension. JAMA. 2004;292:2350–6.
42. Raj MV, Srinivas V, Graham IM, Evans DW. Coexistence of asymmetric septal hypertrophy and aortic valve disease in adults. Thorax. 1979;34:91–5.
43. Pellikka PA, Sarano ME, Nishimura RA, Malouf JF, Bailey KR, Scott CG, Barnes ME, Tajik AJ. Outcome of 622 adults with asymptomatic, hemodynamically significant aortic stenosis during prolonged follow-up. Circulation. 2005;111:3290–5.
44. Mehta RH, Bruckman D, Das S, Tsai T, Russman P, Karavite D, Monaghan H, Sonnad S, Shea MJ, Eagle KA, Deeb GM. Implications of increased left ventricular mass index on in-hospital outcomes in patients undergoing aortic valve surgery. J Thorac Cardiovasc Surg. 2001;122:919–28.
45. Jilaihawi H, Kar S, Doctor N, Fontana G, Makkar R. Contemporary application of cardiovascular hemodynamics: transcatheter aortic valve interventions. Cardiol Clin. 2011;29:211–22.
46. Suh WM, Witzke CF, Palacios IF. Suicide left ventricle following transcatheter aortic valve implantation. Catheter Cardiovasc Interv. 2010;76:616–20.
47. Kayalar N, Schaff HV, Daly RC, Dearani JA, Park SJ. Concomitant septal myomectomy at the time of aortic valve replacement for severe aortic stenosis. Ann Thorac Surg. 2010;89:459–64.
48. Finkelstein A, Keren G, Banai S. Treatment of severe valvular aortic stenosis and subvalvular discrete subaortic stenosis and septal hypertrophy with Percutaneous CoreValve Aortic Valve Implantation. Catheter Cardiovasc Interv. 2010;75:801–3.
49. Moreno R, Calvo L, Garcia E, Dobarro D. Severe septal hypertrophy: is it necessarily a contraindication for the transcatheter implantation of an Edwards-Sapien prosthesis? Rev Esp Cardiol. 2010,63:241–2.
50. Dworakowski R, Wendler O. The transapical route for TAVR. Cardiac Interventions Today: Transcatheter Valve Update. 2011:62–5.
51. Raman SV. The hypertensive heart. An integrated understanding informed by imaging. J Am Coll Cardiol. 2010;55:91–6.
52. Desai MY, Ommen SR, McKenna WJ, Lever HM, Elliott PM. Imaging phenotype versus genotype in hypertrophic cardiomyopathy. Circ Cardiovasc Imaging. 2011;4:156–68.
53. Herrmann S, Stork S, Niemann M, Lange V, Strotmann JM, Frantz S, Beer M, Gattenlohner S, Voelker W, Ertl G, Weidemann F. Low-gradient aortic valve stenosis myocardial fibrosis and its influence on function and outcome. J Am Coll Cardiol. 2011;58:402–12.
54. La Manna A, Sanfilippo A, Capodanno D, Salemi A, Polizzi G, Deste W, Cincotta G, Cadoni A, Marchese A, Figuera M, et al. Cardiovascular magnetic resonance for the assessment of patients undergoing transcatheter aortic valve implantation: a pilot study. J Cardiovasc Magn Reson. 2011;13:82.

18 Extravascular and Extracardiac Findings on MDCT for Transcatheter Aortic Valve Planning

Cameron John Hague

Abstract

Multi-detector computed tomography (MDCT) is an imaging tool which has found a role in the planning of transcatheter aortic valve replacement (TAVR). MDCT provides high-quality images of not only cardiac and vascular findings but also detailed anatomic evaluation of other structures in the thorax, abdomen, and pelvis.

Incidental findings are commonly detected on MDCT exams performed for various indications, including those done for TAVR planning. Such findings are generally categorized according to their potential clinical significance to the patient. The age and level of comorbidity in a TAVR cohort not only increases the likelihood of detecting an incidental finding, but also increases the uncertainty with regard to how such findings, especially those of intermediate clinical significance, are handled.

This chapter provides insight into the basic principles of incidentally detected lesions on MDCT and discusses current management strategies for some of the more commonly encountered incidental lesions in the chest, abdomen, and pelvis.

Keywords

Incidental • Nodule • Lymphadenopathy • Pulmonary embolism • Compression fracture • Pancreatic cyst • Liver • Renal • Breast

Introduction

Multi-detector computed tomography (MDCT) is now a common imaging tool used to aid in the planning of transcatheter aortic valve replacement (TAVR). MDCT has found a role in assessment of iliofemoral diameters and tortuosity, as well as in delineating the complex anatomy of the aortic annulus, as described in other chapters of this text.

MDCT for this purpose involves image acquisition during the arterial phase of iodinated contrast injection, with *z*-axis coverage from the thoracic inlet to the level of the lesser trochanters. Images are reconstructed at full field of view and subsequently reviewed. The acquired data set provides a detailed anatomic evaluation of the thorax, abdomen, and pelvis.

Evaluation of the anatomic areas covered by MDCT for TAVR planning can result in the detection of unrelated or unexpected pathologies, commonly referred to as "incidentalomas" [1]. Recent improvements in spatial and contrast resolution of this modality have enabled the detection of small lesions with high sensitivity, with a resultant increase in the detection of incidental findings [2].

The Basics of Incidental Findings

Incidental findings may be divided into three categories based on their likelihood of significance. Findings may be classified into categories of major, moderate or minor significance [3]. Major findings are those felt to be of definite clinical relevance to the patient. This category can be subdivided

C.J. Hague, MD, FRCPC
Department of Radiology, St. Paul's Hospital,
1081 Burrard Street, Vancouver, BC V6Z 1Y6, Canada
e-mail: cjhague75@gmail.com

J.K. Min et al. (eds.), *Multimodality Imaging for Transcatheter Aortic Valve Replacement*,
DOI 10.1007/978-1-4471-2798-7_18, © Springer-Verlag London 2014

into findings highly likely to have an acute impact on patient care (i.e., acute pulmonary embolism) and those which are non-acute but are likely to mandate a change in patient management (i.e., incidentally detected lung carcinoma). Moderate findings would be incidental findings of uncertain clinical relevance to the patient (i.e., 1.5 cm pancreatic cyst, 7 mm soft tissue lung nodule) or abnormalities which may or may not affect the patient in the future (i.e., gallstones). This category tends to be most problematic, as findings in this category generally require further workup, but without the certainty of a change in patient outcome. Minor findings are considered to be definitively benign and are not felt to require any follow-up (i.e., simple renal cysts or completely calcified lung nodules).

It is an important first principle when an incidental finding is detected to search the patient's record for any prior imaging of this area. The ability to document long-term stability of an abnormality detected on MDCT supports a benign natural history. This fairly simple step can alleviate much patient concern and cost when a decision is made with regard to the significance of such a finding.

In all body areas there are findings which help to establish a definitive diagnosis without further work-up. Where applicable such findings will be discussed later in this text.

Lesions of high clinical significance such as pulmonary embolism or lung lesions felt to represent malignancy should prompt contact with the referring physician.

The cost-effectiveness of dealing with incidental findings is an important consideration. As many of these findings are those of "indeterminate" significance, further work-up is often suggested by the interpreting physician, increasing cost to the health-care system or individual [4].

Unfortunately, recommendations with regard to evaluation of incidental findings are supported by little hard evidence [1]. This lack of evidence makes the management of incidental findings, particularly those in the moderate category, extremely difficult.

Relevance of Incidental Findings in TAVR Patients

Recent published data suggests that over 34 % of patients referred for MDCT before TAVR have significant incidental findings, with a rate of malignancy of 4.2 % [5]. Additionally, it has been demonstrated previously that patient age is a major factor in the frequency with which incidental findings are detected on CT studies [5, 6].

It has been suggested that patient life expectancy be an important consideration when determining recommendations for follow-up and further management of incidental findings on CT examinations [1]. The patients in the Partner Trial cohort B had a median age of over 83 years. Currently, patients of this age range represent the majority of individuals being screened for TAVR. The patients treated with medical therapy and balloon valvuloplasty within the Partner B cohort experienced an all-cause mortality of 50 and 68 % at 1- and 2-year follow-up respectively [7, 8]. It could be argued that there are few if any findings, apart from those demanding acute action, that would be considered clinically significant in such a patient population. Even metastatic non-small cell lung carcinoma (which has a median survival of 6 months) takes on a different connotation in such a cohort. The potential flaw with this line of thinking is partly explained by the success of TAVR. Although no long-term data is currently available with regard to outcomes in patients undergoing a TAVR, early results are promising. In the Partner B cohort, there was a 20 % reduction in all-cause mortality with TAVR with a greater relative risk reduction at 2 years [8, 9]. By altering the natural history of aortic stenosis, many incidental findings noted on MDCT for TAVR workup become potentially more significant as these patients live longer lives. The implications of such findings in high-risk surgical patients and, even more so, in intermediate risk patients are uncertain. It does seem clear that with changing demographics and risk of those being evaluated and screened for TAVR, a thoughtful approach to incidental findings must be taken.

Technical Considerations When Detecting Extravascular and Extracardiac Findings

Given the large *z*-axis coverage of an MDCT for TAVR planning, many different body areas and organ systems are imaged, increasing the chance that an incidental lesion will be detected. The use of iodinated contrast is also a consideration when evaluating abnormalities, particularly with regard to the solid abdominal organs. The timing of the scan in relation to IV contrast administration plays an important role in lesion characterization. MDCT performed for TAVR is timed to maximize contrast within the arterial vascular system. This timing is too early to allow for optimal enhancement of the solid visceral organs [6, 10].

Evaluation of the Chest and Body Wall

Lesions within the subcutaneous tissues and hernias are often discovered on MDCT examinations covering the chest, abdomen, and pelvis and are usually benign [3]. An exception to this is the detection of soft tissue lesions in the breast. MDCT is relatively poor in its ability to characterize a breast mass as benign or malignant [11, 12]. Soft tissue lesions seen in the breast parenchyma are a frequent occurrence when imaging the chest with MDCT, approaching nearly 8 % in an elderly (mean age 73 years, range 50–86 years) female cohort, with 25–30 % of these lesions being malignant [11]. The likelihood that a breast lesion detected on MDCT represents carcinoma increases with patient age [13]. The presence of spiculation of the soft tissue focus and detection of

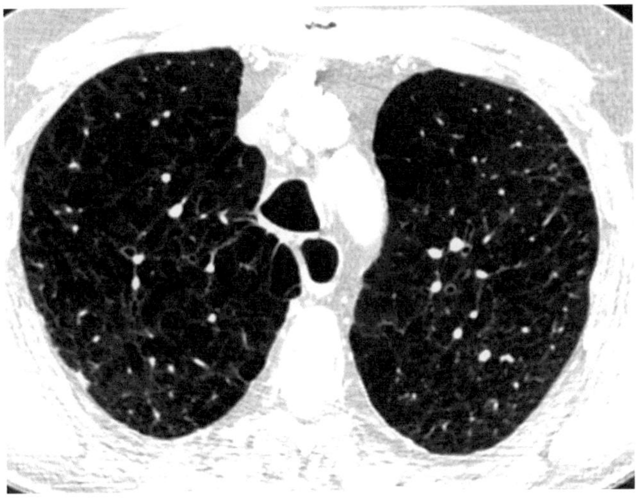

Fig. 18.1 A 72-year-old male, with a 40 pack-year smoking history. MDCT demonstrates severe centrilobular emphysema on the lung algorithm image

axillary adenopathy are strongly suggestive of malignancy [12]. While MDCT displays limited ability to characterize primary breast lesions, a search for metastatic spread of breast carcinoma to lymph nodes, lungs, bones, and solid organs should be undertaken when a lesion is identified [14]. It is important to assess the breast parenchyma when included in the field of view of a CT examination and recommend referral to a dedicated breast imaging center when lesions are detected (Fig. 18.1).

Evaluation of Bony Structures

Incidentally discovered thoracolumbar vertebral compression fractures are common, and often underreported, seen in 9–35 % of MDCT evaluations, with the incidence largely related to patient age and gender (Fig. 18.2) [15, 16]. It is valuable to assess the thoracolumbar spine using a bone reconstruction algorithm in the sagittal plane to avoid missing mild or even moderate compression fractures. Seemingly innocuous, such fractures have shown an association with significant morbidity and mortality [17]. The risk of subsequent vertebral and hip fractures rises significantly [18]. Correlation with bone mineral density is recommended in this setting. The institution of pharmacotherapy, to combat osteoporosis, or vertebroplasty, in the setting of ongoing pain, is a possible treatment option [15].

Pulmonary Evaluation

Evaluation of the lung parenchyma can be divided into assessment of diffuse pathologies such as emphysema or pulmonary fibrosis and detection of focal lesions such as nodules or masses.

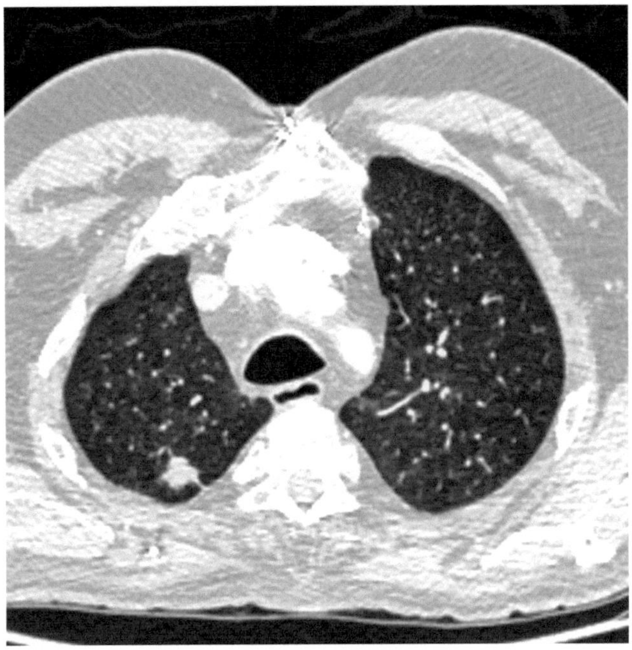

Fig. 18.2 A 60-year-old male patient with a 1.3 cm spiculated right upper lobe lung lesion. This lesion was subsequently biopsied, with pathology in keeping with non-small cell lung cancer (adenocarcinoma)

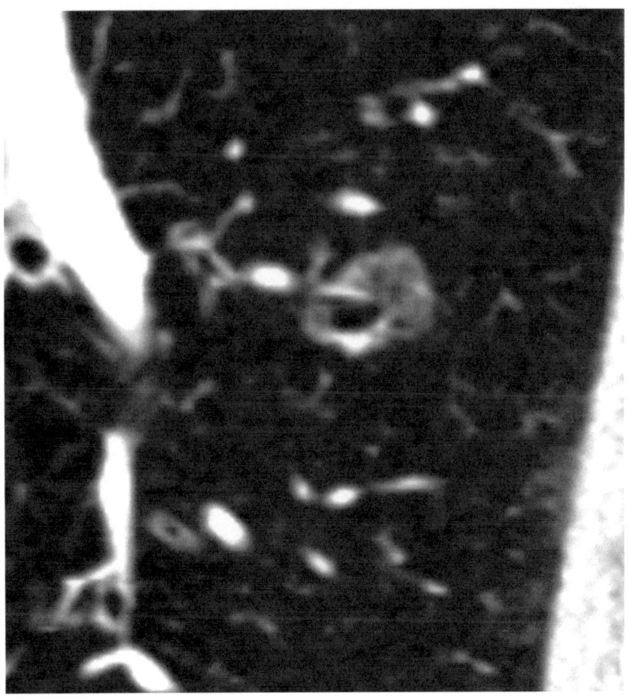

Fig. 18.3 A 79-year-old male, with a 1.6 cm subsolid nodule in the left lower lobe, demonstrating ground glass superiorly and a small solid component inferiorly

Diffuse pathologies such as emphysema increase in incidence with aging (Fig. 18.3). It is estimated that nearly one-third of smokers will develop emphysema by the age of 75, as determined by pulmonary function testing [19]. MDCT is felt to be a more sensitive tool in detection of underlying COPD when compared to standard pulmonary function

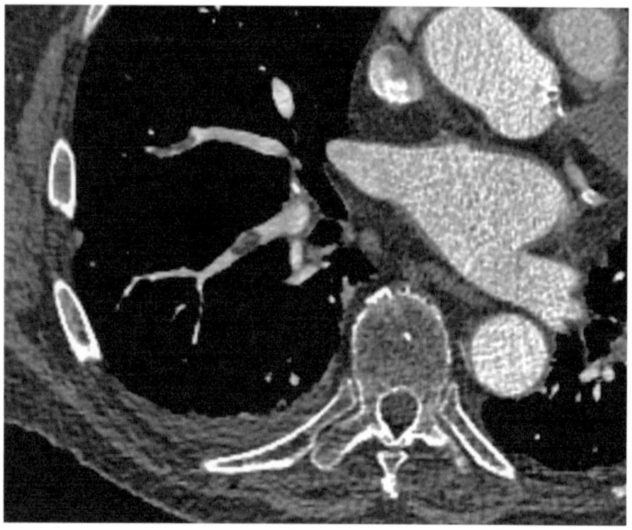

Fig. 18.4 A 71-year-old male patient with acute pulmonary emboli seen in the anterior and lateral segmental vessels to the right lower lobe

testing, although it does remain relatively insensitive to early stages of disease [20].

Pulmonary nodules are a common finding on CT examinations. Depending on the patient population evaluated, they may be detected in up to 51 % of MDCT examinations which image the entire chest [21]. Unlike many incidentally detected findings, well-established guidelines for follow-up of solid pulmonary nodules do exist [22].

There are a number of features which would indicate a nodule is definitively benign. The first of these is the presence of fat attenuation. If a solid lung lesion demonstrates attenuation of –40 to −120 HU, and no history of a primary fat-containing malignancy is present, such a lesion can be considered to be a hamartoma and will not require follow-up imaging [23]. However, as only 50 % of hamartomas will contain measurable fat attenuation on CT, this finding lacks sensitivity. The presence of calcification also helps to suggest a benign etiology. Patterns of calcification that are traditionally linked to benignity are diffuse, central, lamellated, or "popcorn" appearing. Diffuse, central, and lamellated calcification in a nodule is suggestive of a prior granulomatous process. Popcorn-appearing calcification is associated with hamartomas. A perifissural location of a solid nodule, i.e., contact with a fissural surface, is also a feature which suggests benignity [24, 25].

Unfortunately, features of benignity are present in the minority of incidentally discovered nodules (Fig. 18.4). Most lesions therefore must be considered to be indeterminate in nature. The only current guidelines for their management come from the Fleischner society with follow-up imaging recommended on the basis of nodule size and smoking history. It is important, however, to recognize that these are consensus guidelines, not supported by prospective randomized data. As well, the applicability of these guidelines in a cohort of patients being evaluated for TAVR is unclear [22]. What is known is that nodule size is strongly correlated with risk of malignancy, with nodules of <5 mm rarely being malignant (1 %), 5–10 mm nodules are more commonly malignant (6–28 %), and nodules of greater than 20 mm are often malignant (64–82 %) [26].

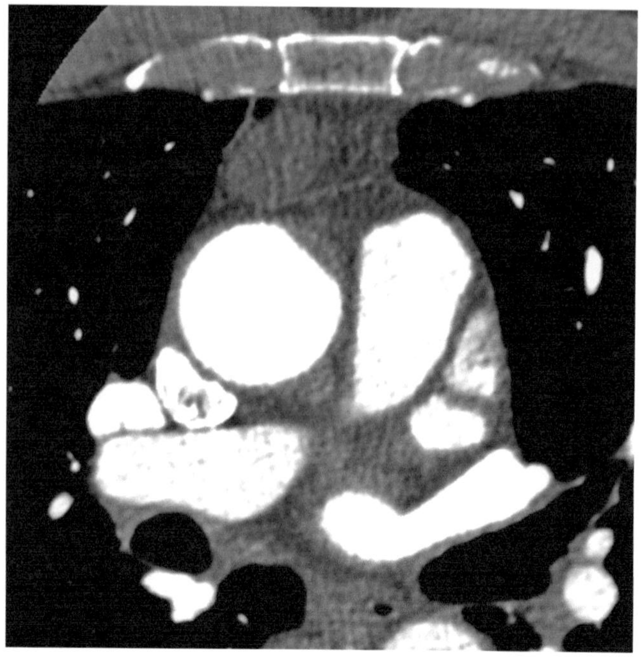

Fig. 18.5 A 78-year-old male, 2.1 cm presumed thymoma, and no associated clinical findings

Subsolid (semisolid and ground glass) nodules present more of a problem as widely accepted guidelines are not yet firmly established (Fig. 18.5). A 2009 paper by Godoy and Naidich provides interim guidelines for the management of subsolid nodules [27]. This paper suggests no follow-up is required for isolated ground glass lesions measuring less than 5 mm. Solitary ground glass lesions measuring 5–10 mm are followed at 3–6 months and if stable at yearly intervals for at least 3 years; if the lesion increases in size, a surgical opinion may be sought. For ground glass lesions greater than 10 mm in size, a follow-up at 3–6 months is recommended; if the lesion persists or increases in size, a surgical opinion is suggested. Mixed ground glass/solid nodules of any size are found to be malignant in up to one-third of cases, and a surgical opinion is suggested when these lesions are found [28]. Importantly, the biology of these lesions is typically indolent, and therefore, their impact on prognosis in the TAVR patient population is unclear. As such, the presence of such a lesion would not likely prevent TAVR. It may be most reasonable to seek a pulmonary referral for patients with such nodules >6 mm in size for risk assessment and to help provide guidance regarding the value of further imaging or biopsy.

Although the phase of contrast on an MDCT for TAVR planning is timed to optimally assess the systemic arterial

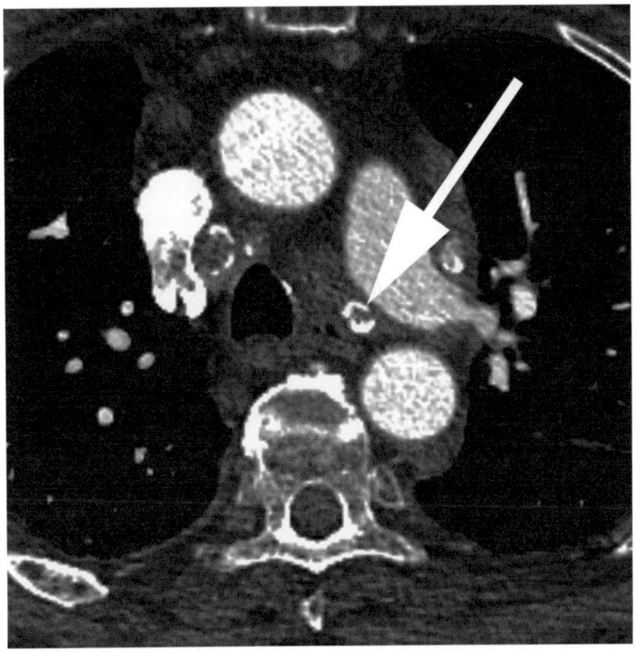

Fig. 18.6 A 82-year-old male, with multiple mediastinal lymph nodes. Some of which demonstrate calcification (*arrow*)

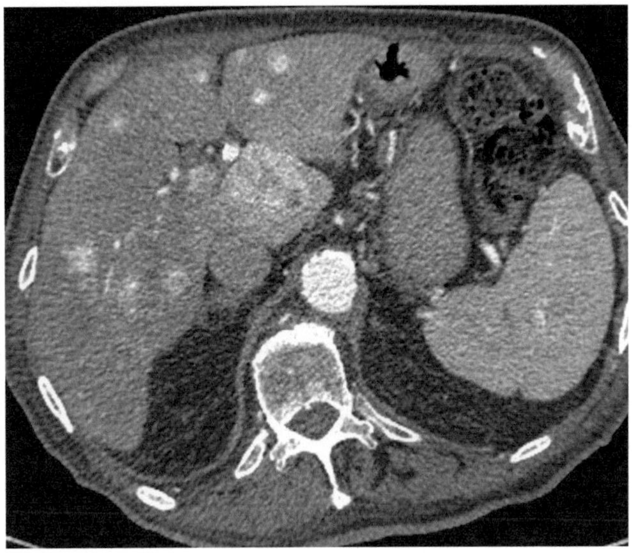

Fig. 18.7 A 85-year-old male patient with multiple avidly enhancing lesions in the liver; an enhancing lesion was also seen in the pancreas (not shown), felt to represent metastatic disease. A remote history of melanoma resection was obtained

structures, there is commonly adequate contrast in the pulmonary arterial system for the evaluation and exclusion of pulmonary emboli (Fig. 18.6). A meta-analysis of incidentally discovered pulmonary emboli suggests a prevalence of 2.6 % [29]. Hospitalization at the time of examination and the presence of cancer were potential predictors of pulmonary emboli (odd ratios 4.27 and 1.80, respectively) [29]. The clinical significance of such findings, especially if the clot burden is small (i.e., only subsegmental), is uncertain. Despite this uncertainty, convincing PE noted on a TAVR screening examination should be reported to the TAVR team on an urgent basis.

Evaluation of the Mediastinum

Incidentally discovered mediastinal lesions on MDCT are rare, occurring in less than 1 % of individuals having MDCT for the purposes of lung cancer screening [30]. In this study by Henschke et al., the most common incidental mediastinal lesion detected were lesions of thymic origin (Fig. 18.7). Thymomas account for the most common primary neoplasm of the mediastinum in patients over 40 year of age [31]. They tend to present in the fifth to sixth decades of life. Management remains controversial; however, surgical resection is suggested with lesions approaching 3 cm, due to propensity for recurrence and increase in technical difficulty in removing larger lesions [32]. Lesions smaller than 3 cm can be followed to ensure stability.

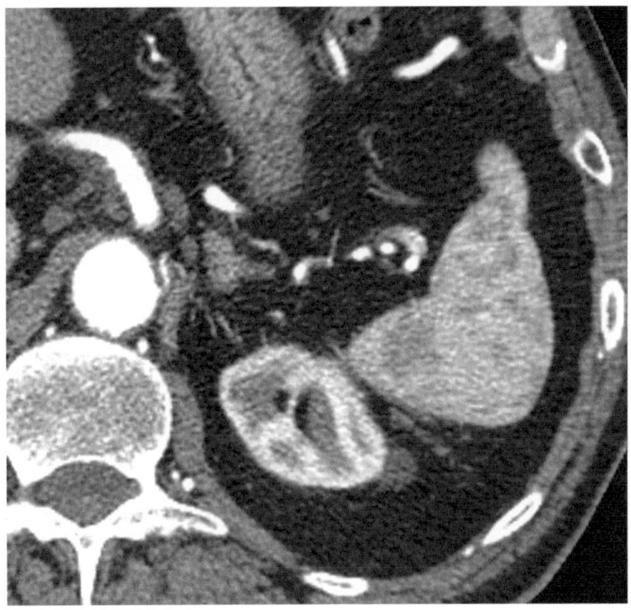

Fig. 18.8 A 67-year-old male patient in which the spleen demonstrates a typical serpiginous-appearing enhancement in the early arterial phase

Incidentally detected mediastinal or hilar adenopathy can be seen in up to 9 % of MDCT examinations of the chest [30]. Lymph nodes in the mediastinum and hilum are considered abnormal or pathologic when their short axis diameter is greater than 1 cm [33]. Evaluation of the lymph nodes for calcification, lung parenchymal findings, and patient history are important first steps in work-up, particularly in regard to discovery of a possible underlying cause (Fig. 18.8) [34].

Size of incidentally detected lymph nodes is correlated with risk of malignancy [35]. A Dutch study indicated that PET was rarely useful in evaluation of incidentally discovered lymph nodes as FDG avidity was demonstrated in 86 % of cases, none of which demonstrated malignancy on biopsy [33]. These researchers conclude that in the absence of a known primary malignancy workup of incidentally discovered adenopathy need not be aggressive, but provide no definitive recommendations with regard to follow-up. Despite the low likelihood of incidentally detected mediastinal adenopathy resulting in an ultimate diagnosis of malignancy if clinical uncertainty persists surgical or transbronchial tissue sampling may be required [34].

Evaluation of the Solid Abdominal Organs

Liver

Liver lesions are commonly identified at autopsy with an estimated prevalence of 50 % [36]. The evaluation and characterization of focal liver lesions on an arterial phase CT examination, such as a TAVR protocol, are fraught with pitfalls. Enhancement characteristics of a liver lesion are important in determination of the underlying pathology. Early arterially enhancing lesions have a broad differential diagnosis, including both benign entities (hemangioma and fibronodular hyperplasia) and lesions with malignant potential or frank malignancy (adenoma, hepatocellular carcinoma, and vascular metastases) (Fig. 18.9). In addition, on early phase examinations, an area of enhancement may represent a vascular shunt, also known as a transient hepatic attenuation difference (THAD). Definitive characterization of focal liver lesions is often not possible owing to the lack of portal venous or delayed phase examination. Another issue with detection of liver lesions on MDCT so soon after contrast has been injected is that lack of enhancement may indicate a truly hypovascular lesion, which may be a cyst (<20 HU), indeterminate solid lesion (>20 HU), or even a hypervascular lesion which is not categorized as such because the phase of contrast is too early for the lesion to demonstrate enhancement.

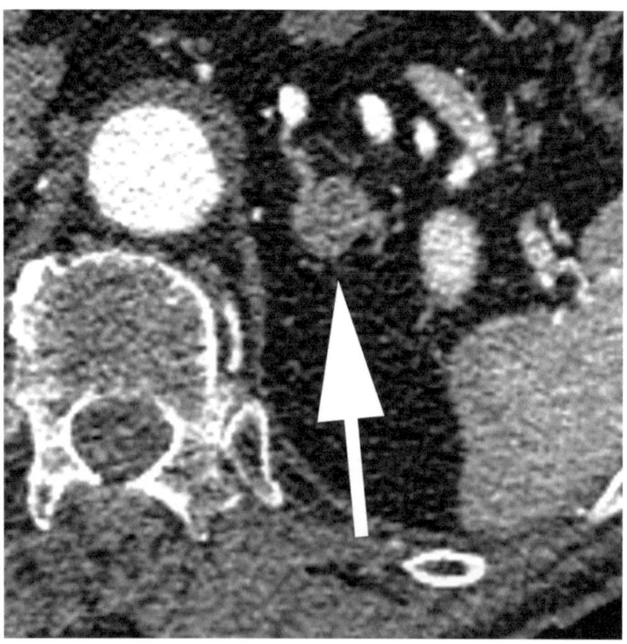

Fig. 18.9 A 84-year-old male patient with a 1.5 cm left adrenal lesion (*arrow*)

The ACR recently provided a guideline position paper for the management of incidentally detected liver lesions [1]. Lesion size, patient demographics, and patient risk are key factors in determining appropriate management. The ACR group uses 40 years of age as a discriminator between low and average risk patients. The high-risk group includes individuals of any age with known primary malignancy, cirrhosis, or other risk factors which predispose to hepatic malignancy such as hepatitis, sclerosing cholangitis, primary biliary cirrhosis, hemochromatosis, hemosiderosis, and hepatic dysfunction. If a lesion is felt to require further workup, modalities besides CT can be employed. Ultrasound is of use if based on the MDCT findings it is felt that the lesion is likely to be cystic in nature; however, if the lesion shows enhancement, ultrasound will have limited specificity compared to MRI. Biopsy of focal liver lesions is generally safe but does have an associated morbidity and mortality of 2–5 and 0.05 %, respectively [37].

In a patient without high-risk clinical features, lesion size and morphology are utilized as the primary discriminating factors. Lesions of any attenuation under 5 mm are not to be followed up and simply referred to as "indeterminate." Lesions 0.5 to 1.5 mm that have no suspicious features (ill-defined margins, enhancement, heterogeneity, enlargement from a prior exam) can be considered benign; lesions in this size range with suspicious features are followed up in 6 months with CT or MR. Lesions 0.5–1.5 mm which enhance avidly and rapidly (i.e., lesions enhancing in the arterial phase) can be considered benign. Lesions over 1.5 cm are considered benign if low attenuation (<20 HU) with no suspicious features. Further evaluation with MRI is suggested in patients over 40 years of age if any suspicious features are present. Avidly enhancing lesions over 1.5 cm may be considered benign in low-risk patients of any age, although, if possible, evaluation with MR may be useful [1].

In high-risk patients, recommendations are to either determine the lesion is benign via further imaging or to obtain a definitive diagnosis via biopsy if the lesion cannot be determined to be nonaggressive and is over 1.5 cm [1].

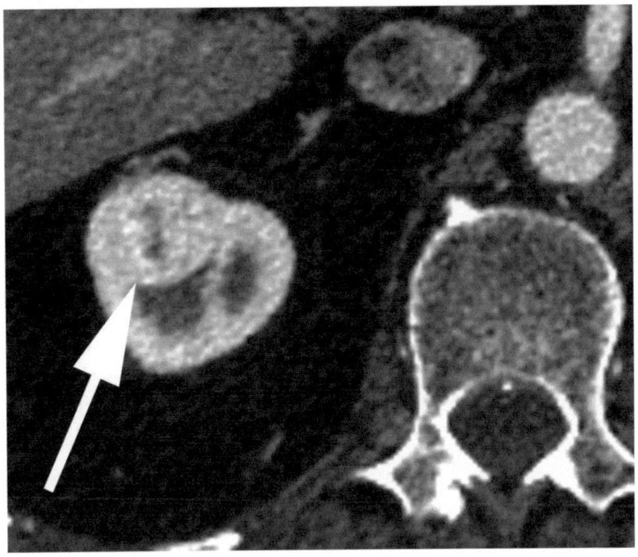

Fig. 18.10 A 88-year-old male patient with a heterogeneous solid right renal lesion measuring 2.5 cm (*arrow*), presumed to represent a renal cell carcinoma

Spleen

The spleen is a particularly difficult solid organ to evaluate on an arterial phase MDCT due to the varied and occasionally bizarre and heterogeneous enhancement during this phase of imaging (Fig. 18.10). Thankfully, the spleen is a rare site of isolated metastatic disease and an uncommon location of primary malignancy. Splenic incidentalomas tend to be rare and when found are usually benign in the absence of a known history of malignancy [38, 39].

Pancreas

Incidentally detected pancreatic lesions pose multiple issues regarding management. Simple cystic lesions are commonly detected in asymptomatic individuals (up to 3 % of abdominal CT examinations) [40]. Additionally, even when not demonstrating concerning morphology (enhancing septa, nodular solid component, associated pancreatic duct dilatation), there is a reasonable chance the lesion will eventually demonstrate malignant pathology [41]. MRI exams of the abdomen detect pancreatic cysts in nearly 20 % of cases [42]. This discrepancy between imaging modalities provides fodder for the argument that such lesions are unlikely to alter mortality.

One explanation for this is that simple cystic pancreatic malignancies grow extremely slowly, if at all. This knowledge of the natural history has lead to the body of evidence that such lesions can be managed with surveillance [43].

Size of a cystic lesion and symptomatology are important factors in determining management. In the absence of symptoms, it is highly likely that a cystic lesion under 3 cm is benign [44]. It is felt that lesions under 2 cm need only be followed up at 1 year to ensure stability. Lesions 2–3 cm should have a noninvasive study (MRI with contrast and MRCP). The ACR's Incidental Findings Committee suggests aspiration can be attempted on lesions greater than 3 cm [1].

While lesions greater than 3 cm may be considered for operative management if they cannot be characterized as a stable IPMN or serous cystadenoma, this recommendation may be at odds with other studies evaluating management of such lesions in patients such as those screened for TAVR. A study by Weinberg et al. suggests that in an older patient cohort management beyond surveillance is a detriment to quality of life for asymptomatic patients with pancreatic cysts [45]. This is an important concept to keep in mind with typical TAVR patients.

Solid pancreatic lesions are generally considered malignant until proven otherwise. Lesions that enhance in the arterial phase would include islet cell tumors and metastatic deposits to the pancreas from a vascular primary tumor (i.e., renal cell or melanoma). A history of a primary malignancy or endocrine symptoms should be elicited when such lesions are discovered incidentally on MDCT.

Adrenals

Incidentally discovered adrenal lesions are common, occurring in up to 7 % of MDCTs which image this area [46]. While the adrenal gland is a common site of metastatic disease, the vast majority of incidentally discovered adrenal lesions, even in patients with known malignancy, are nonhyperfunctioning adrenal adenomas [46]. In patients with no known malignancy, greater than 98 % of incidentally discovered adrenal lesions are benign [47]. If further management is felt to be warranted, the first step would be to evaluate the adrenal lesion for findings that would suggest a specific benign diagnosis, i.e., macroscopic fat to suggest a myelolipoma. Given that a TAVR MDCT is performed with the use of iodinated contrast in the arterial phase, caution should be given with regard to assessment of lesion attenuation (Fig. 18.11). On a non-contrast MDCT, if the adrenal lesion in question is homogeneous and measures less than or equal to 10 HU, it can be assumed to represent a lipid rich adenoma, with no further workup suggested [1]. If the Hounsfield measurement is greater than 10, either an MR or contrast-enhanced CT with washout is performed. Although the washout protocol CT is the ultimate diagnostic imaging tool in assessment of adrenal lesions, MRI can be helpful in this algorithm and is an attractive option, especially in younger patients where radiation dose is a concern. Even in lesions that are not "lipid rich" on the basis of the non-contrast CT,

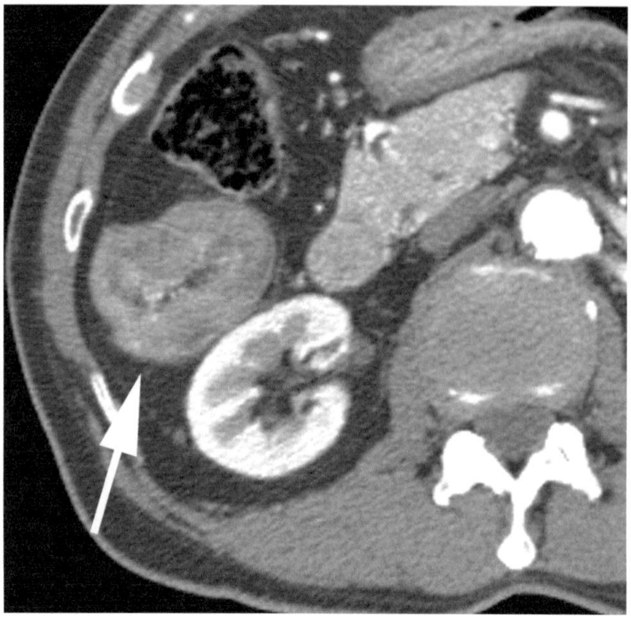

Fig. 18.11 A 84-year-old male patient with marked circumferential thickening of the hepatic flexure of the colon (*arrow*). A colonic adenocarcinoma was subsequently resected

a percentage of them will still demonstrate signal loss on out-of-phase MRI, allowing a diagnosis of an adrenal adenoma to be made with confidence [48].

The contrast washout or "adrenal protocol" CT works on the principle that adrenal adenomas will retain contrast for only a short period of time, as compared to metastatic lesions which demonstrate prolonged contrast retention. An absolute washout of greater than or equal to 60 % (enhanced HU – 15 min delayed HU)/(enhanced HU – unenhanced HU) × 100 or a relative washout value (used when a non-contrast HU is unavailable) greater than or equal to 40 % (enhanced HU – 15 min delayed HU)/enhanced HU × 100 is diagnostic of an adrenal adenoma with a sensitivity and specificity of 98 and 92 %, respectively [49].

Given the compelling data that incidentally detected adrenal lesions <4 cm in size, in the absence of a known malignancy, are almost always benign, the benefit of further work-up and imaging of these lesions in the setting of severe aortic stenosis is almost certainly extremely low [1, 47].

Kidneys

Renal masses are commonly detected incidentally when the abdomen is imaged with MDCT. In general, renal masses should be divided into cystic or solid lesions. Cystic lesions are evaluated according to the time-tested approach outlined by Bosniak [50]. The Bosniak classification of renal cysts includes five categories (Table 18.1). The management decisions are based on not only the morphologic appearances of the lesion, but also the patient's demographics. Patients with limited life expectancy have recommendations that tend to result in less aggressive workup. In general, Bosniak classifications of I and II are benign, not requiring further evaluation. Bosniak IIF lesions have a low likelihood of malignancy but contain some features that would indicate follow-up is necessary. In patients with a limited life expectancy, it is not unreasonable to ignore Bosniak IIF lesions [51]. Bosniak III lesions are indeterminate, and although many lesions in this category are benign, malignancy cannot be excluded on the basis of imaging alone [50]. Percutaneous biopsy of Bosniak III lesions is controversial, but may be a reasonable consideration in a patient with comorbid conditions [52]. In a patient with limited life expectancy it remains a viable option to manage these lesions expectantly [51]. Bosniak IV lesions carry a high risk of malignancy and are managed surgically in a healthy cohort, but may still be managed with active surveillance in a patient with limited life expectancy.

Table 18.1 Bosniak classification system for renal cystic lesions

Bosniak category	Computed tomographic imaging features
I	Thin wall, no septa, no calcification, no solid component, <20 HU
II	Few thin septa, fine calcification, or short segment of bulkier calcification, lesion>20 HU but ≤3 cm with no enhancement
IIF	Multiple thin septa, minimal smooth thickening of the wall or septa, bulky calcification, no measurable enhancement, intrarenal lesion >20 HU and >3 cm
III	Thickened irregular wall or septa. Measurable enhancement, but no nodular solid component
IV	Same as category III but also demonstrating enhancing soft tissue components separate from the wall or septa

Solid renal lesions detected on MDCT are considered malignant until proven otherwise, with some important exceptions. It is essential to assess the lesion in question carefully for the presence of fat attenuation. A noncalcified lesion with internal fat attenuation can be safely considered to be an angiomyolipoma (AML) [1]. Not all angiomyolipomas contain fat detectable with CT or MR. These lesions tend to be hyperdense on non-contrast CT and demonstrate low T2 signal on MR with evidence of loss of signal on out-of-phase gradient imaging. Although a lipid poor AML cannot be definitively diagnosed even with these characteristics, in a patient with significant comorbidities, such morphology may be enough to guide conservative management [53]. As with cystic lesions, solid renal lesions detected incidentally in a patient population with limited life expectancy mandate different management recommendations. In general lesions under 1 cm can be safely observed, lesions above 1.5 cm can be followed, but there is insufficient evidence to be certain this is truly a safe strategy [53]. Biopsy is an option if it felt that operative management may be necessary in such a patient population, although this remains controversial [54]. In our practice, a urology opinion is sought for all Bosniak IV and nonspecific solid lesions to help provide a reasonable management strategy balancing the risk of malignancy and its likely prognosis with the age of the patient and prognosis related to aortic stenosis.

Evaluation of the Hollow Viscous and Retroperitoneum

Non-active diverticular disease of the sigmoid colon is the most common incidentally detected abnormality of the bowel on MDCT exams of the abdomen and pelvis [10]. The incidence of diverticulosis increases with patient age and would be expected to be very common in the TAVR cohort. More concerning bowel pathologies, namely, colon cancer, are also detected incidentally on MDCT. MDCT for evaluation of the abdominal aorta demonstrates colonic malignancy in 0.3 % of cases [6, 10].

Colonic wall thickening is a nonspecific finding; however, in asymptomatic patients colonic malignancy was discovered on endoscopy in 20 % of patients with incidental luminal wall thickening [55]. A separate study diagnosed malignancy at endoscopy in 11 % of asymptomatic patients with wall thickening seen on MDCT involving the colon, with 28 % of patients referred to colonoscopy for thickened bowel have a normal endoscopic evaluation [56]. Referral for endoscopy was felt to be justified given these findings on MDCT in this patient cohort with an average age of the cohorts in these studies of 59 and 69 years, respectively. In general, care must be taken to not construe bowel peristalsis as a focal lesion; however, focal measurable colonic lesions should not be ignored.

Retroperitoneal lesions are not commonly detected as incidental findings on MDCT according to a number of series evaluating the abdominal aorta [6, 10]. With an incidence of less than 1 %, such lesions will not be discussed further here. When discovered solid lesions in the retroperitoneum tend to represent either adenopathy or sarcomatous lesions.

Evaluation of Adnexal Structures

While MDCT is useful for detection of fat attenuation and calcification, when diagnosing an ovarian teratoma, it is otherwise preferable to have adnexal lesions evaluated with either ultrasound or MRI.

Ovarian cancer remains the leading cause of death related to gynecological cancer in North America. Unfortunately, screening has not resulted in improved mortality from this malignancy. One reason for this is that benign adnexal lesions in postmenopausal patients are fairly common (3–4 %), while the incidence of ovarian malignancy discovered either by screening or incidentally is low [57].

A study evaluating incidentally detected ovarian lesions in woman over 50 years of age undergoing a screening CT colonography (CTC) highlights this point [58]. This study detected indeterminate adnexal lesions in 4.1 % of cohort of women with an average age of 57.2 years. None of the indeterminate adnexal lesions resulted in a diagnosis of invasive ovarian cancer at further workup; however, four patients who did not have an adnexal lesion detected on the initial CTC where ultimately diagnosed with ovarian malignancy during follow-up (0.15 %).

Recommendations for work-up of adnexal lesions in patients in the age range in which TAVR is currently performed are problematic. Consensus guidelines for the management of adnexal cystic lesions are available [59]. Although potentially more aggressive than may be necessary, in a female patient with typical demographics of a TAVR candidate, recommending ultrasound evaluation of an incidentally detected adnexal lesion, and subsequently following consensus guidelines, is likely prudent.

Conclusion

Incidental lesions discovered on MDCT are common in patients undergoing evaluation pre-TAVR. Given the limited life expectancy of many patients currently undergoing TAVR, how these findings should be managed remains somewhat confounding. This chapter discusses common incidentally discovered abnormalities on MDCT in numerous body systems and provides general management recommendations, based on current available literature. The approach to incidental findings in this patient population will continue to evolve as the natural history of patients who receive percutaneously placed valves is further delineated and our experience in this field grows.

References

1. Berland L, Silverman SG, Gore RM, Mayo-Smith WW, Megibow AJ, Yee J, et al. Managing incidental findings on abdominal CT: white paper of the ACR incidental findings committee. J Am Coll Radiol. 2010;7:754–73.
2. Berland L. The American College of Radiology strategy for managing incidental findings on abdominal computed tomography. Radiol Clin North Am. 2011;49:237–43.
3. Lumbreras B, Donat L, Hernandez-Aguado I. Incidental findings in imaging diagnostic tests: a systematic review. Br J Radiol. 2010;83: 276–89.
4. Ding A, Eisenberg JD, Pandharipande PV. The economic burden of incidentally detected findings. Radiol Clin North Am. 2011;49: 257–65.
5. Ben-Dor I, Waksman R, Hanna HN, Raizon A, Satler LF, Torquson R, et al. Utility of radiologic review for noncardiac

findings on multislice computed tomography in patients with severe aortic stenosis evaluated for transcatheter aortic valve implantation. Am J Cardiol. 2010;105(10):1461–4.
6. Naidu SG, Hara AK, Brandis AR, Stone WM. Incidence of highly important extravascular findings detected on CT angiography of the abdominal aorta and lower extremities. Am J Roentgenol. 2010; 194:1630–4.
7. Leon MB, Smith CR, Mack M, Miller DC, Moses JW, Svensson LG, et al. Transcatheter aortic-valve implantation for aortic stenosis in patients who cannot undergo surgery. N Eng J Med. 2010;363: 1597–607.
8. Makkar RR, Fontana GP, Jilaihawi H, Kapadia S, Pichard AD, Douglas PS, et al. Transcatheter aortic-valve replacement for inoperable severe aortic stenosis. New Eng J Med. 2012;366: 1696–704.
9. Reynolds MR, Magnuson EA, Lei Y, Leon MB, Smith CR, Svensson LG, et al. Health-related quality of life after transcatheter aortic valve replacement in inoperable patients with severe aortic stenosis. Circulation. 2011;124:1964–72.
10. Iezzi R, Cotroneo AR, Filippone A, Di Fabio F, Merlino B, Bonomo L. Extravascular incidental findings at multislice CT angiography of the abdominal aorta and lower extremities: a retrospective review study. Abdom Imaging. 2007;32:489–94.
11. Hussain A, Gordon-Dixon A, Almusawy H, Sinha P, Desai A. The incidence and outcome of incidental breast lesions detected by computed tomography. Ann R Coll Surg Engl. 2010;92:124–6.
12. Porter G, Steel J, Paisley K, Watkins R, Holgate C. Incidental breast masses detected by computed tomography: are any imaging features predictive of malignancy? Clin Radiol. 2009;64:529–33.
13. Moyle P, Sonoda L, Britton P, Sinnatamby R. Incidental breast lesions detected on CT: what is their significance? Br J Radiol. 2010;83:233–40.
14. Yi JG, Kim SJ, Marom EM, Park JH, Jung SI, Lee MW. Chest CT of incidental breast lesions. J Thorac Imaging. 2008;23(2):148–55.
15. Woo EK, Mansoubi H, Alyas F. Incidental vertebral fractures on multidetector CT images of the chest: prevalence and recognition. Clin Radiol. 2008;63:160–4.
16. Bartalena T, Giannelli G, Rinaldi MF, Rimondi E, Rinaldi G, Sverzellati N, et al. Prevalence of thoracolumbar vertebral fractures on multidetector CT: underreporting by radiologists. Eur J Radiol. 2009;69(3):555–9.
17. Ross PD. Clinical consequences of vertebral fractures. Am J Med. 1997;18(103):30s–43.
18. Lindsay R, Silverman SL, Cooper C, Hanley DA, Barton I, Broy SB, et al. Risk of new vertebral fracture in the year following a fracture. JAMA. 2001;285(3):320–3.
19. Pelkonen M, Notkola IL, Nissinen A, Tukiainen H, Koskela H. Thirty-year cumulative incidence of chronic bronchitis and COPD in relation to 30-year pulmonary function and 40-year mortality: a follow-up in middle-aged rural men. Chest. 2006;130(4):1129–37.
20. Remy-Jardin M, Remy J, Gosselin B, Copin MC, Wurtz A, Duhamel A. Sliding thin slab, minimum intensity projection technique in the diagnosis of emphysema: histopathologic-CT correlation. Radiology. 1996;200(3):665–71.
21. Edey AJ, Hansell DM. Incidentally detected small pulmonary nodules on CT. Clin Radiol. 2009;64:872–84.
22. MacMahon H, Austin JH, Gamsu G, Herold CJ, Jett JR, Naidich DP, et al. Guidelines for management of small pulmonary nodules detected on CT scans: a statement from the Fleischner Society. Radiology. 2005;237(2):395–400.
23. Hansen CP, Holtveg H, Francis D, Rasch L, Bertelsen S. Pulmonary hamartoma. J Thorac Cardiovasc Surg. 1992;104(3):674–8.
24. Ahn MI, Gleeson TG, Chan IH, McWilliams AM, Macdonald SL, Lam S, et al. Perifissural nodules seen at CT screening for lung cancer. Radiol. 2010;254(3):949–56.
25. Xu DM, van der Zaag-Loonen HJ, Oudkerk M, Wang Y, Vliegenthart R, Scholten ET, et al. Smooth or attached solid indeterminate nodules detected at baseline CT screening in the NELSON study: cancer risk during 1 year of follow-up. Radiology. 2009;250(1):264–72.
26. Wahidi MM, Govert JA, Goudar RK, Gould MK, McCrory DC. Evidence for the treatment of patients with pulmonary nodules: when is it lung cancer?: ACCP evidence-based clinical practice guidelines (2nd edition). Chest. 2007;132:94S–107.
27. Godoy MC, Naidich DP. Subsolid pulmonary nodules and the spectrum of peripheral adenocarcinomas of the lung: recommended interim guidelines for assessment and management. Radiology. 2009;253(3):606–22.
28. Henschke CI, Yankelevitz DF, Mircheva R, McGuinness G, McCauley D, Miettinen OS. CT screening for lung cancer: frequency and significance of part solid and nonsolid nodules. Am J Roentgenol. 2002;178(5):1053–7.
29. Dentali F, Ageno W, Becattini C, Galli L, Gianni M, Riva N, et al. Prevalence and clinical history of incidental, asymptomatic pulmonary embolism: a meta-analysis. Thromb Res. 2010;125(6):518–22.
30. Henschke CI, Lee IJ, Wu N, Farooqi A, Khan A, Yankelevitz D, et al. CT screening for lung cancer: prevalence and incidence of mediastinal masses. Radiology. 2006;239(2):586–90.
31. Nasseri F, Eftekhari F. Clinical and radiologic review of the normal and abnormal thymus: pearls and pitfalls. Radiographics. 2010; 30(2):413–28.
32. Davenport E, Malthaner RA. The role of surgery in the management of thymoma: a systematic review. Ann Thorac Surg. 2008;86(2): 673–84.
33. Stigt JA, Boers JE, Oostdijk AH, van den Berg JK, Groen HJM. Mediastinal incidentalomas. J Thorac Oncol. 2011;6:1345–9.
34. Alpert JB, Naidich DP. Imaging of incidental findings on thoracic computed tomography. Radiol Clin North Am. 2011;49(2):267–89.
35. Wiersema MJ, Vazquez-Sequeiros E, Wiersema LM. Evaluation of mediastinal lymphadenopathy with endoscopic US-guided fine-needle aspiration biopsy. Radiology. 2001;219:252–7.
36. Washington K. Masses of the liver. In: Odze R, Goldblum JR, editors. Surgical pathology of the GI tract, liver, biliary tract and pancreas. 2nd ed. New York: Elsevier; 2009. p. 657–789.
37. Appelbaum L, Kane RA, Kruskal JB, Romero J, Sosna J. Focal hepatic lesions: US-guided biopsy-lessons from review of cytologic and pathologic examination results. Radiology. 2009;250:453–8.
38. Ahmed S, Horton KM, Fishman EK. Splenic incidentalomas. Radiol Clin North Am. 2011;49(2):323–47.
39. Ekeh AP, Walusimbi M, Brigham E, Woods RJ, McCarthy MC. The prevalence of incidental findings on abdominal computed tomography scans of trauma patients. J Emerg Med. 2010;38(4):484–9.
40. Laffan TA, Horton KM, Klein AP, Berlanstein B, Siegelman SS, Kawamoto S, et al. Prevalence of unsuspected pancreatic cysts on MDCT. Am J Roentgenol. 2008;191(3):802–7.
41. Levy P, Jouannaud V, O'Toole D, Couvelard A, Vullierme MP, Palazzo L, et al. Natural history of intraductal papillary mucinous tumors of the pancreas: actuarial risk of malignancy. Clin Gastroenterol Hepatol. 2006;4(4):460–8.
42. Zhang XM, Mitchell DG, Dohke M, Holland GA, Parker L. Pancreatic cysts: depiction on single shot fast spin echo MR images. Radiology. 2002;223:547–53.
43. Lahav M, Maor Y, Avidan B, Novis B, Bar-Meir S. Nonsurgical management of asymptomatic incidental pancreatic cysts. Clin Gastroenterol Hepatol. 2007;5(7):813–7.
44. Lee CJ, Scheimann J, Anderson MA, Hines OJ, Reber HA, Farrell J, et al. Risk of malignancy in resected cystic tumors of the pancreas < or = 3 cm in size: is it safe to observe asymptomatic patients? A multi-institutional report. J Gastrointest Surg. 2008; 12(2):234–42.

45. Weinberg BM, Spiegel BM, Tomlinson JS, Farrell JJ. Asymptomatic pancreatic cystic neoplasms: maximizing survival and quality of life using Markov-based clinical nomograms. Gastroenterology. 2010;138(2):531–40.
46. Young Jr WF. Clinical practice. The incidentally discovered adrenal mass. N Engl J Med. 2007;356:601–10.
47. Song JH, Chaudry FS, Mayo-Smith WW. The incidental adrenal mass on CT: prevalence of adrenal disease in 1,049 consecutive adrenal masses in patients with no known malignancy. Am J Roentgenol. 2008;190:1163–8.
48. Haider MA, Ghai S, Jhaveri K, Lockwood G. Chemical shift MR imaging of hyperattenuating (>10HU) adrenal masses: does it still have a role? Radiology. 2004;231(3):711–6.
49. Caoili EM, Korobkin M, Francis IR, Cohan RH, Platt JF, Dunnick NR, et al. Adrenal masses: characterization with combined unenhanced and delayed enhanced CT. Radiology. 2002;222(3):629–33.
50. Israel GM, Bosniak MA. How I do it: evaluating renal masses. Radiology. 2005;236:441–50.
51. Cambpell SC, Novick AC, Beldegrun A, Blute ML, Chow GK, Derweesh IH, et al. Guideline for management of the clinical T1 renal mass. J Urol. 2009;182(4):1271–9.
52. Harisinghani MG, Maher MM, Gervais DA, McGovern F, Hahn P, Jhaveri K, et al. Incidence of malignancy in complex cystic renal masses (Bosniak category III): should imaging-guided biopsy precede surgery? Am J Roentgenol. 2003;180(3):755–8.
53. Silverman SG, Israel GM, Herts BR, Richie JP. Management of the incidental renal mass. Radiology. 2008;249:16–31.
54. Thompson RH, Kurta JM, Kaag M, Tickoo SK, Kundu S, Katz D, et al. Tumor size is associated with malignant potential in renal carcinoma cases. J Urol. 2009;181(5):2033–6.
55. Tellez-Avila FI, Garcia-Osogobio S, Chavez-Tapia NC, Ramirez-Luna MA, Franco-Guzman A, Sosa-Lozano A, et al. Utility of endoscopy in patients with incidental gastrointestinal luminal wall thickening detected with CT. Surg Endosc. 2009; 23(10):2191–6.
56. Moratis D, Singh P, Jayadevan R, Cayten CG. Colonic wall thickening on computed tomography scan and clinical correlation. Does it suggest the presence of an underlying neoplasia? Am Surg. 2006;72(3):269–71.
57. McDonald JM, Modesitt SC. The incidental postmenopausal adnexal mass. Clin Obstet Gynecol. 2006;49(3):506–16.
58. Pickhardt PJ, Hanson ME. Incidental adnexal masses detected at low-dose unenhanced CT in asymptomatic women age 50 and older: implications for clinical management and ovarian cancer screening. Radiology. 2010;257(1):144–50.
59. Levine D, Brown DL, Andreotti RF, Benacerraf B, Benson CB, Brewster WR, et al. Management of asymptomatic ovarian and other adnexal cysts imaged at US. Society of radiologists in ultrasound consensus conference statement. Ultrasound Q. 2010;26(3): 121–31.

19 Transcatheter Aortic Valve Replacement in Patients with Chronic Kidney Disease: Pre-procedural Assessment and Procedural Techniques to Minimize Risk for Acute Kidney Injury

Israel M. Barbash, Danny Dvir, Wm. Guy Weigold, Lowell F. Satler, Ron Waksman, and Augusto D. Pichard

Abstract

Transcatheter aortic valve replacement (TAVR) offers treatment for high-risk patients with severe symptomatic aortic stenosis [1, 2]. Currently, TAVR is performed in high-risk patients with multiple comorbidities and advanced age. These patients frequently have abnormal baseline renal function and are therefore at increased risk for acute kidney injury (AKI) after TAVR due to the significant hemodynamic changes during the procedure and use of contrast agents [3].

AKI following TAVR is a frequent complication that occurs in >10 % of patients. These patients suffer from significantly worse outcome with higher rates of mortality in patients who develop AKI [4–7]. Based on this current evidence, it is imperative to minimize the risks for kidney injury during the TAVR evaluation process and during the TAVR procedure itself. In this chapter, we will summarize and suggest advanced approaches to minimize AKI based on the current evidence base and our own institutional experience.

Keywords

Acute Kidney Injury (AKI) • Iodine • Contrast medium • Contrast induced nephropathy • Low contrast protocols • Direct aortic injection

I.M. Barbash, MD
Department of Interventional Cardiology,
Washington Hospital Center, 110 Irving Street, NW, Suite 4B-1,
Washington, DC 20010, USA

Department of Cath Lab, Washington Hospital Center,
10 Irving St, Washington, DC 20010, USA
e-mail: ibarbash@gmail.com

D. Dvir, MD • W.G. Weigold, MD, FACC, FSCCT
Department of Interventional Cardiology,
Washington Hospital Center, 110 Irving Street,
NW, Suite 4B-1, Washington, DC 20010, USA

Department of Interventional Cardiology,
MedStar Washington Hospital Center,
110 Irving Street, NW, Suite 4B-1, Washington, DC 20010, USA
e-mail: danny.dvir@gmail.com; guy.weigold@medstar.net

L.F. Satler
Department of Interventional Cardiology,
Washington Hospital Center, 110 Irving Street,
NW, Suite 4B-1, Washington, DC 20010, USA

R. Waksman, MD, FACC
Department of Interventional Cardiology,
Washington Hospital Center, 110 Irving Street, NW,
Suite 4B-1, Washington, DC 20010, USA

Department of Cardiology, MedStar Washington Hospital Center,
MedStar Heart Institute, Georgetown University,
110 Irving Street, NW, Suite 4B-1, Washington, DC 20010, USA
e-mail: ron.waksman@medstar.net

A.D. Pichard, MD, FACC (✉)
Department of Interventional Cardiology,
Washington Hospital Center, 110 Irving Street,
NW, Suite 4B-1, Washington, DC 20010, USA

Department of Cardiology, Georgetown University Medical School,
MedStar Washington Hospital Center, Washington, DC, USA
e-mail: guspichard@gmail.com

J.K. Min et al. (eds.), *Multimodality Imaging for Transcatheter Aortic Valve Replacement*,
DOI 10.1007/978-1-4471-2798-7_19, © Springer-Verlag London 2014

Prognostic Significance of AKI

For patients undergoing TAVR, the Valve Academic Research Consortium (VARC) criteria [8] recently defined AKI as a 150–200 % or ≥0.3 mg/dl (≥26.4 mmol/l) increase in serum creatinine when compared to baseline. In an analysis of TAVR patients at our institution, we observed that patients who developed post-procedural AKI according to the VARC criteria had significantly worse outcome, as indicated by longer intensive care unit hospitalization (104 h vs. 29 h; $p<0.001$), need for blood transfusion (63 % vs. 39 %, $p=0.04$), and nonsignificant higher rates of any bleeding (42 % vs. 33 %, $p=0.48$). The in-hospital (21 % vs. 4 %, $p=0.007$) and 30-day mortality (29 % vs. 7 %, $p=0.004$) rates were also significantly higher among AKI patients when compared to patients who did not develop AKI after the procedure, reflecting an almost four- to five-fold increase in mortality [3]. These findings are corroborated by multiple studies [4–7]. These data are the rationale for employing multiple strategies in order to reduce the risks for kidney injury among these high-risk patients.

Our understanding of the pathophysiology of AKI after contrast administration suggests a complex interplay between renovascular and renotubular effects, making it unlikely that a single intervention will be uniformly successful for its prevention. Thus, the recognition of subgroups at high risk for post-procedure AKI is crucial in the management of these patients. In our own experience, we have observed that patients who undergo the transapical approach for TAVR are at significantly increased risk for AKI. One apparent explanation for this observation may relate to a bias related to patient selection for transapical TAVR. Typically, such patients selected for the transapical approach are afflicted with advanced peripheral vascular atherosclerosis with highly calcified, tortuous, and generally smaller aortoiliofemoral vessels. The presence of such advanced peripheral disease may be associated with a higher prevalence of calcium plaques in the aorta and the aortic valve, both of which may embolize to the kidneys during the procedure. Further, simply the presence of renal arterial atherosclerosis may indeed affect the incidence of AKI. Other patient characteristics reported to be associated with increased risk for AKI include elevated baseline creatinine levels, hypertension, chronic lung disease, amount of contrast used, number of blood transfusions, post-procedural thrombocytopenia, and severe inflammatory response syndrome [4, 7, 9, 10].

Pre-procedural Evaluation: Vascular Access

Angiography

Abdominal aortography may serve as an excellent screening tool for patients undergoing TAVR. For current transcatheter heart valve platforms, a minimal luminal diameter required is 6 mm. However, the current Food and Drug Administration-approved balloon-expandable transcatheter heart valve requires larger vessel diameters (>7 mm for the 23-mm valve and >8 mm for the 26-mm valve). Excess vessel tortuosity can prevent the large sheath (22 or 24 F) from advancing into the abdominal aorta.

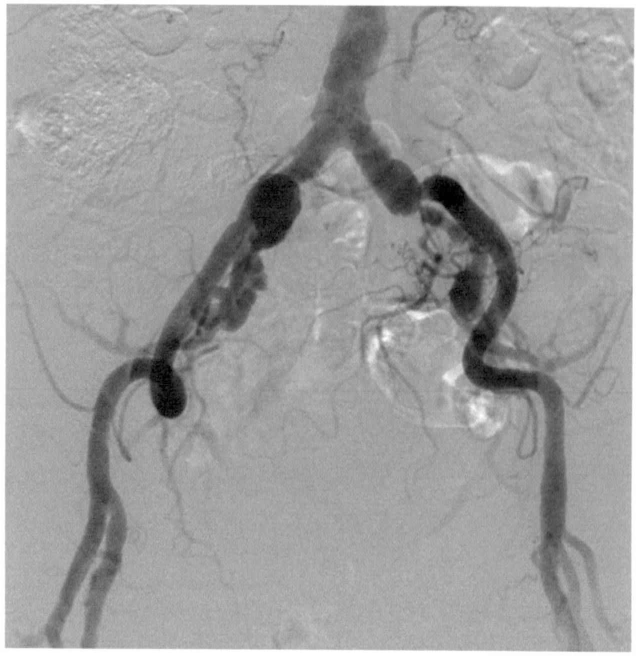

Fig. 19.1 Tortuous iliofemoral arteries by angiography

Tortuosity with large arterial lumens in the absence of calcification typically does not pose a problem when using large sheaths (Fig. 19.1). Thus, tortuosity without calcification that is straightened by a wire does not preclude the procedure. Notably, however, calcification is often not well appreciated by angiography. There are many cases where the aortoiliofemoral angiography demonstrates apparently adequate vessels for percutaneous access, but computed tomography (CT) reveals severe arterial calcification, thereby altering the decision regarding arterial access (Fig. 19.2).

Eltchaninoff et al. [11] suggested an "angiography alone" technique for assessing the suitability of iliac and femoral arteries for TAVR. They evaluated the iliac and femoral arteries of 135 patients by distal aortogram with bilateral iliofemoral runoff in the anteroposterior projection using a low dose of contrast (30 cc). Using a combination of vessel size, tortuosity, and calcification, these authors classified patients as suitable or not for the transfemoral approach. The authors proposed that patients who failed this "screening"—and thus were deemed unsuitable vessels according to the angiography—would not need to undergo CT angiography and, hence, receive additional contrast. These patients would instead be recommended to undergo TAVR via alternative routes.

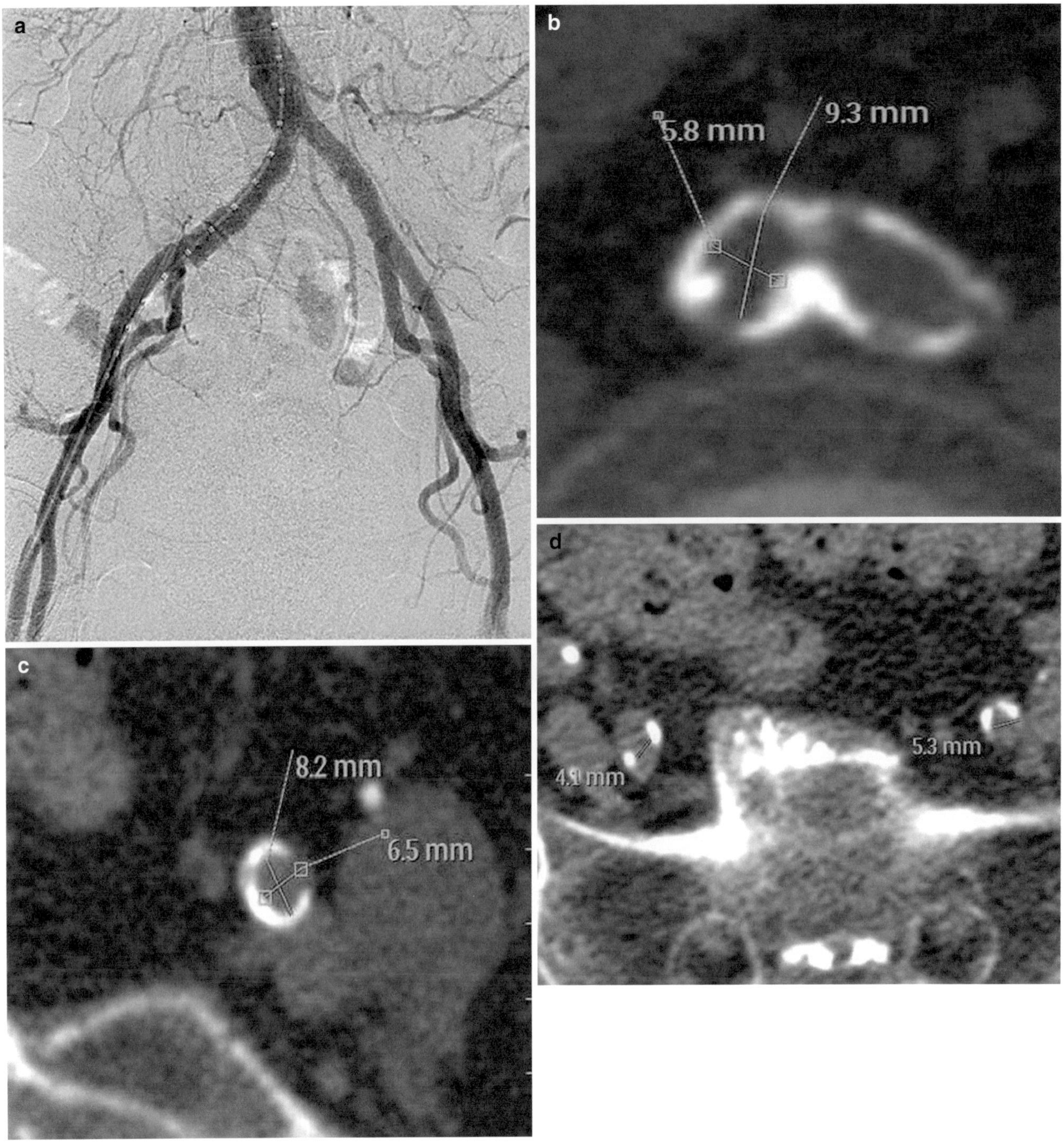

Fig. 19.2 (**a**) Aortoiliofemoral angiogram showing patent arteries with quantitative coronary angiography measurements >7 mm. (**b**) Bifurcation of right and left common iliac arteries showing severe circumferential calcification and small vessel size. (**c**) Circumferential calcification of left external iliac artery. (**d**) Heavy calcification and small lumen of bilateral external iliac arteries

In order to minimize contrast dose by angiographic evaluation, digital subtraction angiography is recommended. This method allows for same or better quality images with smaller amounts of contrast required (10–15 cc) (Fig. 19.3). Vessel diameters are measured with quantitative coronary angiography (QCA) and a reference marker pigtail. Precise vessel measurements are performed in multiple sites in the common femoral, superficial femoral, external, and common iliac arteries.

Rotational digital subtraction angiography is a means to acquire multiple projection views during a single breath-hold injection. Seymour et al. [12] suggested that rotational digital subtraction angiography may provide reliable images of peripheral arteries. In their work, digital subtraction images were acquired every 3.5° in a rotational sweep of 120° to yield 33 projections to assess the renal arteries. The same principle can theoretically be applied to the iliofemoral

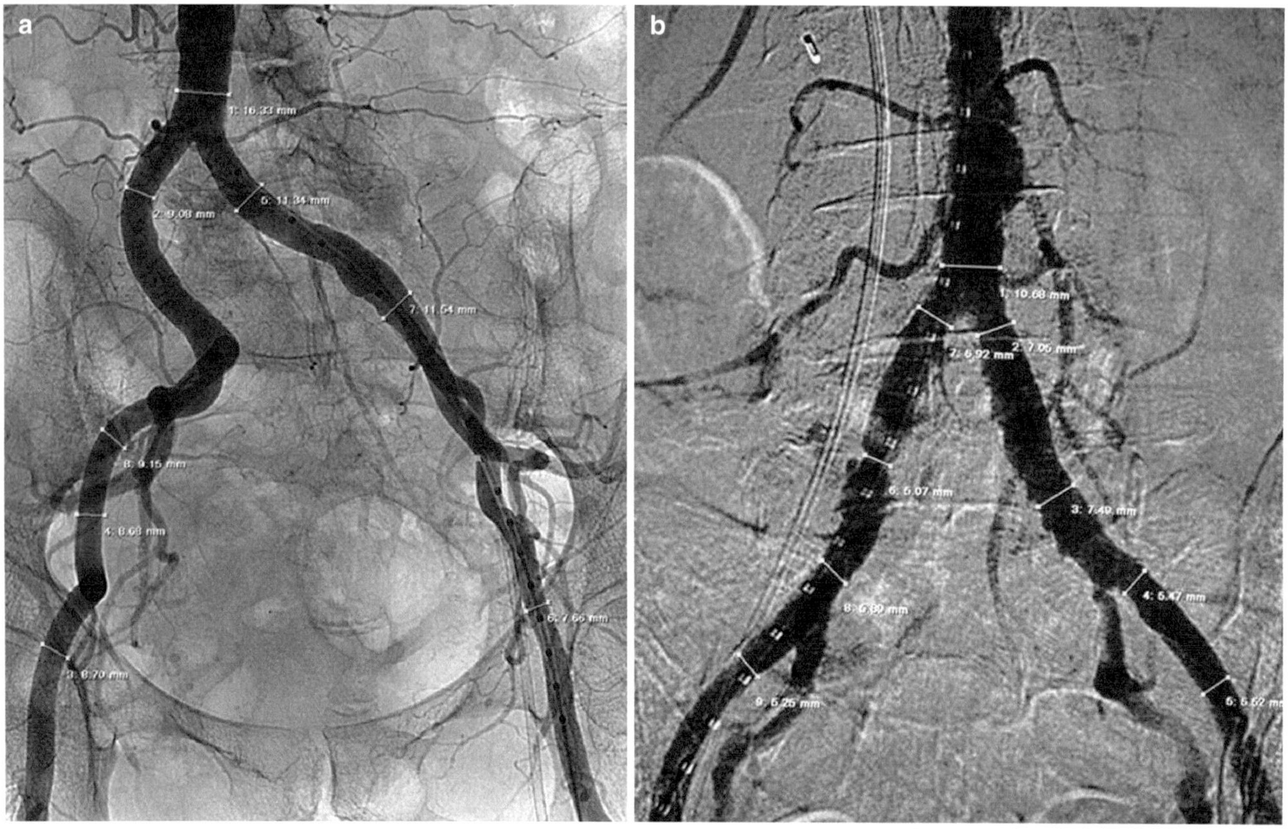

Fig. 19.3 (**a**) Abdominal aortography for measurement of vessel diameters with QCA and a reference marker pigtail. (**b**) Digital subtraction angiography for measurement of vessel diameters with QCA and a reference marker pigtail

arterial tree; however, limitations regarding measurement of lumen caliber and plaque morphology are likely to remain.

CT Angiography

Ultra-Low-Dose Intra-arterial Contrast Injection for Iliofemoral CT Angiography

A new method has been developed to perform CT angiography with significantly low contrast volume [13]. At the completion of the diagnostic cath, a 4-French pigtail catheter is positioned at the abdominal aorta, below the level of the renal arteries, and the patient is transferred to the CT suite. For the CT angiogram, iodinated contrast (iopamidol 370 mmol/ml) is mixed with normal saline in a 1:3 to 1:4 dilution in a single chamber of the power injector, and 40 ml of the contrast/saline mixture is injected through the pigtail catheter at 4 ml/s without a saline chaser. The scanning protocol incorporates a scan delay of 6 s followed by a helical CT of the abdomen and pelvis (64 × 0.625-mm collimation, rotation time 0.75 s, pitch 0.64, 120 kV, 154 mAs). With this technique it is possible to image the entire iliofemoral arterial tree with a very small amount of iodinated contrast (10–15 ml) (Fig. 19.4). Numerous technologic hardware innovations—including volume scanners with a greater number of detector rows, faster rotational speeds, iterative reconstruction method, and dual-energy CT imaging—may enable even lower doses of contrast to be required. Virtual endoscopy with CT is at times useful to estimate the distribution of calcium within the lumen along the vessel being considered for access (Fig. 19.5).

Contrast-Saving Scanning Protocols

Technological advances in computed tomography imaging have improved spatial and temporal resolution without compromising on image quality (Box 19.1). These accomplishments were achieved through increases in the numbers of detectors and improved sampling capabilities in the *z-direction*. Improvements in image reconstruction, such as the development of iterative reconstruction techniques [14] and multisegment reconstruction, have been shown to further enhance the signal-to-noise ratios and temporal resolution of cardiac computed tomography. Dual-source CT, which is constructed on the basis of two X-ray tubes and two detectors mounted on the CT gantry, with a mechanical offset of 90°, minimizes the limitations in temporal resolution of standard multidetector CT without the need for a faster gantry rotation. Using dual-

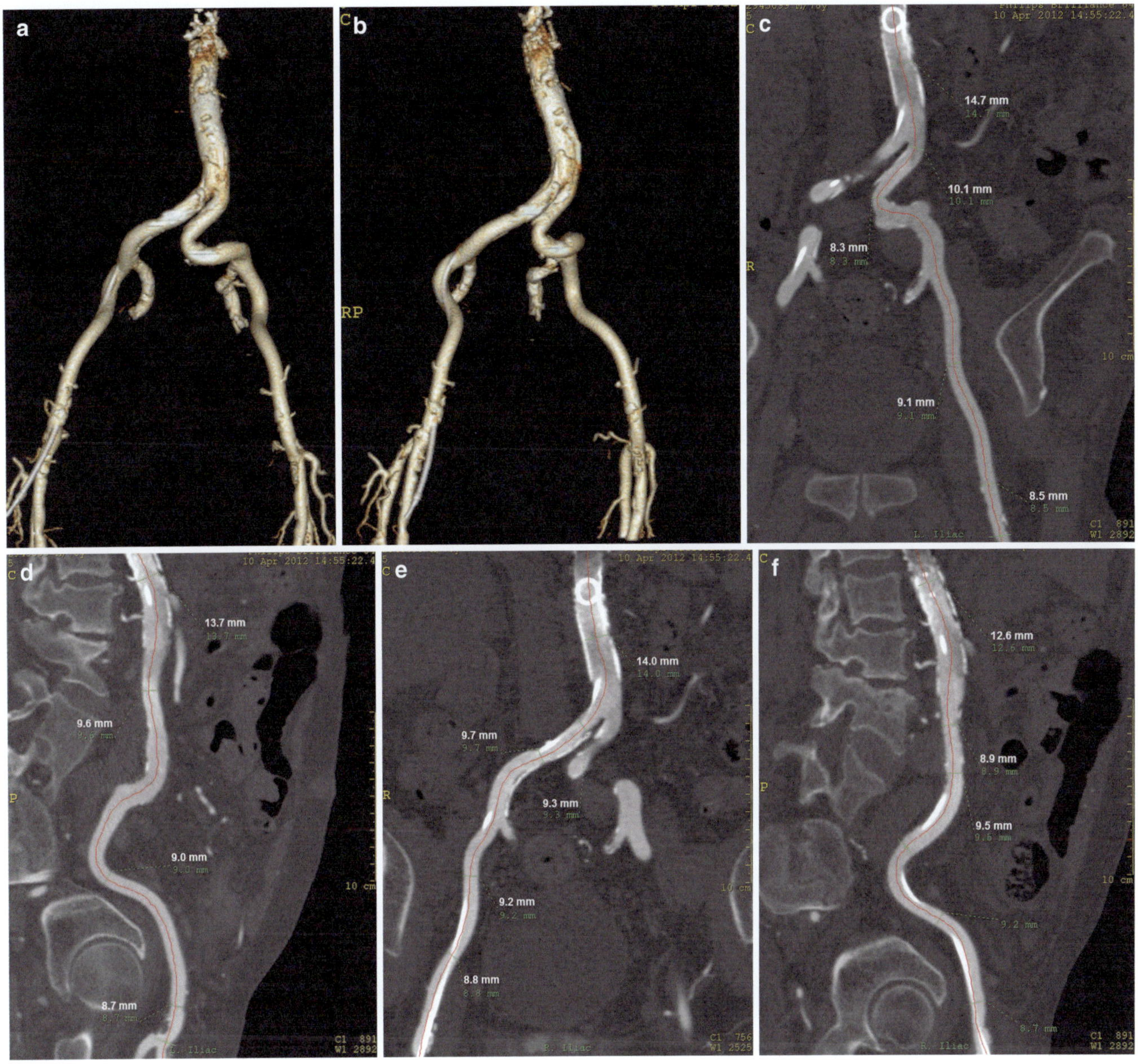

Fig. 19.4 (**a**) Images obtained with 10 cc of contrast injected in the abdominal aorta with a 4 F pigtail, AP view. (**b**) Right anterior oblique vie of the aortoiliofemoral arteries. This allows reconstructions in multiple views, which allows accurate measurements of the vessel diameters and the assessment of the calcification level. (**c**) Multiplanar reformation (MPR) of the left iliac artery in AP view. (**d**) MPR of the left iliac artery in lateral view. (**e**) MPR of the right iliac artery in AP view. (**f**) MPR of the right iliac artery in lateral view

Box 19.1 Reduced Iodinated Contrast CT Protocols

Direct intra-aortic injection	4 Fr catheter inserted in infrarenal aorta Possible to perform iliofemoral assessment with 10–15 cc contrast
High-pitch helical CT	Short acquisition time significantly lowers contrast volume
Dual energy CT	Monochromatic energy imaging may increase signal, thereby reducing contrast load

source CT, Blanke et al. [15] were able to effectively study the aortic root anatomy and iliofemoral vasculature in a single acquisition using a single shot of 110–130 cc iodinated contrast and combined ECG-assisted scanning of the thorax and non-ECG-assisted scanning of the abdomen. Their experience indicates that adequate images could be achieved in nearly all patients using this method. Wuest et al. [16] further enhanced this protocol by using high-pitch spiral CT, which allows high-resolution imaging of large anatomical volumes in a short acquisition time. This technique also allows for the injection of significantly lower volumes of iodinated contrast (40 cc),

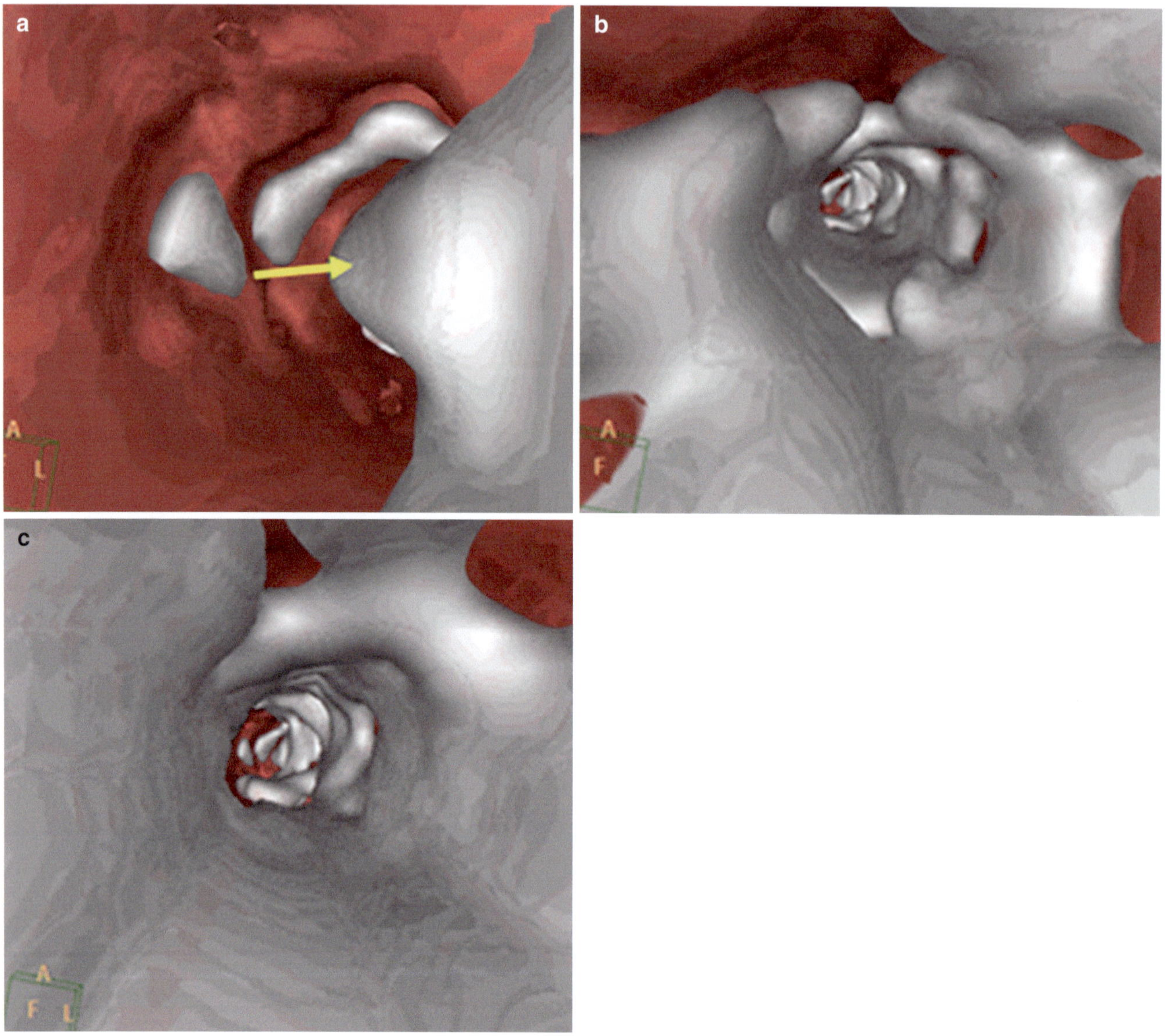

Fig. 19.5 Virtual endoscopy with CT. (**a**) Vessel with small amount of calcium (*arrow*). (**b**) High amount of calcium with concentric arcs of calcium. (**c**) Severe circumferential calcification

which may be advantageous in patients with renal insufficiency or in high-risk AKI patients. Using high-pitch spiral CT, Wuest et al. were able to obtain all the standard aortic root and iliofemoral measurements required for the TAVR procedure.

Non-contrast CT

Non-contrast CT is very important for quantifying the amount of calcification in both longitudinal and axial views. In order to assess amount of calcification, the cursor is moved in a stepwise fashion (millimeter by millimeter) in search of significantly calcified areas. Significant calcification, especially in long arterial segments, does not allow for straightening. In addition, it is imperative to assess calcium distribution and localization at the puncture site since one of the most frequent modes of failure of percutaneous closure devices is when the device is deployed through a calcified vessel wall. Severe calcification at the bifurcation of internal and external iliac arteries is of special concern since this area has no yield for expansion or movement, that is, the internal iliac anchors the bifurcation.

"Blooming," or partial volume, artifacts are frequent in non-contrast CT due to limited spatial resolution. Blooming artifacts require minimization in order to perform adequate vessel measurements and to quantify the calcification extent.

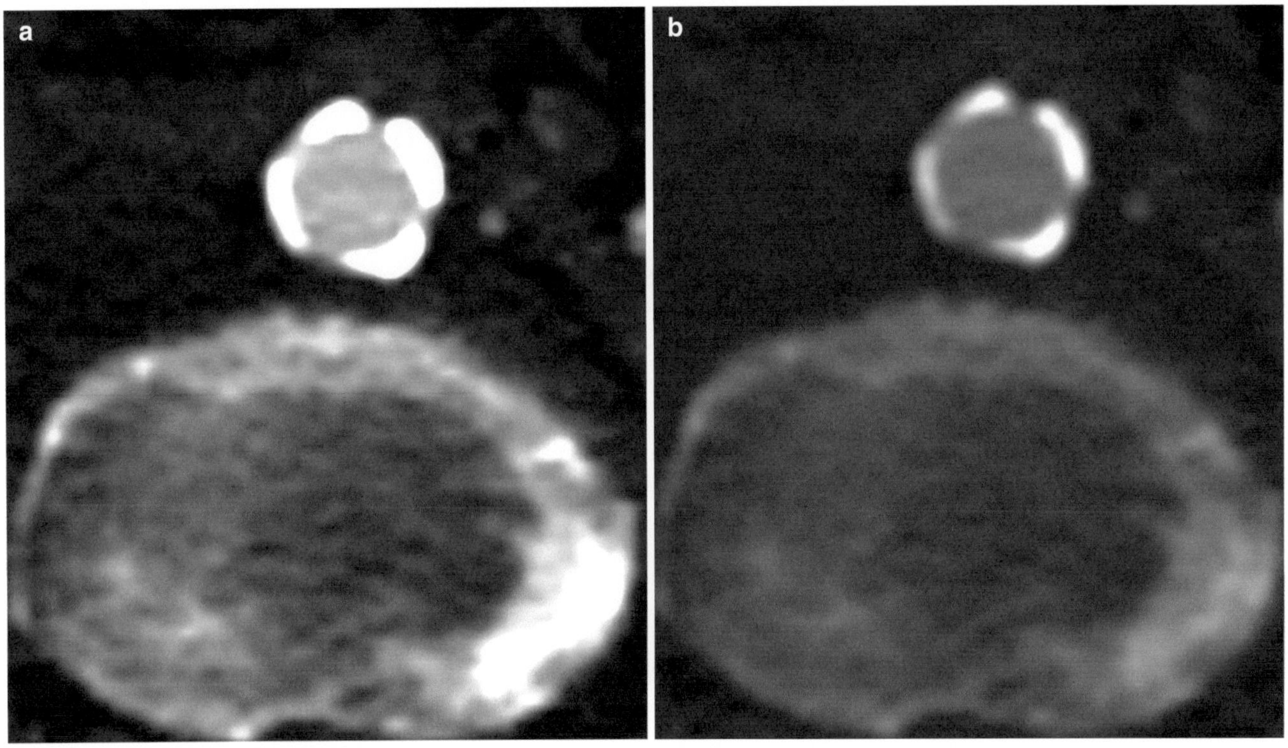

Fig. 19.6 High-level partial volume or "blooming" artifact that (**a**) distorts vessel diameter measurement and evaluation of calcium severity. Reducing the degree blooming (**b**) allows for more precise measurements

The dimensions can change significantly after correction (Fig. 19.6).

Several institutions assess the size of the iliofemoral arteries using non-contrast CT. Such an approach is not recommended, however, since the accuracy of measuring vessel size, especially in inexperienced hands, is limited and is a potential hazard for vascular complications during the procedure.

Intravascular Ultrasound

Intravascular ultrasound (IVUS) of the iliofemoral vessels can be used when there is a discrepancy in the angiography and CT results. IVUS is an excellent tool to measure vessel diameter and has been shown to significantly decrease the use of iodinated contrast (Fig. 19.7) [17]. However, this imaging modality has several limitations. IVUS does not allow for satisfactory calcification analysis and it may provide poor imaging in severely tortuous iliac arteries due to the position of the ultrasound probe within the artery lumen. In our institution, when high-quality CT images are available, IVUS images do not add appreciably useful additional information and, therefore, are used sparingly.

Pre-procedural Evaluation: Aortic Valve Annulus Sizing

While gated CT angiography protocols are gaining acceptance for aortic valve annulus sizing as a pre-procedural planning tool [18], this modality requires the administration of large amounts of iodinated contrast and is thus not recommended for patients with renal insufficiency. An alternative screening tool which in our experience is sufficient in the majority of the cases is to assess the sub-annular diameter, left ventricular outflow tract in two-dimensional (2D) transthoracic echocardiography. In cases where this measurement is borderline or is technically difficult, transesophageal echocardiography is recommended. The perpendicular axis of the annulus using three-dimensional (3D) and/or biplane imaging is determined. Using these techniques, the diameter or perimeter of the aortic annulus is measured. It should be noted, however, that while 2D and 3D measurements are well correlated, 3D measurements, when compared to 2D measurements, typically yield more than 1-mm differences in mean dimensions [19].

Kempfert et al. [20] showed that end-systolic maximal annular diameter of the aortic valve was best correlated with direct intraoperative diameters measured after decalcification of the aortic annulus. These measurements also correlated

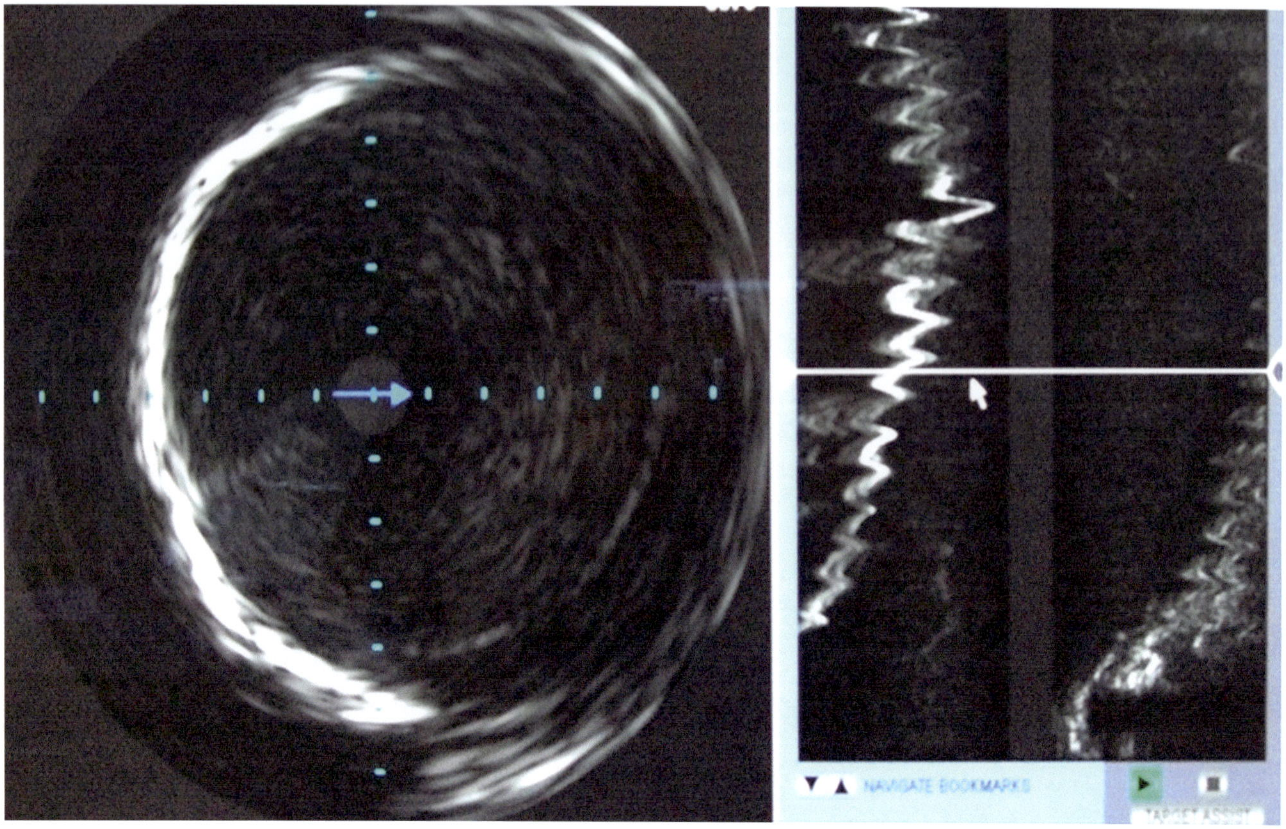

Fig. 19.7 Intravascular ultrasound to assess size and characteristics of iliofemoral vessels

well with CT "effective" diameter. As described above, several CT techniques are currently available to minimize contrast dose [15, 16].

Procedural Techniques

Generally, TAVR procedures do not require large amounts of iodinated contrast. The components of the procedure that typically require iodinated contrast injections are vascular access, aortic root angiogram to determine the perpendicular angulation for valve deployment, valve deployment for final positioning, post-deployment valve assessment, and the final iliofemoral assessment to exclude vascular access injury. There are various techniques that can be undertaken to perform any of these procedural stages without injecting contrast or with minimization of the amount of the injected contrast as outlined in Table 19.1.

General Measures to Decrease Risk for Nephropathy

To minimize risk of contrast-induced nephropathy (CIN), several methods can be employed. One potentially useful strategy is to increase urine output before, during, and after contrast media exposure. To facilitate this, patients should be hydrated the night prior to the procedure. In addition, immediately prior to TAVR, patients can be administered 1 l of 5 % dextrose to increase renal blood flow, which has been shown to reduce a rise in post-procedural creatinine [21]. The contrast can be diluted by 50 % with normal saline in order to decrease the total iodinated contrast load. The RenalGuard system has shown promise in this area by assisting in the creation and maintenance of high urine output, thereby preventing contrast agents from "clogging" renal tubules and limiting toxin exposure to the kidneys. This is achieved by automated matched fluid replacement in real time to reduce side effects associated with over- or under-hydration. Preliminary data to support the protective role of this system can be seen in the Induced Diuresis with Matched Hydration Compared to Standard Hydration for Contrast Induced Nephropathy Prevention (MYTHOS) trial, which randomized 157 patients to RenalGuard versus standard intravenous hydration. A significant increase in the incidence of CIN was seen in all patients (5 % vs. 16 %, respectively, $p=0.028$), including elective percutaneous coronary intervention patients and patients with non-ST elevation myocardial infarction [22].

The role and efficacy of pretreatment with antioxidants such as *N*-acetylcysteine or of agents that induce urinary alkalization (such as sodium bicarbonate) remains at best unclear. A large randomized trial, Evaluation of Sodium Bicarbonate

Table 19.1 Contrast volume usage throughout the TAVR procedure

Procedure stage	Typical amount of iodinated contrast (ml)	Alternative "contrast-saving" techniques
Arterial access	15	Ultrasound-guided puncture
		Co-registration with pre-procedural CTA using HeartNavigator (5 ml ×2 injection for registration)
		Use of road-mapping feature (5 ml injection)
Valve deployment angulation	25	Co-registration with pre-procedural CTA using HeartNavigator (5 ml ×2 injection for registration)
		Performance of rotational aortogram during the initial diagnostic cath
Valve deployment	Variable	Two-step valve deployment (balloon-expandable valve)
		Use of HeartNavigator
		Use of Paieon system
		Use of a pigtail catheter positioned at the annulus level
Assessment of AI post-valve deployment	15	Echocardiography
		Hemodynamics
Final iliofemoral angiogram	10	Selective ipsilateral injection (8 ml)

to Reduce the Incidence of Contrast Induced Chronic Kidney Injury in Patients with Kidney Disease (BOSS), is currently underway to assess this approach. In the few trials that have evaluated the use of *N*-acetylcysteine, divergent results have been observed, with meta-analyses confirming the significant heterogeneity in these trials resulted and the inability to broadly interpret their results [23, 24].

In our own institution, we employ a two-phase valve deployment model, which has proven to be contrast saving. In stage one, the balloon is inflated to one-third of its volume, and a small contrast volume injection is performed. The valve position is then readjusted slightly and finally the valve is then fully deployed. This technique avoids multiple, large-volume aortic root shots aimed at positioning the valve at the right level prior to balloon inflation.

Imaging Methods to Decrease Need for Contrast

There are several co-registration products that assist the operator in identifying the aortic valve plane, choosing the appropriate valve size and the final positioning and deployment of the valve.

The C-THV (Paieon Inc., Park Afek, Israel) is a real-time angiography-based system, designed to facilitate TAVR in multiple steps (Fig. 19.8) [25]. First, it facilitates determination of the optimal valve deployment projection. The system has unlimited number of pairs of C-arm angulations which are orthogonal to the axial plane of the aortic valve, and is calculated using two aortograms with low contrast volume injections. This system also facilitates device-size selection, tracking, and positioning of the valve in real time by displaying a real-time marker of the annulus over the x-ray fluoroscopy. This system may also assist in post-deployment analysis by assessing whether or not the valve stent is fully expanded. Using this system, the operator may save in contrast volume when determining the best deployment projection and during the valve deployment.

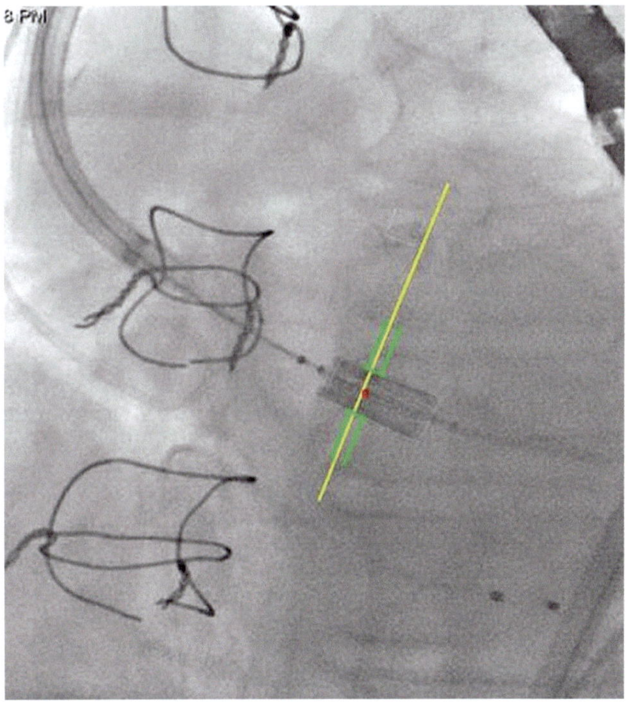

Fig. 19.8 C-THV (Paieon Inc., Park Afek, Israel) is a real-time angiography-based system, designed to facilitate transcatheter aortic valve implantation

Two additional products can register a previously acquired CT angiography 3D volume dataset to the live fluoroscopy: syngo Aortic ValveGuide (Siemens, Erlangen, Germany) [https://www.medical.siemens.com/webapp/wcs/stores/servlet/PSOptionProductDisplayView?catalogId=−1&catTree=100010,1007660,12751,1038666&langId=−1&productId=204641&productType=6&storeId=10001&et_cid=HTML_

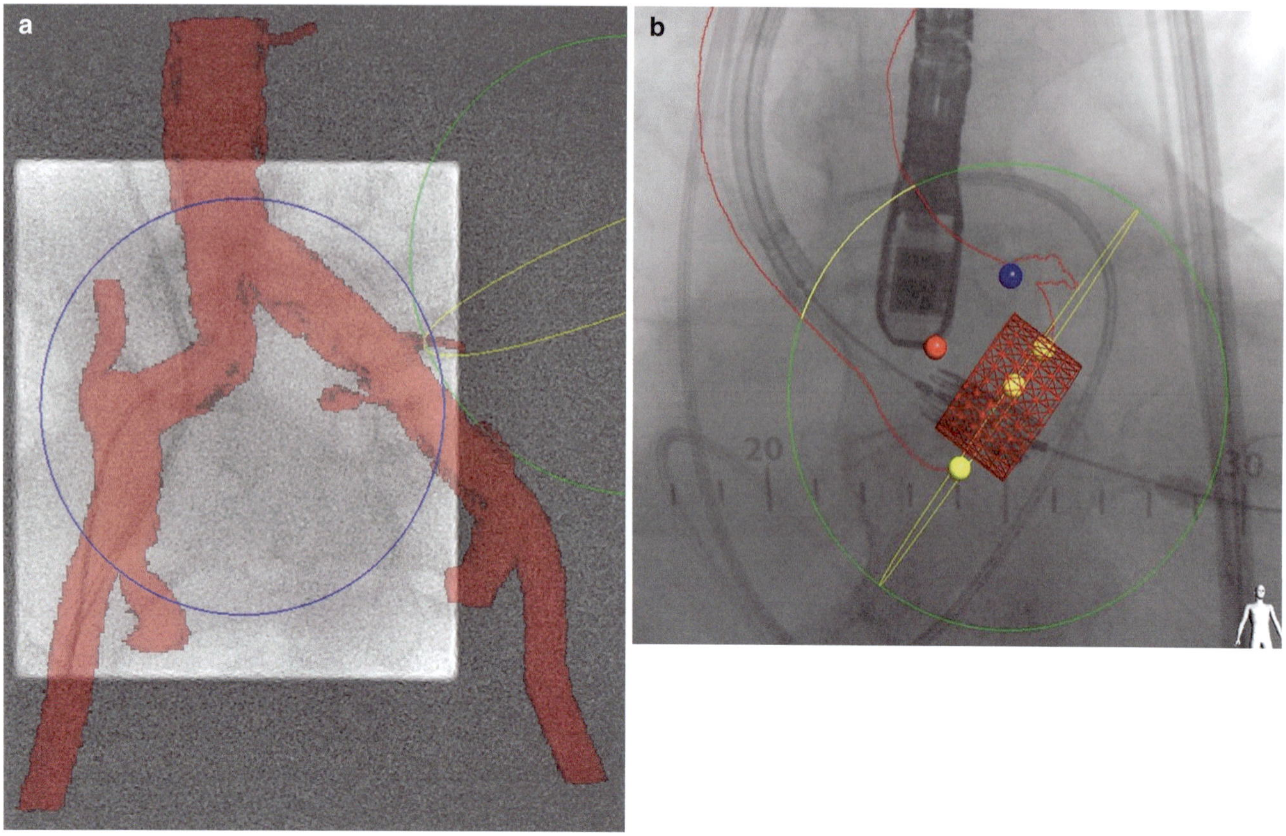

Fig. 19.9 HeartNavigator can assist in achieving vascular access by showing the vessel anatomy over the fluoroscopy images (**a**) and by facilitating the positioning of the transcatheter heart valve (**b**)

Gilkramina_20120301&et_lid=click+here&stc=] and HeartNavigator (Phillips, Andover, MA) [http://www.healthcare.philips.com/us_en/products/interventional_xray/product/interventional_cardiac_surgery/interventional_tools/heartnavigator/] (Fig. 19.9). This is achieved by two small volume contrast angiograms of the aortic root and manual co-registration of the datasets based on anatomic landmarks. By these methods, the operator is able to identify the precise location of the annulus and can position the valve more accurately with less need for additional injections of iodinated contrast. While these products prove useful in clinical use, associated significant limitations should be noted. First, the need to perform two separate iodinated contrast injections during the process of image registration may increase the volume of contrast needed and, hence, the risk of AKI. Additionally, the current versions of the available products are not gated with diaphragmatic movement or with heart contraction; thus their accuracy may be limited in this respect.

Alternative Imaging Modalities That Eliminate Use of Contrast

The CoreValve self-expandable valve and the SAPIEN XT balloon-expandable valve stent frame are composed of nitinol, which creates small artifact in a real-time magnetic resonance imaging environment. This allows for the potential deployment of these transcatheter valves under real-time MRI. The obvious advantages of this approach, beyond eliminating exposure to radiation, are the ability to deploy the valve under clear visualization of the surrounding soft tissue and without the use of iodinated contrast material. This approach would obviously be advantageous in patients with renal insufficiency. The current data evaluating the efficacy of this technique is limited currently to series of experimental animal experiments demonstrating the potential feasibility of this approach [26].

References

1. Leon MB, Smith CR, Mack M, Miller DC, Moses JW, Svensson LG, Tuzcu EM, Webb JG, Fontana GP, Makkar RR, Brown DL, Block PC, Guyton RA, Pichard AD, Bavaria JE, Herrmann HC, Douglas PS, Petersen JL, Akin JJ, Anderson WN, Wang D, Pocock S. Transcatheter aortic-valve implantation for aortic stenosis in patients who cannot undergo surgery. N Engl J Med. 2010; 363:1597–607.
2. Smith CR, Leon MB, Mack MJ, Miller DC, Moses JW, Svensson LG, Tuzcu EM, Webb JG, Fontana GP, Makkar RR, Williams M, Dewey T, Kapadia S, Babaliaros V, Thourani VH, Corso P, Pichard AD, Bavaria JE, Herrmann HC, Akin JJ, Anderson WN, Wang D, Pocock SJ. Transcatheter versus surgical aortic-valve replacement in high-risk patients. N Engl J Med. 2011;364:2187–98.

3. Barbash IM, Ben-Dor I, Dvir D, Maluenda G, Xue Z, Torguson R, Satler LF, Pichard AD, Waksman R. Incidence and predictors of acute kidney injury following transcatheter aortic valve replacement. Am Heart J. 2012;163(6):1031–6.
4. Aregger F, Wenaweser P, Hellige GJ, Kadner A, Carrel T, Windecker S, Frey FJ. Risk of acute kidney injury in patients with severe aortic valve stenosis undergoing transcatheter valve replacement. Nephrol Dial Transplant. 2009;24:2175–9.
5. Nuis RJ, Van Mieghem NM, Tzikas A, Piazza N, Otten AM, Cheng J, van Domburg RT, Betjes M, Serruys PW, de Jaegere PP. Frequency, determinants, and prognostic effects of acute kidney injury and red blood cell transfusion in patients undergoing transcatheter aortic valve implantation. Catheter Cardiovasc Interv. 2011;77:881–9.
6. Sinning JM, Ghanem A, Steinhauser H, Adenauer V, Hammerstingl C, Nickenig G, Werner N. Renal function as predictor of mortality in patients after percutaneous transcatheter aortic valve implantation. JACC Cardiovasc Interv. 2010;3:1141–9.
7. Van Linden A, Kempfert J, Rastan AJ, Holzhey D, Blumenstein J, Schuler G, Mohr FW, Walther T. Risk of acute kidney injury after minimally invasive transapical aortic valve implantation in 270 patients. Eur J Cardiothorac Surg. 2011;39:835–42; discussion 842–3.
8. Leon MB, Piazza N, Nikolsky E, Blackstone EH, Cutlip DE, Kappetein AP, Krucoff MW, Mack M, Mehran R, Miller C, Morel MA, Petersen J, Popma JJ, Takkenberg JJ, Vahanian A, van Es GA, Vranckx P, Webb JG, Windecker S, Serruys PW. Standardized endpoint definitions for transcatheter aortic valve implantation clinical trials: a consensus report from the valve academic research consortium. J Am Coll Cardiol. 2011; 57:253–69.
9. Bagur R, Webb JG, Nietlispach F, Dumont E, De Larochelliere R, Doyle D, Masson JB, Gutierrez MJ, Clavel MA, Bertrand OF, Pibarot P, Rodes-Cabau J. Acute kidney injury following transcatheter aortic valve implantation: predictive factors, prognostic value, and comparison with surgical aortic valve replacement. Eur Heart J. 2010;31:865–74.
10. Elhmidi Y, Bleiziffer S, Piazza N, Hutter A, Opitz A, Hettich I, Kornek M, Ruge H, Brockmann G, Mazzitelli D, Lange R. Incidence and predictors of acute kidney injury in patients undergoing transcatheter aortic valve implantation. Am Heart J. 2011;161:735–9.
11. Eltchaninoff H, Kerkeni M, Zajarias A, Tron C, Godin M, Sanchez Giron C, Baala B, Cribier A. Aorto-iliac angiography as a screening tool in selecting patients for transfemoral aortic valve implantation with the Edwards SAPIEN bioprosthesis. EuroIntervention. 2009;5:438–42.
12. Seymour HR, Matson MB, Belli AM, Morgan R, Kyriou J, Patel U. Rotational digital subtraction angiography of the renal arteries: technique and evaluation in the study of native and transplant renal arteries. Br J Radiol. 2001;74:134–41.
13. Joshi SB, Mendoza DD, Steinberg DH, Goldstein MA, Lopez CF, Raizon A, Weissman G, Satler LF, Pichard AD, Weigold WG. Ultra-low-dose intra-arterial contrast injection for iliofemoral computed tomographic angiography. JACC Cardiovasc Imaging. 2009;2:1404–11.
14. Hara AK, Paden RG, Silva AC, Kujak JL, Lawder HJ, Pavlicek W. Iterative reconstruction technique for reducing body radiation dose at ct: feasibility study. AJR Am J Roentgenol. 2009; 193:764–71.
15. Blanke P, Euringer W, Baumann T, Reinohl J, Schlensak C, Langer M, Pache G. Combined assessment of aortic root anatomy and aortoiliac vasculature with dual-source ct as a screening tool in patients evaluated for transcatheter aortic valve implantation. AJR Am J Roentgenol. 2010;195:872–81.
16. Wuest W, Anders K, Schuhbaeck A, May MS, Gauss S, Marwan M, Arnold M, Ensminger S, Muschiol G, Daniel WG, Uder M, Achenbach S. Dual source multidetector ct-angiography before transcatheter aortic valve implantation (tavi) using a high-pitch spiral acquisition mode. Eur Radiol. 2012;22:51–8.
17. Kawasaki D, Fujii K, Fukunaga M, Fujii N, Masutani M, Kawabata ML, Tsujino T, Ohyanagi M, Masuyama T. Preprocedural evaluation and endovascular treatment of iliofemoral artery disease without contrast media for patients with pre-existing renal insufficiency. Circ J. 2011;75:179–84.
18. Jilaihawi H, Kashif M, Fontana G, Furugen A, Shiota T, Friede G, Makhija R, Doctor N, Leon MB, Makkar RR. Cross-sectional computed tomographic assessment improves accuracy of aortic annular sizing for transcatheter aortic valve replacement and reduces the incidence of paravalvular aortic regurgitation. J Am Coll Cardiol. 2012;59(14):1275–86.
19. Husser O, Rauch S, Endemann DH, Resch M, Nunez J, Bodi V, Hilker M, Schmid C, Riegger GA, Luchner A, Hengstenberg C. Impact of three-dimensional transesophageal echocardiography on prosthesis sizing for transcatheter aortic valve implantation. Catheter Cardiovasc Interv. 2012;956–63.
20. Kempfert J, Van Linden A, Lehmkuhl L, Rastan AJ, Holzhey D, Blumenstein J, Mohr FW, Walther T. Aortic annulus sizing: echocardiographic vs. computed tomography derived measurements in comparison with direct surgical sizing. Eur J Cardiothorac Surg. 2012;42(4):627–33.
21. Clavijo LC, Pinto TL, Kuchulakanti PK, Torguson R, Chu WW, Satler LF, Kent KM, Suddath WO, Waksman R, Pichard AD. Effect of a rapid intra-arterial infusion of dextrose 5% prior to coronary angiography on frequency of contrast-induced nephropathy in high-risk patients. Am J Cardiol. 2006;97:981–3.
22. Marenzi G, Ferrari C, Marana I, Assanelli E, De Metrio M, Teruzzi G, Veglia F, Fabbiocchi F, Montorsi P, Bartorelli AL. Prevention of contrast nephropathy by furosemide with matched hydration: the mythos (induced diuresis with matched hydration compared to standard hydration for contrast induced nephropathy prevention) trial. JACC Cardiovasc Interv. 2012;5:90–7.
23. Briguori C, Colombo A, Violante A, Balestrieri P, Manganelli F, Paolo Elia P, Golia B, Lepore S, Riviezzo G, Scarpato P, Focaccio A, Librera M, Bonizzoni E, Ricciardelli B. Standard vs double dose of n-acetylcysteine to prevent contrast agent associated nephrotoxicity. Eur Heart J. 2004;25:206–11.
24. Kshirsagar AV, Poole C, Mottl A, Shoham D, Franceschini N, Tudor G, Agrawal M, Denu-Ciocca C, Magnus Ohman E, Finn WF. N-acetylcysteine for the prevention of radiocontrast induced nephropathy: a meta-analysis of prospective controlled trials. J Am Soc Nephrol. 2004;15:761–9.
25. Dvir D, Kornowski R. Percutaneous aortic valve implantation using novel imaging guidance. Catheter Cardiovasc Interv. 2010; 76:450–4.
26. Kahlert P, Parohl N, Albert J, Schafer L, Reinhardt R, Kaiser GM, McDougall I, Decker B, Plicht B, Erbel R, Eggebrecht H, Ladd ME, Quick HH. Real-time magnetic resonance imaging-guided transarterial aortic valve implantation: in vivo evaluation in swine. J Am Coll Cardiol. 2012;59:192–3.

Transcatheter Aortic Valve Replacement and Adverse Cerebrovascular Events

20

Brian G. Hynes and Josep Rodés-Cabau

Abstract

The rapid clinical expansion of transcatheter aortic valve replacement (TAVR) has established a paradigm shift in the management of patients with severe aortic valve stenosis [1]. Patients deemed to be at prohibitive or at high risk of adverse outcomes with open surgical aortic valve replacement (SAVR) may now be assessed for suitability for valve replacement employing a less invasive approach. However, recent data have raised concerns in relation to the risk of related stroke [2]. The occurrence of a major adverse cerebrovascular event (CVE) following TAVR remains one of the most frequent and feared complications associated with this procedure [1, 3]. In this chapter we explore the current data both in relation to TAVR-related major stroke as well as silent cerebrovascular ischemic events. The timing of neurological events and their prognostic implications are also examined. Furthermore, potential mechanisms of TAVR-related cerebrovascular injury are described, in addition to efforts to minimize their occurrence. Finally the role of imaging modalities in the diagnosis, management, and prevention of TAVR-associated adverse CVE is highlighted.

Keywords

Transcatheter aortic valve implantation • Transcatheter aortic valve replacement • Stroke • Cerebral magnetic resonance imaging • Atrial fibrillation

Introduction

The rapid clinical expansion of transcatheter aortic valve replacement (TAVR) has established a paradigm shift in the management of patients with severe aortic valve stenosis [1]. Patients deemed to be at prohibitive or at high risk of adverse outcomes with open surgical aortic valve replacement (SAVR) may now be assessed for suitability for valve replacement employing a less invasive approach. However, recent data have raised concerns in relation to the risk of related stroke [2]. The occurrence of a major adverse cerebrovascular event (CVE) following TAVR remains one of the most frequent and feared complications associated with this procedure [1, 3]. In this chapter we explore the current data both in relation to TAVR-related major stroke as well as silent cerebrovascular ischemic events. The timing of neurological events and their prognostic implications are also examined. Furthermore, potential mechanisms of TAVR-related cerebrovascular injury are described, in addition to efforts to minimize their occurrence. Finally the role of imaging modalities in the diagnosis, management, and prevention of TAVR-associated adverse CVE is highlighted.

B.G. Hynes, MB • J. Rodés-Cabau, MD (✉)
Department of Interventional Cardiology
and Structural Heart Disease,
Quebec Heart and Lung Institute, Laval University,
2725 chemin Ste-Foy G1V 4G5,
Quebec City, QC, Canada
e-mail: josep.rodes@criucpq.ulaval.ca

J.K. Min et al. (eds.), *Multimodality Imaging for Transcatheter Aortic Valve Replacement*,
DOI 10.1007/978-1-4471-2798-7_20, © Springer-Verlag London 2014

TAVR and CVE

During the early development and evolution of TAVR, the rates of procedure-related stroke varied considerably from under 4 to 10 % [4, 5]. It is likely that outcomes in these small series were influenced by a multitude of factors that arise as a function of the introduction of any new invasive procedure. Chief among these are issues pertaining to the operator-related learning curve with any novel procedure, TAVR system design evolution, and ever-improving periprocedural patient management. Following these initial TAVR reports, several large multicenter registries were carried out, including approximately 4,000 patients considered nonoperable, or at very high risk, for SAVR. Findings from the largest recent multicenter registries of TAVR reported in the past few years [6–17] are summarized in Table 20.1. Most patients included in these registries were octogenarians and had several comorbidities leading to a high-risk clinical profile (mean logistic EuroSCORE >20 %). The mean stroke rate following TAVR at 30 days reported in these registries was ~3.5 %, ranging from 0.6 to 5 %. This is in agreement with the 3.2 % rate reported in a recent meta-analysis that included more than 10,000 TAVR patients [3]. It is important to note that there has been no standardization among these studies for definitions of cerebrovascular complications associated with TAVR. This may have played a role in the differentially reported stroke rates observed among TAVR registries. In an effort to standardize data reporting, a recently formed multi-specialty committee, the Valve Academic Research Consortium (VARC), drew up guidelines defining recommended clinical endpoints for TAVR studies [18]. Those in relation to CVE are outlined in Table 20.2.

The PARTNER trial, to date, remains the only prospective randomized trial of TAVR. PARTNER included two differentiated cohorts of patients: (1) those considered to be nonoperable (i.e., comorbidities leading to a predicted risk of 50 % or more, of either death by 30 days after surgery or a serious irreversible morbidity; patients with comorbidities leading to a life expectancy <1 year were excluded, $n=358$) [19] and (2) those considered to be at high surgical risk (i.e., predicted risk of operative mortality ≥15 % as determined by the trial site surgeon and cardiologist; guideline = STS score ≥10, $n=699$) [20]. The Edwards SAPIEN valve was used in all cases. The PARTNER trial showed, in the nonoperable cohort, the superiority of TAVR vs. medical treatment with balloon aortic valvuloplasty [BAV] (mortality at 1-year follow-up of 30.7 % vs. 50 %, $p<0.001$) and the non-inferiority of TAVR vs. SAVR in the high-risk cohort (mortality at 1-year follow-up of 24.2 % vs. 26.8 %, $p=0.44$). However, the trial revealed a higher rate of cerebrovascular events in the TAVR group with respect to the medical treatment and SAVR groups. A summary of the results regarding the CVE in the PARTNER trial at 30-day and at 1-year follow-up is shown in Fig. 20.1.

The incidence of late (>30 days) ischemic stroke after TAVR (~2 %/year) was similar to that observed after SAVR and medical treatment in a similar population of elderly and high-risk patients with severe aortic stenosis, strongly suggesting the lack of a late prothrombotic effect associated with transcatheter valves [19, 20]. A substudy of the PARTNER trial showed that a higher atherosclerotic burden and previous CVE were the factors associated with late CVE after TAVR [21]. On the other hand, an excess of late hemorrhagic strokes was observed in the TAVR group compared with the medical treatment group in the PARTNER trial [22], highlighting the potential importance of excessive antithrombotic treatment to these late events after TAVR.

Cerebral Ischemic Defects Following TAVR

Clinically silent cerebrovascular injury resulting from TAVR has come to the fore following a series of studies evaluating cerebral ischemic events using diffusion-weighted magnetic resonance imaging (DW MRI) (Table 20.3, Figs. 20.2 and 20.3). An initial study by Kahlert et al. [23] compared 32 patients undergoing transfemoral (TF) TAVR (22 with the Edwards SAPIEN valve [Edwards Lifesciences Inc., Irvine, CA] and 10 with the CoreValve [Medtronic, Minneapolis, MN]) to historical SAVR controls ($n=21$) (Table 20.3). Patients underwent DW MRI at baseline, a mean of 3.4 (2.5–4.4) days, and again at 3 months post-index procedure. All patients were assessed by an experienced neurologist using both the National Institutes of Health Stroke Scale (NIHSS) and the Mini Mental State Examination (MMSE). Successful valve implantation was achieved in all TAVR patients with no obvious adverse neurologic event during the periprocedural period. No change was noted in the NIHSS scale or MMSE score of any of these patients. Repeat DW MRI post TAVR however demonstrated new hyperintense lesions in 86 % of the Edwards SAPIEN and 80 % of CoreValve TAVR patients. There were significantly fewer patients with new lesions in the control SAVR group (48 %, $p=0.016$). These new lesions were typically identified in both hemispheres reflecting a probable embolic cause. Among individuals with new cerebral lesions, lesion size was significantly smaller in the TAVR groups compared with the SAVR patients. At 3 months, no new DW MRI findings or changes in clinical or neurocognitive testing were noted. Indeed, the authors reported that 80 % of post-TAVR lesions had no residual signal change on repeat DW MRI at the 3-month interval.

Table 20.1 Overview of large recent TAVI registries/series

Study	Approach	TAVI System	Mean age	Logistic EuroSCORE %	Periprocedure/30-day stroke %	30-day mortality	1-year stroke%	1-year survival
Piazza et al. [6] Europe (51 sites) $n=646$	TF: 646	CoreValve®	TF: 81.0	TF: 23.1 ± 13.8	TF: 1.9	TF: 8.0	N/A	N/A
Rodés-Cabau et al. [7] Canada (6 sites) $n=339$	TF: 162 TA: 177	Cribier-Edwards: 57 Edwards SAPIEN®: 275 Edwards SAPIEN XT®: 7	TF: 83 TA: 80	Overall: 27.7 ± 16.3 TF: 25.8 ± 14.9 TA: 29.4 ± 17.2	Overall: 2.3 TF: 3.0 TA: 1.7	Overall: 10.4 TF: 9.5 TA: 11.3	N/A	Overall: 76 TF: 75 TA: 78
Thomas et al. [7] Europe (32 sites) $n=1038$	TF: 463 TA: 575	Edwards SAPIEN®	TF: 81.7 TA: 80.7	TF: 25.7 ± 14.5 TA: 29.1 ± 16.3	Overall: 2.5 TF: 2.4 TA: 2.6	Overall: 8.5 TF: 6.3 TA: 10.3	Overall: 5.5	Overall: 76.1 TF: 81.1 TA: 72.1
Eltchaninoff et al. [9] France (16 sites) $n=244$	TF Edwards: 95 TA Edwards: 71 TF CoreValve®: 66 SC CoreValve®: 12	Edwards SAPIEN®: 166 CoreValve®: 78	Overall: 82.3 TF Edwards: 83.2 TA Edwards: 82.1 TF CoreValve®: 82.5 SC CoreValve®: 75.5	Overall: 25.6 ± 11.4 TF Edwards: 25.6 ± 11.3 TA Edwards: 26.8 ± 11.6 TF CoreValve®: 24.7 ± 11.2 SC CoreValve®: 24.6 ± 14.5	Overall: 3.6 TF Edwards: 4.2 TA Edwards: 2.8 TF CoreValve®: 4.5 SC CoreValve®: 0	Overall: 12.7 TF Edwards: 8.4 TA Edwards: 16.9 TF CoreValve®: 15.1 SC CoreValve®: 8.3	N/A	N/A
Zahn et al. [11] Germany (22 sites) $n=697$	TF: 644 SC: 22 TA: 26 Tao: 5	Edwards SAPIEN®: 109 CoreValve®: 588	Overall: 81.4	Overall: 20.5 ± 13.2	Overall: 2.8	Overall: 12.4	N/A	N/A
Bosmans et al. [12] Belgium (15 sites) $n=328$	TF/TA Edwards: 187 TF CoreValve®: 141	Edwards SAPIEN®: 187 CoreValve®: 141	Overall: 83 TF/TA Edwards: 83 TF CoreValve®: 82	Overall: 28 ± 16 TF/TA Edwards: 30 ± 16 TF CoreValve®: 25 ± 15	Overall: 5.0 TF/TA Edwards: 5.0 TF CoreValve®: 4.0	Overall: 11.0 TF/TA Edwards: 12.0 TF CoreValve®: 11.0	N/A	TF Edwards : 82 TF/TA Edwards: 63 TF CoreValve®: 79
Tamburino et al. [13] Italy (14 sites) $n=663$	TF: 599 SC: 64	CoreValve®	Overall: 81	Overall: 23.0 ± 13.7	Overall: 1.2	Overall: 5.4	Overall: 2.5	Overall: 85
Moat et al. [14] United Kingdom (25 sites) $N=870$	TF: 599 Other approaches: 271	Edwards SAPIEN®: 410 CoreValve®: 452	Overall: 81.9 TF: 81.7 Other routes: 82.3 CoreValve®: 81.3 Edwards: 82.6	Overall: 18.5 (11.7–27.9) TF: 17.1 (11, 25.5) Other routes: 21.4 (14.4, 33.6) CoreValve®: 18.1 (11.1, 27.9) Edwards: 18.5 (12.4, 27.7)	Overall: 4.1 TF: 4.0 Other routes: 4.1 CoreValve®: 4.0 Edwards: 4.2	Overall: 7.1 TF: 5.5 Other routes: 10.7 CoreValve®: 5.8 Edwards: 8.5	N/A	Overall: 78.6 TF: 81.5 Other routes: 72.3 CoreValve®: 78.3 Edwards: 79.4

(continued)

Table 20.1 (continued)

Study	Approach	TAVI System	Mean age	Logistic EuroSCORE %	Periprocedure/30-day stroke %	30-day mortality	1-year stroke%	1-year survival
Gilard et al. [15] France (34 sites) *n* = 3195	TF: 2361 TA: 567 SC: 184 Other approaches: 83	Edwards SAPIEN®: 2107 CoreValve®: 1043 Other systems : 45	Overall: 82.7 TF: 83 TA: 81.5 SC: 82.2 Edwards SAPIEN®: 82.9 CoreValve®: 82.3	Overall: 21.9 ± 14.3 TF: 21.2 ± 14.7 TA: 24.8 ± 14.7 SC: 20.3 ± 15.2 Edwards SAPIEN®: 22.2 ± 14.3 CoreValve®: 21.3 ± 14.3	Overall: 3.4	Overall: 9.7 TF: 8.5 TA: 13.9 SC: 10.1 Edwards SAPIEN®: 9.6 CoreValve®: 9.4	Overall: 4.1	Overall: 24.0 TF: 21.7 TA: 32.3 SC: 25.1 Edwards SAPIEN®: 24.0 CoreValve®: 23.7
Wendler [16] Europe (94 sites) *n* = 2600	TF Edwards: 1694 TA Edwards: 906	Edwards SAPIEN XT®	TF: 81.9 TA: 80.2	TF: 19.9 ± 12.0 TA: 21.8 ± 13.8	TF: 2.3 TA: 2.1	TF: 4.3 TA: 9.9	NA	NA
Linke et al. [17] Europe, Asia, South America (44 sites) *n* = 1015	CoreValve®: 1015	CoreValve®	Overall: 81	Overall: 19.2 ± 12.4	Overall: 2.9	Overall: 4.5	NA	NA

TA transapical, *TF* transfemoral, *SC* subclavian, *TAO* transaortic

Ghanem et al. [24] performed a pilot study involving 22 patients to prospectively assess clinically silent and overt cerebral embolic events in the setting of TF TAVR. Cerebral DW MRI was carried out before, within 3 days post and at 3 months after valve implantation. Three patients (10 %) had a new neurological abnormality on examination post TAVR, but symptoms resolved in two. At the time of the first post-TAVR neuroimaging study, 72.7 % of patients had new ischemic lesions compared to baseline.

Table 20.2 VARC stroke definitions [15]

Stroke diagnostic criteria
Rapid onset of a focal or global neurological deficit with at least one of the following:
Change in level of consciousness, hemiplegia, hemiparesis, numbness or sensory loss affecting one
Side of the body, dysphasia or aphasia, hemianopia, amaurosis fugax, or other neurological signs or
Symptoms consistent with stroke
Duration of a focal or global neurological deficit ≥24 h; OR <24 h, if therapeutic intervention(s) were performed (e.g., thrombolytic therapy or intracranial angioplasty); OR available neuroimaging documents a new hemorrhage or infarct; OR the neurological deficit results in death
No other readily identifiable nonstroke cause for the clinical presentation (e.g., brain tumor, trauma, infection, hypoglycemia, peripheral lesion, pharmacological influences)
Confirmation of the diagnosis by at least one of the following:
Neurology or neurosurgical specialist
Stroke definitions
Transient ischemic attack:
New focal neurological deficit with rapid symptom resolution (usually 1–2 h), always within 24 h
Neuroimaging without tissue injury
Stroke:
(diagnosis as above, preferably with positive neuroimaging study)
Minor—Modified Rankin score 2 at 30 and 90 days†
Major—Modified Rankin score 2 at 30 and 90 days

Modified Rankin score assessments should be made by qualified individuals according to a certification process. If there is discordance between the 30 and 90 day Modified Rankin scores, a final determination of major versus minor stroke will be adjudicated by the neurology members of the clinical events committee

It had been suggested that the transapical (TA) approach may potentially minimize cardioembolic event rates as this method minimizes the need for extensive catheter manipulation within the aortic arch. Arnold et al. [25] performed a similar assessment using cerebral DW MRI in 25 patients undergoing TA TAVR with the Edwards SAPIEN system. Valve implantation was successful in all patients; however, neurological abnormalities were evident post procedure on clinical examination in five patients, one of who developed a major stroke. Analysis of DW MRI revealed new embolic lesions in 68 % of the patients, with more than one lesion in the majority. In those patients with new lesions, the posterior circulation territory was involved in greater than 50 % of cases. Rodés-Cabau et al. [26] compared the incidence of acute cerebral ischemic injury in those undergoing TAVR (employing the Edwards SAPIEN or SAPIEN XT valve) via the TF and the TA approach. In this multicenter study, 60 patients (TF: 29, TA: 31) underwent cerebral DW MRI prior to and within 6 days following TAVR. Additional neurologic and cognitive evaluation was performed at the same intervals as neuroimaging, using the NIHSS and MMSE tests. One patient in each group had clinical evidence of a stroke within 24 h of valve insertion. Up to 68 % of patients had new ischemic lesions on DW MRI post TAVR with a median number of three lesions per patient (range 1–36). Of those with new lesions, 76 % were multiple and 73 and 66 % involved both cerebral hemispheres and circulation (anterior and posterior) territories, respectively. Of note, most (91 %) lesions were

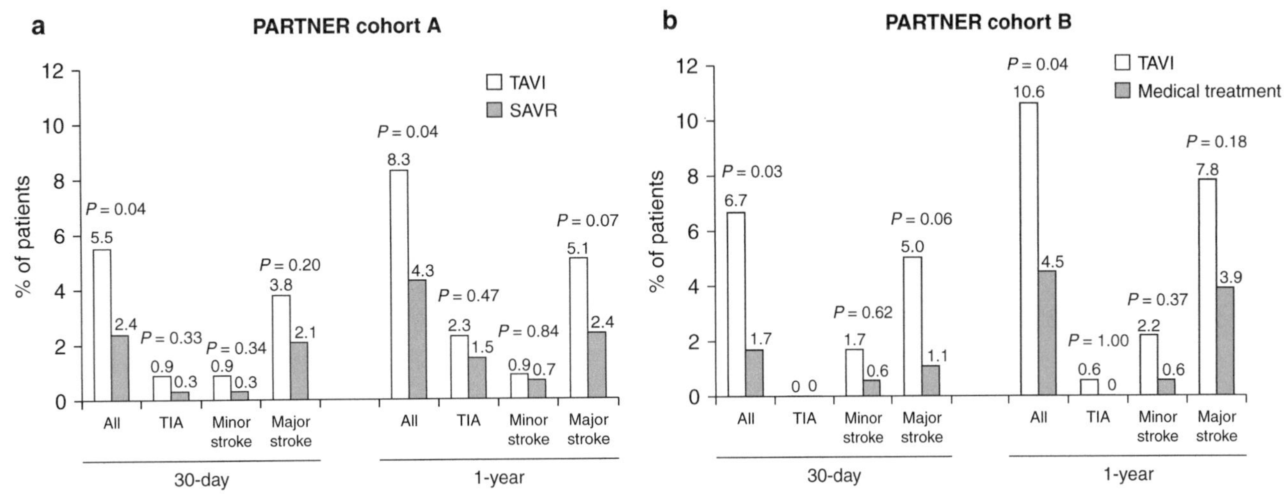

Fig. 20.1 Cerebrovascular events in the PARTNER trial at 30-day and at 1-year follow-up in the nonoperable cohort (**a**) and the high-risk cohort (**b**)

Table 20.3 Diffusion-weighted magnetic resonance imaging studies post transcatheter aortic valve implantation

Study	*n*	Valve type	Approach	Ischemic defects	Median number of lesions	Cognitive/neurologic assessment	Cognitive/neurologic assessment results	Stroke
Kahlert et al. [23]	32	Edwards SAPIEN ($n=22$) CoreValve ($n=10$)	TF	Edwards: 86 % CoreValve: 80 %	Edwards: 4 (2.1–6.0) CoreValve: 2.6 (0.3–4.9)	NIHSS, MMSE, mRS	No change	Overall: 0 %
Ghanem et al. [24]	22	CoreValve	TF	73 %	2.5 (1.0–5.5)	NIHSS, NSE	Neurologic impairment: 3 (10 %)	3.6 %
Rodés-Cabau et al. [26]	60	Edwards SAPIEN	TF ($n=29$) TA ($n=31$)	TF: 66 % TA: 71 %	Overall: 3 (2–8) TF: 3 (1–7) TA: 4 (2–9)	NIHSS, MMSE	No change	Overall: 3.3 % TF: 1.6 % TA: 1.6 %
Fairbairn et al. [27]	31	CoreValve	TF	77 %	2 (1–5)	NIHSS	No change	6.0 %
Arnold et al. [25]	25	Edwards SAPIEN	TA	68 %	N/A	Standardized clinical assessment	Neurologic impairment: 5 (20 %)	4.0 %

TA transapical, *TF* transfemoral, *NIHSS* National Institutes of Health Stroke Scale, *MMSE* Mini Mental State Examination, *mRS* modified Rankin Scale, *NSE* neuron-specific enolase

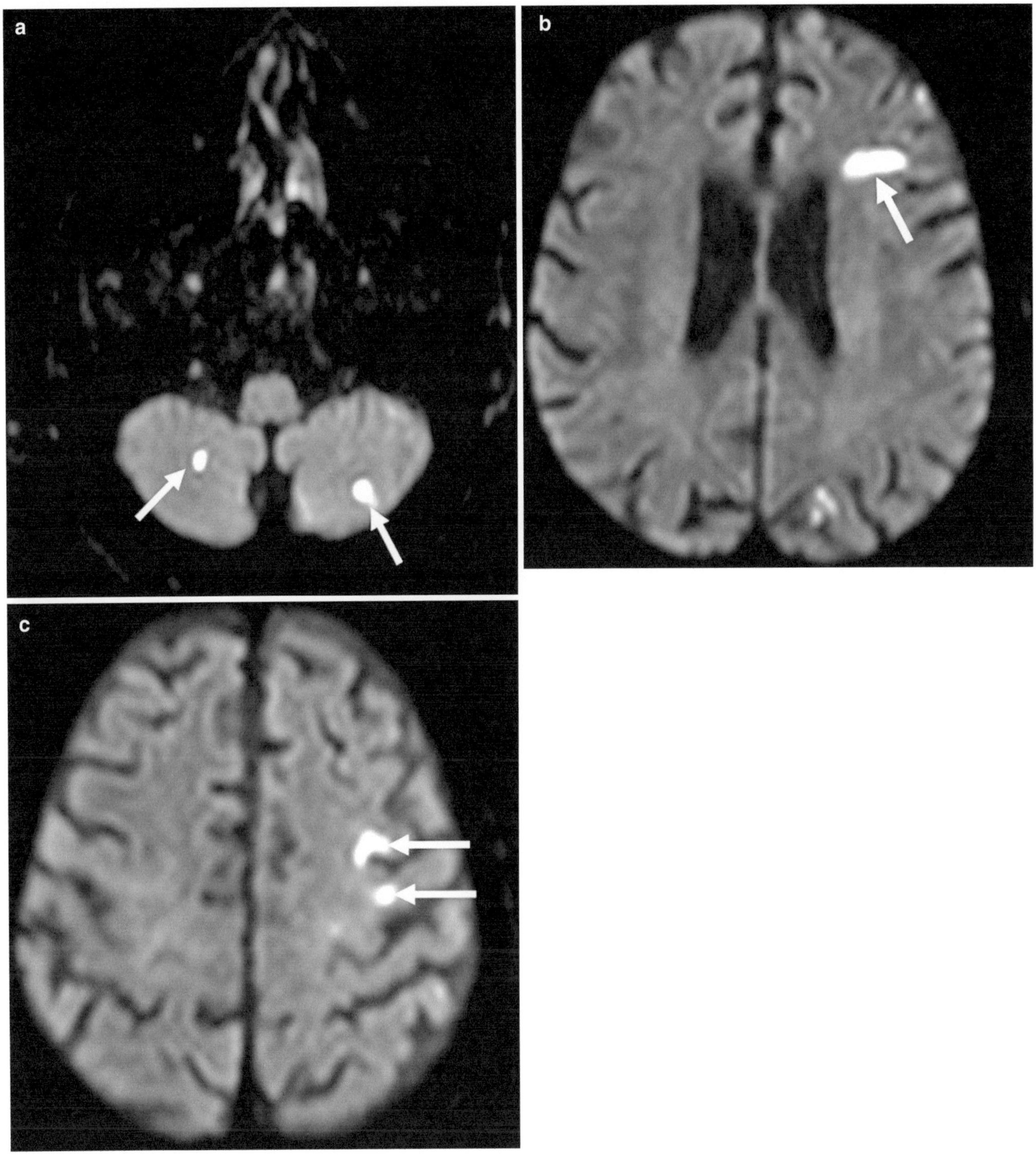

Fig. 20.2 Diffusion-weighted magnetic resonance imaging (DW MRI) images following transapical transcatheter aortic valve implantation (TA TAVI) in an 83-year-old patient showing multiple acute ischemic lesions in the left and right cerebellum (**a**, *white arrows*) and left frontal territory (**b** and **c**, *white arrows*) (Reproduced from Rodés-Cabau et al. with the permission of author and publisher)

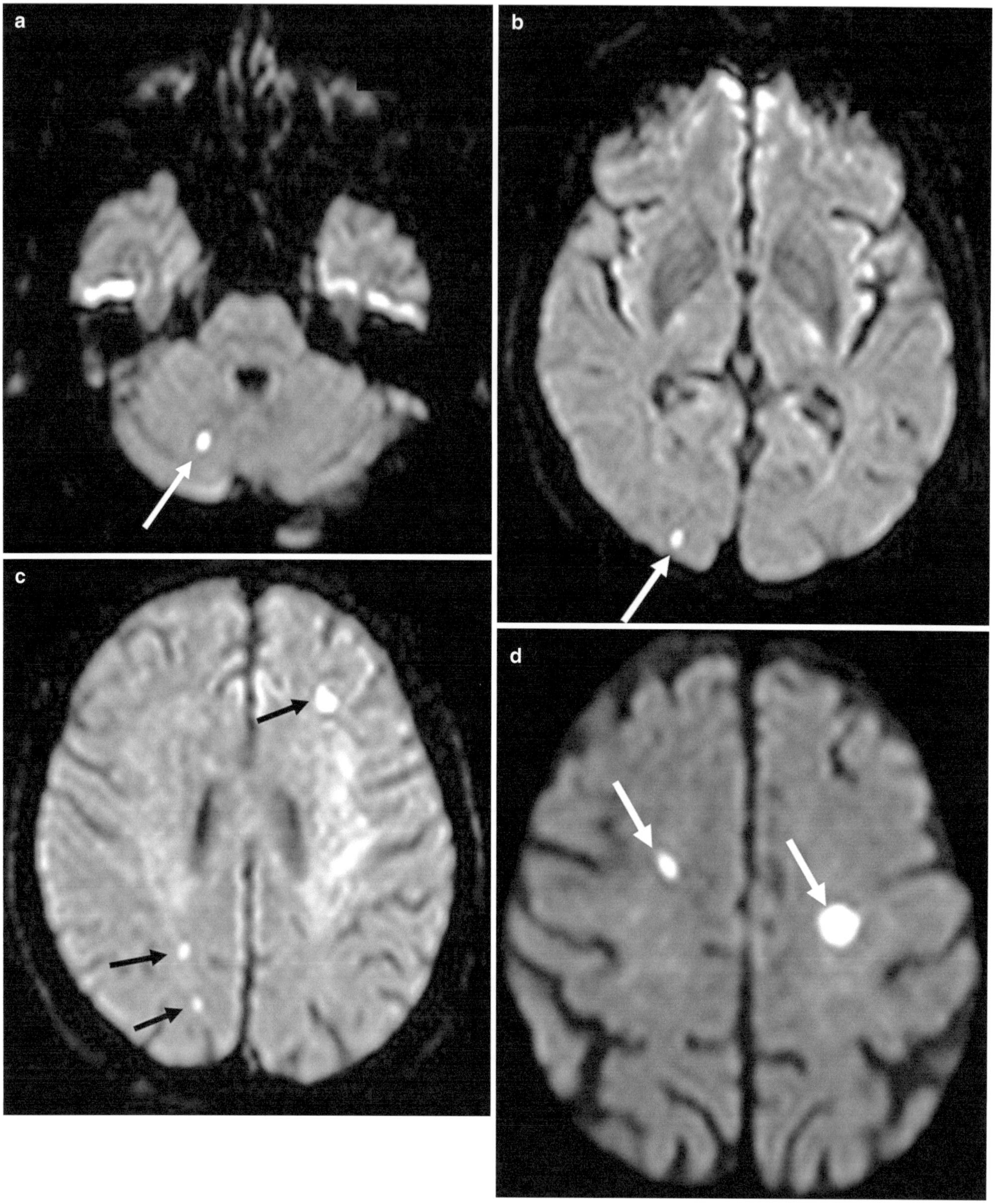

Fig. 20.3 Diffusion-weighted magnetic resonance imaging (DW MRI) images following transfemoral transcatheter aortic valve implantation (TF TAVI) in an 86-year-old patient showing multiple acute ischemic lesions in the right cerebellum (**a**, *white arrow*), right occipital territory (**b**, *white arrow*), left frontal and right parietal territories (**c**, *black arrows*), and left and right frontal superior territories (**d**, *white arrows*) (Reproduced from Rodés-Cabau et al. with the permission of author and publisher)

small (<1 cm). There were no significant differences between groups with regard to the incidence of new ischemic lesions between the TF (66 %) and TA (71 %) approaches. Finally, no interval changes in NIHSS and MMSE test scores were recorded following TAVR.

Fairbairn et al. [27] examined quality of life data in addition to performing DW MRI pre and post TAVR with the CoreValve system in 31 AS patients. Two (6 %) patients were diagnosed clinically with stroke as a consequence of the procedure. DW MRI confirmed up to 26 new ischemic lesions in both of these. Overall, new cerebral ischemic lesions were seen in 24 (77 %) patients, with the infarcts distributed evenly between both hemispheres. The mean number of new lesions per patient was 4.2±6.5 with a mean infarcted tissue volume of 2.05±3.5 ml. The authors demonstrated that increasing age and aortic arch atheroma burden were independent predictors of new ischemic lesions post TAVR. General health status and quality of life improved at 30 days post TAVR with no functional cognitive decline recorded.

The significance of clinically silent cerebrovascular ischemic events post TAVR remains unclear. As detailed above DW MRI evaluation has shown that between 68 and 86 % of TAVR patients have evidence of acute ischemic insults [23–27]. General population studies have found that the prevalence of silent brain infarcts increases with age and may be as high as 28 %, fivefold more common than stroke [28–30]. Though the consequences of silent cerebral ischemia are not fully elucidated, they have been associated with visual defects, motor abnormalities, cognitive decline, and altered mood [31]. Further studies will have to elucidate the real clinical consequences of these DW MRI defects following TAVR procedures.

Pathophysiology of Cerebroembolic Events During TAVR (Box 20.1)

Box 20.1 Potential Etiologies of Cerebroembolic Events During TAVR

- Aortic arch manipulation
- Cerebral emboli (gaseous or thrombotic)
- Showering of calcium during balloon aortic valvuloplasty
- Balloon post-dilatation
- Hypoperfusion
- Atrial fibrillation

Aortic Arch Manipulation

Given the complexities of the TAVR procedure and the often coexistent multiple patient comorbidities, inadvertent cerebral embolization may result from a multitude of events. For instance, left heart catheterization alone via the TF approach, wherein a stenosed calcified aortic valve is crossed in its retrograde fashion, has been shown to result in frequent cerebroemboli [32]. Omran et al. [32] described the occurrence of clinically apparent stroke in 3 % and cerebral DW MRI changes consistent with acute ischemic lesions in 22 %, following retrograde AV crossing. Several studies employing cerebral DW MRI have shown asymptomatic ischemic lesions due to cardiac catheterization with an incidence ranging from 5 % to the 22 % of the aforementioned work [32–34]. Clinically overt stroke has been reported in 0.44 % of patients undergoing PCI and was associated with diabetes mellitus, hypertension, prior stroke, or renal failure [35]. However, age has been shown to influence this rate with one study showing a more than doubling of the stroke rate in patients older than 80 years (0.58 % vs. 0.23 %, $p<0.001$) [36]. Perhaps of even more relevance to TAVR are the associations between aortic atheroma, aortic scraping during catheter manipulation, and release of microemboli [37–39]. Cerebral emboli may also be gaseous or originate from thrombi formed on the catheter or introducer sheath surface, in addition to displaced endovascular atheroma. The very large sheaths necessary for TAVR make smooth transitioning through the peripheral vasculature especially challenging. Furthermore, even with meticulous catheter preparation and flushing, air emboli are commonly observed using transesophageal echocardiography. A significant potential also exists with these catheters for air entrainment leading to large gaseous emboli [40].

Balloon Aortic Valvuloplasty

BAV is an important step during TAVR to facilitate delivery of the undeployed valve. A study using computed tomography alone described radiographic evidence of new cerebral ischemia in 3 out of 26 patients following BAV [41]. A more recent series looked at outcomes following BAV in 262 high- risk patients (mean logistic EuroSCORE 45.6±21.6) and reported a stroke rate that was close to 2 % [42]. TAVR also necessitates at least one to two AV dilations depending on the use of self-expandable or balloon-expandable valves, respectively, and this carries the risk of releasing calcific valve particles intra-arterially that may result in cerebrovascular embolization. Kahlert et al. [43] detailed intraoperative transcranial Doppler (TCD) ultrasound findings of both middle cerebral arteries in 46 patients during TAVR (TF 32, TA 14). The results of this study showed that though high-intensity transient signals (HITS) can occur almost at any time during the TAVR procedure, the greatest number seem to occur during actual valve positioning and implantation.

Similarly Drews et al. [44] performed TCD ultrasonography of both middle cerebral arteries in 50 patients undergoing TA TAVR. The greatest number of HITS and microembolic signals were detected during BAV and with passage of the undeployed valve. Szeto et al. [45] employed TCD ultrasonography to evaluate 28 patients who underwent TAVR with a balloon-expandable valve by TF or TA approach. The main results of this study showed that most HITS occurred during wire manipulation in the aortic arch and with valve deployment. No significant difference in the number of HITS was seen between TF and TA approaches.

These TCD studies provide important insight into the mechanisms of cerebral emboli during TAVR procedures and strongly suggest that most embolic episodes occur during the interaction between the transcatheter valve prosthesis and the native aortic valve (valve positioning and deployment). This might explain the lack of observed differences in adverse cerebrovascular events, between the TF and TA approaches. This is despite the operator, when using the TA approach, being able to minimize the manipulation of large catheters in the ascending aorta and the lack of any engagement with the aortic arch. Miller et al. [21] recently reported the results of a PARTNER substudy primarily focusing on neurological events. Interestingly, the acute cerebrovascular events were associated with smaller valve areas, which are usually associated with a higher degree of valve calcification [46, 47].

Balloon Post-Dilation

Nombella-Franco et al. [48] found that patients undergoing TAVR with more extensive native valve calcification were more likely to require balloon post-dilation (BPD) for aortic regurgitation. In addition they reported that higher stroke rates in patients needing BPD ($n=59$) compared to those who did not have significant paravalvular leak post TAVR ($n=152$). Analysis of valve calcification was performed using thoracic CT three-dimensional multiplanar reconstruction. A calcium volume cutoff of 2,242 mm^3 was the most powerful predictor of the need for BPD with a sensitivity and specificity of 78 and 65 %, respectively (area under ROC curve, 0.74; 95 % CI, 0.65–0.84; $p<0.0001$). Patients who required BPD had higher cerebrovascular event rates (11.9 % vs. 2.0 %, $p=0.006$), with the majority of these occurring within 24 h of TAVR. A 30-day stroke rate of 10.2 % ($n=6$) was documented in the BPD group, while the corresponding value was 1.9 % ($n=3$), $p=0.016$, for those patients who did not undergo BPD.

Hypoperfusion

Another potentially important contributor to ischemic brain injury during TAVR is hypoperfusion, which may occur at a number of stages during valve implantation. For instance, BAV and deployment of the balloon-expandable valves are routinely done during rapid right ventricular pacing to prevent device ejection. These episodes may induce cerebral ischemia in watershed territories as well as impair the washout of dislodged microemboli. Indeed, it has been shown that the combination of hypoperfusion and cerebral emboli often coexists in a number of clinical situations such as cardiac surgery [49]. Transitory poor cerebral perfusion may accentuate the microembolic ischemic effects by reducing the effectiveness of the circulation to wash out debris promptly.

Timing of CVE

From the data that currently exists, it appears that a significant risk of stroke persists beyond the immediate periprocedural period. Combined data from the Canadian Registry [7] and PARTNER Cohort B [19] (nonoperable patients with severe AS) reveals that 13 of the 22 stroke events that were reported by 30 days in both of these studies occurred in the 24-h to 30-day period post TAVR. Tay et al. [50] showed similar results in a single-center series including 253 patients. The variability in the timing of stroke occurrence following TAVR suggests that mechanisms other than catheter-induced cerebral embolization or native valve dilation resulting in embolic debris may be at play. Miller et al. [21] showed that cerebrovascular events occurring after the periprocedural period were mostly related to higher atherosclerotic burden, with patients who suffered late strokes exhibiting higher rates of extensive peripheral arterial disease that had necessitated a TA approach. In addition these patients were found to have had a higher rate of stroke in the 6–12-month period prior to their TAVR procedure.

Atrial Fibrillation

A further potential etiological factor of stroke is TAVR-associated atrial fibrillation. Recently our group described the incidence and prognostic value of new-onset atrial fibrillation after TAVR [51]. In a series of 138 patients undergoing

TAVR, almost 32 % developed new-onset AF at a median of 48 h post valve implantation. A higher incidence was seen in the TA approach (37 % vs. 15.8 %, $p=0.019$), and new-onset AF was associated with a higher stroke and systemic embolism rate at 30 days (13.6 % vs. 3.2 %, $p=0.021$). Importantly, new-onset atrial fibrillation was found to be the strongest predictor of cardioembolic events occurring after the first 24 h following the procedure, suggesting again that the mechanisms of acute (<24 h) vs. subacute (>24 h) stroke post TAVR are probably different. Similarly, Nuis et al. reported a 4.4-fold increase in the rate of stroke in patients undergoing TAVR who had a diagnosis of atrial fibrillation [52]. In their analysis of 214 patients who had TAVR using the Medtronic CoreValve system, the overall incidence of cerebrovascular events was 9 % of which more than half occurred more than 24 h post valve implantation.

Other Factors Contributory to CVE

Finally, given the baseline profile of TAVR patients, it would appear that their elevated risk of stroke intraoperatively and beyond the periprocedural period may be influenced by several non-TAVR-related characteristics. For instance, intraoperative and postoperative stroke rates were found to be both increased by older age, small body surface area, previous stroke, preoperative AF, and use of hypothermic circulatory arrest in a large series of isolated or repeat CABG [53]. Similarly, data from SAVR has shown that risk factors such as age >75 years at time of surgery, diabetes mellitus, previous stroke, and carotid artery stenosis increase adverse CVE rates during long-term follow-up [54]. Patients without these risk factors had CVE rates of 1.37 % per patient-year vs. 5.18 % per patient-year in those with more than one risk factor.

Prognostic Value of Cerebrovascular Events Following TAVR

Data from non-TAVR patients show that severe stroke carries a grave prognosis with a 30-day mortality rate of approximately 58 % in those requiring mechanical ventilation [55]. Also, several studies have demonstrated the poor outcomes of patients who suffer a stroke following a cardiovascular intervention. Melby et al. [56] examined outcomes in 245 octogenarians who underwent SAVR alone or with CABG. Patients who suffered a perioperative stroke had significantly higher 30-day mortality rates (38 % vs. 9 %; OR, 11.3; 95 % CI, 1.7–75.1; $p=0.019$). Tarakji et al. [53] also showed that post CABG patients who experienced a stroke experienced a significantly higher hospital mortality rate (19 % (95 % CI, 16–22 %) vs. 3.7 % (95 % CI, 3.1–4.5 %), $p<0.001$), a finding that persisted after propensity adjustment for preoperative factors.

Stroke arising from catheter-based interventions is also a potentially catastrophic event. Hamon et al. [39] demonstrated an increased relative risk of mortality of 9.95 (95 % CI 5.73–17.27, $p<0.00001$) in pooled data analysis evaluating PCI-related stroke. Although the corresponding data for TAVR-associated stroke remains very limited, some studies have provided important data regarding its prognostic value. Tamburino et al. found that intraprocedural stroke was a predictor of increased 1-year mortality (HR 15.76, CI 3.27–75.9, $p=0.001$) in a study of 663 patients undergoing CoreValve TAVR [13]. Periprocedural major stroke was also associated with a higher mortality at 2-year follow-up in the PARTNER trial [57]. A meta-analysis of 53 TAVR studies including more than 10,000 patients found that stroke was associated with a greater than 3.5-fold higher 30-day mortality compared to those without stroke (25.5±21.9 % vs. 6.9±4.2 %) [3].

Prevention of TAVR-Associated Cerebrovascular Ischemic Injury

Minimizing the risk of TAVR-related stroke is extremely important to ensure overall success of the procedure. Although there is a paucity of hard data to guide the clinician in this rapidly evolving field, it would appear prudent to attempt to apply knowledge obtained from established percutaneous and open surgical procedures. Techniques to reduce TAVR-associated stroke begin with the patient's pre-procedural assessment. Although potential TAVR patients have, by their nature, significant risk factors for CVE, a thorough evaluation with multimodality imaging may aid risk stratification and guide the approach to valve delivery. For instance, significant atheroma burden in the aortic arch may favor a TA approach, conceptually reducing stroke risk, although this has not been backed up by DW MRI and clinical results to date (Table 20.3). Patients are usually pretreated with single (aspirin) or dual (aspirin + clopidogrel) antiplatelet therapy, and the strict monitoring of intraprocedural anticoagulation is vital ensuring the target activated clotting time (>300 s) is maintained. Cardiac anesthesia plays a vital role in preserving hemodynamic stability and minimizing periods of hypo- or hypertension. Overvigorous BAV prior to valve insertion should probably be avoided. Likewise balloon post-dilation following valve implantation should also probably be limited to those cases with moderate-to-severe residual paravalvular aortic regurgitation. Meticulous attention must be paid to thorough sheath and catheter flushing, in addition to valve preparation, to reduce thrombus formation and gaseous embolization. Where possible, every effort must be made to employ a technique of smooth transitioning when exchanging and upsizing equipment within the vasculature.

Embolic Protection Devices (EPD)

The need to reduce TAVR-associated stroke has spurned significant research and the development of new embolic protection devices (EPD) during TAVR (Table 20.4). Nietlispach et al. [58] described their initial experience with the Embrella Embolic Deflector (Edwards Lifesciences, Irvine, CA) in three TF TAVR patients (Edwards SAPIEN valve) and one BAV patient. This device consists of a nitinol-mounted deflecting membrane composed of heparin-coated polyurethane with a pore size of 100 μm. Initial animal work showed it was effective in deflecting emboli ranging in size from 150 to 600 μm away from the carotid circulation [59]. Retrieved particulate matter was reduced in the carotid filtration circuit from 19 % (during unprotected aortic injection of prepared human atheroma) to 1.3 % with Embrella usage ($p<0.001$). During the initial clinical study, the device was successfully deployed in all patients via the right radial artery, with the concept of shielding the brachiocephalic and left common carotid arteries from emboli. No clinically overt strokes were found, but post procedure DW MRI revealed a new ischemic lesion in the BAV patient. Inherent limitations of the device include a potential lack of coverage of the left vertebral arterial system. In addition, different aortic arch types that may impair its ability to deflect emboli may affect the conformity of the device. Recapture of the device may inadvertently lead to cerebral showering at the end of the procedure. Nonetheless, further refinements to this technique may offer a modality of significantly reducing brain injury. A prospective randomized trial (PROTAVR) is planned to demonstrate the efficacy of this device in reducing cerebral ischemic defects as evaluated by MRI.

Another cerebral EPD in evolution is the SMT Embolic Deflection Device (SMT Research and Development Ltd., Herzliya, Israel), which has been designed to deflect debris from all three great aortic arch vessels and is deployed via the transfemoral route (Table 20.4). The first-in-human experience including 15 patients showed the feasibility and safety of this device and suggested a reduction on the number of cerebral ischemic events as evaluated by MRI [60].

Another embolic protection device is the Claret dual filter system (Claret Medical Inc, CA USA) which is deployed via the radial approach but functions by capturing and retaining debris within the proximal brachiocephalic and left common carotid arteries (Table 20.4). Naber et al. described the use of the Claret CE Pro EPD in patients undergoing TAVR at three centers [61]. Successful deployment of the device via the right radial or brachial artery into the aortic arch was achieved in 35 out of 40 patients. Technical success with regard to delivery of both the proximal and distal embolic protection filters improved from 60 % with the first-generation device to almost 90 % for the newer model. Of note, 36 patients had embolic protection of the left common carotid performed using a separate commercially available carotid EPD. Macroscopic debris was seen in 19 of the 35 patients, following recapture and retrieval of the device post TAVR. Two patients had documented major stroke one at 4 h and the second on day 27 post TAVR. At 30 days post procedure, 1 patient also had a minor stroke recorded. Despite improvement with a second-generation device, limitations remain with regard to access site complications, delivery within tortuous vasculature, and provision of complete cerebrovascular protection.

Persistence of CVE Risk Following TAVR

It is also worth noting that the risk of stroke, though highest in the periprocedural period, persists following successful TAVR (Fig. 20.4). The optimal drug therapy post TAVR also remains unclear, with little scientific data to guide the physician. Most operators routinely continue dual antiplatelet therapy (aspirin and clopidogrel) for a number of months, and this has been the recommended therapy by the ACCF/AATS/SCAI/STS Expert Consensus Document on TAVR and the Canadian Cardiovascular Society statement on TAVR [62, 63]. A small randomized trial comparing aspirin vs. aspirin plus clopidogrel following TAVR with the CoreValve system showed no differences in stroke CVE rate between groups [64]. Another randomized trial is currently ongoing in Canada comparing these two strategies (ARTE trial: Clinicaltrials.gov NCT01559298). Also, the potential usefulness of short-term anticoagulation therapy (warfarin or the novel anticoagulation agents) in this setting will merit further exploration. Notably, the clinical characteristics of the current patients undergoing TAVR pose significant challenges to adjust optimal antithrombotic therapy following TAVR. It is likely unrealistic to expect a single antithrombotic regime to fit all patients undergoing TAVR. The ultimate goal would be to recommend a scientifically proven (instead of empirical) regimen based upon a better understanding of the pathophysiology of acute and late CVE, tailored to patient's age, risk factors, and occurrence of periprocedural complications.

Table 20.4 Embolic protection devices

Device	Approach	Device positioning	Mechanism of action	Pore size (μm)	Catheter size (F)
Embrella 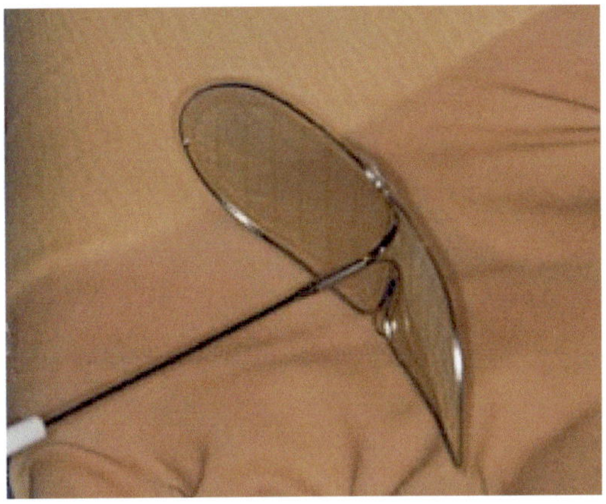	Radial	Aortic arch (covering brachiocephalic and left carotid arteries)	Deflection of embolic material	100	6
SMT 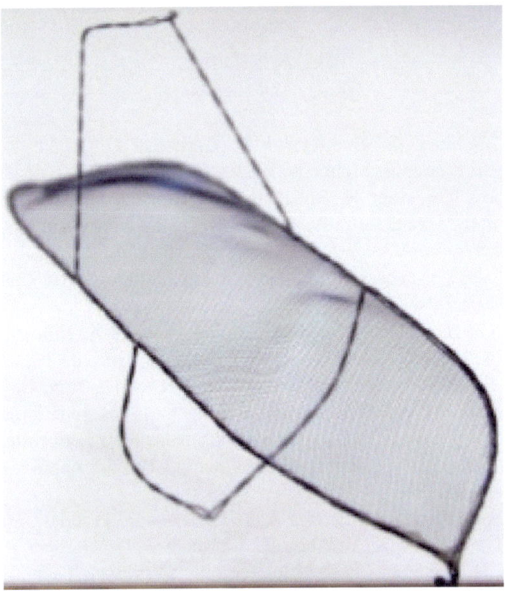	Femoral	Aortic arch (covering brachiocephalic, left carotid, and left subclavian arteries)	Deflection of embolic material	~200	9
Claret Medical 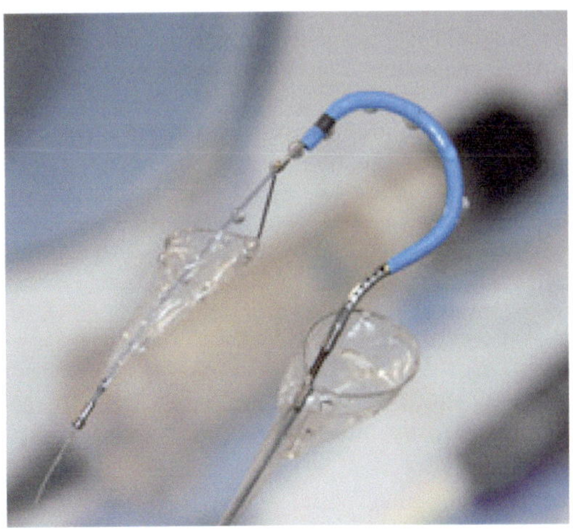	Radial	Brachiocephalic trunk Left common carotid (covering brachiocephalic and left carotid arteries)	Capture of embolic material	140	6

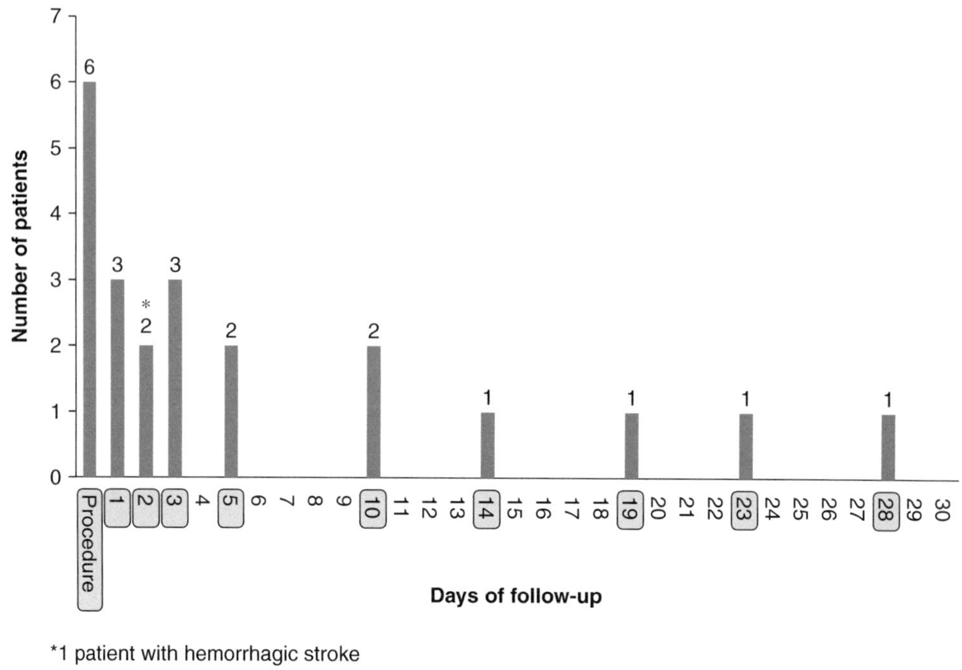

Fig. 20.4 Timing of stroke within the 30 days following TAVI (Data from the PARTNER trial nonoperable cohort [19] and the Multicenter Canadian Experience [7])

Conclusion

TAVR represents an exciting novel therapy. Continued refinement of the valve systems, procedural techniques, and periprocedural care will aid its successful utilization in patients with severe aortic stenosis. It is hoped that future studies will address current limitations particularly with regard to reducing procedure-related adverse cerebrovascular events. A better understanding of the pathophysiologic mechanisms involved in these events will be key to implement the appropriate preventive measures.

Acknowledgment We want to thank Mélanie Côté, MSc, from the Quebec Heart and Lung Institute for her help with the preparation of the tables and figures.

References

1. Rodés-Cabau J. Transcatheter aortic valve implantation: current and future approaches. Nat Rev Cardiol. 2011;9:15–29.
2. Schaff HV. Transcatheter aortic-valve implantation – at what price? N Engl J Med. 2011;364(23):2187–98.
3. Eggebrecht H, Schmermund A, Voigtlander T, Kahlert P, Erbel R, Mehta RH. Risk of stroke after transcatheter aortic valve implantation (TAVR): a meta-analysis of 10,037 published patients. EuroIntervention. 2012;15:129–38.
4. Cribier A, Eltchaninoff H, Tron C, Bauer F, Agatiello C, Nercolini D, Tapiero S, Litzler PY, Bessou JP, Babaliaros V. Treatment of calcific aortic stenosis with the percutaneous heart valve: mid-term follow-up from the initial feasibility studies: the French experience. J Am Coll Cardiol. 2006;47:1214–23.
5. Grube E, Schuler G, Buellesfeld L, Gerckens U, Linke A, Wenaweser P, Sauren B, Mohr FW, Walther T, Zickmann B, Iversen S, Felderhoff T, Cartier R, Bonan R. Percutaneous aortic valve replacement for severe aortic stenosis in high-risk patients using the second- and current third-generation self-expanding CoreValve prosthesis: device success and 30-day clinical outcome. J Am Coll Cardiol. 2007;50:69–76.
6. Piazza N, Grube E, Gerckens U, den Heijer P, Linke A, Luha O, Ramondo A, Ussia G, Wenaweser P, Windecker S, Laborde JC, de Jaegere P, Serruys PW. Procedural and 30-day outcomes following transcatheter aortic valve implantation using the third generation (18 Fr) corevalve revalving system: results from the multicentre, expanded evaluation registry 1-year following CE mark approval. EuroIntervention. 2008;4:242–9.
7. Rodés-Cabau J, Webb JG, Cheung A, Ye J, Dumont E, Feindel CM, Osten M, Natarajan MK, Velianou JL, Martucci G, DeVarennes B, Chisholm R, Peterson MD, Lichtenstein SV, Nietlispach F, Doyle D, DeLarochelliere R, Teoh K, Chu V, Dancea A, Lachapelle K, Cheema A, Latter D, Horlick E. Transcatheter aortic valve implantation for the treatment of severe symptomatic aortic stenosis in patients at very high or prohibitive surgical risk: acute and late outcomes of the multicenter Canadian experience. J Am Coll Cardiol. 2010;55:1080–90.
8. Thomas M, Schymik G, Walther T, Himbert D, Lefevre T, Treede H, Eggebrecht H, Rubino P, Michev I, Lange R, Anderson WN, Wendler O. Thirty-day results of the SAPIEN aortic Bioprosthesis European Outcome (SOURCE) Registry: a European registry of transcatheter aortic valve implantation using the Edwards SAPIEN valve. Circulation. 2011;122:62–9.
9. Thomas M, Schymik G, Walther T, Himbert D, Lefèvre T, Treede H, Eggebrecht H, Rubino P, Colombo A, Lange R, Schwarz RR, Wendler O. One-year outcomes of cohort 1 in the Edwards SAPIEN Aortic Bioprosthesis European Outcome (SOURCE) registry: the European registry of transcatheter aortic valve implantation using the Edwards SAPIEN valve. Circulation. 2012; 124:425–33.

10. Eltchaninoff H, Prat A, Gilard M, Leguerrier A, Blanchard D, Fournial G, Iung B, Donzeau-Gouge P, Tribouilloy C, Debrux JL, Pavie A, Gueret P. Transcatheter aortic valve implantation: early results of the FRANCE (FRench Aortic National CoreValve and Edwards) registry. Eur Heart J. 2011;32(2):191–7.
11. Zahn R, Gerckens U, Grube E, Linke A, Sievert H, Eggebrecht H, Hambrecht R, Sack S, Hauptmann KE, Richardt G, Figulla HR, Senges J. Transcatheter aortic valve implantation: first results from a multi-centre real-world registry. Eur Heart J. 2011;32(2): 198–204.
12. Bosmans JM, Kefer J, De Bruyne B, Herijgers P, Dubois C, Legrand V, Verheye S, Rodrigus I. Procedural, 30-day and one year outcome following CoreValve or Edwards transcatheter aortic valve implantation: results of the Belgian national registry. Interact Cardiovasc Thorac Surg. 2011;12(5):762–7.
13. Tamburino C, Capodanno D, Ramondo A, Petronio AS, Ettori F, Santoro G, Klugmann S, Bedogni F, Maisano F, Marzocchi A, Poli A, Antoniucci D, Napodano M, De Carlo M, Fiorina C, Ussia GP. Incidence and predictors of early and late mortality after transcatheter aortic valve implantation in 663 patients with severe aortic stenosis. Circulation. 2011;123:299–308.
14. Moat NE, Ludman P, de Belder MA, Bridgewater B, Cunningham AD. Long term outcomes following transcatheter aortic valve implantation in high risk patients with severe aortic stenosis. The UK TAVR Registry. J Am Coll Cardiol. 2011;58(20): 2130–8.
15. Gilard M, Eltchaninoff H, Iung B, Donzeau-Gouge P, Chevreul K, Fajadet J, Leprince P, Leguerrier A, Lievre M, Prat A, Teiger E, Lefevre T, Himbert D, Tchetche D, Carrié D, Albat B, Cribier A, Rioufol G, Sudre A, Blanchard D, Collet F, Dos Santos P, Meneveau N, Tirouvanziam A, Caussin C, Guyon P, Boschat J, Le Breton H, Collart F, Houel R, Delpine S, Souteyrand G, Favereau X, Ohlmann P, Doisy V, Grollier G, Gommeaux A, Claudel JP, Bourlon F, Bertrand B, Van Belle E, Laskar M, FRANCE 2 Investigators. Registry of transcatheter aortic-valve implantation in high-risk patients. N Engl J Med. 2012;366(18):1705–15.
16. Wendler O. The Multicenter SOURCE XT TAVR Registry. Presented at EuroPCR 2012, Paris, 17 May 012.
17. Linke A, Gerckens U, Wenaweser P, Tamburino C, Bosmans J, Brecker S, Bauernschmitt R. Treatment of high risk aortic stenosis patients with transcatheter Medtronic CoreValve implantation: results from the international multicenter ADVANCE study. J Am Coll Cardiol. 2012;59(13s1):E8–E8. doi:10.1016/S0735-1097(12)60009-6.
18. Leon MB, Piazza N, Nikolsky E, Blackstone EH, Cutlip DE, Kappetein AP, Krucoff MW, Mack M, Mehran R, Miller C, Morel MA, Petersen J, Popma JJ, Takkenberg JJ, Vahanian A, van Es GA, Vranckx P, Webb JG, Windecker S, Serruys PW. Standardized endpoint definitions for Transcatheter Aortic Valve Implantation clinical trials: a consensus report from the Valve Academic Research Consortium. J Am Coll Cardiol. 2011;57(3): 253–69.
19. Leon MB, Smith CR, Mack M, Miller DC, Moses JW, Svensson LG, Tuzcu EM, Webb JG, Fontana GP, Makkar RR, Brown DL, Block PC, Guyton RA, Pichard AD, Bavaria JE, Herrmann HC, Douglas PS, Petersen JL, Akin JJ, Anderson WN, Wang D, Pocock S, PARTNER Trial Investigators. Transcatheter aortic-valve implantation for aortic stenosis in patients who cannot undergo surgery. N Engl J Med. 2010;363:1597–607.
20. Smith CR, Leon MB, Mack MJ, Miller DC, Moses JW, Svensson LG, Tuzcu EM, Webb JG, Fontana GP, Makkar RR, Williams M, Dewey T, Kapadia S, Babaliaros V, Thourani VH, Corso P, Pichard AD, Bavaria JE, Herrmann HC, Akin JJ, Anderson WN, Wang D, Pocock SJ. Transcatheter versus surgical aortic-valve replacement in high-risk patients. N Engl J Med. 2011; 364(23):2187–98.
21. Miller DC, Blackstone EH, Mack MJ, Svensson LG, Kodali SK, Kapadia S, Rajeswaran J, Anderson WN, Moses JW, Tuzcu EM, Webb JG, Leon MB, Smith CR, PARTNER Trial Investigators and Patients; PARTNER Stroke Substudy Writing Group and Executive Committee. Transcatheter (TAVR) versus surgical (AVR) aortic valve replacement: occurrence, hazard, risk factors, and consequences of neurologic events in the PARTNER trial. J Thorac Cardiovasc Surg. 2012;143(4):832–843.e13.
22. Makkar RR, Fontana GP, Jilaihawi H, Kapadia S, Pichard AD, Douglas PS, Thourani VH, Babaliaros VC, Webb JG, Herrmann HC, Bavaria JE, Kodali S, Brown DL, Bowers B, Dewey TM, Svensson LG, Tuzcu M, Moses JW, Williams MR, Siegel RJ, Akin JJ, Anderson WN, Pocock S, Smith CR, Leon MB, PARTNER Trial Investigators. Transcatheter aortic-valve replacement for inoperable severe aortic stenosis. N Engl J Med. 2012;366(18): 1696–704.
23. Kahlert P, Knipp SC, Schlamann M, Thielmann M, Al-Rashid F, Weber M, Johansson U, Wendt D, Jakob HG, Forsting M, Sack S, Erbel R, Eggebrecht H. Silent and apparent cerebral ischemia after percutaneous transfemoral aortic valve implantation: a diffusion-weighted magnetic resonance imaging study. Circulation. 2010;121(7):870–8.
24. Ghanem A, Muller A, Nahle CP, Kocurek J, Werner N, Hammerstingl C, Schild HH, Schwab JO, Mellert F, Fimmers R, Nickenig G, Thomas D. Risk and fate of cerebral embolism after transfemoral aortic valve implantation: a prospective pilot study with diffusion-weighted magnetic resonance imaging. J Am Coll Cardiol. 2010;55(14):1427–32.
25. Arnold M, Schulz-Heise S, Achenbach S, Ott S, Dorfler A, Ropers D, Feyrer R, Einhaus F, Loders S, Mahmoud F, Roerick O, Daniel WG, Weyand M, Ensminger SM, Ludwig J. Embolic cerebral insults after transapical aortic valve implantation detected by magnetic resonance imaging. JACC Cardiovasc Interv. 2010;3(11): 1126–32.
26. Rodés-Cabau J, Dumont E, Boone RH, Larose E, Bagur R, Gurvitch R, Bedard F, Doyle D, De Larochelliere R, Jayasuria C, Villeneuve J, Marrero A, Cote M, Pibarot P, Webb JG. Cerebral embolism following transcatheter aortic valve implantation: comparison of transfemoral and transapical approaches. J Am Coll Cardiol. 2011;57(1):18–28.
27. Fairbairn TA, Mather AN, Bijsterveld P, Worthy G, Currie S, Goddard AJ, Blackman DJ, Plein S, Greenwood JP. Diffusion-weighted MRI determined cerebral embolic infarction following transcatheter aortic valve implantation: assessment of predictive risk factors and the relationship to subsequent health status. Heart. 2012;98(1):18–23.
28. Price TR, Manolio TA, Kronmal RA, Kittner SJ, Yue NC, Robbins J, Anton-Culver H, O'Leary DH. Silent brain infarction on magnetic resonance imaging and neurological abnormalities in community-dwelling older adults. The Cardiovascular Health Study. CHS Collaborative Research Group. Stroke. 1997;28(6): 1158–64.
29. Di Carlo A, Launer LJ, Breteler MM, Fratiglioni L, Lobo A, Martinez-Lage J, Schmidt R, Hofman A. Frequency of stroke in Europe: a collaborative study of population-based cohorts. ILSA Working Group and the Neurologic Diseases in the Elderly Research Group. Italian Longitudinal Study on Aging. Neurology. 2000;54(11 Suppl 5):S28–33.
30. Longstreth Jr WT, Bernick C, Fitzpatrick A, Cushman M, Knepper L, Lima J, Furberg CD. Frequency and predictors of stroke death in 5,888 participants in the Cardiovascular Health Study. Neurology. 2001;56(3):368–75.

31. Vermeer SE, Longstreth Jr WT, Koudstaal PJ. Silent brain infarcts: a systematic review. Lancet Neurol. 2007;6(7):611–9.
32. Omran H, Schmidt H, Hackenbroch M, Illien S, Bernhardt P, von der Recke G, Fimmers R, Flacke S, Layer G, Pohl C, Luderitz B, Schild H, Sommer T. Silent and apparent cerebral embolism after retrograde catheterisation of the aortic valve in valvular stenosis: a prospective, randomised study. Lancet. 2003;361(9365): 1241–6.
33. Hamon M, Gomes S, Oppenheim C, Morello R, Sabatier R, Lognone T, Grollier G, Courtheoux P. Cerebral microembolism during cardiac catheterization and risk of acute brain injury: a prospective diffusion-weighted magnetic resonance imaging study. Stroke. 2006;37(8):2035–8.
34. Lund C, Nes RB, Ugelstad TP, Due-Tonnessen P, Andersen R, Hol PK, Brucher R, Russell D. Cerebral emboli during left heart catheterization may cause acute brain injury. Eur Heart J. 2005;26(13):1269–75.
35. Dukkipati S, O'Neill WW, Harjai KJ, Sanders WP, Deo D, Boura JA, Bartholomew BA, Yerkey MW, Sadeghi HM, Kahn JK. Characteristics of cerebrovascular accidents after percutaneous coronary interventions. J Am Coll Cardiol. 2004;43(7):1161–7.
36. Batchelor WB, Anstrom KJ, Muhlbaier LH, Grosswald R, Weintraub WS, O'Neill WW, Peterson ED. Contemporary outcome trends in the elderly undergoing percutaneous coronary interventions: results in 7,472 octogenarians. National Cardiovascular Network Collaboration. J Am Coll Cardiol. 2000;36(3):723–30.
37. Keeley EC, Grines CL. Scraping of aortic debris by coronary guiding catheters: a prospective evaluation of 1,000 cases. J Am Coll Cardiol. 1998;32(7):1861–5.
38. Khoury Z, Gottlieb S, Stern S, Keren A. Frequency and distribution of atherosclerotic plaques in the thoracic aorta as determined by transesophageal echocardiography in patients with coronary artery disease. Am J Cardiol. 1997;79(1):23–7.
39. Hamon M, Baron JC, Viader F. Periprocedural stroke and cardiac catheterization. Circulation. 2008;118(6):678–83.
40. Berry C, Cartier R, Bonan R. Fatal ischemic stroke related to nonpermissive peripheral artery access for percutaneous aortic valve replacement. Catheter Cardiovasc Interv. 2007;69(1):56–63.
41. Davidson CJ, Skelton TN, Kisslo KB, Kong Y, Peter RH, Simonton CA, Phillips HR, Behar VS, Bashore TM. The risk for systemic embolization associated with percutaneous balloon valvuloplasty in adults. A prospective comprehensive evaluation. Ann Intern Med. 1988;108(4):557–60.
42. Ben-Dor I, Pichard AD, Satler LF, Goldstein SA, Syed AI, Gaglia Jr MA, Weissman G, Maluenda G, Gonzalez MA, Wakabayashi K, Collins SD, Torguson R, Okubagzi P, Xue Z, Kent KM, Lindsay J, Waksman R. Complications and outcome of balloon aortic valvuloplasty in high-risk or inoperable patients. JACC Cardiovasc Interv. 2010;3(11):1150–6.
43. Kahlert P. Cerebral embolization during transcatheter aortic valve implantation (TAVR): a transcranial Doppler study. Circulation. 2010;122(21_meeting abstracts).
44. Drews T, Pasic M, Buz S, Unbehaun A, Dreysse S, Kukucka M, Mladenow A, Hetzer R. Transcranial Doppler sound detection of cerebral microembolism during transapical aortic valve implantation. Thorac Cardiovasc Surg. 2011;59(4):237–42.
45. Szeto WY. Cerebral embolic exposure during transfemoral and transapical transcatheter aortic valve replacement. J Card Surg. 2011;26:348–54.
46. Messika-Zeitoun D, Aubry MC, Detaint D, Bielak LF, Peyser PA, Sheedy PF, Turner ST, Breen JF, Scott C, Tajik AJ, Enriquez-Sarano M. Evaluation and clinical implications of aortic valve calcification measured by electron-beam computed tomography. Circulation. 2004;110(3):356–62.
47. Cueff C, Serfaty JM, Cimadevilla C, Laissy JP, Himbert D, Tubach F, Duval X, Iung B, Enriquez-Sarano M, Vahanian A, Messika-Zeitoun D. Measurement of aortic valve calcification using multislice computed tomography: correlation with haemodynamic severity of aortic stenosis and clinical implication for patients with low ejection fraction. Heart. 2011;97(9):721–6.
48. Nombela-Franco L, Rodés-Cabau J, Delarochellière R, Larose E, Doyle D, Villeneuve J, Bergeron S, Bernier M, Amat-Santos IJ, Mok M, Urena M, Rheault M, Dumesnil J, Côté M, Pibarot P, Dumont E. Predictive factors, efficacy, and safety of balloon post-dilation after transcatheter aortic valve implantation with a balloon-expandable valve. JACC Cardiovasc Interv. 2012;143(4):832–43.
49. Caplan LR, Hennerici M. Impaired clearance of emboli (washout) is an important link between hypoperfusion, embolism, and ischemic stroke. Arch Neurol. 1998;55(11):1475–82.
50. Tay EL, Gurvitch R, Wijesinghe N, Nietlispach F, Wood D, Cheung A, Ye J, Lichtenstein SV, Carere R, Thompson C, Webb JG. A high-risk period for cerebrovascular events exists after transcatheter aortic valve implantation. JACC Cardiovasc Interv. 2011;4(12):1290–7.
51. Amat-Santos IJ, Rodés-Cabau J, Urena M, DeLarochellière R, Doyle D, Bagur R, Villeneuve J, Côté M, Nombela-Franco L, Philippon F, Pibarot P, Dumont E. Incidence, predictive factors and prognostic value of new-onset atrial fibrillation following transcatheter aortic valve implantation. J Am Coll Cardiol. 2012; 59:178–88.
52. Nuis RJ, Van Mieghem NM, Schultz CJ, Moelker A, van der Boon RM, van Geuns RJ, van der Lugt A, Serruys PW, Rodés-Cabau J, van Domburg RT, Koudstaal PJ, de Jaegere PP. Frequency and causes of stroke during or after transcatheter aortic valve implantation. Am J Cardiol. 2012;109(11):1637–43.
53. Tarakji KG, Sabik 3rd JF, Bhudia SK, Batizy LH, Blackstone EH. Temporal onset, risk factors, and outcomes associated with stroke after coronary artery bypass grafting. JAMA. 2011;305(4): 381–90.
54. Gulbins H, Florath I, Ennker J. Cerebrovascular events after stentless aortic valve replacement during a 9-year follow-up period. Ann Thorac Surg. 2008;86(3):769–73.
55. Holloway RG, Benesch CG, Burgin WS, Zentner JB. Prognosis and decision making in severe stroke. JAMA. 2005;294(6):725–33.
56. Melby SJ, Zierer A, Kaiser SP, Guthrie TJ, Keune JD, Schuessler RB, Pasque MK, Lawton JS, Moazami N, Moon MR, Damiano Jr RJ. Aortic valve replacement in octogenarians: risk factors for early and late mortality. Ann Thorac Surg. 2007;83(5):1651–6; discussion 1656–7.
57. Kodali SK, Williams MR, Smith CR, Svensson LG, Webb JG, Makkar RR, Fontana GP, Dewey TM, Thourani VH, Pichard AD, Fischbein M, Szeto WY, Lim S, Greason KL, Teirstein PS, Malaisrie SC, Douglas PS, Hahn RT, Whisenant B, Zajarias A, Wang D, Akin JJ, Anderson WN, Leon MB, PARTNER Trial Investigators. Two-year outcomes after transcatheter or surgical aortic-valve replacement. N Engl J Med. 2012;366: 1686–95.
58. Nietlispach F, Wijesinghe N, Gurvitch R, Tay E, Carpenter JP, Burns C, Wood DA, Webb JG. An embolic deflection device for aortic valve interventions. JACC Cardiovasc Interv. 2010;3: 1133–8.
59. Carpenter JP, Carpenter JT, Tellez A, Webb JG, Yi GH, Granada JF. A percutaneous aortic device for cerebral embolic protection during cardiovascular intervention. J Vasc Surg. 2011;54(1):174–181. e171.
60. Onsea K, Agostoni P, Samim M, Voskuil M, Kluin J, Budde R, Hendrikse J, Ramjankhan F, van Klarenbosch J, Doesburg P, Sieswerda G, Stella P. First-in-man experience with a new embolic

deflection device in transcatheter aortic valve interventions. EuroIntervention. 2012;8:51–6.

61. Naber CK, Ghanem A, Abizaid AA, Wolf A, Sinning JM, Werner N, Nickenig G, Schmitz T, Grube E. First-in-man use of a novel embolic protection device for patients undergoing transcatheter aortic valve implantation. EuroIntervention. 2012;8:43–50.
62. Holmes Jr DR, Mack MJ, Kaul S, Agnihotri A, Alexander KP, Bailey SR, Calhoon JH, Carabello BA, Desai MY, Edwards FH, Francis GS, Gardner TJ, Kappetein AP, Linderbaum JA, Mukherjee C, Mukherjee D, Otto CM, Ruiz CE, Sacco RL, Smith D, Thomas JD. 2012 ACCF/AATS/SCAI/STS expert consensus document on transcatheter aortic valve replacement. J Am Coll Cardiol. 2012;59(13):1200–54.
63. Webb J, Rodés-Cabau J, Fremes S, Pibarot P, Ruel M, Ibrahim R, Welsh R, Feindel C, Lichtenstein S. Transcatheter aortic valve implantation: a Canadian Cardiovascular Society position statement. Can J Cardiol. 2012;28(5):520–8.
64. Ussia GP, Scarabelli M, Mulè M, Barbanti M, Sarkar K, Cammalleri V, Immè S, Aruta P, Pistritto AM, Gulino S, Deste W, Capodanno D, Tamburino C. Dual antiplatelet therapy versus aspirin alone in patients undergoing transcatheter aortic valve implantation. Am J Cardiol. 2011;108(12):1772–6.

Aortoiliofemoral Assessment: MDCT

21

Theodore Blake and Dominik Fleischmann

Abstract

Multidetector computed tomography (MDCT) angiography of the iliofemoral access arteries is a critical step in patient selection for transcatheter aortic valve replacement. Vascular complications are the largest single source of procedure-related morbidity and mortality. Arterial stenosis, extreme tortuosity, and circumferential or horseshoe calcification are associated with poor outcomes and may preclude retrograde femoral access. MDCT provides high-resolution volumetric datasets which allow the generation of multiplanar and volume-rendered reconstructions for comprehensive visual assessment and provides the input data for accurate quantitative assessment of vessel geometry to avoid a mismatch between the access vessels and the large vascular access sheaths employed.

Keywords

Transcatheter aortic valve repair • CT angiography • CT screening • Multidetector CT • Iliofemoral vascular access • Complication rates • Vascular tortuosity • Vascular calcification • Vascular stenosis • Curved planar reconstructions

Background

In 2002, the first transcatheter aortic valve replacement (TAVR) was performed in a human subject via an antegrade right femoral vein approach [1]. The initial published case series similarly utilized antegrade femoral venous access [2]. However, the antegrade venous approach is associated with high technical complexity requiring transseptal puncture, dilation of the interatrial septum, and passage of large diameter catheters through the mitral valve. Possible complications of this technique include pericardial tamponade relating to transseptal puncture and dilation, transient mitral insufficiency causing procedural hemodynamic instability, and the potential for anterior mitral leaflet injury while the mitral valve is cannulated. Atrial and ventricular arrhythmias are also common during an antegrade venous approach [3].

Over the subsequent decade, tens of thousands of transcatheter aortic valves have been placed worldwide utilizing a variety of access sites. The first retrograde femoral arterial TAVR was placed in 2004, following procedural failure of the antegrade venous approach [4]. A retrograde approach has also been described with access obtained via a surgical cutdown of the left axillary artery or via the ascending aorta through a right anterior minithoracotomy [5]. Despite this, femoral arterial access has arisen as the preferred access site for a retrograde approach, with direct transapical access having supplanted the femoral vein as the preferred antegrade approach in patients deemed unsuitable for femoral arterial access.

T. Blake, BSc, MD, FRCPC
Department of Radiology, Stanford University Hospital, 1130 Welch Rd, Apartment 326, Palo Alto, CA 94304, USA

Department of Radiology, Stanford University School of Medicine, 300 Pasteur Drive, Room S-072, Stanford, CA 94305-5105, USA
e-mail: theob@stanford.edu

D. Fleischmann, MD (✉)
Department of Radiology, Stanford University School of Medicine, 300 Pasteur Drive, Room S-072, Stanford, CA 94305-5105, USA
e-mail: d.fleischmann@stanford.edu

J.K. Min et al. (eds.), *Multimodality Imaging for Transcatheter Aortic Valve Replacement*, DOI 10.1007/978-1-4471-2798-7_21, © Springer-Verlag London 2014

Table 21.1 Vascular access site and access-related complications according to Valve Academic Research Consortium definitions [6, 7]

Major vascular complications
1. Any thoracic aortic dissection
2. Access site or access-related vascular injury (dissection, stenosis, perforation, rupture, arteriovenous fistula, pseudoaneurysm, hematoma, irreversible nerve injury, or compartment syndrome) leading to either death, need for significant blood transfusions (≥4 units), unplanned percutaneous or surgical intervention, or irreversible end-organ damage (e.g., hypogastric artery occlusion causing visceral ischemia or spinal artery injury causing neurological impairment)
3. Distal embolization (non-cerebral) from a vascular source requiring surgery or resulting in amputation or irreversible end-organ damage
Minor vascular complications
1. Access site or access-related vascular injury (dissection, stenosis, perforation, rupture, arteriovenous fistula or pseudoaneurysms requiring compression or thrombin injection therapy, or hematomas requiring transfusion of ≥2 but <4 units) not requiring unplanned percutaneous or surgical intervention and not resulting in irreversible end-organ damage
2. Distal embolization treated with embolectomy and/or thrombectomy and not resulting in amputation or irreversible end-organ damage
3. Failure of percutaneous access site closure resulting in interventional (e.g., stent graft) or surgical correction and not associated with death, need for significant blood transfusions (≥4 units), or irreversible end-organ damage

Complications of Retrograde Femoral Access

Reported complications of iliofemoral TAVR access include dissection, rupture, or complete avulsion of the iliac arteries and are mainly attributable to the large diameter of the sheaths employed. Additional complications related to arterial puncture include postoperative bleeding, hematoma, pseudoaneurysm, arteriovenous fistula, and nerve injury. In an effort to improve the quality of clinical research and to enable meaningful comparisons between clinical trials, TAVR-related complications have recently been defined by the 2011 Valve Academic Research Consortium (VARC) consensus report [6, 7]. The definitions of vascular complications are based on the reporting standards of the Society of Vascular Surgery for complications following endovascular aortic graft repair, with an extended definition of "access site" to also include any location (arterial or venous) traversed by a guidewire, catheter, or sheath including the left ventricular apex and aorta (Table 21.1). Vascular complications are dichotomized as major and minor, and VARC major vascular complications are associated with increased rates of in-hospital and 30-day mortality as well as longer hospital stays, while VARC minor vascular complications are not [8].

Complication Rates

Reported vascular complication rates associated with percutaneous aortic valve placement have ranged widely from 1.9 to 30.7 % [6, 9–19] that may be, in part, due to the lack of standardized definitions for vascular complications in TAVR in the past. For example, many studies have reported only complications requiring further surgical or percutaneous intervention. A meta-analysis of 16 outcome studies employing the VARC criteria published 15 months following their release showed an 11.9 % incidence of major vascular complications (range 5.0–23.3 %), a 9.7 % incidence of minor vascular complications (range 5.6–28.3 %), with a composite incidence of any vascular complication 18.8 % (range 9.5–51.6 %) [20].

Early percutaneous heart valve systems required 22–25 F sheaths to accommodate the large catheters used for valve delivery and were associated with rates of major bleeding as high as 50 % [21]. Several subsequent trials have demonstrated that patients with either a femoral or apical access site complication have 30-day mortality rates twice that of other individuals undergoing the procedure [9, 16]. Given these dangers, great effort has gone into identifying risk factors for vascular complication, and routine screening has been implemented with respect to iliofemoral vascular access. Newer low profile systems have been designed to be compatible with smaller 18 F sheaths in an effort to decrease the incidence of access vessel injury as well as the number of patients that may be precluded from having a transarterial TAVR due to small-caliber iliofemoral vessels [22].

Several large outcome studies suggest that vascular complications are the most common major adverse event seen in association with TAVR [9, 16, 23, 24]. These studies report vascular complication occurring in 10–23 % of procedures performed via femoral arterial approach with access site complications occurring in 13–18 % of such procedures after MDCT screening. Notably, procedures performed via the transapical approach demonstrate similar rates of access site complication.

It appears that with experience, and perhaps more stringent patient selection, vascular complication rates may decrease over time. The frequency of vascular complications decreases with operator experience, 12–4.5 % after 300 cases in one series [23]. This study also demonstrated that access site complication rates were significantly lower with a surgical cutdown of the femoral artery than when a percutaneous closure device was employed (5.9 % vs. 16.8 %) [23]. In contrast, when a fully percutaneous procedure is performed routinely, VARC vascular complication rates have been shown to decrease from 32 to 9 % with increased user experience [25]. This has been attributed to more careful patient selection based, in part on findings from MDCT, as well as increased experience with percutaneous vascular closure techniques.

Risk Factors for Vascular Injury

The experience from endovascular aneurysm repair (EVAR) would suggest that patients at the greatest risk of complication resulting in iliofemoral vessel injury are those with excessive iliac tortuosity, circumferential vessel wall calcification, significant occlusive disease, and small-caliber vessels [26]. Using these guidelines, it has been suggested that 32–35 % of patients at high surgical risk for surgical aortic valve repair (SAVR) have at least one criterion unsuitable for iliofemoral access by MDCT evaluation [24, 27].

Recent work employing MDCT screening prior to retrograde iliofemoral access confirmed that moderate to severe arterial calcification is associated with a threefold increase in vascular complications (29 % vs. 9 %), and the presence of a minimal arterial lumen diameter less than that of the external sheath is associated with a fourfold increase in vascular complications (23 % vs. 5 %) [28]. A systematic analysis assessing arterial minimum lumen diameter in relation to the external sheath diameter has revealed that a sheath to femoral artery ratio (SFAR) of 1.05 or greater is predictive of VARC vascular complications and 30-day mortality [8]. Subgroup analysis of the sample population further demonstrated that this threshold may be more lenient (SFAR = 1.10) if there is no calcification of the iliofemoral vessels and conversely, stricter (SFAR = 1.00) in the presence of mild to severe calcification.

When vascular access is established for a TAVR procedure, the femoral arteries are sequentially dilated to allow passage of the sheath through the iliac arteries and into the aorta. Experience has shown that a long sheath extending directly from the femoral artery to the aorta is preferred over a short sheath as catheter introduction into the iliac arteries has been associated with iliac arterial dissection [3].

The minimum diameter of the iliofemoral arteries used for vascular access should ideally exceed that of the introducer sheath. However, short segments of narrowing in relatively compliant arteries (those without extensive calcification or atheroma) can usually be safely cannulated if they are no more than 1–2 mm smaller in diameter than the delivery system [22, 27]. Occlusive femoral sheaths have been associated with adherence of the vascular endothelium to the sheath itself resulting in complete arterial avulsion upon withdrawal of the sheath. Heavy circumferential (>60 %) calcification of the common iliac arteries has also been shown to be associated with arterial hemorrhage. If the introduction sheath is occlusive, this may not become apparent until the time of sheath removal [3].

Device Sizes

In order to evaluate iliofemoral access, it is of fundamental importance to understand the delivery devices used, including a working knowledge of their materials and diameters. Conventional nomenclature for the sizing of catheters uses the French system (Fr) to describe their outer diameter. Access sheaths are also described using the French system, although the French value assigned to a sheath refers to the maximum catheter size that will fit within its lumen. It does not relate to the outer diameter of the sheath, which is the diameter of interest when evaluating the size of the iliofemoral vessels. To predict size mismatch between the external device diameter and the arterial luminal diameter requires familiarity with the sheath systems employed. This in turn may depend on the implanted valve prosthesis size. Delivery system profiles have decreased since the first transcatheter valve was placed in 2002 (Table 21.2) and it is expected that this trend will continue as newer systems are developed. The newest generation of sheaths employed with Edwards Sapien XT system is a 16 F expandable

Table 21.2 Component profile and desired minimum arterial diameter by MDCT measurement of the most common current and historic balloon-mounted and self-expandable stents used for retrograde femoral access

–	Valve size (mm)	Delivery system	Nominal sheath diameter (F)	Outer diameter (mm)	Desired mean arterial diameter (mm)[b]
Cribier Edwards (2002)	23	–	22	8.4	8.0
	26		24	9.2	8.8
Edwards SAPIEN (2005)	23	RetroFlex 3	22	8.4	8.0
	26		24	9.2	8.8
Edwards SAPIEN XT (2009)	23	NovaFlex	18	7.2	6.9
	26		19	7.5	7.1
Edwards SAPIEN XT (2011)	23	NovaFlex + (eSheath)	16	6.7	6.4
	26		18	7.2	6.9
			20	8.0	7.6
CoreValve 1st Generation (2004)	21	–	25	9–10	–
CoreValve 2nd Generation (2005)	21	–	21	~8	–
CoreValve 3rd Generation (2006)	26	Large Check Flow Introducer System[a]	18	7.3	6.9
	29		18	7.3	6.9
	31 (2011)		18	7.3	6.9

[a]Cook Medical, Bloomington, Indiana
[b]Based upon a sheath to femoral artery ratio (SFAR) of 1.05 [8]

sheath, which is smaller than the balloon-mounted valve. The sheath expands transiently as the valve is passed through it, recoiling afterwards so as to not become adherent to narrow access vessels. However, decreasing sheath diameters may come at the expense of stiffness of the delivery system. Similar to vessel size, a mismatch between system stiffness and vessel tortuosity may represent a quantifiable risk.

Assessment of Iliofemoral Vessels

Early series utilizing both the balloon expandable Edwards valve (Edwards Lifesciences, Irvine, California) and the self-expandable CoreValve ReValving system (Medtronic Core Valve, Irvine, California) were performed in 2005–2006 [3, 21]. These initial series used single plane angiography as the primary modality to assess luminal patency of the iliofemoral access vessels. There are inherent limitations to this method which include the inability to adequately assess the 3D nature of vascular tortuosity and the eccentricity of occlusive disease [29]. The burden of atherosclerotic plaque and vascular calcification may also be underestimated. These limitations may have contributed to high complication rates in early series.

Current angiographic practice employs dual-plane angiography and MDCT, or MDCT alone, for iliofemoral evaluation. MDCT is increasingly being recognized as the de facto gold standard as it is the only technique capable of accurately quantifying minimum vessel diameter, calcification, and tortuosity. Angiographic evaluation of iliac vessels is a useful adjunct to coronary angiography in patients for whom only non-contrast MDCT can be obtained. It has been shown that a standardized approach to patient screening and selection with MDCT reduces morbidity and mortality rates from vascular injury [25].

Intravascular ultrasound (IVUS) could also possibly be used to gauge luminal diameter and plaque burden; however, it is unable to accurately gauge the degree of vascular calcification or provide any practical information on vessel tortuosity. IVUS and magnetic resonance angiography for iliofemoral evaluation is discussed in later chapters.

Multidetector Row CT Angiography

MDCT has evolved considerably since its first inception in 1991 [30] and has had a tremendous impact on vascular imaging. The introduction of multiple-detector-row CT with increasing numbers of detector channels and faster gantry rotation speeds has virtually replaced diagnostic catheter angiography in almost all vascular territories. The synchronization of CT data acquisition with the patient's electrocardiogram (ECG) – first conceived in the 1970s – became a clinical reality with MDCT. This capability is now widely available on 64-detector-row or higher CT systems for imaging the coronary arteries but has been used extensively for preoperative and postoperative imaging of the aortic valve and root as well [31, 32].

CT Angiography for TAVR Planning

The three essential components for cardiovascular CT and CT angiography (CTA) are (a) a high-resolution volumetric CT acquisition, (b) synchronized with contrast medium enhancement of the target vasculature, and (c) 3D (or 4D) image post-processing. If the ascending aorta, aortic root, and heart are of particular diagnostic importance, the thoracic portion of the CT angiographic acquisition is acquired using ECG gating to suppress cardiac motion and pulsation artifacts. This technique – which also used for the preoperative assessment of patients with aortic root aneurysms and acute aortic syndromes – is described in greater detail elsewhere [31, 32].

CT Protocol

Our own institution's acquisition protocol for evaluation of patients being considered for TAVR consists of a non-contrast-enhanced acquisition through the chest, abdomen, and pelvis, followed by a contrast-enhanced CT angiographic acquisition of the chest, abdomen, and pelvis using a single injection of contrast medium and a single breath-hold (Fig. 21.1). Depending on the scanner used, there is a brief interscan delay of up to 4 s between the EKG-gated thoracic and non-gated abdominal and pelvic acquisitions. The total scan time with a 64-channel CT system is in the order of 15–20 s.

Non-contrast images are reconstructed with a section thickness of 2.5–3.0 mm. The contrast-enhanced data are typically reconstructed with a section thickness of 1 mm (0.5–1.25 mm) and at a section spacing of 1 mm or less. In-plane resolution is 512 × 512. An example of scanning parameters for a 64-channel MDCT scanner is shown in Table 21.3.

Contrast Medium

Our contrast medium injection technique follows the basic principles of arterial contrast medium dynamics, as described in greater detail elsewhere [33]. We employ a single injection of non-ionic contrast medium (370 mg I/mL) for the duration of the scan time plus the interscan time, with the injection flow rates based on patient weight. Examples of our protocol are seen in Table 21.4.

In patients with decreased renal function (eGFR 30–60 mL/min), we employ lower iodine concentration contrast medium (300 mg I/mL) and reduced contrast medium volumes. At times, we acquire the data without contrast medium. Low contrast medium volume techniques for patients undergoing TAVR treatment planning CT scans is discussed in other chapters.

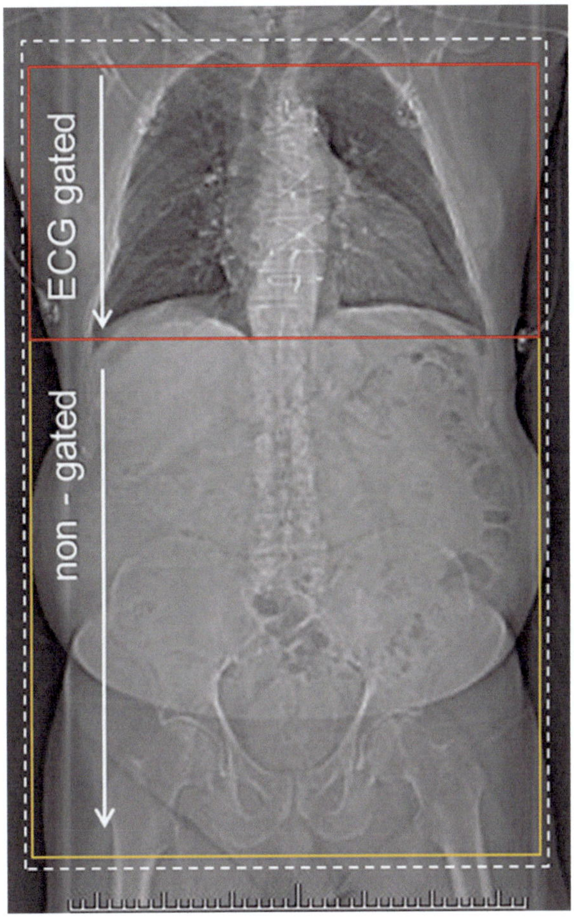

Fig. 21.1 CT angiography for transcatheter aortic valve replacement. Scanning range, thoracic portion (indicated by *red box*) acquired with ECG gating, abdominal portion non-gated (*yellow box*). Both acquisitions are obtained with a single contrast bolus. Total scan time (breath-hold) ~15–20 s

Visualization and Interpretation (Box 21.1)

Box 21.1 MDCT Arterial Visualization: Tips and Tricks

Arterial lumen diameter	Transverse source image viewing should not be used
	Most accurate measures from multiplanar reformats and orthogonal views
	Most accurate method to identify vessel borders is full width at half maximum (FWHM)
	Select optimal window width and level settings for calcified vessels
Vessel wall calcifications	Luminal diameter assessments need to be interpreted in conjunction with arterial calcifications
	Vessel wall calcification involve >180° of arterial wall circumference ('horseshoe calcification') should be noted
Artery tortuosity	Severe tortuosity = >90° between common and external illiac arteries should be noted
	Curvature of centerline can be expressed as inverse of curvature radius

Image interpretation begins with a review of the transverse (axial) source images, which remain the basis for diagnostic evaluation of vascular and important incidental nonvascular findings (Fig. 21.2). We, and others, have observed solid organ cancers (lung, kidney, bladder, and pancreas) and metastatic disease in patients evaluated for TAVR, although the frequency of potentially important incidental findings in this typically elderly population has not yet been determined.

Assessment of vascular findings requires interactive interrogation of the volumetric datasets on a powerful post-processing workstation or server. 3D volume-rendered (VR) images of the iliofemoral vessels are particularly helpful for visualization of vessel tortuosity and their relationships to surrounding anatomy (Fig. 21.3a–c). We have found that in addition to standard vascular VR settings, applying a template that increases translucency of the intravascular contrast medium but maintains full opacity of calcification aids greatly in the characterization of calcific plaques (Fig. 21.3d–f).

For evaluation of the vessel lumen – notably in the presence of vessel wall calcifications or eccentric disease – 2D cross-sectional viewing is typically required, which can include viewing of transverse source images, multiplanar reformations, and the so-called curved planar reformats (CPRs). Curved planar reformations are longitudinal cross sections through an artery of interest and require the extraction of the vascular centerline – either manually or fully automated. CPRs allow for the most comprehensive visualization of diseased arteries, as well as automated generation of cross-sectional images orthogonal to the vessel centerline [34, 35] (Fig. 21.4). Interpretation of abnormal findings on reformatted images should always be done in conjunction with transverse source images to avoid misinterpretation of stenosis from artifacts or high vessel tortuosity. Also, if automated centerline extraction is used, then the centerline should be reviewed to confirm that it has tracked correctly, with adjustments being made as necessary. Vascular centerlines are not only used for visualization – in the form of CPRs and orthonormal cross sections – but centerlines also serve as the input function for quantitative assessment of vessel diameters and curvature.

Arterial Lumen Diameter Measurements

A preliminary assessment of arterial luminal diameters can be performed manually on transverse source CT images on a PACS viewing station or post-processing workstation. Because most arteries are oriented obliquely relative to the transverse image plane, only the short axis measurement of an arterial cross section can be used to estimate the lumen size (see Fig. 21.2). If appropriately measured arterial diameters on transverse images are clearly larger than the delivery system being used, this simple manual assessment is adequate for TAVR access planning in patients with

Table 21.3 Sample MDCT scanning parameters[a] for TAVR candidate screening

	Scan I – non-contrast	Scan II – angiogram
Section thickness (mm)	3	1.0
Reconstruction interval (mm)	3	0.7
Tube voltage/current (eff. mAs)	120 kV/200	Gated: 120 kV/320 Non-gated: 120 kV/219
Detector configuration (mm)	2×32×0.6	2×32×0.6
Scan range	Above aortic arch to the lesser trochanter	Gated: Above the aortic arch to diaphragm Non-gated: Diaphragm to lesser trochanter
Total scan time (s)	~12	Gated chest: ~15 Interscan delay: 4 Abdomen: ~7
Scanning delay	6 s (automated breathing instructions)	Minimum (automated bolus triggering from region of interest in ascending aorta)
Contrast medium	–	370 mg I/mL preferred 300 mg I/mL if azotemic
Injection parameters	–	Biphasic – See Table 21.4
Reconstruction phases (gated portion)	–	Best diastolic (automated selection, usually ~65–70 % RR): entire scan range Best systolic (~30–40 % RR): entire scan range 0–90 % RR (10 phases): heart and ascending aorta

A non-contrast examination is obtained of the entire scan range followed by an EKG-gated thoracic and non-gated abdominal and pelvic CTA utilizing a single contrast injection and breath-hold

[a]Used with Siemens Sensation 64

Table 21.4 Biphasic body weight-based MDCT angiogram injection protocol for TAVR candidate screening which consists of EKG-gated thoracic and non-gated abdominal and pelvic scans

Weight (kg)	Phase I (5 s)	Phase II (total scan time – 5 s)[a] (mL/s)
<55	4.0 mL/s (20 mL)	3.2
<65	4.5 mL/s (23 mL)	3.6
65–85	5.0 mL/s (25 mL)	4.0
>85	5.5 mL/s (28 mL)	4.4
>95	6.0 mL/s (30 mL)	4.8

A high initial injection rate is followed by a lower sustained rate to achieve bright vessel opacification with moderate contrast volumes. All other acquisition and reconstruction parameters are as in Table 21.3

[a]The second phase is followed by a saline flush of 45 mL

elongated and tortuous arteries, calcified and non-calcified atherosclerotic plaque, and eccentric luminal narrowing; however, transverse source image viewing not only is very tedious but also should be considered inadequate.

More accurate measurements of lumen diameters can be obtained on multiplanar reformations that are orthogonal to the arterial centerline and provide the true long and short axis diameters of a vessel (with circular or elliptical cross section). Modern workstations can automatically extract vessel centerlines and display the orthogonal planes that allow manual or automated measurements orthogonal to the vessel at every point regardless of vessel obliquity (see Fig. 21.4).

Manual measurements are usually performed by placing electronic calipers at the vessel borders. It is important to realize that the apparent size of a vessel depends on the display window and level settings. The most accurate way to identify vessel borders on CT images is to use the full width at half maximum (FWHM) as a threshold, which can be selected manually on an attenuation profile across the vessel, or this can be incorporated into automated algorithms as well.

One important pitfall for vessel lumen assessment occurs in the presence of arterial wall calcifications. The high attenuation of calcium together with the limited spatial resolution of the imaging system results in a zone of increased attenuation surrounding the pixels containing the calcification (so-called "blooming" or partial volume effect), which makes calcifications appear larger than they are when standard display window settings are used – resulting in overestimation of plaque size and luminal stenosis. The selection of a wide display window width ("bone window") or – again – use of FWHM to identify best likelihood of the vessel can help in this setting.

The combination of curved planar and orthogonal reformations can be used to gauge not only the diameter of a stenosis but its length as well. This is important when deciding if a stenosis is short enough to be crossed when the vascular lumen diameter is less than that of the external sheath. Additionally, CPRs can be used to great effect in

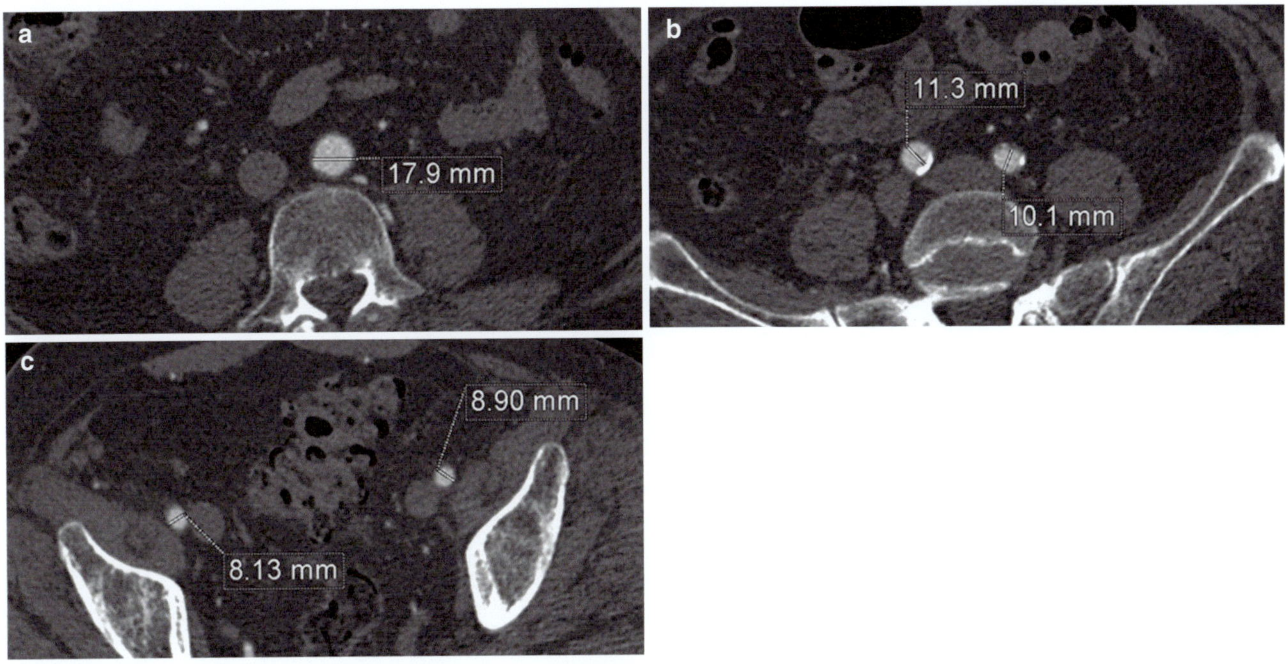

Fig. 21.2 Axial image interpretation. Transverse source CT images with two-dimensional measurements of the aorta (**a**), common iliac (**b**), and external iliac (**c**) arteries. The axial dataset is interpreted initially as it yields potentially important information about the surrounding thoracic, abdominal, and pelvic structures in addition to the angiographic data. Arterial diameter measurements on the transverse images should only be made through the short axis of an arterial cross section, because more often than not the vessel will be running obliquely through the scan plane, and any other measured diameter would overestimate the vessel diameter

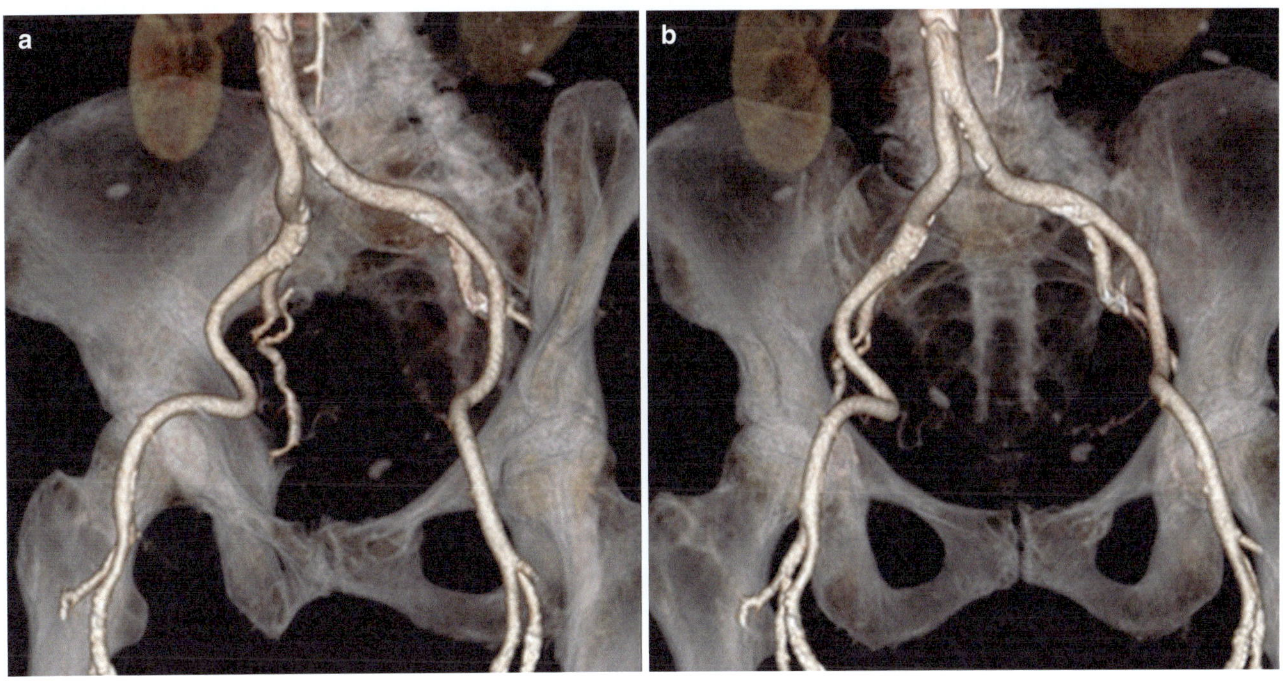

Fig. 21.3 Volume rendering. Volume rendering (VR) allows for interactive interrogation of aorta and pelvic vessels. Adjustment of the volume rendering transfer function parameters allows visualization of anatomy with semitransparent display of bony landmarks in the background, (**a**–**c**) or highlighting vessel wall calcifications (**d**–**f**)

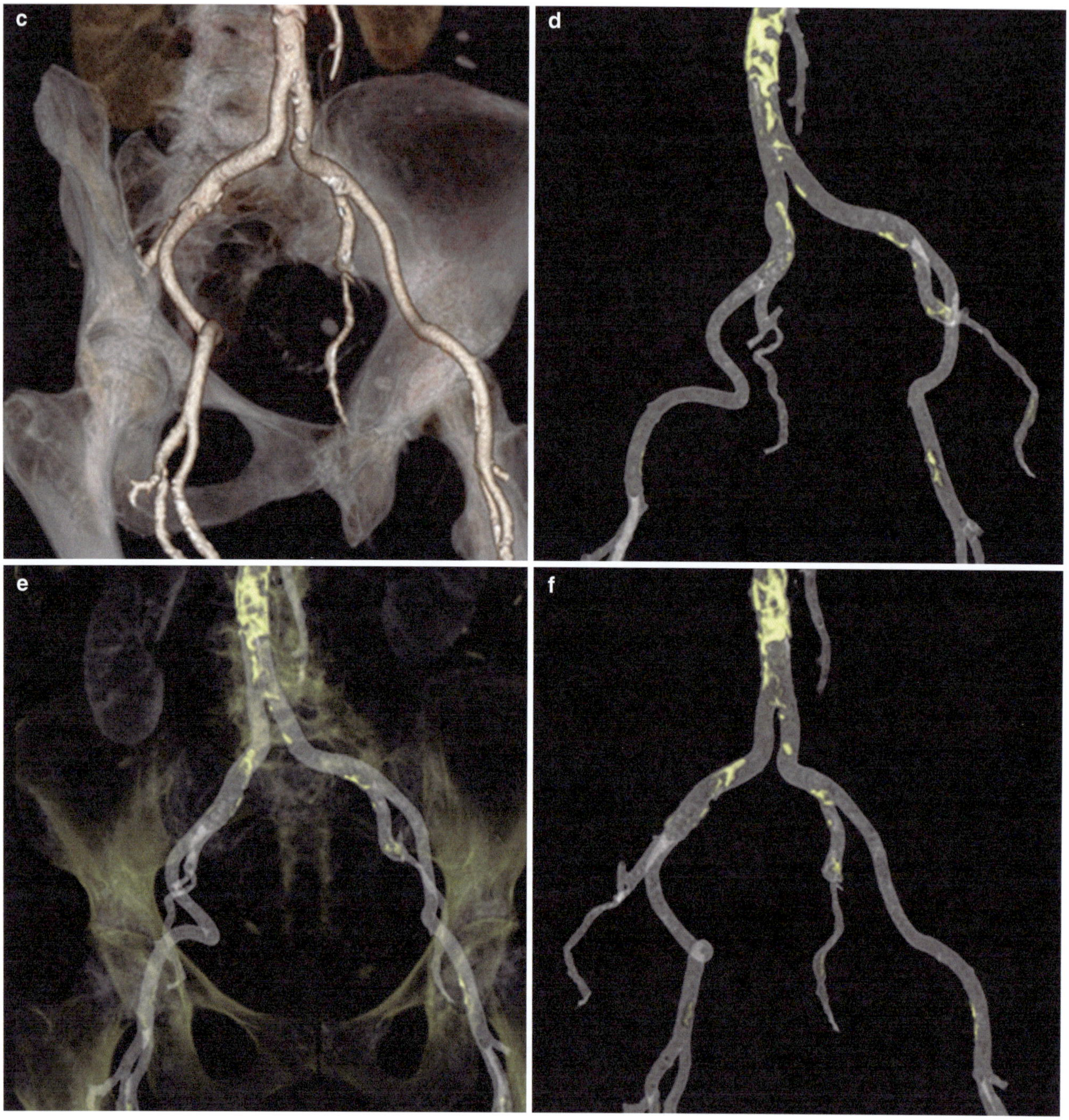

Fig. 21.3 (continued)

characterizing unanticipated vascular findings such as iliac artery dissection which may preclude vascular access (Fig. 21.5).

Assessment of Vessel Wall Calcifications

Access vessel luminal diameter assessments need to be interpreted in conjunction with arterial calcifications [36], notably if the lumen diameter is equal to or smaller than the delivery system. When short focal narrowing of the arterial lumen is caused by non-calcified plaque or by partially calcified plaque, the risk of complications does not seem to be increased. However, if vessel wall calcification involves more than 180° of arterial wall circumference ("horseshoe calcification") or even the complete circumference, such stenosis has a higher risk of complication [36] (Fig. 21.6).

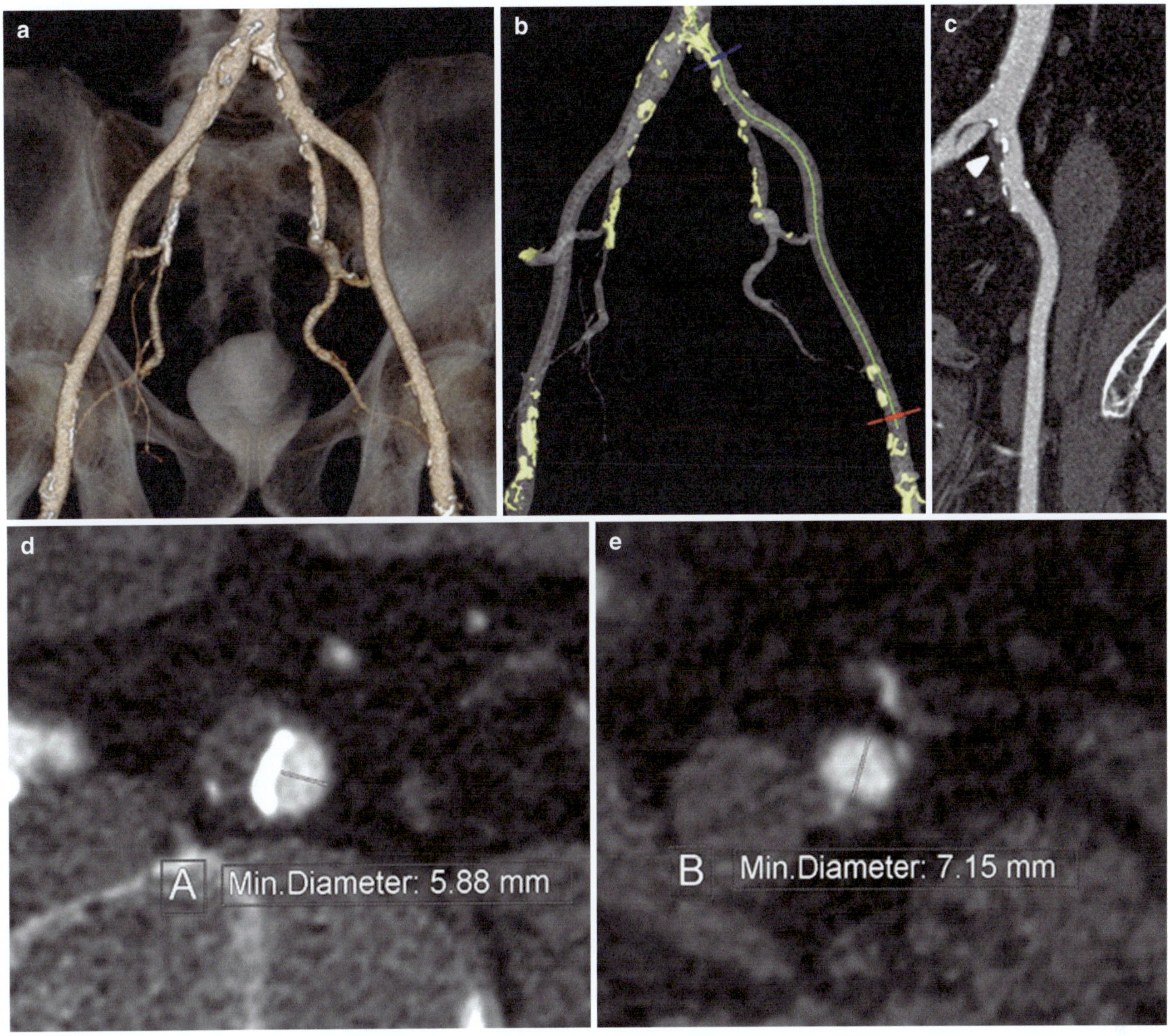

Fig. 21.4 Curved planar reformat evaluation and orthogonal measurement. Volume-rendered reconstruction or the aortoiliofemoral arteries of a 75-year-old man in AP projection (**a**) demonstrate non-tortuous iliofemoral arteries bilaterally with mild narrowing at the origin of the left common iliac. Calcification-rendered reconstruction (**b**) with overlaid centerline (*green line*) also reveals a possible horseshoe calcification at the level of the narrowing (*blue marker*). A sagittal (**c**) curved planar reformat (CPR) shows that the automated extraction of the centerline is in the mid vessel throughout and does not require adjustment. (**d**) An orthogonal measurement taken at the level of the focal stenosis (*blue marker* in **b**) reveals a minimum luminal diameter of less than 6 mm. The calcification at this level is shown to be linear and not horseshoe as suspected. (**e**) Distally an orthogonal measurement at the level of the common femoral artery (*red marker* in **b**) is greater than 7 mm in size

Assessment of Iliac Artery Tortuosity

The tortuosity of vascular structures cannot be assessed on transverse source images and generally requires a 3D display from multiple viewing angles. Anterior-posterior and 45°RAO and 45°LAO projections are the minimum required to allow for a qualitative visual assessment of iliac tortuosity (Fig. 21.7). There does not appear to be a standard by which iliofemoral tortuosity is described in the setting of TAVR planning, although an angle >90° between the common and external iliac arteries has been used to characterize severe tortuosity [27].

Iliofemoral arterial tortuosity is not necessarily a contraindication for femoral access, but typically the less tortuous delivery route is chosen. Even significant arterial kinks can straighten out with regular 0.035 in. guide wires or stiff Lunderquist or Amplatz wires (Fig. 21.8). Despite this, sheaths can become kinked in steep bends which may block passage of the valve delivery system up into the aorta and may require removal of the whole assembly, including sheath.

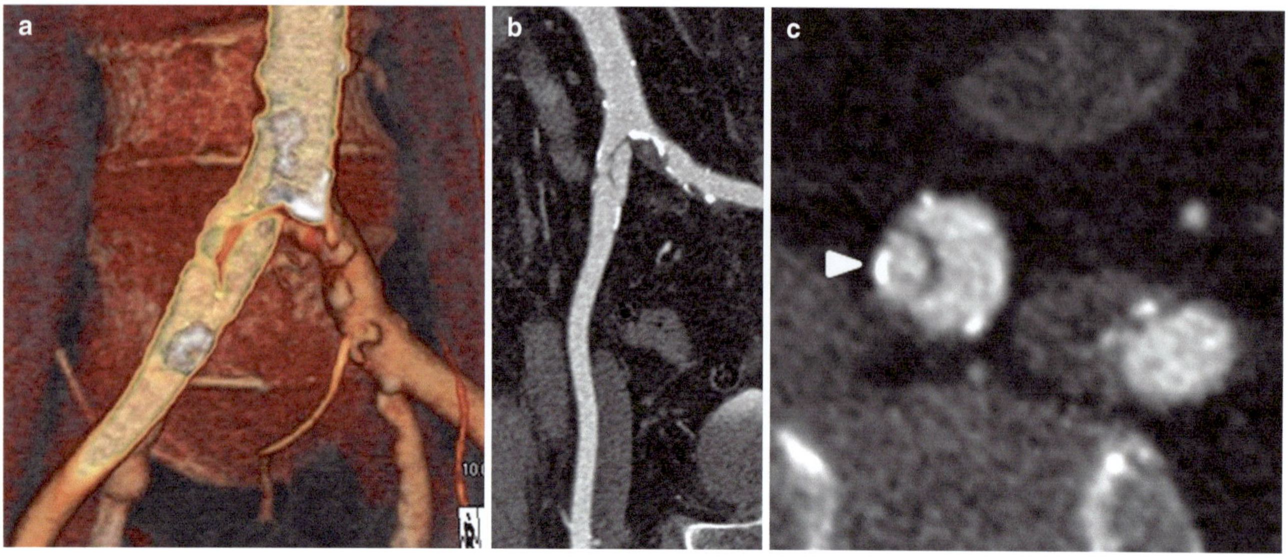

Fig. 21.5 Focal stenosis of left, and focal dissection of right common iliac artery. A 75-year-old man (same individual as in Fig. 21.5) being evaluated for TAVR. An endoluminal VR reconstruction (**a**) of the right common iliac reveals a focal dissection present at the vessel origin with the dissection flap open distally. A curved planar view (**b**) and an orthogonal cross section (**c**) show the limited extent of the dissection and the diminutive true lumen (*arrow head* in **c**). With foreknowledge of a stenosis of the proximal left common iliac (seen in **b**) and the limited right-sided "windsock" type dissection, the angiographer was able to steer a guidewire past the dissection flap for sheath placement and deploy a valve without complication

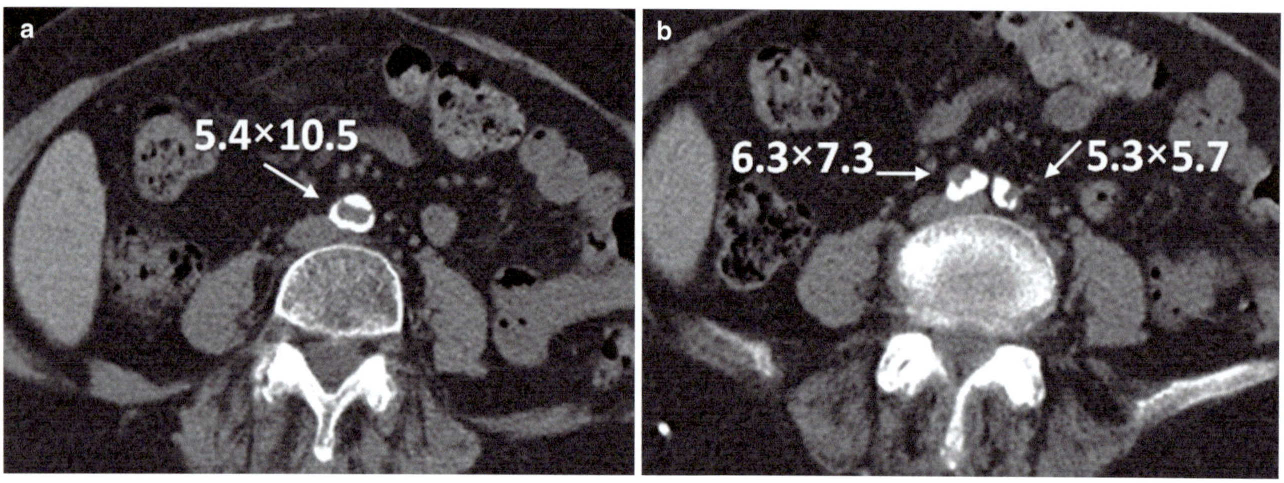

Fig. 21.6 Unsuitable iliofemoral access vessels: small calcified arteries. Axial images of the aorta (**a**) and common iliac arteries (**b**) of an 84-year-old woman with severe AS. Given that the aorta and both iliac arteries are small with diffuse heavily calcification, this patient was considered too high risk for transfemoral access and subsequently underwent successful transapical TAVR

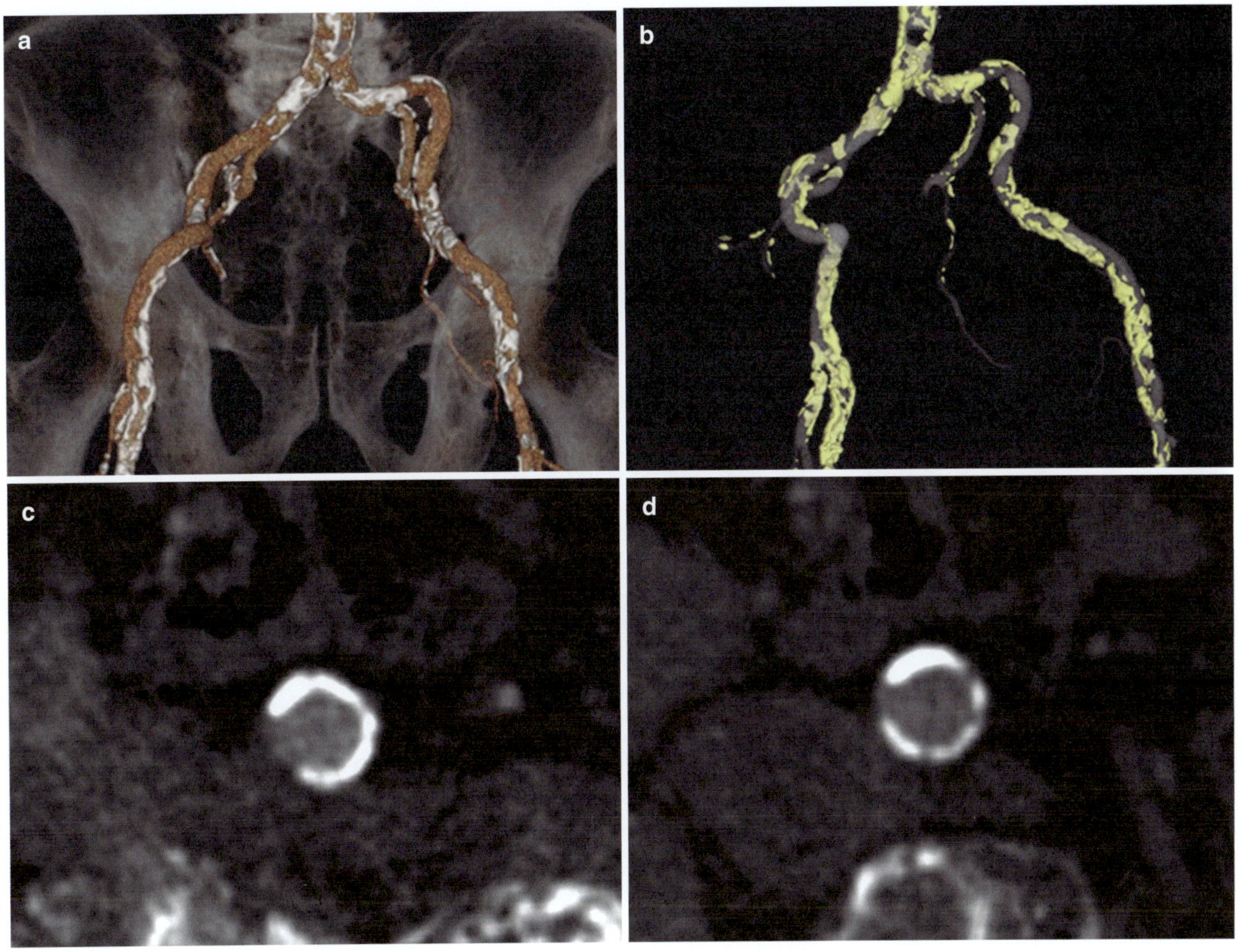

Fig. 21.7 Iliofemoral vessels unsuitable for access: tortuous and calcified arteries. An AP volume-rendered (**a**) and a 45° RAO calcification-rendered (**b**) reconstruction demonstrate aortoiliofemoral calcification and tortuosity. The use of calcification-rendered reconstructions clearly demonstrates the magnitude of the vascular calcification which precludes retrograde femoral access. Orthogonal cross sections of the proximal right common iliac artery show areas of horseshoe (**c**) and near circumferential (**d**) calcification. This individual was subsequently selected for transapical access (not shown)

The seemingly simple task of visually identifying the more tortuous of the two iliofemoral access routes is not always easy to achieve when compared to more accurate quantitative measurements of vascular curvature [37]. The curvature of an arterial centerline can be expressed as the inverse of the curvature radius and plotted as a function along the length of the centerline path (Fig. 21.9). Quantitative assessment of iliac artery tortuosity has been shown to correlate with iliac artery dissections in the setting of abdominal aortic endovascular aneurysm repair [37], but no such data exist for TAVR femoral access planning at this point.

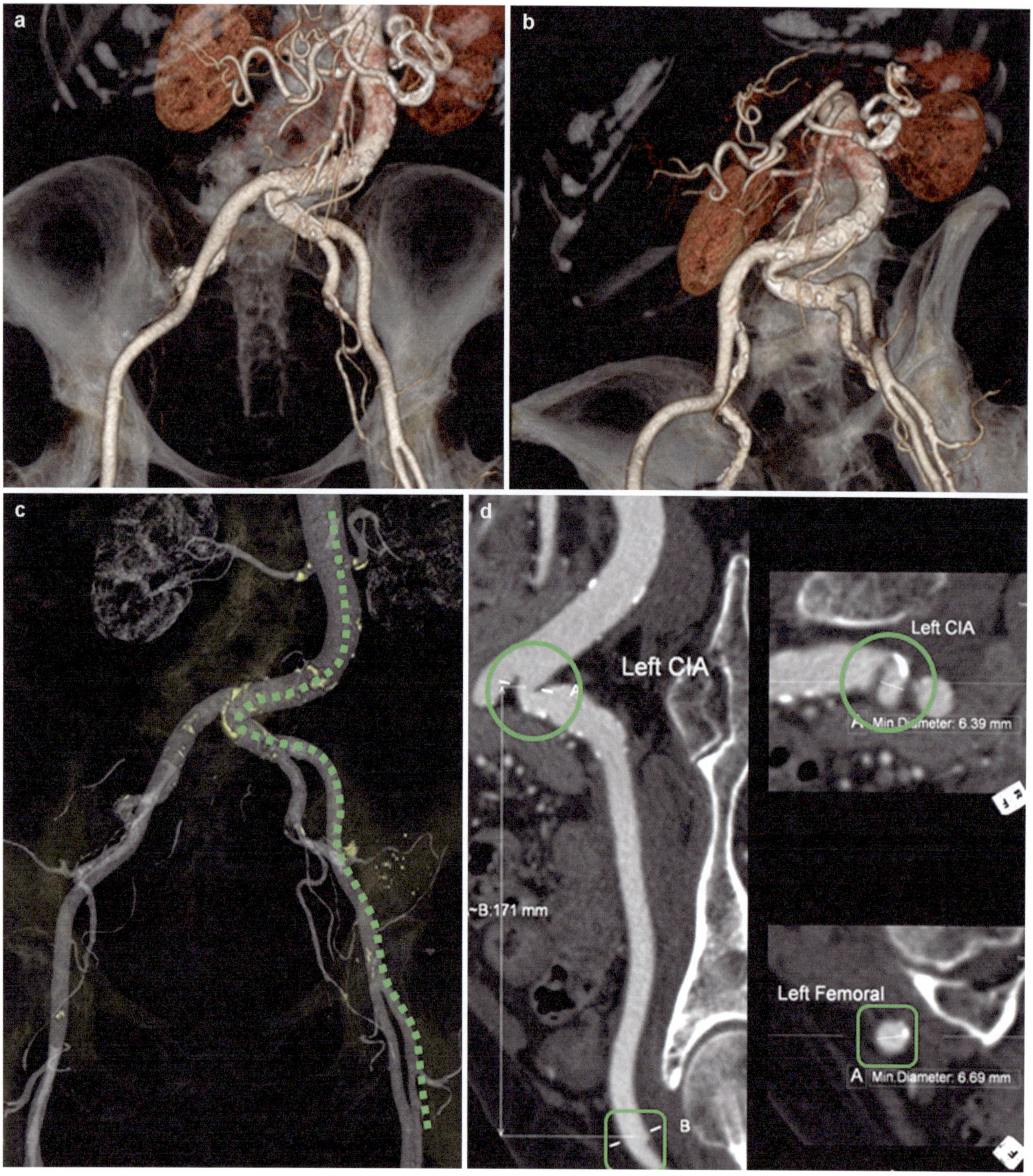

Fig. 21.8 Severe tortuosity of the left common iliac origin. Volume-rendered AP (**a**) and cranially inclined LAO (**b**) reconstructions of the iliofemoral vessels in an 89-year-old woman being screened for TAVR. There is marked tortuosity and kinking of the left common iliac origin which arises at an acute angle from the aorta. After centerline extraction (**c** – *green dotted line*) a CPR is generated to further evaluate the vessel (**d**). An orthogonal reconstruction at the level of the vascular kink (**d** *inset – green circle*) shows that the minimum diameter (6.4 mm) is narrower than the common femoral artery distally (6.7 mm) (**d** *inset – green square*). Although the caliber, tortuosity, and degree of calcification would otherwise not preclude vascular access on the left side, the right side was selected for access sheath deployment to avoid the risk of vascular injury

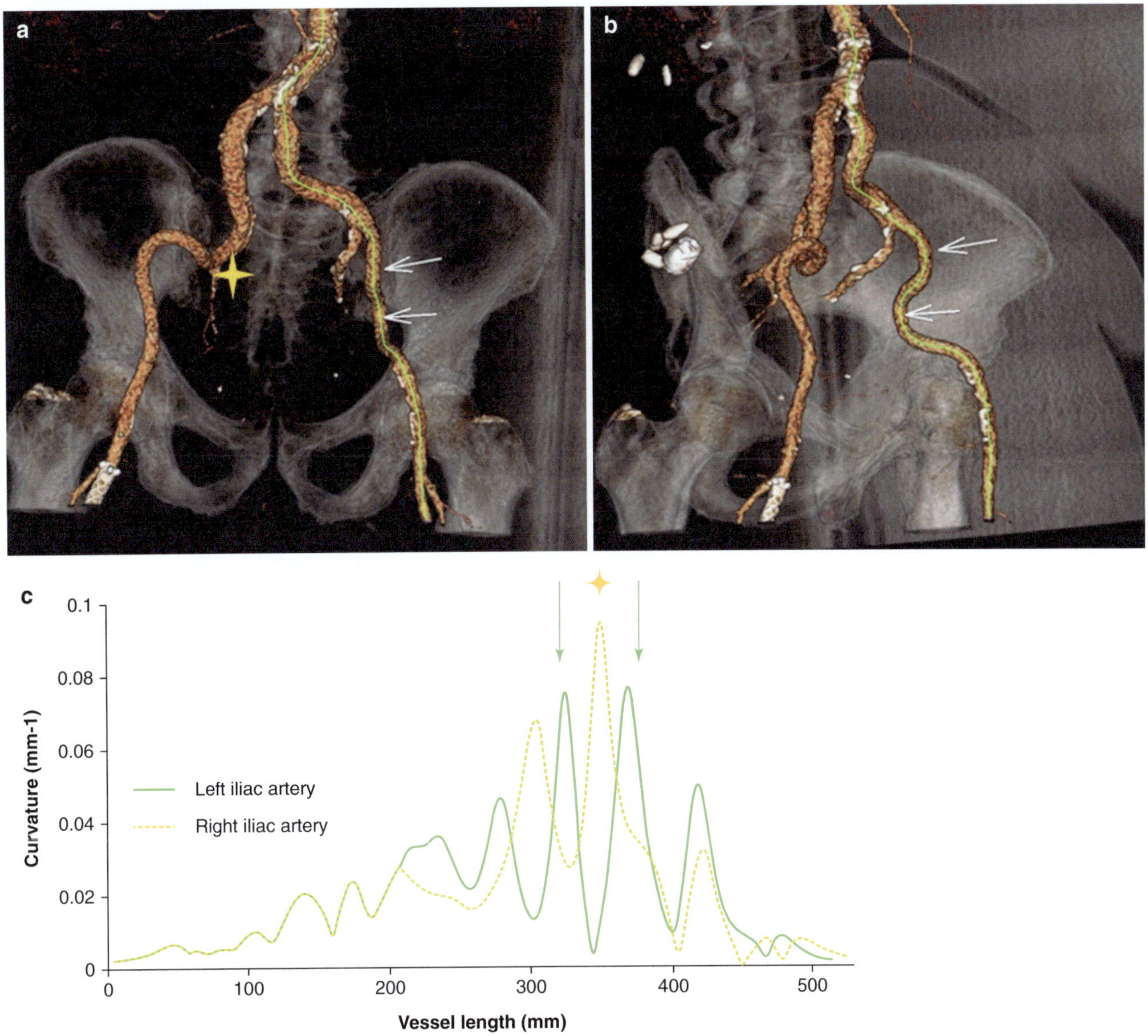

Fig. 21.9 Quantitative assessment of iliac artery curvature. AP (**a**) volume-rendered image of the aortoiliofemoral arteries in a 76-year-old man undergoing TAVR shows severe tortuosity of the right external iliac artery (*asterisk*). Note, that the apparently straight left external iliac artery in (**a**) is in fact tortuous as well in an RAO view (**b**). This is confirmed by measurement of the curvature which shows two curvature maxima in (**c**) for the left iliac artery (*arrows*). Transfemoral TAVR was successfully performed without complications over a stiff wire (not shown) introduced on the left. (Figure **c** courtesy of Kelly Suh, PhD)

Conclusion

Over the past decade multidetector CT angiography has become an integral part of patient selection and treatment planning for transcatheter aortic valve replacement. Procedural complication rates can be minimized through the use of high-resolution MDCT angiography and post-processing software. With the ability to create volume rendered, MPR, CPR, and orthogonal reconstructions – which allow the assessment of tortuosity, vessel lumen, and mural calcification – MDCT has become the standard of reference. Automated and quantitative tools may further improve the utility of MDCT in patient selection and treatment planning.

References

1. Cribier A, Eltchaninoff H, Bash A, Borenstein N, Tron C, Bauer F, et al. Percutaneous transcatheter implantation of an aortic valve prosthesis for calcific aortic stenosis: first human case description. Circulation. 2002;106(24):3006–8. Epub 2002/12/11.

2. Cribier A, Eltchaninoff H, Tron C, Bauer F, Agatiello C, Sebagh L, et al. Early experience with percutaneous transcatheter implantation of heart valve prosthesis for the treatment of end-stage inoperable patients with calcific aortic stenosis. J Am Coll Cardiol. 2004;43(4):698–703. Epub 2004/02/21.
3. Webb JG, Chandavimol M, Thompson CR, Ricci DR, Carere RG, Munt BI, et al. Percutaneous aortic valve implantation retrograde from the femoral artery. Circulation. 2006;113(6):842–50. Epub 2006/02/08.
4. Hanzel GS, Harrity PJ, Schreiber TL, O'Neill WW. Retrograde percutaneous aortic valve implantation for critical aortic stenosis. Catheter Cardiovasc Interv. 2005;64(3):322–6. Epub 2005/03/01.
5. Bruschi G, De Marco F, Fratto P, Oreglia J, Colombo P, Botta L, et al. Alternative approaches for trans-catheter self-expanding aortic bioprosthetic valves implantation: single-center experience. Eur J Cardiothorac Surg. 2011;39(6):e151–8. Epub 2011/03/05.
6. Leon MB, Piazza N, Nikolsky E, Blackstone EH, Cutlip DE, Kappetein AP, et al. Standardized endpoint definitions for transcatheter aortic valve implantation clinical trials: a consensus report from the Valve Academic Research Consortium. Eur Heart J. 2011;32(2):205–17. Epub 2011/01/11.
7. Leon MB, Piazza N, Nikolsky E, Blackstone EH, Cutlip DE, Kappetein AP, et al. Standardized endpoint definitions for Transcatheter Aortic Valve Implantation clinical trials: a consensus report from the Valve Academic Research Consortium. J Am Coll Cardiol. 2011;57(3):253–69. Epub 2011/01/11.
8. Hayashida K, Lefevre T, Chevalier B, Hovasse T, Romano M, Garot P, et al. Transfemoral aortic valve implantation new criteria to predict vascular complications. JACC Cardiovasc Interv. 2011; 4(8):851–8. Epub 2011/08/20.
9. Thomas M, Schymik G, Walther T, Himbert D, Lefevre T, Treede H, et al. Thirty-day results of the SAPIEN aortic Bioprosthesis European Outcome (SOURCE) Registry: a European registry of transcatheter aortic valve implantation using the Edwards SAPIEN valve. Circulation. 2010;122(1):62–9. Epub 2010/06/23.
10. Van Mieghem NM, Nuis RJ, Piazza N, Apostolos T, Ligthart J, Schultz C, et al. Vascular complications with transcatheter aortic valve implantation using the 18 Fr Medtronic CoreValve System: the Rotterdam experience. EuroIntervention. 2010;5(6):673–9. Epub 2010/02/10.
11. Tchetche D, Dumonteil N, Sauguet A, Descoutures F, Luz A, Garcia O, et al. Thirty-day outcome and vascular complications after transarterial aortic valve implantation using both Edwards Sapien and Medtronic CoreValve bioprostheses in a mixed population. EuroIntervention. 2010;5(6):659–65. Epub 2010/02/10.
12. Sharp AS, Michev I, Maisano F, Taramasso M, Godino C, Latib A, et al. A new technique for vascular access management in transcatheter aortic valve implantation. Catheter Cardiovasc Interv. 2010;75(5):784–93. Epub 2010/01/06.
13. Piazza N, Grube E, Gerckens U, den Heijer P, Linke A, Luha O, et al. Procedural and 30-day outcomes following transcatheter aortic valve implantation using the third generation (18 Fr) corevalve revalving system: results from the multicentre, expanded evaluation registry 1-year following CE mark approval. EuroIntervention. 2008;4(2):242–9. Epub 2008/12/30.
14. Tamburino C, Capodanno D, Ramondo A, Petronio AS, Ettori F, Santoro G, et al. Incidence and predictors of early and late mortality after transcatheter aortic valve implantation in 663 patients with severe aortic stenosis. Circulation. 2011;123(3):299–308. Epub 2011/01/12.
15. Lefevre T, Kappetein AP, Wolner E, Nataf P, Thomas M, Schachinger V, et al. One year follow-up of the multi-centre European PARTNER transcatheter heart valve study. Eur Heart J. 2011;32(2):148–57. Epub 2010/11/16.
16. Rodes-Cabau J, Webb JG, Cheung A, Ye J, Dumont E, Feindel CM, et al. Transcatheter aortic valve implantation for the treatment of severe symptomatic aortic stenosis in patients at very high or prohibitive surgical risk: acute and late outcomes of the multicenter Canadian experience. J Am Coll Cardiol. 2010;55(11):1080–90. Epub 2010/01/26.
17. Ducrocq G, Francis F, Serfaty JM, Himbert D, Maury JM, Pasi N, et al. Vascular complications of transfemoral aortic valve implantation with the Edwards SAPIEN prosthesis: incidence and impact on outcome. EuroIntervention. 2010;5(6):666–72. Epub 2010/02/10.
18. Webb JG, Altwegg L, Boone RH, Cheung A, Ye J, Lichtenstein S, et al. Transcatheter aortic valve implantation: impact on clinical and valve-related outcomes. Circulation. 2009;119(23):3009–16. Epub 2009/06/03.
19. Bleiziffer S, Ruge H, Mazzitelli D, Hutter A, Opitz A, Bauernschmitt R, et al. Survival after transapical and transfemoral aortic valve implantation: talking about two different patient populations. J Thorac Cardiovasc Surg. 2009;138(5):1073–80. Epub 2009/09/22.
20. Genereux P, Head SJ, Van Mieghem NM, Kodali S, Kirtane AJ, Xu K, et al. Clinical outcomes after transcatheter aortic valve replacement using valve academic research consortium definitions: a weighted meta-analysis of 3,519 patients from 16 studies. J Am Coll Cardiol. 2012;59(25):2317–26. Epub 2012/04/17.
21. Grube E, Laborde JC, Gerckens U, Felderhoff T, Sauren B, Buellesfeld L, et al. Percutaneous implantation of the CoreValve self-expanding valve prosthesis in high-risk patients with aortic valve disease: the Siegburg first-in-man study. Circulation. 2006;114(15):1616–24. Epub 2006/10/04.
22. Masson JB, Kovac J, Schuler G, Ye J, Cheung A, Kapadia S, et al. Transcatheter aortic valve implantation: review of the nature, management, and avoidance of procedural complications. JACC Cardiovasc Interv. 2009;2(9):811–20. Epub 2009/09/26.
23. Lange R, Bleiziffer S, Piazza N, Mazzitelli D, Hutter A, Tassani-Prell P, et al. Incidence and treatment of procedural cardiovascular complications associated with trans-arterial and trans-apical interventional aortic valve implantation in 412 consecutive patients. Eur J Cardiothorac Surg. 2011;40(5):1105–13. Epub 2011/04/26.
24. Himbert D, Descoutures F, Al-Attar N, Iung B, Ducrocq G, Detaint D, et al. Results of transfemoral or transapical aortic valve implantation following a uniform assessment in high-risk patients with aortic stenosis. J Am Coll Cardiol. 2009;54(4):303–11. Epub 2009/07/18.
25. Toggweiler S, Gurvitch R, Leipsic J, Wood DA, Willson AB, Binder RK, et al. Percutaneous aortic valve replacement: vascular outcomes with a fully percutaneous procedure. J Am Coll Cardiol. 2012;59(2):113–8. Epub 2012/01/10.
26. Murray D, Ghosh J, Khwaja N, Murphy MO, Baguneid MS, Walker MG. Access for endovascular aneurysm repair. J Endovasc Ther. 2006;13(6):754–61. Epub 2006/12/13.
27. Kurra V, Schoenhagen P, Roselli EE, Kapadia SR, Tuzcu EM, Greenberg R, et al. Prevalence of significant peripheral artery disease in patients evaluated for percutaneous aortic valve insertion: preprocedural assessment with multidetector computed tomography. J Thorac Cardiovasc Surg. 2009;137(5):1258–64. Epub 2009/04/22.
28. Leipsic J, Wood DA, Gurvitch R, Hague CJ. Multidetector computed tomography to facilitate transcatheter aortic valve implantation. Curr Cardiovasc Imaging Rep. 2011;4(6):457–67.
29. Rubin GD, Paik DS, Johnston PC, Napel S. Measurement of the aorta and its branches with helical CT. Radiology. 1998;206(3): 823–9. Epub 1998/03/12.
30. Rubin GD, Dake MD, Napel SA, McDonnell CH, Jeffrey RB. Three-dimensional spiral CT angiography of the abdomen: initial clinical experience. Radiology. 1993;186(1):147–52.
31. Fleischmann D, Liang DH, Mitchell RS, Miller DC. Pre- and postoperative imaging of the aortic root for valve-sparing aortic

root repair (V-SARR). Semin Thorac Cardiovasc Surg. 2008;20(4):365–73.
32. Fleischmann D, Mitchell RS, Miller DC. Acute aortic syndromes: new insights from electrocardiographically gated computed tomography. Semin Thorac Cardiovasc Surg. 2008;20(4):340–7.
33. Fleischmann D. CT angiography: injection and acquisition technique. Radiol Clin North Am. 2010;48(2):237–47, vii. Epub 2010/07/09.
34. Kanitsar A, Fleischmann D, Wegenkittl R, Felkel P, Groeller E, editors. CPR – curved planar reformation. IEEE Visualization. Boston: IEEE Computer Society; 2002.
35. Roos JE, Fleischmann D, Koechl A, Rakshe T, Straka M, Napoli A, et al. Multipath curved planar reformation of the peripheral arterial tree in CT angiography. Radiology. 2007;244(1):281–90.
36. Bloomfield GS, Gillam LD, Hahn RT, Kapadia S, Leipsic J, Lerakis S, et al. A practical guide to multimodality imaging of transcatheter aortic valve replacement. JACC Cardiovasc Imaging. 2012;5(4):441–55. Epub 2012/04/14.
37. Tillich M, Bell RE, Paik DS, Fleischmann D, Sofilos MC, Logan LJ, et al. Iliac arterial injuries after endovascular repair of abdominal aortic aneurysms: correlation with iliac curvature and diameter. Radiology. 2001;219(1):129–36. Epub 2001/03/29.

22 Aortoiliofemoral Assessment: MRA

Chesnal D. Arepalli and Stamatios Lerakis

Abstract

Transcatheter aortic valve replacement (TAVR) is an undergoing evaluation for the treatment of inoperable or high-risk severe aortic stenosis (AS) patients. Patients with symptomatic, severe AS are at high risk for conventional surgical aortic valve replacement procedures. One of the alternate ways of managing these patients is through TAVR. Several studies on post TAVR patients with a follow-up interval up to 2 years showed significant clinical benefit, improvements in exercise capacity and in quality of life. Proper patient selection is key to optimize successful clinical outcomes. A number of imaging modalities are available for patient screening. One of them is magnetic resonance imaging (MRI). MRI provides morphological information, functional status, pre-operative planning and thus plays a role in selection of patients. It is ideally suited for patients with renal insufficiency as evaluation could be done without contrast administration. MRI may prove to be a useful alternative for TAVR evaluation and is particularly beneficial to patients with underlying chronic kidney disease.

Keywords

MRI • MRA • TAVR • Aortoiliofemoral imaging • Aortic stenosis

Abbreviations

3D	3 dimension
AR	Aortic regurgitation
AS	Aortic stenosis
CE	Contrast enhanced
CS	Cross section
DSA	Digital subtraction angiography
EuroSCORE	European system for cardiac operative risk evaluation
FISP	Fast imaging with steady-state precession
Gd	Gadolinium
GFR	Glomerular filtration rate
HASTE	Half-fourier acquisition single-shot turbo spin echo
HLA	Horizontal long axis
HOCM	Hypertrophic obstructive cardiomyopathy
IVS	Interventricular septum

C.D. Arepalli, MD (DNB)
Department of Radiology and Imaging Sciences, Division of Cardiothoracic Imaging, Emory University School of Medicine, 1365 Clifton Rd NE – Suite AT 309, Atlanta, GA 30322, USA
e-mail: carepal@emory.edu, chesnaldey@yahoo.com

S. Lerakis, MD, FACC, FAHA (✉)
Department of Medicine, Radiology and Imaging Sciences, Division of Cardiology, Emory University School of Medicine, 1365 Clifton Road NE – Suite AT-503, Atlanta, GA 30322, USA

Department of Biomedical Engineering, Emory University and Georgia Institute of Technology, 1365 Clifton Road NE – Suite AT-503, Atlanta, GA 30322, USA
e-mail: sleraki@emory.edu

J.K. Min et al. (eds.), *Multimodality Imaging for Transcatheter Aortic Valve Replacement*,
DOI 10.1007/978-1-4471-2798-7_22, © Springer-Verlag London 2014

LCCA	Left common carotid artery
LV	Left ventricle
LVEF	Left ventricle ejection fraction
LVOT	Left ventricle outflow tract
MDCT	Multidetector computerized tomography
MIP	Maximum intensity projection
MPR	Multiplanar reconstruction
MRA	Magnetic resonance angiography
MRI	Magnetic resonance imaging
NSF	Nephrogenic systemic fibrosis
PC	Phase contrast
ROI	Region of interest
SA	Short axis
SNR	Signal-to-noise ratio
SoV	Sinus of Valsalva
SSFP	Steady-state free precession
STJ	Sinotubular junction
STS	Society of Thoracic Surgeons
TAVR	Transcatheter aortic valve replacement
VLA	Vertical long axis
VRT	Volume-rendered technique
π	Pi

Introduction

Transcatheter aortic valve replacement (TAVR) is an undergoing evaluation for the treatment of inoperable or high-risk severe aortic stenosis (AS) patients. Patients with symptomatic, severe AS are at high risk for conventional surgical aortic valve replacement procedures and at least one-third of these patients is denied surgery and is medically managed [1–4]. However, significant lower survival rates are observed in medically managed patients [2, 5, 6]. One of the alternate ways of managing these patients is through TAVR. Several studies on post TAVR patients with a follow-up interval up to 2 years showed significant clinical benefit and improvements in exercise capacity and in quality of life [7–12]. TAVR was first done in 2002 [13] and has been an important breakthrough procedure. To date over 60,000 patients have undergone this procedure, and multiple trials and registries are trying to determine the procedural feasibility and improve the outcomes of the procedure with none or minimal complications. Proper patient selection is key to optimize clinical outcomes. A number of imaging modalities are available for patient screening. Each modality has its own advantages and limitations and they should be used synergistically to gain all the information needed for adequate patient screening and evaluation. One of these—magnetic resonance imaging (MRI)—may prove to be a useful alternative, particularly to patients with underlying chronic kidney disease.

Magnetic Resonance Angiography

MRI is based on the detection of signals from hydrogen nuclei, which are prevalent in the human body. When a patient enters a scanner, hydrogen nuclei align with and rotate, or precess, about the axis of the field of the magnet. The precession of these hydrogen nuclei can be disturbed through the application of additional smaller magnetic field pulses. By applying these radiofrequency pulses in a controlled manner in the form of "pulse sequences," images can be produced through the feedback of signals received based on the spatial distribution of the spins within the body with high spatial resolution [14]. Magnetic resonance angiography (MRA) has shown high diagnostic accuracy as compared to standard digital subtraction angiography (DSA) [15–19]. There are certain advantages of MRA over DSA, which is seldom used solely for diagnostic purposes (Table 22.1). MRA has thus become the modality of choice at many centers for evaluation of central and peripheral vessels. MRA technical parameters and their limitations are beyond the scope of this chapter. Nevertheless, treating physicians need to be aware of various options that are available in evaluation of symptomatic and often low cardiac output TAVR patients. This chapter herein reviews the types of MRA, the various indications and contraindications of MRA in TAVR patients, CMR protocols, and the preprocedural systematic evaluation of aortoiliofemoral MRA.

Contrast-Enhanced MRA

In contrast-enhanced (CE) MRA, gadolinium (Gd) compounds are routinely used although, at times, other contrast agents like super paramagnetic iron oxide and chromium-labeled red blood cells can also be used. Prince et al. [20] first introduced first-pass CE-MRA in 1993. Gadolinium contrast agents, based on their pharmacological properties, result in significant T1 relaxation (shortened 10–25-fold) which results in significant signal production. Technological advancements have resulted in reliable, faster, and dynamic acquisition protocols that have significantly advanced the capabilities of MR

Table 22.1 Advantages of MR angiography

1. Non-ionizing radiation
2. Noninvasive method
3. Image acquisition in any plane
4. Vessel analysis and flow quantification especially in stenotic areas in terms of peak velocity and pressure gradient
5. Ability to evaluate adjacent extravascular structures
6. Ability to acquire images without contrast administration
7. Ability to repeat acquisition, if necessary

angiography. Serial scan technique, time-resolved MRA, can be implemented that can provide a dynamic assessment of the vasculature as in DSA. This technique lessens the need for precise bolus timing and at the same time provides physiological information. In addition, time-resolved sequences allow for reduced volumes of Gd contrast for imaging. Gd compounds that are used at present are also less nephrotoxic and result in a reduced burden of hypersensitivity reactions than computed tomographic iodinated contrast media and thus are well tolerated by most patients [21–23].

Gadolinium Contrast Agents Safety Issues

Gadolinium administration has been associated with low incidence of nephrogenic systemic fibrosis (NSF). This condition following CE MRI has been observed exclusively in patients whose renal function is compromised. Grobner et al. [24] first identified this association in 2006 after which several studies confirmed this association and virtually with all types of Gd contrast agents [25–31]. NSF is a debilitating disorder resulting in fibrosis of the skin, connective tissue, and occasionally of internal organs associated with a high morbidity and mortality. As Gd compounds have been implicated in NSF, the disease entity has been thoroughly investigated and guidelines to help reduce the likelihood and impact of NSF have been proposed. Adherence to these guidelines has drastically reduced the incidence of NSF [32–34]. Current recommendations are to avoid injection of Gd contrast agents in patients with reduced glomerular filtration rate (GFR) <30 ml/min/1.73 m^2. If MRA is necessary, contrast agents with predominant hepatic clearance or non-enhanced MRA should be considered.

Non-enhanced MRA

Non-Gd enhanced MRA is a viable alternative in patients whose renal functional parameters are compromised [35–37]. Blood flow can cause signal loss or gain on different types of MRA sequences. This property can be utilized to produce inherent endogenous contrast between stationary tissue and flow of blood in vessels to produce black-blood or bright-blood imaging. Black-blood imaging relies on flow-related signal loss, whereas bright-blood imaging relies on flow-related enhancement. Various MRA techniques and their major advantages and disadvantages are mentioned in Table 22.2.

Indications of MRA Pertinent to TAVR Patients

The utility of MRA as applied to TAVR patients is manifold. The indications for use include the following: to delineate relevant vascular anatomy; to identify the presence and extent of atherosclerotic disease, stenosis, thromboembolic occlusion, or any extrinsic compression over the major vessels/vascular pathways; and to identify the presence, location, and extent of vascular abnormalities (e.g., aneurysms, dissections,

Table 22.2 MRA techniques: advantages and disadvantages

MRA technique	Advantages	Disadvantages
Contrast enhanced MRA	1. Not flow dependent 2. Very high SNR 3. Rapid acquisition 4. Large field of acquisition	1. Contrast administration 2. Allergies to contrast agent 3. Bolus timing issues 4. Expensive
Non-contrast enhanced MRA		
A. Black-blood imaging	1. No contrast 2. No over estimation of stenosis 3. Evaluation of vessel wall pathology 4. Evaluation of extravascular structures	1. Under estimation of stenosis 2. Air or bone may simulate blood flow
B. Bright-blood imaging		
1. Time of flight	1. No contrast 2. Flow direction known	1. Sensitive to patient motion 2. Signal loss in complex flow pattern 3. Tends to overestimate stenosis 4. Long acquisition times
2. Phase contrast	1. No contrast 2. High SNR 3. Excellent intrinsic background signal suppression 4. Directional flow and quantification	1. Velocity related aliasing
3. SSFP/true FISP	1. Not dependent on flow to generate vascular contrast 2. Fast acquisition 3. Breath holding not mandatory	1. Sensitive to motion 2. Fat appears as bright signal

MRA magnetic resonance angiography, *SNR* signal-to-noise ratio, *SSFP* steady-state free precession, *True FISP* fast imaging with steady precession arteriovenous malformations, vasculitis) (Figs. 22.1, 22.2, and 22.3). For all TAVR patients, care should be taken to avoid performing MRI/MRA when contraindicated (Box 22.1).

An example of a MRA protocol for TAVR and the steps involved in acquiring images are listed in Table 22.3. Baseline cardiovascular functional parameters like LVEF, end-diastolic volume, end-systolic volume, and stroke volume are calculated by acquiring SSPE cine images from base to apex either in short axis (SA) or in horizontal long axis (HLA) (4 chamber) views. These views also easily identify the presence of any thrombus or mass within the left ventricle.

An optimal arterial MRA acquisition requires patient preparation, screening the patients for any contraindications to MRA, injection of adequate amount of contrast, and more importantly to time the study while the contrast is in transit in the arterial vessels. In doing so the protocol allows for isolation of the contrast within the arterial system. At our institution, during performance of the scan, we define the true orthogonal anatomical plane of the aortic valve from contrast-enhanced MRA images. Balanced SSFP (True FISP) cine images are acquired: few slices above, through and below the aortic valve plane. These views help in determining the number of valve leaflets, assessing the leaflets mobility, any commissural fusion or bulky mass, or vegetations on the aortic valve. This view also helps in calculating the area of stenosis. Using the same MRA source images, we also obtain a cross-sectional images of aorta and pulmonary artery (just above their respective valves). The images obtained are used to derive flow-related measurements through phase contrast (PC) angiography.

MRA Technique

Herein listed are the steps to acquire MRA images that we employ at our institution. First, we acquire pre-contrast MRA images or mask images. This is obtained to know the proper anatomic coverage, to plan the field of view, to identify unwanted artifacts occurring over the region of interest

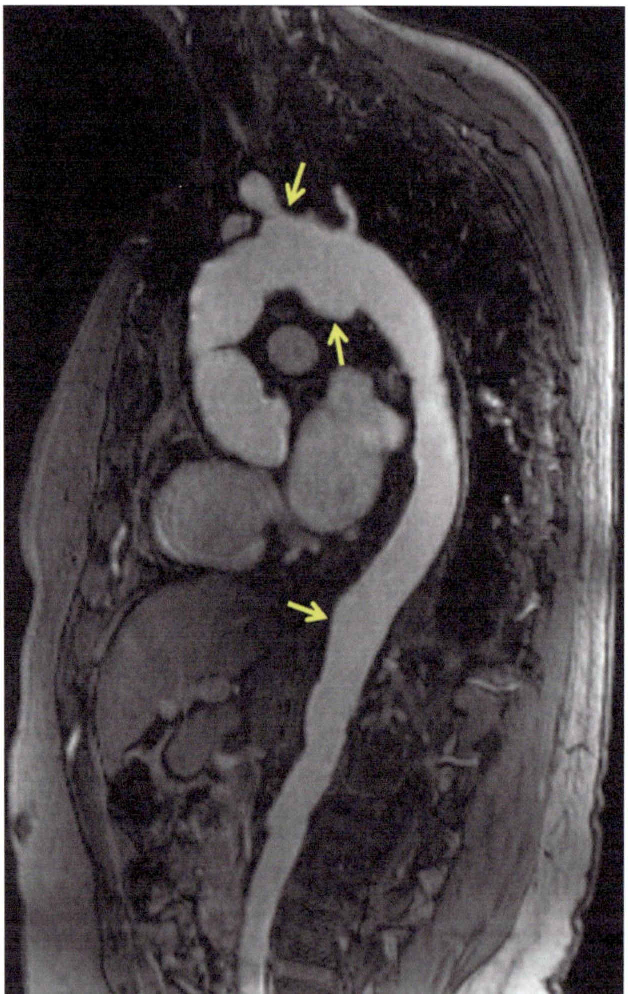

Fig. 22.1 Sagittal oblique MRA of thoracoabdominal aorta shows multiple saccular aneurysms (*arrows*)

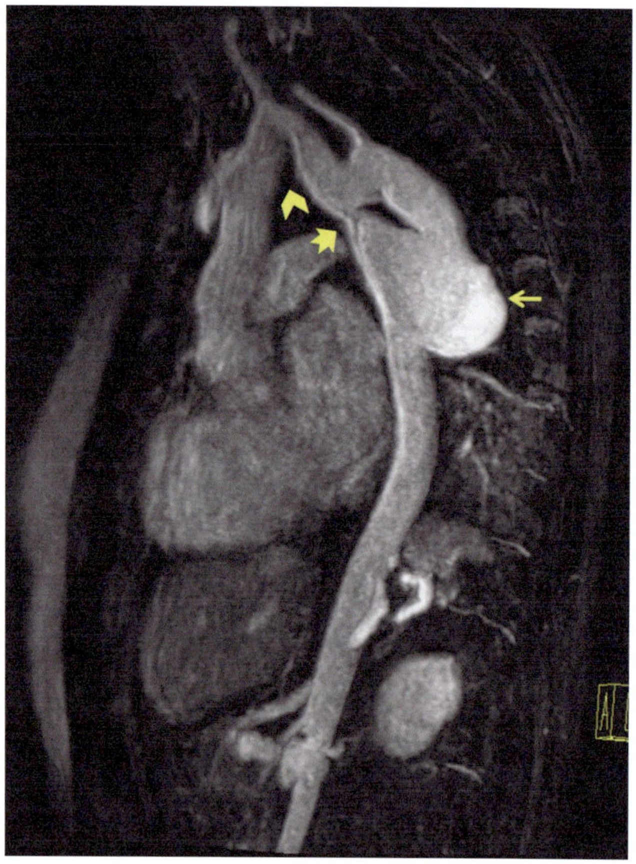

Fig. 22.2 Sagittal oblique MRA of thoracoabdominal region shows coarctation of aorta (*notched arrow*) and a large saccular aneurysm (*straight arrow*) in the proximal portion of left subclavian artery. Note the steep angle narrowing/kink (*chevron*) in the aortic arch. Coarctation of aorta is a contraindication to transfemoral approach. Even if coarctation is not seen, navigation through steep angle of arch is difficult in this patent

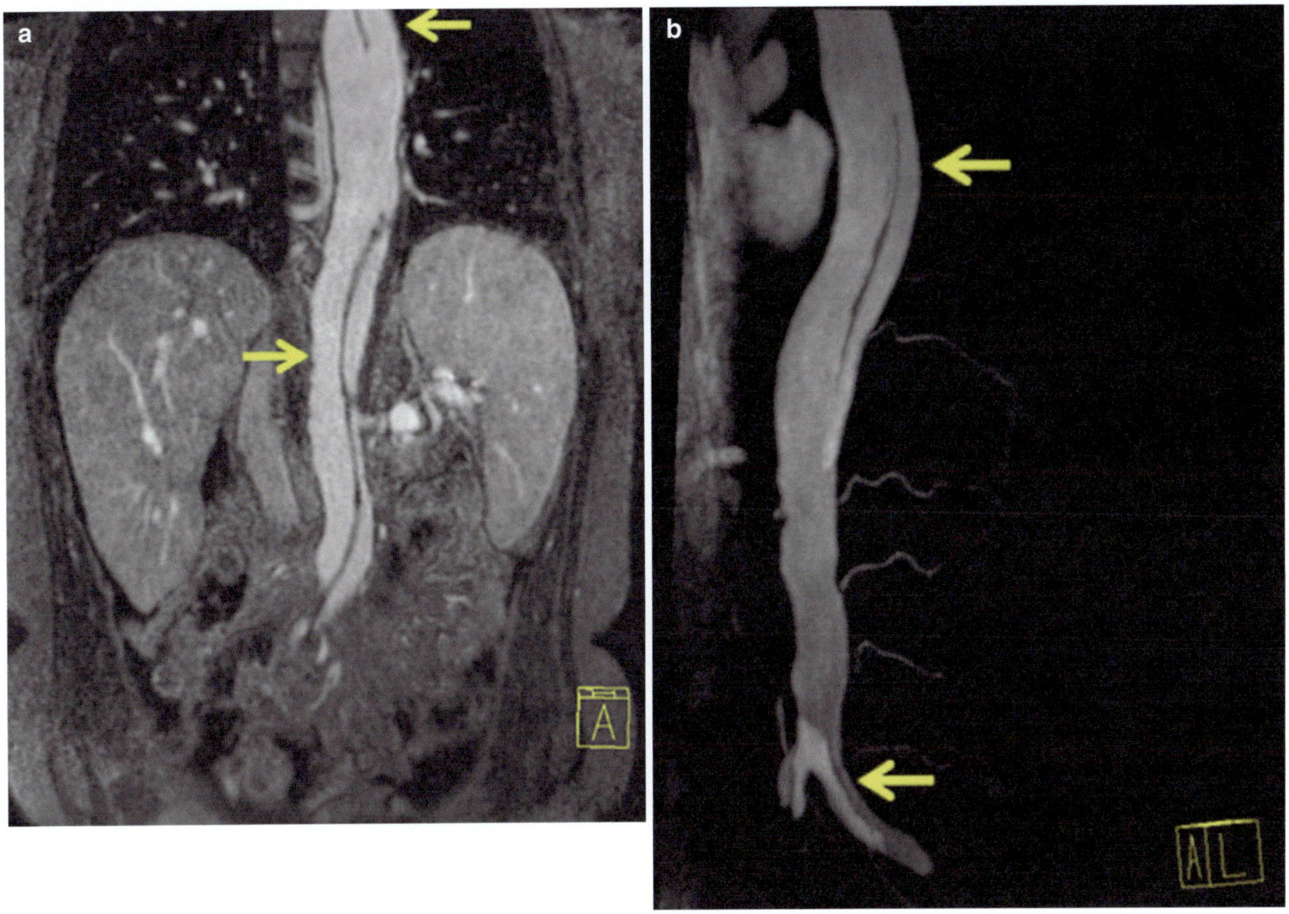

Fig. 22.3 Coronal (**a**) and sagittal (**b**) MRA shows Stanford type B dissection in thoracoabdominal region extending into bilateral common iliac arteries. All these pathologies (Figs. 22.1 to 22.3) affect the vascular access pathway

Box 22.1 Contraindications to MRI and MRA

Non-contrast

Severely claustrophobic patient
Presence of implantable stimulator devices
Presence of non-compatible aneurysmal clips
Presence of haemostatic surgical clips
Presence of pacemaker (relative)

Contrast

Patient at risk of allergy to gadolinium compounds
Patients known to have nephrogenic systemic fibrosis
Renal compromised patients (GFR < 30 ml/min/1.73 m^2)

MRI magnetic resonance imaging, *MRA* magnetic resonance angiography, *GFR* glomerular filtration rate

Table 22.3 Cardiac MRI protocol and MRA technique

Cardiac MRI protocol
1. Localizer scans
2. HASTE axial and coronal slices
3. True FISP cine vertical long axis (VLA), horizontal long axis (HLA), short axis (SA) views, and left ventricular inflow and outflow tract (LVOT) views
4. MRA acquisition*
5. Short axis stack of left ventricle
6. Delayed contrast enhancement images
7. Flow quantification across aorta and pulmonary artery
8. Optional images (T1W, cine views across the aortic root)
*MRA acquisition
1. Premask images
2. Arterial contrast MRA and time-resolved MRA
3. Subtracted images
4. Image post processing (MPR, MIP, VRT etc.)

Abbreviations: *HASTE* half-fourier acquisition single shot turbo spin echo, *FISP* fast imaging with steady state precession, *MPR* multiplanar reconstruction, *MIP* maximum intensity projection, *VRT* volume rendered technique

(ROI), and to familiarize the pattern of breath hold technique to be followed and the expected length of breath hold. Second, we acquire MRA source images and time-resolved MRA. This is followed by administration of contrast agent @ 0.1 mmol/kg body weight and saline flush of 20–30 ml. Source images are obtained in identical fashion to mask image. Usually a series of three to four MRAs can be obtained with the same or on different imaging planes over a period of time, that is, time-resolved MRA, thus providing 4D spatial and temporal vascular imaging [38, 39]. Third, we perform subtracted MRA. Subtraction of pre- and post-contrast 3D

MRA data can be done to provide images without any noisy background tissue and thus improving the resolution of MRA. This method is successful only if the two data sets have identical imaging parameters and spatial orientation. Misregistration of two data sets might lead to poor image quality and artifacts. Next, we perform image post-processing. For assessing the aortic root and the aortoilio-femoral vasculature, an MRA series which shows good luminal enhancement of the vessels is selected. At our institution, we routinely use a dedicated offline 3D workstation. Workstations with similar post-processing tools are available from different vendors. 3D volumetric source or subtracted images are evaluated in multiple planes and are post processed further to highlight the ROI. Importantly, high quality source MRA images are essential to ensure accurate diagnoses as all post-processing tools rely on adequate image quality. If doubt exists or if subtracted images are not of diagnostic quality, MRA interpreting physicians should rely on the source images rather than on subtracted images.

Various post-processing tools are used to analyze the 3D volumetric data [40–42]. Some of the most commonly used tools include multiplanar reformation (MPR), maximum intensity projection (MIP), and volume-rendered techniques (VRT).

Multiplanar Reformat (MPR)

MPR is a post-processing tool where the volumetric data is automatically arranged in three orthogonal planes, namely, axial (or transverse), coronal, and sagittal planes. MPR tool is unique as it allows image processing in any desired plane (Fig. 22.4). By toggling the imaging planes to the axis of a vessel, a profile and enface viewing plane can be obtained for assessment of vascular structures. This is especially helpful in evaluating structures that are oriented obliquely to the standard orthogonal planes. Slice thickness can be manipulated so as to visualize a large field of view albeit with slight decrease in spatial resolution. Advanced software algorithms provide curved MPR option. Curved MPR helps in laying out any curved vessel flat in a 2D plane. It can also be rotated 360° for easy assessment of vessel analysis. This is especially helpful in assessing a real versus pseudostenosis within a tortuous vessel.

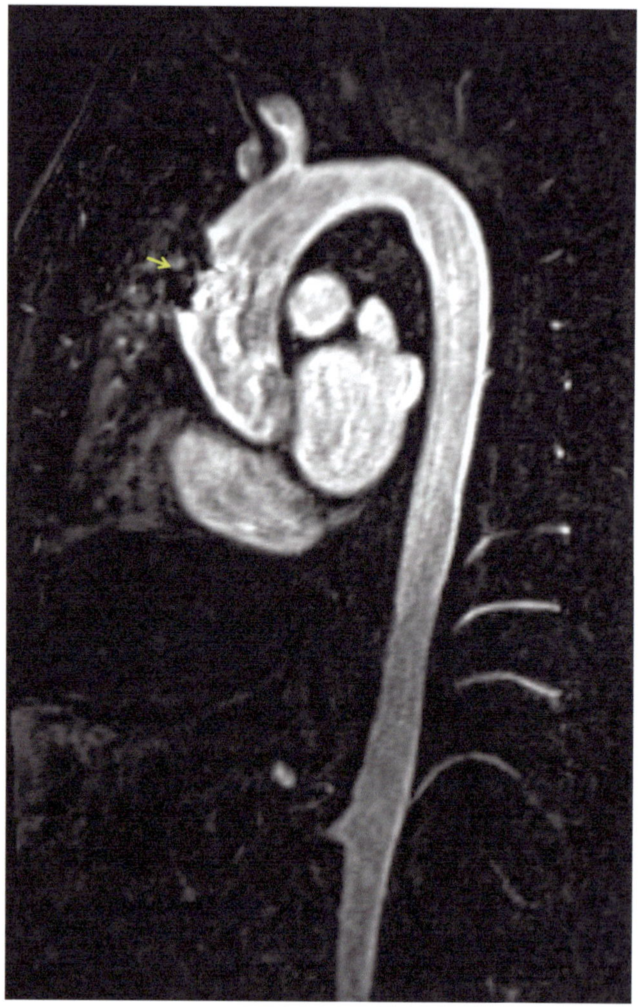

Fig. 22.4 Multiplanar reformation (MPR) of thoraco-abdominal MRA displays a large field of view of vascular structures in a single image. Dark signal metallic artifact in ascending aorta is due to previous bypass surgery

Maximum Intensity Projection (MIP)

MIP is the simplest and most widely used post-processing technique. In this algorithm, a set of parallel rays is projected on to the chosen viewing plane. The rays in their pathway take into consideration only the maximum signal intensity present in the voxel and the low intensity signals are discarded. The end result is a 3D volumetric data with brightest signal projected as a 2D image. This is useful for visualizing the entire vascular tree but with the expense of loss of depth projection (Fig. 22.5). To overcome this, MIP images are rotated in multiple imaging planes to gain an appreciation of the spatial relationship of the various structures being analyzed. The interpreting physician must be aware that any other entities with high signal intensity may also project within the plane of the vasculature and act to obscure it. This is of particular concern when images are significantly degraded by background noise. As a result, MIP imaging is more helpful when background noise has been adequately subtracted from the mask images.

Volume Rendering Technique (VRT)

VRT images allow for analyses of the voxels in the entire volume of data and provide depth information. It assigns a color based on each voxel's signal intensity and opacity on a scale of 0–100 % (Fig. 22.6).

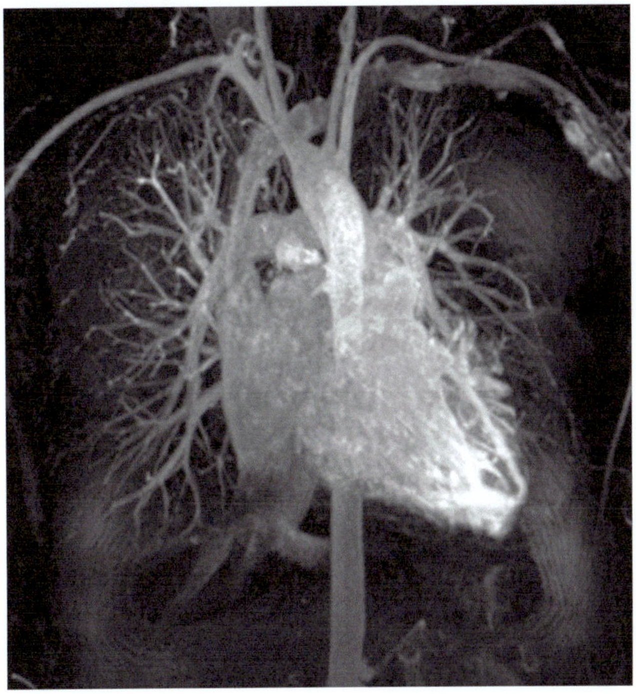

Fig. 22.5 Maximum intensity projection (MIP) of chest vasculature in coronal view shows only the brightest intensity areas and loss of depth information

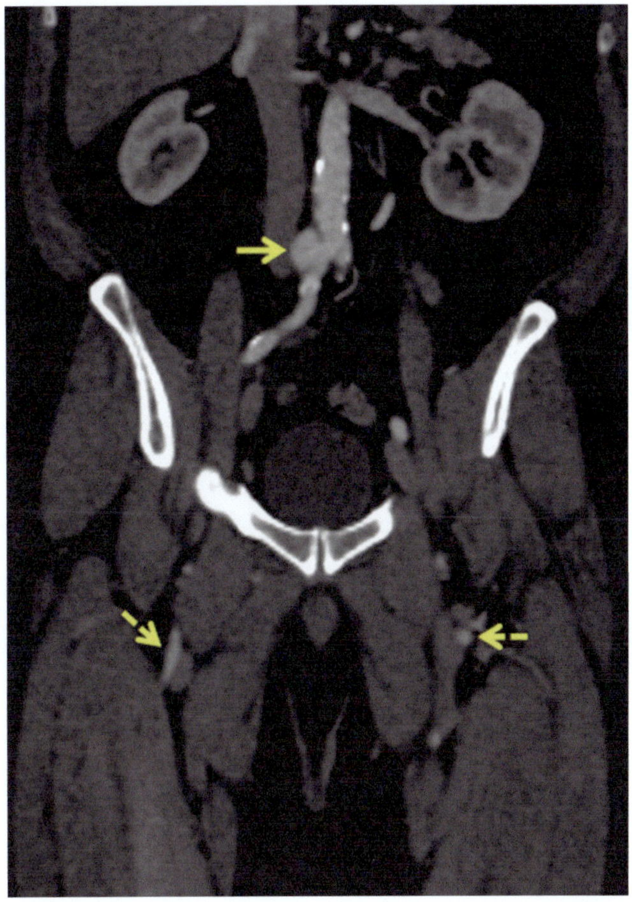

Fig. 22.7 Abdomino-pelvic coronal multiplanar reformatted (MPR) image shows saccular aneurysm (*straight arrow*) arising from right common iliac artery (CIA), just distal to aortic bifurcation. Nonvisualized left CIA and distal half of right CIA with reconstitution as superficial femoral arteries (*dotted arrows*). In this case, as the femoral arterial entry site is bilaterally blocked, alternate vascular pathways need to be considered

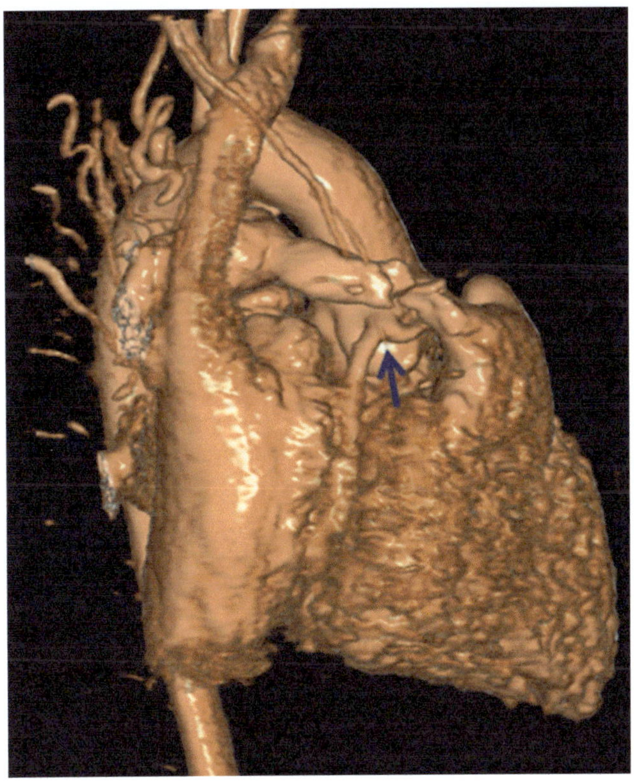

Fig. 22.6 Volume rendering technique (VRT) displays a 3D object with preservation of depth information. Note the well-visualized anomalous origin of LAD from RCA (*blue arrow*)

Anatomical Areas of Interest for TAVR Screening

There are a number of potential vascular and valvular pitfalls that are encountered during TAVR, and dedicated imaging may allow for greater focus during pre-procedural screening to overcome those pitfalls. These include site of access, wherein the proceduralist may encounter difficulty in puncture of the entry site (Fig. 22.7) and difficulty in passing the delivery catheter and the device due to small luminal diameter (Figs. 22.8 and 22.9), tortuous vasculature, atherosclerotic calcific disease, perforation or dissection, or thromboembolism in the aortoiliofemoral arterial segments.

Further, the proceduralist may encounter unfavorable anatomy causing "device-aortic root complex" mismatch. These anatomic characteristics include low-lying coronary ostia, bulky calcified aortic leaflets, aortic root morphology that may increase the risk of aortic rupture/dissection or

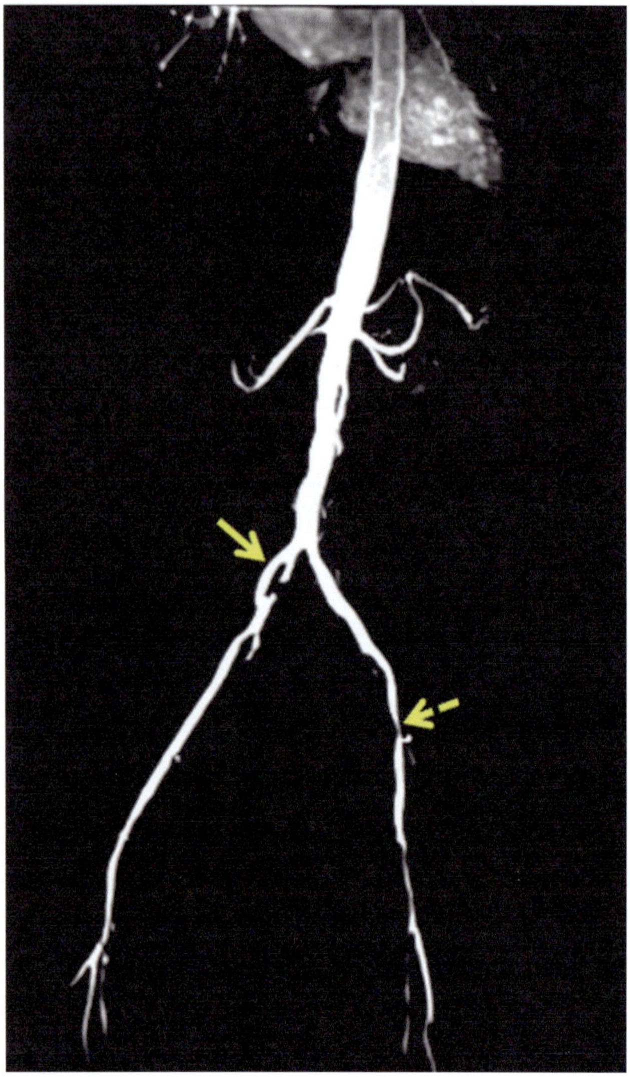

Fig. 22.8 Coronal maximum intensity projection (MIP) of abdominal aortoiliac arterial system. There is focal dilatation of right CIA with disrupted intimal flap within (*straight arrow*). Note on left side, there is diffuse narrowing of left CIA and tight stenosis of left femoral artery (*dotted arrow*)

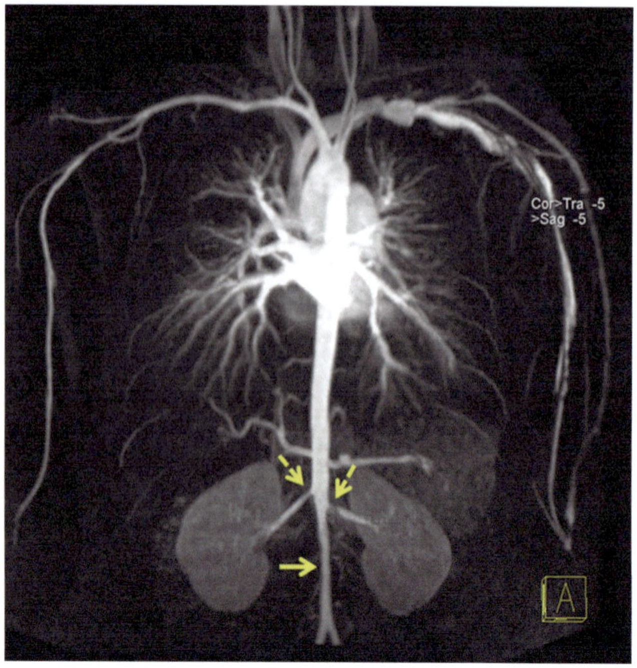

Fig. 22.9 Coronal MIP of thoraco-abdominal aorta shows narrowing of the infrarenal abdominal aorta (*straight arrow*). It is difficult to navigate the catheter in this condition. Note also the bilateral renal artery stenosis (*dotted arrows*)

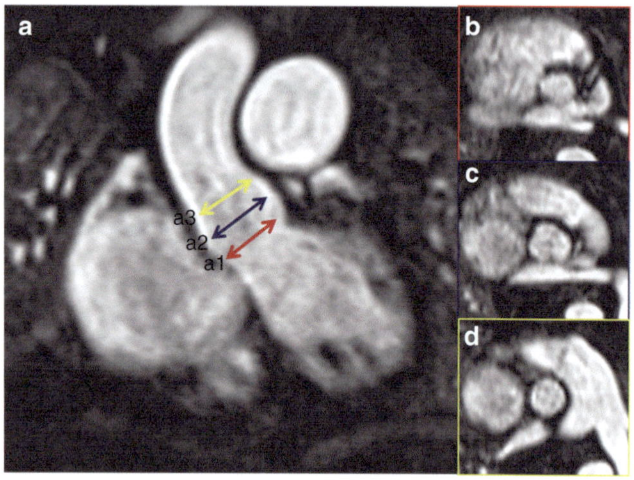

Fig. 22.10 Thoracic aorta: Coronal oblique (illustrated) and sagittal oblique (not illustrated) views are used in measuring the diameters at various levels: (a1) Aortic annulus (*red arrow*), (a2) Sinus of Valsalva [SoV] (*blue arrow*), and (a3) Sinotubular junction (STJ) (*yellow arrow*). Corresponding cross-sectional diameters of a1, a2, and a3 are depicted in b, c, and d, respectively

paravalvular aortic regurgitation (AR), and cardiac morphology that may increase the risk of cardiac perforation or tamponade.

Imaging by MRA may also aid in the decisions of valve positioning. Commonly encountered complications for which comprehensive MRA evaluation may help to avoid include low-lying device implantation resulting in impingement on the LVOT causing atrioventricular block, damage to mitral valve apparatus, high-lying device implantation, or under-expansion of the device that can lead to embolization of device. Conversely, over-expansion of device may lead to aortic rupture/dissection, cardiac perforation, or tamponade.

Aortic Root Assessment

The aortic root is a complex 3D structure [43, 44]. It involves the aortic annulus, the aortic valve leaflets, and the sinotubular junction (STJ) (Fig. 22.10). The proper assessment of aortic root is the principal step for a successful TAVR

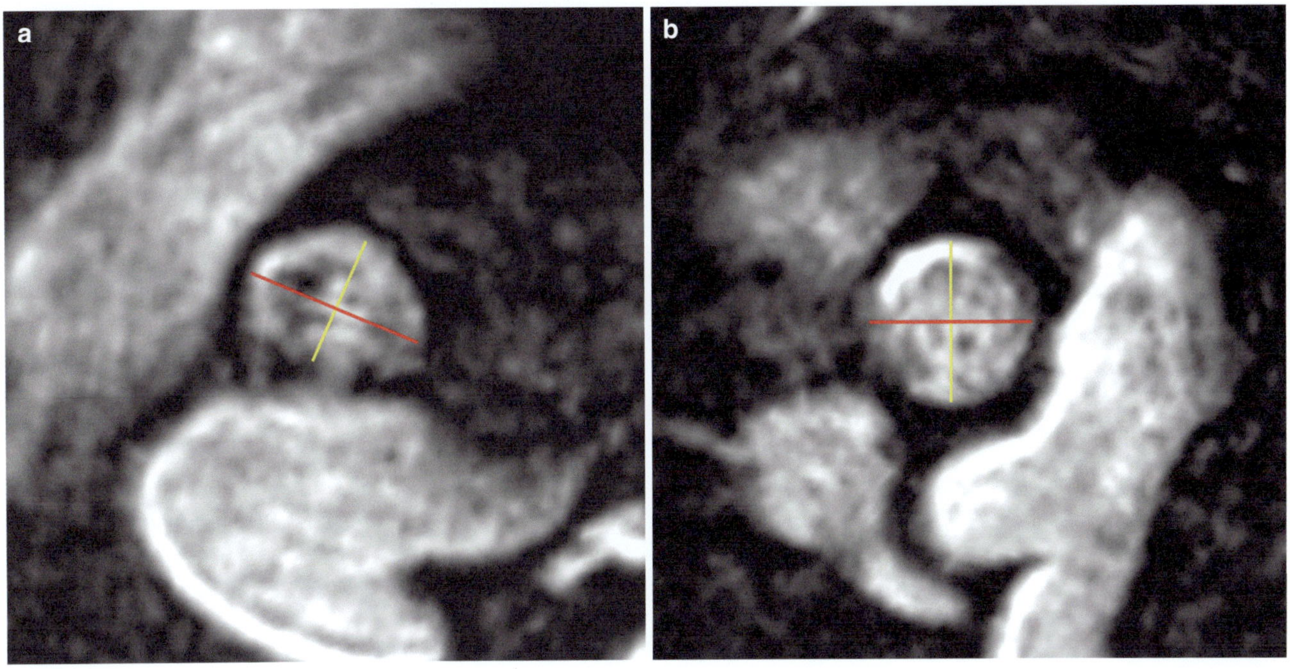

Fig. 22.11 Variable aortic root morphology. Note the (a) oval shape at aortic annulus with major and minor axes (red and blue lines respectively), and (b) near circular shape of aorta at STJ

procedure as it determines the device size. It is important to obtain true measurements along orthogonal planes. While assessing 3D images, reference planes should center on the ROI so that true cross-sectional (CS) plane is obtained to measure the diameter or the area for calculation. Valve sizing and positioning requires understanding the morphology of the aortic root and precise evaluation of each of abovementioned structures.

Aortic Annulus

Aortic annular measurements play a critical role in selection of proper device size for implantation and is the most crucial factor for a successful outcome. Mismatch between annulus measurement and prosthesis are a major source of complications. Placement of oversized valve may lead to catastrophic rupture of aortic root or to cardiac tamponade. Incorrect valve sizing has shown to be the most common cause of postoperative paravalvular PAR [45–47]. Although several studies have demonstrated that moderate to severe AR is independently associated with late mortality rate [48–50], a more recent study indicates that even mild AR is linked to increased late mortality [51]. It is now well known that the aortic annulus geometry is more often elliptical rather than circular in shape (Fig. 22.11) [52, 53]. No single diameter adequately characterizes the 3D geometry of this fairly uniform non-circular structure. As such, a number of measurements have been proposed for annular assessment with MRI including the mean diameter, area, and or the perimeter of the aortic annulus.

Aortic Sinuses

The aortic root bulges outwards to form three aortic sinuses or the sinus of Valsalva (SoV). Measurements of the maximal width of sinus are chosen for procedural planning. Crawford et al. [54], based on echocardiographic study, have concluded that aortic root dilatation is common in AS patients but a small annulus is unusual in AS. Small aortic roots are more common in women. In a study of AS patients, 27 % of the women and 19 % of men did not have aortic root geometry that fulfills the current requirements for TAVR [55].

Sinotubular Junction (STJ)

The STJ is the narrowest part of the ascending aorta above the sinuses. It is usually circular in shape. The measurement of STJ greater than 40 mm indicates dilatation. Annular dilatation is frequently accompanied by STJ dilatation [56]. This aspect also needs to be taken into consideration when planning for TAVR. Similarly to the STJ measurement, the cross-sectional diameter of the ascending aorta is valuable when implanting a longer valve.

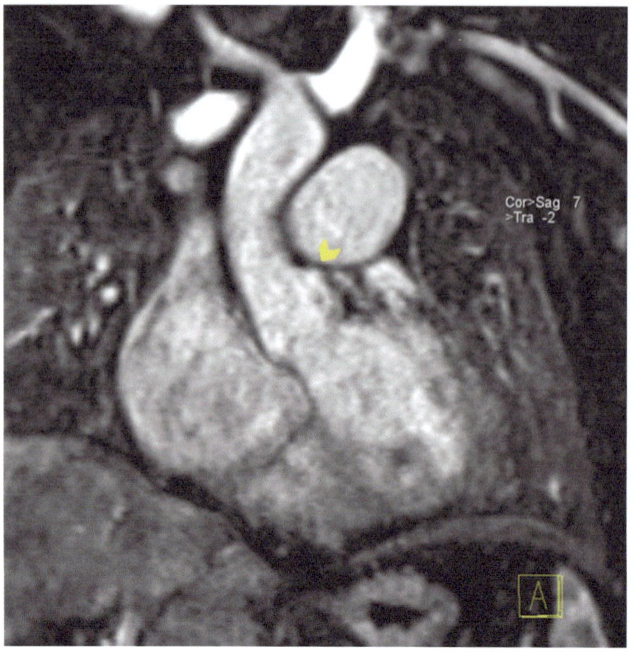

Fig. 22.12 12 Coronary oblique image of ascending aorta shows low-lying left coronary ostium (*chevron*). Height of coronary ostia measured 8 mm. Normal height is usually above 13 mm. Low-lying coronary ostia predisposes to coronary occlusion either due to device or due to native valve leaflets

Depth of Sinus of Valsalva (SoV)

The depth of sinus of Valsalva relative to the aortic valve plane is obtained from the coronal or sagittal oblique images. It extends from aortic annulus to STJ. This is an important measurement for both the balloon-expandable and self-expanding prosthesis. A lesser depth of the SoV might lead to placement of the ventricular portion of the valve prosthesis lower in the LVOT leading to conduction abnormalities.

Coronary Artery Height

The heights of the right and left coronary ostia relative to the aortic annulus are also measured in coronal or sagittal oblique views by adjusting the reference planes. During implantation, low-lying coronary ostia (Fig. 22.12) or bulky heavily calcified cusps may potentially occlude the right or left coronary ostia. Coronary ostial occlusion, although relatively uncommon (<1 %), needs to be anticipated as it can cause myocardial infarction and death. The coronary cutoff height of 11–14 mm has been proposed depending on the type and size of the prosthesis used. From the same views, the length of the corresponding cusp can be measured.

Left Ventricular and Three-Chamber View Measurements

The long axis views for assessment are the vertical long axis (2 chamber), horizontal long axis (4 chamber), and left ventricular outflow tract (3 chamber) views. These views are obtained either as true FISP images or can be obtained from post-processing of 3D MRA data. Scrolling through long axis views easily identifies the presence or absence of any thrombus or mass within the LV (Fig. 22.13a, b). The presence of interventricular septal (IVS) hypertrophy and any subaortic annulus stenosis is clearly visualized in LVOT plane. IVS > 17 mm is a contraindication for implantation of CoreValve. Presence of hypertrophic obstructive cardiomyopathy (HOCM) is an absolute contraindication to both CoreValve and Edwards SAPIEN valve prostheses (Fig. 22.14).

Left Ventricular–Aorta Angle

The left ventricular (LV)-aortic root angle is the angle subtended between the LV inflow and outflow and is measured from the 3-chamber view. LV inflow bisects through the center of mitral valve and LV apex. LV outflow longitudinal axis is extended on to LV chamber through the center of the aortic valve. In transapical procedures, this angle will help guide the direction of the delivery system from the mini thoracotomy access region to the aortic valve. It is difficult to access and is more prone for complications in an extremely steep angle presentation (Fig. 22.15). It was also observed that patients having steep LV-aortic root angle have a higher LVOT gradient [57]. Therefore, alternative approaches such as the transaortic pathway need to be considered. Steep angle cutoff values are not yet established and prospective longitudinal studies will probably address those.

A retrospective study analyzed the LVOT-ascending aorta angle measurement in Medtronic CoreValve implanted devices [58]. It revealed increased LVOT-ascending aorta angle is associated with increased risk of significant AR. This angle needs to be assessed in a standardized manner to plan for the operative procedure [59].

Assessment of Aortoiliofemoral Arterial Segment

In addition to assessment of the aortic valvular complex, a thorough evaluation of the vascular access is needed to help guide the procedure. Hayashida et al. [60] and others have concluded that major vascular complications increase 30-day mortality. Accurate evaluation of the aortoiliofemoral

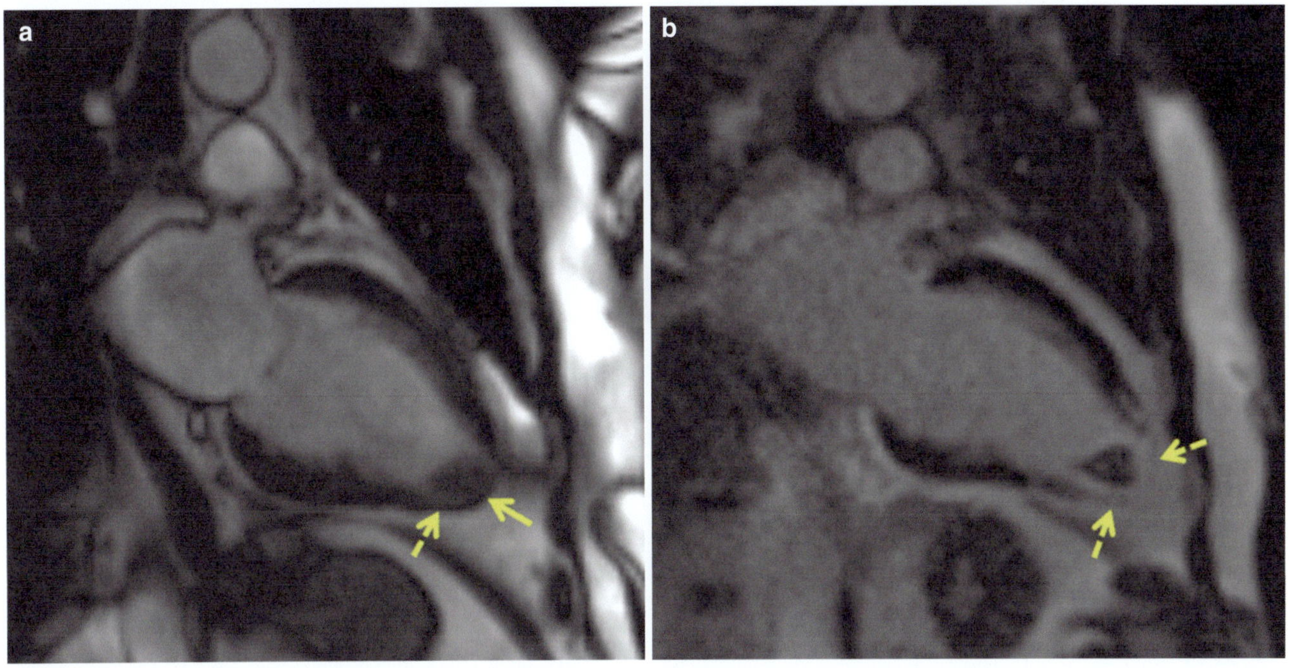

Fig. 22.13 Left ventricular apical thrombus. (**a**) True FISP 2-chamber view of left ventricle (LV) shows a well-defined, round mass in the apical region (*straight arrow*) with surrounding thin walled myocardium (*dotted arrow*). (**b**) Delayed contrast enhancement (DCE) of the same view shows enhancement of apical myocardium, suggestive of fibrosis due to previous myocardial infarction. There is no DCE of the apical mass, suggestive of a thrombus. The presence of apical thrombus is a contraindication for TAVR procedure

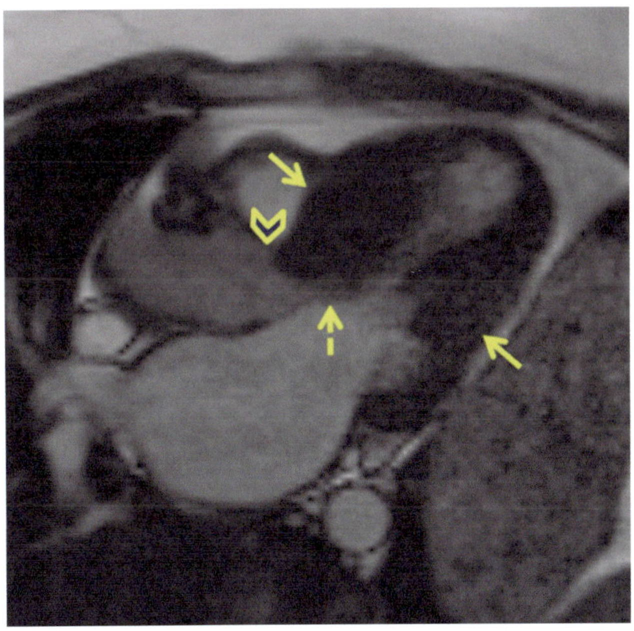

Fig. 22.14 Intraventricular septal hypertrophy (IVSH). True FISP cine snapshot images of LVOT show abnormally increased thickness of septal myocardium (*straight arrows*), (measured ~23 mm) in a case of hypertrophic obstructive cardiomyopathy (HOCM). Note narrowed LV cavity due to grossly thickened basal septal myocardium. IVSH > 17 mm is a contraindication for CoreValve device. Note also the septal anterior motion of mitral valve (*dotted arrow*) and how IVSH impinges on aortic annulus (*chevron*)

segments has a major role in avoiding complications. With MRI, various MIP and VRT techniques can provide an overall orientation of the vessel distribution.

Aortic Arch Geometry/Morphology

A good view of the ascending arch and descending thoracic aorta is obtained in the sagittal oblique view. In a meta-analysis study, procedural stroke (<24 h) occurred in 1.5 % [61]. Cerebrovascular event rates within 30 days of TAVR range from 1 to 7 % [61–64]. Most of these are assumed to be due to embolic events. Vascular access pathway is evaluated for ulcers, stenosis, occlusion, aneurysm, dissections, or any extrinsic compression on the lumen.

The aortic arch is observed for any coarctation, kinking, or for steep angulations. The evaluation of the aortic arch geometry is important to predict procedural complexity and help guide the placement of thromboembolic deflection devices when they are being considered. The aortic arch can be graded in three different ways [65]. At our institution, we follow the classification described by Madhwal et al. [66]. The vertical distance from the origin of the innominate artery to the top of the arch determines the arch type. In Type 1, the distance is <1 diameter of the left common carotid artery (LCCA); in Type 2, the distance is between

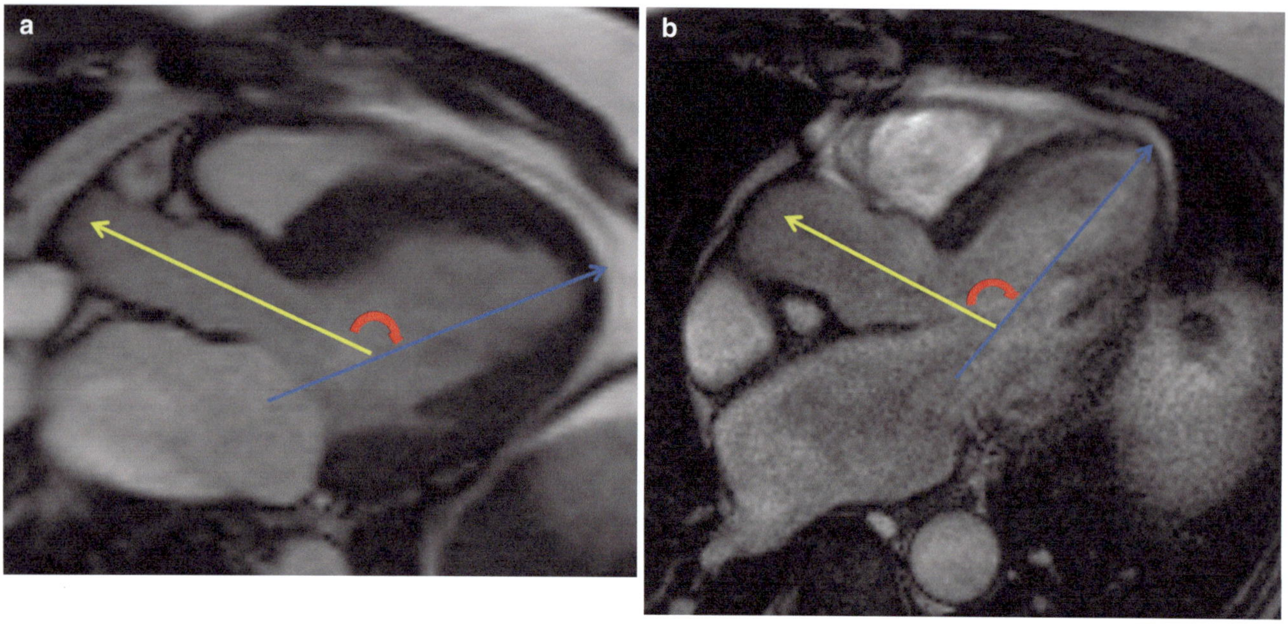

Fig. 22.15 Angle between LV inflow (blue arrow passing through the centre of mitral valve and LV apex) and LV outflow (yellow line passing through the centre of aortic valve and intersecting the blue line) impacts the TAVR procedure to be adopted. Two different TAVR patients; (a) LV – AoR angle (*red arrow*) is obtuse where as it is near perpendicular in (b). Almost perpendicular angle between the LV and AoR makes it difficult to place TAVR device

1 and 2 diameters; and in Type 3, the distance is >2 diameters of LCCA is Type 3 arch (Fig. 22.16a–c). Among the three types, Type 3 arch is the most difficult one to navigate through the catheter.

Multiple measurements are taken at the level of proximal ascending thoracic aorta (just before the arch vessels origin), mid-arch, proximal descending thoracic aorta, and distal descending thoracic aorta at the level of the diaphragm. Note is made of any stenosis or tortuosity of the aorta, any dissections, intramural hematomas, or ulcers anywhere within the thoracic aorta.

Iliofemoral Assessment

Iliofemoral arterial assessment will determine the eligibility for a transfemoral approach for the TAVR. In a study of 100 patients with critical aortic stenosis, at least one-third of patients had unfavorable iliofemoral anatomy and majority of those patients had a minimal luminal diameter of <8 mm [67]. A high prevalence of peripheral arterial disease in TAVR cohort mandates a thorough assessment of iliofemoral anatomy. Vessels are also evaluated for ulcers, stenosis, occlusion, aneurysm, dissections, or any extrinsic compression on the lumen. Luminal diameters are measured in true cross-sectional view at multiple levels: at the iliac artery bifurcation, at the external iliac artery origin, and at the femoral artery. The presence of atherosclerotic disease, whether isolated, diffuse, or circumferential, is noted. Hayashida et al. [60] introduced the concept of sheath to femoral artery ratio to predict major TAVR vascular complications. Further, any undue tortuosity of the vessel of more than 135° confounds the transfemoral approach. It is prudent to project the 3D MRA in VRT or MIP mode and overlay this data on the background bony structures so that an exact reference point for vascular access can be planned.

Conclusion

MRI and 3D MRA have excellent spatial and contrast resolution providing precise measurements of both the aortic annulus and vascular access that often obviates the need for diagnostic catheter-based angiography and can be performed without the use of radiation or iodinated contrast. Further, non-contrast enhanced MRA is a viable alternative in patients whose renal function is compromised. As TAVR procedures become more available, MRA may grow in its utility to provide pre-, intra-, and post-procedural evaluation of patients undergoing TAVR.

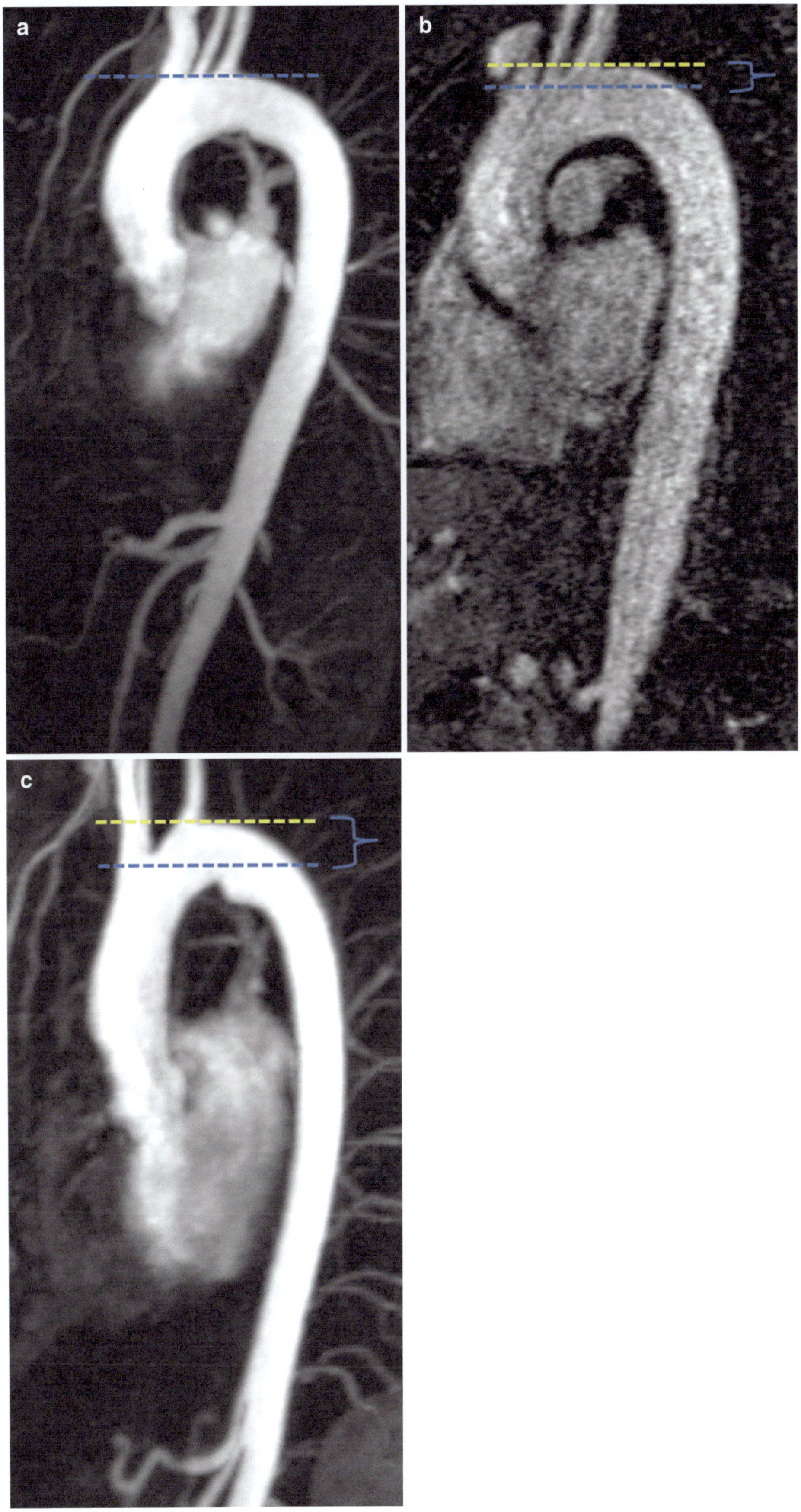

Fig. 22.16 Aortic arch geometry. Comparison of left common carotid artery (LCCA) diameter and the vertical distance between the origin of innominate artery (*blue horizontal dotted line*) and top of the aortic arch (*yellow horizontal dotted line*) in parasagittal view is used to classify aortic arch types. (**a**) Type 1; distance is less than one diameter of LCCA. (**b**) Type 2; distance is between 1 and 2 diameters of LCCA. (**c**) Type 3; distance is greater than 2 diameters of LCCA. Note: Type 3 arch shows a narrow angle of aortic arch. Navigating the catheter through the arch becomes increasingly difficult from Type 1–3

References

1. Iung B, Cachier A, Baron G, Messika-Zeitoun D, Delahaye F, Tornos P, et al. Decision-making in elderly patients with severe aortic stenosis: why are so many denied surgery? Eur Heart J. 2005;26(24):2714–20. Epub 2005/09/06.
2. Chitsaz S, Jaussaud N, Chau E, Yan KS, Azadani AN, Ratcliffe MB, et al. Operative risks and survival in veterans with severe aortic stenosis: surgery versus medical therapy. Ann Thorac Surg. 2011;92(3):866–72. Epub 2011/08/30.
3. Bouma BJ, van Den Brink RB, van Der Meulen JH, Verheul HA, Cheriex EC, Hamer HP, et al. To operate or not on elderly patients with aortic stenosis: the decision and its consequences. Heart. 1999;82(2):143–8. Epub 1999/07/20.
4. Pai RG, Kapoor N, Bansal RC, Varadarajan P. Malignant natural history of asymptomatic severe aortic stenosis: benefit of aortic valve replacement. Ann Thorac Surg. 2006;82(6):2116–22. Epub 2006/11/28.
5. Varadarajan P, Kapoor N, Bansal RC, Pai RG. Survival in elderly patients with severe aortic stenosis is dramatically improved by aortic valve replacement: Results from a cohort of 277 patients aged > or =80 years. Eur J Cardiothorac Surg. 2006;30(5):722–7. Epub 2006/09/05.
6. Kojodjojo P, Gohil N, Barker D, Youssefi P, Salukhe TV, Choong A, et al. Outcomes of elderly patients aged 80 and over with symptomatic, severe aortic stenosis: impact of patient's choice of refusing aortic valve replacement on survival. QJM. 2008;101(7):567–73. Epub 2008/04/30.
7. Gotzmann M, Hehen T, Germing A, Lindstaedt M, Yazar A, Laczkovics A, et al. Short-term effects of transcatheter aortic valve implantation on neurohormonal activation, quality of life and 6-minute walk test in severe and symptomatic aortic stenosis. Heart. 2010;96(14):1102–6. Epub 2009/11/04.
8. Ussia GP, Barbanti M, Cammalleri V, Scarabelli M, Mule M, Aruta P, et al. Quality-of-life in elderly patients one year after transcatheter aortic valve implantation for severe aortic stenosis. EuroIntervention. 2011;7(5):573–9. Epub 2011/09/21.
9. Goncalves A, Marcos-Alberca P, Almeria C, Feltes G, Hernandez-Antolin RA, Rodriguez E, et al. Quality of life improvement at midterm follow-up after transcatheter aortic valve implantation. Int J Cardiol. 2013;162(2):117–22. Epub 2011/06/04.
10. Bagur R, Rodes-Cabau J, Dumont E, Larochelliere RD, Doyle D, Bertrand OF, et al. Exercise capacity in patients with severe symptomatic aortic stenosis before and six months after transcatheter aortic valve implantation. Am J Cardiol. 2011;108(2):258–64. Epub 2011/05/07.
11. Buellesfeld L, Gerckens U, Schuler G, Bonan R, Kovac J, Serruys PW, et al. 2-year follow-up of patients undergoing transcatheter aortic valve implantation using a self-expanding valve prosthesis. J Am Coll Cardiol. 2011;57(16):1650–7. Epub 2011/04/16.
12. Lange R, Bleiziffer S, Mazzitelli D, Elhmidi Y, Opitz A, Krane M, et al. Improvements in transcatheter aortic valve implantation outcomes in lower surgical risk patients: a glimpse into the future. J Am Coll Cardiol. 2012;59(3):280–7. Epub 2011/12/27.
13. Cribier A, Eltchaninoff H, Bash A, Borenstein N, Tron C, Bauer F, et al. Percutaneous transcatheter implantation of an aortic valve prosthesis for calcific aortic stenosis: first human case description. Circulation. 2002;106(24):3006–8. Epub 2002/12/11.
14. Prince MR, Meaney JF. Expanding role of MR angiography in clinical practice. Eur Radiol. 2006;16 Suppl 2:B3–8. Epub 2006/06/28.
15. Willinek WA, von Falkenhausen M, Born M, Gieseke J, Holler T, Klockgether T, et al. Noninvasive detection of steno-occlusive disease of the supra-aortic arteries with three-dimensional contrast-enhanced magnetic resonance angiography: a prospective, intra-individual comparative analysis with digital subtraction angiography. Stroke. 2005;36(1):38–43. Epub 2004/12/01.
16. Deutschmann HA, Schoellnast H, Portugaller HR, Preidler KW, Reittner P, Tillich M, et al. Routine use of three-dimensional contrast-enhanced moving-table MR angiography in patients with peripheral arterial occlusive disease: comparison with selective digital subtraction angiography. Cardiovasc Intervent Radiol. 2006;29(5):762–70. Epub 2006/04/21.
17. Berg F, Bangard C, Bovenschulte H, Hellmich M, Nijenhuis M, Lackner K, et al. Feasibility of peripheral contrast-enhanced magnetic resonance angiography at 3.0 Tesla with a hybrid technique: comparison with digital subtraction angiography. Invest Radiol. 2008;43(9):642–9.
18. Bui BT, Miller S, Mildenberger P, Sam 2nd A, Sheng R. Comparison of contrast-enhanced MR angiography to intraarterial digital subtraction angiography for evaluation of peripheral arterial occlusive disease: results of a phase III multicenter trial. J Magn Reson Imaging. 2010;31(6):1402–10. Epub 2010/06/01.
19. Lin J, Li D, Yan F. High-resolution 3D contrast-enhanced MRA with parallel imaging techniques before endovascular interventional treatment of arterial stenosis. Vasc Med. 2009;14(4):305–11. Epub 2009/10/08.
20. Prince MR, Yucel EK, Kaufman JA, Harrison DC, Geller SC. Dynamic gadolinium-enhanced three-dimensional abdominal MR arteriography. J Magn Reson Imaging. 1993;3(6):877–81. Epub 1993/11/01.
21. Prince MR, Arnoldus C, Frisoli JK. Nephrotoxicity of high-dose gadolinium compared with iodinated contrast. J Magn Reson Imaging. 1996;6(1):162–6. Epub 1996/01/01.
22. Hoffmann U, Fischereder M, Reil A, Fischer M, Link J, Kramer BK. Renal effects of gadopentetate dimeglumine in patients with normal and impaired renal function. Eur J Med Res. 2005;10(4):149–54. Epub 2005/06/11.
23. Kane GC, Stanson AW, Kalnicka D, Rosenthal DW, Lee CU, Textor SC, et al. Comparison between gadolinium and iodine contrast for percutaneous intervention in atherosclerotic renal artery stenosis: clinical outcomes. Nephrol Dial Transplant. 2008;23(4):1233–40. Epub 2008/02/08.
24. Grobner T. Gadolinium–a specific trigger for the development of nephrogenic fibrosing dermopathy and nephrogenic systemic fibrosis? Nephrol Dial Transplant. 2006;21(4):1104–8. Epub 2006/01/25.
25. Marckmann P, Skov L, Rossen K, Dupont A, Damholt MB, Heaf JG, et al. Nephrogenic systemic fibrosis: suspected causative role of gadodiamide used for contrast-enhanced magnetic resonance imaging. J Am Soc Nephrol. 2006;17(9):2359–62. Epub 2006/08/04.
26. Mendoza FA, Artlett CM, Sandorfi N, Latinis K, Piera-Velazquez S, Jimenez SA. Description of 12 cases of nephrogenic fibrosing dermopathy and review of the literature. Semin Arthritis Rheum. 2006;35(4):238–49. Epub 2006/02/08.
27. Wiginton CD, Kelly B, Oto A, Jesse M, Aristimuno P, Ernst R, et al. Gadolinium-based contrast exposure, nephrogenic systemic fibrosis, and gadolinium detection in tissue. AJR Am J Roentgenol. 2008;190(4):1060–8. Epub 2008/03/22.
28. Perez-Rodriguez J, Lai S, Ehst BD, Fine DM, Bluemke DA. Nephrogenic systemic fibrosis: incidence, associations, and effect of risk factor assessment – report of 33 cases. Radiology. 2009;250(2):371–7. Epub 2009/02/04.
29. Bryant 2nd BJ, Im K, Broome DR. Evaluation of the incidence of nephrogenic systemic fibrosis in patients with moderate renal insufficiency administered gadobenate dimeglumine for MRI. Clin Radiol. 2009;64(7):706–13. Epub 2009/06/13.
30. Hoppe H, Spagnuolo S, Froehlich JM, Nievergelt H, Dinkel HP, Gretener S, et al. Retrospective analysis of patients for development of nephrogenic systemic fibrosis following conventional angiography

using gadolinium-based contrast agents. Eur Radiol. 2010;20(3):595–603. Epub 2009/09/18.

31. Chrysochou C, Buckley DL, Dark P, Cowie A, Kalra PA. Gadolinium-enhanced magnetic resonance imaging for renovascular disease and nephrogenic systemic fibrosis: critical review of the literature and UK experience. J Magn Reson Imaging. 2009;29(4):887–94. Epub 2009/03/24.
32. Altun E, Martin DR, Wertman R, Lugo-Somolinos A, Fuller 3rd ER, Semelka RC. Nephrogenic systemic fibrosis: change in incidence following a switch in gadolinium agents and adoption of a gadolinium policy–report from two U.S. universities. Radiology. 2009;253(3):689–96.
33. Martin DR, Krishnamoorthy SK, Kalb B, Salman KN, Sharma P, Carew JD, et al. Decreased incidence of NSF in patients on dialysis after changing gadolinium contrast-enhanced MRI protocols. J Magn Reson Imaging. 2010;31(2):440–6. Epub 2010/01/26.
34. Wang Y, Alkasab TK, Narin O, Nazarian RM, Kaewlai R, Kay J, et al. Incidence of nephrogenic systemic fibrosis after adoption of restrictive gadolinium-based contrast agent guidelines. Radiology. 2011;260(1):105–11. Epub 2011/05/19.
35. Blankholm AD, Ringgaard S. Non-contrast-enhanced magnetic resonance angiography: techniques and applications. Expert Rev Cardiovasc Ther. 2012;10(1):75–88. Epub 2011/12/14.
36. Miyazaki M, Akahane M. Non-contrast enhanced MR angiography: established techniques. J Magn Reson Imaging. 2012;35(1):1–19. Epub 2011/12/17.
37. Miyazaki M, Sugiura S, Tateishi F, Wada H, Kassai Y, Abe H. Non-contrast-enhanced MR angiography using 3D ECG-synchronized half-Fourier fast spin echo. J Magn Reson Imaging. 2000;12(5):776–83. Epub 2000/10/26.
38. Korosec FR, Frayne R, Grist TM, Mistretta CA. Time-resolved contrast-enhanced 3D MR angiography. Magn Reson Med. 1996;36(3):345–51. Epub 1996/09/01.
39. Krishnam MS, Tomasian A, Lohan DG, Tran L, Finn JP, Ruehm SG. Low dose, time-resolved, contrast-enhanced 3D MR angiography in cardiac and vascular diseases: correlation to high spatial resolution 3D contrast-enhanced MRA. Clin Radiol. 2008;63(7):744–55. Epub 2008/06/17.
40. John NW, McCloy RF. Navigating and visualizing three-dimensional data sets. Br J Radiol. 2004;77 Spec No 2:S108–13. Epub 2005/01/29.
41. Pavone P, Luccichenti G, Cademartiri F. From maximum intensity projection to volume rendering. Semin Ultrasound CT MR. 2001;22(5):413–9. Epub 2001/10/23.
42. Luccichenti G, Cademartiri F, Pezzella FR, Runza G, Belgrano M, Midiri M, et al. 3D reconstruction techniques made easy: know-how and pictures. Eur Radiol. 2005;15(10):2146–56. Epub 2005/04/06.
43. Anderson RH. Clinical anatomy of the aortic root. Heart. 2000;84(6):670–3. Epub 2000/11/18.
44. Piazza N, de Jaegere P, Schultz C, Becker AE, Serruys PW, Anderson RH. Anatomy of the aortic valvar complex and its implications for transcatheter implantation of the aortic valve. Circ Cardiovasc Interv. 2008;1(1):74–81. Epub 2008/08/01.
45. Tarantini G, Gasparetto V, Napodano M, Fraccaro C, Gerosa G, Isabella G. Valvular leak after transcatheter aortic valve implantation: a clinician update on epidemiology, pathophysiology and clinical implications. Am J Cardiovasc Dis. 2011;1(3):312–20. Epub 2012/01/19.
46. Yan TD, Cao C, Martens-Nielsen J, Padang R, Ng M, Vallely MP, et al. Transcatheter aortic valve implantation for high-risk patients with severe aortic stenosis: A systematic review. J Thorac Cardiovasc Surg. 2010;139(6):1519–28. Epub 2009/10/23.
47. Masson JB, Kovac J, Schuler G, Ye J, Cheung A, Kapadia S, et al. Transcatheter aortic valve implantation: review of the nature, management, and avoidance of procedural complications. JACC Cardiovasc Interv. 2009;2(9):811–20. Epub 2009/09/26.
48. Abdel-Wahab M, Zahn R, Horack M, Gerckens U, Schuler G, Sievert H, et al. Aortic regurgitation after transcatheter aortic valve implantation: incidence and early outcome. Results from the German transcatheter aortic valve interventions registry. Heart. 2011;97(11):899–906. Epub 2011/03/15.
49. Takagi K, Latib A, Al-Lamee R, Mussardo M, Montorfano M, Maisano F, et al. Predictors of moderate-to-severe paravalvular aortic regurgitation immediately after CoreValve implantation and the impact of postdilatation. Catheter Cardiovasc Interv. 2011;78(3):432–43. Epub 2011/07/28.
50. Tamburino C, Capodanno D, Ramondo A, Petronio AS, Ettori F, Santoro G, et al. Incidence and predictors of early and late mortality after transcatheter aortic valve implantation in 663 patients with severe aortic stenosis. Circulation. 2011;123(3):299–308. Epub 2011/01/12.
51. Kodali SK, Williams MR, Smith CR, Svensson LG, Webb JG, Makkar RR, et al. Two-year outcomes after transcatheter or surgical aortic-valve replacement. N Engl J Med. 2012;366(18):1686–95. Epub 2012/03/27.
52. O'Brien B, Schoenhagen P, Kapadia SR, Svensson LG, Rodriguez L, Griffin BP, et al. Integration of 3D imaging data in the assessment of aortic stenosis: impact on classification of disease severity. Circ Cardiovasc Imaging. 2011;4(5):566–73. Epub 2011/07/09.
53. Ng AC, Delgado V, van der Kley F, Shanks M, van de Veire NR, Bertini M, et al. Comparison of aortic root dimensions and geometries before and after transcatheter aortic valve implantation by 2- and 3-dimensional transesophageal echocardiography and multislice computed tomography. Circ Cardiovasc Imaging. 2010;3(1):94–102. Epub 2009/11/19.
54. Crawford MH, Roldan CA. Prevalence of aortic root dilatation and small aortic roots in valvular aortic stenosis. Am J Cardiol. 2001;87(11):1311–3. Epub 2001/05/30.
55. Bahlmann E, Nienaber CA, Cramariuc D, Gohlke-Baerwolf C, Ray S, Devereux RB, et al. Aortic root geometry in aortic stenosis patients (a SEAS substudy). Eur J Echocardiogr. 2011;12(8):585–90. Epub 2011/04/22.
56. Matalanis G. Valve sparing aortic root repairs – an anatomical approach. Heart Lung Circ. 2004;13 Suppl 3:S13–8. Epub 2005/12/15.
57. Kwon DH, Smedira NG, Popovic ZB, Lytle BW, Setser RM, Thamilarasan M, et al. Steep left ventricle to aortic root angle and hypertrophic obstructive cardiomyopathy: study of a novel association using three-dimensional multimodality imaging. Heart. 2009;95(21):1784–91. Epub 2009/06/25.
58. Sherif MA, Abdel-Wahab M, Stocker B, Geist V, Richardt D, Tolg R, et al. Anatomic and procedural predictors of paravalvular aortic regurgitation after implantation of the Medtronic CoreValve bioprosthesis. J Am Coll Cardiol. 2010;56(20):1623–9. Epub 2010/11/06.
59. del Valle-Fernandez R, Jelnin V, Panagopoulos G, Dudiy Y, Schneider L, de Jaegere PT, et al. A method for standardized computed tomography angiography-based measurement of aortic valvar structures. Eur Heart J. 2010;31(17):2170–8. Epub 2010/05/27.
60. Hayashida K, Lefevre T, Chevalier B, Hovasse T, Romano M, Garot P, et al. Transfemoral aortic valve implantation new criteria to predict vascular complications. JACC Cardiovasc Interv. 2011;4(8):851–8. Epub 2011/08/20.
61. Eggebrecht H, Schmermund A, Voigtlander T, Kahlert P, Erbel R, Mehta RH. Risk of stroke after transcatheter aortic valve implantation (TAVI): a meta-analysis of 10,037 published patients. EuroIntervention. 2012;8(1):129–38. Epub 2012/03/07.
62. Hynes BG, Rodes-Cabau J. Transcatheter aortic valve implantation and cerebrovascular events: the current state of the art. Ann N Y Acad Sci. 2012;1254(1):151–63. Epub 2012/05/03.

63. Grube E, Schuler G, Buellesfeld L, Gerckens U, Linke A, Wenaweser P, et al. Percutaneous aortic valve replacement for severe aortic stenosis in high-risk patients using the second- and current third-generation self-expanding CoreValve prosthesis: device success and 30-day clinical outcome. J Am Coll Cardiol. 2007;50(1):69–76. Epub 2007/07/03.
64. Webb JG, Altwegg L, Boone RH, Cheung A, Ye J, Lichtenstein S, et al. Transcatheter aortic valve implantation: impact on clinical and valve-related outcomes. Circulation. 2009;119(23):3009–16. Epub 2009/06/03.
65. Demertzis S, Hurni S, Stalder M, Gahl B, Herrmann G, Van den Berg J. Aortic arch morphometry in living humans. J Anat. 2010;217(5):588–96. Epub 2010/10/29.
66. Madhwal S, Rajagopal V, Bhatt DL, Bajzer CT, Whitlow P, Kapadia SR. Predictors of difficult carotid stenting as determined by aortic arch angiography. J Invasive Cardiol. 2008;20(5):200–4. Epub 2008/05/08.
67. Kurra V, Schoenhagen P, Roselli EE, Kapadia SR, Tuzcu EM, Greenberg R, et al. Prevalence of significant peripheral artery disease in patients evaluated for percutaneous aortic valve insertion: preprocedural assessment with multidetector computed tomography. J Thorac Cardiovasc Surg. 2009;137(5):1258–64. Epub 2009/04/22.

Aortoiliofemoral Angiography and IVUS

23

Amar Krishnaswamy and E. Murat Tuzcu

Abstract

Transcatheter aortic valve replacement (TAVR) is a revolutionary treatment modality that has proven efficacy in patients with symptomatic, severe aortic stenosis (AS). While there are a number of methods for implantation of the stented valve, the transfemoral (TF) route has emerged as the "default" for patients with appropriate vascular access. Appropriate patient selection, as well as the ability to perform TF-TAVR successfully and minimize the risk of vascular complications, rests on a thorough pre-procedural analysis of the aortoiliofemoral system. This is generally accomplished using all or a combination of the following multimodality imaging: angiography, intravascular ultrasound (IVUS), and multidetector computed tomography (MDCT). We will concentrate this chapter on the analysis of angiography and IVUS.

Keywords

Transcatheter aortic valve replacement (TAVR) • Transfemoral (TF) • Iliofemoral angiography • Intravascular ultrasound (IVUS) • Patient assessment

Requirements for Available Devices

There are currently two widely available devices for TF-TAVR, the Edwards SAPIEN (Edwards Lifesciences, Irvine, CA) and the CoreValve ReValving system (Medtronic, Minneapolis, MN). The first-generation SAPIEN is a balloon-expandable, bovine pericardial valve mounted within a stainless steel stent and is approved for commercial use in the USA. It is available in 23- and 26-mm sizes, which require 22 F and 24 F delivery sheaths, respectively. The smaller valve requires a vessel minimal luminal diameter (MLD) of 7 mm for its delivery sheath and the larger device 8 mm [1].

A. Krishnaswamy, MD • E.M. Tuzcu, MD (✉)
Department of Cardiovascular Medicine, Cleveland Clinic, 9500 Euclid Avenue, Desk J2-3, Cleveland, OH 44195, USA
e-mail: krishna2@ccf.org; tuzcue@ccf.org

The second-generation SAPIEN XT is available for use in Europe and Canada and in the USA is implanted under the auspices of the PARTNER II trial and its registries. In contrast to the original device, the XT is mounted on a nitinol stent. Due to changes in stent and delivery system design, the XT can be implanted via an 18 F or 19 F delivery sheath (for 23- and 26-mm valves, respectively). The required MLD for the XT is 6 mm for the smaller valve and 6.5 mm for the larger size, which has greatly reduced the incidence of vascular complications in a number of series.

The CoreValve is widely used in Europe and Canada and in the USA is implanted under the CoreValve Pivotal US Trial. It is a trileaflet porcine pericardial valve mounted within a self-expanding nitinol frame and is available in 23-, 26-, and 29-mm sizes. All of the valves are delivered via an 18 F sheath system that requires an MLD of 6 mm.

J.K. Min et al. (eds.), *Multimodality Imaging for Transcatheter Aortic Valve Replacement*, DOI 10.1007/978-1-4471-2798-7_23, © Springer-Verlag London 2014

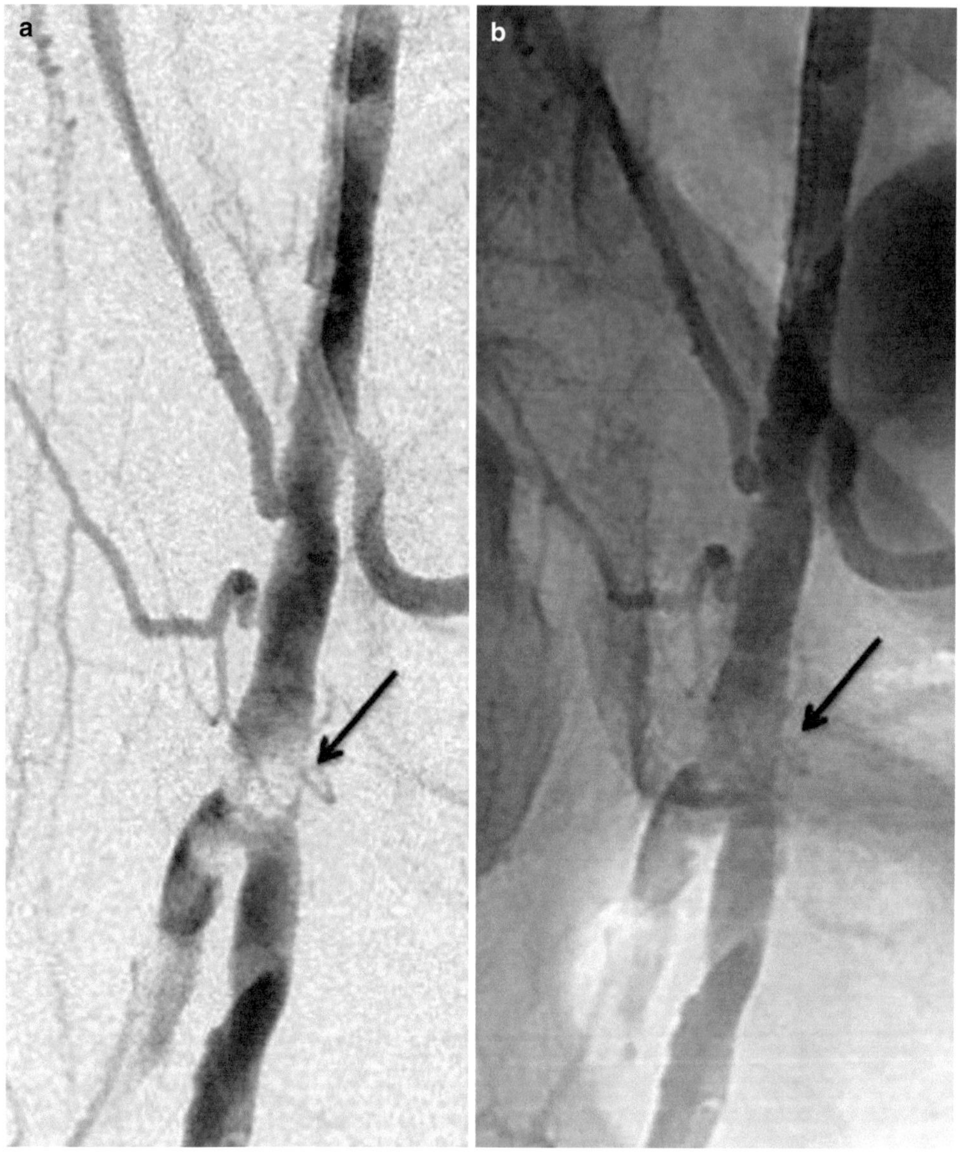

Fig. 23.1 Digital subtraction angiography (**a**) provides a more accurate characterization of vessel lumen and calcification (*arrow*) than routine angiography (**b**) in this patient with severe, calcified distal right common femoral artery disease

Angiographic Procedure

Aortoiliofemoral angiography is often used as an initial screening modality for patients being considered for TF-TAVR. We prefer the use of digital subtraction angiography (DSA) as it allows the operator to minimize contrast dye and often provides a more precise assessment of the vascular lumen than routine angiography alone (Fig. 23.1).

A complete angiographic study includes an image of the entire aortoiliofemoral tree, with additional assessment as necessary. The initial image is best obtained in the anteroposterior (AP) projection, with a field of view large enough to include the aortic bifurcation and the femoral heads (Fig. 23.2). A power injector is often used along with a sidehole catheter (pigtail, straight flush, etc.) placed just below the renal arteries, though hand injection also provides reasonable imaging if DSA is used. A 50/50 mixture of contrast/saline is adequate and is injected at 10 cc/s for 2 s.

To more closely interrogate the iliac system, especially the bifurcation of the external and internal iliac arteries, contralateral oblique views should be obtained (i.e., LAO projection to visualize the right iliac system) (Fig. 23.3). Injection can be accomplished using a catheter placed at the ostium iliac contralateral to the sheath insertion or with a catheter placed in the midportion of the common iliac artery ipsilateral to sheath insertion. If a more clear delineation of the common femoral system is needed, the ipsilateral oblique view should be obtained (i.e., RAO projection for the right common femoral) (Fig. 23.4).

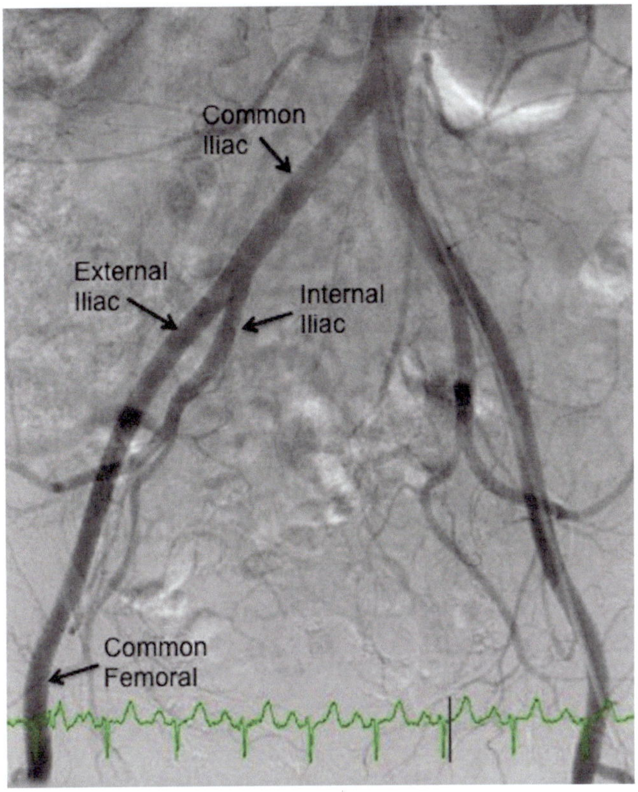

Fig. 23.2 Aortoiliofemoral system (AP projection)

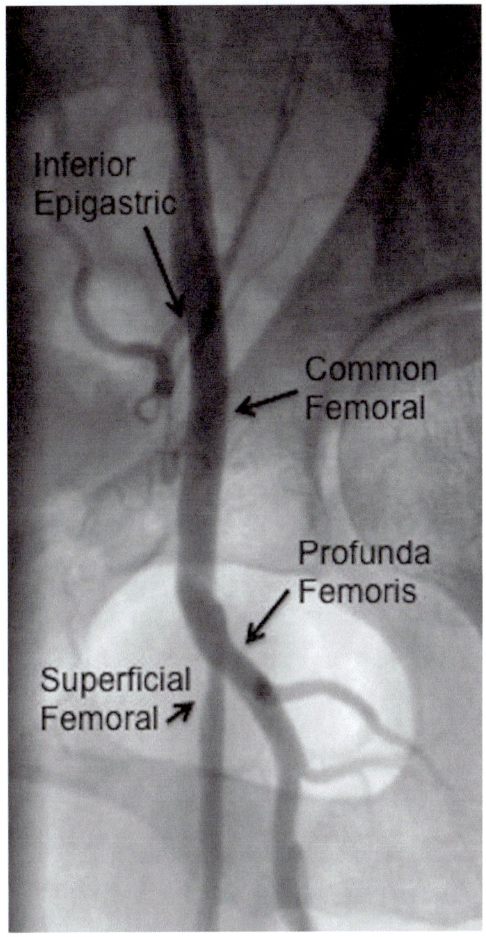

Fig. 23.4 Left common femoral artery (LAO projection)

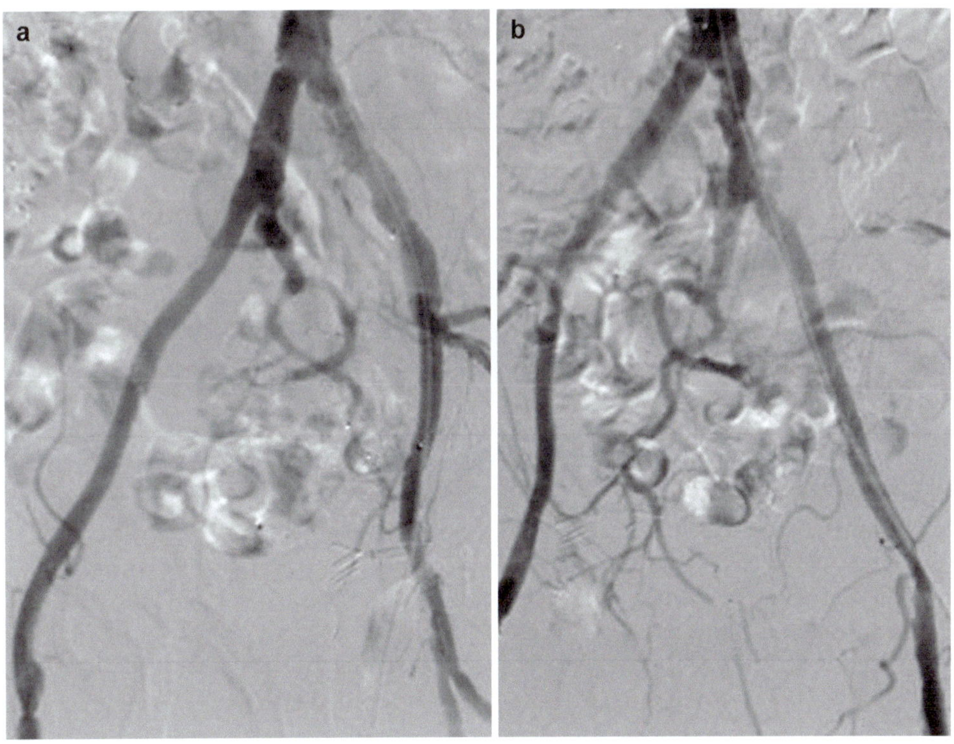

Fig. 23.3 Contraleteral oblique views of the iliac system. (**a**) LAO projection of the right iliacs. (**b**) RAO projection of the left iliacs

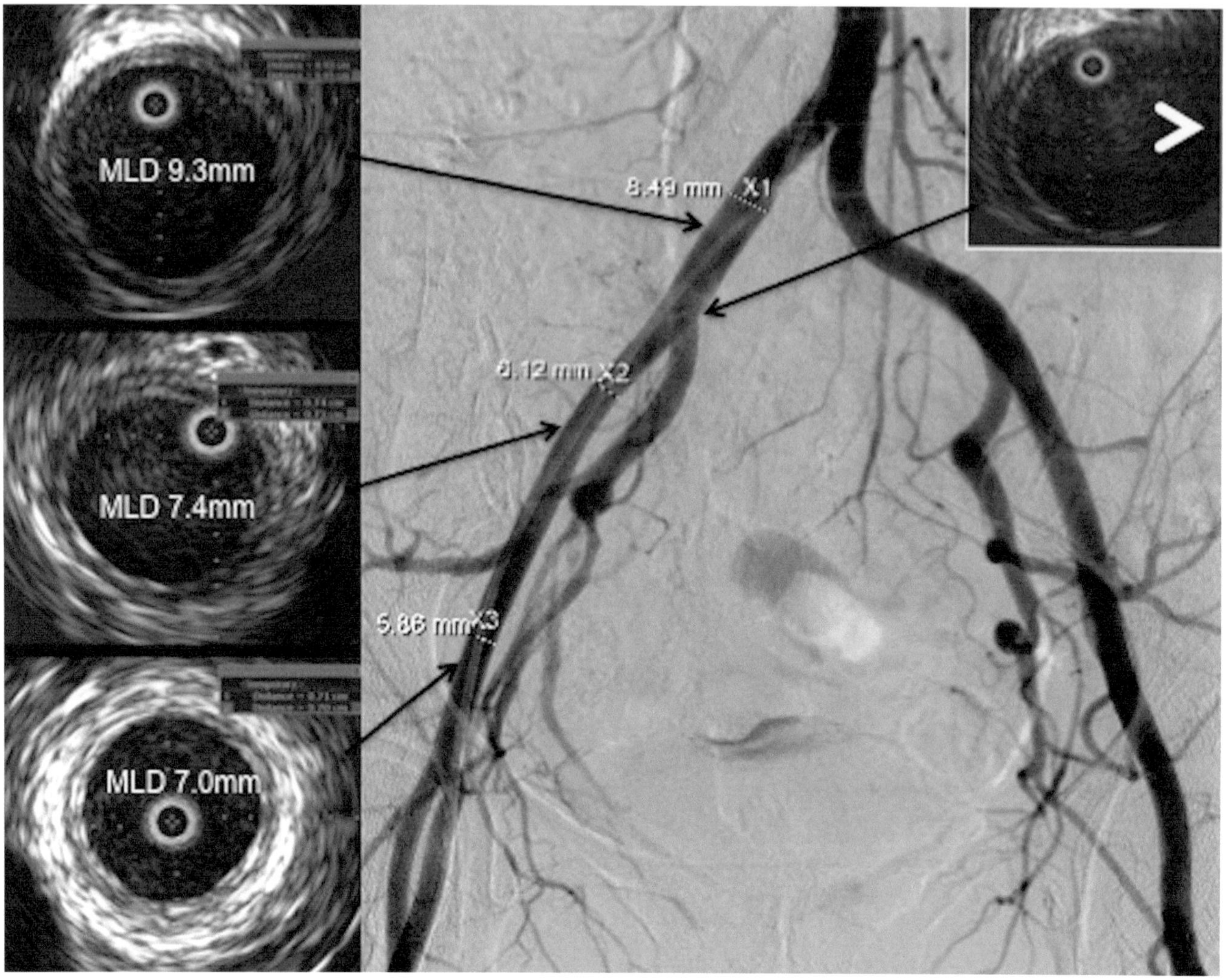

Fig. 23.5 IVUS imaging of the iliofemoral tree. Representative sections confirm adequate lumen diameter for TF-TAVR. Anatomic localization is facilitated by the identification of side branches on the IVUS (*white arrowhead*)

Angiographic Assessment

While angiography was once the reference standard for pre-TAVR assessment, it has been since supplanted by 3-D imaging modalities such as MDCT. Nevertheless, since most patients with symptomatic, severe AS present for coronary angiography, simultaneous pelvic angiography can delineate the appropriate subsequent treatment pathway. The angiogram must be assessed for vessel diameter, calcification, and tortuosity. If patients meet clearly meet criteria for TF-TAVR, further evaluation may not be necessary, thereby avoiding costly testing that also requires additional time, radiation exposure, and contrast dye utilization. Similarly, patients with obvious limitations to the TF approach may be directed toward a work-up for alternative access or surgical AVR. Certainly, a number of patients may not fall in to either group, requiring additional evaluation with IVUS and/or MDCT.

Vessel Size

The requirements for vessel size (MLD) are delineated above. Operators in Europe and Canada use the SAPIEN XT or CoreValve, each of which requires in MLD of 6 mm. In the USA, operators still use the first-generation SAPIEN device for commercial implantation, which requires an MLD of 7 mm for the 23 mm valve and 8 mm for the 26 mm valve. In addition to a qualitative assessment of iliofemoral size, precise measurements can be made using quantitative software that is available in most catheterization laboratories (Fig. 23.5). In patients with borderline size, evaluation with IVUS can be considered (discussed below).

It should be noted that although the instructions for use (IFU) suggest relatively liberal MLD sizing criteria, more restrictive criteria for sizing, especially early in the learning

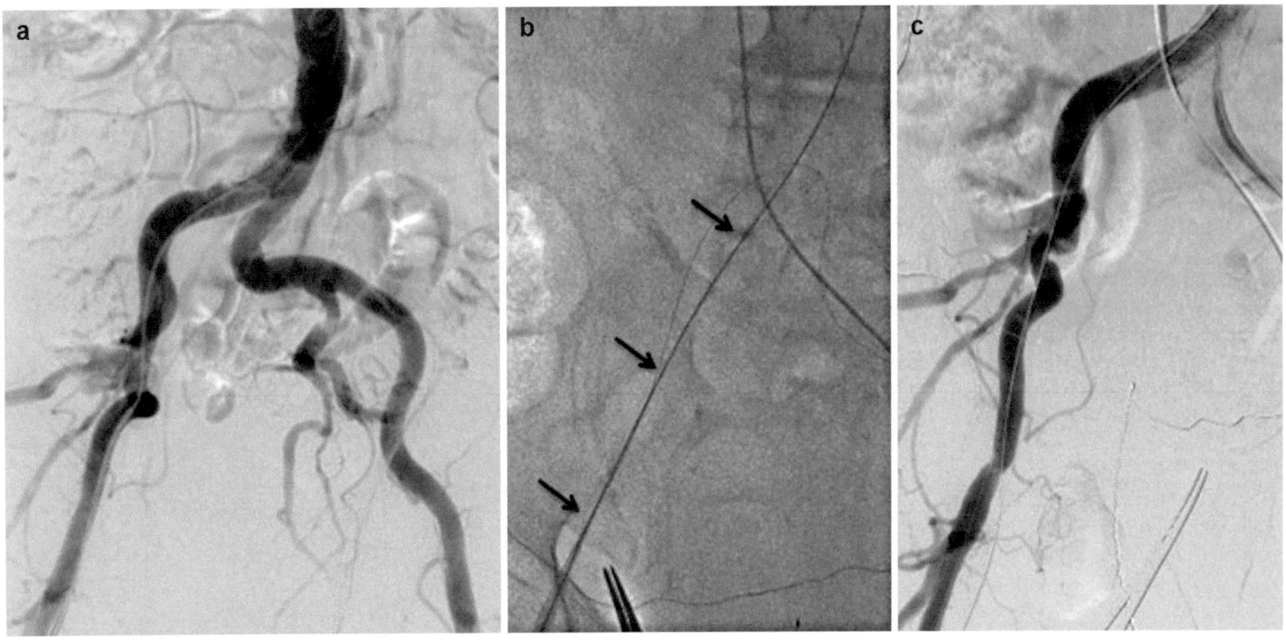

Fig. 23.6 Severe tortuosity in the right iliac system is straightened by a stiff Lunderquist wire. (**a**) Pelvic angiogram (AP projection); (**b**) Lunderquist takes a straight trajectory through the right iliac system (*arrows*); (**c**) Angiography shows that though the vessel itself is not straight with the wire, TF-TAVR is possible given the size of the artery and the straightness of the wire

curve for implantation, is reasonable. Furthermore, patients with a calcified iliofemoral system require an even greater MLD to perform the procedure safely. Hayashida and colleagues demonstrated that a novel indicator, the sheath-to-femoral-artery ratio (SFAR), was a stronger predictor of major vascular complications with TF-TAVR than the size of the arteries or sheath alone, with a threshold value of >1.05 predictive of major vascular complications [2]. In their analysis, when the SFAR was taken together with calcification, the MLD for noncalcified vessels was 6.5 and 6.8 mm for 18- and 19-Fr sheaths, respectively, and 7.2- and 7.5 mm for calcified vessels. This distinction, that a larger lumen is necessary for safe insertion in the presence of calcification, is an important point to remember when assessing MLD for TF-TAVR.

Vessel Tortuosity

Tortuosity of the pelvic vessels is assessed using the following well-accepted scoring criteria: (0) no significant angulation (no tortuosity); (1) 30–60° angulation (mild tortuosity); (2) 60–90° angulation (moderate tortuosity); and (3) >90° angulation (severe tortuosity) [3]. It is generally accepted that angulation <90° is reasonable for TF-TAVR.

If the pelvic angiogram shows significant tortuosity, it may be reasonable to advance a stiff wire (Amplatz Super Stiff wire or Lunderquist wire, Cook Medical, Bloomington, IN) to the aorta to determine whether the tortuosity can be straightened (Fig. 23.6). If so, TF-TAVR may still be possible. It is important to realize, though, that the straight appearance of the stiff guidewire does not necessarily imply that the vessel itself is straight; rather, the wire takes a "straight" path by apposing to the inside edge of each curve (Fig. 23.6c). Therefore, it is still possible to traumatize the edge of the vessel with the delivery sheath; this is especially true in tortuous vessels with significant calcification. It is also important to remember that when the pelvic angiogram is conducted via femoral access with a pigtail catheter in the descending aorta, tortuosity on the access side may be underestimated due to the straightening effect of the catheter itself.

Vessel Calcification

Similar to assessing tortuosity, calcification is also classified using a semi-qualitative scale: (0) no calcification, (1) mild discrete calcification, (2) moderate calcification, and (3) severe calcification [3]. Calcification that is not at either extreme of the spectrum (i.e., none or extremely severe) can be difficult to properly characterize using angiography or fluoroscopy alone, and adjunctive imaging using IVUS (discussed below) or MDCT is necessary. These modalities also allow a more precise quantification of calcification by

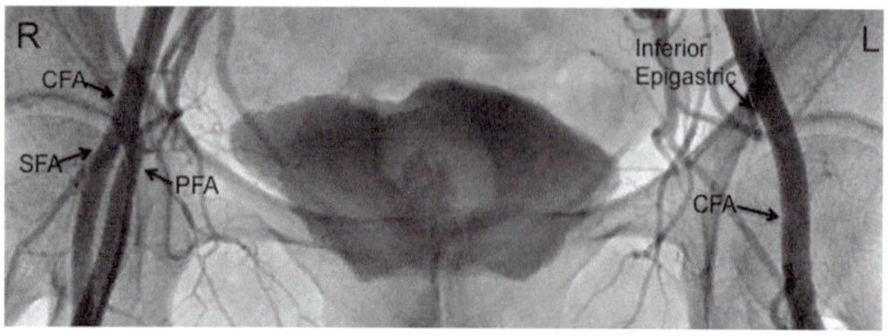

Fig. 23.7 High bifurcation of the CFA. Bifurcation of the right CFA is at the top of the femoral head, providing a very small area for sheath insertion below the pelvic brim. The left CFA is therefore better suited for TF-TAVR access. *CFA* common femoral artery, *SFA* superficial femoral artery, *PFA* profunda femoral artery

reporting the degree of circumferential calcium; greater than 270° is a relative contraindication to the TF approach unless the vessel lumen is very large. Angiographically, a calcium score of 2 or less implies feasibility for TF-TAVR, with the abovementioned caveat regarding the need for larger MLD in vessels with significant calcification. It is important to realize, however, that angiography alone is a very poor indicator of the degree of iliofemoral calcification. For instance, in a study of 93 patients from our institution undergoing angiography for PAD, Arthurs and colleagues demonstrated that calcification was graded as severe in 40 % of patients based on angiography, but only 7 % of patients based upon IVUS [4].

Planning Access

Procedural planning consists not only of assessing vessel size, tortuosity, and calcification (all with an eye toward advancing the large delivery sheath) but also the appropriate location of entry at the CFA. In order to deploy closure devices, entry must be at the CFA, not below its bifurcation in the SFA or profunda. To minimize the risks of retroperitoneal bleeding in case of closure device failure, the arteriotomy should be below the inferior epigastric artery and below the level of the pelvic brim (so that the artery can be compressed against the pelvis if necessary). Pre-procedural fluoroscopy and angiography therefore provide the operator the ability to plan the site of arterial access for the TF-TAVR (Figs. 23.7, 23.8, and 23.9).

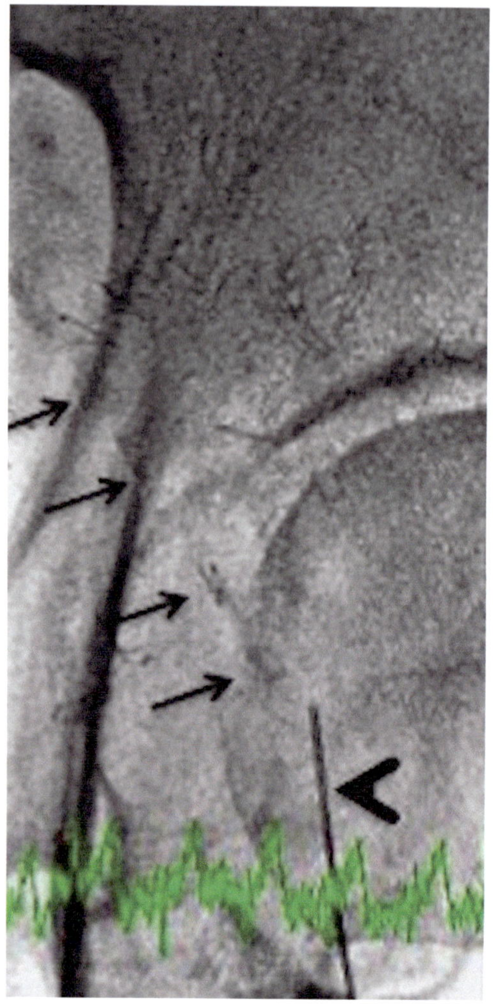

Fig. 23.8 CFA calcification. Fluoroscopy reveals significant calcification of the common femoral artery (*arrows*), prompting needle access distal to the calcified portion of the vessel (*arrowhead*)

IVUS Procedure

There are three available devices for IVUS: the Eagle Eye Platinum and Vision PV 0.18 catheters (Volcano Corporation, Rancho Cordova, CA) and the iCross catheter (Boston Scientific, Natick, MA). The Eagle Eye provides an imaging depth of 20 mm, accommodates an 0.014″ guidewire, and can be passed via a 5-Fr guide. The Vision catheter provides an imaging depth of up to 24 mm and accommodates an 0.018″ guidewire but requires a 6-Fr guide. Similarly, the iCross catheter requires a 6-Fr guide but accommodates only an 0.014″ guidewire.

To perform the IVUS procedure, we typically advance a 0.014″ coronary guidewire to the mid-SFA on the side contralateral to sheath insertion via an IMA (or similar) diagnostic catheter. The catheter is removed, and the IVUS catheter is advanced directly through the femoral sheath and over the wire to the contralateral CFA. Given the brief nature of the procedure and large vessel diameter, anticoagulation is usually not necessary. Images are recorded

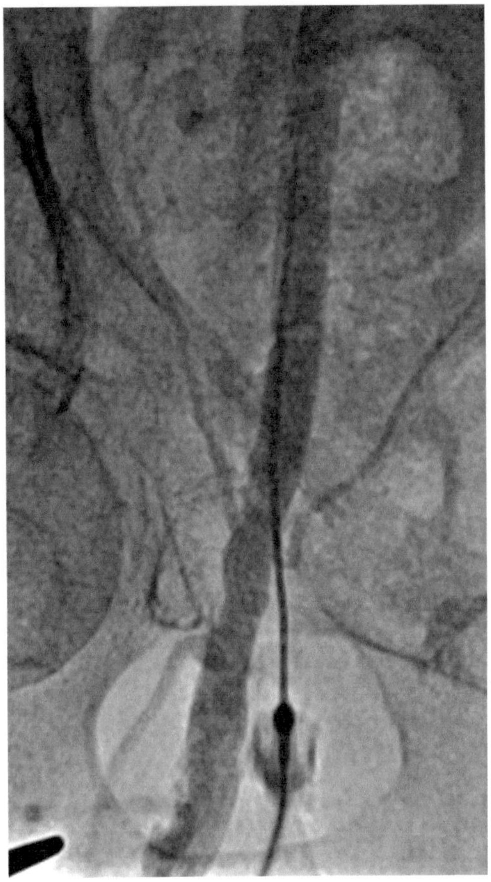

Fig. 23.9 Low inferior epigastric artery. Arterial access for TF-TAVR would be safest at a point near the bottom of the femoral head in this patient

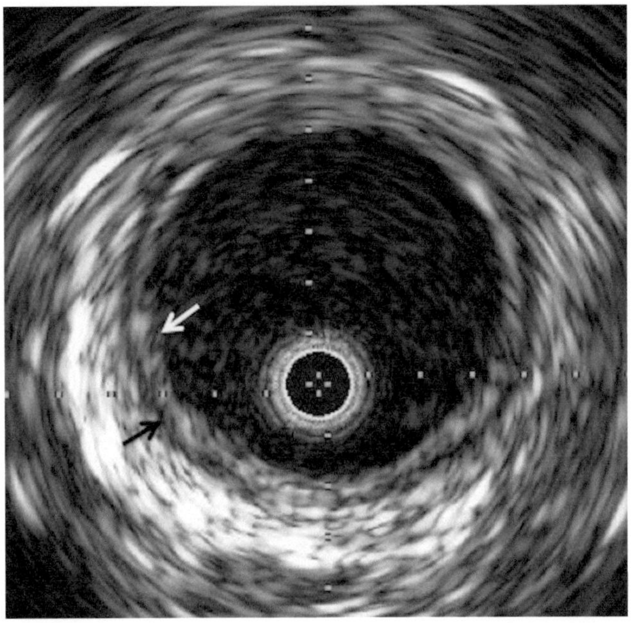

Fig. 23.10 IVUS of the external iliac artery. The intima is shown by the *white arrow* and the media by the *black arrow*. Lumen size is defined by the distance from intima to intima through the middle of the vessel

during manual or automatic pullback, with bookmarks made at the points of major branches (i.e., CFA bifurcation, iliac bifurcation, aortic bifurcation) for easier review.

IVUS Assessment

Intravascular ultrasound is an invasive imaging modality that provides a high degree of structural detail (Fig. 23.10). As with angiography, vessel size and calcification are assessed by IVUS. In addition to a subjective evaluation, precise measurements can be made using automatic or manual planimetry.

If the MLD derived from the angiogram is borderline for TF-TAVR and the operator believes that assessment with IVUS would be helpful to determine whether further testing and evaluation for TF-TAVR (i.e., MDCT) is necessary, then performing the procedure is reasonable (Fig. 23.5). The MLD of a vessel is measured in a direct line that intersects the middle of the vessel lumen. As the artery may not be an exact circle, it is important to obtain multiple measurements at various angles through the center of the artery. It is also important to realize that the IVUS image, similar to the echocardiogram when used for aortic annular assessment, is highly dependent on the angle of the ultrasound beam to the structure being imaged. In a highly tortuous vessel, it is possible that the IVUS beam will cut the vessel at an angle, and not perpendicular to its axis, thereby providing an MLD that is much larger than reality. When compared with angiography, IVUS provides similar luminal diameter measurement [4]. Therefore, if there is a significant discrepancy between angiography and IVUS in assessing lumen size, further evaluation must be performed and the IVUS measurement alone cannot be considered reliable.

IVUS provides a more precise quantification of vessel calcification than angiography or fluoroscopy alone. Similar to the analysis of MDCT images, IVUS images can be assessed for the degree of circumferential calcification (Fig. 23.11). Calcification >270° may be considered prohibitive to the TF approach and certainly implies the need for a greater MLD than would be considered in a noncalcified vessel (as discussed above).

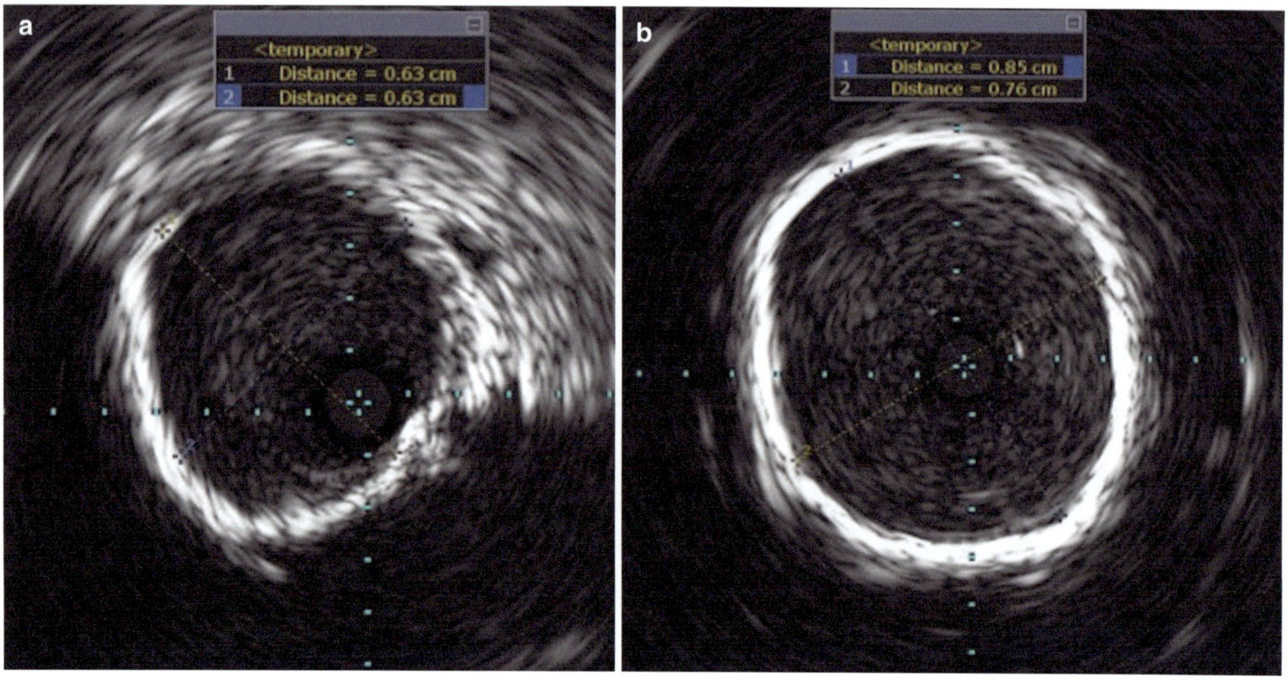

Fig. 23.11 IVUS demonstrating external iliac artery calcification. (**a**) Calcification is seen from 3 to 10 o'clock, resulting in shadowing behind the calcium and an inability to image. Size and calcification were prohibitive to TF-TAVR in this patient. (**b**) Circumferential calcification creates shadowing around the entire vessel and was prohibitive to TF-TAVR

Box 23.1 Angiography and IVUS Arterial Visualization

Arterial characteristics	Visualization and interpretation
Arterial lumen diameter	IVUS considered for borderline size vessels
	More restrictive criteria for sizing considered early in learning curve
	Sheath-to-femoral artery ratio (SFAR) >1.05 predictive of major vascular complications
Vessel wall calcifications	Angiography alone is poor indicator of degree of iliofemoral calcification
	Horseshoe calcification (>270°) is relative contraindication to transfemoral TAVR
	Calcium score ≤2 by angiography implies feasibility for transfemoral TAVR
Artery tortuosity	Tortuosity definitions: angle between common and external iliac arteries
	Mild tortuosity = 30–60°
	Moderate tortuosity = 60–90°
	Severe tortuosity = >90°
	Consider stiff wire to determine whether tortuosity can be straightened

IVUS intravascular ultrasound, *TAVR* transcatheter aortic valve replacement, *SFAR* sheath-to-femoral artery ratio

Conclusion

Transfemoral TAVR has proven to be a tremendous resource for patients with severe AS who are unable to undergo surgical AVR or those with high surgical risk. In order to perform the procedure safely, with a specific eye toward avoidance of vascular complications, a careful assessment of the iliofemoral system is necessary. While MDCT has emerged as the gold-standard tool for this analysis, angiography and IVUS still hold an important place in patient screening. This is in large part due to the fact that in certain patients (i.e., significantly small vessel lumen, severe diffuse calcification, severe tortuosity that does not straighten), angiography and/or IVUS may abrogate the need for further testing that is not only costly but also results in increased radiation and contrast dye exposure. As most patients with severe AS undergo diagnostic coronary angiography during their evaluation, additional iliofemoral angiography is easily accomplished and can be quite helpful.

References

1. Instructions for Use: Edwards SAPIEN Transcatheter Heart Valve with the RetroFlex 3 Delivery System. http://wwwfdagov/downloads/AdvisoryCommittees/CommitteesMeetingMaterials/MedicalDevices/MedicalDevicesAdvisoryCommittee/CirculatorySystemDevicesPanel/UCM262938pdf
2. Hayashida K, Lefevre T, Chevalier B, et al. Transfemoral aortic valve implantation new criteria to predict vascular complications. JACC Cardiovasc Interv. 2011;4:851–8.
3. Eltchaninoff H, Kerkeni M, Zajarias A, et al. Aorto-iliac angiography as a screening tool in selecting patients for transfemoral aortic valve implantation with the Edwards SAPIEN bioprosthesis. EuroIntervention. 2009;5:438–42.
4. Arthurs ZM, Bishop PD, Feiten LE, Eagleton MJ, Clair DG, Kashyap VS. Evaluation of peripheral atherosclerosis: a comparative analysis of angiography and intravascular ultrasound imaging. J Vasc Surg. 2010;51:933–8; discussion 9.

Aortic Annular Geometry and Sizing: Echocardiography

24

Gerald S. Bloomfield, Zainab Samad, and Pamela S. Douglas

Abstract

A complete and accurate assessment of the aortic annulus and the surrounding structures is accomplished non-invasively by on organized echocardiographic approch employing a variety of techniques. An approch with transthoracic and transesophageal imaging modalities using two-and three-dimensional image acquisition can completely inform the geometry, size and hemodyamic characteristics of the aortic annulus structures in preparation for transcatheter aortic valve replacement (TAVR). In addition to addressing the role of echocardiography for aortic annular geometry and sizing, this chapter also includes important considerations such as appreciation of the many anatomical structures that make up the aortic annular complex, the optimal imaging windows and views to appropriately interrogate structures, consideration of the limitations of echocardiography and appreciation of instances when another imaging modality may be appropriate. The goal of a full and accurate assessment of the aortic annular complex is to ensure patient suitability for TAVR, inform device size selection, alert the operator to potential complications and ultimately to ensure a safe transcatheter heart valve deployment.

Keywords

Transcatheter aortic valve replacement • Transthoracic echocardiography • Transesophageal echocardiography • Aortic annulus • Sizing

Introduction

Echocardiographic imaging of the aortic valve, annulus, and surrounding structures prior to TAVR informs patient selection and many subsequent aspects of TAVR patient care. In addition to the hemodynamic information, a full preprocedural echocardiographic assessment for a TAVR candidate will include anatomic assessments and linear measurements utilizing transthoracic and transesophageal approaches and employing two-dimensional and three-dimensional techniques. This chapter outlines the components of the aortic annulus and discusses the importance of assessing their size and position as it relates to a TAVR candidate. We first discuss the structure of the aortic annular complex. We then present the importance of assessing each component of the aortic annular complex: the aortic annulus, the aortic valve leaflets, the coronary ostia, the sinotubular junction and

G.S. Bloomfield, MD, MPH (✉) • P.S. Douglas, MD
Department of Medicine, Duke University Medical Center, 2400 Pratt Street, Durham, NC 27705, USA

Division of Cardiovascular Medicine, Duke University Medical Center, Durham, NC, USA

Duke Clinical Research Institute, 2400 Pratt Street, Room 0311 Terrace Level, Durham, NC 27705, USA
e-mail: gerald.bloomfield@duke.edu; pamela.douglas@duke.edu

Z. Samad, MD, MBBS, MHS
Department of Medicine, Duke University Medical Center, 2400 Pratt Street, Durham, NC 27705, USA

Department of Medicine/Radiology, Duke University, 200 Trent Drive, Room 3447A, Duke South, Durham, NC 27710, USA
e-mail: zainab.samad@duke.edu

J.K. Min et al. (eds.), *Multimodality Imaging for Transcatheter Aortic Valve Replacement*, DOI 10.1007/978-1-4471-2798-7_24, © Springer-Verlag London 2014

proximal aorta, as well as concomitant cardiac and aortic root pathology. Recommendations for imaging each component is provided for transthoracic and transesophageal echocardiography and for three-dimensional imaging when possible. We briefly compare the performance of other noninvasive imaging modalities to echocardiography where data are available and explain the limitations of echocardiography for assessing each component. The advantages of echocardiography, however, for annular geometry and sizing are many and include its near universal access inside and outside of major TAVR centers, affordability, lack of exposure to radiation, lack of need for potentially nephrotoxic intravenous contrast and its established role in TAVR clinical trials.

Normal Aortic Root Anatomy

Knowledge of the three-dimensional geometry and derived linear dimensions of the aortic root complex and the relationships between its various parts is critical to the use of echocardiography for optimal patient selection and procedural guidance, both of which are essential to TAVR procedural success. The aortic root complex consists of the aortic annulus, valvular leaflets, interleaflet triangles, coronary ostia, sinuses of Valsalva, sinotubular junction, and proximal aorta and is contiguous with the left ventricular outflow tract (LVOT). During embryonic development, the cardiac outflow tract and aortic root derive from the truncus arteriosus and separate after a series of ridges and septae are formed, fused, and ultimately folded to form the outflow tracts and great vessels [1]. The normal adult root complex is located rightward and posterior relative to the right ventricular infundibulum and abuts the mitral valve annulus and the muscular and membranous portions of the ventricular septum. Piazza et al. have described the aortic root complex as being composed of three elliptical rings and one crown-like ring: the virtual basal annulus, the anatomic annulus, the sinotubular junction, and a crown-like ring demarcated by the hinges of the leaflets [2]. From caudal to cranial, the *virtual basal annulus* is what is measured routinely as the aortic annulus in standard transthoracic echocardiographic assessment [3]. This ring is defined by the attachment point ("hinge point") of the aortic valve cusps within the LVOT. The *anatomic annulus* is located where the muscular arterial aortic root joins the muscular interventricular septum anteriorly and the fibrous skeleton of the mitral valve apparatus posteriorly and leftward. The superior most ring is the outlet of the aortic root into the ascending aorta – *the sinotubular junction* (*STJ*). This ring is demarcated by the sinus ridge cranial to the three aortic sinuses and the beginning of the tubular ascending aorta. The *crown-like ring* structure is created by the shape of the aortic leaflets attached throughout the length of the aortic root. The leaflets and rings together form a three-dimensional, oval-shaped three-pronged coronet with three anchor points at the nadir of each aortic cusp rather than a cylindrical structure. The "aortic annulus" measurement by all modalities is assessed at the lowest hinge point of the aortic valve (AoV) leaflets at the virtual basal plane in systole [4].

The normal aortic root has a consistent shape with varying size throughout the cardiac cycle. Owing to pressure changes throughout the cardiac cycle and ventricular geometry, the dimensions of the aortic root complex not only are altered during the cardiac cycle, but the components change size at varying rates and even in different directions. During diastole the radius of the plane of the aortic leaflet commissures decreases while the basal annulus dimension increases. During systole, the radius of the commissures increases and the basal annulus decreases in size [5]. The complex nature of aortic root function is further demonstrated by the relative change in size of different parts. Thubrikar et al. demonstrated using animal studies that in systole the commissures (superiorly placed within the three-pronged coronet) expand by 12–16 % [6, 7], while the virtual basal ring moves inward by 16 % [8]. In addition, the interleaflet distance decreases in systole causing a change in the geometry of the open valve from conical to coronet [5]. The annulus complex also moves in the cranio-caudal plane throughout the cardiac cycle with cranial movement in early systole and caudal descent during the remainder of systole reaching a nadir position during isovolumic relaxation [9].

Echocardiographic Assessment of the Aortic Annulus

Correct measurement of the aortic annulus is crucial to TAVR as it determines eligibility for the procedure, device selection, and device sizing and guides procedural planning. Clinical trials of the Edwards SAPIEN™ transcatheter heart valve (THV) exclude patients with an annular size <18 mm or >25 mm, while the Medtronic CoreValve® trial excludes patients with an annular size <20 mm or >29 mm by echocardiography [10, 11]. Further, both these trials rely primarily on echocardiographic measurements for device sizing rather than other modalities. Undersizing of the prosthetic device in relation to the annulus can lead to device migration, paravalvular regurgitation, or potentially patient-prosthesis mismatch (PPM) [12]. Uncontrolled or excessive oversizing of the prosthesis may lead to peripheral vascular or aortic root injury or may impair THV function related to redundancy of THV leaflet tissue [2].

TTE

Annular sizing by transthoracic echocardiography (TTE) has been the gold standard for TAVR clinical trials and clinical practice and can be performed satisfactorily in most patients [3, 4, 10]. The annular diameter is typically measured in systole from a parasternal long-axis window, often zoomed on the LVOT (Fig. 24.1). Owing to improvements in image processing and resultant improved resolution, it is possible to measure the annular dimension from the tissue-blood to blood-tissue interfaces at the insertion points of the aortic valve cusps rather than distance between leading edge echoes which has been previously recommended [13]. The "annulus" in this view is a nonanatomic structure (i.e., the virtual basal ring) and is defined by the distance from the basal attachment of the right coronary cusp to the left or noncoronary commissure using two-dimensional imaging. The orientation of the typical two-dimensional transthoracic echocardiographic view displays a relative sagittal plane measurement of the aortic annulus that approximates the minor axis of the elliptically shaped annulus as measured by other imaging modalities. As such, the distance from the hinge point of the right coronary cusp to the left-noncoronary commissure does not correspond to the maximum diameter of the annulus [2, 3] (Fig. 24.2a, b). The maximal diameter is measured at the time of maximal valve opening rather than in diastole. M-mode measurements are not recommended for annular measurements in adults due to undersizing that has been observed at the sinuses of Valsalva (SoV) when compared to two-dimensional imaging [14]. The resolution currently available for three-dimensional transthoracic imaging is usually not adequate for annular sizing but can illustrate important anatomic relationships.

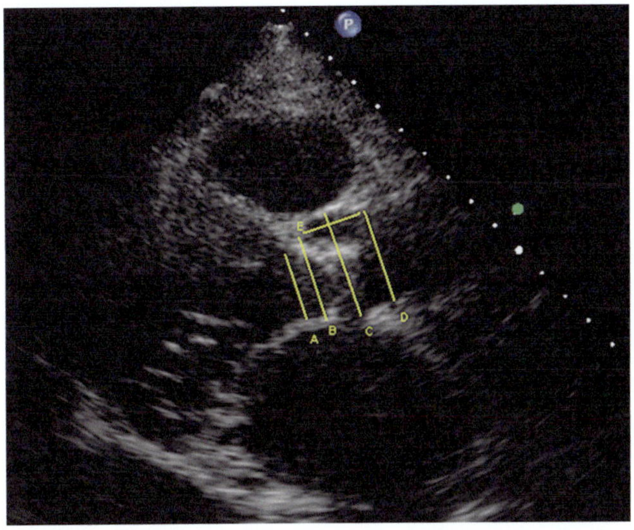

Fig. 24.1 Two-dimensional transthoracic echocardiogram using a parasternal long-axis view of the aortic root demonstrating a thickened, bright aortic valve. The aortic dimensions shown here include diameter of the left ventricular outflow tract (*yellow line A*), diameter of the aortic annulus (*yellow line B*), diameter of the aortic sinus (*yellow line C*), diameter of the aortic sinotubular junction (*yellow line D*), and sinotubular height (*yellow line E*)

TEE

Transesophageal echocardiography (TEE) is useful for technically complicated or challenging cases, when annular size is uncertain or close to established cutoffs and for determining the number of cusps when transthoracic imaging is equivocal [3, 9, 15]. A mid-esophageal long-axis image at 120–140° traditionally provides adequate views of the LVOT

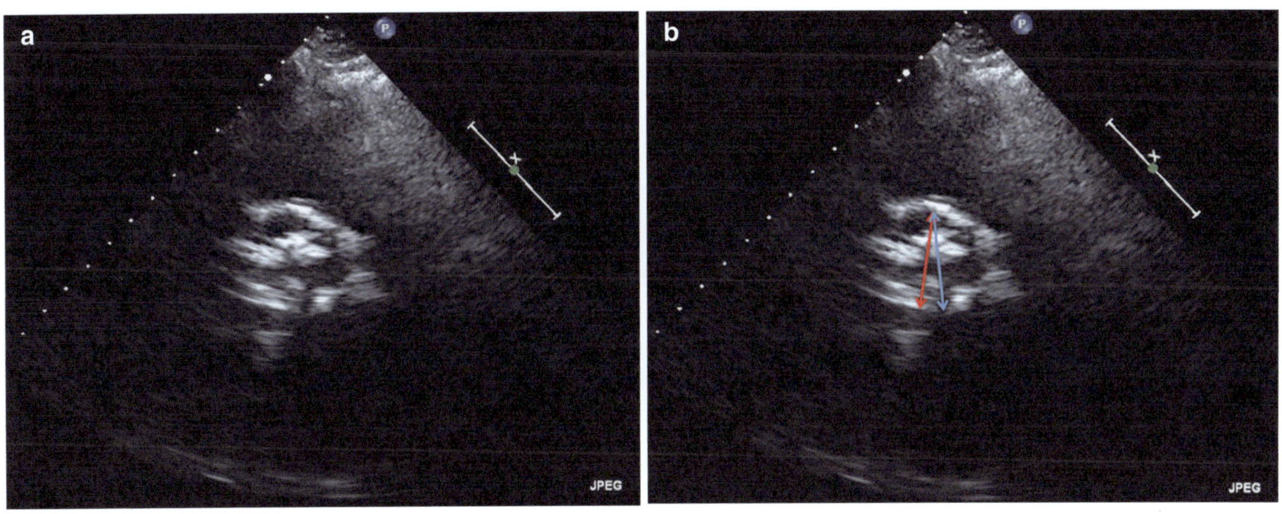

Fig. 24.2 Two-dimensional transthoracic echocardiogram from the parasternal short-axis window of the aortic root demonstrating maximal valve opening in systole. (**a**) Although there is heavy calcification, TTE is usually adequate to identify the number of aortic cusps, three in this image. (**b**) The annular distance as measured by transthoracic echocardiography does not correspond to the maximum diameter of the annulus. In this short-axis image, the *red double arrow* corresponds to the annular dimension as measured from the parasternal long-axis view. The full diameter of the outflow tract (*blue double arrow*) is shown in this short-axis image

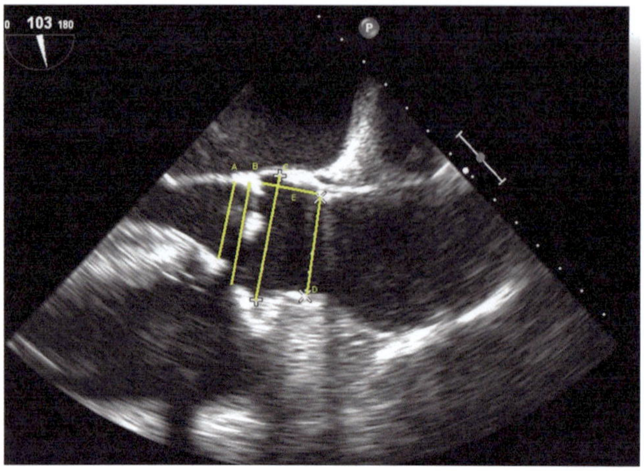

Fig. 24.3 Two-dimensional transesophageal echocardiogram showing a long-axis view of the aortic root demonstrating a thickened and bright aortic valve. In this view, the following aortic dimensions are shown: diameter of the left ventricular outflow tract (*yellow line A*), diameter of the aortic annulus (*yellow line B*), diameter of the aortic sinuses (*yellow line C*), diameter of the aortic sinotubular junction (*yellow line D*), and sinotubular height (*yellow line E*). Calcification of the aortic annulus may make measurement difficult

and annulus in a sagittal plane similar to TTE (Fig. 24.3). Single-plane short-axis views at 35–60° can also demonstrate the shape of the annulus but should not be used in isolation due to limitations in identifying the identical plane obtained from long-axis views. Employing biplane imaging to obtain a short-axis image, however, augments the usefulness of this view to demonstrate the elliptical shape of the annulus (Fig. 24.4a–c). TEE-based annular measurements generally correlate with TTE ($r=0.89$) although TTE-based measurements are usually larger with mean difference of 0.22 mm and absolute difference between TEE and TTE of 0.6 ± 0.8 mm [16]. TEE measurements demonstrate higher intra- and interobserver concordance than TTE and computed tomography and have been shown to alter prosthesis selection in 16 % of cases compared to dual-source computed tomography [17, 18].

Comparison to Other Noninvasive Imaging Modalities

There is no gold standard for noninvasive assessment of aortic annulus dimensions. Whether it is TTE, TEE, or another noninvasive method, the ultimate decision will fall to the operator depending on local expertise and availability. Each technique has its advantages and disadvantages [4]. It is important, however, to recognize the unique characteristics of echocardiography. The sagittal plane measurement by TTE and TEE usually approximates the minor axis of the elliptically shaped annulus as measured by multi-detector computed tomography (MDCT) scanning. The difference between MDCT and TTE (1.22 ± 1.3 mm) or TEE (1.52 ± 1.1 mm) is larger than the difference between TTE and TEE [16]. In addition, traditional TTE or TEE measurement of the annulus uses long-axis images of the aorta in which the cusp opening is centered in the aorta; however, this view does not bisect the aorta at its largest dimension but rather images a plane just lateral to the maximum dimension which may cause significant underestimation of the true maximal annular diameter [2]. This is the most likely cause of undersizing of the annulus by echocardiographic measurement. Preprocedural MDCT-based measurements of annular diameter and post-procedural comparisons of THV area to annulus area predict paravalvular aortic regurgitation slightly better than TEE annular diameter (area under the curve: 0.81 compared to 0.70, respectively) [19]. Newer MDCT-based approaches which employ three-dimensionally derived cross-sectional measurements of the aortic annulus affect device sizing and patient selection and reduces paravalvular aortic regurgitation for the Edwards SAPIEN™ THV compared to traditional two-dimensional TEE [20]. This underscores the added value of routinely employing three-dimensional techniques for aortic annulus sizing such as by MDCT, cardiac magnetic resonance imaging (CMR) [21], or three-dimensional TEE [18, 22].

Echocardiography, however, has limitations in some patients being considered for TAVR. Most notable is the acoustic shadowing that can obscure interpretation of the annular complex due to heavily calcified aortic leaflets or root. With TEE, mitral annular calcification can also cause acoustic shadowing over the LVOT. In addition, with two-dimensional imaging, the imaging field is in a single plane that can lead to different measurements compared to three-dimensional real-time imaging and multiplanar reconstruction which allows complete morphologic analysis [23].

Echocardiographic Assessment of the Aortic Leaflets

The major implications of aortic leaflet morphology for TAVR are related to the number of cusps present, the degree of leaflet calcification, and the height of the leaflets with respect to the coronary ostia. The latter is addressed in a separate section. Bicuspid aortic valves are considered a contraindication for TAVR due to concerns of poor seating, asymmetrical stent expansion, and/or paravalvular aortic regurgitation due to severe distortion of the native valve leaflets [10, 11]. Although there are now numerous reports of successful TAVR procedures in patients with congenitally bicuspid aortic valves [24–28], incomplete deployment may lead to aortic regurgitation or impairment of valvular function [29].

Echocardiography can evaluate the extent, location, and distribution of AoV calcification and provide important information helpful for the success of TAVR. Severe, asymmetric calcification of the AoV leading to asymmetry of leaflet excursion may also result in incomplete expansion of the THV, limited orifice size and paravalvular regurgitation. One grading system used for surgical AVR which discriminates calcium being confined to leaflet tips (mild), calcium extending from the leaflet tips to the leaflet bases (moderate), and bulky calcification that extended from tip to base in all three leaflets (severe) has shown modest correlation with the actual weight of the excised

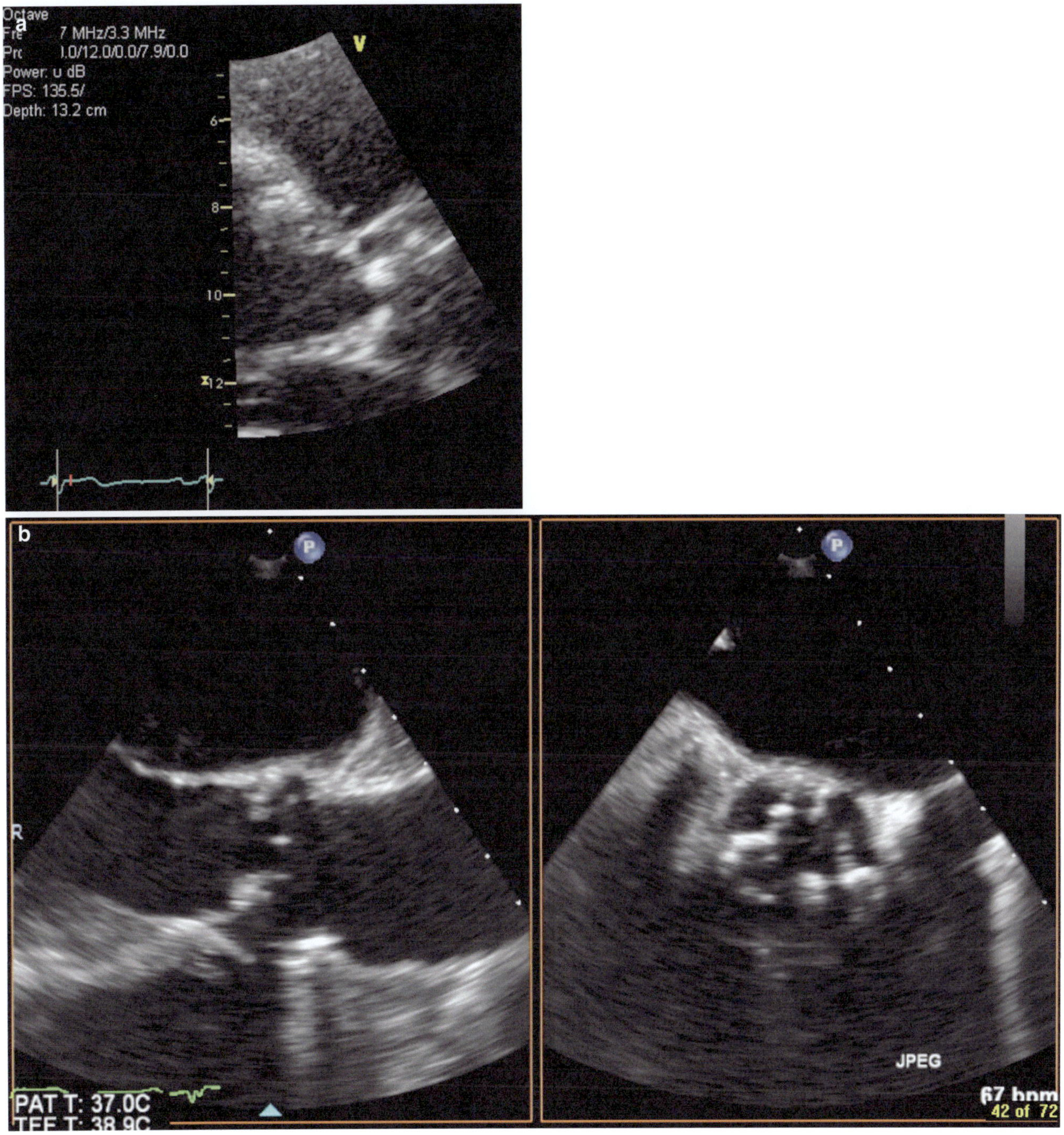

Fig. 24.4 Use of biplane imaging to view the true elliptical shape of the aortic annulus. (**a**) Two-dimensional transthoracic echocardiogram of left parasternal long-axis view of aortic root showing calcified aortic leaflets. (**b**) Two-dimensional transesophageal echocardiogram biplane images showing the aortic root in long axis and short axis. (**c**) Three-dimensional transesophageal echocardiogram full-volume data set cropped to show the aortic root in the same patient from (a) and (b)

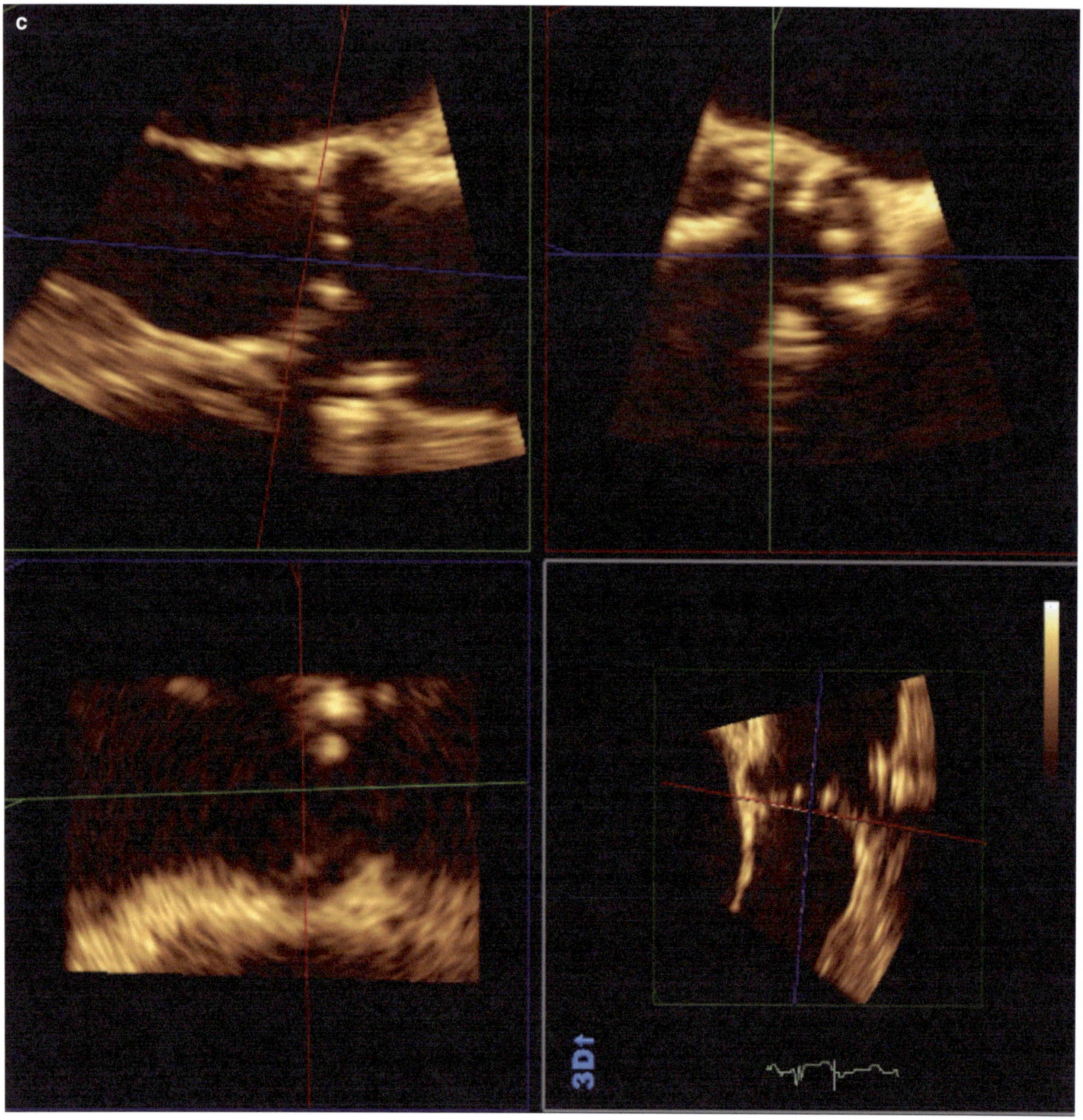

Fig. 24.4 (continued)

native valve (Box 24.1) [30]. Bulky AoV calcification is a risk factor for left main coronary artery occlusion during THV deployment, and in rare cases, with creation of a membranous septal defect due to inferior displacement of extensive annular or basal leaflet calcifications during stent expansion [31]. Valvular calcification poses a risk with either the SAPIEN™ or CoreValve® THV; however, positioning of the CoreValve® is more independent of valvular calcification owing to its constrained waist and larger length.

Box 24.1 Echocardiographic Grading of Aortic Valve Calcium

Aortic Valve Calcification Grading System (adapted from that used for surgical aortic valve replacement)

Mild	Calcium being confined to leaflet tips
Moderate	Calcium extending from the leaflet tips to the leaflet bases
Severe	Bulky calcification that extended from tip to base in all three leaflets

TTE

TTE is usually adequate to identify the number of aortic cusps and to quantify severity, location, and symmetry of calcification (see Fig. 24.2a). A long-axis parasternal view of the LVOT and aorta is used to identify the severity of calcification and overall valve mobility. While the right coronary cusp and left or noncoronary commissure are visible in the traditional long-axis view, short-axis views of the aortic valve from the parasternal or subcostal window are also often necessary to identify the exact number of cusps, location of calcification, and commissural fusion, if present.

TEE

It must be noted that significant AoV calcification may limit further analysis by TTE due to acoustic shadowing. If this is the case, TEE may be helpful [32]. A mid-esophageal short-axis image at 35–60° or biplane imaging from the long-axis image traditionally provides adequate views of the aortic cusps and commissures. In addition to classifying calcification, valve opening (e.g., concentric, eccentric) should also be described. The role of three-dimensional transesophageal echocardiography in the preprocedural assessment is still evolving but has mostly involved providing an accurate depiction of the annulus and measurement of the annular-coronary ostial distance and, less often, providing an assessment of the aortic cusps when TTE is indeterminate. Limitations related to acoustic shadowing by calcium deposits also apply to imaging of the aortic leaflets especially if the calcification extends into the annulus, the sinuses of Valsalva, and mitral annulus. Image acquisition from deep gastric views allows the operator to avoid shadowing from calcification in the aortic annulus and ascending aorta but does not usually overcome shadowing from calcification of the mitral valve apparatus. Resolution is also decreased compared to esophageal views because of the valve's greater distance from the transducer.

Comparison to Other Noninvasive Imaging Modalities

There are few published direct comparisons between various noninvasive multimodality imaging techniques for assessment of the aortic leaflets themselves. However, given that calcification and morphology are major aspects of this component of the aortic annular complex, there are strengths and limitations that deserve consideration. Severe and bulky calcification of the aortic leaflets and annulus may render echocardiography and CMR unreliable, while less severe calcification may not pose as much limitation [33]. CMR delineates calcium as a low signal permitting visualization of the valve but may limit the ability to perform precise measurements [34]. MDCT, on the other hand, allows imaging of the exact location and quantification of calcification that may aid in prognosis of patients with aortic stenosis (AS) and planning for TAVR [35, 36]. The choice of modality must also take into consideration comorbidities such as renal dysfunction, dye allergy, arrhythmias, and pulmonary disease as these may limit the use of potentially nephrotoxic intravenous contrast, ECG gating, and breath holds for MDCT and CMR, respectively.

Echocardiographic Assessment of the Coronary Ostia

Coronary artery compromise is an important but fortunately infrequent complication of TAVR occurring in <1 % of patients in clinical trials and single-center reports [37, 38]. The SAPIEN™ Aortic Bioprosthesis European Outcome (SOURCE) Registry reported a 0.6 % incidence of coronary obstruction over 30 days in their post-marketing registry [39]. The possible mechanisms for coronary ostial obstruction during TAVR have been described and include (1) impingement of the coronary ostia by the THV support structure; (2) inappropriately high positioning of the sealing cuff of the THV; (3) embolization of atheroma, calcium, thrombus, air, or vegetation; (4) an oversized THV; (5) aortic root dissection; and (6) displacement of the native and bulky aortic leaflets towards the coronary ostia (Box 24.2) [37, 40–42]. Webb described risk factors for coronary ostial obstruction which include a low-lying coronary ostium <10–12 mm from the basal leaflet insertion to the coronary ostium, bulky calcification of native leaflets, and a narrow aortic root [42]. These risk factors have been present in many of the reported cases of coronary ostial obstruction during TAVR [41, 43] although no definite criteria exist to exclude patients on the basis of risk for coronary obstruction.

Box 24.2 Possible Mechanisms for Coronary Ostial Obstruction During TAVR

1. Impingement of the coronary ostia by the THV support structure
2. Inappropriately high positioning of the sealing cuff of the THV
3. Embolization of atheroma, calcium, thrombus, air or vegetation
4. Oversized THV
5. Aortic root dissection
6. Displacement of the native and bulky aortic leaflets towards the coronary ostia

THV transcatheter heart valve

The normal adult aortic cusps vary in height even in apparently tricuspid valves without congenital malformation. Vollebergh et al. described the natural variation in leaflet height with right, noncoronary, and left coronary leaflets measuring on average 14.1, 14.1, and 14.2 mm, respectively. In adults with calcific AS, the average right, noncoronary, and left coronary leaflet heights are slightly smaller: 13.9, 13.6, and 14.0 mm, respectively [44]. Minimum recommended annular-ostial heights for the 23 and 26 mm SAPIEN™ THVs are >10 and >11 mm, respectively [4], although some suggest a more cautious approach using >14 mm as a general guideline for a safe annular-ostial distance [31]. The annular-ostial height is not relevant for the CoreValve® THV because of its unique structure and constrained waist which sits within the SoV to avoid "jailing" the coronary ostia [3]. For the self-expanding valve, however, the height of the SoV is an important consideration, with a preferred SoV height of >15 mm. SoV heights of <10 mm are generally considered so low as to preclude successful THV implantation [45].

TTE/TEE

On the basis of the likely mechanisms of coronary ostial obstruction and to minimize the risk, echocardiography can provide important preprocedural information. It is crucial to know the distance from the virtual basal ring ("aortic annulus") to the ostia of the left and right coronary arteries and to compare this with the length of the cusps. TTE is inferior to TEE in this regard due to low resolution and limited views of the cusps and coronary ostia in the long axis. Two-dimensional TEE is able to define the annular-ostial distance and length of the right coronary cusp using a mid-esophageal long-axis view of the LVOT and aortic root. This is best achieved in the long-axis view of the LVOT slightly off-axis to show the right coronary ostium and proximal right coronary artery. For the left main coronary ostium, three-dimensional TEE is required as the left main ostium lies in the coronal plane that cannot be imaged using standard two-dimensional TEE imaging. By using a three-dimensional full-volume data set of the aortic root complex and multiplanar reconstruction, the left annular-ostial and cusp length can be acquired (Fig. 24.5a, b).

Comparison to Other Noninvasive Imaging Modalities

Aortic cusp length and annular-ostial height can be measured noninvasively using echocardiography, CMR, and MDCT [46]. Severe calcification may cause acoustic shadowing with TTE. Moreover, severe calcification can cause a signal void with CMR, leaving MDCT scanning or TEE as noninvasive imaging methods of choice for determining annular-ostial height and leaflet length. There have been no trials comparing various noninvasive imaging modalities in assessing the relationship of measures of annular-ostial height with clinical outcomes.

Echocardiographic Assessment of the Sinotubular Junction and Proximal Aorta

The sinotubular junction (STJ) describes the upper most ring of the aortic root complex representing the interface between the aortic root and the tubular ascending aorta and plays an important role in maintaining competence of implanted prosthetic valves [47]. Echocardiographic studies demonstrate the dynamic nature of the aortic root during the cardiac cycle with the STJ width increasing by 3.4 ± 1.9 mm from diastole to systole [48]. Echocardiographic and *ex vivo* studies have also demonstrated that the STJ and ascending aorta are usually larger in patients with calcific AS compared to patients with normally functioning valves with a mean difference of 1.3 mm [2, 49]. For TAVR, STJ width and the presence and degree of calcification appear to be critical and may be related to the incidence of patient-prosthesis mismatch (PPM) [50, 51]. Small and heavily calcified STJs may predispose patients to balloon migration, THV embolization, or aortic root rupture during implantation of the THV and is associated with more severe atherosclerotic aortic arch disease [3, 52–54]. Although consideration of the STJ width and degree of calcification appear critical for correct and lower-risk positioning, quantitative data on the impact of the STJ and tubular aorta size and morphology on TAVR outcomes are limited [55].

TTE

Two-dimensional TTE images should be used to visualize the aortic root in different views in varying intercostal spaces and at different distances from the left sternal border. Right parasternal views, with the patient in a right lateral decubitus position, can also be useful to focus on the root including the STJ. In the long-axis view from parasternal views (i.e., corresponding to the sagittal plane by other noninvasive modalities), the STJ is measured in a similar manner to the aortic annulus and SoV from tissue-blood interface to blood-tissue interface (see Fig. 24.1). Significant calcification may limit accurate measurement by TTE.

TEE

The thoracic aorta is generally better imaged using TEE as it lies in the near field of the transducer. The STJ can be seen in the mid-esophageal long-axis view between 120 and 140° or slightly higher in the esophagus depending on the orientation of the heart and aorta.

Comparison to Other Noninvasive Imaging Modalities

Noninvasive imaging assessment of the STJ varies significantly depending on the modality. Two-dimensional TTE measurements of the STJ and ascending aorta are usually significantly smaller than CMR-based measurements [34]. While MDCT and CMR measurements of the STJ and ascending aorta are usually in close agreement, the agreement between TTE and either noninvasive method is poor. For the STJ, Jabbour et al. described 95 % limits of agreement for the largest measurement of −4.7 to 3.1 mm comparing CMR to MDCT, −8.4 to 7.0 mm comparing CMR to TTE, and −9.0 to 9.1 mm comparing MDCT to TTE [56]. Poor agreement

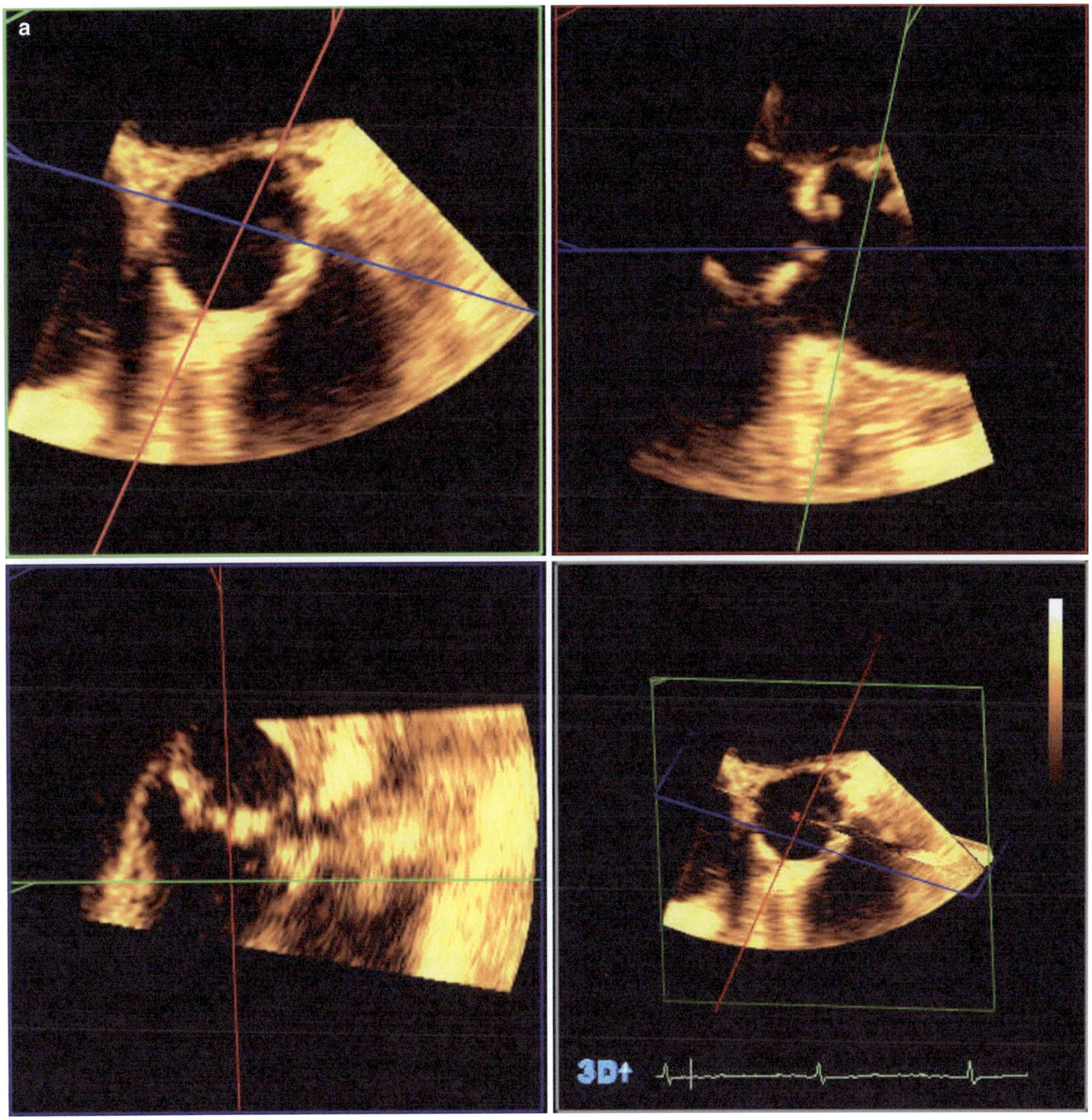

Fig. 24.5 Three-dimensional transesophageal echocardiography used to identify the relationship between the aortic valve and left coronary ostium. (**a**) Full-volume data set acquired by transesophageal echocardiography cropped to show the aortic root and the origin of the left coronary artery. (**b**) The full-volume data set from 6A has been cropped to show the origin of the left coronary artery. *Yellow line D1* represents left coronary leaflet length, and *Green line D2* represents distance from leaflet insertion to left coronary artery ostium

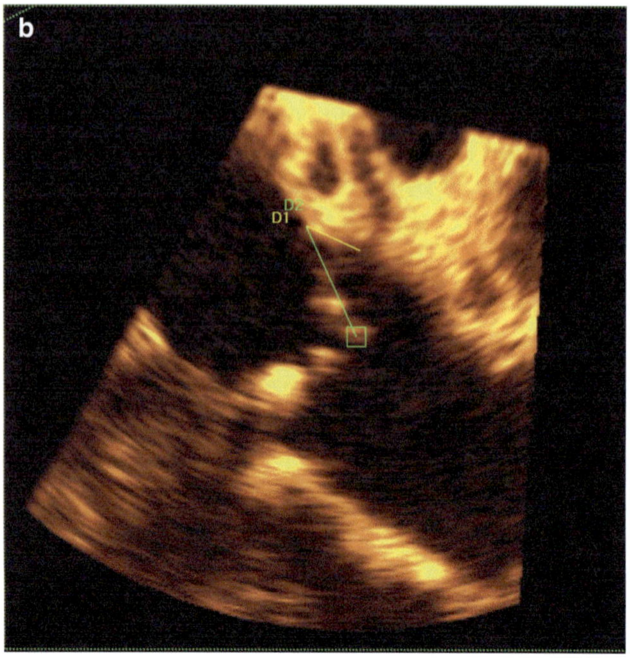

Fig. 24.5 (continued)

between CMR and MDCT scanning with TTE was also found comparing the ascending aorta in that study; however, MDCT- and TTE-based measurements of a dilated sinotubular junction or ascending aorta (i.e., as with aortic aneurysm) are comparable [57]. TEE, while not a routine part of TAVR preprocedural assessment in all centers, provides more reliable measurements of the STJ and tubular aorta than TTE [58]. Little data exists with direct comparisons between MDCT, CMR, echocardiography, and angiography for sizing of the STJ and proximal aorta in relation to clinical outcomes. Despite these shortcomings, outcomes have been excellent when echocardiographic assessments of the aortic root have been used and are comparable to those obtained using MDCT scanning [16]. Systematic comparisons of the accuracy and TAVR-related clinical implications of different multimodality techniques measuring the STJ and ascending aorta are needed.

Echocardiographic Assessment of Concomitant Cardiac and Aortic Root Pathology

Anterior Mitral Valve Leaflet

The aortic annulus is in close proximity to the mitral valve apparatus with the majority of the noncoronary leaflet and a portion of the left coronary leaflet in fibrous continuity with the anterior mitral valve leaflet. The two interleaflet triangles abutting the noncoronary leaflet are also in fibrous continuity with the right and left fibrous trigones, the anterior mitral valve annulus (the aorto-mitral curtain), and a portion of the membranous septum. Anterior mitral valve morphology is especially important to characterize in the preprocedural phase in order to avoid unintentional impingement of the anterior leaflet with placement of the THV too low within the ventricle [52]. Moreover, dense calcification within the aorto-mitral curtain or mitral annular calcification may increase the risk of paravalvular regurgitation due to asymmetric expansion of the THV [59].

Mitral Regurgitation

Most (76 %) patients with severe AS have some degree of mitral regurgitation (MR), and moderate-to-severe MR is seen in 22–48 % of patients undergoing TAVR [10, 40, 60]. Most of these patients have organic as opposed to functional MR [61]. During implantation, the guidewire or introducer sheath may interfere with the mitral subvalvular apparatus and cause or worsen the degree of MR. Worsening MR is included in the differential diagnosis of acute hemodynamic instability during implantation, and as such the operator should be aware of any baseline mitral insufficiency. Therefore, determining the presence, nature, and degree of MR should also be a routine aspect of the TAVR preprocedural assessment. This is usually adequately achieved with two-dimensional transthoracic echocardiography imaging of the left atrium, mitral valve, left ventricle, and pulmonary veins using two-dimensional, color, and spectral Doppler in standard manner to characterize MR [62]. TEE with biplane or full-volume three-dimensional image acquisition may be particularly helpful intraprocedurally to identify the situation when the guidewire is caught within the mitral subvalvular apparatus.

Septal Thickness and Ventricular Thrombus

Both self-expandable and balloon-expandable THVs extend their lower edge into the LVOT. Abnormalities within this region should be identified during the preprocedural assessment in order for the operator to be able to anticipate and take steps to minimize complications (Fig. 24.6). A marked upper septal bulge, for example, protruding into the LVOT, may create a significant challenge to the proper seating of the THV and may risk repositioning after cessation of the pacing runs [4]. A prominent septal bulge has also been associated with atrioventricular (AV) block and need for pacemaker implantation post-TAVR [63, 64]. Hemodynamically significant LVOT obstruction due to septal hypertrophy is a contraindication to TAVR; however, there are reports of successful implantations performed with modifications of the THV for such patients [65].

Morphology of the LVOT is usually adequately visualized with two-dimensional TTE imaging of the LVOT in the long

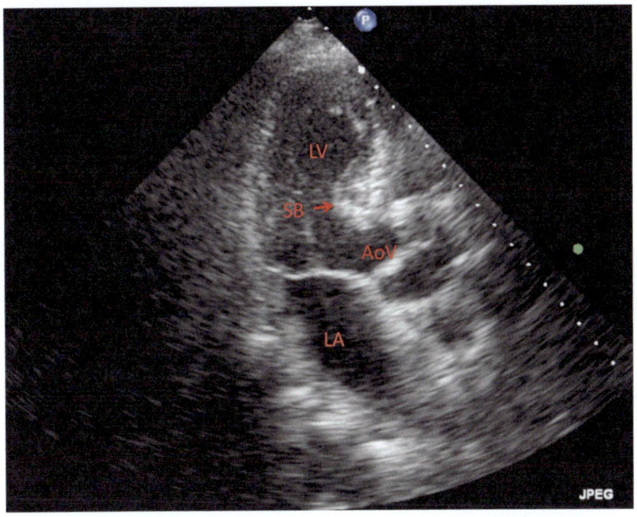

Fig. 24.6 Two-dimensional transthoracic echocardiogram in an apical long-axis view of the left ventricle demonstrating a prominent septal bulge in the left ventricular outflow tract. *LV* left ventricle, *LA* left atrium, *AoV* aortic valve, *SB* septal bulge

axis from a parasternal window. Apical windows utilizing off-axis views can also further delineate the relationships between the LVOT, anterior mitral leaflet, and aortic root. Left ventricular thrombus, another contraindication to TAVR, must also be excluded.

Comparison to Other Noninvasive Imaging Modalities

Anterior Mitral Valve Leaflet

The anterior mitral valve leaflet can be visualized noninvasively by MDCT, CMR, fluoroscopy, and echocardiography. As it relates to TAVR, the presence and degree of calcification in and around the mitral valve and the relationship of the anterior mitral valve leaflet to the LVOT are important to evaluate in the preprocedural stage. MDCT may likely be the modality of choice for quantifying calcification barring motion artifacts, significant arrhythmia, or other potential limitations of MDCT. CMR can display the presence of calcification as well which is represented by a low signal. The ability to obtain morphologic as well as hemodynamic information related to mitral valve function in real time without the added time necessary for post-processing is a significant advantage of echocardiography compared to MDCT or CMR. Similar to MDCT and CMR, TEE using multiplanar reconstruction of three-dimensional data sets allow for complete visualization and offline manipulation of the images to inform the anatomic relationships between the mitral leaflets and LVOT [66].

Mitral Regurgitation

Echocardiography is the gold standard noninvasive imaging modality for evaluating valve defects including MR. The near universal access to echocardiography for TAVR candidates and the ability to visualize regurgitant jet flows in real time with excellent temporal resolution probably contribute to the general clinical acceptance of echocardiography for MR. TTE is adequate for qualitative and semiquantitative assessments of MR; however, when available, TEE is preferred especially when planning interventions [67]. Two-dimensional TEE underestimates effective orifice area (by 0.13 cm^2), regurgitant volume (by 21.6 %), and overall severity of MR as compared with three-dimensional TEE [66]. Three-dimensional TEE underestimates regurgitant volume compared to CMR (by 1.2 %) but to a lesser degree than two-dimensional TEE compared to CMR (by 21.3 %) [66]. MDCT and CMR are unique, however, in that they both can provide high-precision measures of left ventricular volumes and quantifying total stroke volume, mitral regurgitant volume, and regurgitant fraction [68]. While CMR does allow for direct visualization of retrograde flow over the mitral valve, MDCT does not and this limits its clinical acceptance in quantifying MR. Moreover, regurgitant flow data obtained by MDCT and CMR may be inconclusive due to poor signal-to-noise ratio, false ECG triggering, or motion artifacts [68]. Echocardiographic assessments of MR may be limited by the patient's body habitus or coexisting lung disease resulting in suboptimal acoustic windows and technically limited studies [69]; however, semiquantitative echocardiographically determined severity of MR remains the gold standard and predicts clinical events [70].

Septal Thickness

Left ventricular septal thickness is usually assessed by echocardiography prior to TAVR [64, 71]; however, the role of MDCT is emerging. MDCT-based measurements of septal thickness, for example, predict AV block post-TAVR [63]. It is not clear whether the relationship between the measurements of septal thickness by MDCT and outcomes is unique to MDCT as similar findings have been observed with echocardiography [71]. Direct comparisons of various imaging modalities performance for septal thickness in relation to TAVR clinical outcomes are lacking; however, studies of normal and athletic hearts show that echocardiography tends to overestimate interventricular septum thickness compared to CMR (by up to 1.7 mm) [72, 73] and MDCT (by up to 2.2 mm) [74, 75]. One explanation for this discrepancy is that trabeculations, if present, are better excluded from the interventricular septal measurement by MDCT and CMR than by echocardiography and differences in spatial and temporal resolution [72, 76].

Left Ventricular Thrombus

In clinical practice, echocardiography is most often used to detect left ventricular thrombus. Diagnostic yield is improved when the study is performed specifically to detect left ventricular thrombus and when sonographic intravenous contrast is used [77, 78]. While left ventricular thrombi may also be detected by MDCT [79, 80], there are more data available comparing echocardiography to CMR [81–84]. Weinsaft et al. demonstrated a low sensitivity (33 %) and positive predictive value (29 %) for echocardiography compared to CMR which improved marginally when LV thrombus was the indication for the echocardiogram [83]. For the TAVR candidate in whom the detection of left ventricular thrombus determines eligibility for the procedure, the operator should not rely on suboptimal echocardiographic images but must perform another diagnostic test such as a contrast-enhanced echocardiogram, CMR, or MDCT when there is a suspicion for a left ventricular thrombus.

Summary

A full assessment of the aortic root complex is a mandatory part of the noninvasive imaging assessment prior to TAVR. This assessment can be achieved by multimodality echocardiographic imaging using a combination of two- and three-dimensional imaging obtained by transthoracic and transesophageal echocardiography. Most of the components of the aortic valve and root can be excellently characterized with TTE, as has been done in TAVR clinical trials (e.g., aortic annulus size, number of leaflets). However, TEE is more reliable for evaluating other aspects such as aortic leaflet length, coronary ostial height, the proximal aorta, and when TTE images are technically limited due to body habitus, poor acoustic imaging windows, or when calcification prohibits a detailed examination. In addition to the aortic root complex, adjacent structures such as the mitral valve and LVOT must also be considered as they can impact the feasibility and success of TAVR. When echocardiographic imaging is limited (most often by acoustic shadowing by calcium), other imaging modalities such as MDCT or CMR can be considered. Barring poor diagnostic images, echocardiography will often provide a thorough, minimally invasive method to obtain important information about aortic root geometry and size with the aim of ensuring a safe deployment of the THV.

References

1. Abdulla R, Blew GA, Holterman MJ. Cardiovascular embryology. Pediatr Cardiol. 2004;25:191–200.
2. Piazza N, de Jaegere P, Schultz C, Becker AE, Serruys PW, Anderson RH. Anatomy of the aortic valvar complex and its implications for transcatheter implantation of the aortic valve. Circ Cardiovasc Interv. 2008;1:74–81.
3. Zamorano JL, Badano LP, Bruce C, et al. EAE/ASE recommendations for the use of echocardiography in new transcatheter interventions for valvular heart disease. J Am Soc Echocardiogr. 2011;24: 937–65.
4. Bloomfield GS, Gillam LD, Hahn RT, et al. A practical guide to multimodality imaging of transcatheter aortic valve replacement. JACC Cardiovasc Imaging. 2012;5:441–55.
5. Thubrikar M, Piepgrass WC, Shaner TW, Nolan SP. The design of the normal aortic valve. Am J Physiol. 1981;241:H795–801.
6. Brewer RJ, Deck JD, Capati B, Nolan SP. The dynamic aortic root. Its role in aortic valve function. J Thorac Cardiovasc Surg. 1976; 72:413–7.
7. Thubrikar M, Harry R, Nolan SP. Normal aortic valve function in dogs. Am J Cardiol. 1977;40:563–8.
8. Thubrikar M, Nolan SP, Bosher LP, Deck JD. The cyclic changes and structure of the base of the aortic valve. Am Heart J. 1980;99: 217–24.
9. Nakai H, Takeuchi M, Yoshitani H, Kaku K, Haruki N, Otsuji Y. Pitfalls of anatomical aortic valve area measurements using two-dimensional transoesophageal echocardiography and the potential of three-dimensional transoesophageal echocardiography. Eur J Echocardiogr. 2010;11:369–76.
10. Leon MB, Smith CR, Mack M, et al. Transcatheter aortic-valve implantation for aortic stenosis in patients who cannot undergo surgery. N Engl J Med. 2010;363:1597–607.
11. clinicaltrials.gov. Safety and efficacy study of the Medtronic CoreValve® system in the treatment of symptomatic severe aortic stenosis in high risk and very high risk subjects who need aortic valve replacement. 2012. http://www.clinicaltrials.gov/show/NCTQ1531374. Last accessed 29 Jun 2013.
12. Détaint D, Lepage L, Himbert D, et al. Determinants of significant paravalvular regurgitation after transcatheter aortic valve: implantation impact of device and annulus discongruence. JACC Cardiovasc Interv. 2009;2:821–7.
13. Lang RM, Bierig M, Devereux RB, et al. Recommendations for chamber quantification: a report from the American Society of Echocardiography's Guidelines and Standards Committee and the Chamber Quantification Writing Group, developed in conjunction with the European Association of Echocardiography, a branch of the European Society of Cardiology. J Am Soc Echocardiogr. 2005;18:1440–63.
14. Roman MJ, Devereux RB, Kramer-Fox R, O'Loughlin J. Two-dimensional echocardiographic aortic root dimensions in normal children and adults. Am J Cardiol. 1989;64:507–12.
15. Zoghbi WA, Chambers JB, Dumesnil JG, et al. Recommendations for evaluation of prosthetic valves with echocardiography and doppler ultrasound: a report From the American Society of Echocardiography's Guidelines and Standards Committee and the Task Force on Prosthetic Valves, developed in conjunction with the American College of Cardiology Cardiovascular Imaging Committee, Cardiac Imaging Committee of the American Heart Association, the European Association of Echocardiography, the Japanese Society of Echocardiography and the Canadian Society of Echocardiography. J Am Soc Echocardiogr. 2009;22:975–1014.
16. Messika-Zeitoun D, Serfaty J-M, Brochet E, et al. Multimodal assessment of the aortic annulus diameter: implications for transcatheter aortic valve implantation. J Am Coll Cardiol. 2010;55: 186–94.
17. Hutter A, Opitz A, Bleiziffer S, et al. Aortic annulus evaluation in transcatheter aortic valve implantation. Catheter Cardiovasc Interv. 2010;76:1009–19.
18. Altiok E, Koos R, Schröder J, et al. Comparison of two-dimensional and three-dimensional imaging techniques for measurement of aortic annulus diameters before transcatheter aortic valve implantation. Heart. 2011;97:1578–84.
19. Willson AB, Webb JG, Labounty TM, et al. 3-dimensional aortic annular assessment by multidetector computed tomography predicts moderate or severe paravalvular regurgitation after transcatheter aortic valve replacement: a multicenter retrospective analysis. J Am Coll Cardiol. 2012;59:1287–94.

20. Jilaihawi H, Kashif M, Fontana G, et al. Cross-sectional computed tomographic assessment improves accuracy of aortic annular sizing for transcatheter aortic valve replacement and reduces the incidence of paravalvular aortic regurgitation. J Am Coll Cardiol. 2012;59:1275–86.
21. Koos R, Altiok E, Mahnken AH, et al. Evaluation of aortic root for definition of prosthesis size by magnetic resonance imaging and cardiac computed tomography: implications for transcatheter aortic valve implantation. Int J Cardiol. 2012;158(3):353–8.
22. Ng ACT, Delgado V, van der Kley F, et al. Comparison of aortic root dimensions and geometries before and after transcatheter aortic valve implantation by 2- and 3-dimensional transesophageal echocardiography and multislice computed tomography. Circ Cardiovasc Imaging. 2010;3:94–102.
23. Wood DA, Tops LF, Mayo JR, et al. Role of multislice computed tomography in transcatheter aortic valve replacement. Am J Cardiol. 2009;103:1295–301.
24. Wijesinghe N, Ye J, Rodés-Cabau J, et al. Transcatheter aortic valve implantation in patients with bicuspid aortic valve stenosis. JACC Cardiovasc Interv. 2010;3:1122–5.
25. Ferrari E, Locca D, Sulzer C, et al. Successful transapical aortic valve implantation in a congenital bicuspid aortic valve. Ann Thorac Surg. 2010;90:630–2.
26. Chiam PT, Chao VT, Tan SY, et al. Percutaneous transcatheter heart valve implantation in a bicuspid aortic valve. JACC Cardiovasc Interv. 2010;3:559–61.
27. Delgado V, Tops LF, Schuijf JD, et al. Successful deployment of a transcatheter aortic valve in bicuspid aortic stenosis: role of imaging with multislice computed tomography. Circ Cardiovasc Imaging. 2009;2:e12–3.
28. Kochman J, Huczek Z, Koltowski L, Michalak M. Transcatheter implantation of an aortic valve prosthesis in a female patient with severe bicuspid aortic stenosis. Eur Heart J. 2012;33:112.
29. Zegdi R, Ciobotaru V, Noghin M, et al. Is it reasonable to treat all calcified stenotic aortic valves with a valved stent? Results from a human anatomic study in adults. J Am Coll Cardiol. 2008;51: 579–84.
30. Babaliaros VC, Liff D, Chen EP, et al. Can balloon aortic valvuloplasty help determine appropriate transcatheter aortic valve size? JACC Cardiovasc Interv. 2008;1:580–6.
31. Masson J-B, Kovac J, Schuler G, et al. Transcatheter aortic valve implantation: review of the nature, management, and avoidance of procedural complications. JACC Cardiovasc Interv. 2009;2: 811–20.
32. Unsworth B, Malik I, Mikhail GW. Recognising bicuspid aortic stenosis in patients referred for transcatheter aortic valve implantation: routine screening with three-dimensional transoesophageal echocardiography. Heart. 2010;96:645.
33. Tuzcu EM, Kapadia SR, Schoenhagen P. Multimodality quantitative imaging of aortic root for transcatheter aortic valve implantation: more complex than it appears. J Am Coll Cardiol. 2010; 55:195–7.
34. Paelinck BP, Van Herck PL, Rodrigus I, et al. Comparison of magnetic resonance imaging of aortic valve stenosis and aortic root to multimodality imaging for selection of transcatheter aortic valve implantation candidates. Am J Cardiol. 2011;108:92–8.
35. Messika-Zeitoun D, Aubry M-C, Detaint D, et al. Evaluation and clinical implications of aortic valve calcification measured by electron-beam computed tomography. Circulation. 2004;110: 356–62.
36. Mizia-Stec K, Pysz P, Jasiński M, et al. Preoperative quantification of aortic valve stenosis: comparison of 64-slice computed tomography with transesophageal and transthoracic echocardiography and size of implanted prosthesis. Int J Cardiovasc Imaging. 2012;28(2): 343–52.
37. Leon MB, Piazza N, Nikolsky E, et al. Standardized endpoint definitions for transcatheter aortic valve implantation clinical trials: a consensus report from the Valve Academic Research Consortium. J Am Coll Cardiol. 2011;57:253–69.
38. Lefèvre T, Kappetein AP, Wolner E, et al. One year follow-up of the multi-centre European PARTNER transcatheter heart valve study. Eur Heart J. 2011;32:148–57.
39. Thomas M, Schymik G, Walther T, et al. Thirty-day results of the SAPIEN aortic Bioprosthesis European Outcome (SOURCE) Registry: a European registry of transcatheter aortic valve implantation using the Edwards SAPIEN valve. Circulation. 2010;122:62–9.
40. Webb JG, Pasupati S, Humphries K, et al. Percutaneous transarterial aortic valve replacement in selected high-risk patients with aortic stenosis. Circulation. 2007;116:755–63.
41. Kapadia SR, Svensson L, Tuzcu EM. Successful percutaneous management of left main trunk occlusion during percutaneous aortic valve replacement. Catheter Cardiovasc Interv. 2009;73: 966–72.
42. Webb JG. Coronary obstruction due to transcatheter valve implantation. Catheter Cardiovasc Interv. 2009;73:973.
43. Webb JG, Chandavimol M, Thompson CR, et al. Percutaneous aortic valve implantation retrograde from the femoral artery. Circulation. 2006;113:842–50.
44. Vollebergh FE, Becker AE. Minor congenital variations of cusp size in tricuspid aortic valves. Possible link with isolated aortic stenosis. Br Heart J. 1977;39:1006–11.
45. John M, Liao R, Zheng Y, et al. System to guide transcatheter aortic valve implantations based on interventional C-arm CT imaging. Med Image Comput Comput Assist Interv. 2010;13:375–82.
46. Lu T-LC, Huber CH, Rizzo E, Dehmeshki J, von Segesser LK, Qanadli SD. Ascending aorta measurements as assessed by ECG-gated multi-detector computed tomography: a pilot study to establish normative values for transcatheter therapies. Eur Radiol. 2009;19:664–9.
47. Maselli D, De Paulis R, Scaffa R, et al. Sinotubular junction size affects aortic root geometry and aortic valve function in the aortic valve reimplantation procedure: an in vitro study using the Valsalva graft. Ann Thorac Surg. 2007;84:1214–8.
48. Park J-S, Choi Y-W, Shin J-S, et al. Validation of three-dimensional echocardiography for quantification of aortic root geometry: comparison with multi-detector computed tomography. J Cardiovasc Ultrasound. 2011;19:128–33.
49. Stolzmann P, Knight J, Desbiolles L, et al. Remodelling of the aortic root in severe tricuspid aortic stenosis: implications for transcatheter aortic valve implantation. Eur Radiol. 2009;19:1316–23.
50. Ewe SH, Muratori M, Delgado V, et al. Hemodynamic and clinical impact of prosthesis-patient mismatch after transcatheter aortic valve implantation. J Am Coll Cardiol. 2011;58:1910–8.
51. Jilaihawi H, Chin D, Spyt T, et al. Prosthesis-patient mismatch after transcatheter aortic valve implantation with the Medtronic-Corevalve bioprosthesis. Eur Heart J. 2010;31:857–64.
52. Jayasuriya C, Moss RR, Munt B. Transcatheter aortic valve implantation in aortic stenosis: the role of echocardiography. J Am Soc Echocardiogr. 2011;24:15–27.
53. Svensson LG, Dewey T, Kapadia S, et al. United States feasibility study of transcatheter insertion of a stented aortic valve by the left ventricular apex. Ann Thorac Surg. 2008;86:46–54; discussion 54–5.
54. Finkelhor RS, Youssefi ME, Mohan SK, Bahler RC. Aortic sinotubular junction calcium as a marker of severe aortic atherosclerosis. Am J Cardiol. 1998;82:1549–52, A8.
55. Schoenhagen P, Tuzcu EM, Kapadia SR, Desai MY, Svensson LG. Three-dimensional imaging of the aortic valve and aortic root with computed tomography: new standards in an era of transcatheter valve repair/implantation. Eur Heart J. 2009;30:2079–86.
56. Jabbour A, Ismail TF, Moat N, et al. Multimodality imaging in transcatheter aortic valve implantation and post-procedural aortic

regurgitation: comparison among cardiovascular magnetic resonance, cardiac computed tomography, and echocardiography. J Am Coll Cardiol. 2011;58:2165–73.
57. Tamborini G, Galli CA, Maltagliati A, et al. Comparison of feasibility and accuracy of transthoracic echocardiography versus computed tomography in patients with known ascending aortic aneurysm. Am J Cardiol. 2006;98:966–9.
58. Bridgman PG, Bloomfield P, Reid JH, Mankad PS. Prediction of stentless aortic bioprosthesis size with transesophageal echocardiography and magnetic resonance imaging. J Heart Valve Dis. 1997;6:487–9.
59. Delgado V, Ng ACT, Shanks M, et al. Transcatheter aortic valve implantation: role of multimodality cardiac imaging. Expert Rev Cardiovasc Ther. 2010;8:113–23.
60. Tzikas A, Piazza N, van Dalen BM, et al. Changes in mitral regurgitation after transcatheter aortic valve implantation. Catheter Cardiovasc Interv. 2010;75:43–9.
61. Hekimian G, Detaint D, Messika-Zeitoun D, et al. Mitral regurgitation in patients referred for transcatheter aortic valve implantation using the edwards sapien prosthesis: mechanisms and early postprocedural changes. J Am Soc Echocardiogr. 2012;25:160–5.
62. Zoghbi WA, Enriquez-Sarano M, Foster E, et al. Recommendations for evaluation of the severity of native valvular regurgitation with two-dimensional and Doppler echocardiography. J Am Soc Echocardiogr. 2003;16:777–802.
63. Romero M, Pan M, Espejo S, et al. Interventricular septal morphology as a new predictor of AV-block after transcatheter aortic valve implantation. Circulation. 2011;124:1–1.
64. Piazza N, Nuis R-J, Tzikas A, et al. Persistent conduction abnormalities and requirements for pacemaking six months after transcatheter aortic valve implantation. EuroIntervention. 2010;6:475–84.
65. Moreno R, Calvo L, García E, Dobarro D. Severe septal hypertrophy: is it necessarily a contraindication for the transcatheter implantation of an Edwards-Sapien prosthesis? Rev Esp Cardiol. 2010;63:241–2.
66. Shanks M, Siebelink H-MJ, Delgado V, et al. Quantitative assessment of mitral regurgitation: comparison between three-dimensional transesophageal echocardiography and magnetic resonance imaging. Circ Cardiovasc Imaging. 2010;3:694–700.
67. Macnab A, Jenkins NP, Bridgewater BJM, et al. Three-dimensional echocardiography is superior to multiplane transoesophageal echo in the assessment of regurgitant mitral valve morphology. Eur J Echocardiogr. 2004;5:212–22.
68. Lembcke A, Wiese TH, Enzweiler CNH, et al. Quantification of mitral valve regurgitation by left ventricular volume and flow measurements using electron beam computed tomography: comparison with magnetic resonance imaging. J Comput Assist Tomogr. 2003;27:385–91.
69. Shah DJ. Functional valve assessment: the emerging role of cardiovascular magnetic resonance. Methodist Debakey Cardiovasc J. 2010;6:15–9.
70. Enriquez-Sarano M, Avierinos J-F, Messika-Zeitoun D, et al. Quantitative determinants of the outcome of asymptomatic mitral regurgitation. N Engl J Med. 2005;352:875–83.
71. Jilaihawi H, Chin D, Vasa-Nicotera M, et al. Predictors for permanent pacemaker requirement after transcatheter aortic valve implantation with the CoreValve bioprosthesis. Am Heart J. 2009;157:860–6.
72. Prakken NHJ, Teske AJ, Cramer MJ, et al. Head-to-head comparison between echocardiography and cardiac MRI in the evaluation of the athlete's heart. Br J Sports Med. 2012;46(5):348–54.
73. Scharhag J, Urhausen A, Schneider G, Rochette V, Kramann B, Kindermann W. Left ventricular mass in endurance-athletes with athlete's heart and untrained subjects–comparison between different echocardiographic methods and MRI. Z Kardiol. 2003;92:309–18.
74. Stolzmann P, Scheffel H, Trindade PT, et al. Left ventricular and left atrial dimensions and volumes: comparison between dual-source CT and echocardiography. Invest Radiol. 2008;43:284–9.
75. Malagò R, Tavella D, Mantovani W, et al. MDCT coronary angiography vs 2D echocardiography for the assessment of left ventricle functional parameters. Radiol Med. 2011;116:505–20.
76. Lin FY, Devereux RB, Roman MJ, et al. Cardiac chamber volumes, function, and mass as determined by 64-multidetector row computed tomography: mean values among healthy adults free of hypertension and obesity. JACC Cardiovasc Imaging. 2008;1:782–6.
77. Visser CA, Kan G, David GK, Lie KI, Durrer D. Two dimensional echocardiography in the diagnosis of left ventricular thrombus. A prospective study of 67 patients with anatomic validation. Chest. 1983;83:228–32.
78. Mansencal N, Nasr IA, Pillière R, et al. Usefulness of contrast echocardiography for assessment of left ventricular thrombus after acute myocardial infarction. Am J Cardiol. 2007;99:1667–70.
79. Tehrani F, Eshaghian S. Detection of left ventricular thrombus by coronary computed tomography angiography. Am J Med Sci. 2009;338:167–8.
80. Tasu JP, Pellerin D, Karila-Cohen D, Delfressy JF, Bléry M. Images in cardiovascular medicine. Computed tomography and magnetic resonance imaging of left ventricular thrombus. Circulation. 2001;103:e8–9.
81. Srichai MB, Junor C, Rodriguez LL, et al. Clinical, imaging, and pathological characteristics of left ventricular thrombus: a comparison of contrast-enhanced magnetic resonance imaging, transthoracic echocardiography, and transesophageal echocardiography with surgical or pathological validation. Am Heart J. 2006;152:75–84.
82. Weinsaft JW, Kim RJ, Ross M, et al. Contrast-enhanced anatomic imaging as compared to contrast-enhanced tissue characterization for detection of left ventricular thrombus. JACC Cardiovasc Imaging. 2009;2:969–79.
83. Weinsaft JW, Kim HW, Crowley AL, et al. LV thrombus detection by routine echocardiography: insights into performance characteristics using delayed enhancement CMR. JACC Cardiovasc Imaging. 2011;4:702–12.
84. Mollet NR, Dymarkowski S, Volders W, et al. Visualization of ventricular thrombi with contrast-enhanced magnetic resonance imaging in patients with ischemic heart disease. Circulation. 2002;106:2873–6.

Aortic Annular Geometry and Sizing: CT

25

Reza Arsanjani, Jonathon Leipsic, Daniel S. Berman, and James K. Min

Abstract

Calcified aortic stenosis is the most common valvular heart disease in the elderly and is associated with significant morbidity and mortality after the onset of symptoms. Surgical aortic valve replacement (SAVR) improves symptoms and survival, however many patients with severe aortic stenosis do not undergo SAVR due to multiple coexisting comorbidities. Transcatheter aortic valve replacement (TAVR) has recently emerged as a novel method to treat these selected high-risk patients with aortic stenosis. Moderate or severe paravalvular aortic regurgitation (PAR) is significantly higher for high-risk TAVR patients compared to surgical patients and is an independent predictor of short-, mid-, and long-term mortality. PAR following TAVR has been shown to be related to prosthesis-annulus incongruence, highlighting the importance of appropriate annular measurements, especially given that current TAVR devices are limited to specific annular sizes. Multiple imaging modalities have been used to measure aortic annulus. This chapter focuses on anatomy of aortic annulus, comparison of different imaging modalities, clinical significance, and our recommendations for measuring aortic annulus using multi-detector computed tomography (MDCT).

Keywords

Aortic annulus • Multimodal imaging • Transcatheter aortic valve replacement • Computed tomography • Echocardiogram correlation

Introduction

Calcified aortic stenosis (AS), either due to calcification of a normal trileaflet or congenital bicuspid valve, is the most common valvular heart disease, affecting 2–4 % of adults over age 65 in the USA alone [1, 2]. The natural history of aortic stenosis involves a prolonged latent period with relatively low rate of morbidity and mortality; however, after the onset of symptoms, the prognosis significantly worsens [1]. Without an intervention, the average survival following the onset of symptoms, including angina, syncope, or heart failure, is 2–3 years [1, 3–5], with a high risk of sudden death. The onset of symptoms underscores a critical point in management of aortic stenosis, where aortic valve replacement is the only effective treatment [1].

Surgical aortic valve replacement (SAVR) improves symptoms and survival [6–8]; therefore, surgery is virtually indicated in all symptomatic patients with severe AS [1].

R. Arsanjani, MD
Division of Cardiology, Department of Medicine, Cedars-Sinai Medical Center, David Geffen UCLA School of Medicine, Los Angeles, CA, USA

J. Leipsic, MD, FRCPC, FSCCT
Division of Cardiology, Department of Radiology, University of British Columbia, St. Paul's Hospital, Vancouver, BC, Canada

D.S. Berman, MD
Departments of Imaging and Medicine, Cedars-Sinai Medical Center, Cedars-Sinai Heart Institute, David Geffen UCLA School of Medicine, Los Angeles, CA, USA

J.K. Min, MD, FACC, FSCCT (✉)
Weill Cornell Medical College, NewYork-Presbyterian Hospital, New York, NY, USA
e-mail: jkm2001@med.cornell.edu

J.K. Min et al. (eds.), *Multimodality Imaging for Transcatheter Aortic Valve Replacement*, DOI 10.1007/978-1-4471-2798-7_25, © Springer-Verlag London 2014

Table 25.1 Anatomic requirements for currently available valves

	Edwards Sapien XT	Medtronic CoreValve
Annulus size and prosthetic valve size	18–22 mm ➔ 23 mm valve	20–23 mm ➔ 26 mm valve
	21–25 mm ➔ 26 mm valve	24–27 mm ➔ 29 mm valve
	25–27 mm ➔ 29 mm valve	
Sinus of Valsalva diameter	N/A	>27 mm
Sinotubular junction diameter	N/A	<43 mm
Distance to the coronary ostia	>10 mm	>10 mm

N/A not applicable

Although the operative mortality rate is relatively low, with the average perioperative mortality for isolated AVR ranging between 3 and 4 % and those for combined AVR and CABG ranging between 5 and 7 % [9–11], many patients with severe aortic stenosis do not undergo SAVR due to multiple coexisting comorbidities [12–14]. Unfortunately, there are no medical therapies that prolong life for these patients, and approximately 50 % will die within the first 2 years [1]. Transcatheter aortic valve replacement (TAVR) has recently emerged as a novel method to treat these selected high-risk patients with aortic stenosis, with more than 15,000 patients undergoing TAVR worldwide as of early 2010 [15].

While SAVR imparts higher incidence of major bleeding and new-onset atrial fibrillation, TAVR is associated with a higher incidence major vascular complications and major strokes. In addition, moderate or severe paravalvular aortic regurgitation at 1 year was significantly greater for high-risk TAVR patients compared to surgical patients (7.0 % vs. 1.9 %, $p<0.001$) [16]. In the follow-up of these high-risk patients, moderate or severe paravalvular aortic regurgitation (PAR) persisted at 2 years in the TAVR patients (6.9 % vs. 0.9 %, $p<0.001$) [16]. Importantly, prior studies have demonstrated that significant PAR is an independent predictor of short-, mid-, and long-term mortality [16–18].

Notably, PAR following TAVR has been shown to be related to prosthesis-annulus incongruence, highlighting the importance of appropriate annular measurements [19]. In addition, oversizing can lead to vascular complications as well as difficulty in crossing the native aortic valve with the delivery system [20]. These findings are particularly important, given that current TAVR devices are limited to specific annular sizes (Table 25.1). Multiple imaging modalities have been used to measure aortic annulus. This chapter focuses on the anatomy of aortic annulus, comparison of different imaging modalities, clinical significance, and our recommendations for measuring aortic annulus using multi-detector computed tomography (MDCT) as it pertains to TAVR procedure.

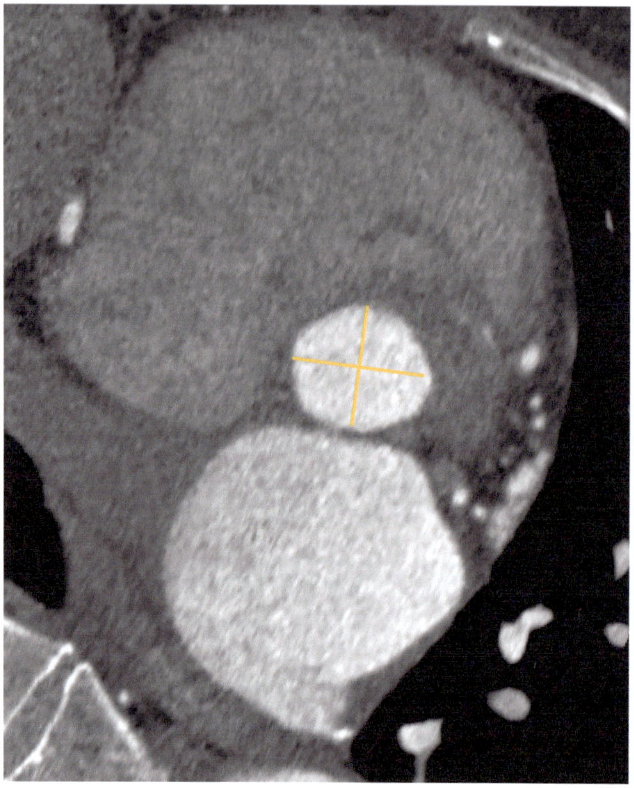

Fig. 25.1 Double oblique transverse reconstruction of the aortic root below the commissural insertion in an 83-year-old female with severe aortic stenosis, demonstrating an elliptical structure (the *yellow lines* demonstrate the minimal and maximal annular diameter)

Aortic Annulus Anatomy

The aortic annulus is an elliptoid structure that is a part of the fibrous skeleton of the heart, which functions to support the valve and the aortic root against high pressures that occur during left ventricular systole (Fig. 25.1). The aortic annulus is a complex three-dimensional structure, which is usually described as semilunar and crown-like [21, 22] (Fig. 25.2). The aortic valve leaflets are attached throughout the length of the aortic root, forming the "three-pronged coronet," while the hinges form the supporting structure creating a crown-like ring [22] (Fig. 25.3). The base of this crown represents the inlet from the left ventricular outflow tract into the aortic root [22], and the top of the crown represents the outlet of the aortic root into the descending aorta [22]. The aortic annulus measurement, regardless of modalities used, is assessed at the base of the crown in systole.

The ring of collagenous tissue that forms the aortic annulus ring surrounds and supports the aortic orifice. The non-coronary and left coronary leaflets are parts of the fibrous tissue, which along with the anterior leaflet of mitral valve, form the fibrous trigones [22]. These trigones anchor the

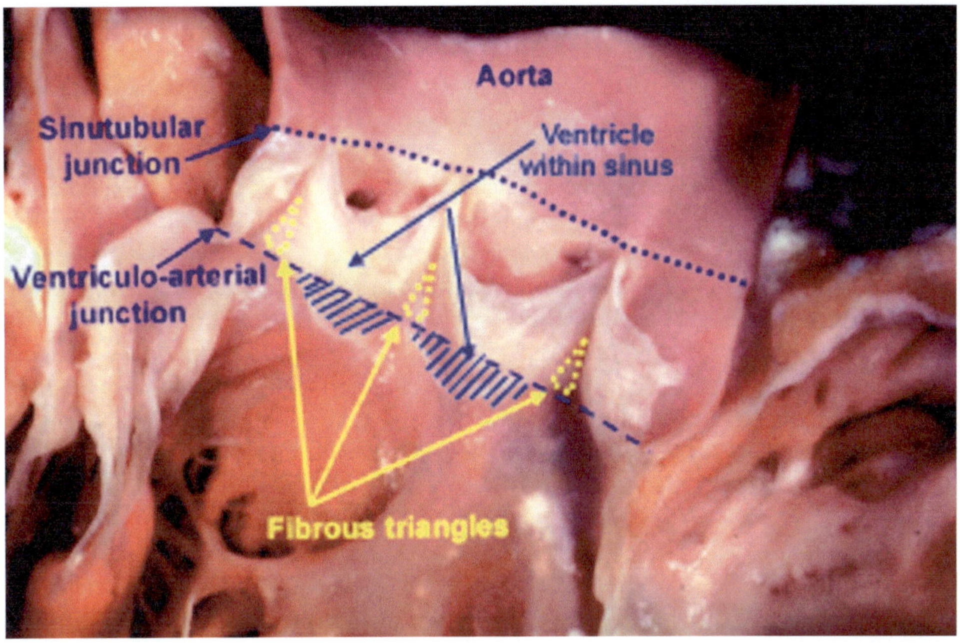

Fig. 25.2 The aortic root has been opened through a longitudinal incision across the area of aortic-mitral valvar continuity and spread open to show the semilunar attachments of the valvar leaflets

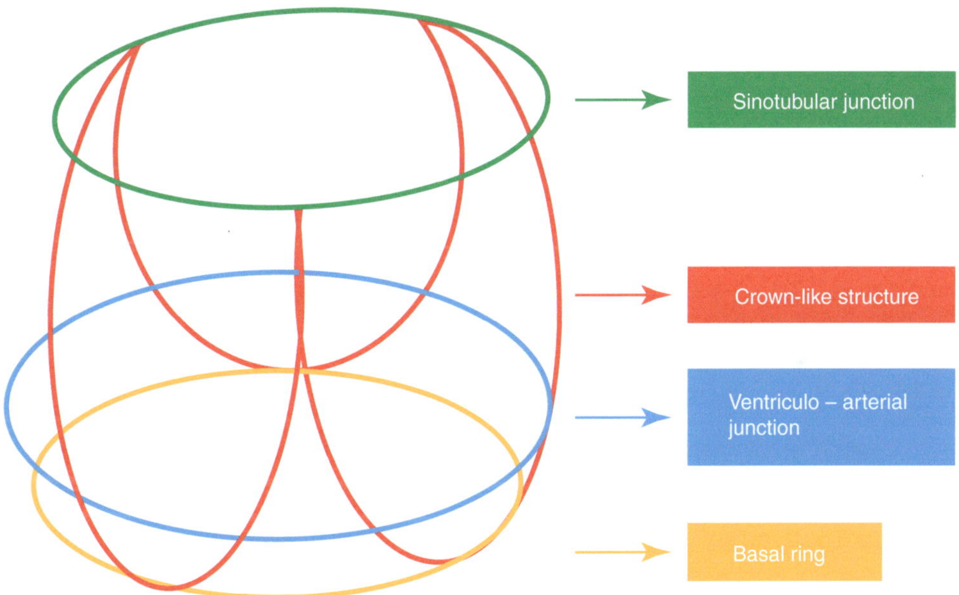

Fig. 25.3 Diagram of aortic root anatomy showing its considerable length along with coronet shape and location of various annular planes

roof of the left ventricle to the aortic-mitral valvular unit. This complex anatomy along with its obliquely aligned and ovoid structure leads to obstacles in performing measurements using different imaging modalities.

Aortic Annulus Measurement: Comparison of Different Imaging Modalities

Traditionally, two-dimensional (2D) echocardiography has been the most utilized method for measuring aortic annulus based on its availability. The current American Society of Echocardiography and European Association of Echocardiography recommend measuring the aortic annulus from inner edge to inner edge in mid-systole using parasternal long-axis view on the transthoracic echocardiography (TTE) while zooming in on the left ventricular outflow tract (LVOT) [23]. In addition, the aortic annulus can be measured at the long axis (120° view) using 2D transesophageal echocardiography (TEE). Unfortunately, despite its wide availability, 2D TTE and TEE have several limitations, including diameter measurements being based on a single annular plane as well as the assumption of circular annular geometry, when in fact the annular geometry is often oval in shape.

A recent study by Ng et al. compared the 2D circular, 3D circular, 3D planimetered annular, and LVOT areas by TEE, with MDCT planimetered areas used as a "gold standard" in 53 patients undergoing TAVR with the Edwards Sapien valve for treatment of severe symptomatic AS [24]. The mean MDCT planimetered annular area (4.65 ± 0.82 cm^2) before TAVR was significantly higher than 2D TEE circular (3.89 ± 0.74 cm^2, $p<0.001$), 3D TEE circular (4.06 ± 0.79 cm^2, $p<0.001$), and 3D TEE planimetered annular areas (4.22 ± 0.77 cm^2, $p<0.001$). The 3D TEE planimetered annular areas had the best agreement with respective MDCT planimetered areas.

These investigators also assessed the clinical significance of underestimating the aortic annular cross-sectional areas and noted that based on recalculated preoperative aortic valve areas using 3D TEE circular, 3D TEE planimetered, and MDCT planimetered annular areas, a respective 10, 25, and 25 % of patients were recategorized into moderate aortic stenosis based on current guidelines [24]. Furthermore, it was also noted that following TAVR, the MDCT planimetered (4.65 ± 0.82 vs. 4.20 ± 0.46 cm^2, $p<0.001$) and 3D TEE planimetered (4.22 ± 0.77 vs. 3.62+0.43 cm^2, $p<0.001$) annular areas decreased, due to the "new effective" aortic annulus, assuming the internal dimensions of the circular prosthetic valve. Finally, Ng et al. noted that although 3D TEE can avoid the circular geometric assumptions made by 2D and 3D circular measurements (by directly performing planimetry of the cross-sectional annular/LVOT areas), it still underestimated annular areas by up to 10 % compared to respective MDCT planimetered areas, based on the CT's superior spatial signal-to-noise ratio [24].

Two additional studies also compared echocardiography versus MDCT with direct intraoperative sizing. Kempfert et al. assessed aortic annular size in 26 patients with severe AS undergoing standard SAVR [25]. They measured maximal, minimal, and mean diameter using MDCT, as well as measuring "effective diameter." The "effective diameter" was defined as the diameter of a circle with the exact same area as the measured area of the annular circumference reconstructed from the MDCT data set. They noted the best agreement between intraoperative direct sizing and MDCT effective diameter as well as end-systolic echocardiographic diameters, although the MDCT effective diameter was larger. However, they noted that in patients with oval-shaped annulus, the MDCT effective diameter had the best agreement in intraoperative sizing [25]. A second study by Dashkevich et al. compared aortic annular diameter measured with MDCT and TEE versus direct intraoperative measurements using a Hegar dilator, in 33 patients with severe aortic stenosis undergoing SAVR [26]. They found that the calculated average diameter by MDCT correlated very well with intraoperative measurements ($r=0.923$, $p<0.001$) and with the size of implanted valve ($r=0.867$, $p<0.001$), while correlation of TEE and intraoperative measurements was only satisfactory ($r=0.523$, $p=0.002$) [26]. They also noted that TEE tended to underestimate the dimensions of aortic annulus.

The aortic annulus is routinely larger when measured by MDCT compared to 2D or 3D TEE measurements. Further, the discordance between MDCT and TTE or TEE is greater than the differences between TTE and TEE [27]. The differences in size could be related to geometrical assumptions by echocardiography that the aortic annulus is circular. A study by Tops et al. evaluated aortic annulus diameter in 169 patients, who had undergone 64-slice MDCT for evaluation of coronary artery disease [28]. They noted that in 47 % of patients the difference between coronal and sagittal diameters was ≥3 mm, indicating an oval-shaped aortic annulus [24]. Another study by Delgado et al. also noted significant difference between mean coronal (25.1 ± 2.4 mm) and sagittal (22.9 ± 2.0 mm) diameter ($p<0.001$) in 53 patients with severe aortic stenosis undergoing TAVR [29].

However, it is important to note that the aortic annulus is a dynamic structure and is noted to become less ellipsoidal and more circular during systole [30]. A study by Hamdan et al. evaluated the deformation dynamics of the aortic annulus in 35 patients with aortic stenosis and 11 normal subjects undergoing 256-slice computed tomography [30]. They noted that in both subjects with normal and stenotic valves, the minimum diameter increased in systole and the ellipticity index decreased. However, despite these dynamic changes, the perimeter increase was negligible in patients with calcified valves (0.56 ± 0.85 %; $p<0.001$) and small even in normal subjects (2.2 ± 2.2 %; $p=0.01$). These findings are consistent with another study by Bertaso et al., which also demonstrated a small (<1 mm) but statistically significant difference in aortic annulus dimensions between diastole and systole in patients with severe AS referred for TAVR [31].

In addition to its dynamic nature across the cardiac cycle, the annular size is also dependent on left ventricular function [32]. Ng et al. compared mean aortic annular diameter and geometries between 90 patients with severe AS and 111 controls based on MDCT measurements [32]. It was noted that patients with severe AS had similar aortic annular dimensions and geometries when compared to controls, even after correcting for baseline differences in age and body surface area (BSA). However, severe AS patients with LV dysfunction [left ventricular ejection fraction (LVEF) <50 %] had significantly larger mean aortic annular diameter (26.4 ± 1.9 vs. 24.5 ± 2.1 mm, $p<0.001$) compared with patients with preserved LVEF [32]. The authors noted that male gender and larger body surface area were independent determinants of larger aortic annulus diameter.

Clinical Significance: Aortic Annulus Measurement by MDCT

Despite absolute differences in between aortic annular measurements between MDCT, TTE, and TEE, the significance of these differences as well as impact on procedural success remains unclear. Traditionally, aortic annulus measurements are performed using 2D TTE and TEE. Messika-Zeitoun et al. analyzed how the annulus diameter measurements using different imaging modalities might influence the TAVR strategy based on manufacturer's recommendation in 45 patients with severe AS referred for TAVR [27]. As previously mentioned, although the overall correlation between the methods was good, the difference between MDCT and TTE or TEE was larger than the differences between TTE and TEE. Furthermore, even though the overall agreement between TTE and TEE was good (kappa = 0.68), the TAVR would have been different in 17 % of patients. The agreement between MDCT and TTE or TEE was significantly lower (kappa = 0.28 and 0.27, respectively); however, the decision based on MDCT measurements would have modified TAVR strategy in ≥40 % of patients [27]. Thirty-four patients underwent implantation based on TEE, which was successful in all but one patient with moderate to severe regurgitation.

Multiple studies have evaluated the correlation between the degree of PAR and the aortic annulus measurement using MDCT. Buzzatti et al. assessed the role of CT for evaluation of the degree of aortic regurgitation in 115 patients undergoing TAVR [33]. They noted that significant aortic regurgitation was directly related to annulus diameters, especially maximum and minimum diameters. Prosthesis-annulus oversizing, defined as the ratio between prosthesis size and mean annular size, was associated with a reduction in PAR, with a cutoff of 7 % as the limit below which the degree of aortic regurgitation increased. Another study by Wilson et al. analyzed 3D aortic annular dimension using MDCT for prediction of paravalvular aortic regurgitation following TAVR in 109 consecutive patients undergoing TAVR with a balloon-expandable aortic valve [34]. Moderate or severe PAR was again noted to be associated with prosthesis undersizing, defined as the prosthesis diameter minus mean diameter. They also found that the aortic valve prosthesis was undersized relative to MDCT-derived mean diameter and area in 35.3 and 45.1 % of cases, respectively [34]. In addition, the authors noted that oversizing of the prosthesis may reduce the risk of moderate or severe PAR. A third study by Jilaihawi et al. evaluated the discriminatory value of MDCT annular measures for post-TAVR paravalvular aortic regurgitation compared to 2D echocardiographic measures [35]. They noted that maximal diameter minus prosthesis size based on MDCT had the highest discriminatory value for PAR (receiver-operating characteristic area under the curve = 0.82, 95 % confidence interval: 0.69–0.94; $p < 0.001$), while traditional echocardiographic measures were nondiscriminatory [35]. The authors also noted that the prospective application of a MDCT-guided annular sizing approach resulted in less moderate or severe PAR after TAVR than traditional echocardiographic measures (7.5 % vs. 21.9 %; $p = 0.045$). The authors concluded that 3D cross-sectional measures using CT, should be the new gold standard for aortic annular evaluation for TAVR.

The aforementioned studies highlight several important features about aortic annular measurements using MDCT. MDCT angiography produces isotropic images that can be reconstructed in any 2D plane, including those traditionally used for measurement of aortic annulus by TTE or TEE, although MDCT measurements are generally larger than either TTE or TEE. However, as previously mentioned, aortic annulus is often not circular but rather oval shaped, which might be the reason 3D CT-guided annular sizing outperforms the traditional echocardiography for prediction of PAR post-TAVR. Furthermore, reproducibility of 2D measurements by CT is marginal at best, which can lead to significant issues with annular sizing for TAVR. Therefore, it would be beneficial to evaluate LVOT-aortic annulus geometry using 3D CT annular measurements rather than trying to recreate 2D echo-equivalents. Furthermore, true transaxial images obtained by CT, which are orthogonal to the aortic annulus plane, allow for short-axis and long-axis measurements of annulus. Finally, despite differences between TEE and MDCT, we recommend that both values be reported and considered prior to TAVR in order to reduce the chance for error and provide a more comprehensive definition of the annular size and shape.

MDCT Acquisition Protocol and Image Processing

There are a number of possible scan protocols for TAVR assessment, although we recommend that images be acquired using a ≥64-detector row MDCT. In addition, although beta-blockers are routinely administered prior to MDCT and some patients with severe aortic stenosis might already be established on beta-blockers, we do not routinely provide additional beta-blockers at the time of scanning regardless of baseline heart rate for concerns of induced hypotension [15]. We also recommend retrospective gating—despite the acknowledged higher radiation dose—because it allows for multiphasic reconstruction, which is particularly important in patients undergoing TAVR based on the high prevalence of baseline arrhythmias. In addition, the multiphasic data enabled by retrospective ECG gating enables evaluation of both diastolic and systolic phases, which provide information related to annular size across the cardiac cycle.

MDCT images should be reconstructed in the coronal, sagittal, and transverse (axial) orientation utilizing standard multiplanar reformats, and images should be analyzed using a 3D oblique tool. We recommend to begin analysis in the coronal plane with an axial cutplane rotated in an anti-clockwise direction so that the line runs from a right caudal to a left cranial position. Next, sagittal reconstruction should be performed by vertically orientating the images so that it is orthogonal to the long axis of the aortic annulus. Subsequently, the horizontal line representing the axial cutplane is moved up or down on either sagittal or coronal projection in order to create a double oblique transverse or axial image of the aortic root until most caudal attachments of the three aortic leaflets are identified [15] (Fig. 25.4). It is essential that the inferior aspect of all three aortic cusps

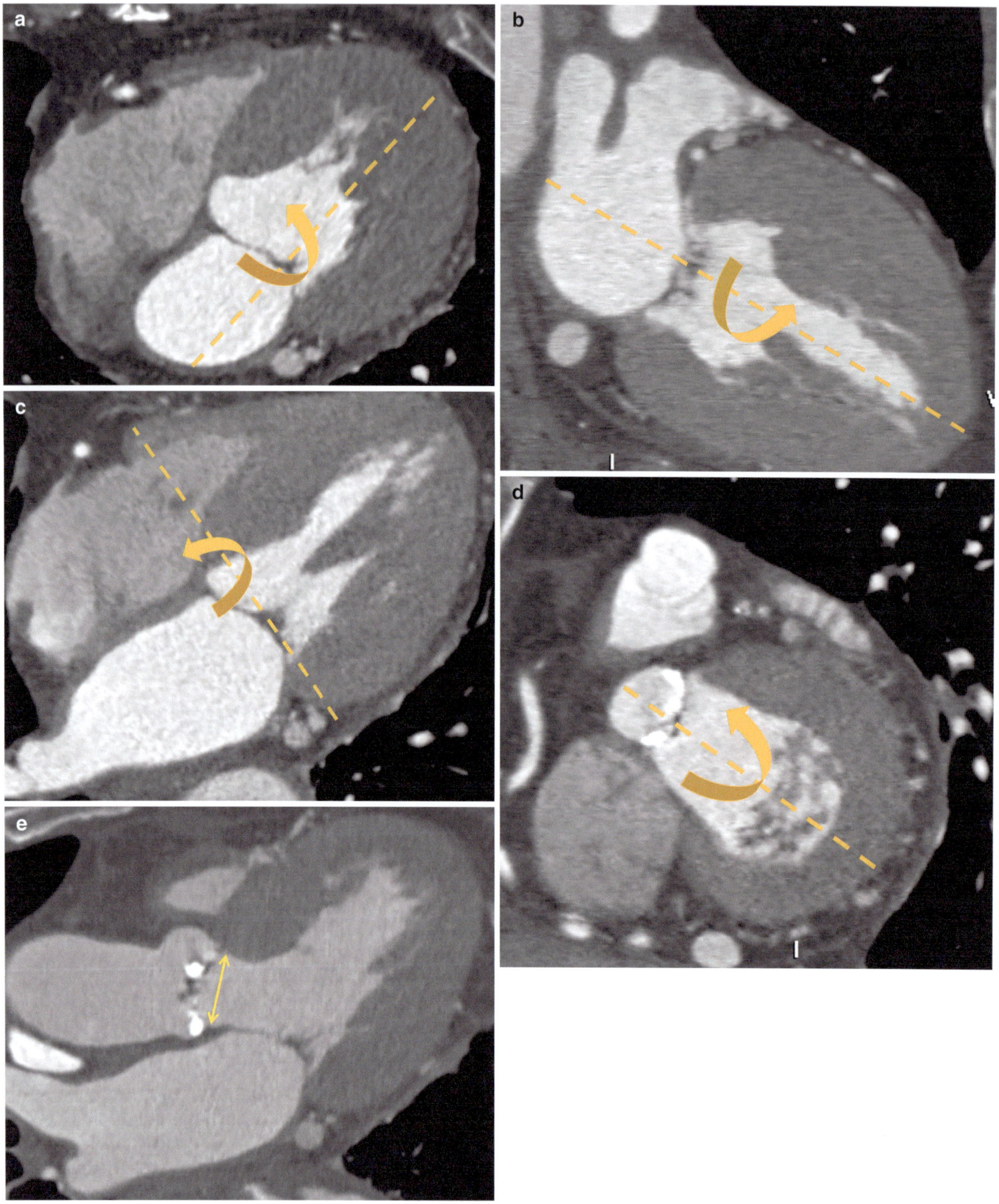

Fig. 25.4 Multiplanar image reconstruction of a gate CT angiogram in a 93-year-old male with severe symptomatic aortic stenosis for the evaluation of the aortic root and annulus. (**a**) The transverse image is initially bisected with an oblique tool through the mitral valve to the ventricular apex (dashed *yellow line* indicates plane of cut with *yellow arrow* indicating direction of cut), resulting in the formation of a vertical long-axis reconstruction. (**b**) The left ventricle is then cut in a plane from the left atrium through the center of the mitral valve through the left ventricular apex, (**c**) resulting in a relative four-chamber reconstruction. (**d**) An oblique tool is then rotated in a perpendicular fashion through interventricular septum in order to create a short-axis projection. (**e**) Finally, a cutplane is placed in an oblique fashion at the base of the short-axis projection out to the left ventricular outflow tract and aorta to create a three-chamber projection (diameter measured at caudal attachment of the leaflets represented by double headed *yellow arrow*)

is identified in the same plane, representing the true double oblique transverse image of the aortic annular plane, which is often nonparallel and oblique to the plane of the aortic valve. It is important to recognize that rapid heart rates and heavy calcification may adversely affect overall image quality, and the annulus measurement is not exempt from these degradations.

Aortic Annulus Measurement

Numerous prior studies have suggested recommendations to aortic annulus measurement using MDCT (including annular assessment in coronal and sagittal views) utilizing three-chamber reconstruction (in a manner replicative of that seen by echocardiography); as well as measuring the maximal and minimal diameter measurement using double oblique transverse imaging. In addition, others have recommended reporting the average of the maximum and minimum diameter measurements. For diameter measures, we also recommend reporting this average because it appears to be most reproducible [36].

Conclusion

Aortic annulus measurement is an essential part of TAVR procedure. MDCT can effectively be used for measuring the aortic annulus with good correlation with 3D TEE, although MDCT measures are routinely larger. MDCT annular measurements can accurately predict annular-prosthesis mismatch as well as PAR and, at times, outperforms echocardiographic measurements. MDCT measurements should routinely be performed prior to TAVR and incorporated as a comprehensive evaluation of patients prior to TAVR.

References

1. Bonow RO, Carabello BA, Kanu C, De Leon Jr AC, Faxon DP, Freed MD, Gaasch WH, Lytle BW, Nishimura RA, O'Gara PT, O'Rourke RA, Otto CM, Shah PM, Shanewise JS, Smith Jr SC, Jacobs AK, Adams CD, Anderson JL, Antman EM, Faxon DP, Fuster V, Halperin JL, Hiratzka LF, Hunt SA, Lytle BW, Nishimura R, Page RL, Riegel B. ACC/AHA 2006 guidelines for the management of patients with valvular heart disease: a report of the American College of Cardiology/American Heart Association Task Force on Practice Guidelines (writing Committee to Revise the 1998 Guidelines for the Management of Patients With Valvular Heart Disease): developed in collaboration with the Society of Cardiovascular Anesthesiologists: endorsed by the Society for Cardiovascular Angiography and Interventions and the Society of Thoracic Surgeons. Circulation. 2006;114(5):e84–231.
2. Freeman RV, Otto CM. Spectrum of calcific aortic valve disease: pathogenesis, disease progression, and treatment strategies. Circulation. 2005;111(24):3316–26.
3. Turina J, Hess O, Sepulcri F, Krayenbuehl HP. Spontaneous course of aortic valve disease. Eur Heart J. 1987;8(5):471–83.
4. Schwarz F, Baumann P, Manthey J, Hoffmann M, Schuler G, Mehmel HC, Schmitz W, Kübler W. The effect of aortic valve replacement on survival. Circulation. 1982;66(5):1105–10.
5. Kelly TA, Rothbart RM, Cooper CM, Kaiser DL, Smucker ML, Gibson RS. Comparison of outcome of asymptomatic to symptomatic patients older than 20 years of age with valvular aortic stenosis. Am J Cardiol. 1988;61(1):123–30.
6. Smith N, McAnulty JH, Rahimtoola SH. Severe aortic stenosis with impaired left ventricular function and clinical heart failure: results of valve replacement. Circulation. 1978;58(2):255–64.
7. Connolly HM, Oh JK, Orszulak TA, Osborn SL, Roger VL, Hodge DO, Bailey KR, Seward JB, Tajik AJ. Aortic valve replacement for aortic stenosis with severe left ventricular dysfunction. Prognostic indicators. Circulation. 1997;95(10):2395–400.
8. Kvidal P, Bergström R, Hörte LG, Ståhle E. Observed and relative survival after aortic valve replacement. J Am Coll Cardiol. 2000;35(3):747–56.
9. Edwards FH, Peterson ED, Coombs LP, DeLong ER, Jamieson WR, Shroyer ALW, Grover FL. Prediction of operative mortality after valve replacement surgery. J Am Coll Cardiol. 2001;37(3):885–92.
10. O'Brien SM, Shahian DM, Filardo G, Ferraris VA, Haan CK, Rich JB, Normand S-LT, DeLong ER, Shewan CM, Dokholyan RS, Peterson ED, Edwards FH, Anderson RP. The Society of Thoracic Surgeons 2008 cardiac surgery risk models: part 2 – isolated valve surgery. Ann Thorac Surg. 2009;88(1 Suppl):S23–42.
11. Shahian DM, O'Brien SM, Filardo G, Ferraris VA, Haan CK, Rich JB, Normand S-LT, DeLong ER, Shewan CM, Dokholyan RS, Peterson ED, Edwards FH, Anderson RP. The Society of Thoracic Surgeons 2008 cardiac surgery risk models: part 3 – valve plus coronary artery bypass grafting surgery. Ann Thorac Surg. 2009; 88(1 Suppl):S43–62.
12. Bach DS, Siao D, Girard SE, Duvernoy C, McCallister Jr BD, Gualano SK. Evaluation of patients with severe symptomatic aortic stenosis who do not undergo aortic valve replacement: the potential role of subjectively overestimated operative risk. Circ Cardiovasc Qual Outcomes. 2009;2(6):533–9.
13. Varadarajan P, Kapoor N, Bansal RC, Pai RG. Clinical profile and natural history of 453 nonsurgically managed patients with severe aortic stenosis. Ann Thorac Surg. 2006;82(6):2111–5.
14. Iung B, Cachier A, Baron G, Messika-Zeitoun D, Delahaye F, Tornos P, Gohlke-Bärwolf C, Boersma E, Ravaud P, Vahanian A. Decision-making in elderly patients with severe aortic stenosis: why are so many denied surgery? Eur Heart J. 2005; 26(24):2714–20.
15. Leipsic J, Gurvitch R, Labounty TM, Min JK, Wood D, Johnson M, Ajlan AM, Wijesinghe N, Webb JG. Multidetector computed tomography in transcatheter aortic valve implantation. JACC Cardiovasc Imaging. 2011;4(4):416–29.
16. Kodali SK, Williams MR, Smith CR, Svensson LG, Webb JG, Makkar RR, Fontana GP, Dewey TM, Thourani VH, Pichard AD, Fischbein M, Szeto WY, Lim S, Greason KL, Teirstein PS, Malaisrie SC, Douglas PS, Hahn RT, Whisenant B, Zajarias A, Wang D, Akin JJ, Anderson WN, Leon MB. Two-year outcomes after transcatheter or surgical aortic-valve replacement. N Engl J Med. 2012;366(18):1686–95.
17. Tamburino C, Capodanno D, Ramondo A, Petronio AS, Ettori F, Santoro G, Klugmann S, Bedogni F, Maisano F, Marzocchi A, Poli A, Antoniucci D, Napodano M, De Carlo M, Fiorina C, Ussia GP. Incidence and predictors of early and late mortality after transcatheter aortic valve implantation in 663 patients with severe aortic stenosis. Circulation. 2011;123(3):299–308.
18. Abdel-Wahab M, Zahn R, Horack M, Gerckens U, Schuler G, Sievert H, Eggebrecht H, Senges J, Richardt G. Aortic regurgitation after transcatheter aortic valve implantation: incidence and early outcome. Results from the German transcatheter aortic valve interventions registry. Heart. 2011;97(11):899–906.

19. Détaint D, Lepage L, Himbert D, Brochet E, Messika-Zeitoun D, Iung B, Vahanian A. Determinants of significant paravalvular regurgitation after transcatheter aortic valve: implantation impact of device and annulus discongruence. JACC Cardiovasc Interv. 2009;2(9):821–7.
20. Blanke P, Reinöhl J, Schlensak C, Siepe M, Pache G, Euringer W, Geibel-Zehender A, Bode C, Langer M, Beyersdorf F, Zehender M. Prosthesis oversizing in balloon-expandable transcatheter aortic valve implantation is associated with contained rupture of the aortic root. Circ Cardiovasc Interv. 2012;5(4):540–8.
21. Anderson RH. Clinical anatomy of the aortic root. Heart. 2000; 84(6):670–3.
22. Piazza N, de Jaegere P, Schultz C, Becker AE, Serruys PW, Anderson RH. Anatomy of the aortic valvar complex and its implications for transcatheter implantation of the aortic valve. Circ Cardiovasc Interv. 2008;1(1):74–81.
23. Baumgartner H, Hung J, Bermejo J, Chambers JB, Evangelista A, Griffin BP, Iung B, Otto CM, Pellikka PA, Quiñones M. Echocardiographic assessment of valve stenosis: EAE/ASE recommendations for clinical practice. J Am Soc Echocardiogr. 2009; 22(1):1–23; quiz 101–2.
24. Ng ACT, Delgado V, Van der Kley F, Shanks M, Van de Veire NRL, Bertini M, Nucifora G, Van Bommel RJ, Tops LF, De Weger A, Tavilla G, De Roos A, Kroft LJ, Leung DY, Schuijf J, Schalij MJ, Bax JJ. Comparison of aortic root dimensions and geometries before and after transcatheter aortic valve implantation by 2- and 3-dimensional transesophageal echocardiography and multislice computed tomography. Circ Cardiovasc Imaging. 2010;3(1):94–102.
25. Kempfert J, Van Linden A, Lehmkuhl L, Rastan AJ, Holzhey D, Blumenstein J, Mohr FW, Walther T. Aortic annulus sizing: echocardiographic vs. computed tomography derived measurements in comparison with direct surgical sizing. Eur J Cardiothorac. 2012. Available at: http://www.ncbi.nlm.nih.gov/pubmed/22402450. Accessed 21 Aug 2012.
26. Dashkevich A, Blanke P, Siepe M, Pache G, Langer M, Schlensak C, Beyersdorf F. Preoperative assessment of aortic annulus dimensions: comparison of noninvasive and intraoperative measurement. Ann Thorac Surg. 2011;91(3):709–14.
27. Messika-Zeitoun D, Serfaty J-M, Brochet E, Ducrocq G, Lepage L, Detaint D, Hyafil F, Himbert D, Pasi N, Laissy J-P, Iung B, Vahanian A. Multimodal assessment of the aortic annulus diameter: implications for transcatheter aortic valve implantation. J Am Coll Cardiol. 2010;55(3):186–94.
28. Tops LF, Wood DA, Delgado V, Schuijf JD, Mayo JR, Pasupati S, Lamers FPL, Van der Wall EE, Schalij MJ, Webb JG, Bax JJ. Noninvasive evaluation of the aortic root with multislice computed tomography implications for transcatheter aortic valve replacement. JACC Cardiovasc Imaging. 2008;1(3):321–30.
29. Delgado V, Ng ACT, Van de Veire NR, Van der Kley F, Schuijf JD, Tops LF, De Weger A, Tavilla G, De Roos A, Kroft LJ, Schalij MJ, Bax JJ. Transcatheter aortic valve implantation: role of multidetector row computed tomography to evaluate prosthesis positioning and deployment in relation to valve function. Eur Heart J. 2010;31(9):1114–23.
30. Hamdan A, Guetta V, Konen E, Goitein O, Segev A, Raanani E, Spiegelstein D, Hay I, Di Segni E, Eldar M, Schwammenthal E. Deformation dynamics and mechanical properties of the aortic annulus by 4-dimensional computed tomography: insights into the functional anatomy of the aortic valve complex and implications for transcatheter aortic valve therapy. J Am Coll Cardiol. 2012;59(2):119–27.
31. Bertaso AG, Wong DTL, Liew GYH, Cunnington MS, Richardson JD, Thomson VS, Lorraine B, Kourlis G, Leech D, Worthley MI, Worthley SG. Aortic annulus dimension assessment by computed tomography for transcatheter aortic valve implantation: differences between systole and diastole. Int J Cardiovasc Imaging. 2012. Available at: http://www.ncbi.nlm.nih.gov/pubmed/22318541. Accessed 21 Aug 2012.
32. Ng ACT, Yiu K-H, Ewe SH, Van der Kley F, Bertini M, De Weger A, De Roos A, Leung DY, Schuijf JD, Schalij MJ, Bax JJ, Delgado V. Influence of left ventricular geometry and function on aortic annular dimensions as assessed with multi-detector row computed tomography: implications for transcatheter aortic valve implantation. Eur Heart J. 2011;32(22):2806–13.
33. Buzzatti N, Maisano F, Latib A, Cioni M, Taramasso M, Mussardo M, Colombo A, Alfieri O. Computed tomography-based evaluation of aortic annulus, prosthesis size and impact on early residual aortic regurgitation after transcatheter aortic valve implantation. Eur J Cardiothorac Surg. 2012. Available at: http://www.ncbi.nlm.nih.gov/pubmed/22551969. Accessed 22 Aug 2012.
34. Willson AB, Webb JG, Labounty TM, Achenbach S, Moss R, Wheeler M, Thompson C, Min JK, Gurvitch R, Norgaard BL, Hague CJ, Toggweiler S, Binder R, Freeman M, Poulter R, Poulsen S, Wood DA, Leipsic J. 3-dimensional aortic annular assessment by multidetector computed tomography predicts moderate or severe paravalvular regurgitation after transcatheter aortic valve replacement: a multicenter retrospective analysis. J Am Coll Cardiol. 2012;59(14):1287–94.
35. Jilaihawi H, Kashif M, Fontana G, Furugen A, Shiota T, Friede G, Makhija R, Doctor N, Leon MB, Makkar RR. Cross-sectional computed tomographic assessment improves accuracy of aortic annular sizing for transcatheter aortic valve replacement and reduces the incidence of paravalvular aortic regurgitation. J Am Coll Cardiol. 2012;59(14):1275–86.
36. Gurvitch R, Webb JG, Yuan R, Johnson M, Hague C, Willson AB, Toggweiler S, Wood DA, Ye J, Moss R, Thompson CR, Achenbach S, Min JK, Labounty TM, Cury R, Leipsic J. Aortic annulus diameter determination by multidetector computed tomography: reproducibility, applicability, and implications for transcatheter aortic valve implantation. JACC Cardiovasc Interv. 2011;4(11): 1235–45.

Coaxial Angle Prediction for TAVR: CT

26

Mathew Brooks and Ronen Gurvitch

Abstract

Procedural success in transcatheter aortic valve replacement (TAVR) depends on precise positioning and deployment of the valve in the three-dimensional aortic annulus and root. Fluoroscopy is the imaging modality typically relied on during valve positioning and deployment in TAVR. Accurate coaxial positioning of the valve with this method is best achieved by selecting a fluoroscopic deployment projection that is perpendicular to the native aortic valve plane. The use of a suboptimal "off-axis" fluoroscopic deployment projection may result in incorrect valve positioning and in turn lead to paravalvular aortic regurgitation, valve embolization, coronary ostium obstruction, heart block, or interference with the mitral valve apparatus [1–3]. Traditionally the native aortic plane has been assessed by invasive aortic root angiography, often requiring a number of aortograms be performed until a satisfactory projection is obtained. Frequently, however, such perpendicular projections are difficult to determine with significant contrast media utilized in attempts to do so in patients who often have significant renal dysfunction. More recently, multislice computed tomography (MDCT) has emerged as an accurate and practical alternative to repeated aortograms, providing operators with precise implant projections that can be determined prior to the procedure (Box 26.1). This chapter will outline the practical uses of MSCT to help predict the correct implant projection and review the available evidence with this technique.

Keywords

Transcatheter valve implantation • Angle prediction • Computed tomography

Introduction

Procedural success in transcatheter aortic valve replacement (TAVR) depends on precise positioning and deployment of the valve in the three-dimensional aortic annulus and root. Fluoroscopy is the imaging modality typically relied on during valve positioning and deployment in TAVR. Accurate coaxial positioning of the valve with this method is best achieved by selecting a fluoroscopic deployment projection that is perpendicular to the native aortic valve plane. The use of a suboptimal "off-axis" fluoroscopic deployment projection may result in incorrect valve positioning and in turn lead to paravalvular aortic regurgitation, valve embolization, coronary ostium obstruction, heart block, or interference with the mitral valve apparatus [1–3]. Traditionally the native aortic plane has been assessed by invasive aortic root angiography, often requiring a number of aortograms be performed until a satisfactory projection is obtained. Frequently, however, such perpendicular projections are difficult to determine with significant contrast media utilized in attempts to do so in patients who often have significant renal dysfunction. More recently, multislice computed tomography (MDCT) has emerged as an accurate and practical alternative to repeated aortograms, providing operators with precise implant projections that can be determined prior to the procedure (Box 26.1). This chapter will outline the practical uses of MSCT to help predict the correct implant projection and review the available evidence with this technique.

M. Brooks, MD, MBBS, FRACP
R. Gurvitch, MD, MBBS, FRACP (✉)
Department of Cardiology, Royal Melbourne Hospital, Grattan Street, Parkville, Melbourne, VIC 3050, Australia
e-mail: ronen_gurvitch@yahoo.com.au

J.K. Min et al. (eds.), *Multimodality Imaging for Transcatheter Aortic Valve Replacement*, DOI 10.1007/978-1-4471-2798-7_26, © Springer-Verlag London 2014

Box 26.1 MDCT Angle Prediction for TAVR

- CT studies have shown that the average line of perpendicularity runs from a RAO-caudal projection with zero-crossings at approximately 10–15° caudal and 10–15° LAO.
- One method for generating an optimal co-axial angle is to start by placing a point on the inferior most aspect of each aortic valve cusp.
- Care must be taken to identify the most inferior margin of each aortic cusp from the orthogonal projection of the root.
- Angles are determined manually by rotating the three dimensional (3D) aortic reconstruction to discern the appropriate projection.
- An angle is deemed appropriate when the triangle is no longer evident; that is, when it appears as a single line.
- Advantages: Reduction in procedure time, procedural contrast volume, and fluoroscopic time used for the procedure.

Native Aortic Valve Plane

The native aortic valve is typically orientated in a left oblique plane with slight anterior angulation. As a result when assessing for suitable fluoroscopic deployment projections, right anterior oblique (RAO) views tend to require caudal angulation, and left anterior oblique (LAO) views require some cranial angulation to achieve perpendicularity with the native aortic valve plane. MSCT and C-arm CT studies have shown that the average line of perpendicularity runs from a RAO-caudal projection with zero crossings at approximately 10–15° caudal and 10–15° LAO, before continuing with increasing cranial requirement for steeper LAO projections (Fig. 26.1) [4, 5]. The precise degree of caudal and cranial angulation required at each LAO or RAO point varies between patients, necessitating the need for individualized assessment. Evaluation of the native aortic valve plane has conventionally been carried out by performing repeated aortic root angiograms. Multiple orthogonal aortic root angiograms are performed until a suitable projection perpendicular to the valve plane is found (Fig. 26.2). In general, aortic root angiograms may begin at either straight caudal 10° or LAO 10° with small adjustments made accordingly, reflecting the average line of perpendicularity. Despite this, it is rare to find a satisfactory projection with the first or second aortic root angiogram, and in some patients, finding an appropriate plane can be difficult to achieve. This is particularly so with extreme or unusual aortic valve and root angulation such as in patients with musculoskeletal abnormalities, kyphoscoliosis, or horizontal or unfolded aortas. Furthermore, heavily calcified aortic valve leaflets may obscure the remaining cusps, making accurate visualization of the valve plane difficult. In these difficult cases, additional contrast (approximately 10–15 ml per repeated aortic root angiogram), time

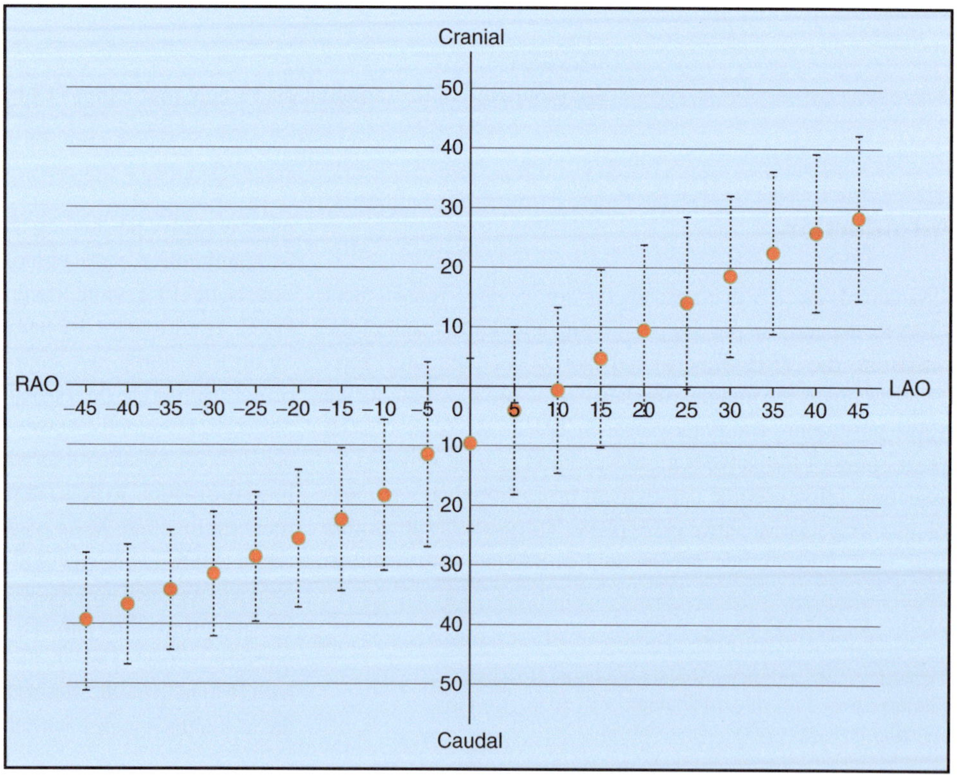

Fig. 26.1 "Line of perpendicularity." This curve demonstrates the average caudal or cranial angulation required across the RAO to LAO spectrum to achieve perpendicularity to the valve plane

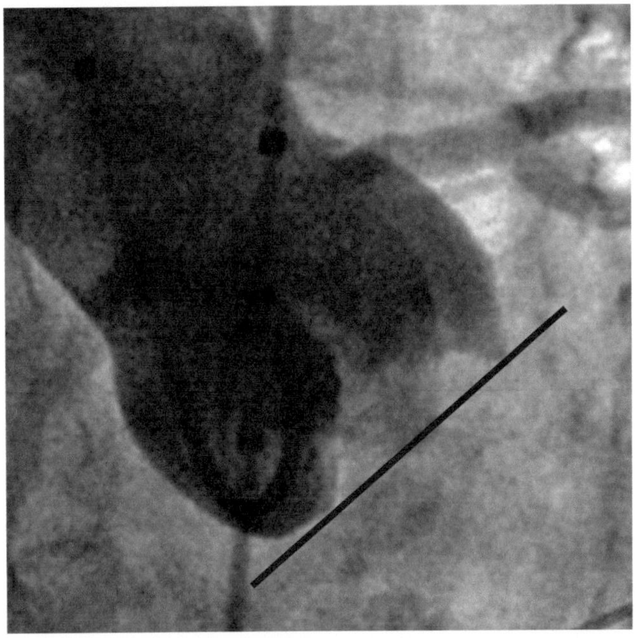

Fig. 26.2 Determination of the correct aortic valve plane. A fluoroscopic projection where the inferior margins of the three sinuses of Valsalva provide a perpendicular view to the aortic valve plane (*black line*)

and radiation exposure is required. In some cases, despite additional attempts, an acceptable projection cannot be found. MDCT is an alternative method that enables prediction of optimal fluoroscopic deployment projections, with data that can be extrapolated from routine MDCT studies prior to TAVR. Both MSCT and more recently C-arm CT have been used for this purpose with their ability to accurately predict deployment projections now demonstrated in small studies [4–6].

Multislice Computed Tomography

Image Acquisition

Multislice computed tomography (MSCT) uses three-dimensional volume-rendered transparent reconstructions of the thoracic aorta. Reconstructions are produced on workstations from double oblique transverse images (Fig. 26.3). Projections perpendicular to the native aortic valve plane are found by placing a point on the inferior most aspect of each aortic valve cusp. From these points, a triangular trace can be created. Particular attention must be paid to determining the most inferior margin of each aortic cusp from the orthogonal projection of the root. If the inferior margin is chosen erroneously for one or more aortic cusps, the valve plane chosen may be incorrect. Angles at present are determined manually by rotating the three-dimensional aortic reconstructions to discern the appropriate projection. An angle is deemed appropriate when the triangle is not evident and is replaced by a line, suggesting that the three placed points are in line. A contrast volume of between 80 and 120 ml is usually required for image acquisition, which includes imaging of the peripheral vasculature.

Predictive Accuracy

Preliminary studies evaluating the ability of MSCT to accurately predict optimal fluoroscopic deployment projections have been promising. *Kurra* et al. conducted a small prospective study comparing MSCT-generated predictive angles with conventional angiography. The degree of cranial and caudal angulation required to obtain an optimal projection angle in both LAO 40° and RAO 20° projections was assessed using both modalities. A suitable deployment projection could be found in all patients with the use of MSCT and in 38 of 40 patients using conventional angiography. The degree of cranial angulation required in the LAO view was not significantly different between the two modalities (cranial: 25 ± 9 vs. 23 ± 8, $p = 0.214$). A small but significant difference in the degree of caudal angulation required in the RAO projection was demonstrated between conventional angiography and matched MSCT images (caudal 21 ± 9 vs. $29 \pm 10°$, $p = 0.002$), but no post-deployment assessment was made for either modality to determine accuracy.

The accuracy of MSCT compared with conventional angiography in determining optimal angiographic deployment projections has to date only been evaluated in one study [4]. Twenty patients who underwent TAVR with pre-procedural MSCT angle prediction were compared with a proceeding consecutive cohort of 20 patients that underwent TAVR with conventional angiographic angle prediction. Baseline characteristics were well matched in both groups. Post-deployment accuracy of each predicted fluoroscopic projection was classified as excellent, satisfactory, or poor (as defined in Fig. 26.4). When MSCT was used, an excellent or satisfactory final valve implant projection angle was achieved in 18 cases (90 %) versus 13 cases (65 %) when conventional angiography was used. While statistical significance was not achieved ($p = 0.06$), a strong trend was observed favoring MSCT. Given that both TAVR and the utilization of MSCT to generate predictive angiographic deployment projection are relatively new technologies, larger studies assessing the role of MSCT are yet to be conducted and furthermore, no outcome data is currently available.

Additional Advantages

The use of MSCT to generated predictive angles offers additional advantages. In TAVR patients, MSCT has a

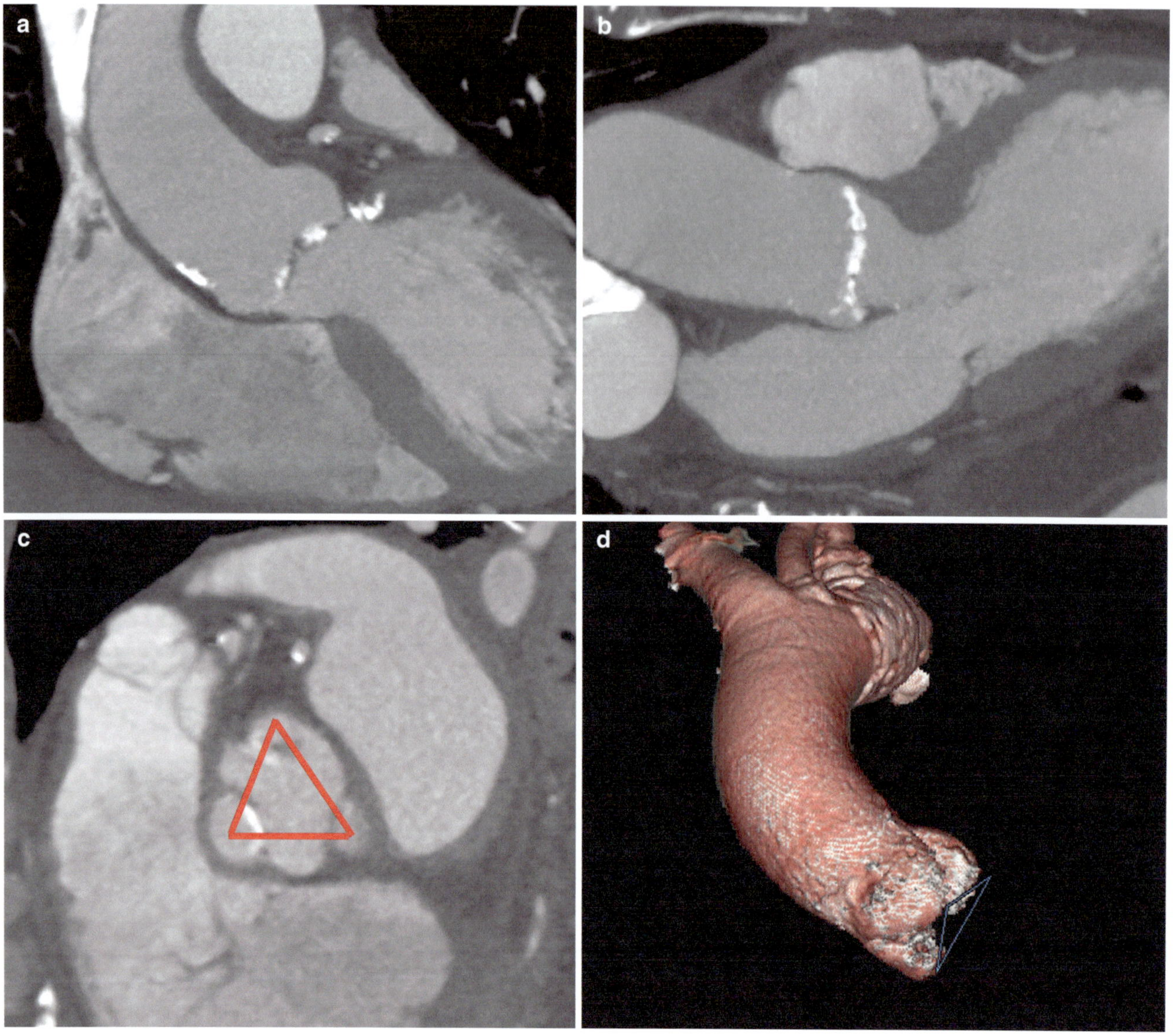

Fig. 26.3 Stepwise approach to construction of a three-dimensional volume-rendered image of the aortic root. The aorta is bisected from a routine coronal projection (**a**) to create a sagittal oblique multiplanar reformat (**b**). From the sagittal oblique, an orthogonal projection of the root (**c**) is acquired using the standard oblique workstation tool. After scrolling to the most inferior margins of the aortic cusps on the orthogonal projection of the root, points are deposited on these most inferior margins and linked in a *triangular fashion* (**d**). A three-dimensional volume-rendered image of the ascending aorta is then created with the *triangle* in place

well-established role in pre-procedural assessment and planning [7–11]. MSCT provides detailed assessment of:

- Aortic valve characteristics (annulus size, leaflet number, and degree of calcification which can be used in conjugation with echocardiography derived data)
- Annulus to coronary artery ostium height
- Iliofemoral arterial anatomy (aiding in determining suitability for transfemoral approach)

Given the important and near universal pre-procedural use of MSCT, concurrent assessment of the optimal angiographic deployment projections during the MSCT scan is appealing. Pre-procedural determination of an optimal MSCT-generated predictive angle will reduce procedural time and contrast volume particularly in patients whom the native aortic valve plane is significantly varied from that normally observed. The three-dimensional nature of the MSCT image set allows for endless reformations of potential fluoroscopic deployment projections for any LAO and RAO angulation. In some cases, this may provide timely practical benefits with regard to radiation, equipment, and ergonomics. For example, if in the cranial-caudal axis, a very steep caudal angle (>40) is predicted for a given patient, this may be difficult to achieve given the constraints of the patient's body and the table.

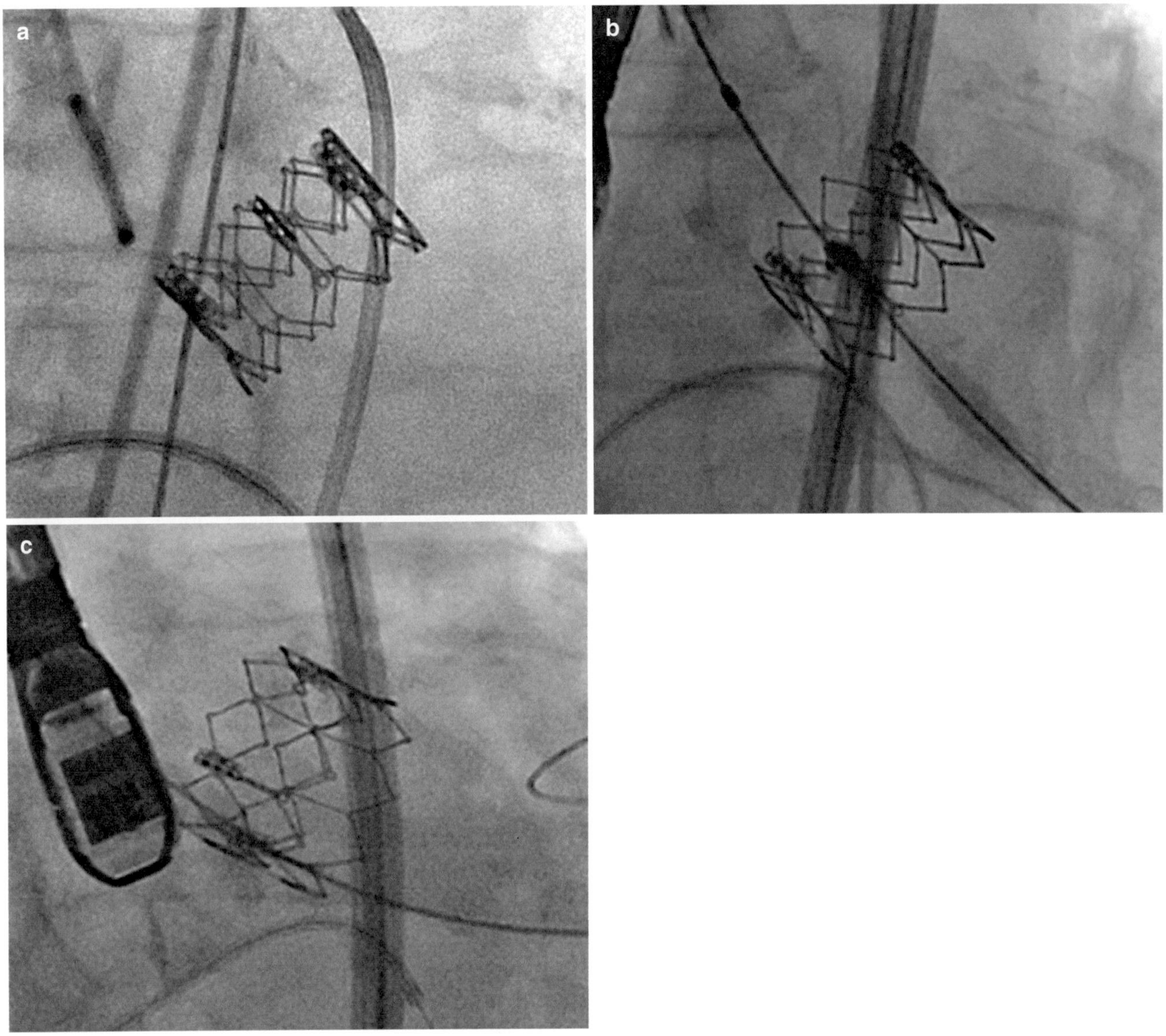

Fig. 26.4 Accuracy of angiographic projection of valve deployment. (**a**) Excellent—superior struts line up perfectly. (**b**) Satisfactory—superior valve struts project differently but within the height of a cell. (**c**) Poor—superior valve struts project in different planes, with a distance greater than the height of a cell

Limitations

While preliminary studies have highlighted the potential advantages of using MSCT-generated predictive angles, limitations exist and sole reliance on this technology in all comers cannot be advised. The quality of the MSCT images obtained, unsurprisingly, strongly influences the predictive accuracy of this modality and must be taken into account by TAVR operators. Significant motion or calcification artifact, poor contrast opacification, and suboptimal image gating can degrade MSCT image quality. Through assigning the MSCT-generated predictive angles a Likert score of 1–3 based on image quality and reporter confidence, *Gurvitch* et al. demonstrated that predictive accuracy is proportional to image quality [4]. When the confidence grade was poor, in 73 % of cases, the predicted angles would have resulted in suboptimal deployment angles. When the confidence grade was high however, >90 % of angles were excellent or satisfactory. While the use of this method of assessment was in its beginnings at the time this study was performed, the incidence of suboptimal projections was not insignificant (occurring in 15 of the 60 generated predictive angles), and furthermore in 95 % of cases, all Likert scores were either the same or within 1 score for all projections. This has important implications for the widespread use of such technology, especially during the learning curve of each center. TAVR operators should be aware that

MSCT-generated predictive angles should be used with caution when the source of MSCT images is suboptimal. In addition, prediction error with MSCT may occur if significant variation in patient positioning exists between MSCT and the TAVR procedure. The contrast load required is also problematic in patients with significant preexisting renal impairment.

C-Arm CT

Image Acquisition

C-arm CT enables three-dimensional reconstructions to be generated from images obtained during C-arm rotational aortic root angiography. Radiographic contrast is injected through a pigtail catheter placed in the aortic root during the rotational aortic root angiography acquisition. Immediately before and during injection, breath hold and rapid ventricular pacing is initiated. The volume data set can be reconstructed on a dedicated workstation. A contrast volume of between 20 and 32 ml is typically required. Post automatic depiction of the aortic valve cusps, a circle is created indicating the aortic valve plane. As with MSCT, the aortic root reconstruction is rotated until the circle appears as a straight line, indicating a view perpendicular to the valve.

Predictive Accuracy

At present, trial data evaluating the role of C-arm CT for angle prediction is limited with only one, nonrandomized trial published to date. *Binder* et al. evaluated C-arm CT for prediction of the optimal deployment angle and compared it with MSCT [5]. C-arm CT was able to provide adequate image quality for reproducible angle predictions in 97.5 % of cases (39 of the 40 patients enrolled). Image acquisition was safe with no significant complications, particularly from the rapid ventricular pacing or contrast load, observed. Significant correlation between C-arm CT and MSCT was found for predictions of perpendicular valve view angles ($r=0.682$, $p<0.001$). The correlation was significant for angles close to midsagittal projections as well as for extreme RAO/LAO angulations. Accuracy was determined by drawing regression lines of the predicted angles for each patient and method and calculating the shortest distance to the post-deployment perpendicular prosthesis projection. Both modalities were highly accurate with deviation from the regression line of predicted angles to the post-deployment prosthesis view which was small ($5.1 \pm 4.6°$ for C-arm CT and $7.9 \pm 4.9°$ for MDCT $p=0.01$). The regression lines were parallel, but the lines of the C-arm CT were shifted approximately 3° more caudal to the MSCT lines, which the authors suggested may be caused by patient positioning.

Given the ability to perform C-arm CT on the table during the TAVR procedure, it eliminates any potential error related to variation in patient position, which can occur with MSCT. Furthermore, lower contrast volume is required (typically 20–32 ml), which is of particular relevance in patients with significant renal dysfunction.

Conclusion

In TAVR, the use of a fluoroscopic projection perpendicular to the native aortic valve plane is important in achieving accurate valve positioning and deployment. While repeated invasive aortic root angiography has traditionally been used, CT has emerged as a promising and practical alternative. Preliminary studies have demonstrated that pre-procedural MSCT and C-arm CT are accurate and safe in predicting optimal angiographic deployment projections and may indeed be superior to conventional aortic root angiography. Pre-procedural angle prediction with the use of CT reduces the number of aortograms required, therefore shortening both procedural time and contrast usage. The predictive accuracy of MSCT is, however, poor in patients whom suboptimal MSCT image quality is obtained. Larger randomized controlled trials are required to further evaluate including assessment of outcome data between the various modalities.

References

1. Wong DR, Ye J, Cheung A, Webb JB, Carera RG, Lichtenstein SV. Technical considerations to avoid pitfalls during transapical aortic valve implantation. J Thorac Cardiovasc Surg. 2010;140:196–202.
2. Al Ali AM, Altwegg L, Horlick EM, et al. Prevention and management of transcatheter balloon-expandable aortic valve malposition. Catheter Cardiovasc Interv. 2008;72:573–8.
3. Massoon JB, Kovac J, Schuler G, et al. Transcatheter aortic valve implantation: review of the nature, management, and avoidance of procedural complications. J Am Coll Cardiol Intv. 2009;2:811–20.
4. Gurvitch R, Wood DA, Leipsic J, et al. Multislice computed tomography for prediction of optimal angiographic deployment projections during transcatheter aortic valve implantation. J Am Coll Cardiol Intv. 2010;3:1157–65.
5. Binder RK, Leipsic J, Wood DA, et al. Prediction of optimal deployment projection for transcatheter aortic valve replacement: angiographic 3-dimensional reconstruction of the aortic root versus multidetector computed tomography. Circ Cardiovasc Interv. 2012;5:247–52.
6. Kurra V, Kapadia SR, Tuzcu EM, et al. Pre-procedural imaging of aortic root orientation and dimension: comparisons between X-ray angiographic planar imaging and 3-dimensional multidetector row computed tomography. J Am Coll Cardiol Intv. 2010;3:105–13.
7. Ng AC, Delgado V, Van der Kley F, et al. Comparison of aortic root dimensions and geometries before and after transcatheter aortic valve implantation by 2- and 3-dimensional transesophageal echocardiography and multislice computed tomography. Circ Cardiovasc Imaging. 2010;3:94–102.

8. Wood DA, Tops LF, Mayo JR, et al. Role of multislice computed tomography in transcatheter aortic valve replacement. Am J Cardiol. 2009;103:1295–301.
9. Tops LF, Wood DA, Delgado V, et al. Noninvasive evaluation of the aortic root with multislice computed tomography implications for transcatheter aortic valve replacement. J Am Coll Cardiol Img. 2008;1:321–30.
10. Leipsic J, Wood DA, Manders D, et al. The evolving role of MDCT in transcatheter aortic valve replacement: a radiologists' perspective. AJR Am J Roentgenol. 2009;193:W214–9.
11. Leipsic J, Hague CJ, Gurvitch R, et al. MDCT to guide transcatheter aortic valve replacement and mitral valve repair. Cardiol Clin. 2012;30(1):147–60.

Use of Multidetector Computed Tomography for Planning Transcatheter Aortic Valve Sizing

27

Adam Berger, Alexander Bruce Willson, James K. Min, Daniel Grafstein, and Jonathon Leipsic

Abstract

Computed tomography (CT) has an increasingly important role in transcatheter aortic valve replacement (TAVR), offering noninvasive three-dimensional measurements of the aortic annulus which are used for transcatheter heart valve (THV) sizing. Accurate valve sizing is vital to reduce the risk of complications with TAVR, particular paravalvular aortic regurgitation, aortic annular rupture, and coronary occlusion. In this chapter, we review the anatomy of the aortic annulus, the historical move towards three-dimensional annular measurement, how to incorporate these measurements into valve sizing, and future perspectives of CT-based valve sizing.

Keywords

Aortic valve • Transcatheter heart valve • Stenosis • Regurgitation Doppler echocardiography • Computed tomography • Cardiac magnetic resonance

A. Berger, MBBS, MPH
Department of Medical Imaging, St Paul's Hospital UBC, Vancouver, BC, Canada

Division of Cardiology, Department of Radiology, University of British Columbia, St. Paul's Hospital, 1081 Burrard St, Vancouver, BC V6S 1Y6, Canada

A.B. Willson, MBBS (Hons), MPH, FRACP
Division of Cardiology, Department of Radiology, University of British Columbia, St. Paul's Hospital, 1081 Burrard St, Vancouver, BC V6S 1Y6, Canada

Department of Cardiology, Nambour General Hospital, Hospital Road, Nambour, QLD 4560, Australia
e-mail: alwillson77@hotmail.com

J.K. Min, MD, FACC, FSCCT
Weill Cornell Medical College, NewYork-Presbyterian Hospital, New York, NY, USA
e-mail: jkm2001@med.cornell.edu

D. Grafstein, MD
Department of Medical Imaging, St Paul's Hospital UBC, Vancouver, BC, Canada

J. Leipsic, MD, FRCPC, FSCCT (✉)
Division of Cardiology, Department of Radiology, University of British Columbia, St. Paul's Hospital, 1081 Burrard St, Vancouver, BC V6S 1Y6, Canada
e-mail: jleipsic@providencehealth.bc.ca

Abbreviations

AVR	Aortic valve replacement
MDCT	Multidetector computed tomography
PAR	Paravalvular regurgitation
TAVR	Transcatheter aortic valve replacement
TEE	Transesophageal echocardiography
THV	Transcatheter aortic valve
TTE	Transthoracic echocardiography

Introduction

Computed tomography (CT) has an increasingly important role in transcatheter aortic valve replacement (TAVR), offering noninvasive three-dimensional measurements of the aortic annulus which are used for transcatheter heart valve (THV) sizing. Accurate valve sizing is vital to reduce the risk of complications with TAVR, particular paravalvular aortic regurgitation, aortic annular rupture, and coronary occlusion. In this chapter, we review the anatomy of the aortic annulus, the historical move towards three-dimensional annular measurement, how to incorporate

J.K. Min et al. (eds.), *Multimodality Imaging for Transcatheter Aortic Valve Replacement*, DOI 10.1007/978-1-4471-2798-7_27, © Springer-Verlag London 2014

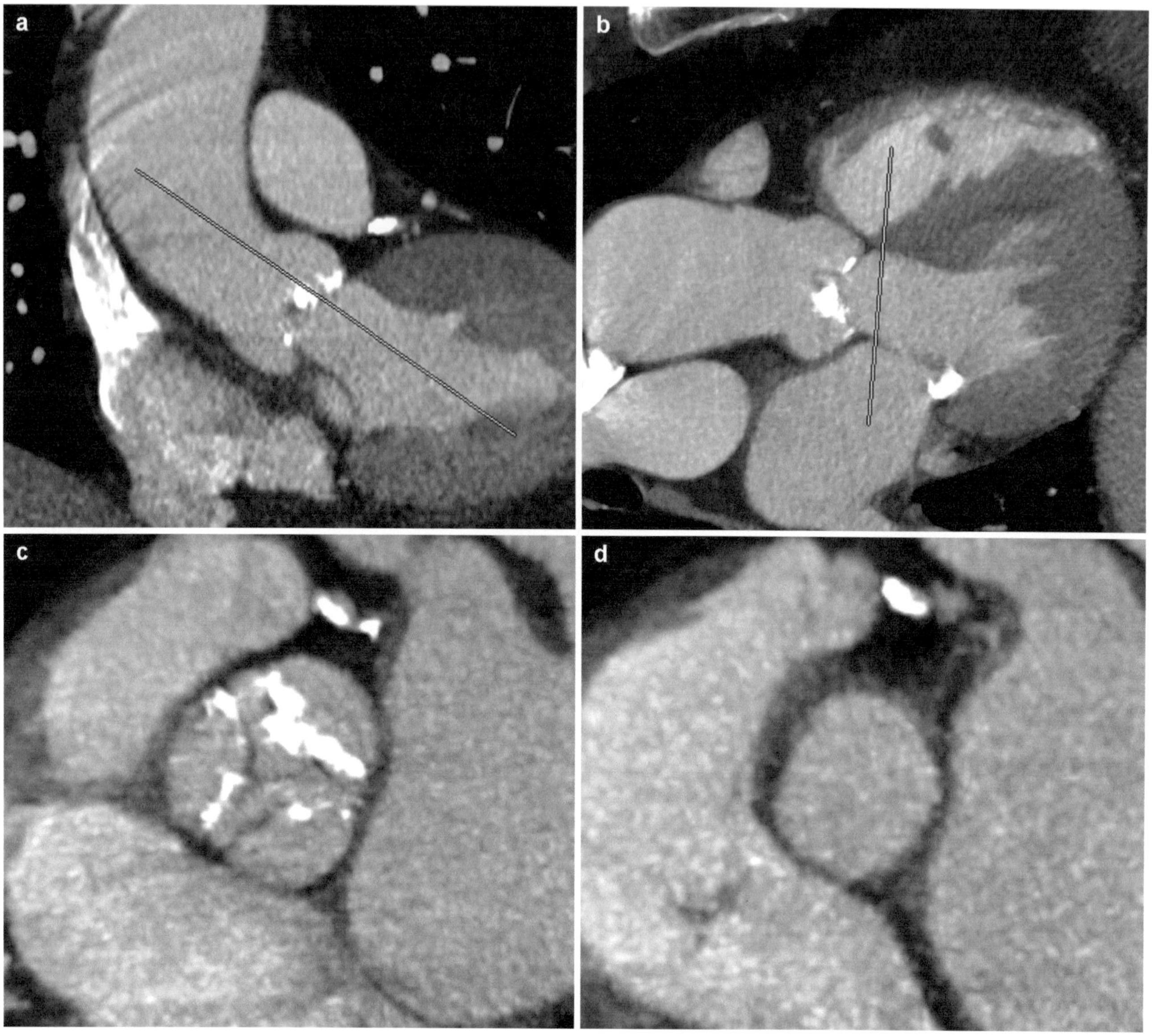

Fig. 27.1 Reconstructing a double oblique transverse image of the basal ring from an MDCT in an 82-year-old male patient with severe symptomatic AS. From the coronal projection (**a**), a vertically oriented oblique tool is placed to produce a sagittal oblique reconstruction of the ascending aorta. A transverse or axial cut plane is then placed on the sagittal reconstruction (**b**) at the level of the commissures. This transverse cut plane yields a double oblique transverse image of the aortic root (**c**). The dataset is then scrolled up or down until the most caudal attachments of the aortic valve are identified (**d**). The nadirs of all three cusps must be identified on the one transverse image, ensuring the appropriate plane for assessment of the aortic annulus. Not uncommonly, these simple four steps yield only a double oblique transverse image of two of the aortic cusps, and it may often require the further rotation of the sagittal oblique projection until the third cusp comes into view

these measurements into valve sizing, and future perspectives of CT-based valve sizing.

Aortic Root Anatomy

The aortic root is the direct continuation of the left ventricular outflow tract and extends from the basal attachment of the aortic valve cusps within the left ventricle itself to their peripheral attachment at the level of the sinotubular junction. The root is widest at the midpoints of the sinuses and smaller at the basal attachment of the leaflets and the sinotubular junction [1, 2]. The semilunar leaflet insertions take the form of a three-pronged coronet rather than forming a ring as implied by the term "annulus." The base of the crown can be thought of as a virtual ring, formed by the most basal attachment points of the three cusps (Fig. 27.1) [1, 2].

Although much was known about the anatomical configuration of the annulus, insight into the in vivo anatomy of the aortic valvular complex—previously available only from surgical or pathological observation of a non-beating heart—only became possible with modern three-dimensional imaging techniques [2]. The aortic annulus has been shown to be noncircular on both 3D transesophageal echocardiography (3D TEE)

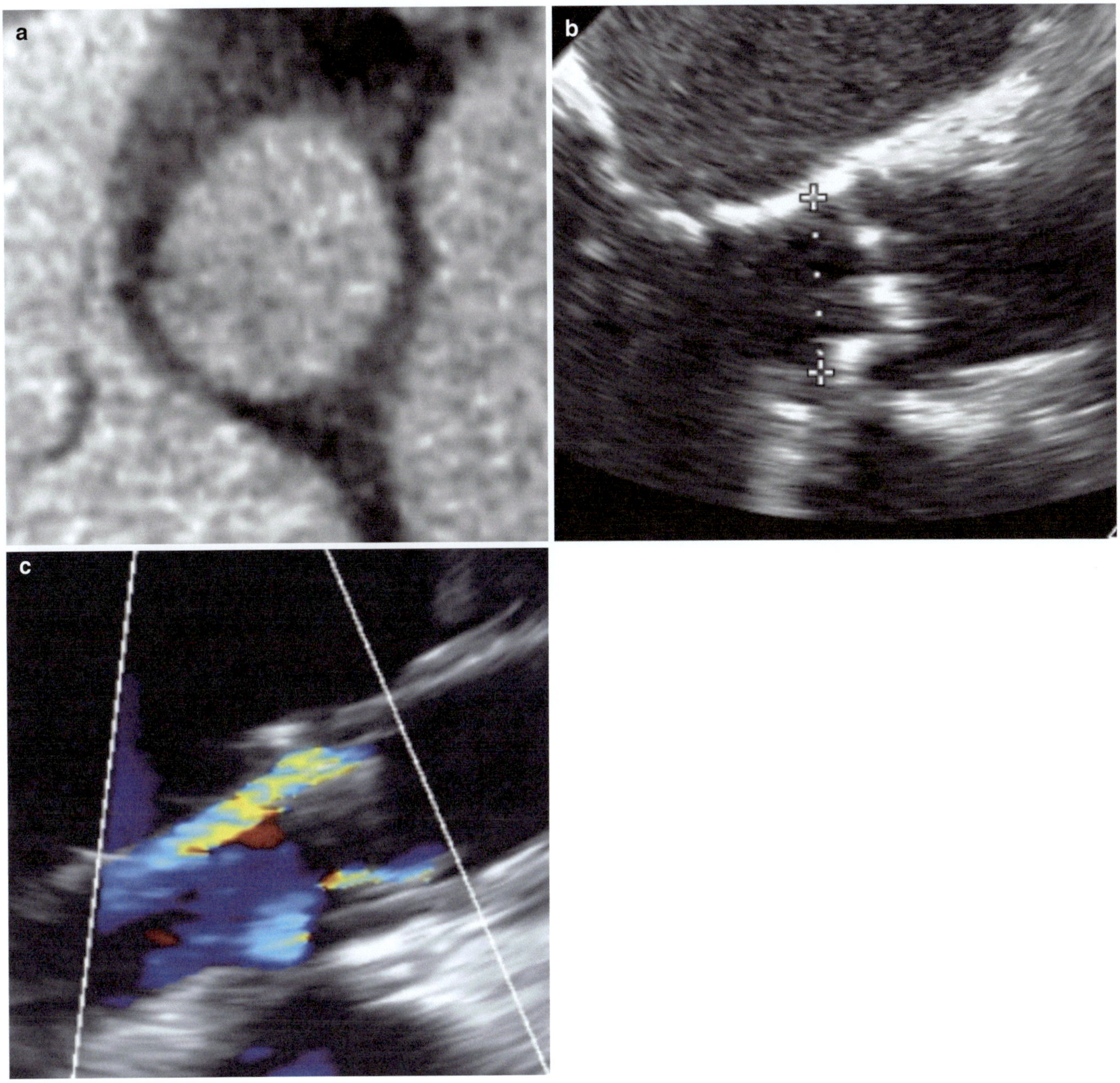

Fig. 27.2 Representative images of the basal ring in a 78-year-old male patient with aortic stenosis. The annulus was deemed too large for a balloon-expandable prosthesis with a mean diameter of 30.7 mm (short axis of 27.9 mm and long axis of 33.5 mm) (**a**) and an area of 8.04 cm^2 (**b**). The 29-mm SAPIEN XT has a nominal area of 6.6 cm^2 which is clearly too small for this annulus and would result in approximately 17 % undersizing of the annulus. The post-TAVR TTE shows the resultant moderate paravalvular regurgitation (**c**)

and multidetector computed tomography (MDCT) [3–5]. As a result of this elliptical configuration, the aortic annulus does not lend itself to accurate evaluation by a two-dimensional imaging modality that measures an axial diameter.

The aortic root is dynamic, with the aortic annulus subject to pulsatile changes of the cardiac cycle and contour deformity related to movement of the aorto-mitral continuity and dynamic left atrial volume and pressure changes [6, 7]. Subsequent changes in geometry and dimensions have to be considered when selecting a THV size and historically have been underappreciated by two-dimensional imaging.

Aortic Annulus Measurement with Computed Tomography

Enabled by the isotropic voxels acquired with CT, the aortic annulus can be assessed in its true plane at the level of the basal ring. When the plane of the aortic annulus is achieved, it can be measured in a number of ways. Most commonly, the long axis (maximum) and the short axis (minimum) are measured allowing for the calculation of a mean diameter. Planimetry can also be performed enabling both perimeter and area measurements (Fig. 27.2). Derived diameters can then be calculated based on the formula for the area of a circle or the perimeter of a circle, respectively, although there are real limitations in deriving diameters from these three-dimensional measurements [8, 9].

The above CT measurements have been shown to be highly reproducible with low inter- and intra-observer variability [6, 8]. The area-derived diameter and basal ring average diameters are consistently measured as larger than the corresponding echocardiographic measurements, with a mean difference when compared with TEE-derived diameter of 1.5 ± 1.6 and 1.1 ± 1.7 mm respectively.

Aortic Annular Geometry and THV Sizing: Evolving Role of CT

Noninvasive assessment and measurement of the aortic annulus is essential for the success of TAVR. An undersized valve increases the risk of post-procedural paravalvular aortic regurgitation, while excessive oversizing may increase the risk of coronary occlusion or annular rupture. Excessive oversizing may also result in embolization, as the valve may not capture appropriately resulting in the so-called melon seeding and subsequent embolization into the aorta particularly in the setting of significant septal hypertrophy. Reproducible and accurate measurements of the aortic annulus allow appropriate selection of THV size (Box 27.1).

Box 27.1 Methods of CT Aortic Annular Sizing

Measure	Recommendation	Used clinically?
Area	Yes	Currently used at certain centers for balloon-expandable valve
Coronal measure	No	Obliquity of aorta different for different individuals
Long-axis diameter	No	Excess variability
Mean diameter	Yes	Currently used at certain centers for balloon expandable valve
Max diameter – stent diameter >4 mm	Yes	Currently used at certain centers for balloon expandable valve
Perimeter	Yes	Currently used a measure for self-expanding valves
Sagittal	No	Obliquity of aorta different for different individuals
Short axis diameter	No	Excess variability

Unlike surgical aortic valve replacement, where prosthesis sizing is performed using a sizing probe under direct visualization, TAVR relies exclusively on pre- and periprocedural imaging for valve selection. Annular measurements have historically been performed using two-dimensional (2D) transthoracic echocardiography (TTE), transesophageal echocardiography (TEE), or calibrated aortic angiography, with discordance between these measurements being common [9, 10]. The noncircular geometry of the aortic annulus results in an underappreciation of annular size when using two-dimensional imaging techniques [6–8]. In a recent analysis performed in 125 patients undergoing TAVR from two sites, the mean difference between the long and short axis of the aortic annulus was 5.5 mm [6].

There has been growing interest in better defining the shape and size of the annulus through the integration of three-dimensional (3D) imaging tools such as CT, magnetic resonance imaging (MRI), and 3D TEE [3]. Annular assessment with 3D TEE has reported larger annular sizes than those observed using traditional 2D TEE [3]. ECG-gated CT was historically performed in patients before TAVR implantation to evaluate peripheral vascular access, annular plane, and coronary height, however, is increasingly being used to measure annular size [4]. Current sizing recommendations and clinical practice are derived from the currently available randomized data [9, 10] in which the annular size was estimated using echocardiographic measurements. Clinical outcomes with TEE-based annulus determination and routine oversizing of the valve by 1 to 2 mm have been good, but the burden of post-TAVR moderate or severe paravalvular aortic regurgitation (PAR) remains approximately 10–15 % [11]. The importance of post-TAVR PAR is increasingly recognized as being of great importance with the recently published 2-year PARTNER B outcome data not only suggesting that 40 % of patients alive at 2 years have at least mild PAR, but, perhaps more importantly, that those patients with PAR have a significantly worse prognosis than those without [11]. While PAR may not be exclusively related to undersizing, there is a growing awareness that two-dimensional imaging does not allow for an adequate appreciation of annular geometry and may lead to inappropriate sizing. This issue has led to the exploration of three-dimensional imaging modalities for annular sizing, such as 3D TEE and CT. The hope is that annular measurements acquired using 3D techniques will provide a more global assessment of annular geometry and eccentricity, allow for more accurate sizing of the THV, and thereby reduce the burden of post-TAVR PAR [6, 12]. At present, there are specific annular size limitations for TAVR based on echocardiographic measures of the annulus. For the Edwards SAPIEN valve, the annulus must measure between 18 and 25 mm; for the current generation of CoreValve, the annulus must range between 20 and 27 mm. Recently, both a 20-mm transfemoral and a 29-mm transfemoral/transapical balloon-expandable SAPIEN XT valve have become available.

Proposed CT Sizing Guidelines for Transcatheter Heart Valves

While sizing guidelines with CT remain a goal for TAVR, it must first be recognized that the implications of three-dimensional sizing are different for balloon-expandable and self-expanding prostheses. For the balloon-expandable prosthesis, a CT-based THV sizing scale is a work in progress. This process has largely grown out of retrospective analyses of cohorts with and without PAR in an attempt to better understand appropriate THV sizing. Gurvitch et al. [8] have shown that CT sizing using the mean of basal short- and long-axis diameters could influence or modify TAVR strategy in up to 44 % of patients. Given the success of the procedure, the suggestion of altering sizing in 40–45 % of cases has largely been rejected by the TAVR community. This is almost certainly appropriate given that at present the only randomized data documenting the efficacy of TAVR is based on echocardiographic sizing of the annulus. However, when the THV sizing cutoffs were adjusted to allow for the measured differences in diameters between echocardiographic-derived and CT-derived data, the THV size would have been modified in only 10–12 %.

While the evidence does not yet support the replacement of standard echocardiographic annular measurement with three-dimensional techniques, the analysis of the aortic annulus in its true plane with bidimensional and area-based measurements already provides useful adjunctive data to two-dimensional echocardiographic assessment. While these measurements have not been validated or integrated in randomized trials, they have already proven to be helpful in predicting complications of THV undersizing such as paravalvular leak [6, 12].

For CT measures of the aortic annulus to move beyond interesting additive information, a CT-based sizing scale must be integrated into THV selection. We propose a sizing scale based both on the mean of the short and long axis of the basal ring and the area measurement of the basal ring. In order to minimize the risk of significant PAR, the implanted THV size should be greater than the three-dimensional area of the annulus on CT. In a recent analysis of our cohort, for THVs that were oversized by at least 10 % of the annular area, there were no cases of significant PAR [6]. We recommend making these measurements in end systole comparable to echocardiographic measurements [6] as the area and mean diameter are larger in this phase of the cardiac cycle, although we recognize that the data is evolving and that perimeter measurements may in fact be more stable throughout the cardiac cycle [13]. It has been suggested that sizing based on diastolic measurements may modify sizing in up to 20–25 % of cases depending on the sizing thresholds used [14]. We do note that intentional oversizing may come with a potential cost of coronary occlusion or annular rupture, but this has not been our experience with a historical unintentional oversizing of the area of the basal ring by approximately 5 % over the last 125 cases on the basis of echocardiographic based sizing [14].

Additionally, the fear that CT sizing will result in a greater degree of oversizing may not be well founded, as the limitations of two-dimensional echocardiographic sizing have led to a great deal of variation in annular oversizing with unintentional oversizing of the annular area by as much as 65.6 % and undersizing by as much as 22.8 % [14]. Importantly, there were no cases of coronary occlusion or of annular injury in the cohort analyzed. In addition, in the cases where the prosthesis is oversized, the THVs remain fully expanded, with under expansion only noted once extreme levels of oversizing, in the magnitude of 40–50 %, are reached. Jilawahi and colleagues [12] recently documented similar findings that three dimensionally derived cross-sectional measurements of the aortic annulus were superior to conventional two-dimensional echocardiographic sizing in the prediction of patients with significant PAR. Interestingly, CT cross-sectional assessment of the aortic annulus was reported to affect device sizing and patient selection and to somewhat reduce post-TAVR PAR. Similar to past assessments, CT measurements were reproducible and could be precisely defined with retrospective ECG-gated acquisitions. While this data is quite compelling, the CT sizing cohort was quite small, and the authors do not provide significant details for the integration of CT measures for sizing nor a specific CT sizing scale.

Proposed CT Sizing Guidelines for Balloon-Expandable Valves

Our group has proposed a different sizing guideline (Table 27.1). The recommendation is to select a prosthesis with a cross-sectional area modestly larger than the CT-derived aortic annulus area. A target of 10–15 % area oversizing with upper and lower limits of 20 to 0 % is suggested (Fig. 27.3). The Vancouver CT sizing guidelines target this range of oversizing while being mindful that fully deploying currently available balloon-expandable prosthesis sizes (20, 23, 26, and 29 mm) (Fig. 27.4) would necessitate accepting a broader range of oversizing than is desirable. Since diameter sizing either by direct measurement or through derivation from an area measurement can only provide modest accuracy and reproducibility, we avoided this approach [7].

Table 27.1 demonstrates the percentage of annular oversizing for a given annular area and valve size. For example, if a patient's CT annular area is 3.70 cm^2, then a 23-mm valve (area 4.15 cm^2) is recommended, and this results in oversizing the annulus by 12 %. As highlighted in gray on the sizing

Table 27.1 The Vancouver CT sizing guidelines. The recommendation is to select a prosthesis with a cross-sectional area modestly larger than the aortic annulus. A target of 10–15 % area oversizing with upper and lower limits of 1–20 % is suggested

Annular area (mm^2)	20 mm THV (%)	23 mm THV (%)	26 mm THV (%)	29 mm THV (%)
230	NR			
240	NR (30.9)			
250	25.7			
260	20.8			
270	16.4			
280	12.2			
290	8.3			
300	4.7			
310	1.3	NR		
320	NR (−1.9 %)	29.8		
330		25.9		
340		22.2		
350		18.7		
360		15.4		
370		12.3		
380		9.3		
390		6.5		
400		3.9	NR	
410		1.3	NR (29.5)	
420		NR (−1.1)	26.4	
430			23.5	
440			20.7	
450			18.0	
460			15.4	
470			13.0	
480			10.6	
490			8.4	
500			6.2	
510			4.1	NR
520			2.1	NR (27.0)
530			0.2	24.6
540				22.3
550				20.1
560				17.9
570				15.9
580				13.9
590				12.0
600				10.1
610				8.3
620				6.5
630				4.8
640				3.2
650				1.6
660				0.1
670				NR

Percentage of annular oversizing calculated by nominal external valve area/annular area. The highlighted gray zones represent annular areas where valve selection is challenging. Oversizing the annulus greater than 20 % may increase the risk of annular injury. Options include underfilling the THV balloon, using the smaller valve size and risk paravalvular regurgitation or considering surgical aortic valve replacement

NR not recommended

guidelines table (Table 27.1) (Fig. 27.4), there are some annuli where it is not possible to oversize by less than 20 %. For these patients, our preferred option is to underfill the THV balloon although the impact on valve durability and post-implant THV geometry is unknown. Alternatively, one could opt to choose a smaller prosthesis, but this approach would be associated with a higher attendant risk of paravalvular leak. Finally, consideration might be given to implantation of an alternative transcatheter prosthesis or even to surgical valve replacement. Nominal balloon volumes for the 20-, 23-, 26-, and 29-mm THV are 11, 17, 22, and 33 cc, respectively. The appropriate amount of balloon underfilling when comfortable oversizing is exceeded has not yet been defined. Our initial experiences suggest underfilling the THV balloon by approximately 5–10 % when oversizing by greater than 20 %, but again further refinement is necessary. In addition, like with all aspects of TAVR, there are almost certainly many factors that must be incorporated in the decision-making process including patient age, valvular calcification, bulkiness of the calcification, and calcification of the LVOT. An appreciation that annular sizing, while crucial, is not the only factor which underpins THV choice must also be recognized. The presence of "anatomic modifiers" such as those described above or a potential risk of coronary obstruction may on occasion influence sizing choice. The effect of balloon underfilling on post-implant THV geometry is unknown.

While our preference is for annular area sizing, we do recognize the merits of an annular perimeter sizing approach [15]. The perimeter has been suggested by some to be more impervious to the dynamism of the cardiac cycle [15] with minimal if any intracycle variation. This experience has, however, not been shared with all centers [13, 14]. Blanke et al. reported a 7.4 % difference in the perimeter from peak to trough through the cardiac cycle with largest dimensions noted consistently close to end systole [13]. While the frequency of sizing modification would be lower with perimeter measurements than other parameters, our group has noted similar dynamic changes in the annular perimeter with resultant potential for THV selection modification in 15 % of patients [14]. In addition, the perimeter has not been shown to be measured with the same degree of reproducibility as the annular area or mean diameter particularly across workstation platforms [10]. That being said, whether area or perimeter sizing is selected, both provide significantly deeper understanding of the annular geometry and three-dimensional configuration than traditional two-dimensional echocardiography. This is the real strength of MDCT for TAVR. It yields reproducible three-dimensional measurements of the annulus that afford the operator the ability to make informed and thoughtful decisions regarding THV selection.

This three-dimensional capability of CT is currently being employed for sizing of the self-expandable CoreValve (Medtronic, Minneapolis. MI). The current guidelines for THV selection have in fact transitioned to perimeter-based

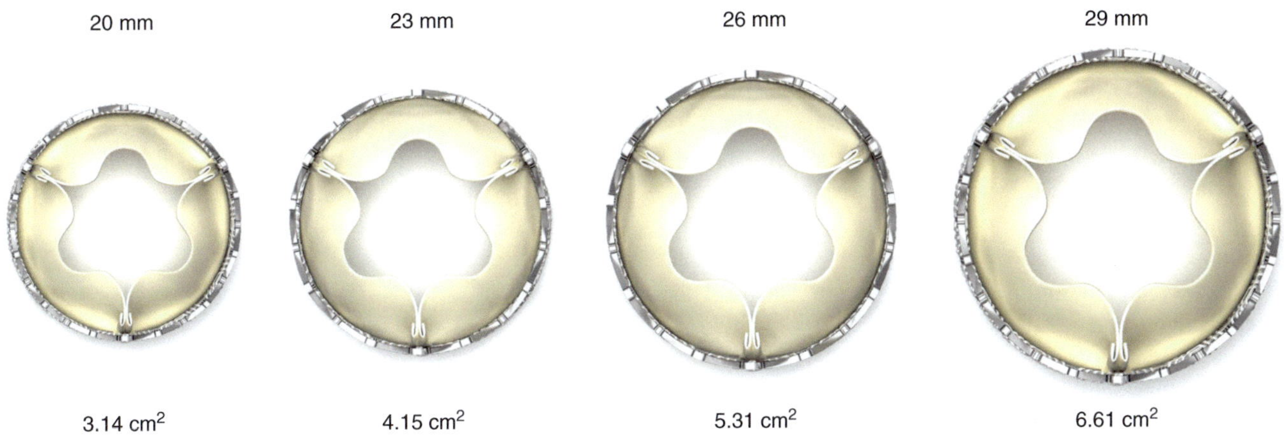

Fig. 27.3 Representative images of an 86-year-old female who underwent TAVR with THV selection made on the basis of echocardiographic measures of the annulus. The basal ring area measured 5.05 cm^2 (**a**) suggesting a 26-mm THV with resultant 5 % oversizing of the annulus. The TTE (**b**) measurement of 21.0 mm suggested a 23-mm THV. A 23-mm THV was placed in this case with resultant moderate to severe paravalvular regurgitation

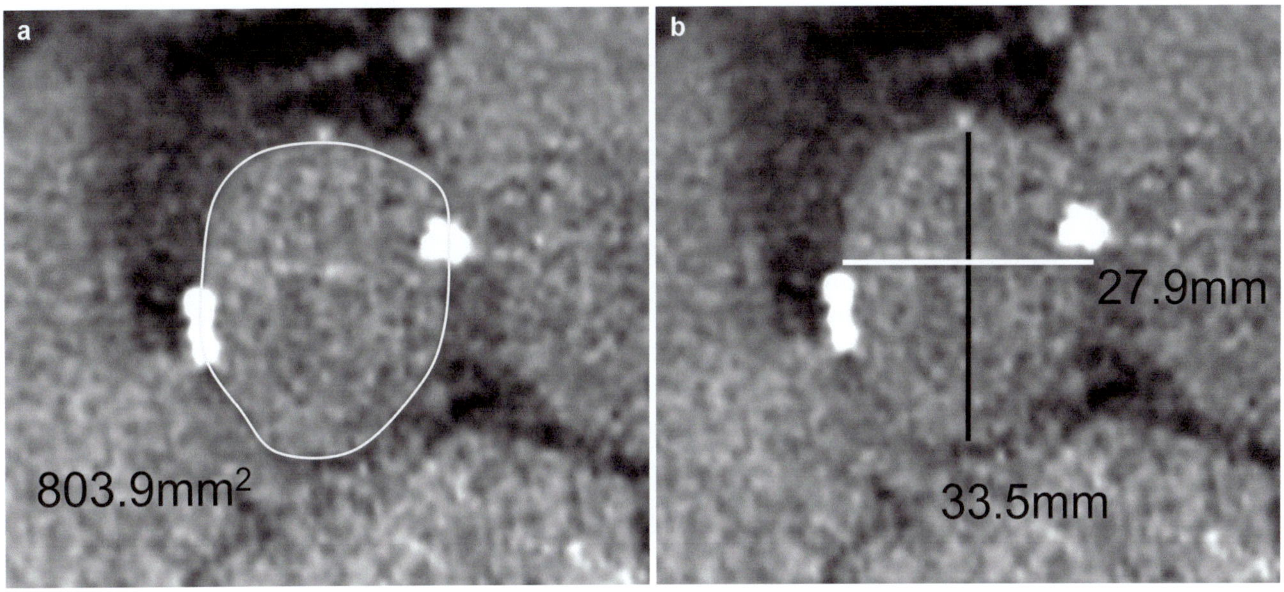

Fig. 27.4 Representative images of the range of balloon-expandable SAPIEN XT (Edwards Lifesciences, Irvine, CA) transcatheter heart valves. Note the significant increase in nominal area between the various valve sizes

CT sizing. Similar to our proposed area sizing, the circumference/perimeter of the annulus is integrated into valve selection. The self-expandable prosthesis is then chosen with a target of 10–15 % oversizing of the native annular perimeter/circumference (Table 27.2).

Table 27.2 Current sizing recommendations for a self-expanding transcatheter heart valve platform (CoreValve, Medtronic, Minneapolis, Minnesota)

Valve size (mm)	Diameter range (mm)	Perimeter range (mm)	Area range (mm^2)
23	18–20	56.5–62.8	254.5–314.2
26	20–23	62.8–72.3	314.2–415.5
29	23–27	72.3–84.8	415.5–572.6
31	26–29	81.7–91.1	530.9–660.5

Practical Applications of CT Measurements for Annular Sizing

The practical application of this CT experience, with both the balloon-expandable and self-expanding platform, remains somewhat limited at present, owing to the limited valve sizes. Imagers and proceduralists alike should understand and consider the potential implications of CT-based sizing and the increase in THV nominal area when going from the smaller to larger THV. Taking the Edwards balloon-expandable valve, for example, upsizing from a 23-mm to a

26-mm balloon-expandable THV is associated with an exponential 28 % increase in external valve area, and increasing from a 26- to 29-mm valve is associated with a further 25 % increase. These rather large incremental changes in THV area make it difficult to appropriately size borderline cases. Consider, for example, an annular area of 4.30 cm^2. The annulus would appear too large for a 23-mm (4.15 cm^2) balloon-expandable THV with a risk of significant PAR; however, a 26-mm prosthesis would result in 24 % oversizing of the annulus, which may be unacceptably high for the proceduralist. This example highlights the important fact that, at present, THV selection remains a multifactorial decision based on a number of clinical and imaging factors and that imaging tools such as CT or echocardiography can simply provide guidance for THV selection.

Future Directions

CT annular sizing is undergoing significant refinement and is on the cusp of more broad adoption with a number of prospective studies being undertaken to assess its impact on PAR and procedural complications such as root injury. A deeper understanding of the potential impact of dynamic changes of the annulus on annular sizing and THV selection is also being sought. The aortic root is subject to dynamic and cyclical changes in cardiac filling and deformation, resulting in cross-sectional area and diameter changes throughout the cardiac cycle. Two components affect dynamic cross-sectional geometry. Stretch of the confining anatomic structures around the annulus leads to a simultaneous increase in area and perimeter during systole. However, flattening of the aorto-mitral junction during diastole with subsequent shortening of short-axis dimensions leads to an increase in eccentricity with an overproportional decrease in area compared to perimeter. Given these dynamic changes of the annulus, most centers continue to advocate for annular assessment in systole to ensure that THV selection is based on the largest annular size in an attempt to help mitigate the likelihood of significant PAR. This area would, however, benefit from further study to better understand the implications of THV selection and annular sizing in various points in the cardiac cycle.

The potential strategy of underfilling the expansion balloon at the time of valve deployment to yield a smaller nominal area is another important area requiring further study. While an interesting idea, and one of the few options available at present to help solve the issue of limited valve sizes, the data remains quite limited. Given these limitations, as THV sizing more formally integrates three-dimensional measurements particularly from CT, a more meticulous and granular approach to THV sizing will almost certainly ensue. As a result, it seems likely that a larger number of THV sizes will be introduced allowing for a more accurate and patient-specific selection of valve size.

Finally, new next-generation valves with varied geometry and design are being evaluated. The transferability of any THV sizing scheme, be it from echocardiography or CT on a current-generation valve platform, is uncertain and will require prospective analysis.

References

1. Anderson RH. Clinical anatomy of the aortic root. Heart. 2000; 84(6):670–3.
2. Piazza N, et al. Anatomy of the aortic valvar complex and its implications for transcatheter implantation of the aortic valve. Circ Cardiovasc Interv. 2008;1(1):74–81.
3. Anderson RH, Lal M, Ho SY. Anatomy of the aortic root with particular emphasis on options for its surgical enlargement. J Heart Valve Dis. 1996;5 Suppl 3:S249–57.
4. Leipsic J, et al. Multidetector computed tomography in transcatheter aortic valve implantation. JACC Cardiovasc Imaging. 2011;4(4): 416–29.
5. Webb JG, et al. Transcatheter aortic valve implantation: impact on clinical and valve-related outcomes. Circulation. 2009; 119(23):3009–16.
6. Willson AB, et al. Three-dimensional aortic annular assessment by multidetector computed tomography predicts moderate or severe paravalvular regurgitation after transcatheter aortic valve replacement: a multicenter retrospective analysis. J Am Coll Cardiol. 2012;59:1287–94.
7. Piazza N., Lange R.; Imaging of Valvular Heart Disease: I Can See Clearly Now. Anatomy of the aortic valve. http://org.crsti.dliv2010.s3.amazonaws.com/pdfs/034_Ovality_of_the_aortic_valve_annulus. 2010. Accessed 15, April 2011.
8. Gurvitch R, Webb JG, Yuan R, Johnson M, Hague C, Willson AB, Toggweiler S, Wood DA, Ye J, Moss R, Thompson CR, Achenbach S, Min JK, Labounty TM, Cury R, Leipsic J. Aortic annulus diameter determination by multidetector computed tomography: reproducibility, applicability, and implications for transcatheter aortic valve implantation. JACC Cardiovasc Interv. 2011;4(11):1235–45. doi:10.1016/j.jcin.2011.07.014.
9. Leon MB, et al. Transcatheter aortic-valve implantation for aortic stenosis in patients who cannot undergo surgery. N Engl J Med. 2010;363(17):1597–607. Epub 2010 Sep 22.
10. Smith CR, et al. Transcatheter versus surgical aortic-valve replacement in high-risk patients. Transcatheter aortic-valve implantation for aortic stenosis in patients who cannot undergo surgery. N Engl J Med. 2011;364(23):2187–98. Epub 2011 Jun 5.
11. Kodali SK, Williams MR, Smith CR, et al. Two-year outcomes after transcatheter or surgical aortic valve replacement. N Engl J Med. 2012;366:1686–95. Epub 2012 Mar 26.
12. Jilaihawi H, Kashif M, Fontana G, et al. Cross-sectional computed tomography assessment improves accuracy of aortic annular sizing for transcatheter aortic valve replacement and reduces the incidence of paravalvular aortic regurgitation. J Am Coll Cardiol. 2012;59: 1275–86. Epub 2012 Feb 22.
13. Blanke P, Russe M, Leipsic J, et al. Conformational pulsatile changes of the aortic annulus: impact on prosthesis sizing by computed tomography for transcatheter aortic valve replacement. JACC Cardiovasc Interv. 2012;5:984–94.

14. Willson AB, Webb JG, Freeman M, Wood DA, Gurvitch R, Thompson CR, Moss RR, Toggweiler S, Binder RK, Munt B, Cheung A, Hague C, Ye J, Leipsic J. Computed tomography-based sizing recommendations for transcatheter aortic valve replacement with balloon-expandable valves: comparison with transesophageal echocardiography and rationale for implementation in a prospective trial. J Cardiovasc Comput Tomogr. 2012;6:406–14.
15. Hamdan A, Guetta V, Konen E, Goitein O, Segev A, Raanani E, Spiegelstein D, Hay I, Di Segni E, Eldar M, Schwammenthal E. Deformation dynamics and mechanical properties of the aortic annulus by 4-dimensional computed tomography: insights into the functional anatomy of the aortic valve complex and implications for transcatheter aortic valve therapy. J Am Coll Cardiol. 2012;59(2): 119–27. doi:10.1016/j.jacc.2011.09.045.

Imaging for Transfemoral Versus Transapical Approaches to TAVR: What Differences Are Important?

28

Mark J. Kearns and Anson Cheung

Abstract

Senile degenerative aortic stenosis is the most prevalent valvular disease. The affected patient population is often elderly with significant comorbid disease burden. This chapter's aim is to provide an overview of pre-procedural imaging for TAVR, and to highlight the differences between trans-femoral and trans-apical approaches.

Keywords

Transcatheter • Aortic valve • Transfemoral • Transapical • Imaging • TAVI • TAVR

Introduction

The most frequent valve disease is degenerative aortic stenosis (AS). The affected patient population is often elderly with a significant comorbid disease burden. Symptomatic, severe AS is a class I American Heart Association/American College of Cardiology I indication for surgical aortic valve replacement (AVR) [1]. Despite this recommendation, a large proportion of such patients are either not referred for surgical assessment, or turned down following assessment on the basis that the operative risks are felt to outweigh the benefits.

Over the last decade, transcatheter aortic valve replacement (TAVR) has emerged as a relatively safe and effective treatment option in selected high-risk patients with severe AS who are felt to be unsuitable candidates for surgical AVR. To date, over 50,000 TAVR cases have been performed worldwide, with recent procedural success rates of over 95 % [2, 3] and mortality in the range of 5–18 % [4–10]. Today, TAVR is predominantly performed either retrogradely via the femoral arteries or antegradely via the left ventricular (LV) apex.

M.J. Kearns, BSc, MD (✉) • A. Cheung, MD
Department of Cardiovascular Surgery, St. Paul's Hospital, 484-1081 Burrad Street, Vancouver, BC V6Z 146, Canada
e-mail: kearns.markj@gmail.com; acheung@providenceheatlh.bc.ca

Data from the randomized PARTNER trial is now available, with follow-up out to two years. The PARTNER B cohort demonstrated a 20 % absolute reduction in 1-year all-cause mortality in the TAVR cohort compared with standard medical therapy [11]. These patients were considered to be inoperable. Subsequently the PARTNER A cohort, comprised of patients at high surgical risk, revealed that TAVR is non-inferior to surgical AVR with respect to 1-year all-cause mortality, albeit with an increased risk of stroke at 1 year [12]. The recently published 2-year follow-up data from cohort A [13] continue to support TAVR as an alternative to surgery in high-risk patients.

The goals of imaging in pre-procedural assessment for TAVR were adroitly covered in a recent review by Bloomfield and colleagues [14]. Namely, the imaging aims are to ensure patient suitability for the proposed access site, that the proposed device can be safely and successfully implanted based on available device-anatomic relationships, and to contribute to the development of a procedural plan. Much of the currently reported outcomes data for TAVR were generated using echocardiography and aortoiliofemoral angiography as the imaging modalities to guide pre-procedural assessment. The currently accepted paradigm, however, has evolved to integrate data from multiple imaging modalities to provide patients with a tailored treatment plan, attempting to minimize procedural and peri-procedural adverse events. Herein, we aim to highlight the relevant differences among imaging modalities in pre-procedural TAVR assessment.

J.K. Min et al. (eds.), *Multimodality Imaging for Transcatheter Aortic Valve Replacement*,
DOI 10.1007/978-1-4471-2798-7_28, © Springer-Verlag London 2014

Patient Selection

Patient selection for TAVR involves a multidisciplinary team review. There should be a full appreciation of the patient's clinical comorbidities and the unique challenges they pose prior to the application of TAVR. An attempt is also made to appreciate the procedural risk involved in each proposed case. Several risk scoring systems are available which provide a crude assessment of procedural risk, the most commonly applied ones being the European System for Cardiac Operative Risk Evaluation (EuroSCORE) and the Society of Thoracic Surgeons (STS) score [15, 16]. However, there are many limitations in using these scoring systems as the sole determinant for inclusion for TAVR. Special attention should be given to the degree of cognitive impairment and frailty in potential candidates, as well as the presence of any additional conditions that limit the length and quality of life. Given the advanced age and significant comorbid disease burden in patients who currently receive TAVR therapies, frailty is frequently identified as a coexisting condition. The utility of TAVR must thus be carefully considered on a case-by-case basis [17–20].

Firm indications and contraindications for TAVR have not yet been fully established or promulgated by the major American or European professional societies. It appears generally accepted that TAVR should be reserved for patients with severe symptomatic AS in whom surgery would be high risk or unfeasible. As a general rule, contraindications to TAVR can be seen in Box 28.1 [1, 21, 22, 23]. Contraindications specific to the transfemoral TAVR (TF-TAVR) route include the following: severe calcification, tortuosity, or small diameter (device dependent) of the iliacs; previous aorto-bifemoral bypass grafting; severe ascending and aortic root angulation; heavy burden of ascending and aortic arch atheroma, coarctation; and aortic aneurysm with protruding mural thrombus. Potential contraindications to the transapical TAVR route (TA-TAVR) include previous LV surgery, heavily calcified pericardium, severe respiratory insufficiency, and a non-reachable LV apex.

Box 28.1 General Contraindications to Transfemoral TAVR

- Left ventricular mass, thrombus, or vegetation
- Annular dimension <18 mm or >29 mm for balloon-expandable prostheses
- Annular dimension <20 mm or >27 mm for self-expanding prostheses
- Congenitally unicuspid or bicuspid aortic valves
- Mechanical aortic prosthesis
- Mitral valve prosthesis
- Left ventricular ejection fraction <20 %
- Sub-aortic stenosis
- Left atrial thrombus
- Severe left ventricular hypertrophy
- Ascending aortic diameter <43 mm and sinus of Valsalva width <27 mm (<29 mm valve is used) for self-expanding prostheses

As part of the screening process, various specialized imaging modalities are employed with a view to determining whether the patient is a suitable TAVR candidate. The specific investigations aim to confirm the presence and severity of AS, assess left ventricular function and concomitant valvular lesions, evaluate the coronary arteries, and determine the presence and severity of cerebrovascular disease.

At present, echocardiography is the preferred tool to assess the severity of AS. Doppler echocardiography permits calculation of aortic valve area (AVA), as well as mean and maximum trans-systolic valvular gradients. As defined by current guidelines, severe AS has an associated AVA of <1 cm^2 and/or a mean transvalvular gradient >40 mmHg [24–26]. Transthoracic echocardiography (TTE) is generally performed first, but transesophageal echocardiography (TEE) studies may be required in the case of suboptimal image quality. Echocardiography allows for assessment of the morphology of the aortic valve and root, as well as the extent and location of valve calcifications. The latter is important for identifying factors that may allow avoidance of procedural complications. As an example, bulky valvular calcifications may heighten the risk of improper valve deployment with consequent paravalvular regurgitation (PAR) and is an independent risk factor for embolic stroke and coronary ostial occlusion [27, 28].

Multidetector computed tomography (MDCT) and magnetic resonance imaging (MRI) may serve as an adjunct to echocardiography for analysis of aortic valve morphology [29–31]. There is good agreement between MDCT, MRI, and echocardiography for calculation of AVA and assessing valve anatomy [30]. MDCT can provide excellent visualization and quantification of valve calcifications.

The degree of baseline aortic regurgitation (AR) and mitral regurgitation (MR) should be established by TTE or TEE. Intra-procedural balloon dilation and manipulations within the LV cavity can worsen the degree of AR and/or MR, resulting in hemodynamic instability [32]. LV function is assessed with particular attention also paid to left ventricular mass and morphology. The presence of LVH—particularly superior asymmetric septal hypertrophy—and the angle between the LV and aorta are important for procedural planning.

All TAVR candidates are evaluated for significant coronary artery disease (CAD). Concomitant CAD is common and negatively impacts early and late outcomes, but the majority of CAD in patients undergoing TAVR can be managed conservatively [33, 34]. When revascularization is indicated, the specific approach to treatment should be dictated by the patient's clinical condition and anatomy. Angiography remains the current standard for coronary imaging. While permitting a noninvasive method for coronary artery assessment, MDCT is somewhat limited in the current TAVR population, owing to the high burden of calcific coronary atherosclerosis. MDCT does, however, allow accurate assessment of coronary ostial height, as discussed below.

Neurologic events following TAVR are not uncommon due to thromboembolism from the valve site or atherothrombotic emboli from the ascending aorta and arch [1]. The extent of calcification and atheromatous disease of the ascending aorta and arch can be assessed by echocardiography and MDCT, which may allow for enhanced risk stratification for peri- or post-TVAR cerebrovascular events [35]. Refinements in patient selection lower profile delivery systems, and embolic protection devices may serve to lessen adverse neurologic outcomes after TAVR.

Pre-procedural Imaging

The TAVR candidate must submit to comprehensive diagnostic imaging, the results of which are critically relevant to technical aspects of procedural planning. Major issues to be addressed include the route of device delivery, size, and geometry (and anatomic relationships) of the aortic root and ascending aorta, and annular sizing. TF-TAVR is currently the default method of valve delivery unless contraindications exist. In the presence of contraindications to TF-TAVR identified by imaging, an alternative method of valve delivery—typically TA-TAVR—can then be selected. Given the present state wherein TF- and TA-TAVR represent the predominance of delivery methods, this chapter will focus on imaging for these approaches.

Assessment of Aorta and Peripheral Arteries: Aortoiliofemoral Access

Assessment of aortoiliofemoral access fundamentally influences selection of the TF- or TA-TAVR route of delivery. TF access requires a minimum passage—6 mm for the CoreValve and 6–6.5 mm for the Sapien/XT valve—through one femoral, iliac artery, and the aorta [36]. Since vascular access complications with TF-TAVR are relatively high (range 6.3–30.7 %) [11, 37–39] and influenced by various factors, pre-procedural screening is key. This often begins with angiographic assessment of the descending and abdominal aorta, in addition to the iliofemoral arteries to detect stenosis, occlusion, and aneurysmal disease. Angiography, however, is somewhat limited in its capacity to evaluate atheromatous disease, plaque burden, and degree of vessel tortuosity. For this reason, MDCT has become the most relevant imaging modality to assess for feasibility of aortoiliofemoral access, and its standardized application in this context has been shown to reduce mortality rates from vascular injury [40]. MDCT can accurately assess vessel tortuosity, the burden and pattern of calcification, the extent of atheromatous disease, and other high-risk features (including dissections and complex atheromas) [41] (Fig. 28.1).

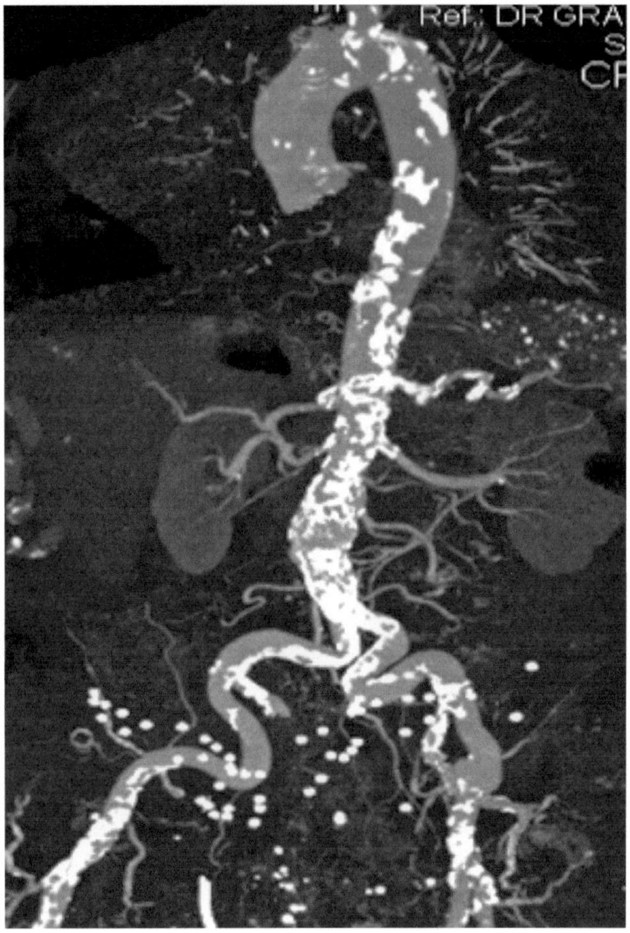

Fig. 28.1 Maximum intensity projection of a multidetector row CT angiogram demonstrating significant aortoiliofemoral calcific atheroma

Recent efforts to minimize the contrast volume to prevent contrast-induced nephropathy associated with aortoiliofemoral imaging have demonstrated feasibility and good image quality. These techniques employ direct injection of dilute contrast media in the infrarenal abdominal aorta [42]. In patients with severe renal insufficiency, non-contrast MRI scans can also image the aortoiliofemoral access sites [43].

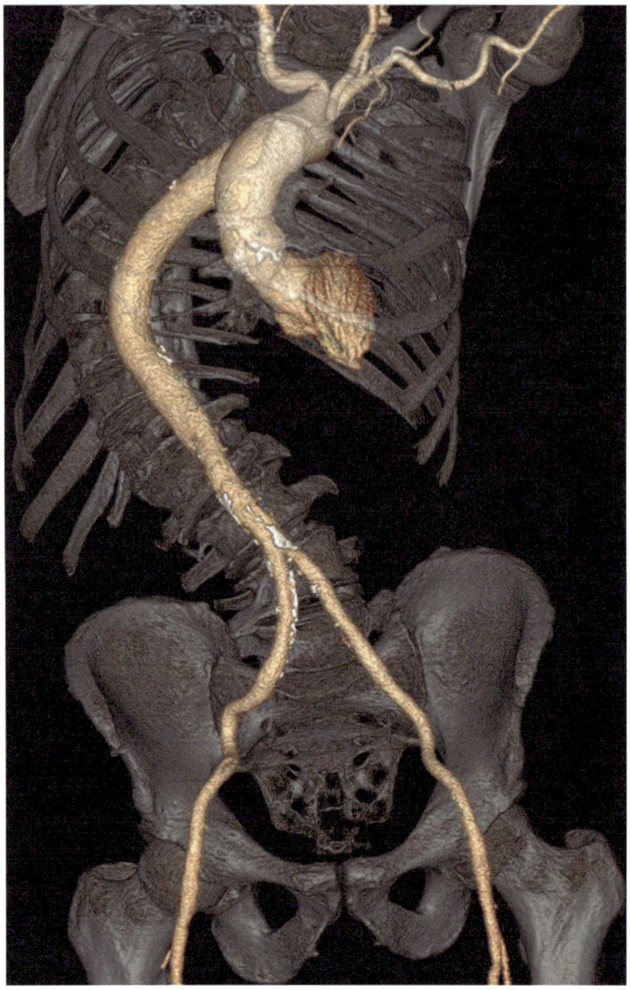

Fig. 28.2 Volume-rendered view of a multidetector row CT angiogram demonstrating significant tortuosity of the thoracoabdominal aorta

In the presence of short segments of compliant artery, the femoral access site can have a smaller diameter than the intended sheath by 1–2 mm, as predicted by MDCT. A sheath-to-femoral-artery ratio of 1.05 or higher is predictive of vascular complications and an increased 30-day mortality [44]. Ultrasound is infrequently used for pre-procedural vascular assessment but may aid in evaluating access vessel characteristics and optimal puncture site at the time of the TAVR. It has been reported that as many as 33 % of patients with critical AS had unfavorable iliofemoral access, with more than three-fourths of those patients having a minimal luminal diameter <8 mm [45, 46]. Circumferential and horseshoe-type calcifications, in association with small and diseased iliofemoral vessels, represent contraindications to the TF approach. When access via the iliofemoral arteries is not possible, other routes are considered [47]. Severe aortic tortuosity may test the length and maneuverability of the TF-TAVR delivery system (Fig. 28.2).

Assessment of Aorta and Peripheral Arteries: Root and Ascending

Aortic root structures, including their dimensions and morphology, are analyzed in detail for all TAVR candidates. In addition to contributing to selection of device type and size, analysis of the root and ascending aorta further contributes to selection of the delivery route. Various features of the root and ascending aorta—including valve cusps, degree and morphology of calcification and atheromatous disease, coronary ostial height, characteristics of the LV outflow tract (LVOT), and the interrelated geometry of these structures—may preclude the use of either TF- or TA-TAVR approaches [36]. These features are also predictive of, in some cases, procedural success and complications. Aortic annular sizing is discussed in detail in the next section.

Echocardiography and MDCT are used to evaluate the extent and locations of annular and leaflet calcifications. Severe calcification can result in acoustic shadowing with echocardiography [14] and renders CMR less suitable due to signal void in such cases. Consequently, MDCT is currently the favored modality for quantifying severity and location of root calcifications. The dimensions and morphology of the root can predict the likelihood of inadequate valve deployment, with consequent risks of paravalvular aortic regurgitation (PAR) and device embolism. The degree and pattern of calcification at the cusps and surrounding structures is also associated with PAR due to asymmetric valve expansion—such as might be the case in the presence of a densely calcified inter-trigonal area—in addition to catastrophic root rupture and cerebral or downstream embolism [48]. Aortic valve calcium scoring prior to TA-TAVR may play a role in predicting post-procedure PAR [49].

Coronary ostial height is assessed by a combination of echocardiography, CMR or MDCT, with a view to ensuring that device deployment will not compromise the coronary ostia from the device itself or displaced debris. TTE and particularly TEE can delineate the distance from the annulus to the right coronary ostium but is limited in detecting the annulus-to-left-coronary distance, which does not lie in a standard echocardiographic plane. Measurements from 3D echocardiographic datasets may be feasible in determining the height of the left coronary ostium.

MDCT provides a comprehensive assessment of coronary ostial height, with an average annulus-to-left-coronary distance of 13.4 ± 3.2 and an annulus-to-right-coronary distance of 13.6 ± 2.8 mm [50]. The distance between the left coronary cusp (LCC) and left coronary ostium is measured from oblique sagittal or coronal projections on MDCT [41]. While it is important to measure coronary ostial height to reduce the risk of ostial obstruction [47], no definite criteria exist to exclude patients on the basis of inadequate height. Nevertheless, a cutoff of 11–14 mm has been proposed, with a height <10 mm potentially suggesting a risk of ostial

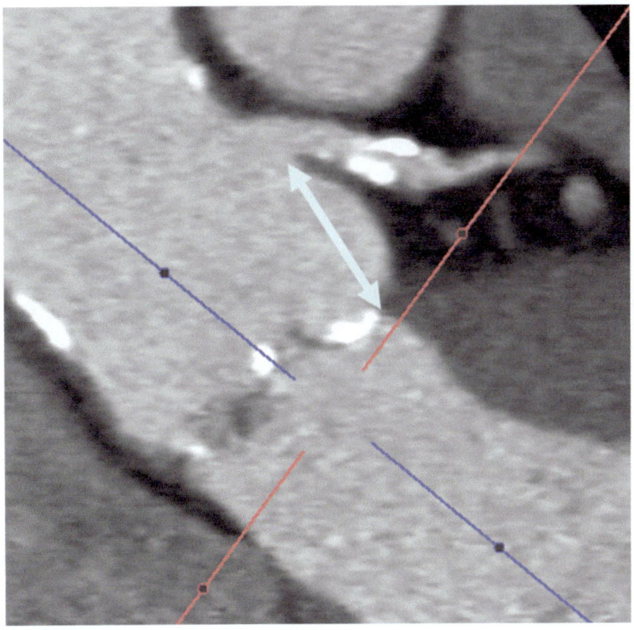

Fig. 28.3 Multiplanar reformat of a multidetector row CT angiogram demonstrating the height from the aortic leaflet insertion point to the left main artery (*double headed arrow*)

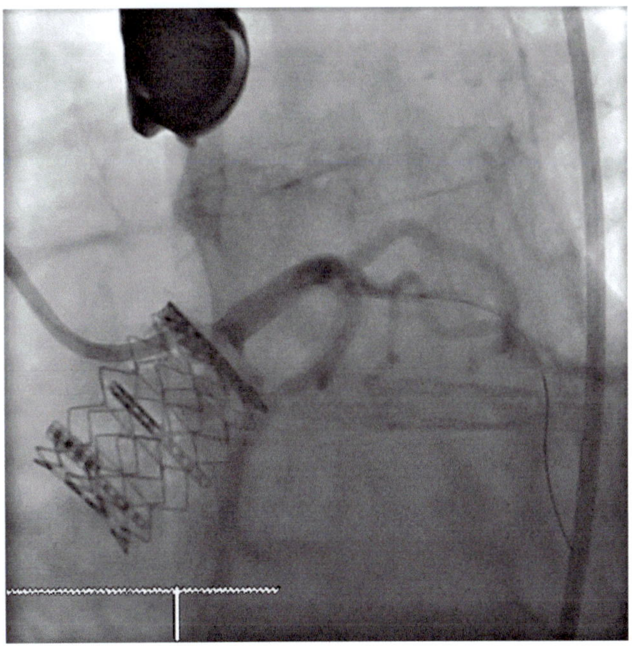

Fig. 28.4 Fluoroscopic projection demonstrating high valve deployment

occlusion [47] (Fig. 28.3). The risk of coronary obstruction is felt to be higher in the setting of heavily and diffusely calcified valve cusps, low-left main height, and patient with narrow aortic sinuses. It is also important to integrate the valve characteristics with a patient's individual anatomy. For example, valve height and its portions that are covered by a skirt of fabric are relevant to note, as excessively high deployment can interfere with coronary flow (Fig. 28.4).

The angulation of the aortic root with respect to the body axis is critical to assess prior to implant. This is done to ensure precise coaxial positioning of the device along the centerline of the aortic annular plane [41]. Because of significant variability in patient anatomy, pre-procedural assessment of root geometry can be helpful in predicting the angle of implant. Traditionally, the orientation of the root has been assessed angiographically, with repeated contrast injections. More recently, MDCT-based reconstructions have been valuable in pre-procedural prediction of the root angle [45, 51]. This has the potential to reduce intra-procedural times, as well as radiation and contrast doses.

Annulus Sizing

The anatomy of the aortic valvar complex has become a subject of revived interest since the development of TAVR as a viable therapy. Emphasis has been placed on the elliptical (rather than circular) nature of the aortic annulus, and its impact on annular measurement and valve sizing. By definition, the annulus is taken as the virtual inferior basal ring measured in systole. An oval shape of the aortic annulus can be appreciated with 3D modalities (3D ECHO, CMR, MDCT), and in approximately 50 % of patients, the mean difference between coronal and sagittal measurements was reported to be 3.0 ± 1.9 mm [52–54]. Despite being the most widely used method of annular sizing, 2D TTE and TEE has been criticized on the basis that it assumes circularity of the annulus and provides an incomplete assessment of annular size. Recently, x-plane echocardiography—wherein two orthogonal views can be simultaneously imaged—further confirms the elliptical nature of the annulus (Fig. 28.5). MDCT-based annular measurements provide short and long axis dimensions of the annulus, also demonstrating its elliptical shape. The mean of these two values (Dmean), as well as the cross-sectional surface area derived diameter (Dcsa) produce the best approximation of a one-dimensional radius for valve sizing [36, 55]. Good agreement between CMR- and MDCT-generated annular measurements has been reported [53, 54, 56]. 3D CMR may be an alternative modality for annular sizing in patients with renal insufficiency.

Annular measurements determine the size of prosthesis that will be implanted. Undersizing is associated with the risks of poor hemodynamics, PAR, valve migration, and embolism. Excessive oversizing can result in catastrophic consequences such as aortic rupture, tamponade, or aortic hematoma [1, 26]. TAVR device deployment relies on some degree of oversizing, as the valves depend on radial forces for secure seating. Approximately one in nine patients undergoing TAVR is left with moderate to severe PAR, which is associated with adverse outcomes [11, 57, 58]. The main causes of PAR after TAVR are valve undersizing and incorrect positioning [59–61]. CT-based sizing guidelines are in

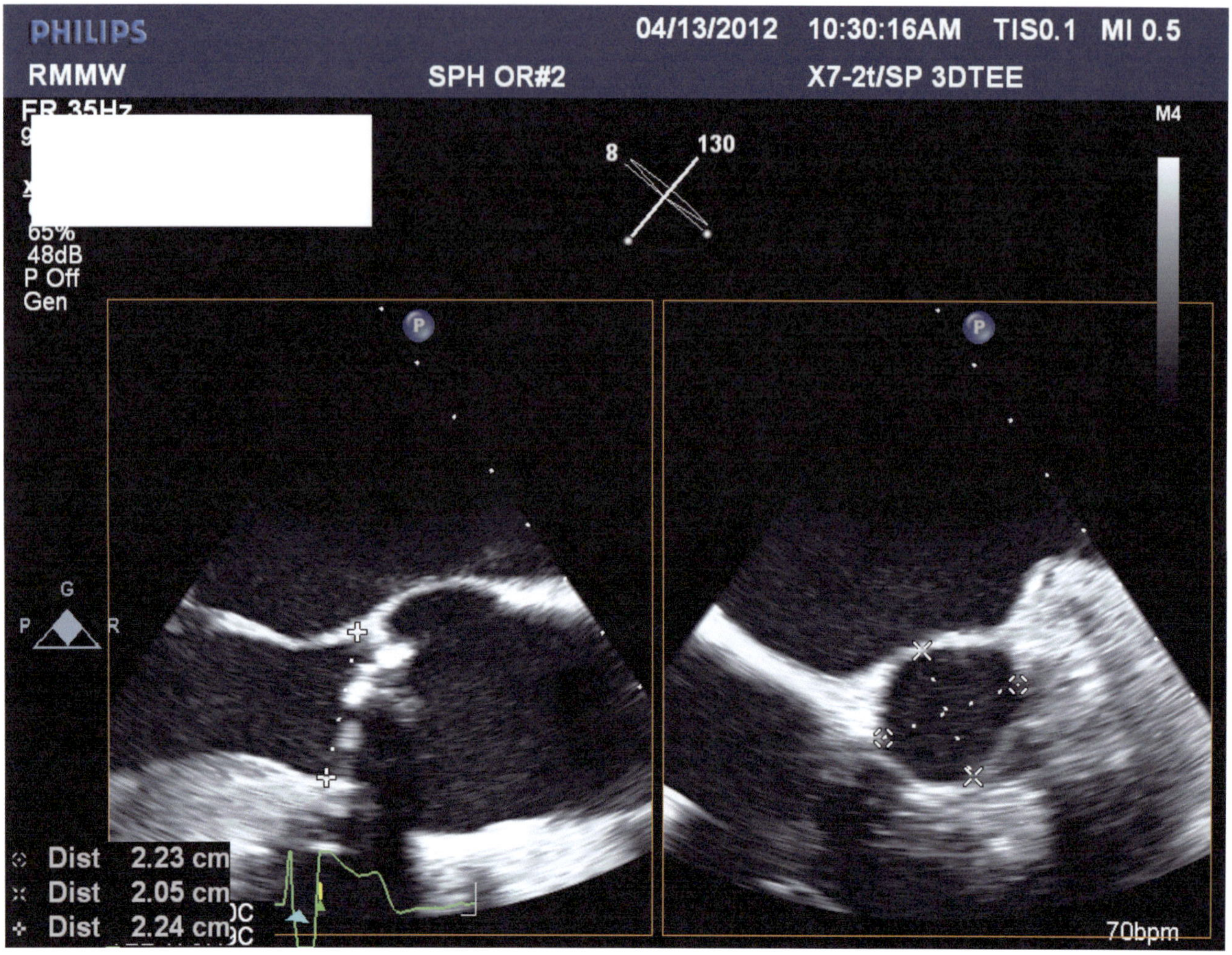

Fig. 28.5 X-plane transesophageal echocardiogram demonstrating two orthogonal views of the aortic valve and annulus

development to integrate 3D CT data into the valve selection process, which is currently based on echocardiographic measurements [14, 26].

There are no fundamental differences between TF- and TA-TAVR, with respect to annular sizing. The main differences in annular sizing relate mainly to the specific imaging modality employed. In general, annulus size as measured by TTE is 1 mm smaller than that measured by TEE. TEE size is generally 1–1.5 mm smaller than that measured by MDCT [41, 54]. As noted, good agreement has been reported between CMR and MDCT.

Summary

TAVR is currently reserved for patients with symptomatic severe AS, in whom surgery is either high risk or unfeasible. Many procedures have been performed to date, with acceptable outcomes. The application of multimodality imaging in patient selection and pre-procedural imaging promises to further refine these steps with the aim of reducing procedural complications and unsatisfactory patient outcomes.

Imaging for the patient selection process is common to both TF- and TA-TAVR approaches. For pre-procedural imaging, annular sizing is also common to both approaches, being used to identify the potential for procedural complications and to size the device. The main imaging differences between TF- and TA-TAVR relate to assessment of the aortoiliofemoral arterial system, and whether the proposed access route would be a suitable one. Size parameters, morphology, and concomitant structural features of the ventricle, root, aorta, and iliofemoral arteries determine suitability for TF- or TA-TAVR.

References

1. Holmes DR, Mack MJ, Kaul S, et al. 2012 ACCF/AATS/SCAI/STS expert consensus document on transcatheter aortic valve replacement. J Am Coll Cardiol. 2012;59:1200–54.
2. Yan TD, Cao C, Martens-Nielsen J, et al. Transcatheter aortic valve implantation for high-risk patients with severe aortic stenosis: a systematic review. J Thorac Cardiovasc Surg. 2010;139:1519–28.

3. Coeytaux RR, Williams JW, Gray RN, Wang A. Percutaneous heart valve replacement for aortic stenosis: state of the evidence. Ann Intern Med. 2010;153:314–24.
4. Grube E, Buellesfeld L, Mueller R, et al. Progress and current status of percutaneous aortic valve replacement: results of three device generations of the CoreValve Revalving system. Circ Cardiovasc Interv. 2008;1:167–75.
5. Cribier A, Eltchaninoff H, Tron C, Bauer F. Treatment of calcific aortic stenosis with the percutaneous heart valve: mid- term follow-up from the initial feasibility studies: the French experience. J Am Coll Cardiol. 2006;47:1214–23.
6. Himbert D, Descoutures F, Al-Attar N, et al. Results of transfemoral or transapical aortic valve implantation following a uniform assessment in high-risk patients with aortic stenosis. J Am Coll Cardiol. 2009;54:303–11.
7. Rodés-Cabau J, Dumont E, De LaRochelliere R, et al. Feasibility and initial results of percutaneous aortic valve implantation including selection of the transfemoral or transapical approach in patients with severe aortic stenosis. Am J Cardiol. 2008;102:1240–6.
8. Zajarias A, Cribier AG. Outcomes and safety of percutaneous aortic valve replacement. J Am Coll Cardiol. 2009;53:1829–36.
9. Webb JG, Altwegg L, Boone RH, et al. Transcatheter aortic valve implantation: impact on clinical and valve-related outcomes. Circulation. 2009;119:3009–16.
10. Piazza N, Grube E, Gerckens U, et al. Procedural and 30-day outcomes following transcatheter aortic valve implantation using the third generation (18 Fr) corevalve revalving system: results from the multicentre, expanded evaluation registry 1-year following CE mark approval. EuroIntervention. 2008;4:242–9.
11. Leon MB, Smith CR, Mack M, et al. Transcatheter aortic-valve implantation for aortic stenosis in patients who cannot undergo surgery. N Engl J Med. 2010;363:1597–607.
12. Smith CR, Leon MB, Mack MJ, et al. Transcatheter versus surgical aortic-valve replacement in high-risk patients. N Engl J Med. 2011;364:2187–98.
13. Kodali SK, Williams MR, Smith CR, et al. Two-year outcomes after transcatheter or surgical aortic-valve replacement. N Engl J Med. 2012;366:1686–95.
14. Bloomfield GS, Gillam LD, Hahn RT, et al. A practical guide to multimodality imaging of transcatheter aortic valve replacement. J Am Coll Cardiol Intv. 2012;5:441–55.
15. Roques F, Nashef SA, Michel P, et al. Risk factors and outcome in European cardiac surgery: analysis of the EuroSCORE multinational database of 19030 patients. Eur J Cardiothorac Surg. 1999;15:816–22.
16. O'Brien SM, Shahian DM, Filardo G, et al. The Society of Thoracic Surgeons 2008 cardiac surgery risk models: part 2—isolated valve surgery. Ann Thorac Surg. 2009;88:S23–42.
17. Lunney JR, Lynn J, Foley DJ, et al. Patterns of functional decline at the end of life. JAMA. 2003;289:2387–92.
18. Consensus statement of the Society of Critical Care Medicine's Ethics Committee regarding futile and other possibly inadvisable treatments. Crit Care Med. 1997;25:887.
19. Lanken PN, Ahlheit BD, Crawford S, et al. Withholding and withdrawing life-sustaining therapy. Am Rev Respir Dis. 1991;144:727–32.
20. McDermid RC, Bagshaw SM. Prolonging life and delaying death: the role of physicians in the context of limited intensive care resources. Philos Ethics Humanit Med. 2009;4:1–7.
21. Vahanian A, Alfieri O, Al-Attar N, et al. Transcatheter valve implantation for patients with aortic stenosis: a position statement from the European Association of Cardio-Thoracic Surgery (EACTS) and the European Society of Cardiology (ESC), in collaboration with the European Association of Percutaneous Cardiovascular Interventions (EAPCI). Eur Heart J. 2008;29:1463–70.
22. Ruel M, Labinaz M. Transcatheter aortic-valve replacement: a cardiac surgeon and cardiologist team perspective. Curr Opin Cardiol. 2010;25:107–13.
23. Delgado V, Tops LF, Schuijf JD, et al. Successful deployment of a transcatheter aortic valve in bicuspid aortic stenosis: role of imaging with multislice computed tomography. Circ Cardiovasc Imaging. 2009;2(2):e12–3.
24. Bonow RO, Carabello BA, Chatterjee K, et al. ACC/AHA 2006 guidelines for the management of patients with valvular heart disease. Circulation. 2006;114:e84–231.
25. Vahanian A, Baumgartner H, Bax J, et al. Guidelines on the Management of Valvular Heart Disease: the task force on the Management of Valvular Heart Disease of the European Society of Cardiology. Eur Heart J. 2007;28:230–68.
26. Zamorano JL, Badano LP, Bruce C, et al. EAE/ASE recommendations for the use of echocardiography in new transcatheter interventions for valvular heart disease. J Am Soc Echocardiogr. 2011;24:937–65.
27. Zegdi R, Ciobotaru V, Noghin M, et al. Is it reasonable to treat all calcified stenotic aortic valves with a valved stent? Results from a human anatomic study in adults. J Am Coll Cardiol. 2008;51:579–84.
28. Webb JG, Chandavimol M, Thompson CR, et al. Percutaneous aortic valve implantation retrograde from the femoral artery. Circulation. 2006;113:842–50.
29. Caruthers SD, Lin SJ, Brown P, et al. Practical value of cardiac magnetic resonance imaging for clinical quantification of aortic valve stenosis: comparison with echocardiography. Circulation. 2003;108:2236–43.
30. Pouleur AC, le Polain de Waroux JB, Pasquet A, et al. Aortic valve area assessment: multidetector CT compared with cine MR imaging and transthoracic and transesophageal echocardiography. Radiology. 2007;244:745–54.
31. Burman ED, Keegan J, Kilner PJ. Aortic root measurement by cardiovascular magnetic resonance: specification of planes and lines of measurement and corresponding normal values. Circ Cardiovasc Imaging. 2008;1:104–13.
32. Jilaihawi H, Kar S, Doctor N, et al. Contemporary application of cardiovascular hemodynamics: transcatheter aortic valve interventions. Cardiol Clin. 2011;29:211–22.
33. Dewey TM, Brown DL, Herbert MA, et al. Effect of concomitant coronary artery disease on procedural and late outcomes of transcatheter aortic valve implantation. Ann Thorac Surg. 2010;89:758–67.
34. Webb J, Cribier A. Percutaneous transarterial aortic valve implantation: what do we know? Eur Heart J. 2011;32:140–7.
35. Furie KL, Kasner SE, Adams RJ, et al. Guidelines for the prevention of stroke in patients with stroke or transient ischemic attack: a guideline for Healthcare Professionals From the American Heart Association/American Stroke Association. Stroke. 2011;42:227–76.
36. Gessat M, Frauenfelder T, Altwegg L, et al. Transcatheter aortic valve implantation. Role of imaging. Aswan Heart Centre Science & Practice Series. 2011;3.
37. Tamburino C, Capodanno D, Ramondo A, et al. Incidence and predictors of early and late mortality after transcatheter aortic valve implantation in 663 patients with severe aortic stenosis. Circulation. 2011;123:299–308.
38. Eltchaninoff H, Prat A, Gilard M, et al. Transcatheter aortic valve implantation: early results of the FRANCE (FRench Aortic National CoreValve and Edwards) registry. Eur Heart J. 2011;32:191–7.
39. Gurvitch R, Wood DA, Tay EL, et al. Transcatheter aortic valve implantation: durability of clinical and hemodynamic outcomes beyond 3 years in a large patient cohort. Circulation. 2010;122:1319–27.
40. Toggweiler S, Gurvitch R, Leipsic J, et al. Percutaneous aortic valve replacement: vascular outcomes with a fully percutaneous procedure. J Am Coll Cardiol. 2012;59:113–8.
41. Leipsic J, Gurvitch R, LaBounty TM, et al. Multidetector computed tomography in transcatheter aortic valve implantation. J Am Coll Cardiol Img. 2011;4:416–29.

42. Nietlispach F, Leipsic J, Al-Bugami S, et al. CT of the ilio-femoral arteries using direct aortic contrast injection: proof of feasibility in patients screened towards percutaneous aortic valve replacement. Swiss Med Wkly. 2009;139:458–62.
43. Swan JS, Kennell TW, Acher CW, et al. Magnetic resonance angiography of aorto-iliac disease. Am J Surg. 2000;180:6–12.
44. Hayashida K, Lefèvre T, Chevalier B, et al. Transfemoral aortic valve implantation: new criteria to predict vascular complications. J Am Coll Cardiol Intv. 2011;4:851–8.
45. Kurra V, Kapadia SR, Tuzcu EM, et al. Pre-procedural imaging of aortic root orientation and dimensions: comparison between X-ray angiographic planar imaging and 3-dimensional multidetector row computed tomography. J Am Coll Cardiol Intv. 2010;3:105–13.
46. Kurra V, Schoenhagen P, Roselli EE, et al. Prevalence of significant peripheral artery disease in patients evaluated for percutaneous aortic valve insertion: preprocedural assessment with multidetector computed tomography. J Thorac Cardiovasc Surg. 2009;137:1258–64.
47. Masson J-B, Kovac J, Schuler G, et al. Transcatheter aortic valve implantation: review of the nature, management, and avoidance of procedural complications. J Am Coll Cardiol Intv. 2009;2:811–20.
48. Delgado V, Ng ACT, Shanks M, et al. Transcatheter aortic valve implantation: role of multimodality cardiac imaging. Expert Rev Cardiovasc Ther. 2010;8:113–23.
49. Haensig M, Lehmkuhl L, Rastan AJ, et al. Aortic valve calcium scoring is a predictor of significant paravalvular aortic insufficiency in transapical-aortic valve implantation. Eur J Cardiothorac Surg. 2012;0:1–8.
50. Akhtar M, Tuzcu EM, Kapadia SR, et al. Aortic root morphology in patients undergoing percutaneous aortic valve replacement: evidence of aortic root remodeling. J Thorac Cardiovasc Surg. 2009;137:950–6.
51. Gurvitch R, Wood DA, Leipsic J, et al. Multislice computed tomography for prediction of optimal angiographic deployment projections during transcatheter aortic valve implantation. J Am Coll Cardiol Intv. 2010;3:1157–65.
52. Ali AMA, Altwegg L, Horlick EM, et al. Prevention and management of transcatheter balloon-expandable aortic valve malposition. Catheter Cardiovasc Interv. 2008;72:573–8.
53. Tops LF, Wood DA, Delgado V, et al. Noninvasive evaluation of the aortic root with multislice computed tomography: implications for transcatheter aortic valve replacement. J Am Coll Cardiol Img. 2008;1:321–30.
54. Messika-Zeitoun D, Serfaty J-M, Brochet E, et al. Multimodal assessment of the aortic annulus diameter: implications for transcatheter aortic valve implantation. J Am Coll Cardiol. 2010;55:186–94.
55. Schultz CJ, Moelker A, Piazza N, et al. Three dimensional evaluation of the aortic annulus using multislice computer tomography: are manufacturer's guidelines for sizing for percutaneous aortic valve replacement helpful? Eur Heart J. 2010;31:849–56.
56. Koos R, Altiok E, Mahnken AH, et al. Evaluation of aortic root for definition of prosthesis size by magnetic resonance imaging and cardiac computed tomography: Implications for transcatheter aortic valve implantation. Int J Cardiol. 2012;158(3):353–8.
57. Willson AB, Webb JG, Labounty TM, et al. 3-dimensional aortic annular assessment by multidetector computed tomography predicts moderate or severe paravalvular regurgitation after transcatheter aortic valve replacement: a multicenter retrospective analysis. J Am Coll Cardiol. 2012;59:1287–94.
58. Abdel-Wahab M, Zahn R, Horack M, et al. Aortic regurgitation after transcatheter aortic valve implantation: incidence and early outcome. Results from the German transcatheter aortic valve interventions registry. Heart. 2011;97:899–906.
59. Detaint D, Lepage L, Himbert D, et al. Determinants of significant paravalvular regurgitation after transcatheter aortic valve implantation: impact of device and annulus discongruence. J Am Coll Cardiol Intv. 2009;2:821–7.
60. Takagi K, Latib A, Al-Lamee R, et al. Predictors of moderate-to-severe paravalvular aortic regurgitation immediately after CoreValve implantation and the impact of postdilatation. Catheter Cardiovasc Interv. 2011;78:432–43.
61. Sherif MA, Abdel-Wahab M, Stöcker B. Anatomic and procedural predictors of paravalvular aortic regurgitation after implantation of the Medtronic CoreValve bioprosthesis. J Am Coll Cardiol. 2010;56:1623–9.

Common Uses of Echocardiography for TAVR

29

Rebecca T. Hahn

Abstract

Recent guidelines and reviews of echocardiographic imaging during transcatheter aortic valve replacement (TAVR) have emphasized the clinical utility of this modality for intra-procedural guidance and risk assessment [1, 2]. At our institution, we currently perform TAVR procedures under general anesthesia with a transesophageal echocardiographic (TEE) probe in place. At this time, we feel this is a vital safeguard for to mitigate intra-procedural and postimplantation complications. Technical advances, such as miniaturization of TEE probes and 3D imaging with intracardiac probes, may change the intra-procedural imaging protocols in the future.

Keywords

Transcatheter aortic valve replacement • Transesophageal echocardiography

Introduction

Recent guidelines and reviews of echocardiographic imaging during transcatheter aortic valve replacement (TAVR) have emphasized the clinical utility of this modality for intra-procedural guidance and risk assessment [1, 2]. At our institution, we currently perform TAVR procedures under general anesthesia with a transesophageal echocardiographic (TEE) probe in place. At this time, we feel this is a vital safeguard for to mitigate intra-procedural and postimplantation complications. Technical advances, such as miniaturization of TEE probes and 3D imaging with intracardiac probes, may change the intra-procedural imaging protocols in the future.

For intra-procedural imaging, a three-dimensional (3D) capable TEE machine is strongly recommended but not required. Recent guidelines for 3D echocardiographic imaging have been published [3] and have been integral to the standardization of 3D image acquisition and display. If a pre-procedural TEE was not performed, then a full TEE protocol is completed with attention to measurements of the LVOT, aortic annulus, aortic root diameter, sino-tubular junction diameter, annulus-to-left main height and annulus-to-right-coronary height. A full understanding of these measurements is essential for prevention and/or anticipation of possible complications following TAVR (Table 29.1). As the pre-procedural echocardiographic assessment has been described in a prior chapter, this current chapter describes the echocardiographic protocols used for intra-procedural guidance during TAVR.

Confirmation of Wire and Catheter Placement

TEE can be used to confirm placement of catheters and wires. Central monitoring catheters placed into the right heart may require imaging during initial internal jugular puncture and insertion of the catheter into the right heart (Fig. 29.1) as described in recent guidelines [4]. Placement of the pacing wire from either superior vena caval or inferior vena caval sites may also require imaging to confirm positioning and document the presence of pericardial effusions.

Numerous potential access sites exist for TAVR, and the function of TEE may change with the TAVR approach. For transapical TAVR, because of the small apical window generated by

R.T. Hahn, MD, FACC, FASE
Department of Medicine, Columbia University Medical Center, New York-Presbyterian Hospital, 177 Fort Washington Avenue, HIP 6-623, New York, NY 10032, USA
e-mail: rth2@columbia.edu

J.K. Min et al. (eds.), *Multimodality Imaging for Transcatheter Aortic Valve Replacement*, DOI 10.1007/978-1-4471-2798-7_29, © Springer-Verlag London 2014

limited thoracotomy, imaging of the left ventricular apex (mid-esophageal view) is useful to ensure optimal location of the apical puncture (Fig. 29.2). A cannulation site in the anterior or anterolateral apex allows for appropriate axial alignment of the initial puncture and wire direction. This is important to avoid entanglement of the wire in the mitral apparatus and position the wire quickly across the aortic valve. Frequently, the location of the apical puncture is dictated by the coronary artery anatomy or abnormal positioning of the heart relative to the thoracotomy. In addition, very small, concentrically hypertrophied, and hyperdynamic ventricles may be particularly problematic. In these patients, problems may not become evident until the larger transcatheter heart valve (THV) and guide catheter are introduced. The size of the device within the small, hyperdynamic ventricle may increase the likelihood of entrapment of a left ventricular mitral chordae. During needle insertion, advancement of the guide wire, and subsequent apical cannulation, imaging of the mitral valve either with color-compare mode or biplane imaging with color Doppler may allow early recognition of valvular compromise (Fig. 29.3).

Table 29.1 Assessment of the aortic valvular complex for prevention and/or anticipation of possible complications following TAVR

Risk assessment	Hemodynamic emergencies
Aortic annulus	Aortic/AV trauma
Aortic root and coronary arteries	Periaortic hematoma
Aortic root morphology	Aortic dissection
Ectopic calcification	Annular rupture
Wire position	Pericardial tamponade
Mitral valve apparatus	Mitral valve compromise
Left ventricular size and function	Left main coronary occlusion
Balloon aortic valvuloplasty	Severe aortic regurgitation
Positioning and deployment of THV	Central regurgitation
Aortic valve, root, and LVOT morphology	Paravalvular regurgitation

Mitral for the more commonly used transfemoral approach, echocardiographic imaging is used for assessing the position and stability of the J-wire within the ventricle. The stability of the wire is integral to maintaining appropriate positioning and stabilization of the transcatheter heart valve deployment catheters. The wire should be well within the body of the ventricle and a curve formed within the apex. If the wire is in the mid-ventricle (Fig. 29.4a) or wrapped around mitral chordae, the proceduralists performing TAVR will frequently reposition. 3D imaging may help localize the cannulation site and guide wire path within the ventricle (Fig. 29.4b).

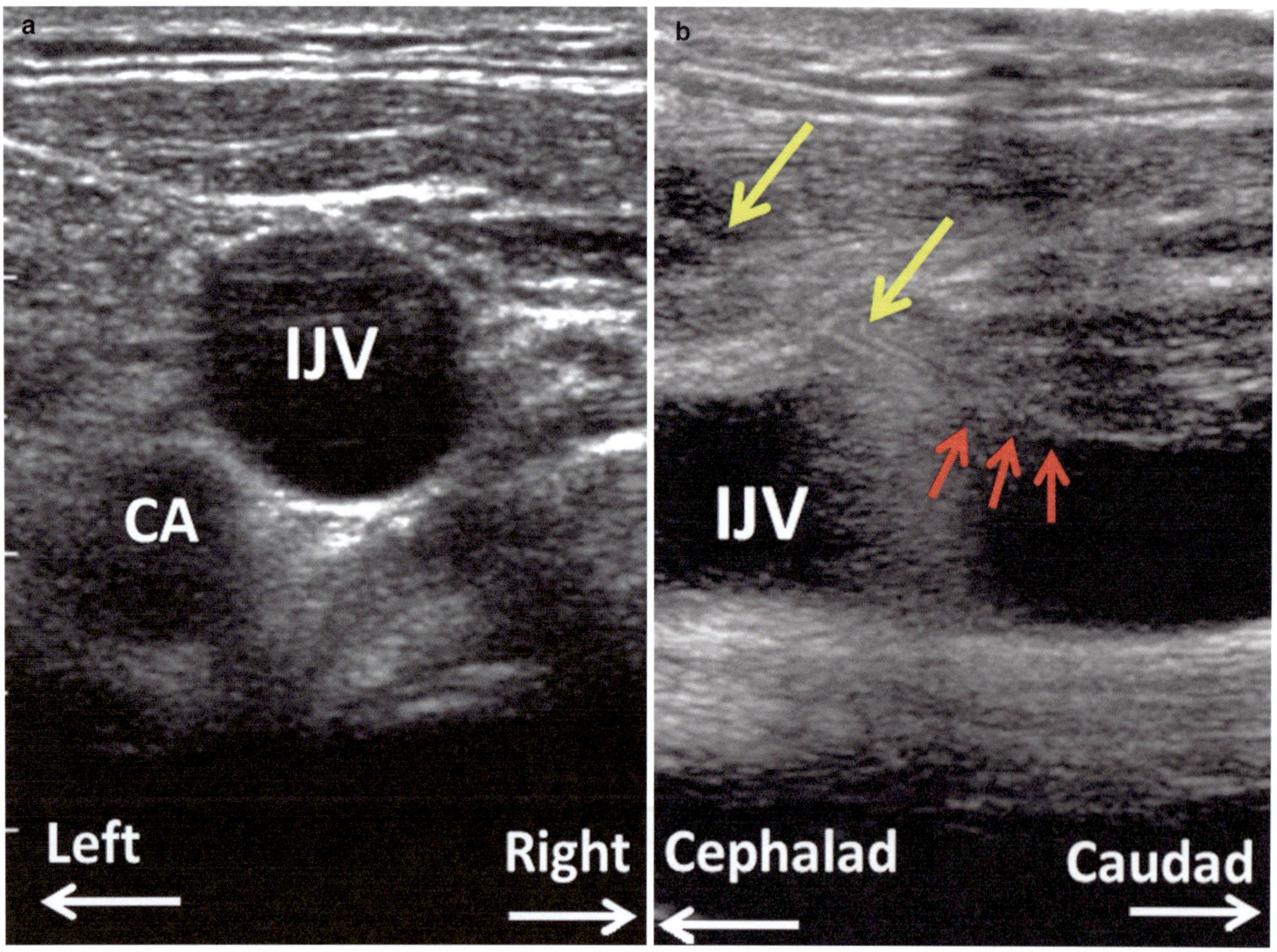

Fig. 29.1 Imaging of the right internal jugular vein for placement of central monitoring catheters may require vascular imaging as well as transesophageal (*TEE*) imaging. (**a**) shows the short-axis view of the right internal jugular vein (*IJV*) and carotid artery (*CA*). (**b**) shows the needle (*yellow arrows*) causing compression (*red arrows*) of the vein just prior to entering the lumen. (**c**) shows TEE imaging of the bicaval view to confirm the entrance of the J-wire (yellow arrows) into the superior vena cava (*blue arrow*) and right atrium (*RA*). *LA* = left atrium

Fig 29.1 (continued)

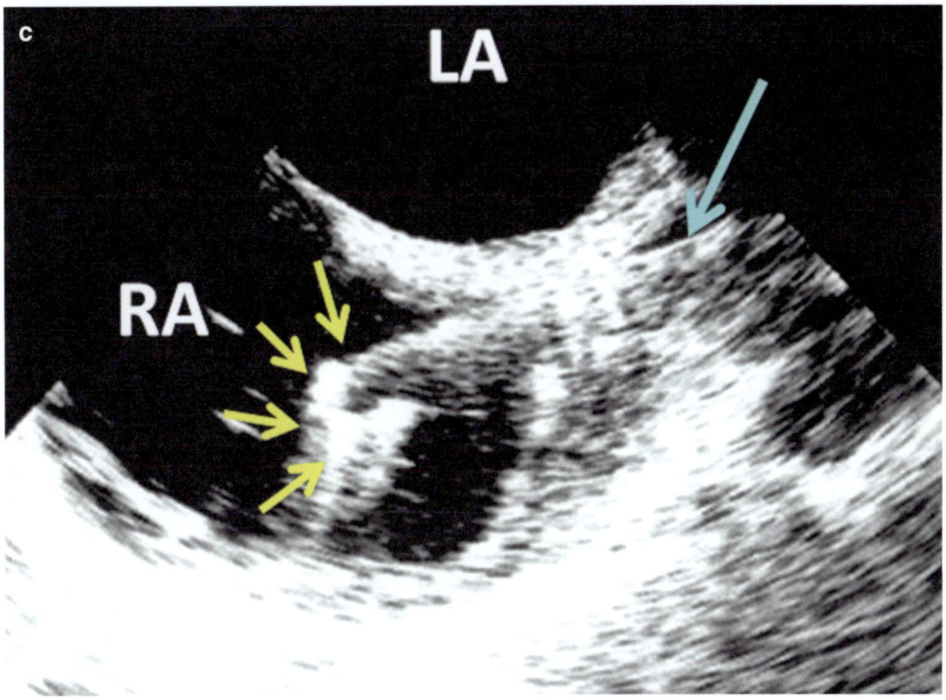

Balloon Aortic Valvuloplasty

Balloon aortic valvuloplasty (BAV) is performed prior to TAVR to increase cusp opening and excursion and to facilitate placement of the THV. BAV however is not without complications, with serious adverse events reported in up to 15.6 % of patients [5]. These may include death, stroke, coronary occlusion, severe aortic regurgitation, resuscitation, cardioversion, tamponade, permanent pacemaker, and severe vascular complications. Echocardiography can be important in assessing the presence of aortic regurgitation and the integrity of the aorta. Acute severe aortic regurgitation may cause severe hemodynamic compromise and necessitate urgent valve implantation. Both valve avulsion (Fig. 29.5) and fixation of the markedly calcified cusps may occur. During BAV, the biplane mode is again utilized with imaging of the mid-esophageal LAX and SAX views of the AV. Following BAV, increase in cusp motion is expected and the severity of AR should be assessed. Although not routinely performed, deep transgastric Doppler can show a reduction in the transsystolic gradient (Fig. 29.6).

Imaging during BAV can also be used for diagnostic purposes. If annular dimension has been difficult to measure, the maximum balloon diameter may also help determine the most appropriate valve size to use. In addition, observing the motion and location of the displaced calcified cusps may help predict complications such as coronary obstruction or aortic root injury.

Positioning of the THV

Intra-procedural echocardiographic imaging is used to confirm THV positioning prior to deployment. Current catheter cone designs stabilize the valve and reduce movement during balloon inflation. Because the lower border of the closed THV cusps sits in the middle of the stent, the valve stent crimped on the balloon should be centered on the aortic annulus (50 % above and below the annulus) or slightly higher in the aorta (60 % above and 40 % below the annulus); however, each case must be individualized depending on the anatomy of the aortic valvar complex. A short aortic root or low-lying position of the left main coronary artery may necessitate a lower position. The crimped stent can usually be differentiated echocardiographically from the underlying balloon (Fig. 29.7a) by angulating the transducer to identify an echodense, sharp-edged structure (as opposed to the heterogeneous appearance of the underlying deflated balloon). Knowing the dimensions of the THV is important in order to center the stent on the annulus. Acoustic shadowing of the annulus on echocardiography due to calcification of the aortic and mitral valves may render identification of the stent difficult. Because the acoustic density of the stent is greater than the balloon, reducing the overall gain may reduce the acoustic noise of the balloon that enhances the borders of the stent. In more difficult cases, live 3D (narrow sector) may enhance imaging of the stent by increasing the "depth of field" (Fig. 29.7b). A test run of rapid pacing allows fine-tuning of the THV position, but a final check is always performed just prior to deployment.

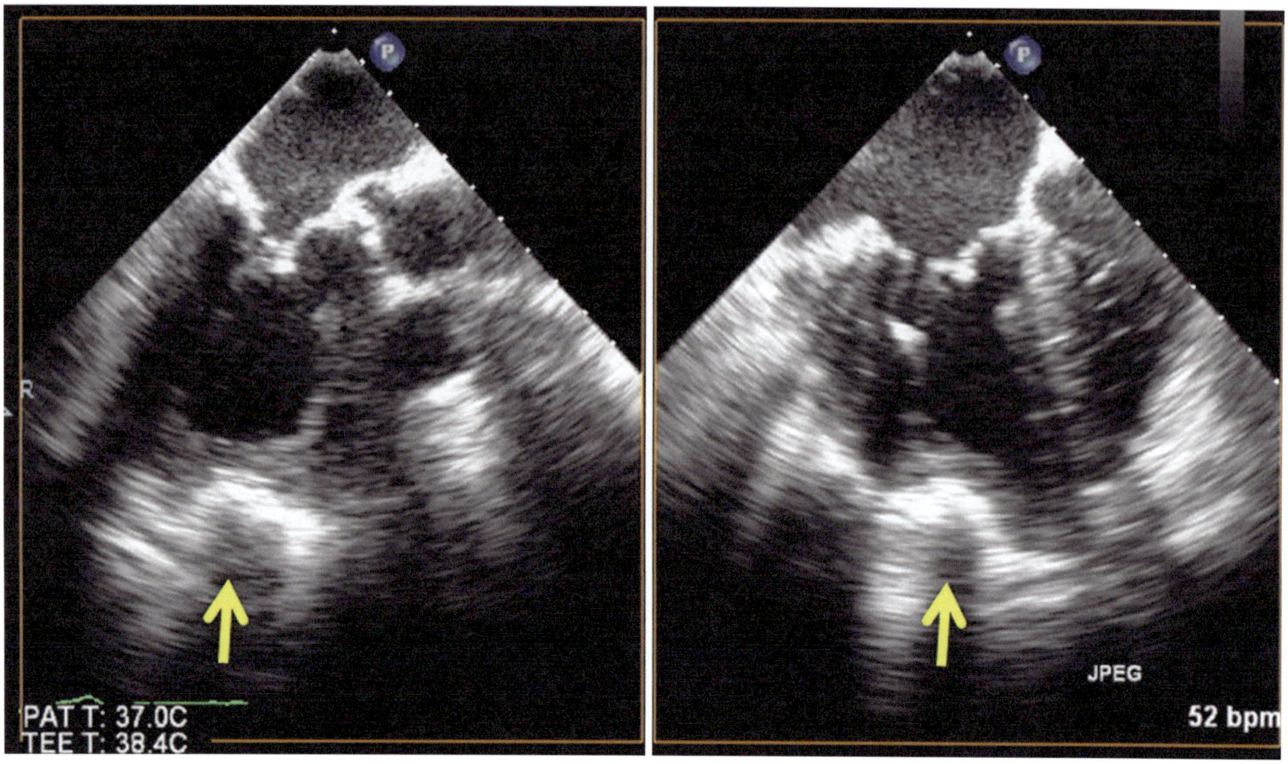

Fig. 29.2 For the transapical approach, localization of the left ventricular apex (mid-esophageal view) is performed using simultaneous multiplane imaging to ensure optimal location of the apical puncture. The *yellow arrow* indicates the surgeon's digit at the proposed site of puncture

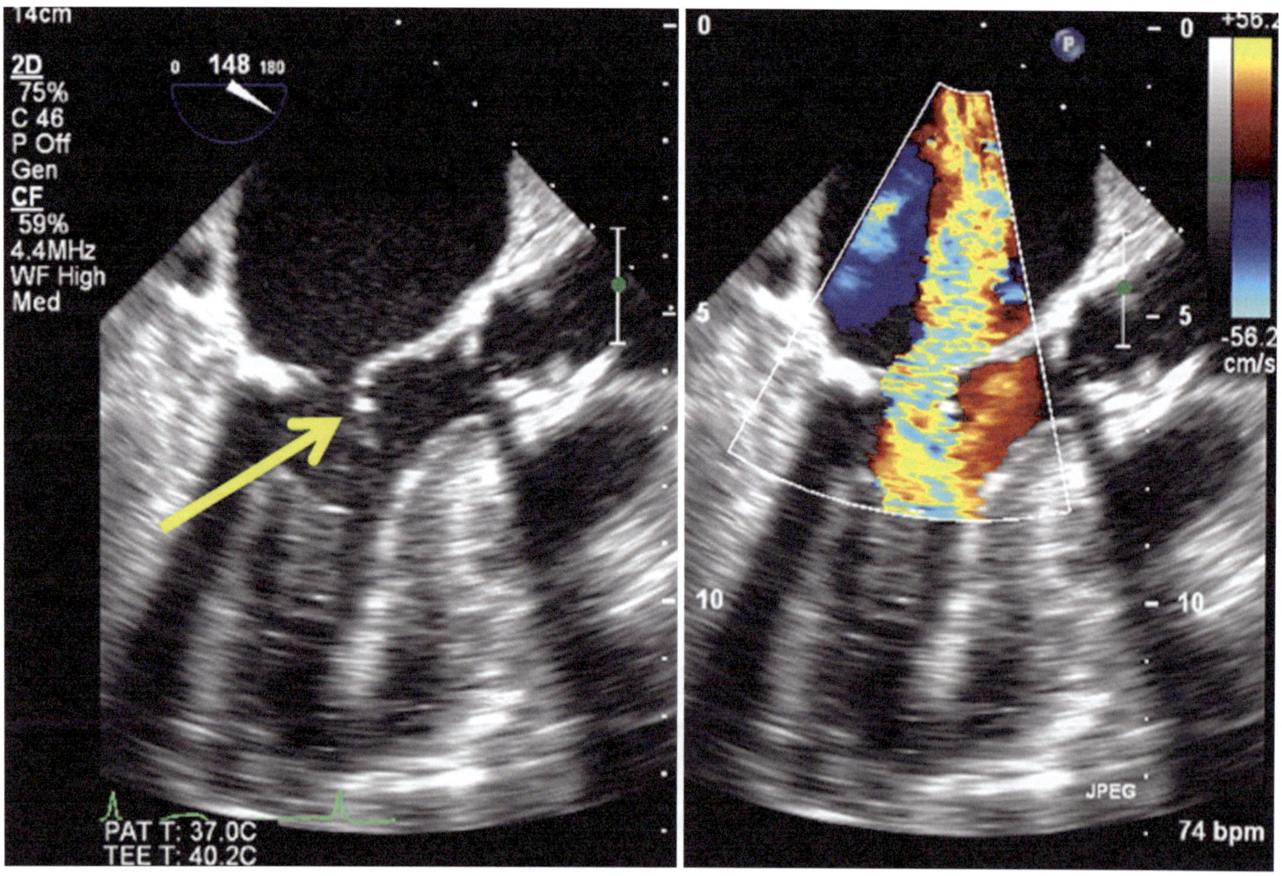

Fig. 29.3 Simultaneous two-dimensional and color Doppler imaging of the mitral valve showing tethering of the mitral leaflet (*yellow arrow*) caused by entrapment of stiff wire following apical cannulation. The color Doppler image suggests severe mitral regurgitation which was not seen at baseline

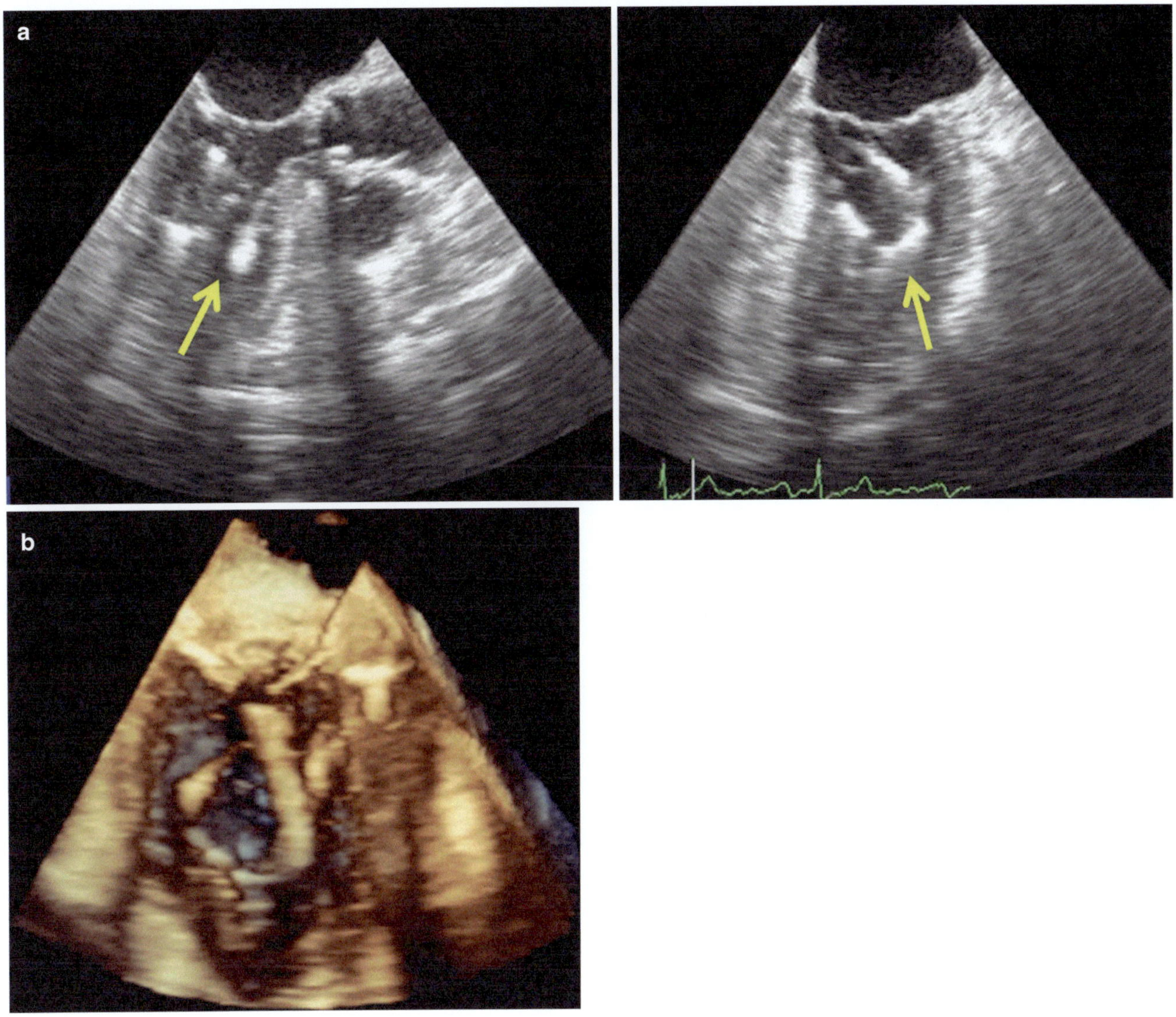

Fig. 29.4 For the transfemoral approach, echocardiographic imaging is used for assessing the position and stability of the J-wire within the ventricle. Panel (**a**) is a biplane image of the J-wire in the mid-ventricle which is a suboptimal position. Three-dimensional imaging (panel **b**) may be helpful in identifying wire position as well as the relationship to the mitral valve apparatus. Arrows in both panels are pointing to the J-wire

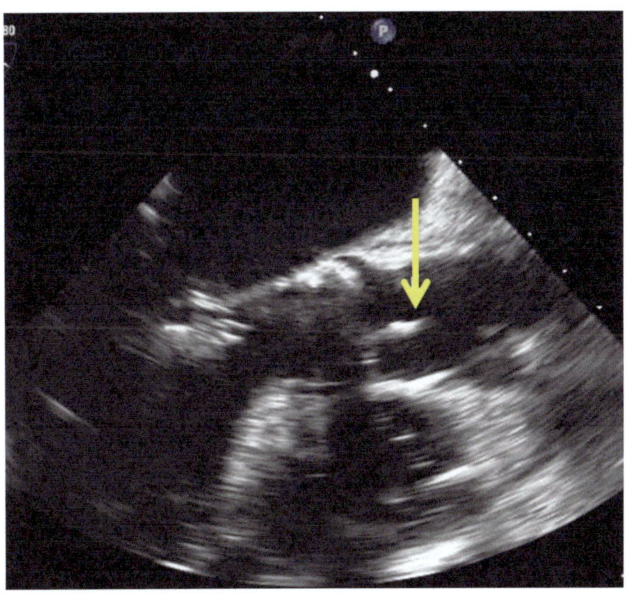

Fig. 29.5 Imaging during balloon aortic valvuloplasty can expeditiously determine the etiology of acute severe aortic regurgitation. In this instance, the *yellow arrow* indicates an avulsed aortic valve cusp

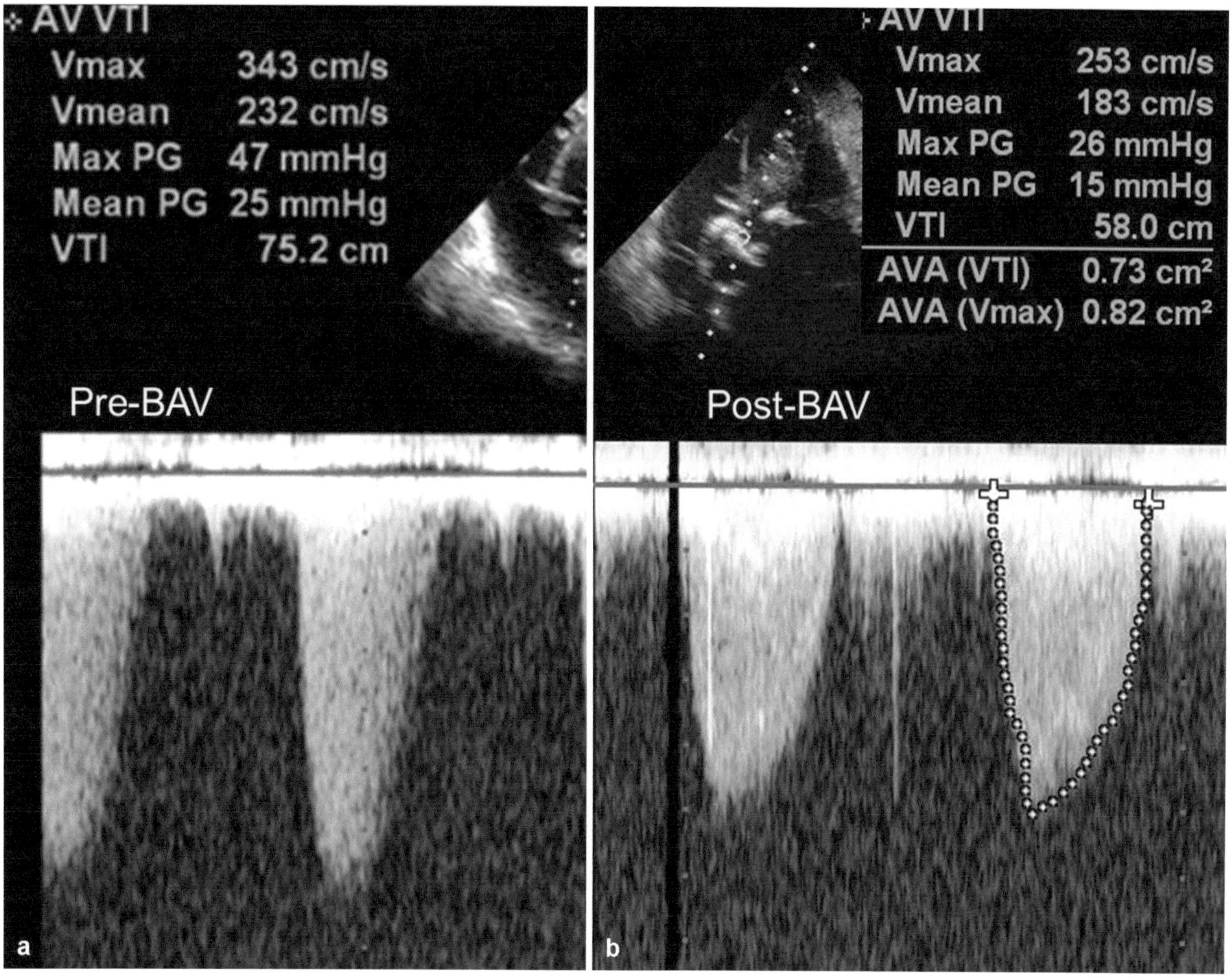

Fig. 29.6 Doppler assessment in pre-balloon valvuloplasty (**a**) suggests a mean aortic valve gradient of 25mm Hg with the post-balloon valvuloplasty doppler assessment (**b**) showing a reduction in the mean pressure to 15 mm Hg.

Intra-procedural Imaging for Complications

Following THV deployment, echocardiographic imaging provides rapid and accurate assessment of procedural success as well as complications. Transcatheter valve position, valve shape, leaflet motion, and gradients can all be assessed with TEE at the time of the procedure. Color flow Doppler imaging provides prompt and precise feedback to the proceduralists about the presence, location, and severity of aortic regurgitation; coronary patency; and mitral valve function. The etiology of any hemodynamic compromise such as from ventricular dysfunction or aortic root catastrophe can be assessed instantly.

Simultaneous multiplanar imaging or biplane imaging is a function of 3D TEE probes and is most useful in post-deployment imaging, both by saving time and increasing the accuracy of the assessment. The long-axis view is best for determining the final valve position (Fig. 29.8); however the short-axis views are vital to assess valve shape (Fig. 29.9) as well as presence and severity of paravalvular and transvalvular aortic regurgitation. Paravalvular regurgitation is best imaged from short-axis views just below the THV skirt (Fig. 29.10). More than mild or mild-moderate aortic regurgitation may often be reduced by a second balloon inflation. In contrast, transvalvular regurgitation should be assessed at the level of THV cusp closure in the middle of the stent (Fig. 29.11). Severe central aortic regurgitation in a well-placed THV should raise the possibility of primary THV failure and may necessitate urgent placement of a second THV. Deep gastric views may also be very helpful in assessing the severity of aortic regurgitation. From this imaging plane, there is no acoustic shadowing of the annulus. Whenever assessing the presence

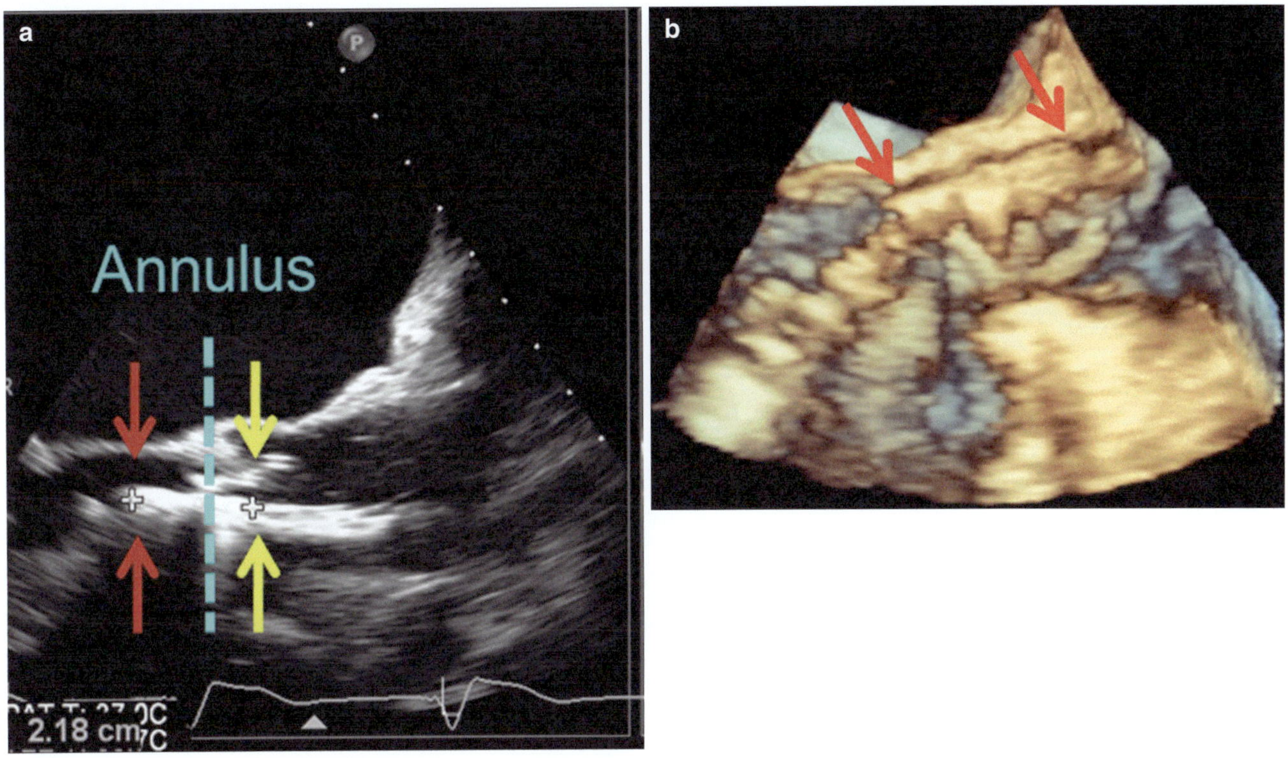

Fig. 29.7 As opposed to the heterogeneous appearance of the underlying deflated balloon, the crimped transcatheter heart valve (between *arrows* in panel **a**) is echodense and straight-edged. In more difficult cases, live 3D (narrow sector) may enhance imaging of the stent *red arrow* by increasing the "depth of field" (**b**)

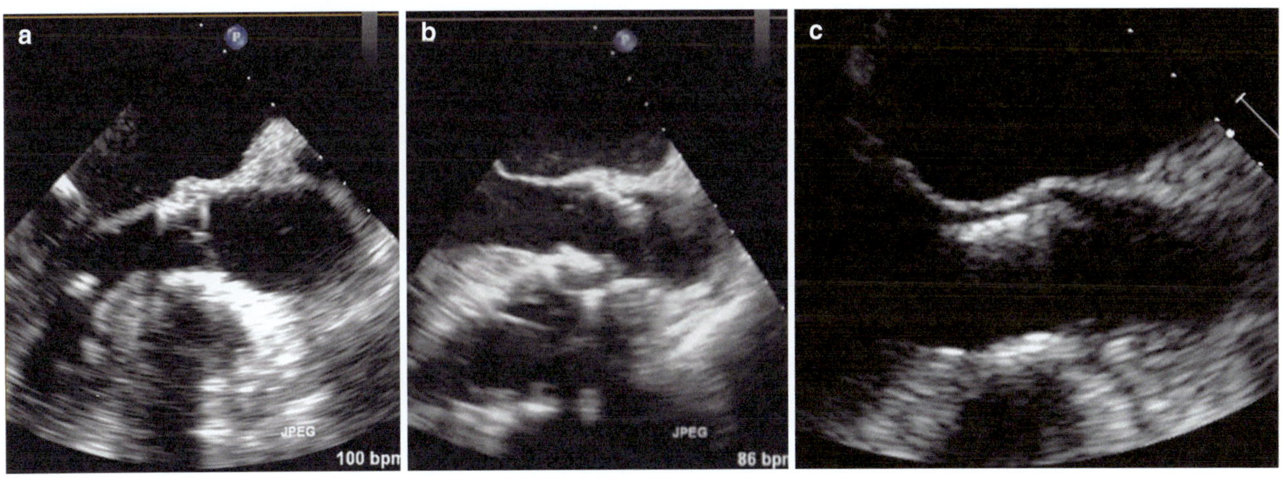

Fig. 29.8 Following valve deployment, the long-axis (sagittal plane) view is most useful for determining the final valve position. Panel (**a**) shows a well-positioned valve. Panel (**b**) shows a superiorly positioned valve (within the aorta). Panel (**c**) shows an apically positioned valve (within the LV)

and severity of aortic regurgitation, multiple views of the annulus should be obtained.

The assessment of hypotension is a particularly important function of intra-procedural echocardiographic imaging. Patency of the coronary arteries should always be assessed immediately following valve deployment in patients dependent upon native coronary artery blood supply. Short-axis images the aortic root at the level of the left main coronary artery can be acquired using 2D or 3D (biplane) imaging and color flow Doppler can be used to assess turbulent flow (Fig. 29.12). A marked reduction in left ventricular size or volume may indicate significant hypovolemia and bleeding. Development of a

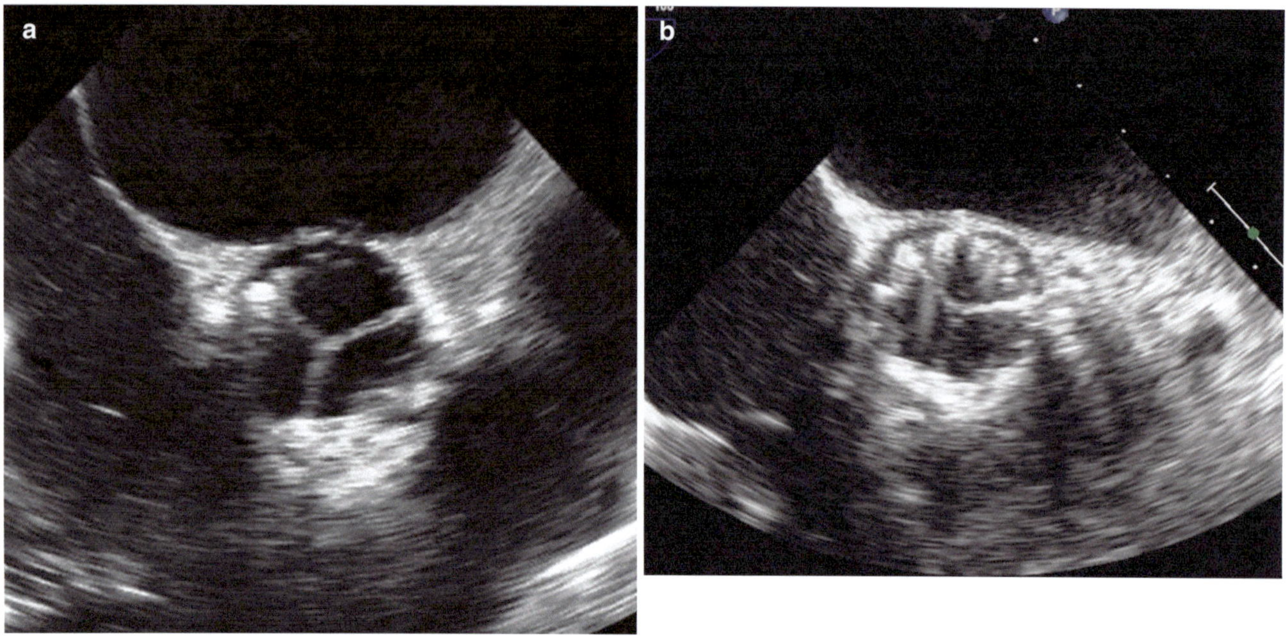

Fig. 29.9 Following valve deployment, the short-axis (transverse plane) view is most useful for determining the valve shape and leaflet motion. Panel (**a**) shows an asymmetric, oval transcatheter valve, whereas Panel (**b**) shows a symmetric, circular transcatheter valve

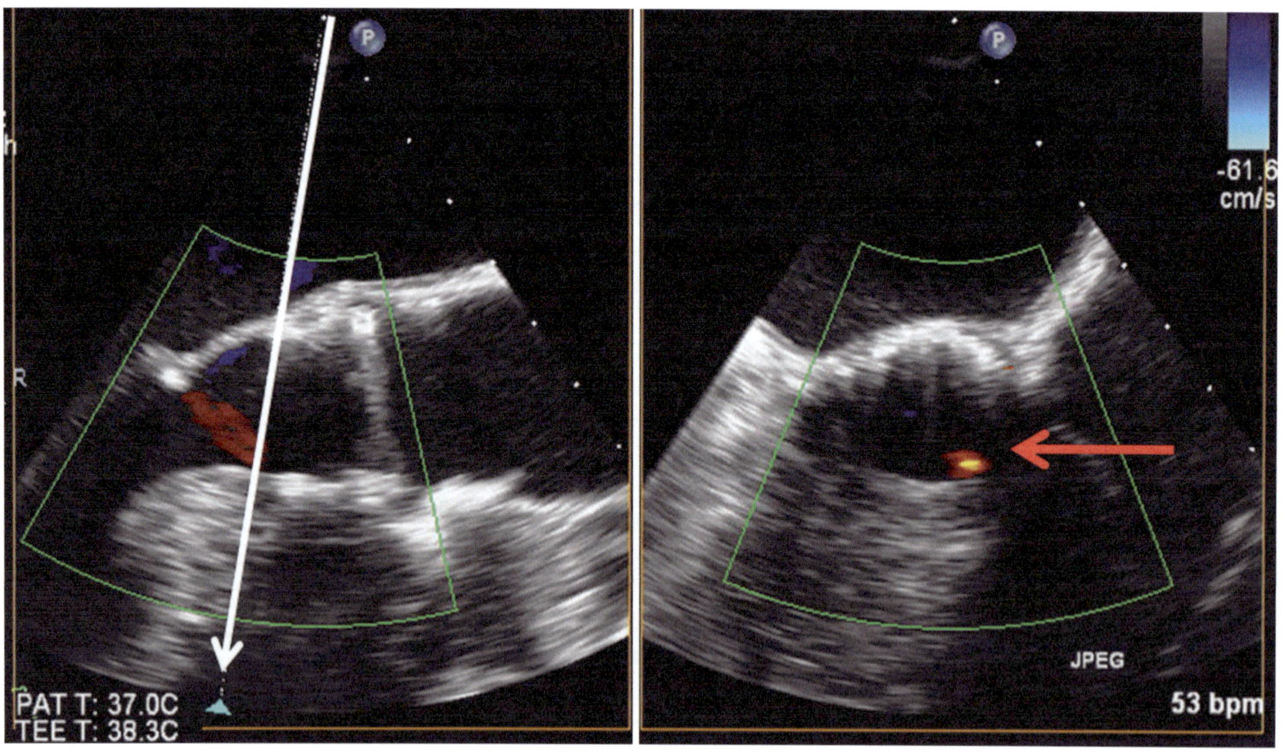

Fig. 29.10 Paravalvular regurgitation is best imaged from short-axis views just below the transcatheter heart valve skirt. In the *left panel* of this biplane image, the *white arrow* shows the location of the orthogonal short-axis image in the *right panel*. In this example, the region just apical to the transcatheter heart valve is ideal for imaging paravalvular regurgitation (*red arrow*)

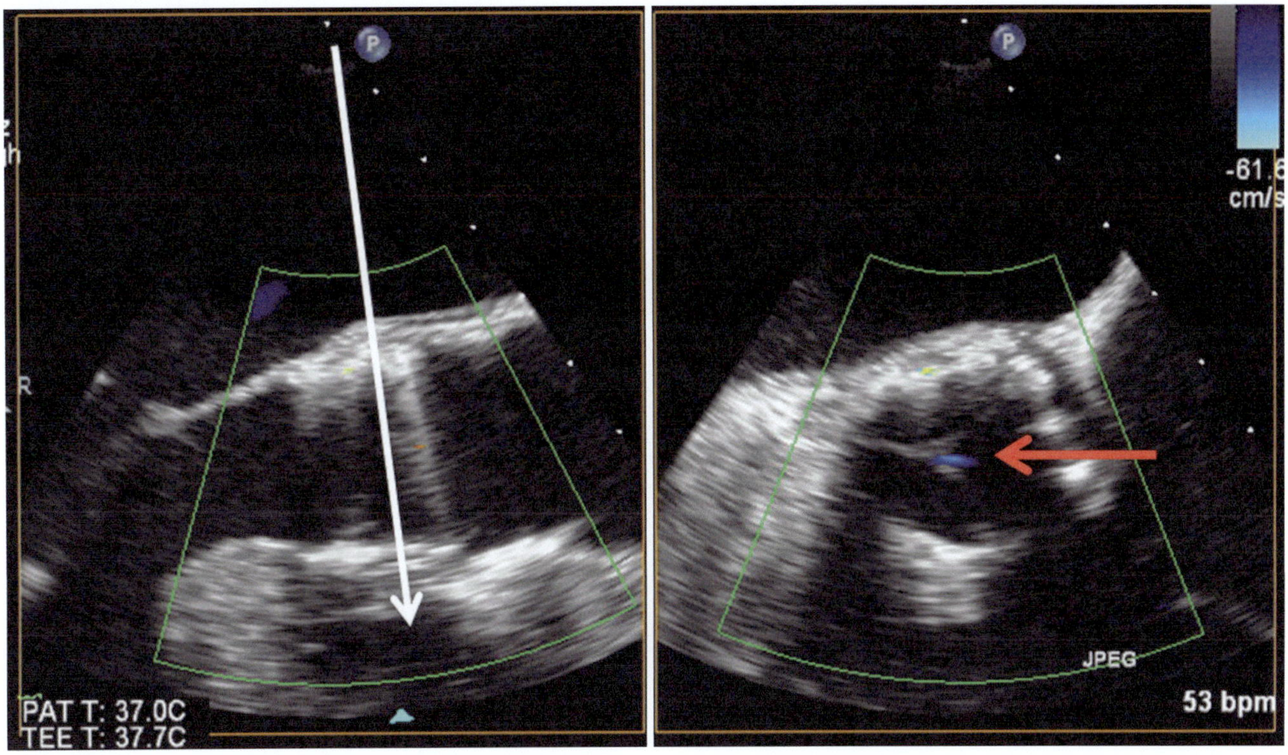

Fig. 29.11 Central regurgitation should be assessed at the level of transcatheter heart valve cusp closure in the middle of the stent. In the *left panel* of this biplane image, the *white arrow* shows the location of the orthogonal short-axis image in the *right panel*. In this example, the closure of the cusps of the transcatheter heart valve is imaged to assess central aortic regurgitation (*red arrow*)

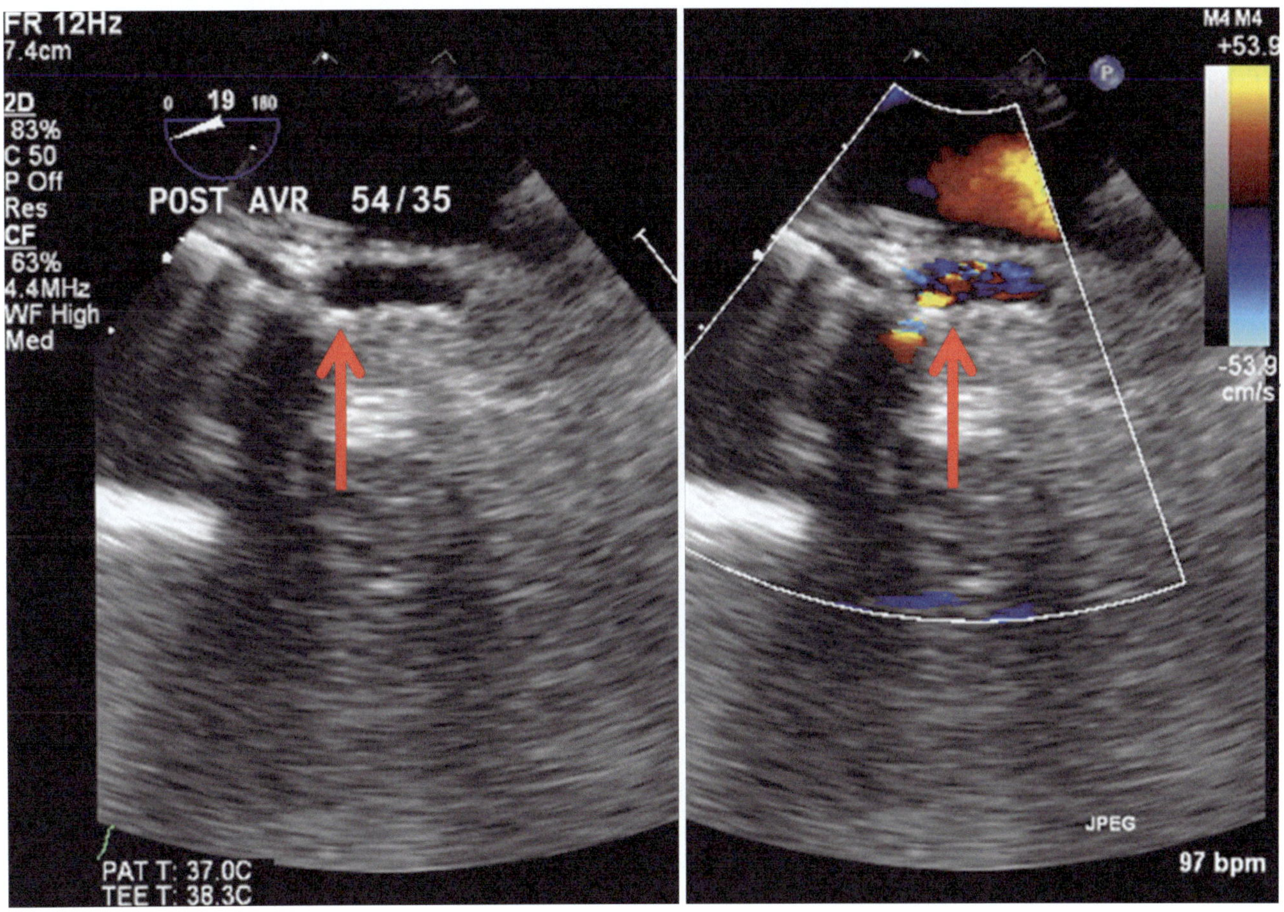

Fig. 29.12 The patency of the coronary arteries should be assessed following deployment of the transcatheter heart valve. In this example of simultaneous 2D and color Doppler imaging of the left main coronary artery, a calcified native left coronary cusp causes significant turbulence within the left main coronary artery (*red arrows*)

large pericardial of pleural effusion may indicate myocardial or aortic rupture.

References

1. Zamorano JL, Badano LP, Bruce C, Chan KL, Goncalves A, Hahn RT, et al. EAE/ASE recommendations for the use of echocardiography in new transcatheter interventions for valvular heart disease. J Am Soc Echocardiogr. 2011;24(9):937–65.
2. Bloomfield GS, Gillam LD, Hahn RT, Kapadia S, Leipsic J, Lerakis S, et al. A practical guide to multimodality imaging of transcatheter aortic valve replacement. JACC Cardiovasc Imaging. 2012;5(4):441–55.
3. Lang RM, Badano LP, Tsang W, Adams DH, Agricola E, Buck T, et al. EAE/ASE recommendations for image acquisition and display using three-dimensional echocardiography. J Am Soc Echocardiogr. 2012;25(1):3–46.
4. Troianos CA, Hartman GS, Glas KE, Skubas NJ, Eberhardt RT, Walker JD, et al. Guidelines for performing ultrasound guided vascular cannulation: recommendations of the American Society of Echocardiography and the Society of Cardiovascular Anesthesiologists. J Am Soc Echocardiogr. 2011;24(12):1291–318.
5. Ben-Dor I, Pichard AD, Satler LF, Goldstein SA, Syed AI, Gaglia Jr MA, et al. Complications and outcome of balloon aortic valvuloplasty in high-risk or inoperable patients. JACC Cardiovasc Interv. 2010;3(11):1150–6.

Angiography and Rotational Angiography for TAVR

30

Benoit Daneault and Jeffrey W. Moses

Abstract

Angiography (or fluoroscopy) is essential for guidance during transcatheter aortic valve replacement (TAVR); however its utility to assess aortic annulus dimension is not well established. Only a few small-scale studies have compared angiographic measurements with other imaging modalities. In general, they have observed moderate correlation with multidetector row CT (MDCT) and transesophageal echocardiography (TEE). However intra- and interobserver reproducibility was only moderate with angiography and inferior to other modalities. Newer technology—such as the Paieon's C-THV system—has been developed to help identify adequate perpendicular views to the annulus to facilitate accurate deployment and has been shown to be effective. Rotational angiography has been recently applied to TAVR, and preliminary data suggest a possible role for evaluation of aortic annulus dimensions as well as enhanced placement accuracy but more robust studies are needed. Rotational angiography has, however, been demonstrated to predict optimal projection angles reliably, with less radiation than MDCT and with limited use of iodinated contrast. These factors suggest the use of angiography and rotational angiography to be useful for assessment of aortic dimension and determination of optimal projection angles.

Keywords

Angiography • Rotational angiography • Paieon's C-THV system • DynaCT • Innova • 3-dimensional angiography (3DA)

Abbreviations

LAO	Left anterior oblique
LVOT	Left ventricular outflow tract
MDCT	Multidetector computed tomography
MRI	Magnetic resonance imaging
RAO	Right anterior oblique
STJ	Sinotubular junction
TAVR	Transcatheter aortic valve replacement
TEE	Transesophageal echocardiogram
THV	Transcatheter heart valve
TTE	Transthoracic echocardiogram
2D	2-dimensional
3D	3-dimensional
3DA	3-dimensional angiography

B. Daneault, MD, FRCPC (✉)
Department of Medicine,
Centre Hospitalier Universitaire de Sherbrooke,
Université de Sherbrooke, 3001, 12e Avenue Nord,
Sherbrooke, QC J1H 5N4, Canada
e-mail: benoit.daneault@usherbrooke.ca

J.W. Moses, MD
Department of Medicine, Columbia University Medical Center,
177 Fort Washington Avenue, New York, NY 10032, USA
e-mail: jm2456@columbia.edu

J.K. Min et al. (eds.), *Multimodality Imaging for Transcatheter Aortic Valve Replacement*,
DOI 10.1007/978-1-4471-2798-7_30, © Springer-Verlag London 2014

Introduction

Fluoroscopy and cine-angiography are the main imaging modalities used during transcatheter aortic valve replacement (TAVR). Angiography is essential to guide femoral access, the manipulation of wires and catheters, and transcatheter heart valve (THV) positioning. They are also useful for the assessment of aortic regurgitation severity, assessment of procedural complications after THV deployment, and guidance of percutaneous access site closure for transfemoral cases. The success of these procedures relies on excellent angiographic imaging.

From early clinical experiences, it has been realized that portable fluoroscopic systems should be avoided since they do not generate images of adequate quality and have been implicated in cases of THV malposition. Angiography and rotational angiography can also be useful for pre-procedural assessment of the aortic valve complex. Recent studies however suggest that three-dimensional (3D) assessment of the annulus is essential to guide valve sizing and placement, and that use of such 3D modalities may help in reducing paravalvular regurgitation [1–4]. This chapter will review the role of angiography, rotational angiography, and adjunctive systems in the evaluation of aortic annular dimensions and optimal projection angle for TAVR.

Angiography and Annular Measurement

The major limitation of angiography for aortic annular assessment is the two-dimensional (2D) aspect of this modality. While aortograms can be performed in multiple projections to assess different aortic planes, this technique may require significant amount of contrast and time and does not allow for a true 3D evaluation of the annulus. Angiographic assessment of the aortic annular dimension has been evaluated and compared to other imaging modalities in limited small studies, with methods used to measure annular dimension inconstant between studies.

Altiok et al. evaluated 49 patients with angiography, MDCT, transthoracic echocardiography (TTE), 2D transesophageal echocardiography (TEE), and 3D TEE [5]. In this study, two angiographic projections and a marked pigtail was used to assess annulus diameter. The sagittal plane was assessed with a 90° left anterior oblique (LAO) view and the coronal plane with a posteroanterior (PA) view. Each aortogram was done using 25 mL of contrast injected at a rate of 14 mL/s. The mean coronal diameter was significantly larger than the sagittal diameter (23.42 ± 2.08 mm vs. 22.54 ± 2.07 mm; $p<0.05$). There was a moderate correlation between measurements obtained by angiography compared to those obtained from MDCT ($r=0.74$ for sagittal plane and $r=0.56$ for coronal plane). Intra- and interobserver reproducibility was high for all other imaging modalities but was only moderate for angiography in the coronal ($r=0.57$ and $r=0.61$ for intra- and interobserver, respectively) and sagittal plane ($r=0.58$ and $r=0.56$).

Similarly, Kurra et al. also evaluated aortic annulus measurements obtained from angiography and compared it to MDCT in 40 patients by an alternate technique [6]. Annular dimensions were obtained from a right anterior oblique (RAO)/caudal and a LAO/cranial projection with coplanar alignment of the annulus. These investigators observed no significant difference in the dimensions obtained from the LAO and RAO projections (2.3 ± 0.4 cm vs. 2.3 ± 0.3 cm; $p=0.67$). When these measures were compared with the corresponding images obtained from MDCT, there was a significant difference in the measures obtained in the RAO projection (2.4 ± 0.3 cm for angiography vs. 2.2 ± 0.3 cm for MDCT; $p=0.029$) and a strong trend for those from the LAO projection (2.3 ± 0.3 cm for angiography vs. 2.4 ± 0.3 cm for MDCT; $p=0.052$). The mean diameter derived from the 2 measures was, however, similar between the two imaging modalities (2.3 ± 0.3 cm for MDCT vs. 2.3 ± 0.4 cm for angiography; $p=1.0$).

In a follow-up study, Tzikas et al. compared angiographic aortic annular measurement to TTE and MDCT in 70 patients [7]. Angiography was performed using a 6 F pigtail catheter in a coplanar view where the three cusps were aligned in the coronal plane and annuli diameters measured. Annuli diameters measured in coronal plane of MDCT (26.3 mm) were larger than with angiography (24.4 mm; $p=$NS) and angiographic diameters were significantly larger than TTE diameters (22.6 mm; $p<0.05$) and MDCT in the sagittal plane (21.8 mm). Correlation between angiography and MDCT in the coronal plane was good ($r=0.76$) but only moderate when compared with TTE ($r=0.57$). Interobserver reproducibility was best with MDCT followed by angiography and TTE.

Finally, Paelinek et al. compared angiography with magnetic resonance imaging (MRI), TEE, and TTE in 28 patients [8]. A marked pigtail positioned in the noncoronary cusp was used, and the angiography was performed in a view aligning all cusps, similar to the latter description. Diameters were measured between the angiographic attachments of the calcified leaflets in systole. MRI, TTE, and TEE measurements were done using the sagittal plane. Unlike other prior studies, these investigators observed smaller annuli with angiography compared to all other modalities ($p<0.001$). The intra- (−0.27 ± 0.39 cm) and interobserver (−0.26 ± 0.44 cm) reproducibility was larger with angiography than with other modalities.

Collectively, angiographic assessment of annular dimension has been studied in limited, small-scale studies, many of which used different techniques to measure aortic annulus diameters. Several lessons have been learned from these early studies; namely, annular diameters are distinctive when obtained in different projection (sagittal vs. coronal).

Dimensions in the coronal plane are larger than in the sagittal plane, consistent with observation from 3D TEE and MDCT. There seems to be moderate correlation between angiography and MDCT when comparing images obtained in the same plane. However, intra- and interobserver reproducibility is only moderate with angiography compared to good with MDCT. It is the authors' belief that 3D modalities such as MDCT are more reliable and robust for planning TAVR treatment.

Angiography and Optimal Projection Angle

Angiography is useful not only to evaluate aortic annulus dimension but also to guide THV implantation. To facilitate optimal positioning of the THV, a perpendicular projection to the annulus plane is essential. This angle has traditionally been located by trial and error with repeated angiograms using 10–15 mL of contrast but has also been evaluated for feasibility in limited study [9].

At present, the Paieon's C-THV system (Paieon, Israel) is a proprietary real-time angiography-based software designed to facilitate TVH implantation. It operates as a stand-alone PC workstation that is connected to the C-arm and hospital image network for image acquisition. An important clinical use for this system is to help the operator find a perpendicular projection for THV implantation. The system is based on two aortograms: a LAO/cranial and a RAO/caudal view (Fig. 30.1). With these two views, the system will generate a series of suitable angles for the operator (Fig. 30.2). This system has been studied by Tzikas et al. on 73 patients [10]. They retrospectively compared the results of the Paieon system with MDCT, wherein the mean difference in angle between both modality was 6.6±4.9°. Notably, the difference was significantly less if the second projection was done in the recommended zone of the system. When evaluated

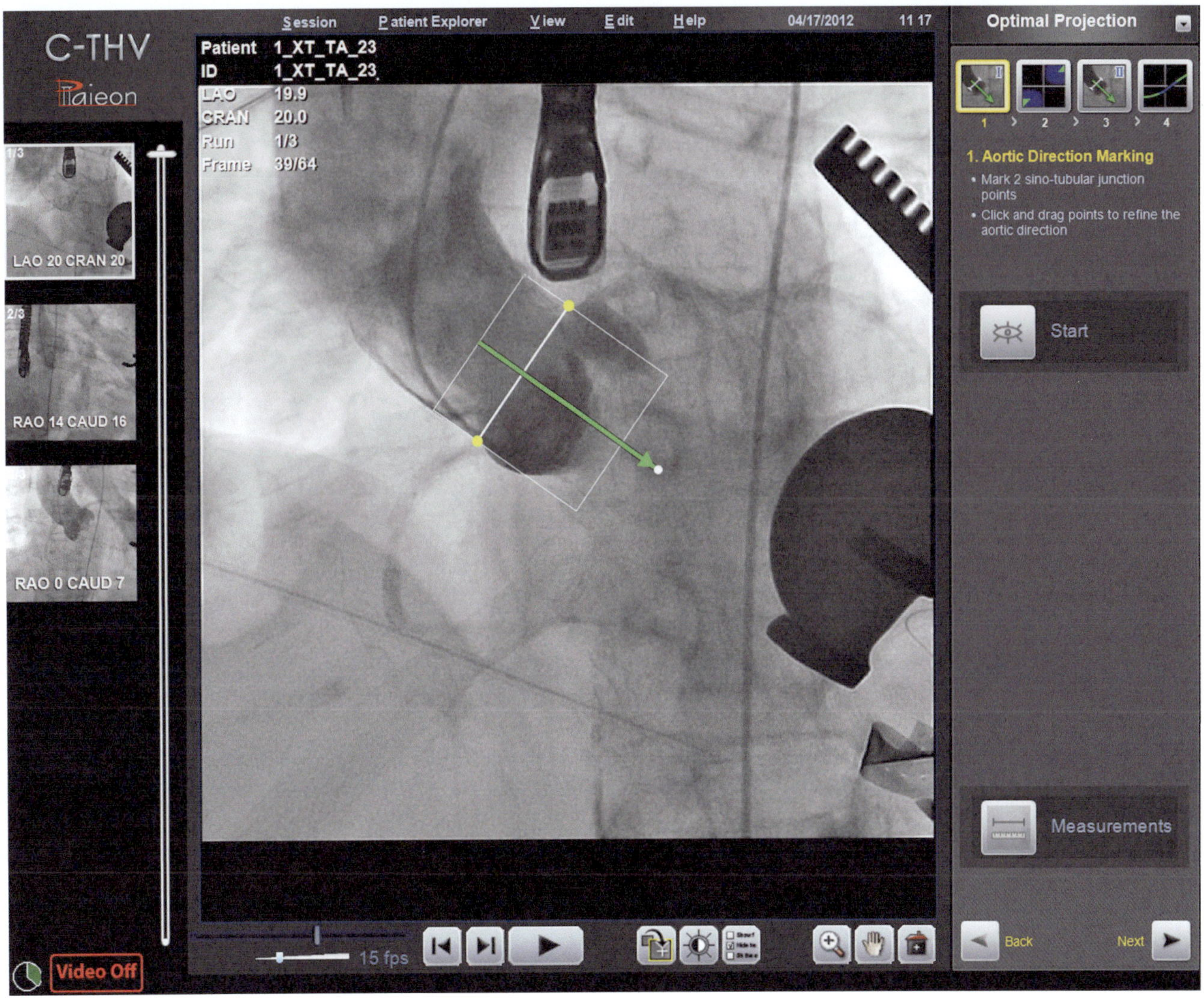

Fig. 30.1 Paieon's C-THV system using first aortogram and marking orientation of the aorta

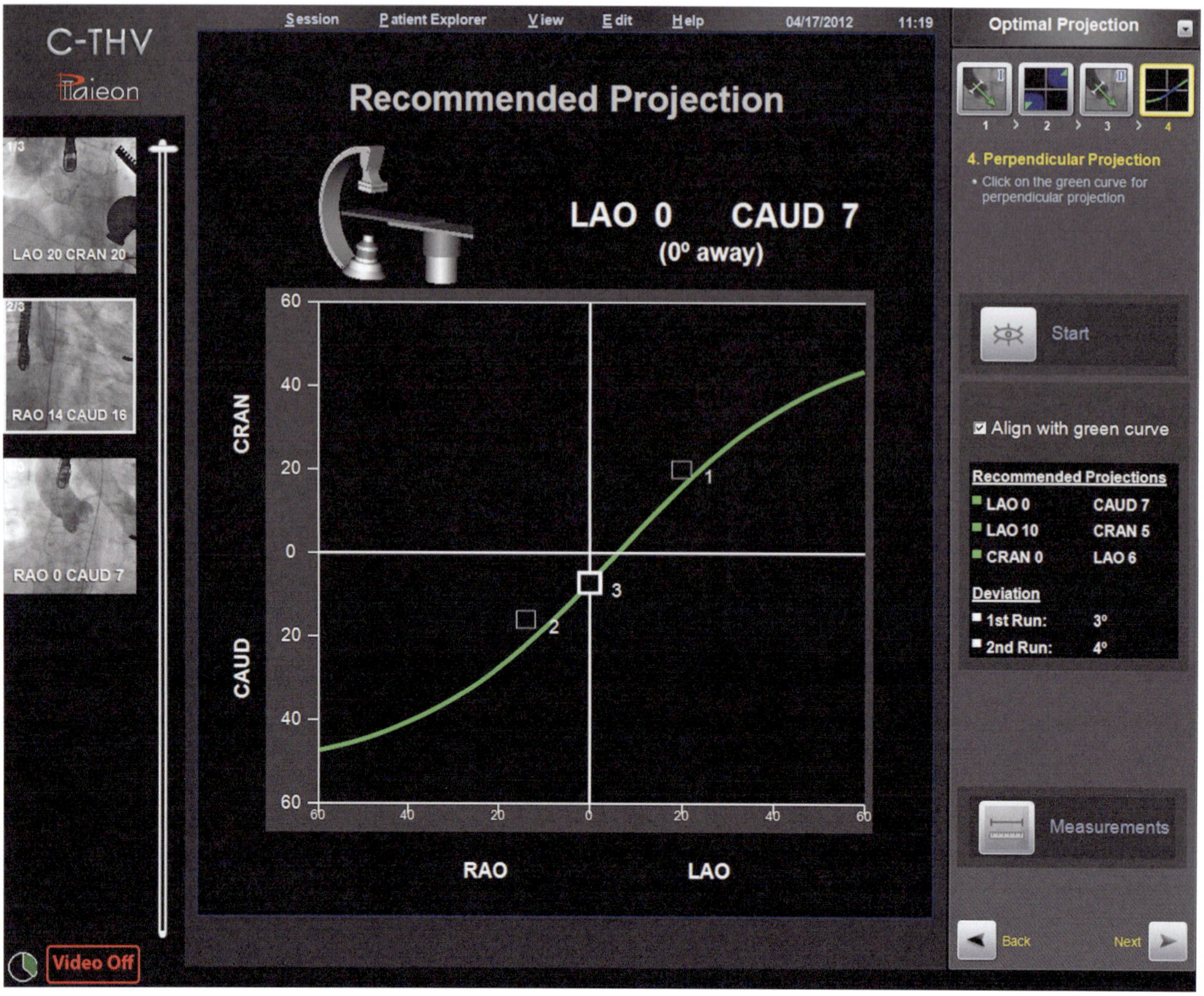

Fig. 30.2 Paieon's C-THV system showing multiple angle of perpendicularity based on two angiograms (#1 and 2). Angiogram #3 is on the curve and represents the projection chosen by the operator

prospectively, the C-THV system was also good at predicting working angle with a mean difference of $5.5 \pm 3.4°$ with the operator's choice.

The C-THV system can also be used as an adjunctive imaging tool during valve positioning. Its ability to track calcification with real-time fluoroscopy allows the system to display a target line representing the aortic annulus plane (Fig. 30.3). During THV positioning, a yellow line denotes the annulus, while two green lines localize to the zone of the THV that is to be positioned at the annular level (Fig. 30.4).

Finally, the C-THV system allows post-deployment measurements in order to assess THV expansion (Fig. 30.5). This modality has not yet been validated clinically although in rare cases has allowed operators to recognize THV under-expansion. Given these attributes, the Paieon system has been used as a research tool to evaluate additional stent expansion after balloon expandable THV post-dilatation [11].

Rotational Angiography

Rotational angiography is a technology that utilizes an X-ray tube and flat panel detector system to acquire and allow construction of 3D images of both vascular and soft tissue structures. This is accomplished by rotating the C-arm around the patient (200–220°) while collecting an array of equally spaced 2D X-ray projection images and then using algorithms to reconstruct a 3D image. This

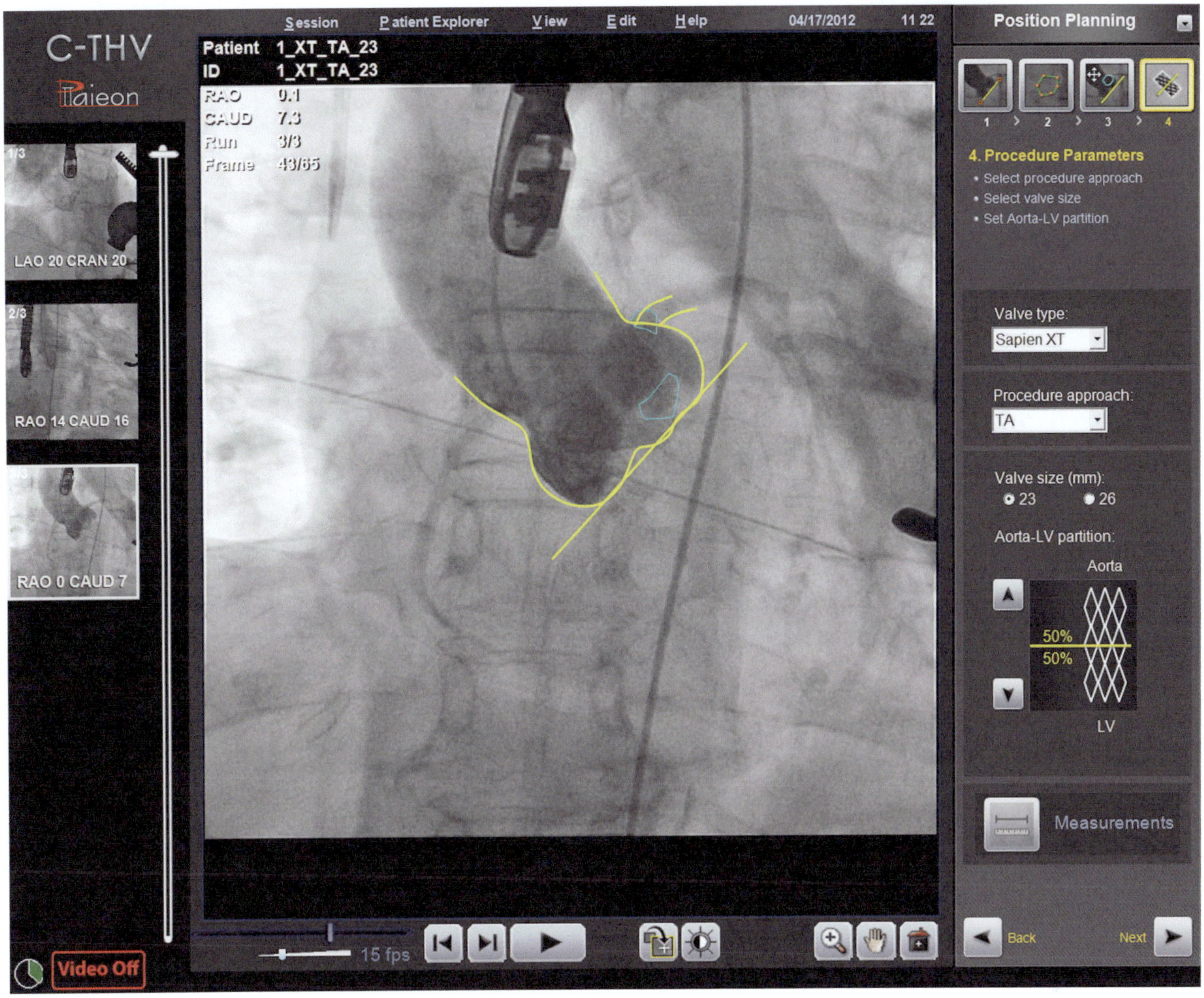

Fig. 30.3 Paieon's C-TVH system showing contour tracking and the annulus target line

technology is now available from many manufacturers of cardiac catheterization laboratory suites: Siemens AG (Erlangen, Germany), GE Healthcare (Chalfont St Giles, UK), and Philips Healthcare (Best, the Netherlands). While this technique was at first limited to imaging high-contrast structures such as bone and contrast-filled vessels, the availability of flat panel detectors has enabled the ability to obtain CT-like images of soft tissue. This technology has recently been adapted for imaging dynamic structures such as the beating heart [12].

This adaptation of rotational angiography to the beating heart consists of making multiple sweeps (as opposed to the single sweep used for imaging static structures) while recording the ECG—such that a single arc of image data can be collected for one phase of the cardiac cycle via retrospective gating—and a 3D image for that phase can then be reconstructed. Rotational angiography has been successful at imaging heart structures including the four cardiac chambers, pulmonary outflow tract, pulmonary veins, and proximal coronary arteries. With the use of rapid ventricular pacing during aortography, single-sweep imaging of the ascending aorta can be performed with excellent resolution. This new technology has now been applied to TAVR. It has been combined with software dedicated to identify the plane of the aortic annulus and aortic dimensions in various packages (Syngo X Workstation, Siemens Healthcare; Innova 3D cardiac, GE Healthcare; HeartNavigator, Philips Healthcare). Evidence of its utility predicting projection angles and for annular dimension assessment is accumulating.

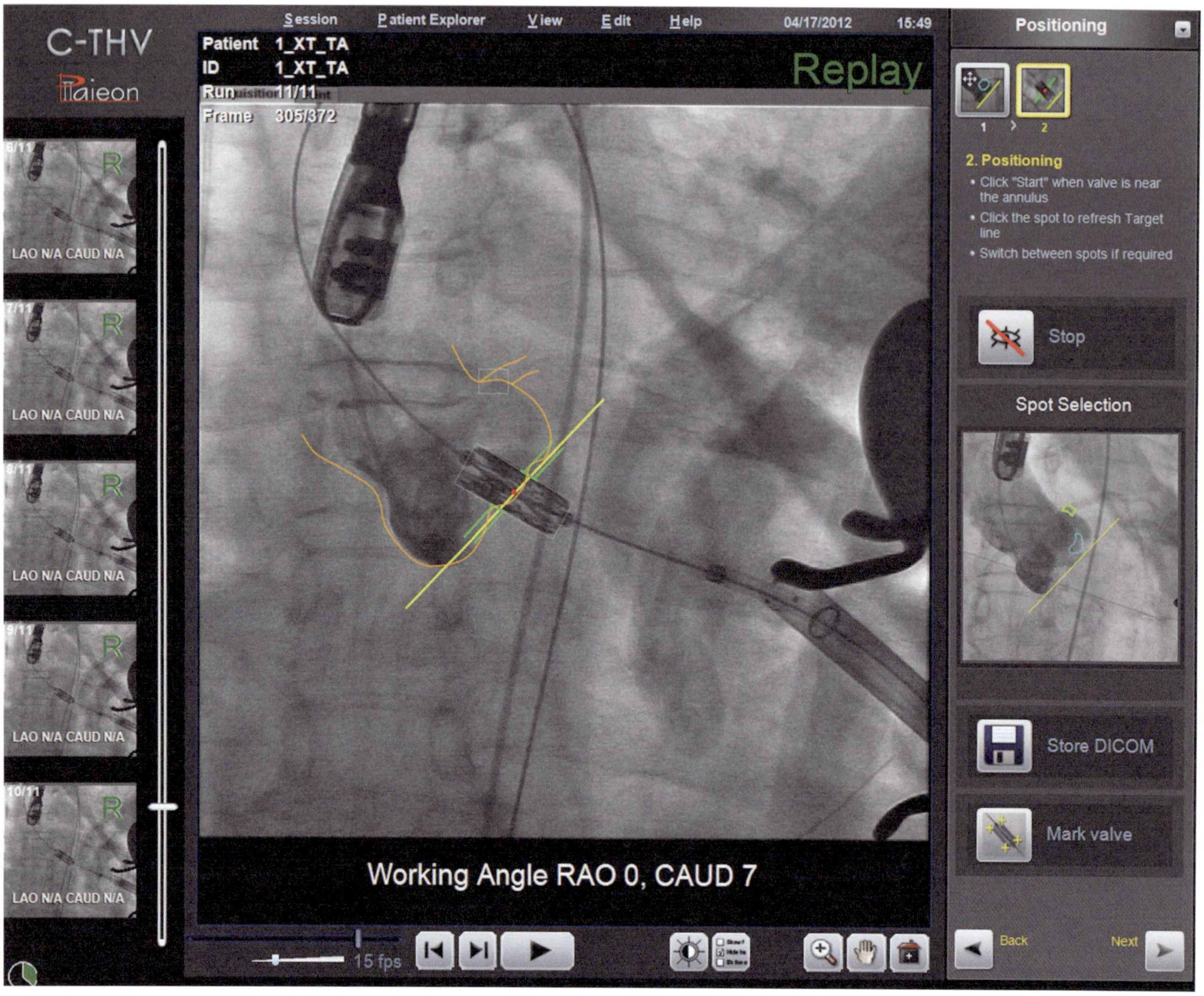

Fig. 30.4 Paieon's C-THV system during THV positioning. The contour of the aorta and the annulus line are shown in *yellow*. The *green lines* represent the middle of the THV, which should be deployed at the level of the aortic annulus. The system allows different configuration of the *green lines* (e.g., 60 % aortic, 40 % ventricular)

Evidence Supporting Use of Rotational Angiography

Bai et al. evaluated radiation dose of MDCT compared to rotational angiography or C-arm CT, or DynaCT (Siemens AG, Erlangen, Germany) [13]. For all scanning protocols evaluated, a significant reduction in organ dose with DynaCT was observed as compared to MDCT with comparable image quality. More recently, Binder et al. evaluated the efficacy of angiographic 3D reconstruction using DynaCT to predict optimal deployment projection for TAVR and compared it with MDCT [14]. 3D angiography (3DA) images were acquired during rapid ventricular pacing (160–180 bpm) and a breath hold. A 6 F pigtail catheter positioned in the non-coronary cusp was used to inject 32 mL of contrast at 8 mL/s (or 20 mL of contrast diluted with 40 mL of normal saline injected at 15 mL/s). Volume sets from rotational angiograms were reconstructed using a dedicated workstation (SyngoX Workstation, Siemens Healthcare, Erlangen, Germany) that automatically depicted the aortic valve cusps and generated a circle indicating the annular plane (Fig. 30.6). Predicted projections were compared with post-deployment projections showing superposition of anterior and posterior stent struts. 3DA was obtained in 40 patients (68 % also had a MDCT) with image quality was inadequate in 1 patient. There was a significant correlation between 3DA and MDCT for prediction of perpendicular views ($r=0.682$; $p<0.001$). The shortest distance from the post-deployment perpendicular prosthesis projection to the regression line was shorter for 3DA ($5.1 \pm 4.6°$) than for MDCT ($7.9 \pm 4.9°$; $p=0.01$).

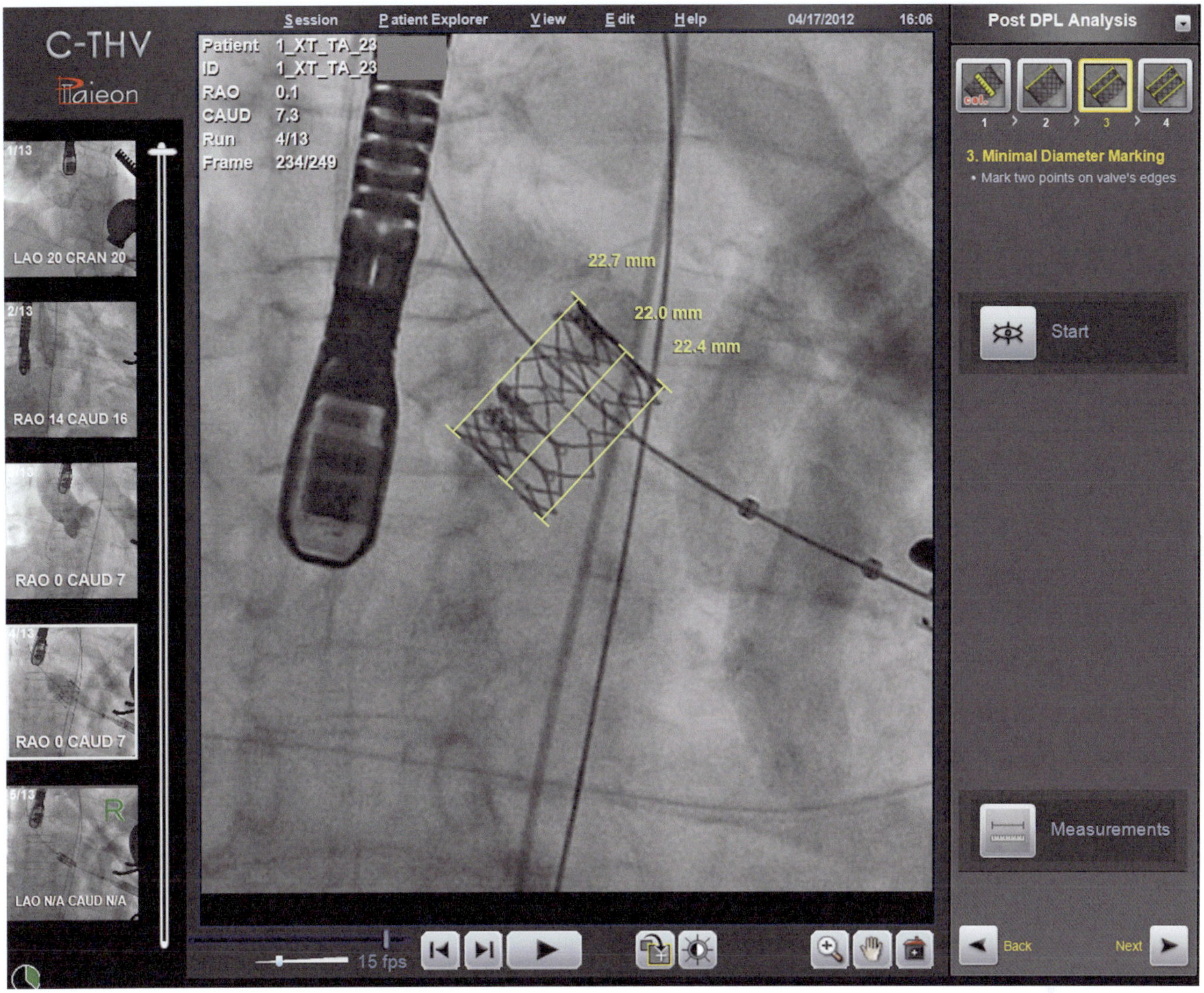

Fig. 30.5 Paieon's C-THV system post-deployment analysis showing inflow, mid, and outflow dimension of the THV stent

Despite these small differences, this study confirmed the feasibility of 3DA to identify a perpendicular angle.

The ability to perform 3DA during the procedure ensures identical patient positioning and may explain the slight superiority compared to MDCT in this study. The Paieon's C-THV system, as mentioned above, has been demonstrated to be helpful to determine perpendicular projections. The 3DA and the Syngo software add to possibility to visualize the geographic position of each cusp, which may help further the operator to pick an adequate projection for THV implantation. Meyhöfer et al. measured aortic annulus diameter using rotational angiography and compared it with TEE in 99 patients [15]. A different fixed C-arm system (Innova 3100^{IQ}, GE Healthcare, Chalfont St Giles, UK) with a square 30 cm flat panel detector to perform the 3D rotational angiography acquisition (Innova 3D Cardiac) (Fig. 30.7) was used. The system records 150 projections at 30 frames per second during the 5 s 200° rotation. Images are automatically sent to the post-processing workstation (Advantage Workstation, Volume Share, GE Healthcare, Chalfont St Giles, UK) and reconstructed in 3D volume. To minimize motion of the cardiac structure and minimize contrast utilization, acquisitions were performed under rapid pacing at 180 beats per minute (bpm) and during a breath hold. Injection of 50 mL of contrast at a rate of 12 mL/s was done with a 5 F pigtail catheter positioned in the ascending aorta. The investigators were able to obtain adequate images to assess annular diameter in all patients. Slightly larger annular dimensions were observed with rotational angiography (22.13 ± 2.09 mm) when compared to TEE (21.58 ± 2.09 mm), while the sinotubular junction (STJ) was similar with both modalities (26.22 ± 2.71 vs. 26.22 ± 2.73) (Fig. 30.8). There was a good correlation between rotational angiography and TEE for annulus and STJ dimensions (r = 0.83).

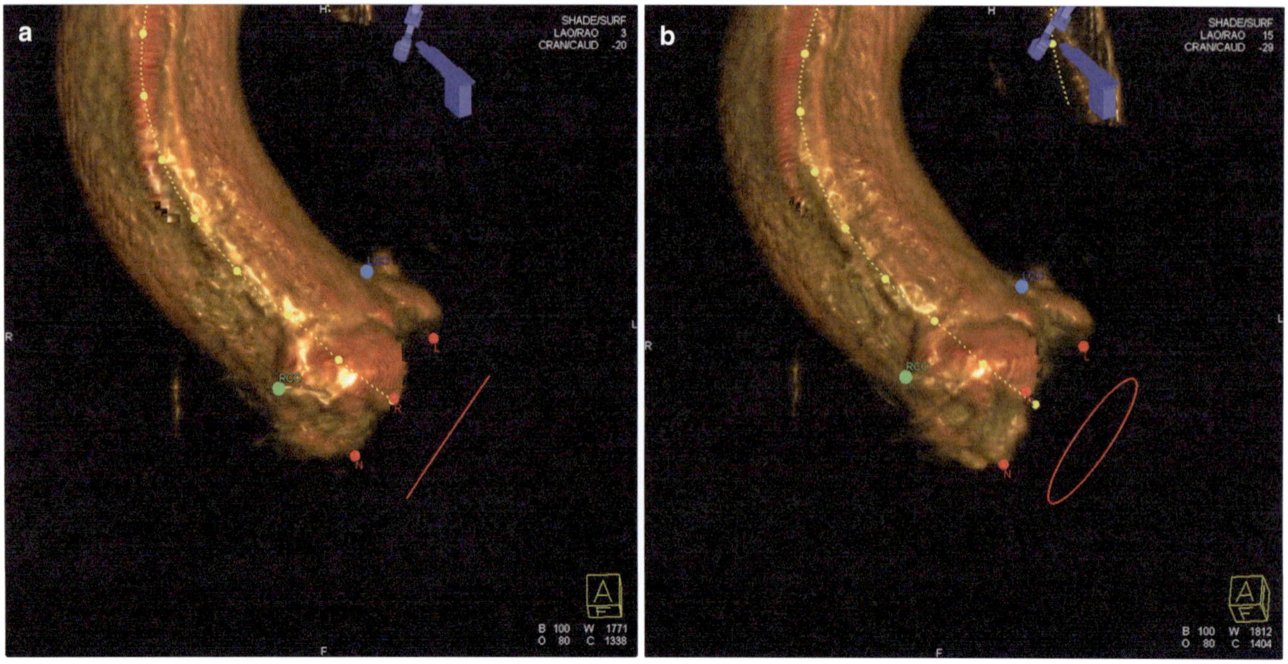

Fig. 30.6 Rotational angiography using DynaCT and the Syngo software for 3D reconstruction. The *red dots* represent the nadir of each cusp. The *blue dot* represents the ostium of the left main coronary artery and the *green dot* the ostium of the right coronary artery. In panel (**a**), all cusps are aligned on the same plane and the *red circle* is seen as a *line*. In panel (**b**), the *circle* is seen since the cusps are not aligned in the same plane

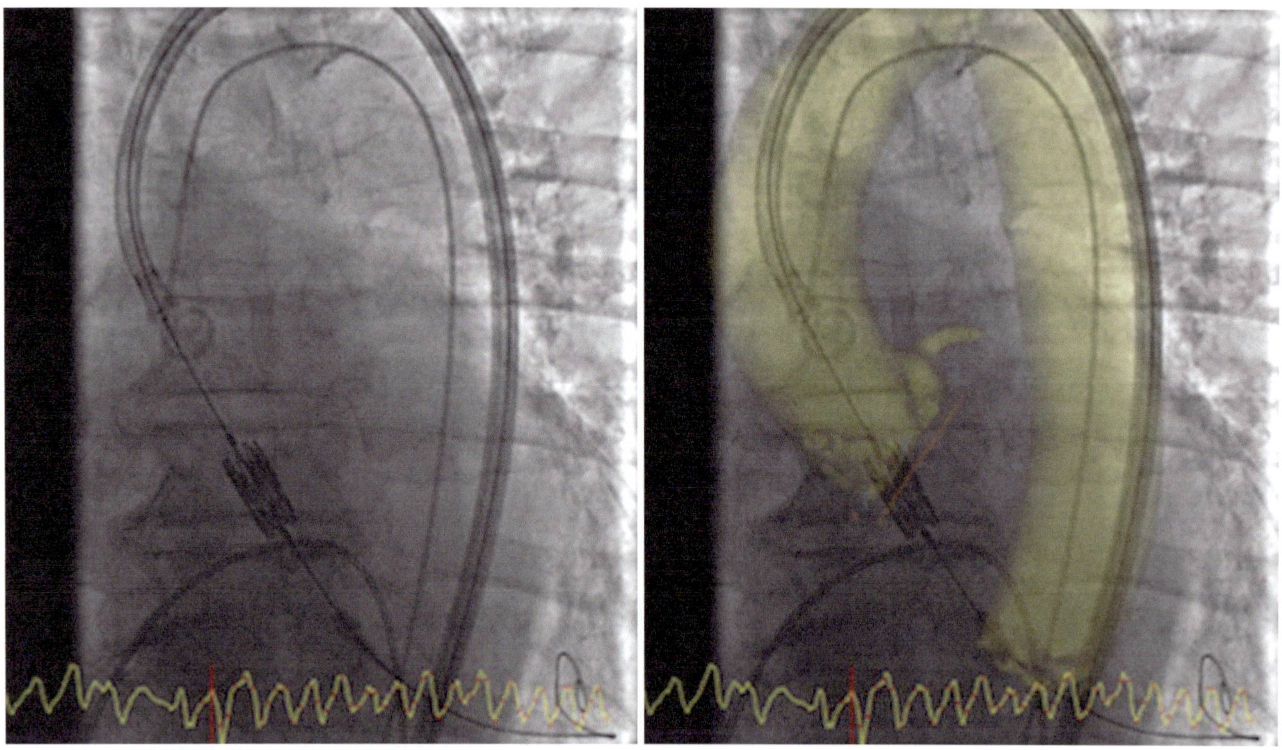

Fig. 30.7 Superimposition of aortic landmark and annulus plane obtained from prior CT scan over live fluoroscopic images using the GE system

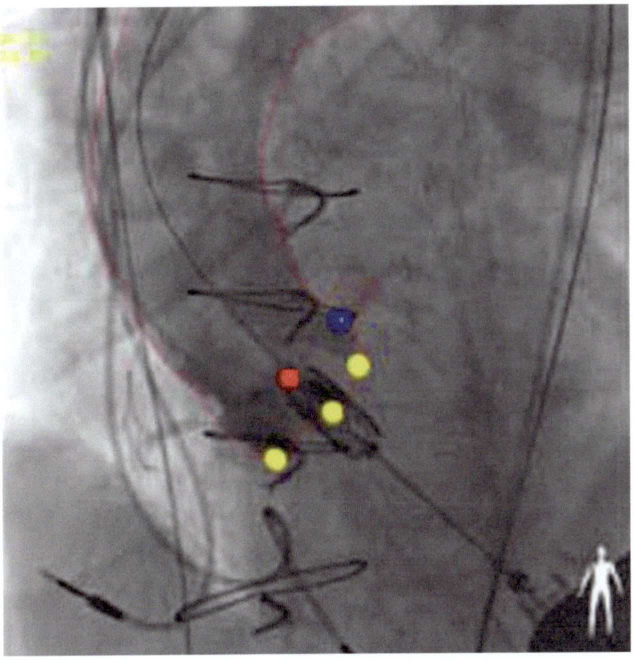

Fig. 30.8 Superimposition of aortic landmark and annulus plane obtained from prior CT scan over live fluoroscopic images using the HeartNavigator (Philips) system. *Yellow dots* represent virtual annular ring, and *blue* and *red dots* represent the origins of the left main and right coronary arteries, respectively

Limitations of Rotational Angiography

While this new technology seems promising for prediction of an optimal projection angles during TAVR procedures, some limitations with regard to aortic annular sizing must be considered. Similar to angiography, the techniques described above evaluate a different anatomical "annulus" than MDCT or TEE since the left ventricular outflow tract (LVOT) is not filled by contrast. Perimeter and area measurements with this technique are subject to significant intra- and interobserver variability owing to no clear anatomical delineation between the nadirs of each cusp. Different imaging protocols may be explored in the future with the pigtail across the aortic valve that would allow for injection of contrast in the LVOT and the aorta during rapid ventricular pacing to assess the ability to reproduce the measures acquired with CT. However, this may compromise the reliable identification of optimal projection angles and may require greater amount of contrast. Further studies comparing rotational angiography to MDCT are warranted before this technique should be adopted as a standard.

Conclusion

There is growing evidence suggesting that 3D assessment of the aortic annulus is essential for appropriate THV selection. Rotational angiography has shown great promise for encouraging this evaluation, but greater clinical evidence and larger scale studies comparing it to commonly used modalities are necessary to support its routine utilization for annular sizing.

References

1. Jilaihawi H, Kashif M, Fontana G, Furugen A, Shiota T, Friede G, et al. Cross-sectional computed tomographic assessment improves accuracy of aortic annular sizing for transcatheter aortic valve replacement and reduces the incidence of paravalvular aortic regurgitation. J Am Coll Cardiol. 2012;59(14):1275–86. Epub 2012/03/01.
2. Willson AB, Webb JG, Labounty TM, Achenbach S, Moss R, Wheeler M, et al. 3-dimensional aortic annular assessment by multidetector computed tomography predicts moderate or severe paravalvular regurgitation after transcatheter aortic valve replacement: a multicenter retrospective analysis. J Am Coll Cardiol. 2012;59(14):1287–94. Epub 2012/03/01.
3. Jabbour A, Ismail TF, Moat N, Gulati A, Roussin I, Alpendurada F, et al. Multimodality imaging in transcatheter aortic valve implantation and post-procedural aortic regurgitation: comparison among cardiovascular magnetic resonance, cardiac computed tomography, and echocardiography. J Am Coll Cardiol. 2011;58(21):2165–73. Epub 2011/11/15.
4. Unbehaun A, Pasic M, Dreysse S, Drews T, Kukucka M, Mladenow A, et al. Transapical aortic valve implantation: incidence and predictors of paravalvular leakage and transvalvular regurgitation in a series of 358 patients. J Am Coll Cardiol. 2012;59(3):211–21. Epub 2012/01/14.
5. Altiok E, Koos R, Schröder J, Brehmer K, Hamada S, Becker M, et al. Comparison of two-dimensional and three-dimensional imaging techniques for measurement of aortic annulus diameters before transcatheter aortic valve implantation. Heart. 2011;97(19):1578–84.
6. Kurra V, Kapadia SR, Tuzcu EM, Halliburton SS, Svensson L, Roselli EE, et al. Pre-procedural imaging of aortic root orientation and dimensions: comparison between X-ray angiographic planar imaging and 3-dimensional multidetector row computed tomography. JACC Cardiovasc Interv. 2010;3(1):105–13.
7. Tzikas A, Schultz CJ, Piazza N, Moelker A, Van Mieghem NM, Nuis R-J, et al. Assessment of the aortic annulus by multislice computed tomography, contrast aortography, and trans-thoracic echocardiography in patients referred for transcatheter aortic valve implantation. Catheter Cardiovasc Interv. 2011;77(6):868–75.
8. Paelinck BP, Van Herck PL, Rodrigus I, Claeys MJ, Laborde J-C, Parizel PM, et al. Comparison of magnetic resonance imaging of aortic valve stenosis and aortic root to multimodality imaging for selection of transcatheter aortic valve implantation candidates. Am J Cardiol. 2011;108(1):92–8.
9. Bagur R, Rodés-Cabau J, Doyle D, De Larochellière R, Villeneuve J, Lemieux J, et al. Usefulness of TEE as the primary imaging technique to guide transcatheter transapical aortic valve implantation. JACC Cardiovasc Imaging. 2011;4(2):115–24.
10. Tzikas A, Schultz C, Van Mieghem NM, de Jaegere PPT, Serruys PW. Optimal projection estimation for transcatheter aortic valve implantation based on contrast-aortography: validation of a Prototype Software. Catheter Cardiovasc Interv. 2010;76(4):602–7.
11. Daneault B, Koss E, Hahn RT, Kodali S, Williams MR, Généreux P, et al. Efficacy and safety of postdilatation to reduce paravalvular regurgitation during balloon-expandable transcatheter aortic valve replacement. Circ Cardiovasc Interv. 2013;6(1):85–91.

12. Lauritsch G, Boese J, Wigstrom L, Kemeth H, Fahrig R. Towards cardiac C-arm computed tomography. IEEE Trans Med Imaging. 2006;25(7):922–34. Epub 2006/07/11.
13. Bai M, Liu B, Mu H, Liu X, Jiang Y. The comparison of radiation dose between C-arm flat-detector CT (DynaCT) and multi-slice CT (MSCT): a phantom study. Eur J Radiol. 2012;81:3577–80.
14. Binder RK, Leipsic J, Wood D, Moore T, Toggweiler S, Willson A, et al. Prediction of optimal deployment projection for transcatheter aortic valve replacement: angiographic 3-dimensional reconstruction of the aortic root versus multidetector computed tomography. Circulation: Cardiovascular Interventions; 2012.
15. Meyhöfer J, Ahrens J, Neuss M, Hölschermann F, Schau T, Butter C. Rotational angiography for preinterventional imaging in transcatheter aortic valve implantation. Catheter Cardiovasc Interv. 2012;79(5):756–65.

Fusion Imaging for TAVR

31

Chad Kliger, Vladimir Jelnin, Gregory P. Fontana, and Carlos E. Ruiz

Abstract

Accurate patient selection, pre-procedural planning, and intra-procedural guidance are paramount for procedural success in transcatheter aortic valve replacement (TAVR). Multimodality imaging plays a pivotal role in each of these steps and is essential for TAVR. Fluoroscopy remains the foundation for imaging guidance of transcatheter therapy; however, it does not provide the spatial information of 3D cardiac anatomy necessary for complex interventional procedures. With recent technologic improvements, the integration of multimodality imaging with fluoroscopy in the catheterization laboratory, also known as fusion imaging, now provides an alternative to traditional fluoroscopically guided catheterization. Multidetector computed tomography and rotational angiography (RA) are currently being utilized. This chapter will describe in detail the current use of fusion imaging in TAVR revealing the technical features, methodology, and potential utility, along with a better understanding of the limitations of this technology and future directions.

Keywords

Multidetector computed tomography • Rotational angiography • Fusion imaging • Computed tomography/fluoroscopy fusion • Rotational angiography/fluoroscopy fusion

Introduction

Accurate patient selection, pre-procedural planning, and intra-procedural guidance are paramount for procedural success in transcatheter aortic valve replacement (TAVR). Multimodality imaging plays a pivotal role in each of these steps and is essential for TAVR. The imaging modalities that have been utilized include fluoroscopy, two- and three-dimensional (2D and 3D) transthoracic and transesophageal echocardiography, multidetector computed tomography (MDCT), and intracardiac echocardiography (ICE) [1]. Each modality provides unique detailed anatomic information and spatial relationships of cardiac structures important in TAVR.

Fluoroscopy remains the foundation imaging modality for guidance of transcatheter heart valve deployment. However, fluoroscopy provides poor characterization of soft tissue or non-radiopaque structures and provides 2D projections of complex 3D anatomy that lack the spatial information necessary for complex interventional procedures. With recent technologic improvements, the integration of multimodality imaging with fluoroscopy in the catheterization laboratory, also known as fusion imaging, now provides an alternative to traditional fluoroscopically guided catheterization. It has the potential to improve procedural efficacy and safety, while reducing radiation exposure, contrast volume requirements, and procedural duration.

The basis of fusion imaging relies on the utilization of 3D data acquisition from CT, rotational angiography, and/or echocardiography. This 3D data can be merged with live

C. Kliger, MD, MS • V. Jelnin, MD • C.E. Ruiz, MD, PhD (✉)
Department of Cardiology, Lenox Hill Heart and Vascular Institute-North Shore/LIJ Health System, 130 East 77th Street, 9th Floor Black Hall, New York, NY 10075, USA
e-mail: ckliger@nshs.edu; vjelnin@nshs.edu; cruiz@nshs.edu

G.P. Fontana, MD
Department of Cardiothoracic Surgery, Lenox Hill Heart and Vascular Institute-North Shore/LIJ Health System, 130 East 77th Street, 9th Floor Black Hall, New York, NY 10021-10075, USA
e-mail: gfontana@nshs.edu

J.K. Min et al. (eds.), *Multimodality Imaging for Transcatheter Aortic Valve Replacement*,
DOI 10.1007/978-1-4471-2798-7_31, © Springer-Verlag London 2014

fluoroscopy to provide a 3D model with important cardiac and surrounding structures identified, while preserving the spatial and temporal resolution essential from fluoroscopy. The fundamental features of fusion imaging for TAVR include the localization of aortic valve anatomy, determination of appropriate transcatheter valve size, identification of optimal X-ray projections for implantation, and guidance for valve deployment.

Currently, multidetector computed tomography and rotational angiography (RA) are the imaging modalities that are being utilized for fusion imaging within the cardiac catheterization laboratory. There are currently two proprietary softwares available that allow MDCT/fluoroscopy and RA/fluoroscopy fusion, respectively: HeartNavigator (Philips Heathcare, Best, Netherlands) and syngo DynaCT (Siemens Medical, Berlin, Germany). Each technology will be described in detail discussing their technical features, methodology, and potential utility in transcatheter aortic valve therapy.

Overview of TAVR

In order to understand the potential of fusion imaging in TAVR, the procedural characteristics and possible complications of this technology require further explanation. Presently, there are two TAVR systems available for clinical use: the balloon-expandable Edwards Sapien valve (Edwards Lifesciences, California, USA) and the self-expandable CoreValve (Medtronic, Minnesota, USA). For the balloon-expandable valve, optimal positioning of the prosthesis for deployment is where half to two-thirds of the stented prosthesis rests on the ventricular side of the aortic annulus (Fig. 31.1a). For the self-expanding valve, optimal placement of the prosthesis is 4–8 mm below the aortic annular plane, with the aortic annulus contact point placed between the first and second joints or nodes (Fig. 31.1b). Acceptable implantation can be defined by any portion of the valve skirt positioned within the determined annular plane, described later in this chapter, and with the central leaflet coaptation line located supra-annular.

Complications related to TAVR can occur if the aortic prosthesis deployment is either too high or too low. High implantation can lead to aortic injury, paravalvular regurgitation, coronary occlusion due to either the stented valve or impingement by the native aortic leaflets, or embolization of the transcatheter valve into the aorta. Low implantation is associated with conduction abnormalities, paravalvular regurgitation, embolization of the transcatheter valve into the left ventricle, or mitral valve dysfunction including regurgitation, perforation, or restricted motion of the anterior mitral leaflet.

Fusion imaging provides the operator with added information to confirm appropriate transcatheter valve sizing, aids in valve positioning and deployment, and improves intra-procedural assessment to help guide the need further for further management. For the balloon-expandable valve, further management may include post-balloon dilatation and/or valve-in-valve placement. For the self-expanding valve, high valve

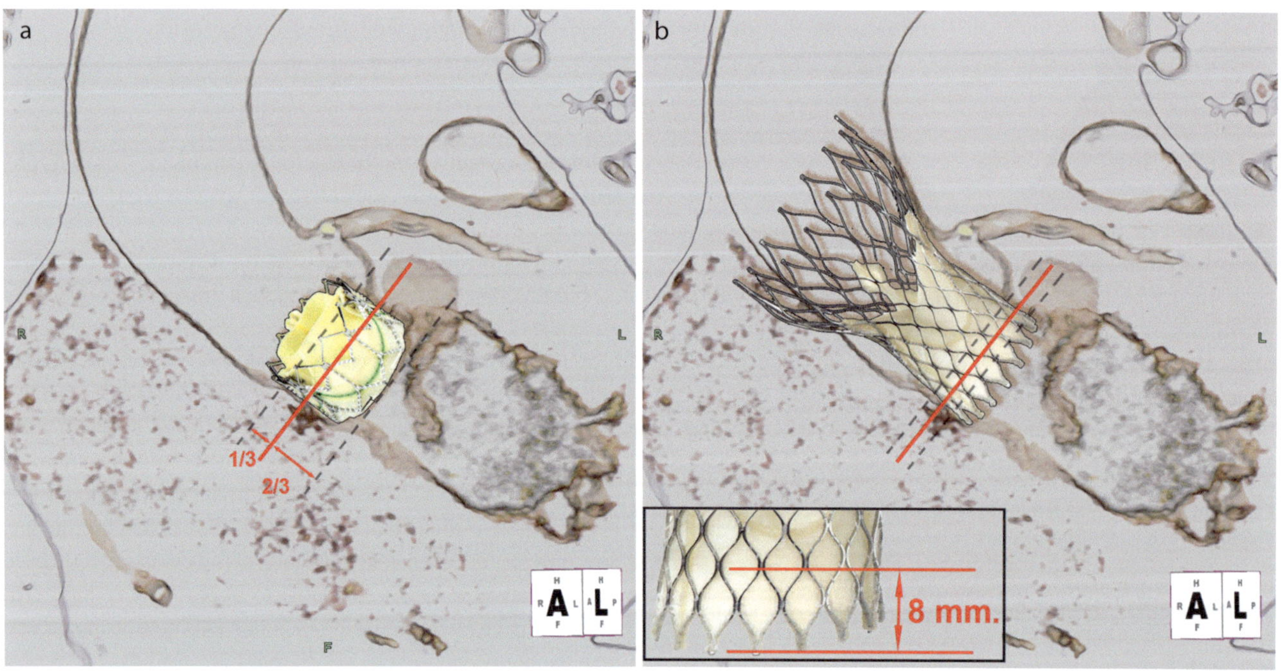

Fig. 31.1 (**a**) Balloon-expandable Edwards Sapien (Edwards Lifesciences, California, USA) and (**b**) self-expanding CoreValve (Medtronic, Minnesota, USA) transcatheter valves with optimal implantation depth where half to two-thirds (Edwards Sapien) and 4–8 mm (CoreValve) of the stented prosthesis rests on the ventricular side of the aortic annulus (*red line*)

implantation necessitates retrieval of the prosthesis assuming it is still attached to the delivery system or valve-in-valve placement once released. Conversely, low implantation requires pulling the prosthesis back if still attached to the delivery system or, when released, snaring and pulling of the valve. Valve-in-valve placement can also be used.

Fundamentals of Fusion Imaging

There are three essential components to fusion imaging: segmentation, registration, and live guidance (Box 31.1). Segmentation, or "post-processing," involves the 3D reconstruction of axial CTA data using volume-rendering techniques. Anatomic structures of the heart are identified on the 3D image, and appropriate landmarks are labeled and measured. Registration entails the adjustment of the 3D CTA images to match the position and the scale of the overlaid fluoroscopic view. This can be performed using either automatic intensity or manual visual matching of the 3D image to 2D fluoroscopy in multiple planes.

Finally, live guidance utilizes the 3D-rendered CT data and displays it in the same perspective as the X-ray system. Rotation of the X-ray camera or movement of the table produces an equivalent movement in the registered overlay projection. Any landmarks placed on the segmented CTA image are fused with live fluoroscopy to assist the operator during the procedure. Segmentation, along with any measurements and planning, can occur prior to the procedure. The remaining components are carried out in the catheterization laboratory.

Computed Tomography in TAVR

Pre-procedural MDCT is performed with any available contemporary single- or dual-source multidetector scanner [2, 3] The protocol for image acquisition varies depending on the scanner but all with the goal of acquiring high-resolution, ECG-gated datasets with the best possible opacification of the thoracic aorta including the aortic valve and coronary arteries. A dedicated protocol, similar to that utilized for coronary computed tomography angiography (CTA), can be employed and modified according to patient size. Collimation is usually submillimeter (0.5–1.0 mm) and at a 0.2–0.35 pitch. Gantry rotation ranges from 0.26 to 0.4 s with the highest rotations speed providing improved temporal resolution with reduced cardiac motion artifact. Tube current ranges from 450 to 800 mA and tube voltage from 80 to 120 kVp, depending on patient size.

Heart rate reduction with beta blockade is not mandatory as compared with coronary CTA. Nonionic contrast media injection of 60–90 mL, depending on patient size, and at a rate of 5–6 mL/s rate provides optimal images. The injection site most commonly used is the antecubital vein, using an 18-gauge angiocath. The timing between the injection of contrast and the beginning of image acquisition should be determined with the aim of peak contrast concentration in the aortic root.

Retrospective ECG gating is predominately used at our institution for acquisition, which provides the entire dataset of images throughout the cardiac cycle. Three-dimensional images are reconstructed using volume-rendering techniques with any available standard reconstruction software (Fig. 31.2a). Adding time, 4D reconstruction is possible when multiple phases are used, typically 10–20 phases with 5–6 % R-R interval increments. Analysis of multiphase data allows for functional cardiac analysis and direct aortic planimetry (Fig. 31.2b). Scrolling through the systolic phases from 20 to 45 % can determine the point of maximal aortic valve opening and the largest aortic valve area.

Curved multiplanar reconstructions (MPR) are performed by tracing a line through the center point of the left ventricular outflow tract, aortic annulus, and proximal ascending aorta, known as the centerline (Fig. 31.2c, d). The annular plane, also termed basal ring, is created by the nadir of the three aortic cusps, perpendicular to the curved MPR line on the ventricular side (Fig. 31.2e). An alternative method to define the basal ring and provide TAVR measurements includes the reconstruction of a double oblique transverse image of the basal ring [2]. Measurements of the short and long axis diameter, mean diameter, area-derived diameter, and perimeter can be obtained and the appropriate respective valve size determined, with the intention of oversizing the valve by 10–20 % [3] (Fig. 31.2f). Additional measurements include the distance from annular plane to the coronary ostia, height and width of the aortic sinuses, and ascending aortic diameter.

MDCT can also be used to determine the optimal C-arm position for valve deployment. Transcatheter valves need to be deployed in a projection that is perpendicular to the native

Box 31.1 Steps to Fusion Imaging for TAVR

Segmentation (Post-processing)	3D reconstruction of axial CT data using volume rendered techniques Anatomic structures of heart identified on 3D image and appropriate landmarks labeled and measured
Registration	Adjustment of 3D CT images to match position and scale of overlaid fluoroscopic view
Live Guidance	Utilization of 3D CT data with display in same perspective as x-ray system Rotation of x-ray camera or movement of table produces an equivalent movement in registered overlay position

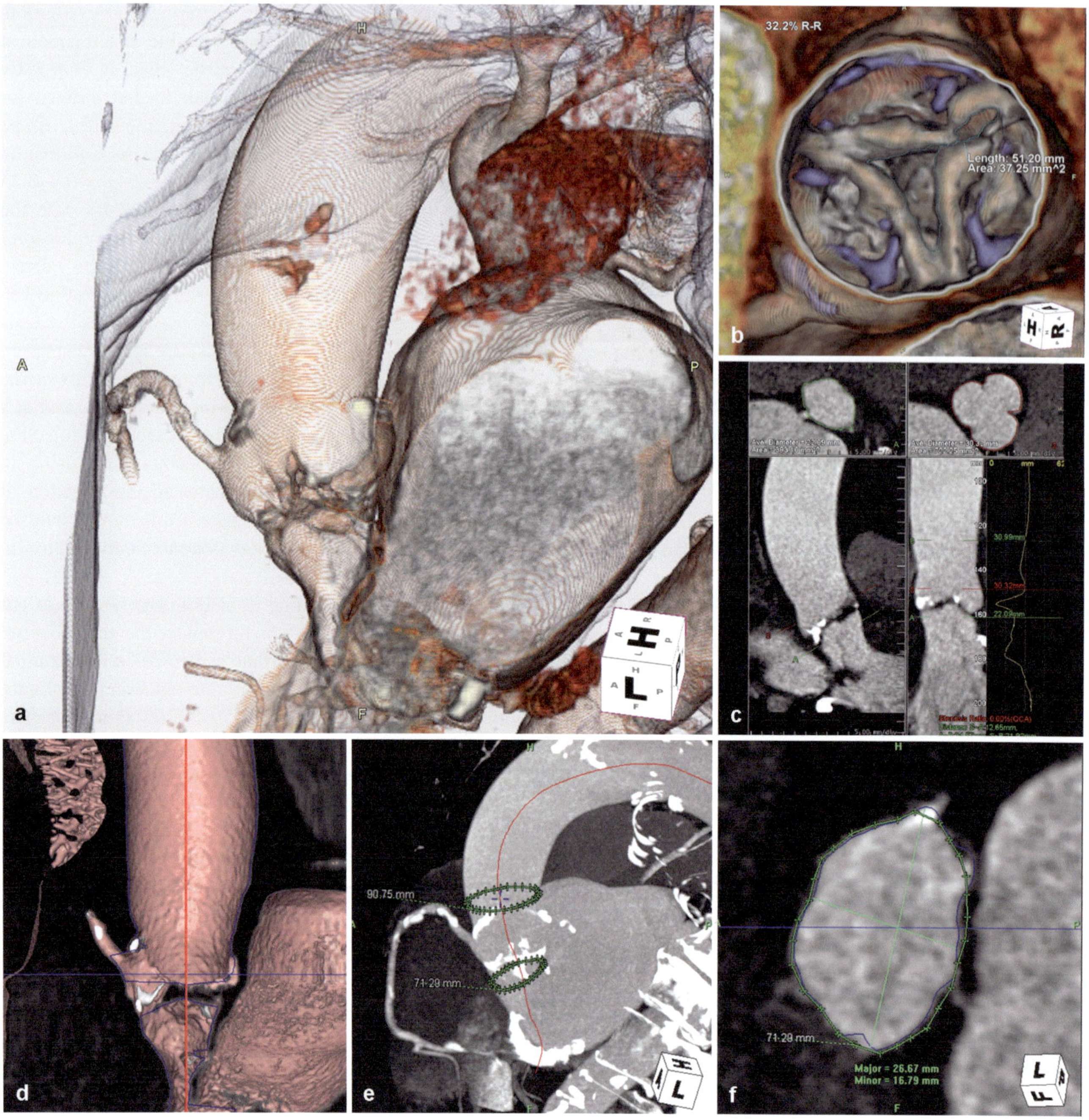

Fig. 31.2 Reconstruction. (**a**) 3D/4D cardiac reconstruction using volume-rendering techniques. (**b**) Direct aortic planimetry at point of maximal aortic valve excursion. (**c**, **d**) Curved multiplanar reconstructions (MPR) performed by tracing a centerline (*red*) through the center of the left ventricular outflow tract, aortic annulus, and ascending aorta. (**e**) The annular plane or basal ring (lower *green circle* in **e**) formed by the nadir of the three aortic cusps, perpendicular to the curved MPR line. (**f**) Measurements of the annular plane can be performed with the appropriate valve size determined (HeartNavigator, Philips Heathcare, Best, Netherlands)

aortic annulus, ensuring coaxial stent position along the centerline. Rotating the 3D volume-rendered reconstructions such that the basal ring becomes a straight line confirms perpendicular projection to the X-ray beam. Multiple appropriate angles can be determined and a "line of perpendicularity" for each patient can be generated along a right anterior oblique (RAO) and caudal to left anterior oblique (LAO) and cranial direction [2].

Rotational Angiography

Intraprocedural 2D rotational angiography can be performed with any image intensifier or flat detector system [4]. The large C-arm sweeps through a wide rotation angle acquiring cine-angiographic images with timed contrast injection. The duration of rotation and trajectory vary depending on the fluoroscopic system utilized. The setup requires first isocentering the patient by visualizing the location of the aortic root in frontal and lateral angulations, with the aortic root brought to the center of the field of view. Contrast injection is performed using a pigtail catheter positioned in the nadir of the noncoronary sinus. The injection rate and volume of contrast varies based on rotational scan duration. The use of diluted contrast of 20–25 mL total injected at a rate of 15–20 mL/s has been reported [4–6]. This reduced contrast volume, compared with CTA, due to local administration may be important in the TAVR population with increased rates of renal insufficiency.

Gantry rotation covers approximately 200° from RAO 100° to LAO 100° at 40° per second. Breath hold and rapid ventricular pacing are utilized to minimize motion of the ascending aorta and reduce flow across the aortic valve during acquisition. X-ray tube voltage, current, and pulse duration are set to provide optimal contrast between the aorta and background structures and to reconstruct the contrast-filled aortic structures. 3D and 4D reconstruction using associated software is then performed with volume-rendering techniques; important structures of interest include the aortic arch, aortic valve leaflets, and the coronary ostia. Because the C-arm performs a much slower rotation than CTA, retrospective ECG gating is used to select the X-ray images acquired during a desired cardiac phase. With fewer images, the potential for more artifacts is possible. Rotational angiography in TAVR can be used for aortic annular anatomic assessment, quantitative analysis using MPR, and procedural guidance, potentially replacing the role of pre-procedural CTA [7].

MDCT/Fluoroscopy Fusion

The HeartNavigator system (Philips Heathcare, Best, Netherlands) is a proprietary software available for MDCT/fluoroscopy fusion imaging in TAVR and utilizes the pre-procedural cardiac CT images [8]. Pre-procedural 2D images are 3D volume-rendered and automatically segmented to identify the aortic root, coronary ostia, the aortic valve, the left ventricle, and the valve plane running through the bottom of the three cusps [9–11] (Fig. 31.3). Segmentation can be manually optimized if necessary. After segmentation, the required X-ray projections are planned by positioning a simulated X-ray view based on 3D-rendered images with the same perspective as that of the C-arm. Views are selected such that the fluoroscopic image is in line with the valve plane. The planned views, typically RAO caudal or LAO cranial, are then stored for use during the procedure. Manual measurements are performed using the automatic detection of the valve plane, which ensures that the measurements are performed without foreshortening (Fig. 31.4).

The patient's position on the X-ray table is then adjusted to achieve the isocenter of the heart in two orthogonal fluoroscopic views. The CT images are registered by using contrast-enhanced fluoroscopy of the aorta in two different views performed 20° apart, by adjusting the position of the overlaid CTA onto the fluoroscopic images (Fig. 31.5a). Registration can also be performed without contrast injection by using "internal markers" such as the bronchi, carina, prosthetic valve frames, vertebrae, or pacemaker wires [12] (Fig. 31.5b). Volume-rendered 3D images of the aorta are replaced with an outlined view of the aorta in order to prevent an obscured view of the fluoro-aortogram. Four views are displayed showing the segmented CT data from different viewpoints. Point-to-point measurements can be performed in any view, and an appropriate valve type and dimension can be selected and confirmed with pre-procedural measurements. Because these measurements are performed in the appropriate plane in the 3D reconstructed model, improved accuracy of measurements may be achieved.

During the procedure, the planned views can be recalled and the C-arm moved automatically to the planned projection. 3D-rendered images are displayed with the same perspective as the X-ray system, and any rotations of the C-arm are congruent with the CT. Fused overlay imaging shows the relation between the transcatheter valve as seen on X-ray with the anatomy as seen on CT (Fig. 31.6). Accurate positioning of the device demands correct alignment of the C-arm with the valve plane, perpendicular to transcatheter delivery and deployment. Slight misalignment can cause aortic foreshortening and may lead to errors in judging the correct location for device deployment with respect to the valve plane. The optimal view for the device placement should also display the origins of the left and right coronary arteries, without overlap from the coronary sinus. Appropriate visualization ensures device implantation away from the coronary ostium, reducing the risk of coronary occlusion.

Pre-procedural cardiac CT can also be fused using the syngo InSpace iPilot system (Siemens Medical, Berlin, Germany). However, performing rotational angiography, DynaCT described below, at the time of the procedure is necessary for improved anatomic definition [13]. Rotational angiography is accomplished during a breath hold without contrast administration. The 3D dataset from the rotational angiography is then registered to the pre-procedural 3D CTA dataset, 3D-3D registration, and overlaid onto the fluoroscopic image. 3D-3D registration requires acquisition of rotational angiography at the identical patient position as pre-procedural CTA for proper fusion.

Rotational Angiography and Fluoroscopy Fusion

The syngo DynaCT system (Siemens Medical, Berlin, Germany) is a proprietary software available for rotational angiography fusion imaging in TAVR and utilizes

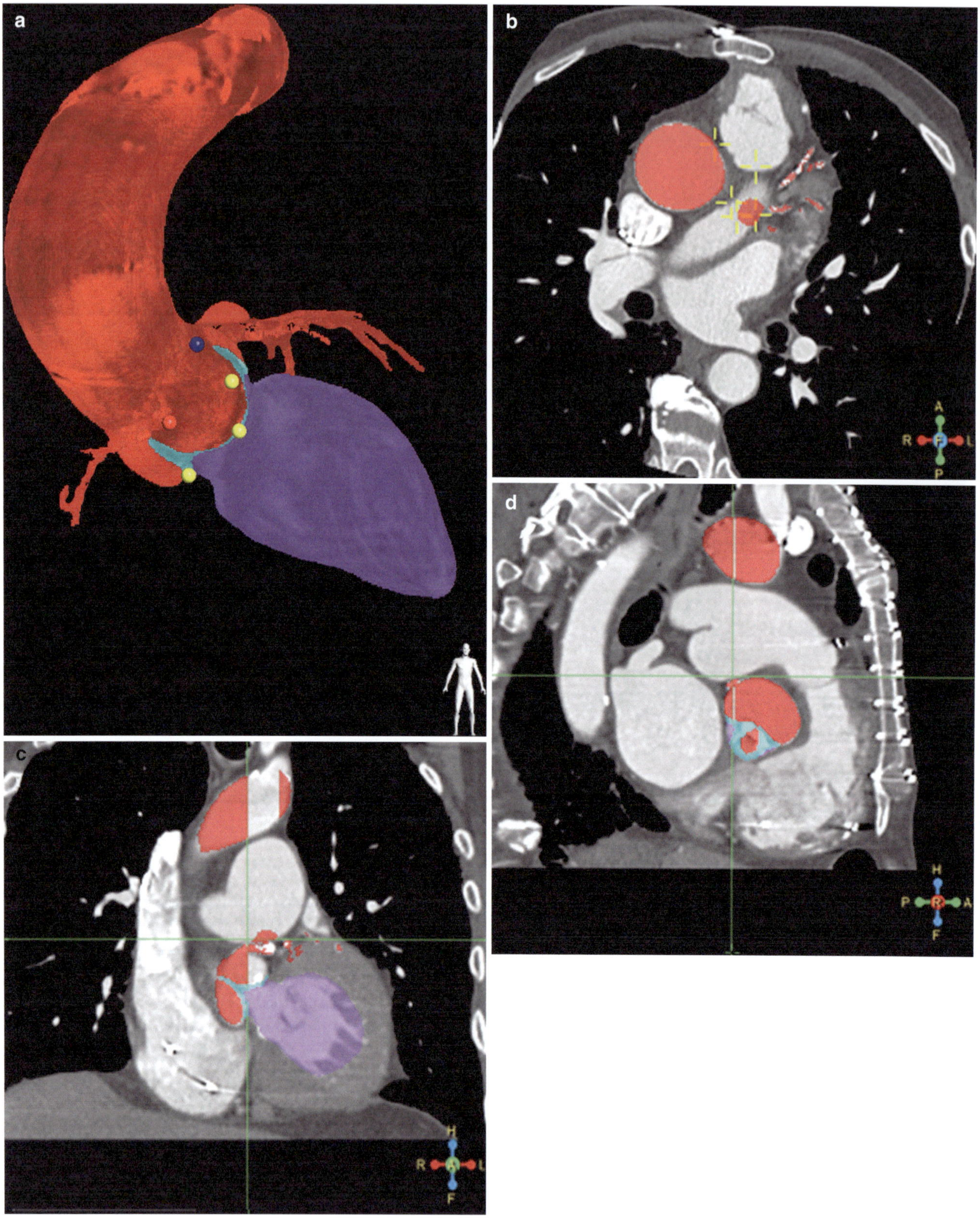

Fig. 31.3 Segmentation. (**a**) Automatic segmentation of 3D volume-rendered images to identify the aortic root and proximal coronary arteries (*red*), left ventricle (*purple*), coronary ostia (*blue dot* - left main coronary artery and *red dot* - right coronary artery), and the nadir of the three coronary cusps (*yellow dots*). Segmentation in axial (**b**), sagittal (**c**), and coronal (**d**) planes are used for editing and confirmation. (HeartNavigator, Philips Heathcare, Best Netherlands)

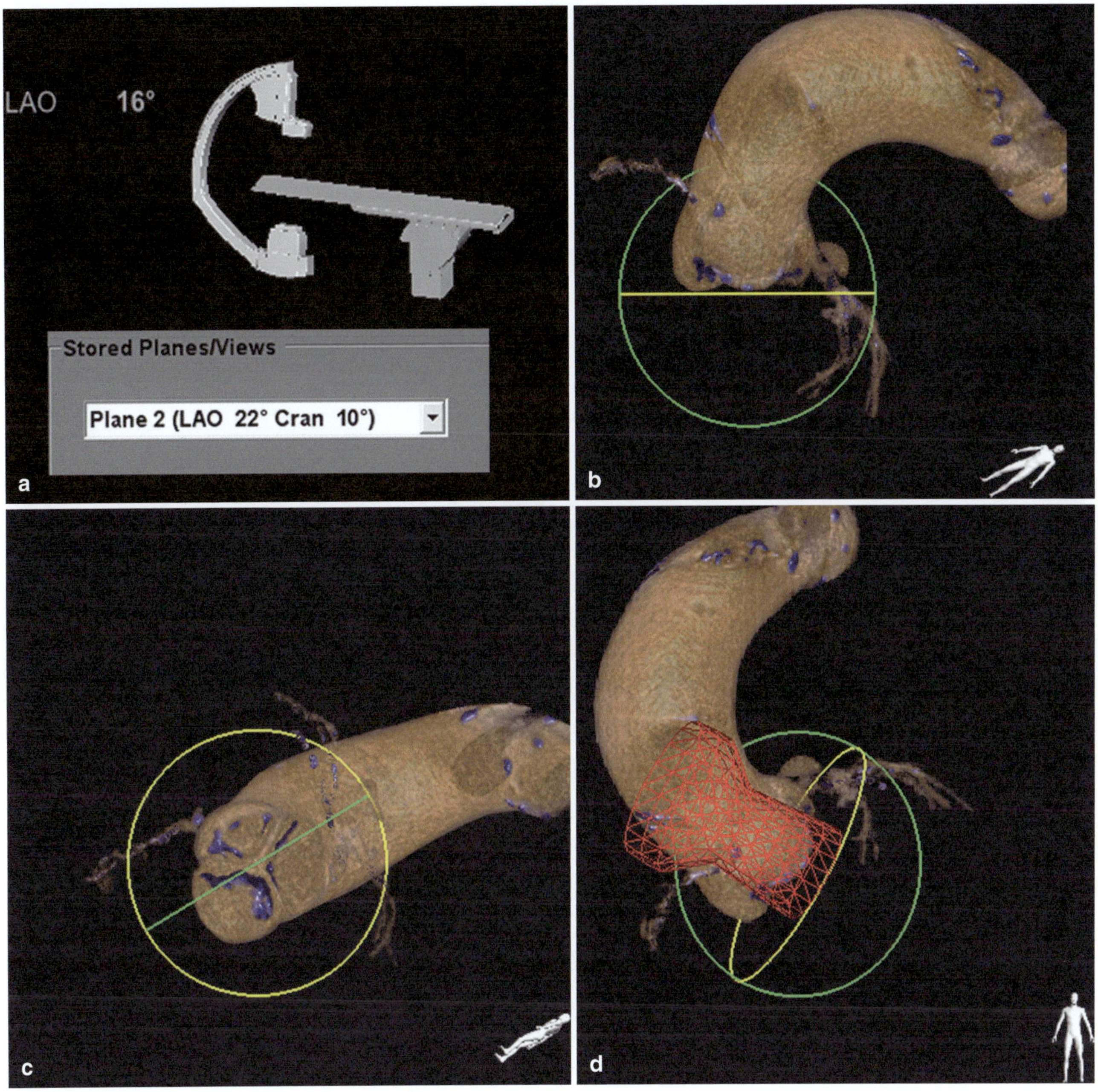

Fig. 31.4 Optimal C-arm position. (**a–c**) Simulated X-ray projections based on 3D-rendered images, with the same perspective as that of the C-arm, allow the selection of fluoroscopic views where the C-arm is perpendicular to the annular plane (*yellow circle* at the nadir of the aortic cusps, *green circle* at a perpendicular plane). (**d**) Computer-generated CoreValve frame (*red*) appropriately positioned below the annular plane (HeartNavigator, Philips Heathcare, Best, Netherlands)

intra-procedural 2D rotational angiography images [4–6, 13–15]. 2D rotational images can be performed on the aortic root by C-arm rotation over 200° in 5 s. 3D and 4D reconstruction using volume-rendering techniques is achieved, and the syngo Aortic ValveGuide (Siemens Medical, Berlin, Germany) segments the aortic root and displays critical landmarks from 3D volume (Fig. 31.7). These landmarks include the lowest point of each aortic cusp, the commissural points, the coronary ostia, and the centerline. A circle parallel to the plane of the three lowest cusp points can be generated discerning the annular plane. With rotation of the C-arm, the circle degenerates into a straight line identifying the angle at which the three lowest points are aligned, the optimal angulation for valve implantation. The height of the aortic annulus to the coronary ostia can be measured to confirm sufficient height for TAVR implantation.

The review of landmarks in three orthogonal planes (axial, sagittal, and coronal) using maximum intensity

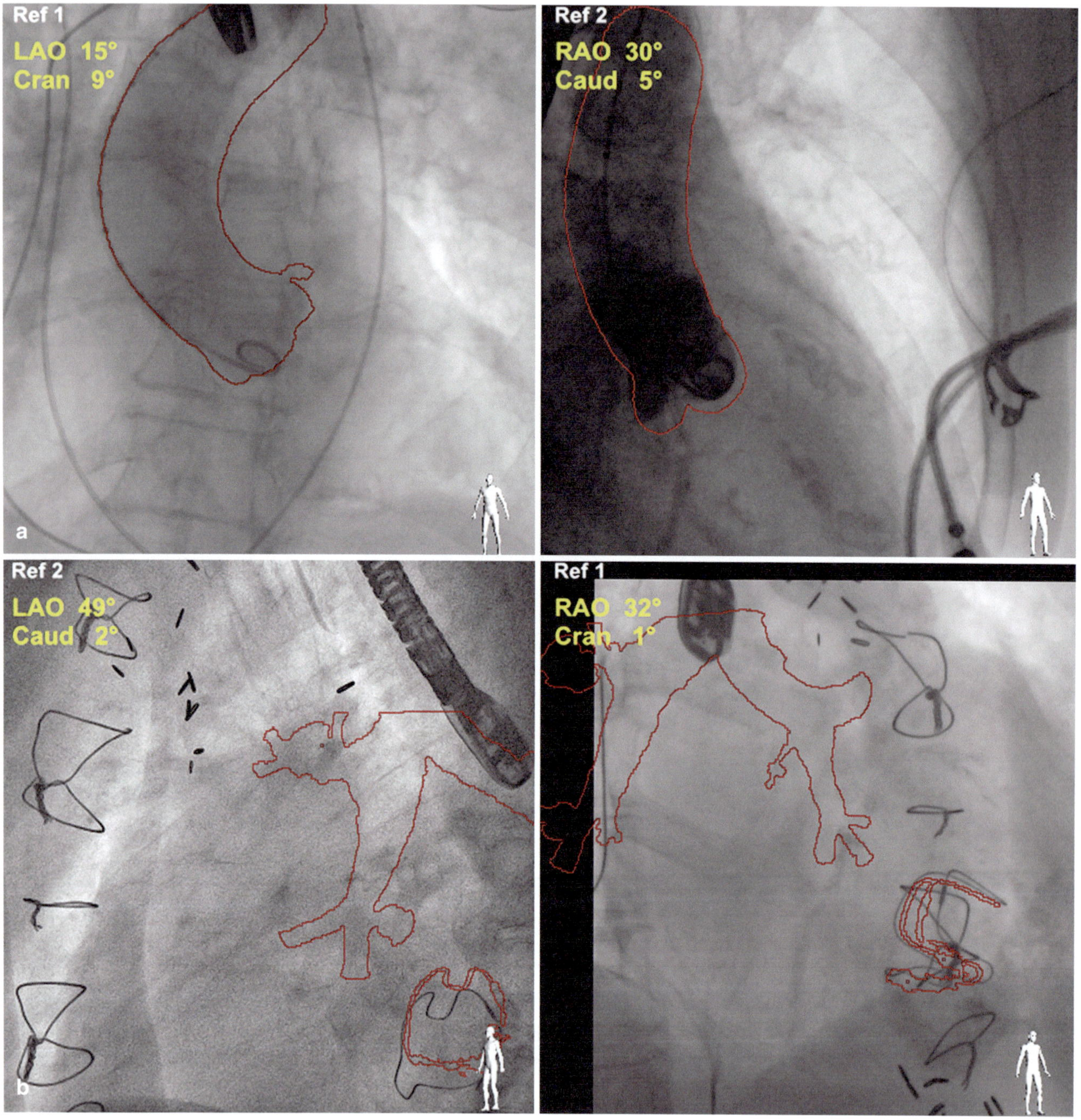

Fig. 31.5 Registration. Adjustment of the 3D computed tomography angiographic images to match the position and scale of the overlayed fluoroscopic view. (**a**) Registration using contrast-enhanced fluoroscopy of the aorta in two different view greater than 20° apart. (**b**) Registration without contrast using "internal markers," bronchi/carina and prosthetic valve (outlined in *red*) (HeartNavigator, Philips Heathcare, Best, Netherlands)

projections (MIP) and in 3D volume rendering allows for editing and confirmation. Once confirmed, the volume-rendered view can be rotated, corresponding to C-arm angulation. In order to overlay the 3D volume images onto live fluoroscopy, the contours of the 3D volume image are identified utilizing edge detection, and the outline of the aortic root only is overlaid onto live fluoroscopy, not to obscure the fluoroscopic image. The 3D volume contour is automatically registered with the fluoroscopic images using syngo iPilot (Siemens Medical, Berlin, Germany) as both images are acquired on the same system and without a change in the patient's position (Fig. 31.8).

Contrast-enhanced 3D rotational angiography can also be performed using the HeartNavigator system (Philips

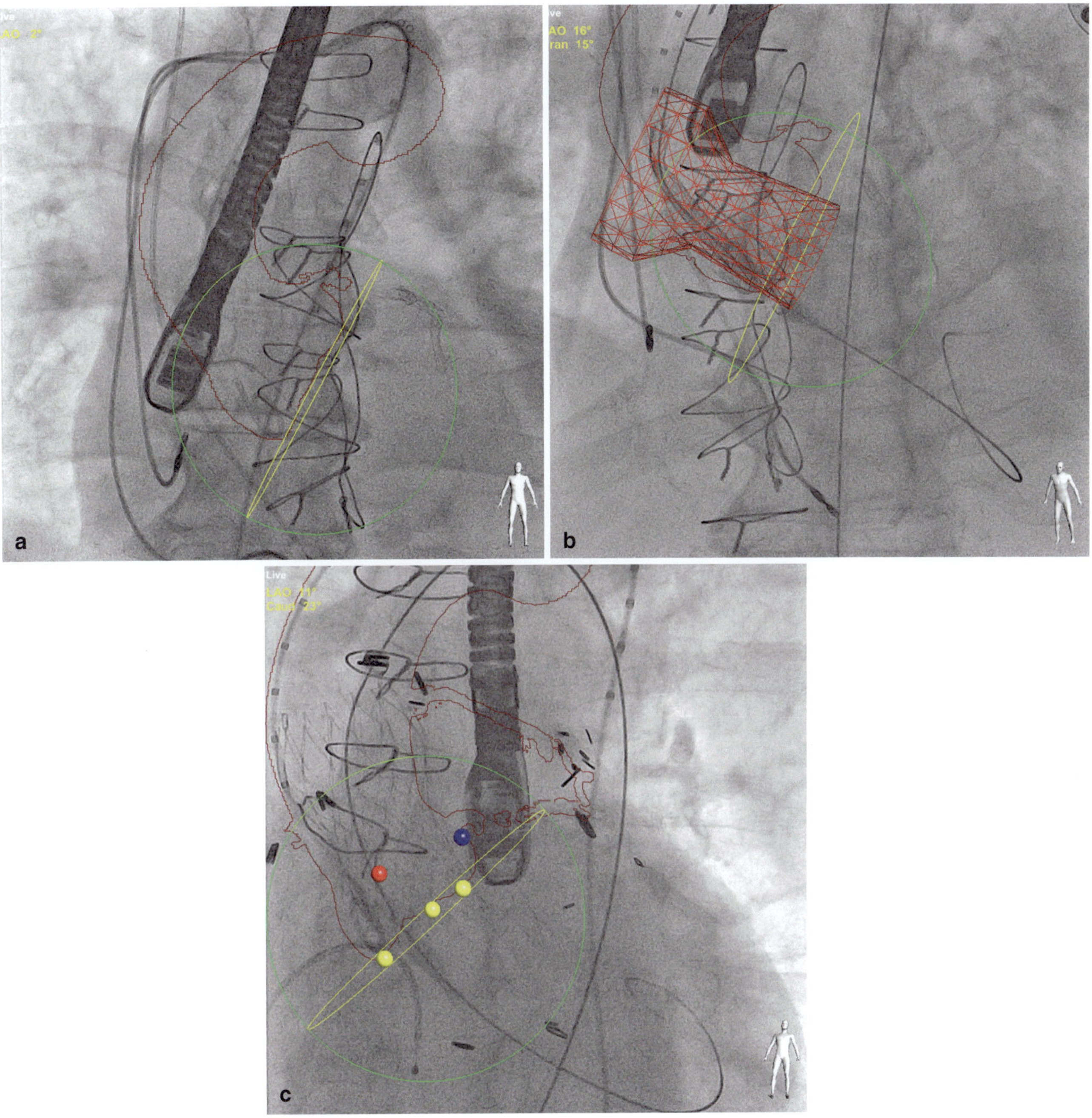

Fig. 31.6 Live guidance. (**a**) Multidetector computed tomography/fluoroscopy fusion imaging with the annular plane (*yellow circle* at the nadir of the aortic cusps) perpendicular to the fluoroscopic view, optimal view. (**b**) Computer-generated CoreValve frame (*red*) appropriately positioned below the annular plane. (**c**) Deployment of CoreValve prosthesis with the annular plane, nadir of aortic cusps (*yellow dots*), coronary ostia (*red* and *blue dots*) identified (HeartNavigator, Philips Heathcare, Best, Netherlands)

Heathcare, Best, Netherlands) with their respective single-plane detector and the same fusion techniques utilized for MDCT/fluoroscopy fusion [14]. Breath-hold acquisitions are obtained with selective contrast injection within the aortic root. Typically, the C-arm rotates 220° around the patient over 4 s. Image reconstruction is performed using their respective software, and the 3D volume datasets are fused using manual registration techniques. Intra-procedural volumetric fusion has been evaluated for the left atrium and pulmonary veins in the setting of pulmonary vein isolation therapy but not yet described in TAVR [16–19]. Similar technology is available by General Electric using their proprietary software, Innova 3D (GE Healthcare, Chalfont St Giles, UK) [14].

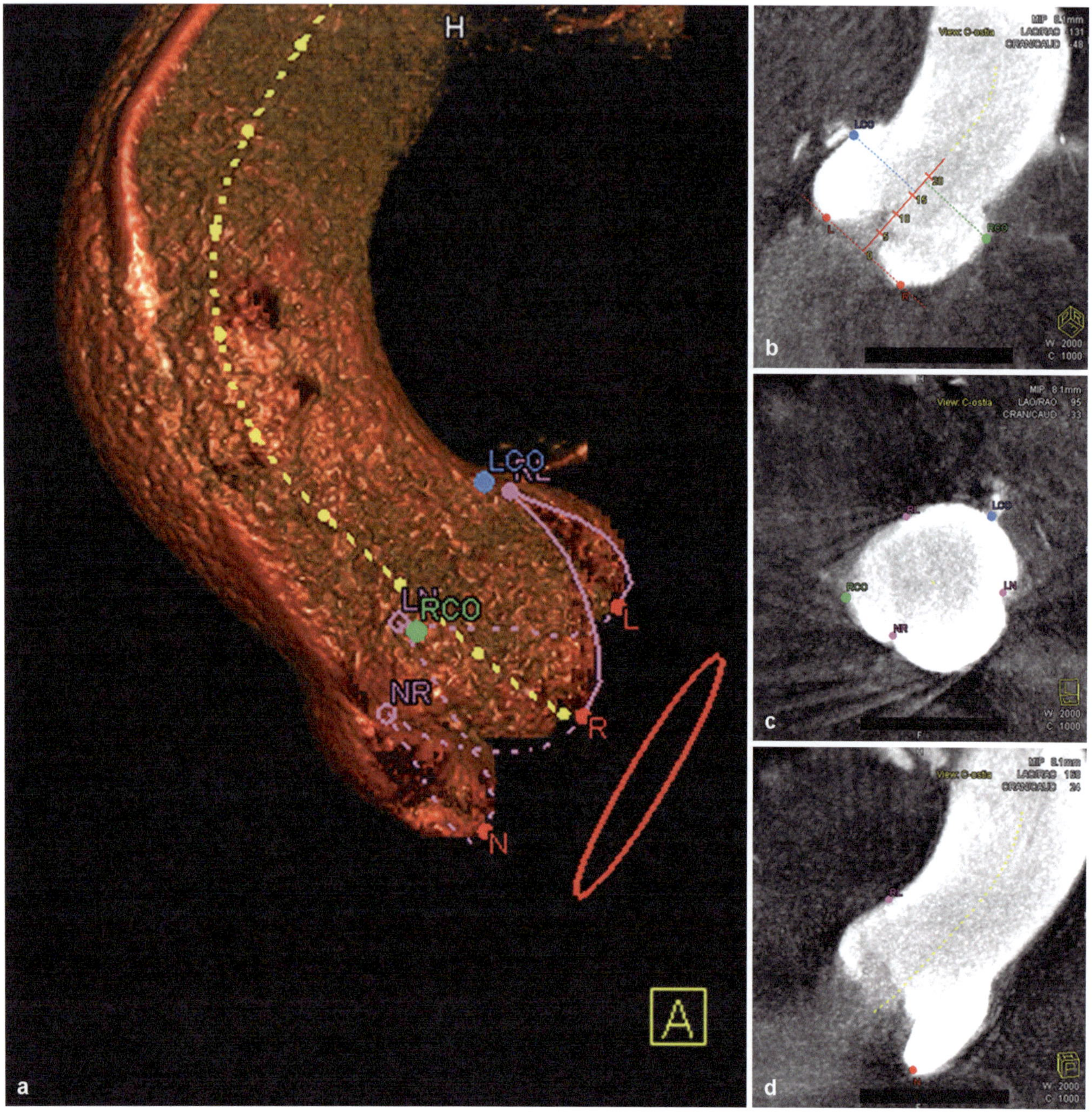

Fig. 31.7 Reconstruction/Segmentation. 3D/4D cardiac reconstruction using volume-rendering techniques and segmentation of the aortic root with critical landmarks displayed on 3D volume (**a**). Ostium of the left main coronary artery (*blue dot*) and right coronary artery (*green dot*), nadir of coronary cusps (*red dots*), commissural points (*pink dots*), centerline (*yellow dashed line*), and a projected circle (*red*) into the left ventricular outflow tract parallel to the annular plane are identified. The landmarks are reviewed in three orthogonal planes for editing and confirmation (**b–d**) (syngo DynaCT/Aortic ValveGuide, Siemens Medical, Berlin, Germany)

Limitations of Current Fusion Imaging

Although overlay technology provides significant potential for TAVR, there are limitations. The use of CT increases radiation exposure for the patient, beyond the dose needed historically for transcatheter therapy. Most TAVR procedures require and/or utilize a pre-procedural cardiac CTA. Exposure in the TAVR population is less of a concern given their advanced age and multiple comorbidities. Cardiac motion and a lack of motion compensation can lead to inaccuracy. Near-term future technology may allow the importation of multiple phases of the cardiac cycle and ECG tracking for adjustments in heart rate.

Factors including patient positioning, volume status, and physiological variation that take place between pre-procedural

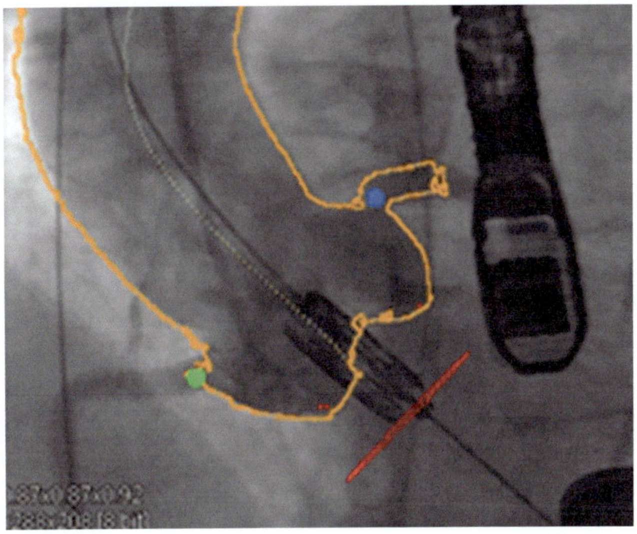

Fig. 31.8 Live guidance. Positioning of an Edwards Sapien valve (Edwards Lifesciences, California, USA) using fusion imaging guidance is shown. An outline of the aortic root (*yellow*) is overlaid onto live fluoroscopy, which is automatically registered to the fluoroscopic image. A projected circle (*red*) into the left ventricular outflow tract parallel to the annular plane becomes a straight line when the C-arm angulation is perpendicular to the field of view. The ostium of the left main coronary artery (*blue dot*) and right coronary artery (*green dot*) is identified (syngo iPilot, Siemens Medical, Berlin, Germany)

imaging and the intervention can also alter the cardiac anatomy and the ability to appropriately register images [12]. Heart muscle is not static and may deform with catheter manipulation. Fusion of procedural rotational angiography can significantly reduce many of these factors. However, the data acquisition requires identical patient positioning to that used during the pre-procedural CTA for proper fusion. In addition, challenges of cardiac motion and reduced tissue contrast resolution in relation to bony structures may limit the utility of rotational angiography [16]. Newer methods for registration include the use of intracardiac ultrasound, which may improve designation and definition of intracardiac landmarks [20].

Future Fusion Technology

3D datasets from MRI can also be utilized for fusion imaging [21]. Registration of CTA and rotational angiography with live fluoroscopy is simpler given that both imaging methods use ionizing radiation. Registration of MRI images is more complex given the differences in image acquisition compared to ionizing radiation techniques but is also possible and has been described with the syngo InSpace iPilot software (Siemens Medical, Berlin, Germany). MRI is able to provide diagnostic-quality 3D images with hemodynamic information and without the need for ionizing radiation.

Intracardiac echocardiography (ICE) has been used to guide transcatheter aortic valve implantation. Newer systems are capable of manually reconstructing a 3D ICE image using multiple 2D image slices. These images can be merged with 3D computed tomography angiography, magnetic resonance imaging, and potentially fluoroscopy providing increased intracardiac detail and real-time more accurate anatomic information.

Achieving 4D ICE would also provide ultrasound images in real time in lieu of post-processing fusion. The AcuNav V (Siemens, Munich, Germany) has been presented and has shown the possibility of obtaining high-resolution volumetric images in real time. Fusion imaging for 4D ICE technology is unclear. However, overlay of real-time 3D TEE volumes onto live fluoroscopy creating echo-fluoroscopic fusion imaging is a possibility and has been described using EchoNav (Philips Heathcare, Best, Netherlands).

Conclusion

Fusion imaging combines the advantages of different imaging modalities to provide improved procedural accuracy and safety. The addition of a third dimension to a fluoroscopic 2D procedure allows for enhanced delineation of complex anatomy and simplified procedural navigation. Despite the described limitations and with improving or alternative fusion modalities, there is significant potential for fusion imaging in transcatheter aortic valve replacement and with other structural heart disease interventions.

References

1. Delgado V, van der Kley F, Schalij MJ, Bax JJ. Optimal imaging for planning and guiding interventions in structural heart disease: a multi-modality imaging approach. European Heart Journal Supplements. 2010;12:E10–23.
2. Leipsic J, Gurvitch R, Labounty TM, Min JK, Wood D, Johnson M, Ajlan AM, Wijesinghe N, Webb JG. Multidetector computed tomography in transcatheter aortic valve implantation. JACC Cardiovasc Imaging. 2011;4:416–29.
3. Gurvitch R, Webb JG, Yuan R, Johnson M, Hague C, Willson AB, Toggweiler S, Wood DA, Ye J, Moss R, Thompson CR, Achenbach S, Min JK, Labounty TM, Cury R, Leipsic J. Aortic annulus diameter determination by multidetector computed tomography: reproducibility, applicability, and implications for transcatheter aortic valve implantation. JACC Cardiovasc Interv. 2011;4:1235–45.
4. John M, Liao R, Zheng Y, Nottling A, Boese J, Kirschstein U, Kempfert J, Walther T. System to guide transcatheter aortic valve implantations based on interventional C-arm CT imaging. Med Image Comput Comput Assist Interv. 2010;13:375–82.
5. Kempfert J, Falk V, Schuler G, Linke A, Merk D, Mohr FW, Walther T. Dyna-CT during minimally invasive off-pump transapical aortic valve implantation. Ann Thorac Surg. 2009;88:2041.
6. Kempfert J, Noettling A, John M, Rastan A, Mohr FW, Walther T. Automatically segmented DynaCT: enhanced imaging during transcatheter aortic valve implantation. J Am Coll Cardiol. 2011;58:e211.

7. Bai M, Liu B, Mu H, Liu X, Jiang Y. The comparison of radiation dose between C-arm flat-detector CT (DynaCT) and multi-slice CT (MSCT): a phantom study. Eur J Radiol. 2012;81(11):3577–80.
8. Schrofel H, Bakker N, van der Boomen R. Transcatheter aortic valve implantation in a hybrid operating room using HeartNavigator. Medicamundi. 2010;53:2–9.
9. Waechter I, Kneser R, Korosoglou G, Peters J, Bakker NH, van der Boomen R, Weese J. Patient specific models for planning and guidance of minimally invasive aortic valve implantation. Med Image Comput Comput Assist Interv. 2010;13:526–33.
10. Ecabert O, Peters J, Schramm H, Lorenz C, von Berg J, Walker MJ, Vembar M, Olszewski ME, Subramanyan K, Lavi G, Weese J. Automatic model-based segmentation of the heart in CT images. IEEE Trans Med Imaging. 2008;27:1189–201.
11. Peters J, Ecabert O, Meyer C, Kneser R, Weese J. Optimizing boundary detection via simulated search with applications to multimodal heart segmentation. Med Image Anal. 2010;14:70–84.
12. Li JH, Haim M, Movassaghi B, Mendel JB, Chaudhry GM, Haffajee CI, Orlov MV. Segmentation and registration of three-dimensional rotational angiogram on live fluoroscopy to guide atrial fibrillation ablation: a new online imaging tool. Heart Rhythm. 2009;6:231–7.
13. Krishnaswamy A, Tuzcu EM, Kapadia SR. Three-dimensional computed tomography in the cardiac catheterization laboratory. Catheter Cardiovasc Interv. 2011;77:860–5.
14. Schwartz JG, Neubauer AM, Fagan TE, Noordhoek NJ, Grass M, Carroll JD. Potential role of three-dimensional rotational angiography and C-arm CT for valvular repair and implantation. Int J Cardiovasc Imaging. 2011;27:1205–22.
15. Juergen M, Johanna A, Michael N, Frank H, Thomas S, Christian B. Rotational angiography for preinterventional imaging in transcatheter aortic valve implantation. Catheter Cardiovasc Interv. 2012;79:756–65.
16. Thiagalingam A, Manzke R, D'Avila A, Ho I, Locke AH, Ruskin JN, Chan RC, Reddy VY. Intraprocedural volume imaging of the left atrium and pulmonary veins with rotational X-ray angiography: implications for catheter ablation of atrial fibrillation. J Cardiovasc Electrophysiol. 2008;19:293–300.
17. Knecht S, Skali H, O'Neill MD, Wright M, Matsuo S, Chaudhry GM, Haffajee CI, Nault I, Gijsbers GH, Sacher F, Laurent F, Montaudon M, Corneloup O, Hocini M, Haissaguerre M, Orlov MV, Jais P. Computed tomography-fluoroscopy overlay evaluation during catheter ablation of left atrial arrhythmia. Europace. 2008;10:931–8.
18. Stevenhagen J, Van Der Voort PH, Dekker LR, Bullens RW, Van Den Bosch H, Meijer A. Three-dimensional CT overlay in comparison to CartoMerge for pulmonary vein antrum isolation. J Cardiovasc Electrophysiol. 2010;21:634–9.
19. Manzke R, Reddy VY, Dalal S, Hanekamp A, Rasche V, Chan RC. Intra-operative volume imaging of the left atrium and pulmonary veins with rotational X-ray angiography. Med Image Comput Comput Assist Interv. 2006;9:604–11.
20. Rossillo A, Indiani S, Bonso A, Themistoclakis S, Corrado A, Raviele A. Novel ICE-guided registration strategy for integration of electroanatomical mapping with three-dimensional CT/MR images to guide catheter ablation of atrial fibrillation. J Cardiovasc Electrophysiol. 2009;20:374–8.
21. Dori Y, Sarmiento M, Glatz AC, Gillespie MJ, Jones VM, Harris MA, Whitehead KK, Fogel MA, Rome JJ. X-ray magnetic resonance fusion to internal markers and utility in congenital heart disease catheterization. Circ Cardiovasc Imaging. 2011;4:415–24.

Valve-in-Valve for Transcatheter Aortic Valve Replacement: Do Imaging Requirements Change?

32

Rohan Poulter, Vinayak Bapat, and David A. Wood

Abstract

Bioprosthetic surgical valves have shorter durability compared to mechanical devices and the risk of reoperation is often prohibitively high. Contemporary transcatheter valves have been, and will continue to be, successfully deployed within failing surgical prostheses utilizing a valve-in-valve technique. Detailed knowledge of the physical characteristics of the in situ surgical prosthesis is crucial for procedural success. Currently, the internal diameter of the surgical valve is the most important dimension used to size transcatheter valves. Unfortunately, there is significant variability in both labeling and reported dimensions between surgical valve manufacturers with no accepted gold standard. Multiple novel transcatheter valve systems are currently being developed for valve-in-valve applications that utilize a variety of innovative sizing criteria. Imaging plays a key role in all aspects of valve-in-valve implantation. Multidetector computed tomography (MDCT) can help size existing surgical prosthesis and is proving invaluable for next-generation device development and refinement. Although echocardiography provides important periprocedural guidance for radiolucent surgical prostheses, a detailed understanding of the radiopaque surgical landmarks is crucial for correct valve-in-valve positioning and thus successful implantation.

Keywords

Bioprosthetic valve • Transcatheter valve • Valve-in-valve • Internal diameter • Fluoroscopic markers

Introduction

Bioprosthetic valves are commonly utilized when there is need to reduce thromboembolic risk and avoid bleeding associated with anticoagulation [1]. However the durability of bioprosthetic valves is less than mechanical prostheses [2, 3] and reoperation for failing bioprostheses is the current standard of care [4–6] (Fig. 32.1). Unfortunately, patients requiring reoperation are at higher risk for adverse events with rates in reported series ranging from 4 to 20 % [7–11]. The use of transcatheter valve technology to treat degenerating surgical bioprostheses (the "valve-in-valve" procedure) has paralleled the growth of transcatheter aortic valve replacement (TAVR) in native valve disease. Multiple case series have reported excellent 30-day outcomes [12–27] and, more recently, the Global

R. Poulter, MD, MBBS, MRCP(UK), FRACP (✉)
Division of Cardiology, Vancouver General Hospital, 9th Floor Diamond Health Care Centre, 2775 Laurel St, Vancouver, BC V6B2W6, Canada
e-mail: poulterr@gmail.com

V. Bapat, FRCS, CTh
Department of Cardiothoracic Surgery, Guys and St. Thomas' Hospital, 6th Floor East Wing, Westminster Bridge Road, London SE1 7EH, UK
e-mail: vnbapat@yahoo.com

D.A. Wood, MD, FRCPC
Division of Cardiology, St. Paul's and Vancouver General Hospital, Diamond Health Care Centre (Cardiology – Level 9), 2775 Laurel St, Vancouver, BC V6B2W6, Canada
e-mail: david.wood@vch.ca

J.K. Min et al. (eds.), *Multimodality Imaging for Transcatheter Aortic Valve Replacement*,
DOI 10.1007/978-1-4471-2798-7_32, © Springer-Verlag London 2014

Valve-In-Valve Registry reported stable hemodynamics and persistent improvement in functional status at 12 months (Fig. 32.2).

It is recognized that the valve-in-valve procedure is technically challenging and requires appropriate case and device selection. Imaging plays a key role in all aspects of valve-in-valve implantation. Multidetector computed tomography (MDCT), echocardiography, and periprocedural angiography to evaluate the radiopaque surgical landmarks are all crucial for correct valve-in-valve sizing and positioning and thus, successful implantation. We will review imaging requirements for valve-in-valve implantation for failed surgical bioprostheses. Valve-in-valve implantation for failed or malpositioned transcatheter valves is a separate topic and not discussed.

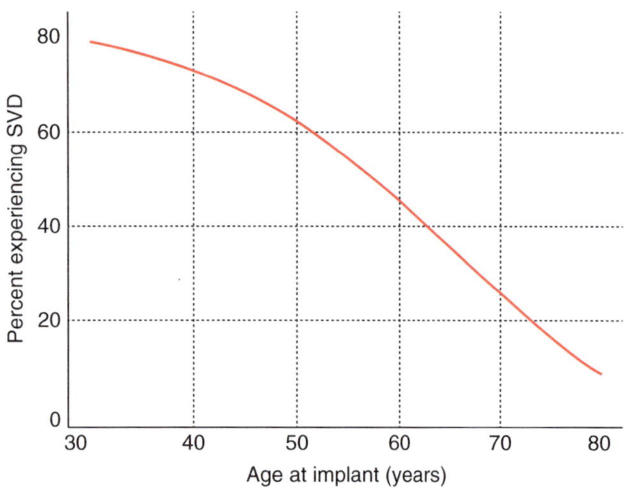

Fig. 32.1 Incidence of structural valve degeneration (*SVD*) with surgical bioprosthetic valves

Surgical Valves

Bioprosthetic surgical valves have consistent, reproducible leaflet kinetics as the leaflets are mounted in a rigid framework. The wide variety of surgical valves available can be broadly classified into stented and stentless devices (Tables 32.1 and 32.2). These groups have unique features that must be considered for valve-in-valve sizing and positioning. Conventional bioprosthetic valves incorporate bovine or porcine pericardium incorporated into a stent frame or stentless conduit.

Stented valves have a support structure composed of various alloys and plastics attached to a basal ring covered by a fabric sewing cuff (Fig. 32.3). The basal ring may be circular or scallop shaped and newer designs incorporate low profiles or supra-aortic design features. The support structures define the internal, outer, and external diameter of the valve. The support structures are generally radiopaque and well visualized on computed tomography during assessment of the internal diameter of the in vivo surgical prosthesis as well as on angiography during positioning and implantation. The rigid frame of most bioprostheses facilitates transcatheter valve positioning and paravalvular sealing while reducing the risk of atrioventricular block, annular rupture, and coronary obstruction. It is important to recognize two important exceptions: the Sorin Mitroflow valve (Sorin, Vancouver, BC, Canada) and the St. Jude Trifecta valve (St. Jude, St. Paul, MN). In contrast to other stented valves, these valves have leaflets mounted outside the stent to maximize the orifice area. During valve-in-valve implantation the leaflets are not constrained by the stent frame and thus may extend to the aortic wall causing obstruction of the coronary ostia.

Stentless valves may be autograft, heterograft, or homograft and are sutured into the aortic root in the

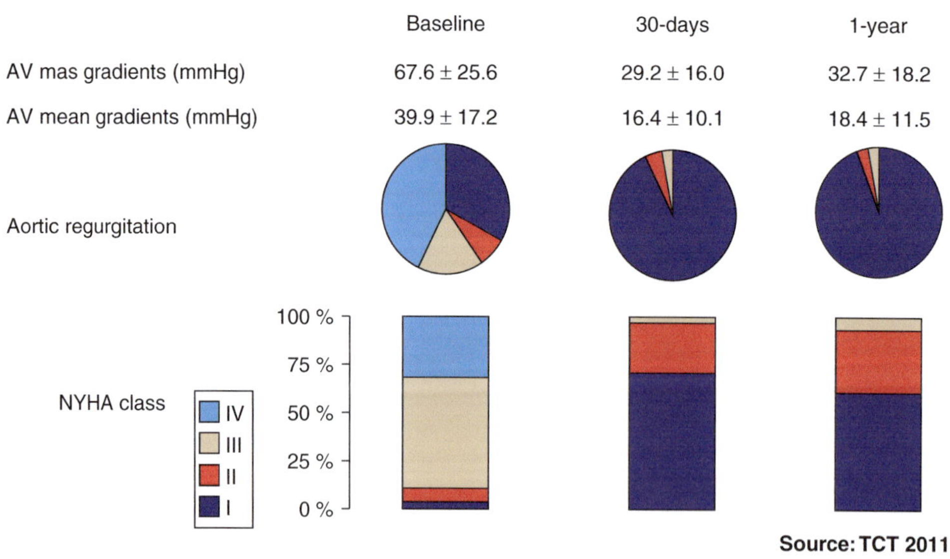

Fig. 32.2 One-year outcome results from the Global Valve-in-Valve Registry ($n=78$). *AV* aortic valve, *NYHA* New York Heart Association (Image courtesy of Dr Danny Dvir, Washington Hospital Center, Washington DC, USA)

Table 32.1 Structural dimensions of stented bioprosthetic valves

Valve label size	Valve type/model (manufacturer)	Sewing ring external diameter, mm	Stent outer diameter, mm	Stent internal diameter, mm	Profile height, mm
18	Soprano (Sorin Biomedica)	26	21	17.8	12
19	Magna (Edwards Lifesciences)	24	19	18	13
	Perimount (Edwards Lifesciences)	26	19	18	14
	Mosaic (Medtronic)	25	19	17.5	13.5
	Hancock Ultra (Medtronic)	24	19	17.5	14
	Mitroflow (Sorin Biomedica)	21	18.6	15.4	11
	Trifecta (St. Jude Medical)	24	19	17	15
	Epic Supra/Biocor Supra (St. Jude Medical)	25	19	19	14
20	Soprano (Sorin Biomedica)	28	23	19.8	14
	Aspire (Vascutek Terumo)	23	20	18.2	16
21	Magna (Edwards Lifesciences)	26	21	20	15
	Perimount (Edwards Lifesciences)	29	21	20	15
	Mosaic/Hancock II (Medtronic)	27	21	18.5	15
	Hancock/Hancock Ultra (Medtronic)	26	21	18.5	
	Mitroflow (Sorin Biomedica)	23	20.7	17.3	13
	Trifecta (St. Jude Medical)	26	21	19	16
	Epic/Biocor (St. Jude Medical)	25	21	19	14
	Aspire (Vascutek Terumo)	24	21	19.2	16
22	Soprano (Sorin Biomedica)	30	25	21.7	15
23	Magna (Edwards Lifesciences)	28	23	22	16
	Perimount (Edwards Lifesciences)	31	23	22	16
	Mosaic/Hancock II (Medtronic)	30	23	20.5	16
	Hancock/Hancock Ultra (Medtronic)	28	23	22	
	Mitroflow (Sorin Biomedica)	26	22.7	19	14
	Trifecta (St. Jude Medical)	28	23	21	17
	Epic/Biocor (St. Jude Medical)	27	23	21	15
	Aspire (Vascutek Terumo)	26	23	21	17
24	Soprano (Sorin Biomedica)	32	27	23.7	16
25	Magna (Edwards Lifesciences)	28	23	22	17
	Perimount (Edwards Lifesciences)	31	23	22	17
	Mosaic/Hancock II (Medtronic)	33	25	22.5	17.5
	Mosaic Ultra/Hancock I Ultra (Medtronic)	30	25	22.5	
	Mitroflow (Sorin Biomedica)	29	25.1	21	15
	Trifecta (St. Jude Medical)	31	25	23	18
	Epic/Biocor (St. Jude Medical)	29	25	23	16
	Epic Supra (St. Jude Medical)	N/A	25	25	
	Aspire (Vascutek Terumo)	28	25	23	18
26	Soprano (Sorin Biomedica)	35	29	25.6	19
27	Magna (Edwards Lifesciences)	32	27	26	18
	Perimount (Edwards Lifesciences)	35	27	26	18
	Mosaic/Hancock II (Medtronic)	36	27	24	18.5
	Mosaic Ultra/Hancock II Ultra (Medtronic)	32	27	24	
	Mitroflow (Sorin Biomedica)	31	27.3	22.9	16
	Trifecta (St. Jude Medical)	33	27	25	19
	Epic/Biocor (St. Jude Medical)	31	27	25	17
	Aspire (Vascutek Terumo)	30	27	25	18
28	Soprano (Sorin Biomedica)	38	31	27.6	19
29	Magna (Edwards Lifesciences)	34	29	28	19
	Perimount (Edwards Lifesciences)	37	29	28	19
	Mosaic/Hancock II (Medtronic)	39	29	26	20
	Mosaic Ultra/Hancock II Ultra (Medtronic)	34	29	26	
	Mitroflow (Sorin Biomedica)	33	29.5	24.7	16
	Trifecta (St. Jude Medical)	35	29	27	20

Table 32.2 Structural dimensions of stentless bioprosthetic valves

Valve label size	Bioprosthesis	Manufacturer	Outer diameter, mm	Internal diameter, mm
19	Freestyle	Medtronic	19	16
	Prima Plus	Edwards Lifesciences	19	16
	3 F Therapeutics	ATS Medical	19	17
	Pericarbon Freedom	Sorin Biomedica	19	17
21	Freestyle	Medtronic	21	18
	Prima Plus	Edwards Lifesciences	21	18
	3 F Therapeutics	ATS Medical	21	19
	Toronto SPV	St. Jude Medical	21	18
	Pericarbon freedom	Sorin Biomedica	21	19
23	Freestyle	Medtronic	23	20
	Prima Plus	Edwards Lifesciences	23	20
	3 F Therapeutics	ATS Medical	23	21
	Toronto SPV	St. Jude Medical	23	20
	Pericarbon Freedom	Sorin Biomedica	23	21
25	Freestyle	Medtronic	25	21
	Prima Plus	Edwards Lifesciences	25	21
	3 F Therapeutics	ATS Medical	25	23
	Toronto SPV	St. Jude Medical	25	21
	Pericarbon Freedom	Sorin Biomedica	25	23

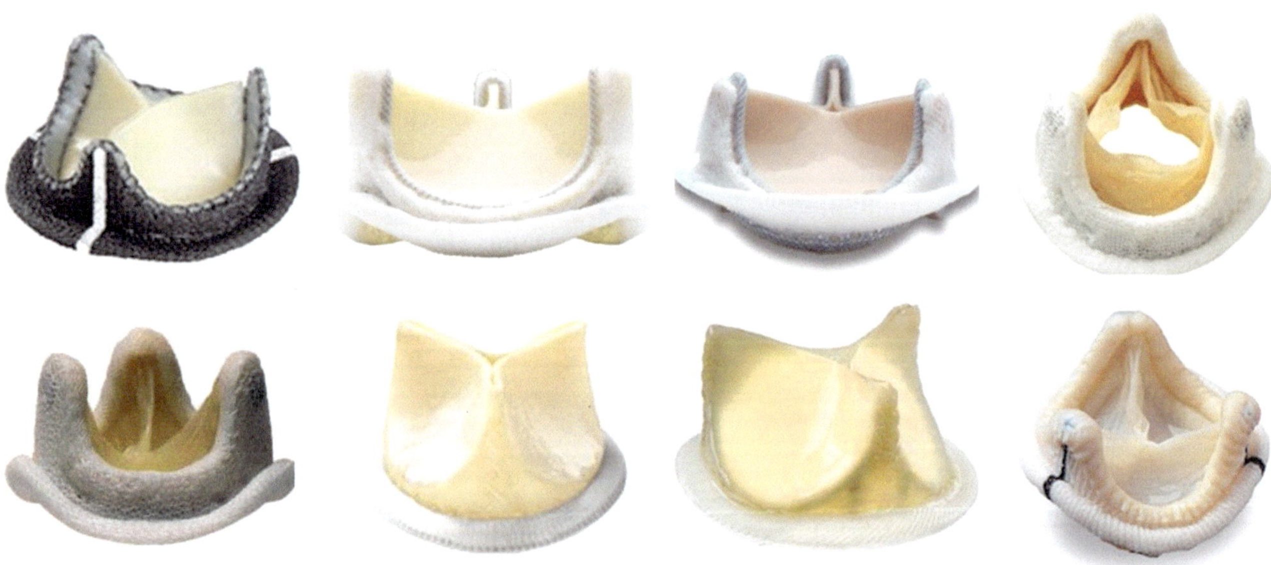

Fig. 32.3 Stented bioprosthetic surgical valves. *Top row* (*left-right*): Soprano (Sorin Biomedica), Magna (Edwards Lifesciences), Perimount (Edwards Lifesciences), Mosaic (Medtronic). *Bottom row* (*left-right*): Hancock Ultra (Medtronic), Mitroflow (Sorin Biomedica), Trifecta (St. Jude Medical), Epic (St. Jude Medical)

position of the native valve, thus eliminating the need for the support structures (Fig. 32.4). However, the stentless valve also lacks radiopaque elements to guide positioning and anchor the new transcatheter valve. Positioning with fluoroscopy relies on the presence of leaflet calcification.

Transcatheter Valves

Currently three transcatheter device systems have been used for valve-in-valve intervention (Fig. 32.5). Importantly these valves differ fundamentally from surgical valves as the leaflet kinematics is determined by valve expansion.

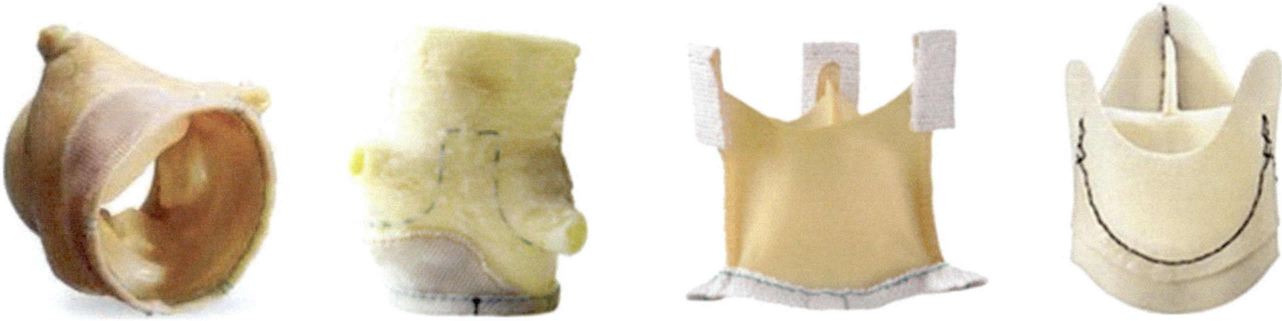

Fig. 32.4 Stentless bioprosthetic surgical valves (*left-right*): Freestyle (Medtronic), Prima Plus (Edwards Lifesciences), 3 F Therapeutics (ATS Medical), Pericarbon Freedom (Sorin Biomedica)

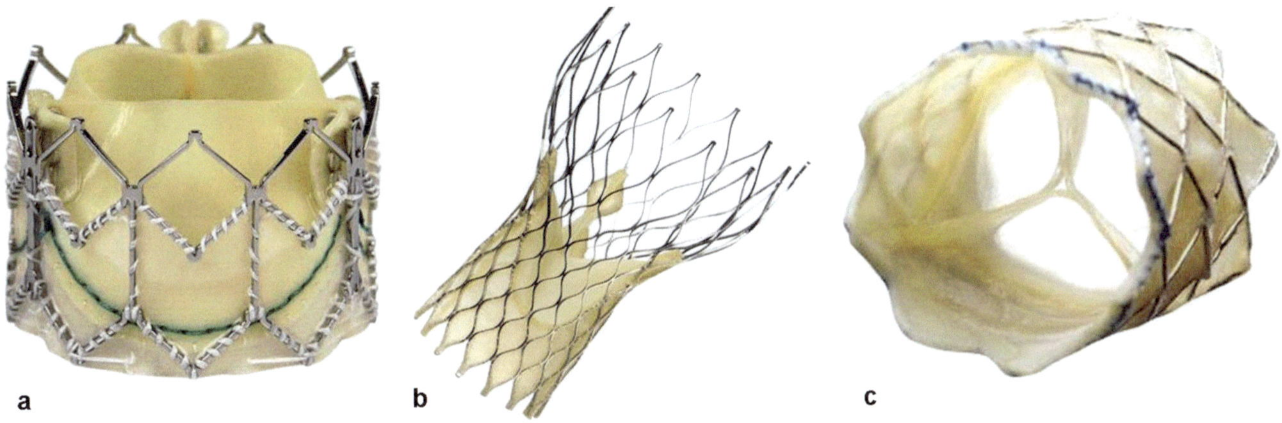

Fig. 32.5 Current transcatheter valve devices used for valve-in-valve implantation. (**a**) SAPIEN XT (Edwards Lifesciences), (**b**) CoreValve (Medtronic), (**c**) Melody (Medtronic)

SAPIEN/XT Balloon Expandable Valves

The Edwards SAPIEN and SAPIEN XT valve is a balloon expandable valve with bovine pericardium leaflets on a radi-opaque cobalt chromium frame. The current SAPIEN XT device is available in 20, 23, 26, and 29 mm sizes and can be implanted in valves with internal diameters of 16–27 mm; however, caution is warranted when implanting within small surgical prostheses as the residual transvalvular gradient can be significant. Small-diameter surgical bioprostheses (particularly ≤19 mm) may not allow for optimal expansion of current transcatheter implants. The strut height of the SAPIEN XT valve post-deployment ranges from 13.5 to 19.1 mm making this device suitable for implantation in all four valve positions.

CoreValve Prostheses

The Medtronic CoreValve has three porcine leaflets mounted on a self-expandable nitinol stent. It is currently available in two sizes: 26 mm (accommodates 20–23 mm diameter) and 29 mm (accommodates 23–27 mm diameter). The valve can only be mounted one way in the restraining sheath, hence the device can only be deployed retrograde. The length of this device makes it unsuitable for implantation in the mitral position.

Melody Valve

The Melody transcatheter valve (Medtronic Inc) is a bovine jugular venous valve attached to a platinum iridium scaffold. Originally designed to treat dysfunctional right ventricular outflow tract conduits, this valve has been deployed in the pulmonic and tricuspid position.

Imaging for Valve Sizing

Surgical stented valves have labeled sizes from 18 to 29 mm and stentless 19–25 mm depending upon the manufacturer. However these sizings are not standardized [28, 29] and may often refer to the internal or outer diameter for stented valves,

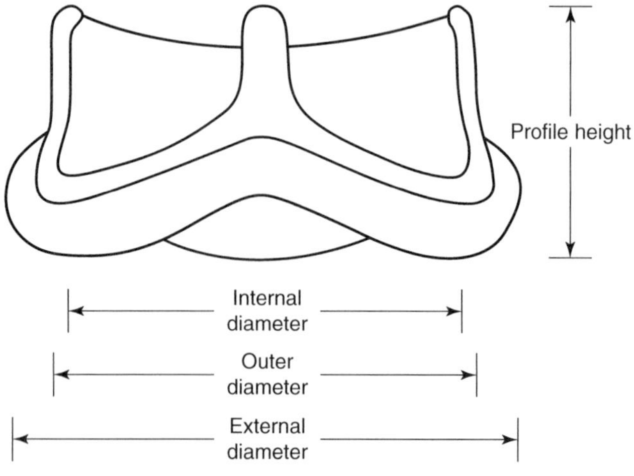

Fig. 32.6 Reference dimensions of surgical bioprosthetic valves

or external diameter for stentless valves (Fig. 32.6). In this regard, operative reports and reference tables of surgical valve dimensions are crucial for planning. In cases where the type of prosthesis is unknown, computed tomography or transesophageal echocardiography may help clarify valve geometry.

The principle of oversizing used in transcatheter intervention of native valve aortic stenosis [30] also applies to valve-in-valve intervention. It is the internal diameter that is most relevant for valve-in-valve therapy as an implant is chosen with a nominal external diameter matching the internal diameter of the failed valve. Importantly, the internal diameter of surgical valves can vary by up to 10 % from the labeled size. Within stented prostheses the sewing ring and stent posts can constrain an oversized transcatheter valve, while stentless valves often need 2–3 mm oversizing to achieve stability. Currently, optimal transcatheter valve function requires expansion of the prosthesis to its nominal dimensions. A transcatheter valve implanted within a smaller surgical prosthesis can be expected to function suboptimally with increased transvalvular gradient, impaired leaflet coaptation, and reduced durability. Matching of an appropriate size transcatheter valve to the surgical valve is thus crucial as excessive oversizing, especially in small-diameter surgical prostheses (<19 mm), may lead to lack of expansion of the transcatheter valve resulting in high-residual transvalvular gradients [31, 32]. While the acceptable boundaries of under-expansion remain undefined, a recent case report utilizing a 20 mm SAPIEN XT valve within a 16 mm internal diameter surgical prosthesis for severe regurgitation resulted in only a modest residual transvalvular gradient. Further study is warranted as there remains limited long-term evidence documenting durability of valve-in-valve implantations.

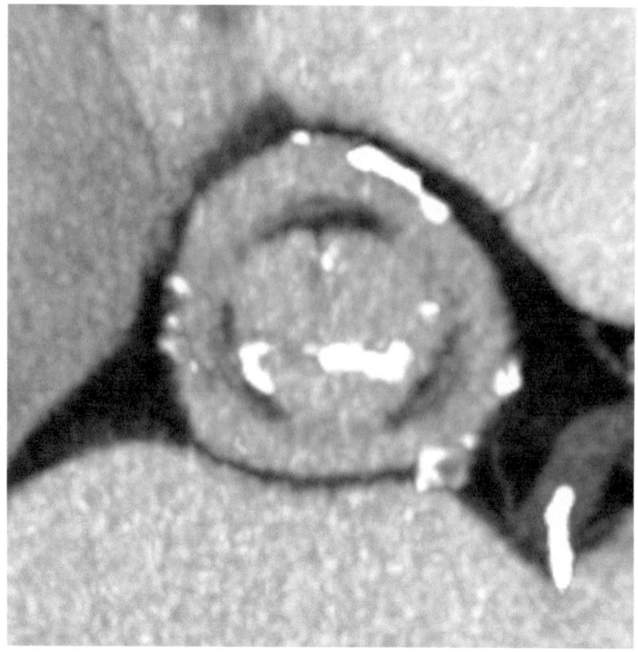

Fig. 32.7 CT multiplanar reformat showing Hancock II bioprosthetic valve in the aortic position. Calcification occurs at points of high stress and is present along the commissures extending to the leaflet insertion points

Imaging the In Vivo Valve

Understanding the mechanism of surgical valve failure is of significant relevance to planning a valve-in-valve procedure. Bioprosthetic valves may fail due to leaflet or non-leaflet pathologies. Leaflet failure is most commonly due to degeneration or calcification. Often as valves degenerate, calcific deposits form within the leaflet tissue at sites of high stress (commissural and leaflet attachment points). Valves with significant calcification or pannus may have reduced internal diameters relative to ex vivo sizing and imaging of the valve to assess leaflet bulkiness, as well as the extent and location of pannus and calcification can be used when considering sizing of the transcatheter valve. Cardiac CT and transesophageal echo are both useful modalities for assessing leaflet morphology (Fig. 32.7).

In addition to stenosis, bioprosthetic valves may develop significant regurgitation due to leaflet degeneration, endocarditis, or paravalvular leaks. The latter must be distinguished from other causes of valvular regurgitation as it cannot be ameliorated by valve-in-valve intervention (Fig. 32.8).

Anatomic Suitability for Valve-in-Valve Procedures

Assessment of the in vivo valve is important for sizing and predicting leaflet function. Adequate expansion, symmetry, and circularity is needed for optimal function [33], and the presence of significant bulkiness or calcification could lead to a suboptimal result. The geometry of the aortic root, the relationship of the prosthesis, and leaflet height in relation to the coronary ostia as well as the size of the sinotubular junction are relevant in pre-procedure planning (Fig. 32.9). Typically, however, as the transcatheter valve is constrained within the structure of the surgical prosthesis, there is less concern with coronary obstruction, annular rupture, and heart block with valve-in-valve implantation compared to native valve intervention (Fig. 32.10).

Imaging for Access and Delivery

Access routes for valve-in-valve intervention are the same as those for conventional TAVR. Both transapical and transfemoral access are currently used for aortic valve-in-valve implantation. Transapical access currently remains the preferred route for mitral valve-in-valve interventions as it provides direct coaxial alignment. A variety of percutaneous and surgical routes have been used for tricuspid and pulmonic valve-in-valve procedures both within native valves and surgically implanted right heart conduits. Regardless of the route selected, coaxial alignment is critical for valve-in-valve implantation success. Surgical bioprosthetic valves have the benefit of radiopaque annular and strut frames [34] making the optimal angle for deployment easier to ascertain than with native valve disease [35, 36] (Figs. 32.11 and 32.12).

Positioning of the new prosthesis is dependent on the model used (Fig. 32.13). The CoreValve may be deployed in a supra-annular position to optimize the hemodynamics. Conversely, the SAPIEN XT must overlap to extend below the bioprosthetic annulus to splay the struts and prevent embolization. As the height of the deployed SAPIEN XT valve may be up to 3 mm shorter than when crimped on the balloon, the positioning must account for the transcatheter valve struts engaging the tissue valve and concertina shortening occurring on the ventricular side. Adequacy of deployment can be determined by intraprocedural TEE, and subsequent TTE and CT (Fig. 32.14).

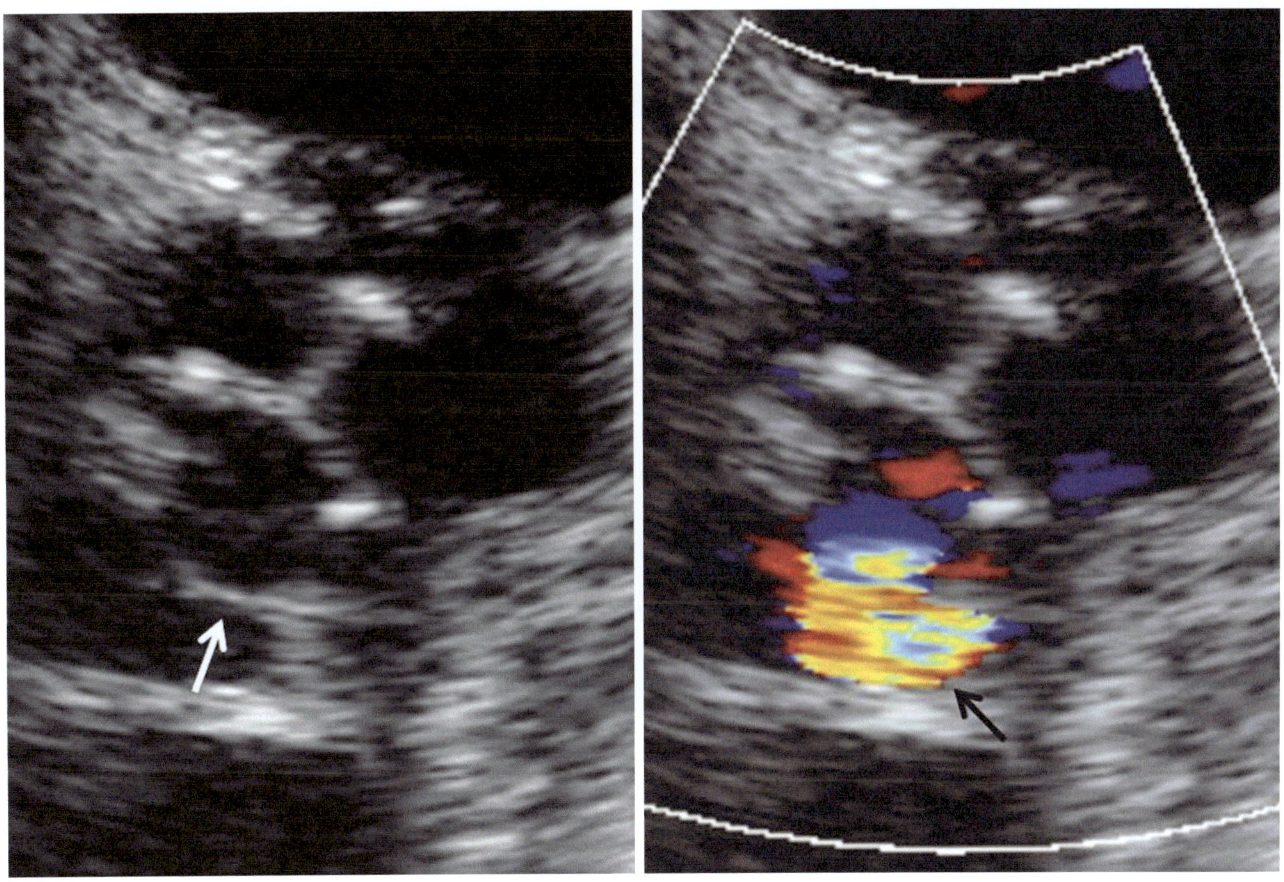

Fig. 32.8 Transesophageal echocardiographic images showing a surgical prosthesis in the aortic position. The sewing ring is visible (*white arrow*) and color flow imaging shows a large paravalvular leak (*black arrow*). Paravalvular leaks cannot be managed with a valve-in-valve procedure

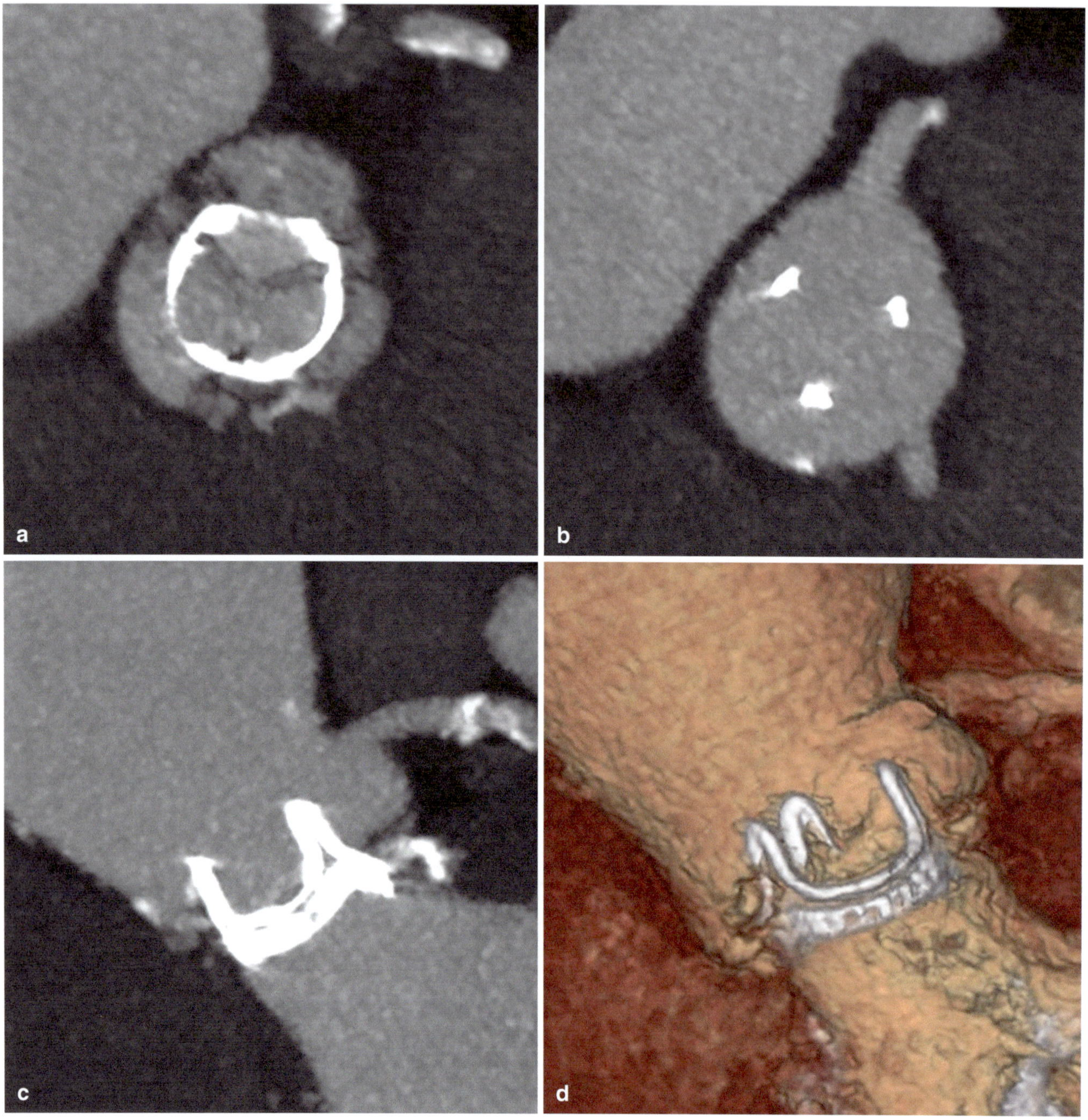

Fig. 32.9 CT assessment of a Perimount bioprosthetic valve. Multiplanar reformats show the annular ring (**a**) and leaflet struts (**b**) with clearance to both the coronary ostia (**b**) and (**c**). 3-D volume rendered reconstruction (**d**) demonstrates the relationship of the valve to structures in the aortic root

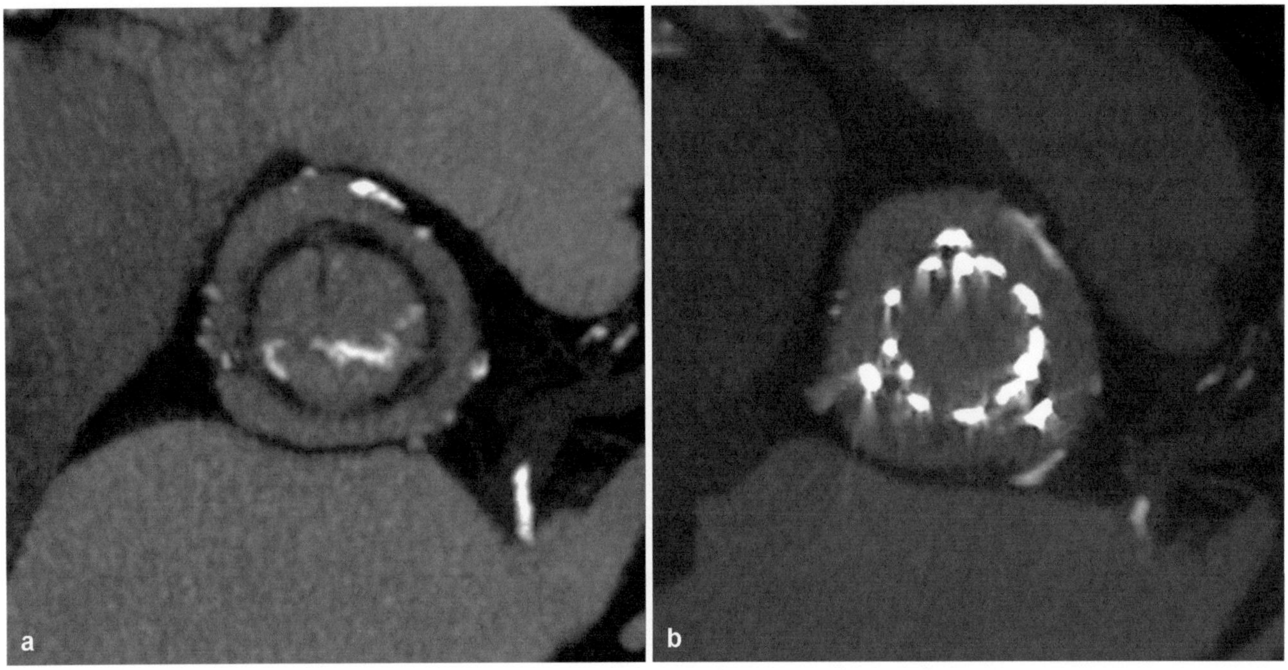

Fig. 32.10 A Hancock II surgical prosthesis (**a**) with the frame of a SAPIEN XT visible within the leaflet struts (**b**)

Novel Transcatheter Systems for Valve-in-valve Implantation

Multiple novel transcatheter valve systems are currently being developed for valve-in-valve applications that utilize a variety of innovative sizing criteria. Although still being refined, these systems will need to be easily deliverable and repositionable while maximizing the effective orifice area and minimizing both the residual gradient and inter- or transvalvular regurgitation. As with existing transcatheter systems, sizing will still be individualized for each patient, taking into consideration the reported internal diameter, patient size, bulkiness of the degenerated valve, nature of the valve failure, and the location of calcification or pannus. MDCT is proving invaluable for next-generation device development and refinement.

Conclusion

Transcatheter valve-in-valve intervention is becoming an acceptable alternative to standard surgical reoperation in select high-risk patients with degenerated surgical bioprostheses. Valve-in-valve procedures can be performed using current transcatheter valve devices using similar access and imaging to native valve interventions. The structural elements of the surgical prosthesis often limit the risk of complications due to coronary obstruction, annular rupture, and atrioventricular heart block. However, optimal transcatheter valve function requires expansion of the prosthesis to its nominal dimensions. Knowledge of the in situ surgical prosthesis is therefore crucial for procedural success. MDCT imaging is useful for identifying and sizing the in vivo surgical prostheses. MDCT also clearly defines adjacent anatomical structures important for valve-in-valve positioning. Echocardiography and angiography provide crucial periprocedural guidance during valve-in-valve implantation within both radiolucent and radiopaque surgical prostheses. Further study is warranted to assess the long-term durability of valve-in-valve implantation within degenerated surgical prostheses in all four valve positions.

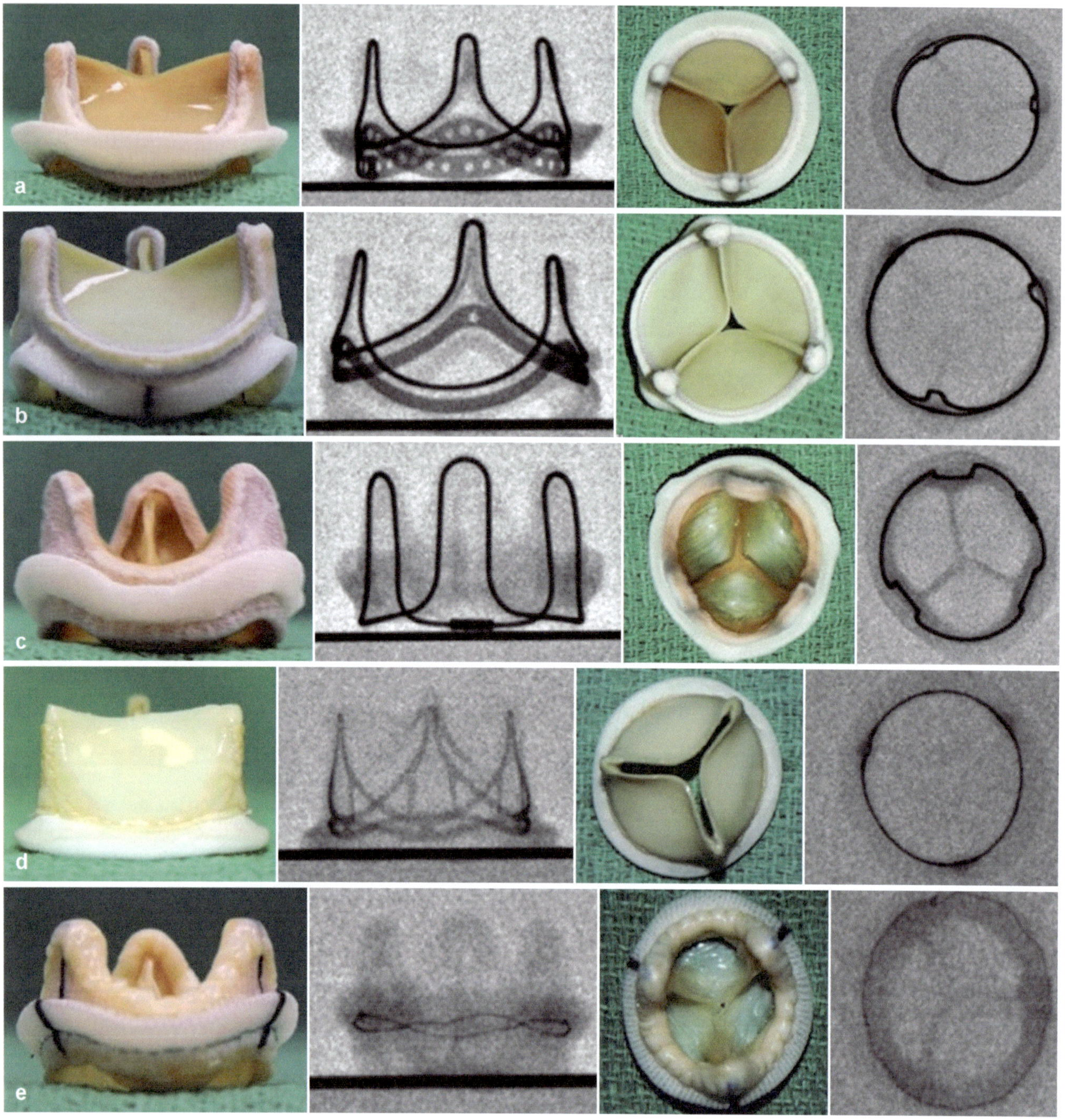

Fig. 32.11 Fluoroscopic appearance of selected bioprosthetic surgical valves. (**a**) Perimount (Edwards Lifesciences), (**b**) Magna (Edward Lifesciences), (**c**) Carpentier-Edwards Porcine (Edwards Lifesciences), (**d**) Trifecta (St. Jude Medical), (**e**) Epic (St. Jude Medical)

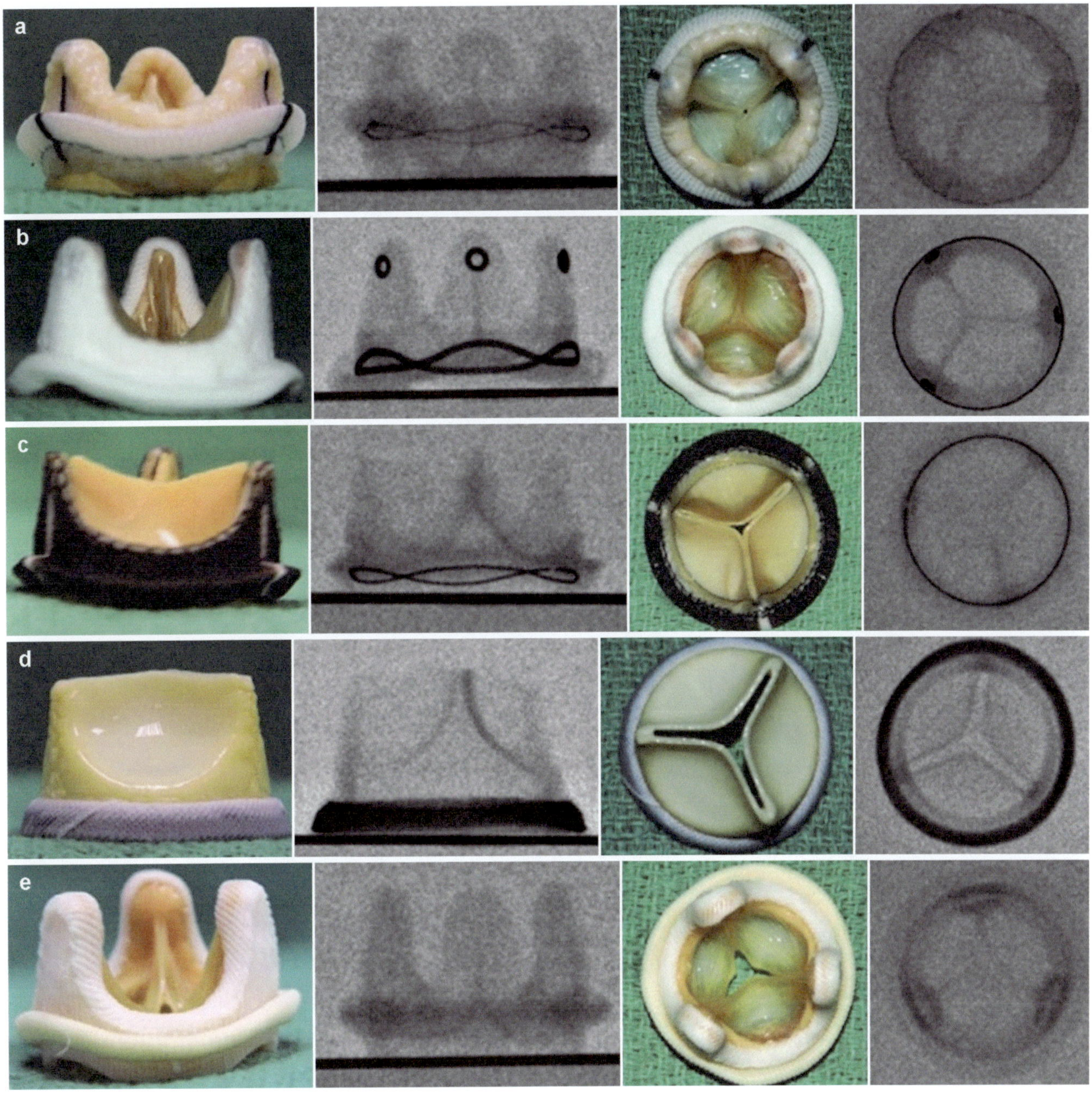

Fig. 32.12 Fluoroscopic appearance of selected bioprosthetic surgical valves. (**a**) Mosaic (Medtronic), (**b**) Hancock II (Medtronic), (**c**) Soprano (Sorin), (**d**) Mitroflow (Sorin), (**e**) Aspire (Vascutek)

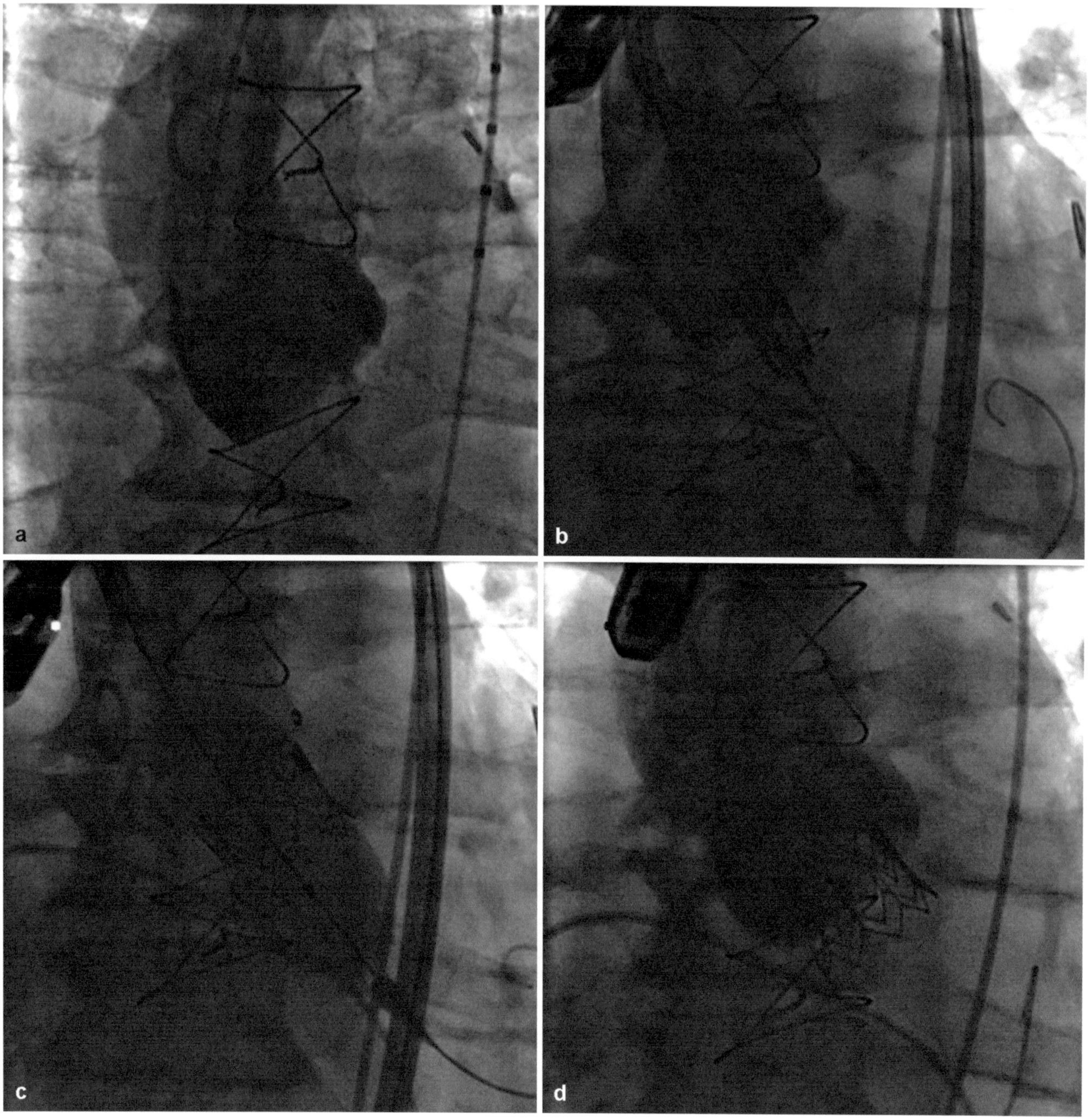

Fig. 32.13 Deployment of a SAPIEN XT inside a Hancock II surgical prosthesis. Injection in the aortic root demonstrates a coaxial angle for deployment. The radiopaque markers of the prosthesis and the cusps of the aortic root are aligned (**a**). The SAPIEN XT is positioned using the markers and aortic cusps as a guide (**b**). The transcatheter valve is deployed (**c**) and repeat injection confirms optimal positioning (**d**). Note the splaying of the frame on the ventricular side

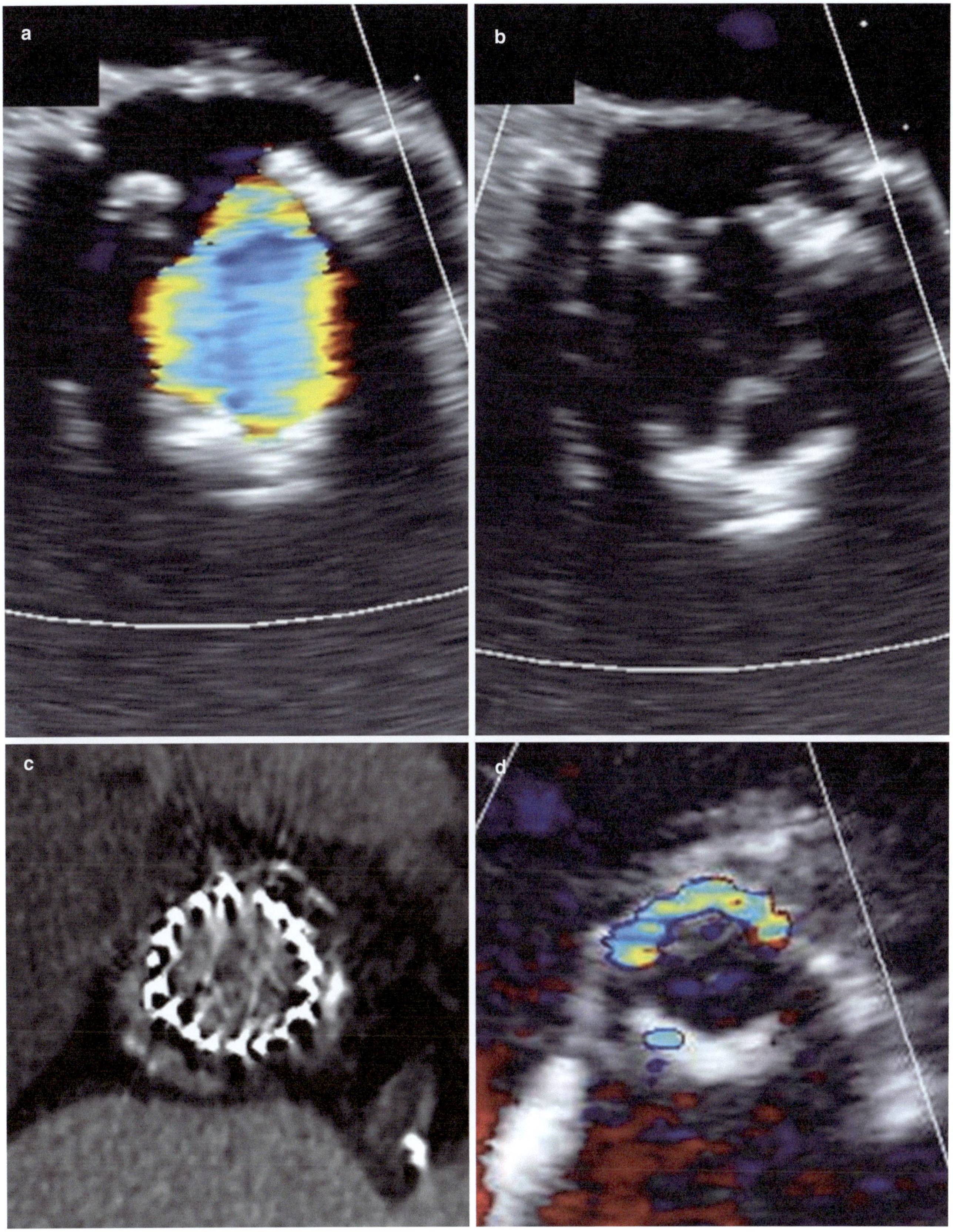

Fig. 32.14 Assessing optimal transcatheter valve-in-valve deployment. Intraprocedural TEE shows good valve orifice (**a**) with no aortic regurgitation (**b**). Subsequent CT shows a well expanded circular frame within the surgical struts (**c**) and transthoracic echocardiography demonstrates mild late paravalvular regurgitation (**d**)

References

1. Ruel M, Chan V, Bedard P, Kulik A, Ressler L, Lam BK, Rubens FD, Goldstein W, Hendry PJ, Masters RG, Mesana TG. Very long-term survival implications of heart valve replacement with tissue versus mechanical prostheses in adults <60 years of age. Circulation. 2007;116(11 Suppl):I294–300.
2. Chikwe J, Filsoufi F. Durability of tissue valves. Semin Thorac Cardiovasc Surg. 2011;23(1):18–23.
3. Grunkemeier GL, Jamieson WR, Miller DC, Starr A. Actuarial versus actual risk of porcine structural valve deterioration. J Thorac Cardiovasc Surg. 1994;108(4):709–18.
4. Balsam LB, Grossi EA, Greenhouse DG, Ursomanno P, Deanda A, Ribakove GH, Culliford AT, Galloway AC. Reoperative valve surgery in the elderly: predictors of risk and long-term survival. Ann Thorac Surg. 2010;90(4):1195–200; discussion 1201.
5. Jones JM, O'Kane H, Gladstone DJ, Sarsam MA, Campalani G, MacGowan SW, Cleland J, Cran GW. Repeat heart valve surgery: risk factors for operative mortality. J Thorac Cardiovasc Surg. 2001;122(5):913–8.
6. Maganti M, Rao V, Armstrong S, Feindel CM, Scully HE, David TE. Redo valvular surgery in elderly patients. Ann Thorac Surg. 2009;87(2):521–5.
7. Leontyev S, Borger MA, Davierwala P, Walther T, Lehmann S, Kempfert J, Mohr FW. Redo aortic valve surgery: early and late outcomes. Ann Thorac Surg. 2011;91(4):1120–6.
8. Beurtheret S, Gariboldi V, Feier H, Grisoli D, Riberi A, Mouly-Bandini A, Metras D, Kerbaul F, Collart F. Short-term results of repeat valve replacement: a predictive factor analysis. J Heart Valve Dis. 2010;19(3):326–32.
9. Lytle BW, Cosgrove DM, Taylor PC, Gill CC, Goormastic M, Golding LR, Stewart RW, Loop FD. Reoperations for valve surgery: perioperative mortality and determinants of risk for 1,000 patients, 1958–1984. Ann Thorac Surg. 1986;42(6):632–43.
10. Piehler JM, Blackstone EH, Bailey KR, Sullivan ME, Pluth JR, Weiss NS, Brookmeyer RS, Chandler JG. Reoperation on prosthetic heart values. Patient-specific estimates of in-hospital events. J Thorac Cardiovasc Surg. 1995;109(1):30–48.
11. Kirsch M, Nakashima K, Kubota S, Houel R, Hillion ML, Loisance D. The risk of reoperative heart valve procedures in Octogenarian patients. J Heart Valve Dis. 2004;13(6):991–6; discussion 996.
12. Boone RH, Webb JG, Horlick E, Benson L, Cao QL, Nadeem N, Kiess M, Hijazi ZM. Transcatheter pulmonary valve implantation using the Edwards SAPIEN transcatheter heart valve. Catheter Cardiovasc Interv. 2010;75(2):286–94.
13. Cerillo AG, Chiaramonti F, Murzi M, Bevilacqua S, Cerone E, Palmieri C, Del Sarto P, Mariani M, Berti S, Glauber M. Transcatheter valve-in-valve implantation for failed mitral and tricuspid bioprosthesis. Catheter Cardiovasc Interv. 2011;78(7):987–95.
14. Cheung AW, Gurvitch R, Ye J, Wood D, Lichtenstein SV, Thompson C, Webb JG. Transcatheter transapical mitral valve-in-valve implantations for a failed bioprosthesis: a case series. J Thorac Cardiovasc Surg. 2011;141(3):711–5.
15. de Weger A, Tavilla G, Ng AC, Delgado V, van der Kley F, Schuijf JD, Bax JJ, Klautz RJ. Successful transapical transcatheter valve implantation within a dysfunctional mitral bioprosthesis. JACC Cardiovasc Imaging. 2010;3(2):222–3.
16. Gotzmann M, Mugge A, Bojara W. Transcatheter aortic valve implantation for treatment of patients with degenerated aortic bioprostheses–valve-in-valve technique. Catheter Cardiovasc Interv. 2010;76(7):1000–6.
17. Kempfert J, Van Linden A, Linke A, Borger MA, Rastan A, Mukherjee C, Ender J, Schuler G, Mohr FW, Walther T. Transapical off-pump valve-in-valve implantation in patients with degenerated aortic xenografts. Ann Thorac Surg. 2010;89(6):1934–41.
18. Khambadkone S, Coats L, Taylor A, Boudjemline Y, Derrick G, Tsang V, Cooper J, Muthurangu V, Hegde SR, Razavi RS, Pellerin D, Deanfield J, Bonhoeffer P. Percutaneous pulmonary valve implantation in humans: results in 59 consecutive patients. Circulation. 2005;112(8):1189–97.
19. Khawaja MZ, Haworth P, Ghuran A, Lee L, de Belder A, Hutchinson N, Trivedi U, Laborde JC, Hildick-Smith D. Transcatheter aortic valve implantation for stenosed and regurgitant aortic valve bioprostheses CoreValve for failed bioprosthetic aortic valve replacements. J Am Coll Cardiol. 2010;55(2):97–101.
20. Maroto LC, Rodriguez JE, Cobiella J, Marcos P. Transapical off-pump aortic valve-in-a-valve implantation in two elderly patients with a degenerated porcine bioprosthesis. Eur J Cardiothorac Surg. 2010;37(3):738–40.
21. McElhinney DB, Hellenbrand WE, Zahn EM, Jones TK, Cheatham JP, Lock JE, Vincent JA. Short- and medium-term outcomes after transcatheter pulmonary valve placement in the expanded multicenter US melody valve trial. Circulation. 2010;122(5):507–16.
22. Montorfano M, Latib A, Chieffo A, Moshiri S, Franco A, Grimaldi A, Alfieri O, Colombo A. Successful percutaneous anterograde transcatheter valve-in-valve implantation in the mitral position. JACC Cardiovasc Interv. 2011;4(11):1246–7.
23. Pasic M, Unbehaun A, Dreysse S, Buz S, Drews T, Kukucka M, Hetzer R. Transapical aortic valve implantation after previous aortic valve replacement: clinical proof of the "valve-in-valve" concept. J Thorac Cardiovasc Surg. 2011;142(2):270–7.
24. Roberts PA, Boudjemline Y, Cheatham JP, Eicken A, Ewert P, McElhinney DB, Hill SL, Berger F, Khan D, Schranz D, Hess J, Ezekowitz MD, Celermajer D, Zahn E. Percutaneous tricuspid valve replacement in congenital and acquired heart disease. J Am Coll Cardiol. 2011;58(2):117–22.
25. Seiffert M, Franzen O, Conradi L, Baldus S, Schirmer J, Meinertz T, Reichenspurner H, Treede H. Series of transcatheter valve-in-valve implantations in high-risk patients with degenerated bioprostheses in aortic and mitral position. Catheter Cardiovasc Interv. 2010;76(4):608–15.
26. Van Garsse LA, Ter Bekke RM, van Ommen VG. Percutaneous transcatheter valve-in-valve implantation in stenosed tricuspid valve bioprosthesis. Circulation. 2011;123(5):e219–21.
27. Webb JG, Wood DA, Ye J, Gurvitch R, Masson JB, Rodes-Cabau J, Osten M, Horlick E, Wendler O, Dumont E, Carere RG, Wijesinghe N, Nietlispach F, Johnson M, Thompson CR, Moss R, Leipsic J, Munt B, Lichtenstein SV, Cheung A. Transcatheter valve-in-valve implantation for failed bioprosthetic heart valves. Circulation. 2010;121(16):1848–57.
28. Christakis GT, Buth KJ, Goldman BS, Fremes SE, Rao V, Cohen G, Borger MA, Weisel RD. Inaccurate and misleading valve sizing: a proposed standard for valve size nomenclature. Ann Thorac Surg. 1998;66(4):1198–203.
29. Shibata T, Inoue K, Ikuta T, Bito Y, Yoshioka Y, Mizoguchi H. Which valve and which size should we use in the valve-on-valve technique for re-do mitral valve surgery? Interact Cardiovasc Thorac Surg. 2009;8(2):206–10.
30. Cribier A, Eltchaninoff H, Tron C, Bauer F, Agatiello C, Nercolini D, Tapiero S, Litzler PY, Bessou JP, Babaliaros V. Treatment of calcific aortic stenosis with the percutaneous heart valve: mid-term follow-up from the initial feasibility studies: the French experience. J Am Coll Cardiol. 2006;47(6):1214–23.
31. Azadani AN, Jaussaud N, Matthews PB, Chuter TA, Ge L, Guy TS, Guccione J, Tseng EE. Aortic valve-in-valve implantation: impact of transcatheter- bioprosthesis size mismatch. J Heart Valve Dis. 2009;18(4):367–73.
32. Azadani AN, Jaussaud N, Matthews PB, Ge L, Chuter TA, Tseng EE. Transcatheter aortic valves inadequately relieve stenosis in small degenerated bioprostheses. Interact Cardiovasc Thorac Surg. 2010;11(1):70–7.

33. Azadani AN, Tseng EE. Transcatheter heart valves for failing bioprostheses: state-of-the-art review of valve-in-valve implantation. Circ Cardiovasc Interv. 2011;4(6):621–8.
34. Bapat V, Mydin I, Chadalavada S, Tehrani H, Attia R, Thomas M. A guide to fluoroscopic identification and design of bioprosthetic valves: a reference for valve-in-valve procedure. Catheter Cardiovasc Interv. 2013;81:853–61.
35. Binder RK, Leipsic J, Wood D, Moore T, Toggweiler S, Willson A, Gurvitch R, Freeman M, Webb JG. Prediction of optimal deployment projection for transcatheter aortic valve replacement: angiographic 3-dimensional reconstruction of the aortic root versus multidetector computed tomography. Circ Cardiovasc Interv. 2012;5:247–52.
36. Gurvitch R, Wood DA, Leipsic J, Tay E, Johnson M, Ye J, Nietlispach F, Wijesinghe N, Cheung A, Webb JG. Multislice computed tomography for prediction of optimal angiographic deployment projections during transcatheter aortic valve implantation. JACC Cardiovasc Interv. 2010;3(11):1157–65.

Intraprocedural Use of Echocardiography for TAVR

33

Jorge Castellanos, Raj Makkar, Hasan Jilaihawi, and Robert J. Siegel

Abstract

Since the advent of transcatheter aortic valve replacement (TAVR) in 2002, more than 20,000 bioprosthetic valves have been deployed in patients with severe aortic stenosis (Jilaihawi, Catheter Cardiovasc Interv 80(1):128–38, 2012). Long-term clinical outcomes data from TAVR underscore the importance of adequately measuring the aortic annulus and having the ability to clearly visualize the relationship between the bioprosthetic valve, the native aortic valve, and surrounding anatomic structures. The development of 3D echocardiography has facilitated the ability to correctly measure the aortic valve annulus in multiple planes and aid in the deployment of the bioprosthetic valve in the catheterization laboratory. This chapter will describe the strengths and limitations of 3D TEE in assessing the aortic valve annulus and any other associated cardiac structures during TAVR.

Keywords

3D echocardiography • 2D echocardiography • TAVR • Transcatheter aortic valve replacement • Bioprosthetic valve

Introduction

Aortic stenosis (AS) is believed to be among the most debilitating valvular pathologies [1]. Its prevalence increases with age, affecting approximately 3 % of the population over the age of 75 [2]. Most patients with AS remain relatively asymptomatic for the majority of their lives, but once symptoms develop, there is a rapid decline in functional status with up to a 50 % mortality rate within the first 2 years [3–6]. A recent retrospective study of 125 patients with severe AS indicates a far worse prognosis for symptomatic patients with AS. The 1-year mortality rates were as high as 62.5 % in patients with evidence of elevated left ventricular (LV) filling pressures measured by echo Doppler ultrasound [7]. Observational studies have shown that surgical replacement of the aortic valve can offer these patients with symptom relief and increases their survival [8–10], but recent data indicate that nearly 30 % of patients with symptomatic aortic stenosis are refused surgical correction of their aortic stenosis due to substantial comorbidities [7, 11–14].

Before the advent of transcatheter aortic valve replacement (TAVR), the management of AS primarily consisted of watchful waiting with serial transthoracic echocardiograms (TTE) and medical management until they developed symptoms or LV dysfunction. The updated 2008 ACC/AHA guidelines for the management of valvular heart disease defines severe AS as a maximum systolic continuous wave Doppler velocity of more than 4 m/s, a mean valve gradient

J. Castellanos, MD, MPP (✉)
Department of Cardiology, Cedars Sinai Medical Center, 8700 Beverly Blvd, Rm 5536B, Los Angeles, CA 90048, USA
e-mail: jorge.castellanos@cshs.org

R. Makkar, MD, FACC • H. Jilaihawi, MD, MRCP
Department of Cardiology, Cedars-Sinai Heart Institute, Cedars-Sinai Medical Center, 8631 West 3rd St, Ste 415, Los Angeles, CA 90048, USA
e-mail: raj.makkar@cshs.org; hasanjilaihawi@gmail.com

R.J. Siegel, MD, FACC, FASE
Department of Cardiology, Cedars Sinai Medical Center, 8700 Beverly Blvd, Rm 523, Los Angeles, CA 90048, USA
e-mail: robertjames.siegel@cshs.org

J.K. Min et al. (eds.), *Multimodality Imaging for Transcatheter Aortic Valve Replacement*, DOI 10.1007/978-1-4471-2798-7_33, © Springer-Verlag London 2014

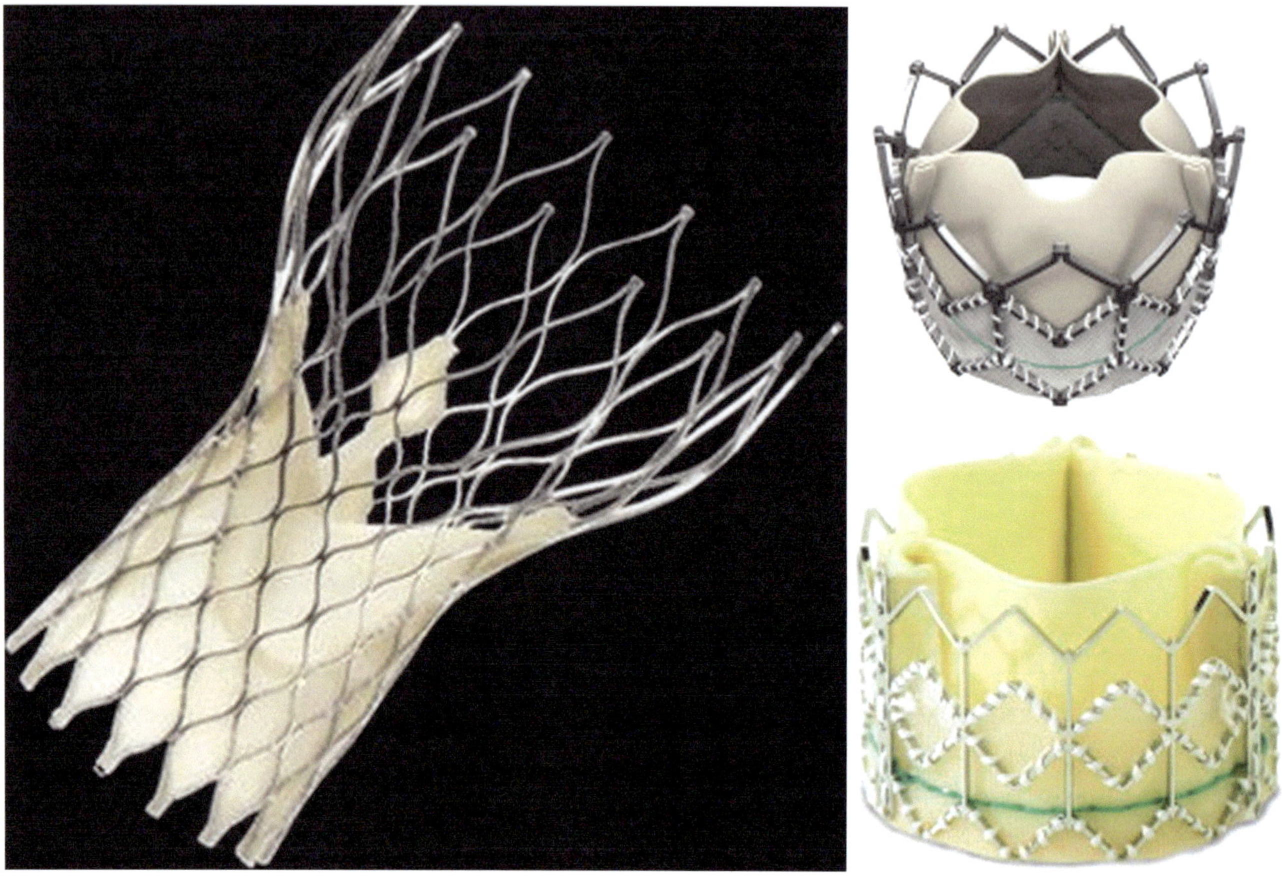

Fig. 33.1 CoreValve (*left*, courtesy of Medtronic). SAPIEN 9000 TFX (*bottom right*) and SAPIEN XT 9300 TFX (*top right*) valves (Adapted with permission from Jayasuriya et al. [27])

of more than 40 mmHg or a calculated aortic valve area of less than 1 cm^2 [15]. Surgical intervention is recommended for patients with severe AS who also have symptoms including chest pain, syncope, shortness of breath, decreased exercise capacity, or left ventricular systolic dysfunction defined as a left ventricular ejection fraction <50 %. For the 30–50 % of patients with symptomatic severe AS not being surgical candidates due to substantial comorbidities [14, 16–18], TAVR has emerged an alternative treatment [7]. Figure 33.1 shows the three types of bioprosthetic aortic valves currently in use, one from Medtronic CoreValve (Luxembourg) and two from Edwards Sapien Valve.

The PARTNER trial, published in 2010, compared TAVR with medical therapy among patients with severe AS considered unsuitable surgical candidates for AVR. The all-cause death rate at 1 year with TAVR was 30.7 % compared to 50.7 % with standard medical therapy. Patients undergoing TAVR experienced improved quality of life as well, with the rate of heart failure symptoms (NYHA Class III or IV) 25.2 % in the TAVR group compared to 58 % in the standard therapy group. However, incidence of early strokes or vascular complications within 30 days of procedural intervention was higher in the TAVR group, although only vascular complications manifested statistically significant differences [3]. Two-year follow-up data from the original PARTNER trial demonstrates the persistence in life-years gained, with mortality in the TAVR group 43.3 % versus 68 % in the standard therapy group. Similarly, rates of rehospitalization for the TAVR patients over a 2-year period were also significantly less than those in the standard therapy group (35 % versus 72.5 %). The rate of strokes over the 2-year follow-up period was 13.8 % for TAVR, and 5.5 % for the standard therapy group, with most of the early TAVR strokes being ischemic and late TAVR strokes being hemorrhagic [22].

Intraprocedural Imaging of the Aortic Valve

Two-dimensional transthoracic echocardiography is used to assess aortic stenosis severity in order to qualify for TAVR placement. Multiple modalities are used in evaluating the severity of AS, including noninvasive and invasive hemodynamic measurements in the echocardiography and catheterization laboratory. Real-time fluoroscopic and transesophageal echocardiographic (TEE) guidance are used to evaluate cardiac function, locate the position of the native valve, and deploy the bioprosthetic valve. But as can be seen in Fig. 33.2, fluoroscopy provides limited information about the severity of aortic stenosis, correct sizing of the aortic annulus, or assessing for cardiac function.

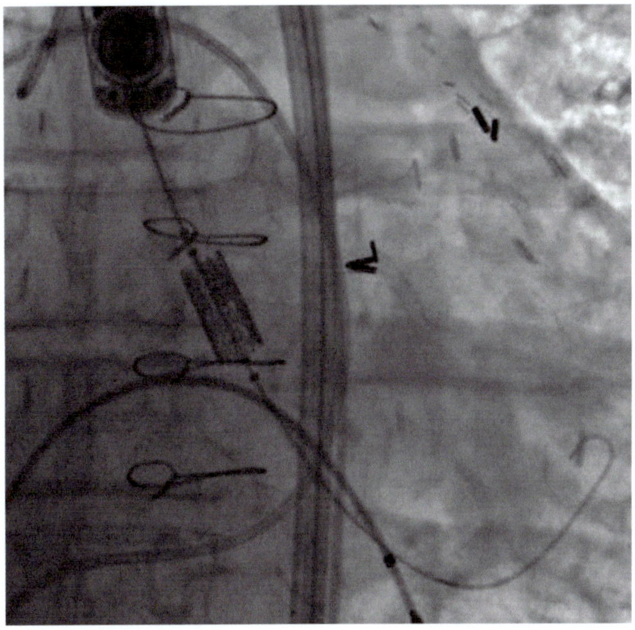

Fig. 33.2 Fluoroscopic view of the Edwards Sapien Valve across the aortic valve pre-deployment. The ability to visualize the aortic valve annulus using fluoroscopy without contrast is limited unless the aortic valve is significantly calcified. In this example, there is limited aortic valve calcification. Transesophageal echo provides valuable supplemental information to guide the operator and possibly limit contrast injections

Both 2D TTE (preprocedurally) and 2D TEE (intraprocedurally) have been used to address these limitations of fluoroscopy, but the appreciation of spatial relationships with 2D echocardiography is limited. Consequently, operators have now started to utilize 3D echocardiography before, during and after the deployment of the bioprosthetic aortic valve to better assess the aortic valve diameter and catheter orientation. The majority of applications for 3D echocardiography have been with TEE given that 3D TTE has very poor resolution, making it of little practical use for pre- or intraprocedural TAVR. 3D TEE imaging offers precise multiplanar dimensional measurements as well as superior anatomic detail of the stenotic valve, aortic root, and subvalvular anatomy, the relationship of the aortic valve and the anterior mitral leaflet (Fig. 33.3a–d), and can identify the distance of the coronary ostia to the aortic annulus. Furthermore, post-deployment, 3D TEE can demonstrate the exact location and severity of a paravalvular or transvalvular leak.

During deployment of the bioprosthetic aortic valve, 2D and 3D TEE along with fluoroscopy are used to verify bioprosthesis positioning in the aortic annulus. Altiok et al., in addition to demonstrating the advantages of 3D imaging in procedural guidance, showed a high degree of correlation between the coronal and sagittal 3D TEE versus multidetector computed tomography (MDCT) aortic annulus diameters (23.6 ± 1.89 mm vs. 23.46 ± 2.07 mm and 22.19 ± 1.96 vs. 22.27 ± 2.01 mm, respectively). Data suggest that 3D cross-sectional measurements using MDCT can be used to accurately assess the annular size of the aortic valve and possibly help reduce the risk of moderate or severe paravalvular aortic regurgitation [19, 20]. Jilaihawi et al. published a single-center retrospective study showing that 3D MDCT was superior to 2D echocardiography for correctly

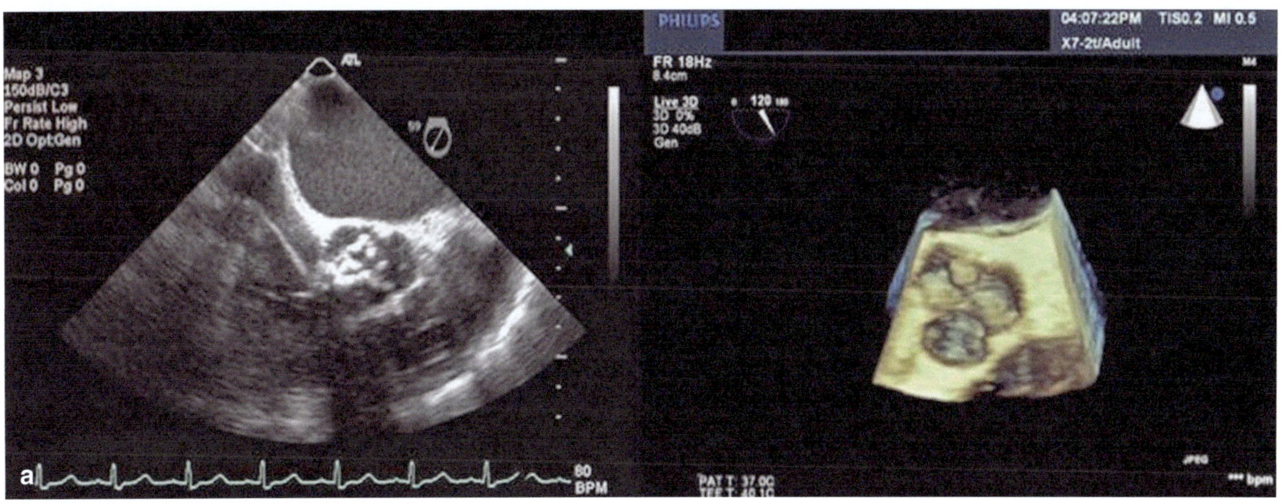

Fig. 33.3 (**a**) Comparison of 2D and 3D TEE short-axis view across the aortic valve. Note how one can better appreciate the anatomic relationship between the calcified aortic cusps and the aortic annulus in the 3D TEE relative to 2D TEE. (**b**) The relationship between the beginning and end of the crimped Sapien valve relative to the native aortic valve is more easily seen in the 3D TEE versus 2D TEE. (**c**) Deployment of the Sapien valve. (**d**) The precise location of the Sapien valve relative to the aortic annulus, left ventricular outflow tract, and the anterior mitral leaflet is more easily seen with the 3D TEE

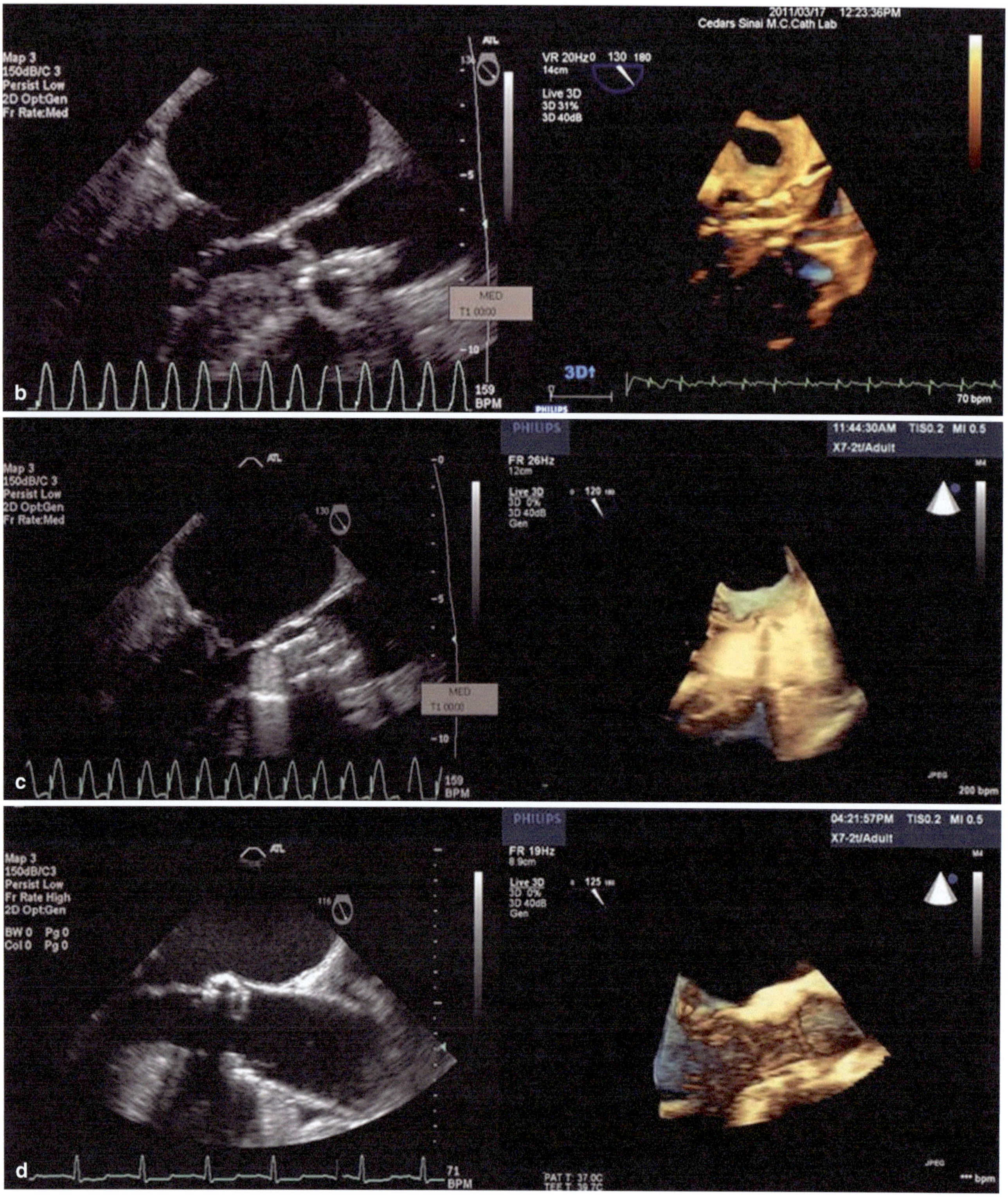

Fig. 33.3 (continued)

sizing the aortic valve annulus for TAVR. They showed a significant decrease in post-TAVR paravalvular aortic regurgitation (PAR) by using multi-slice CT rather than 2D echocardiography to measure the aortic valve annulus [21]. Although these data underscore the superiority of 3D versus 2D imaging modalities, there are still no multicenter randomized studies that compare the clinical outcomes of patients who have their aortic annulus measured with 3D MDCT or 3D TEE versus 2D TEE. These types of studies are necessary because due to a concern that increased prosthesis size generally dictated by cross-sectional imaging may theoretically lead to increased rates of catastrophic aortic annulus rupture or dissection (Table 33.1).

TAVR Pre-deployment

Once a patient has met criteria for TAVR, precise measurements of the aortic annulus are needed in order to correctly size the bioprosthetic valve. As can be appreciated in Fig. 33.4, the aortic valve annulus is usually wider in the coronal cross-section than the sagittal – producing an oval aortic valve annulus. This observation that the aortic valve annulus is oval has been observed in several other studies and has been found to have important clinical outcome implications [23].

Table 33.1 Relative usefulness of TEE versus CT

	2D TEE	3D TEE	MDCT
AS severity	++	+	+/–
Aortic valve morphology	++	++	+[a]
Calcium distribution	+	+	++
Aortic root orientation	––	––	++
Aortic annulus diameter	++	++	++
Aortic root morphology	++	++	++
Coronary ostia to aortic annulus distance	+/–	+	++

Adapted with permission from Bloomfield et al. [29]
–– not useful, +/– limited usefulness, + useful, ++ very useful
[a]Assessment of valve morphology using MDCT is likely to improve over time with advancements in technology

Although there remains controversy surrounding the optimal methodology for measuring the aortic valve annulus, there are several techniques that are currently being used to measure it as there is no gold standard. One of the most common techniques is using 3D TEE multiplane assessment of the aortic annulus, where simultaneous orthogonal views can be obtained in the sagittal and coronal plane during systole (Fig. 33.4). A similar approach is used with 2D TEE, where the sagittal diameter of the aortic valve is measured between the base of the right and noncoronary cusps from a mid-esophageal long-axis view of 110–140 ° during systole. A mid-esophageal short-axis view of 30–60° or an X-plane from the long-axis view is used at obtain the coronal diameter. Once the aortic annulus dimensions are noted, the sinus of Valsalva, the sinotubular junction, and the ascending aorta are also measured.

It is important to correctly measure the sagittal and coronal dimensions of the aortic valve annulus because undersizing of the bioprosthetic valve can lead to significant paravalvular leak, which if greater than mild, is an independent predictor of a twofold increase in late mortality [16, 24]. Furthermore, undersizing of the aortic valve can lead to dislodgement and embolization of the valve, while oversizing can cause aortic annular rupture, quickly evolving to cardiac tamponade and death. Given the higher anatomic spatial relationship of 3D TEE, it is hypothesized that it can better assess the true dimensions of the aortic valve annulus. But

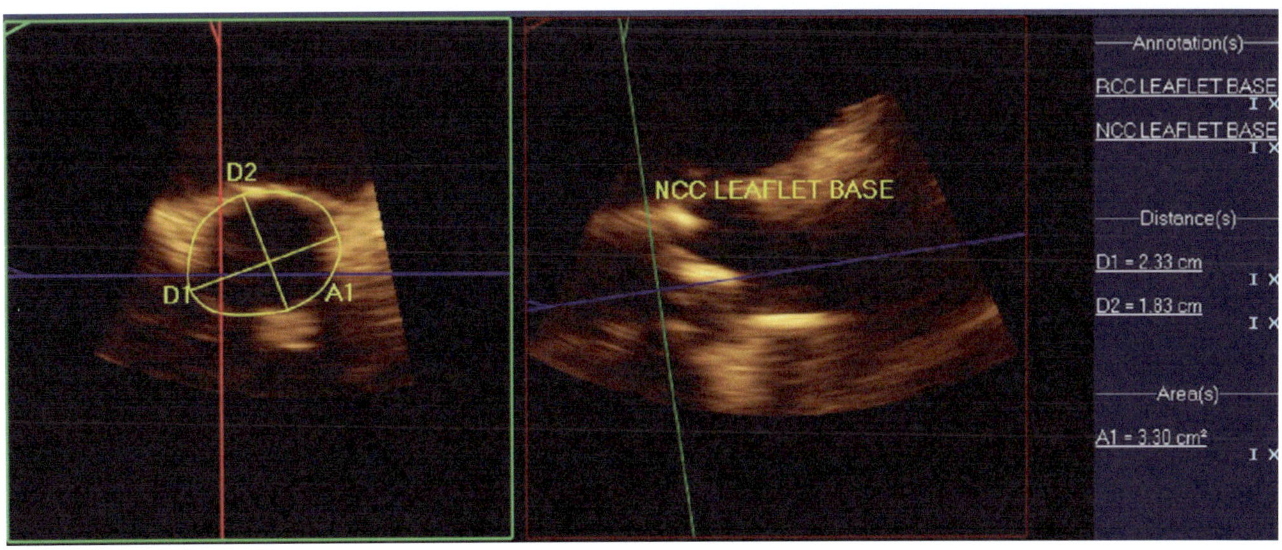

Fig. 33.4 Multiplanar assessment of aortic annulus using 3D TEE: *Left panel* demonstrates short-axis view of the aortic valve. Note the difference in the sagittal and coronal measurements, indicating that the aortic valve annulus is oval. *Right panel* shows an orthogonal measurement of the aortic annulus

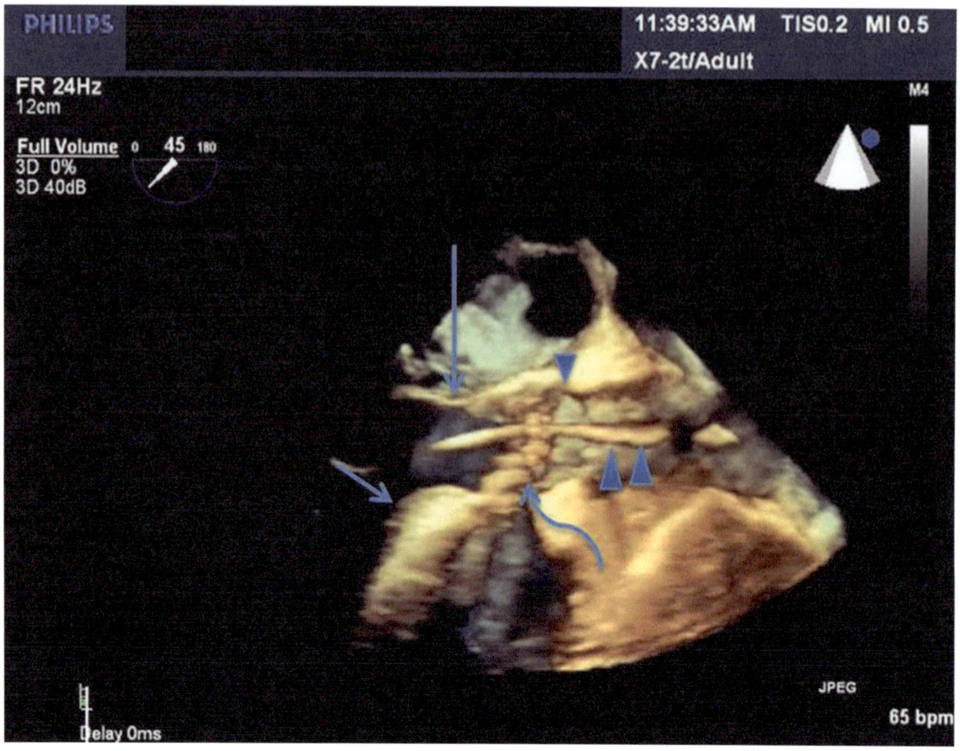

Fig. 33.5 Benefit of 3D TEE long-axis view showing the LVOT, anterior mitral leaflet (*long arrow*), interventricular septum (*short arrow*), aortic valve (*curved arrow*), the TAVR guide catheter (*double arrow-head*), sinotubular junction (*single arrowhead*)

the lack of a gold standard for measuring the aortic valve annulus makes it difficult to study in clinical trials.

The long-axis view is typically the preferred view for imaging during valve implantation. As can be appreciated in Fig. 33.5, a major advantage of 3D TEE is that it can be used to image the aortic valve from the aorta or left ventricular outflow tract, aiding in the assessment of septal hypertrophy as well as evaluating the spatial relationship of the aortic annulus to the anterior mitral leaflet and the interventricular septum.

Most patients with severe aortic stenosis have undergone cardiac remodeling, altering the anatomic relationship of normal cardiac structures. Annular remodeling in aortic stenosis can lead to a decrease in the expected distance from the aortic valve annulus to the coronary ostia. Furthermore, patients with AS often develop left ventricular hypertrophy as a result of chronically elevated left ventricular systolic pressures, resulting in symmetric and asymmetric septal hypertrophy. 3D TEE allows for precise assessment of the spatial relationship between the bioprosthetic valve, the interventricular septum, the coronary ostia, and the anterior mitral leaflet.

A bioprosthetic valve that is deployed too far into the left ventricular outflow tract (LVOT) can embolize into the left ventricle, often requiring open heart surgery to remove it. If the bioprosthetic valve is placed too far into the LVOT, but remains anchored in the annulus, there is the risk that its lateral struts can interfere with proper movement of the anterior mitral leaflet and result in mitral regurgitation. Patients with asymmetric septal hypertrophy may need to have the valve deployed higher in order to avoid the development of aortic subvalvular gradients and under-expansion of the bioprosthetic valve. But deploying a valve too high poses another problem since it can lead to obstruction of the coronary ostia. The distance from the ostium of the left coronary artery to the coronary cusp is of importance because calcium on the coronary cusp adjacent to the coronary ostium can be dislodged into the coronary artery during valve deployment.

TAVR Deployment

Unlike fluoroscopy or 2D TEE, 3D TEE allows for precise identification of several structures relevant to the deployment of the bioprosthetic valve: the aortic annulus, the LVOT, the sinotubular junction, the coronary ostia, intracardiac catheters, and the bioprosthetic valve (Figs. 33.6 and 33.7) [28]. A recent paper by Tamborini et al. suggests that 3D TEE is as precise as 3D CT in assessing the distance from the aortic annulus to the left main coronary ostium [25].

In order to deploy the prosthetic valve, a temporary pacing wire placed in the apex of the right ventricular paces the ventricles at 160–180 BPM, reducing cardiac motion and dramatically decreasing blood flow through the LVOT. At this point, if it is determined that the bioprosthetic aortic valve is still in the correct position, it is rapidly deployed and 2D and 3D TEE can be used to confirm the correct placement and assess for any complications, including pericardial

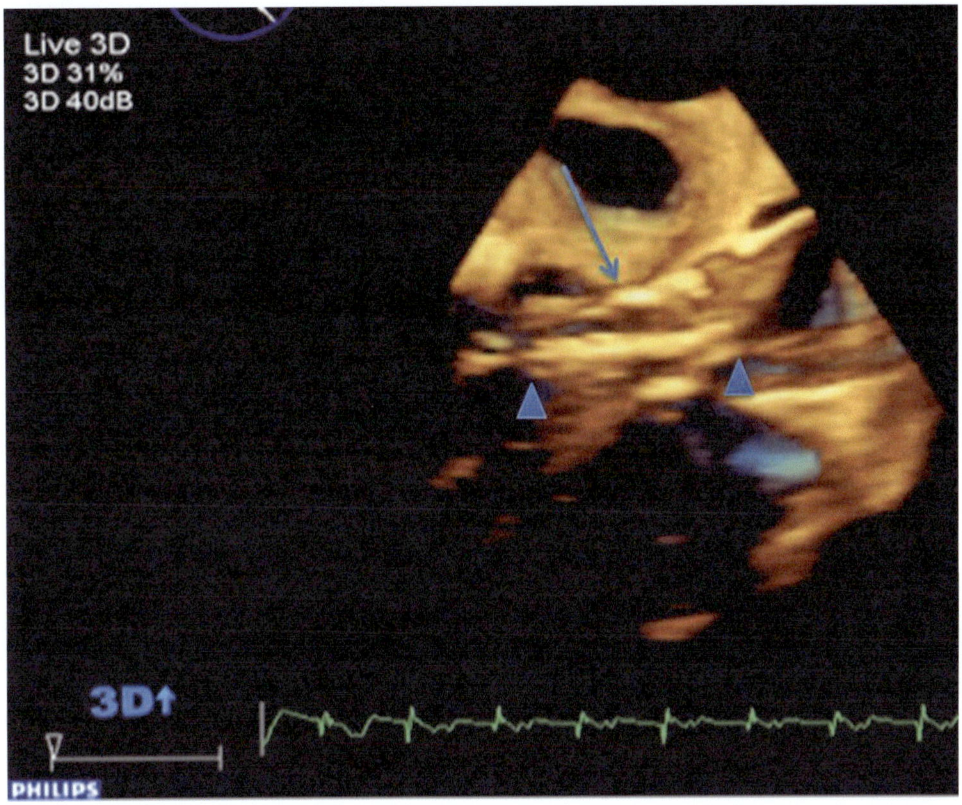

Fig. 33.6 Front and back edge of crimped Edwards Sapien Valve (*arrowheads*), aortic valve annulus (*long arrow*)

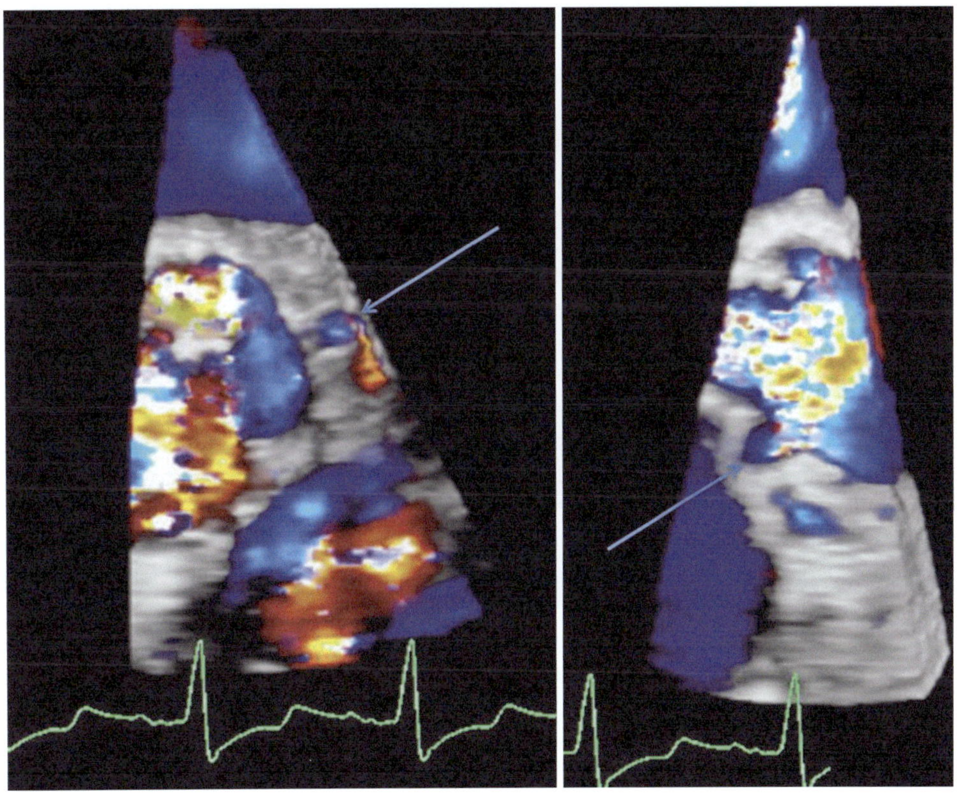

Fig. 33.7 Clear depiction of the left main (*left arrow*) and right coronary artery (*right arrow*) with 3D TEE with color Doppler

tamponade due to annular rupture, pacemaker perforation of the right ventricle, guide wire perforation of the LV, obstruction of coronary artery flow, myocardial stunning, or mitral regurgitation. Optimal deployment of the bioprosthesis is generally considered to be with 60 % of the prosthesis above the annulus and 40 % below the aortic annulus.

Three-dimensional TEE allows for assessing the coaxial relationship of the bioprosthetic valve and the aortic annulus. Deploying the valve misaligned to the center axis of the aortic annulus can lead to angulation of the bioprosthesis, which may contribute to significant paravalvular aortic regurgitation (PAR). Wire manipulation or delivery catheter adjustment can improve the coaxial alignment before deployment. There is usually a small amount of paravalvular aortic regurgitation to be expected because the aortic annulus is oval, calcified, and rigid in most patients, while the bioprosthetic valve is circular. In some cases where there is more than trace PAR, post-deployment balloon dilatation is used to improve apposition of the bioprosthetic valve to the aortic valve annulus and decrease PAR.

TAVR Post-deployment

Once the bioprosthetic valve has been deployed, 3D TEE is used to identify the extent of aortic regurgitation, LV function, malposition of the aortic valve, any evidence of aortic annulus rupture, or pericardial tamponade (Table 33.1). Aortic regurgitation is common post-TAVR. Up to 88 % of cases have PAR, transvalvular regurgitation, or a combination of both [26]. It is important to assess the degree of aortic regurgitation because recent data from the PARTNER trial has shown an association between PAR and mortality. Two-year PARTNER trial data from 699 patients with severe AS who were randomly assigned to surgical versus transcatheter valve replacement clearly indicates a significantly higher mortality rate among patients who underwent TAVR who exhibited mild to severe aortic regurgitation versus none or trace aortic regurgitation. Mild PAR was present in approximately 40 % of TAVR patients at 2-year follow-up, while moderate or severe PAR was present in approximately 7 % of TAVR patients. There was a twofold increase of mortality among patients with mild to severe PAR relative to patients with non- or trace PAR, underscoring the importance of limiting paravalvular leaks by correctly sizing the aortic valve annulus and considering post-deployment dilatation of the bioprosthetic [16].

Although uncommon, transvalvular aortic regurgitation is also a potential complication, but it usually arises from undersizing the aortic valve annulus, which at the time of deployment leads to poor leaflet coaptation. Similarly to PAR, mild to severe transvalvular aortic regurgitation is associated with an increased risk of mortality, but compared to the prevalence of PAR, it is much less common, occurring in approximately 1 % of cases [20].

Table 33.2 TEE for guiding transcatheter aortic valve replacement (AVR)

1. Assessment of aortic annular diameter with 2D and 3D
2. Determine LV and RV systolic function; identifying other associated valve disease or cardiac abnormalities such as severe mitral regurgitation or pericardial effusion
3. Guide and confirm coaxial alignment of the delivery catheter within LVOT and aortic root
4. Identify the ventricular and aortic ends of the prosthesis prior to deployment of valve to align with the aortic valve cusps
5. Optimize bioprosthetic valve position before deployment
6. Assess severity of aortic regurgitation post-valve deployment
7. Assess the complications including LV dysfunction, coronary obstruction, valve embolization, pericardial tamponade, mitral regurgitation, or aortic annular rupture

A poorly seated bioprosthetic aortic valve is a serious complication as it can result in distal embolization into the aorta or if it was placed too proximal into the LVOT, dislodgement into the left ventricular cavity. 3D TEE can quickly assess a malposed bioprosthetic aortic valve by noting the extent and shape of PAR and under-expansion of the stent frame. In these situations, post-deployment balloon inflation with a larger diameter balloon can often improve stent frame expansion and apposition of the aortic valve to the aortic annulus. 3D TEE can also be used to assess any changes in mitral regurgitation, whether as a result of tethering of the anterior mitral leaflet due to a strut of the bioprosthetic valve that is too low into the LVOT or systolic anterior motion of the mitral valve when the left ventricle becomes hyperdynamic as a result of the sudden drop in the transaortic valvular gradient. The latter of these is particularly germane in the presence of severe left ventricular hypertrophy, the so-called suicide ventricle. Table 33.2 summarizes the role that TEE plays in TAVR.

Conclusion

Although 2D echocardiography has greater temporal and spatial resolution than 3D echocardiography, it lacks the imaging characteristics to provide the anatomic relationships that are often helpful during TAVR. Current studies suggest that relative to 2D echocardiography, 3D TEE may more accurately measure and assess the aortic valvar apparatus. Although acoustic artifacts that are commonly present due to calcium deposition in stenotic native aortic valves limit 3D TEE, it has the capacity to view the same object from different angles, helping to decrease the effects calcium may have on viewing key structures. Echocardiography also has the advantage over other imaging methods because it can obtain continuous, real-time imaging of the aortic valve and neighboring structures without any radiation exposure or administration of contrast. Given the increased mortality rate among patients with PAR, 3D TEE can be used to quickly, accurately, and precisely localize a paravalvular leak and take steps to reduce it.

References

1. Jilaihawi H, Chakravarty T, Weiss RE, Fontana GP, Forrester J, Makkar RR. Meta-analysis of complications in aortic valve replacement: comparison of Medtronic-Corevalve, Edwards-Sapien and surgical aortic valve replacement in 8,536 patients. Catheter Cardiovasc Interv. 2012;80(1):128–38. PubMed PMID: 22415849. Epub 2012/03/15. eng.
2. Lindroos M, Kupari M, Heikkila J, Tilvis R. Prevalence of aortic valve abnormalities in the elderly: an echocardiographic study of a random population sample. J Am Coll Cardiol. 1993;21(5):1220–5. PubMed PMID: 8459080. Epub 1993/04/01. eng.
3. Leon MB, Smith CR, Mack M, Miller DC, Moses JW, Svensson LG, et al. Transcatheter aortic-valve implantation for aortic stenosis in patients who cannot undergo surgery. N Engl J Med. 2010;363(17):1597–607. PubMed PMID: 20961243. Epub 2010/10/22. eng.
4. Ross Jr J, Braunwald E. Aortic stenosis. Circulation. 1968;38 (1 Suppl):61–7. PubMed PMID: 4894151. Epub 1968/07/01. eng.
5. Turina J, Hess O, Sepulcri F, Krayenbuehl HP. Spontaneous course of aortic valve disease. Eur Heart J. 1987;8(5):471–83. PubMed PMID: 3609042. Epub 1987/05/01. eng.
6. Kelly TA, Rothbart RM, Cooper CM, Kaiser DL, Smucker ML, Gibson RS. Comparison of outcome of asymptomatic to symptomatic patients older than 20 years of age with valvular aortic stenosis. Am J Cardiol. 1988;61(1):123–30. PubMed PMID: 3337000. Epub 1988/01/01. eng.
7. Biner S, Rafique AM, Goykhman P, Morrissey RP, Naghi J, Siegel RJ. Prognostic value of E/E′ ratio in patients with unoperated severe aortic stenosis. JACC Cardiovasc Imaging. 2010;3(9):899–907. PubMed PMID: 20846623. Epub 2010/09/18. eng.
8. Schwarz F, Baumann P, Manthey J, Hoffmann M, Schuler G, Mehmel HC, et al. The effect of aortic valve replacement on survival. Circulation. 1982;66(5):1105–10. PubMed PMID: 7127696. Epub 1982/11/01. eng.
9. Murphy ES, Lawson RM, Starr A, Rahimtoola SH. Severe aortic stenosis in patients 60 years of age or older: left ventricular function and 10-year survival after valve replacement. Circulation. 1981;64(2 Pt 2):II184–8. PubMed PMID: 7249320. Epub 1981/08/01. eng.
10. Lund O. Preoperative risk evaluation and stratification of long-term survival after valve replacement for aortic stenosis. Reasons for earlier operative intervention. Circulation. 1990;82(1):124–39. PubMed PMID: 2364510. Epub 1990/07/01. eng.
11. Bouma BJ, van Den Brink RB, van Der Meulen JH, Verheul HA, Cheriex EC, Hamer HP, et al. To operate or not on elderly patients with aortic stenosis: the decision and its consequences. Heart. 1999;82(2):143–8. PubMed PMID: 10409526. Pubmed Central PMCID: 1729124. Epub 1999/07/20. eng.
12. Iung B, Cachier A, Baron G, Messika-Zeitoun D, Delahaye F, Tornos P, et al. Decision-making in elderly patients with severe aortic stenosis: why are so many denied surgery? Eur Heart J. 2005;26(24):2714–20. PubMed PMID: 16141261. Epub 2005/09/06. eng.
13. Varadarajan P, Kapoor N, Bansal RC, Pai RG. Clinical profile and natural history of 453 nonsurgically managed patients with severe aortic stenosis. Ann Thorac Surg. 2006;82(6):2111–5. PubMed PMID: 17126120. Epub 2006/11/28. eng.
14. Bach DS, Siao D, Girard SE, Duvernoy C, McCallister Jr BD, Gualano SK. Evaluation of patients with severe symptomatic aortic stenosis who do not undergo aortic valve replacement: the potential role of subjectively overestimated operative risk. Circ Cardiovasc Qual Outcomes. 2009;2(6):533–9. PubMed PMID: 20031890. Epub 2009/12/25. eng.
15. Bonow RO, Carabello BA, Chatterjee K, de Leon Jr AC, Faxon DP, Freed MD, et al. 2008 focused update incorporated into the ACC/AHA 2006 guidelines for the management of patients with valvular heart disease: a report of the American College of Cardiology/American Heart Association Task Force on Practice Guidelines (Writing Committee to revise the 1998 guidelines for the management of patients with valvular heart disease). Endorsed by the Society of Cardiovascular Anesthesiologists, Society for Cardiovascular Angiography and Interventions, and Society of Thoracic Surgeons. J Am Coll Cardiol. 2008;52(13):e1–142. PubMed PMID: 18848134. Epub 2008/10/14. eng.
16. Kodali SK, Williams MR, Smith CR, Svensson LG, Webb JG, Makkar RR, et al. Two-year outcomes after transcatheter or surgical aortic-valve replacement. N Engl J Med. 2012;366(18):1686–95. PubMed PMID: 22443479. Epub 2012/03/27. eng.
17. Iung B, Baron G, Butchart EG, Delahaye F, Gohlke-Barwolf C, Levang OW, et al. A prospective survey of patients with valvular heart disease in Europe: The Euro Heart Survey on Valvular Heart Disease. Eur Heart J. 2003;24(13):1231–43. PubMed PMID: 12831818. Epub 2003/07/02. eng.
18. Pellikka PA, Sarano ME, Nishimura RA, Malouf JF, Bailey KR, Scott CG, et al. Outcome of 622 adults with asymptomatic, hemodynamically significant aortic stenosis during prolonged follow-up. Circulation. 2005;111(24):3290–5. PubMed PMID: 15956131. Epub 2005/06/16. eng.
19. Willson AB, Webb JG, Labounty TM, Achenbach S, Moss R, Wheeler M, et al. 3-dimensional aortic annular assessment by multidetector computed tomography predicts moderate or severe paravalvular regurgitation after transcatheter aortic valve replacement: a multicenter retrospective analysis. J Am Coll Cardiol. 2012;59(14):1287–94. PubMed PMID: 22365423. Epub 2012/03/01. eng.
20. Ng AC, Delgado V, van der Kley F, Shanks M, van de Veire NR, Bertini M, et al. Comparison of aortic root dimensions and geometries before and after transcatheter aortic valve implantation by 2- and 3-dimensional transesophageal echocardiography and multislice computed tomography. Circ Cardiovasc Imaging. 2010;3(1):94–102. PubMed PMID: 19920027. Epub 2009/11/19. eng.
21. Jilaihawi H, Kashif M, Fontana G, Furugen A, Shiota T, Friede G, et al. Cross-sectional computed tomographic assessment improves accuracy of aortic annular sizing for transcatheter aortic valve replacement and reduces the incidence of paravalvular aortic regurgitation. J Am Coll Cardiol. 2012;59(14):1275–86. PubMed PMID: 22365424. Epub 2012/03/01. eng.
22. Makkar RR, Fontana GP, Jilaihawi H, Kapadia S, Pichard AD, Douglas PS, et al. Transcatheter aortic-valve replacement for inoperable severe aortic stenosis. N Engl J Med. 2012;366(18):1696–704. PubMed PMID: 22443478. Epub 2012/03/27. eng.
23. Schoenhagen P, Numburi U, Halliburton SS, Aulbach P, von Roden M, Desai MY, et al. Three-dimensional imaging in the context of minimally invasive and transcatheter cardiovascular interventions using multi-detector computed tomography: from pre-operative planning to intra-operative guidance. Eur Heart J. 2010;31(22):2727–40. PubMed PMID: 20797981. Epub 2010/08/28. eng.
24. Tamburino C, Capodanno D, Ramondo A, Petronio AS, Ettori F, Santoro G, et al. Incidence and predictors of early and late mortality after transcatheter aortic valve implantation in 663 patients with severe aortic stenosis. Circulation. 2011;123(3):299–308. PubMed PMID: 21220731. Epub 2011/01/12. eng.

25. Tamborini G, Fusini L, Gripari P, Muratori M, Cefalu C, Maffessanti F, et al. Feasibility and accuracy of 3DTEE versus CT for the evaluation of aortic valve annulus to left main ostium distance before transcatheter aortic valve implantation. JACC Cardiovasc Imaging. 2012;5(6):579–88. PubMed PMID: 22698526. Epub 2012/06/16. eng.
26. Moss RR, Ivens E, Pasupati S, Humphries K, Thompson CR, Munt B, et al. Role of echocardiography in percutaneous aortic valve implantation. JACC Cardiovasc Imaging. 2008;1(1):15–24. PubMed PMID: 19356400. Epub 2008/01/01. eng.
27. Jayasuriya C, Moss RR, Munt B. Transcatheter aortic valve implantation in aortic stenosis: the role of echocardiography. J Am Soc Echocardiogr. 2011;24:15–27.
28. Lerakis S, Babaliaros VC, Block PC, Junagadhwalla Z, Thourani VH, Howell S, et al. Transesophageal echocardiography to help position and deploy a transcatheter heart valve. JACC Cardiovasc Imaging. 2010;3:219–21.
29. Bloomfield GS, Gillam LD, Hahn RT, Kapadia S, Leipsic J, Lerakis S, et al. A practical guide to multimodality imaging of transcatheter aortic valve replacement. JACC Cardiovasc Imaging. 2012;5(4):441–55. PubMed PMID: 22498335. Epub 2012/04/14. eng.

Complications of TAVR

34

Miriam L. Wheeler and Christopher R. Thompson

Abstract

Echocardiography has continued to play a key role in selection of patients and prosthesis size for transcatheter aortic valve replacement (TAVR), guiding the procedure and assessing its results in intra-procedural and post-procedural imaging. Intra-procedural transesophageal echo allows an opportunity to recognize risk factors for, and minimize, complications related to TAVR. This chapter discusses and describes the echocardiographer's echocardiographic features suggesting high risk for complications and imaging of those complications' role from assisting in prosthesis selection to positioning for deployment and to troubleshooting the hemodynamically unstable patient. Complications include valve embolization, cardiac tamponade, paravalvular aortic regurgitation, aortic root or ventricular septal rupture, coronary obstruction and acute ventricular systolic dysfunction, acute severe mitral regurgitation, and aortic dissection. Late complications such as endocarditis and apical pseudoaneurysm are also discussed.

Keywords

Transcatheter aortic valve replacement (TAVR, TAVI) • Complications • Echocardiography • Paravalvular aortic regurgitation • Aortic root rupture • Aortic annulus • Procedural imaging • Transapical • Valve prosthesis malposition • Embolization

The initial attempts at TAVR were associated with a very high complication rate, many of them vascular and related to the large sheath sizes required to deliver the prosthesis [1, 2]. These complications were carefully documented and analyzed, leading to significant improvements in the delivery apparatus, the prostheses, and the procedure. Furthermore, the complications were published and discussed extensively as part of the training program for new operators [3–5]. These efforts have allowed new programs to commence with excellent results and low complication rates. Despite the best efforts of the entire TAVR team, however, complications of the procedure continue to occur. Prompt recognition of these complications can, in many cases, facilitate rapid intervention to mitigate the progressive consequences of the initial complication. This chapter will focus on echocardiographic recognition of factors likely to result in complications and on the manifestations of the complications of TAVR.

The goal of TAVR is to successfully position and deploy an appropriately sized prosthesis within the left ventricular outflow tract and aortic root thereby increasing the aortic valve orifice. Thus complications of the procedure include damaging vessels, valves, and the heart (including the iliac artery, the aorta, the aortic annulus or root, the anterior mitral valve leaflet, the ventricular septum, and the apex); selecting an inappropriate size of prosthesis resulting in embolization,

M.L. Wheeler, MB, ChB, FRACP (✉)
Division of Cardiology, St. Paul's Hospital Cardiac Echo Lab and the University of British Columbia, 1081 Burrard St, Vancouver V6Z 1Y6, Canada
e-mail: miriamwheeler@hotmail.com

C.R. Thompson, MD, CM, FRCPC (Cardiology)
Division of Cardiology, Department of Medicine, St. Paul's Hospital Cardiac Echo Lab and the University of British Columbia, 1081 Burrard St, Vancouver V6Z 1Y6, Canada

J.K. Min et al. (eds.), *Multimodality Imaging for Transcatheter Aortic Valve Replacement*, DOI 10.1007/978-1-4471-2798-7_34, © Springer-Verlag London 2014

aortic rupture, high implant gradients, or important paravalvular regurgitation; and placing the prosthesis too ventricular resulting in embolization, interference with the anterior mitral leaflet, persistent aortic stenosis, or paravalvular regurgitation or too aortic resulting in embolization, coronary obstruction, or paravalvular regurgitation [3, 4, 6].

Baseline Imaging

Baseline transesophageal imaging should be performed pre-procedure to allow comparison with subsequent images when complications occur. In particular, attention should be paid to left and right ventricular systolic function, regional wall motion abnormalities, aortic regurgitation, mitral regurgitation, and the presence and amount of pericardial fluid. Knowledge of the baseline state is invaluable when the echocardiographer is subsequently asked to troubleshoot unexplained hemodynamic instability.

Prosthesis Sizing

Following assessment of baseline imaging, the focus then turns to the aortic annulus. It is our practice to preselect a device size based on transthoracic echo and CT images and then modify the size if necessary based on the transesophageal measurements of the annulus, sinus shape, sinotubular junction measurement, and aortic leaflet calcium appearance [7, 8].

The aortic annulus is measured in the long-axis view (approximately 120–140°) from the base of the leaflet insertion of the right coronary cusp to the base of the noncoronary cusp insertion at the mitral-aortic intervalvular fibrosa [9, 10]. Accurate identification of these landmarks is crucial both to perform annular measurements for valve sizing and subsequently to accurately recognize the appropriate valve position in relation to the landmarks.

In borderline cases where the annular dimension would support use of either a smaller or larger prosthesis, attention should be made to the degree of calcium present and location of focal calcification, the dimension of the sinus of Valsalva and sinotubular junction, and whether the ratio of the sinus of Valsalva to sinotubular junction suggests "flat sinuses." A larger aortic root may accept the larger prosthesis in borderline cases, whereas marked calcium with flat sinuses of Valsalva is a red flag for subsequent displacement of calcium into the aortic root with increased risk of aortic rupture.

Once the annulus is determined and appropriate prosthesis selected, we have found careful observation of the movement of native valve leaflets and calcium and their relationship to the aorta during balloon valvuloplasty to be very helpful in confirming the appropriate prosthesis size and balloon volume. If there is little margin during inflation of a balloon smaller than that which we intend to use during prosthesis deployment, we choose to use less than nominal balloon volume for the prosthesis selected or to decrease the prosthesis size. Figure 34.1a shows aortic sinus tenting with balloon valvuloplasty, while Fig. 34.1b shows a similar appearance following prosthesis deployment by a balloon with less than nominal volume.

Prosthesis Positioning

Prosthesis positioning and deployment can be straightforward when there are clear angiographic and echocardiographic landmarks, the device is coaxial with the long axis of the left ventricular outflow tract and aortic root, and the echocardiographer and interventional cardiologist agree on the position. It can also be extremely difficult when some of these factors are not present and particularly when either the angiographic or echocardiographic images suggest the position is appropriate and the other modality suggests the position is not correct. A superior TAVR team understands that discrepancies will occur, that when discrepancies occur the "right" answer is the one that results in the best outcome for the patient , and that being "wrong" is an opportunity to discover pitfalls in the current state of knowledge and an opportunity to advance the field and the imaging discipline.

Following balloon valvuloplasty, the prosthesis is then positioned in the ascending aorta prior to crossing the aortic valve. A combined echocardiographic and fluoroscopic approach to prosthesis positioning minimizes risk of a valve being deployed either too aortic or too ventricular. Poor position at deployment results in risk of the prosthesis embolizing, significant paravalvular aortic regurgitation, or malfunction due to suboptimal leaflet capture and interference with the prosthesis [10]. Positioning the prosthesis optimally for deployment requires relatively rapid decision making, as the prosthesis obstructs the critically stenosed aortic valve frequently compromising cardiac output with resultant hypotension.

Fluoroscopic guidance of TAVR aims to place the prosthesis with approximately one-third of the prosthesis ventricular to the base of the aortic cusps [11]. With echocardiographic guidance we aim to have the ventricular end of the prosthesis contact the intervalvular fibrosa just aortic to the hinge point of the anterior mitral leaflet, that is, the junction of the intervalvular fibrosa with the moving portion of the anterior mitral leaflet [9, 10]. Since the intervalvular fibrosa can range from quite lengthy to almost nonexistent, this can result in a long or very short landing zone. Appropriate placement in a short landing zone is demanding, and malplacement is more common with short as compared with normal or lengthy landing zones. If the prosthesis is placed too ventricular ("low"), the valve may embolize,

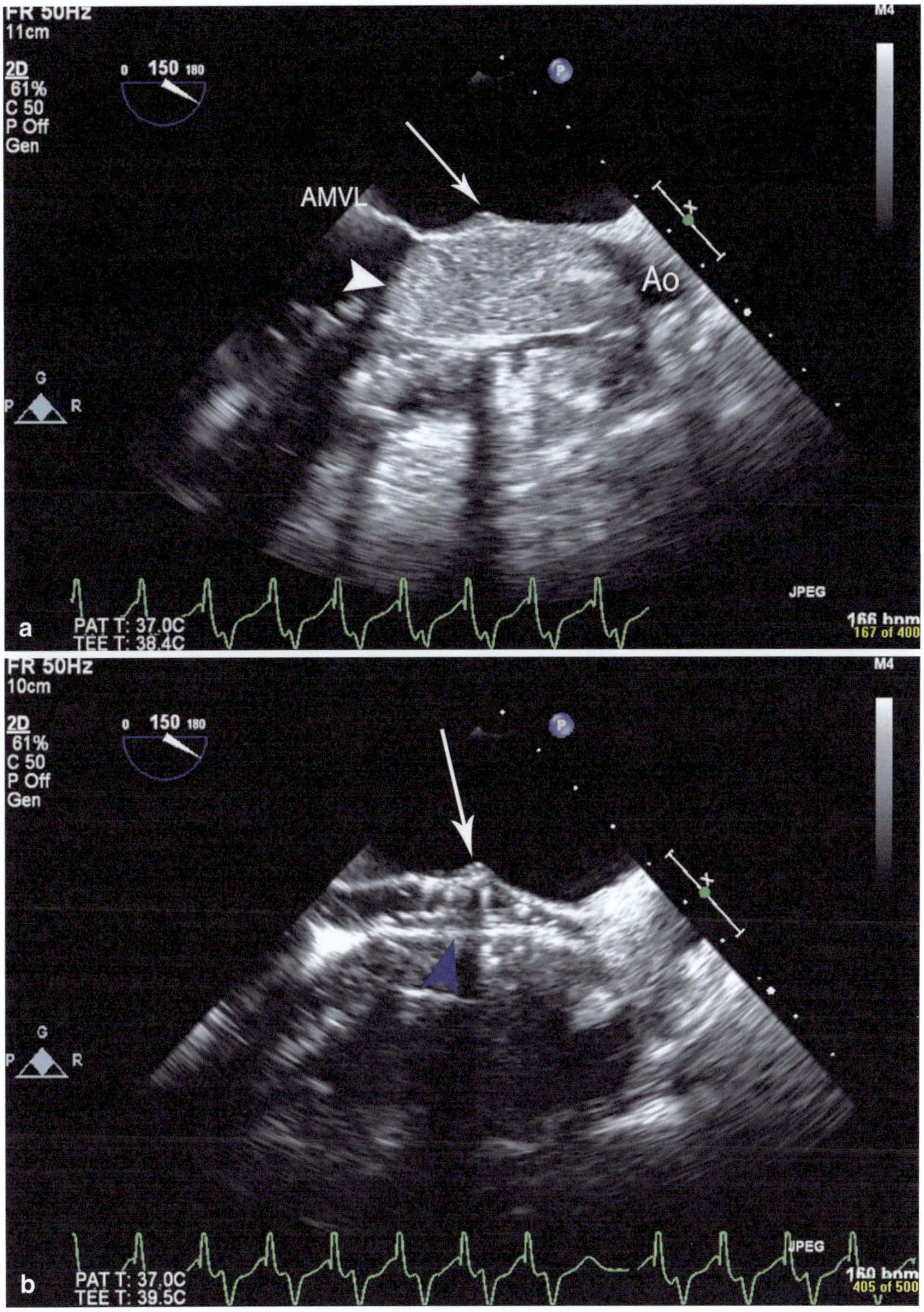

Fig. 34.1 (**a**) Balloon valvuloplasty of the native aortic valve. The balloon filled with diluted radiocontrast is seen extending from the left ventricular outflow tract to the aortic root. The posterior wall of the flat aortic sinus tents to a point (*arrow*) as calcium is displaced by balloon inflation. *AMVL* anterior mitral valve leaflet, *Ao* aorta. (**b**) Following deployment of the aortic prosthesis, the displaced calcium (*arrow*) is seen tenting the posterior aortic sinus. The shaft of the partially collapsed balloon (*blue arrowhead*) and guidewire are seen

interfere with the mitral valve, allow marked regurgitation, or be associated with persistent aortic stenosis if the aortic end of the prosthesis fails to capture the native aortic leaflets and keeps them out of the transvalvular flow path. Figure 34.2 demonstrates both the prosthesis contacting the moving portion of the anterior mitral leaflet and the native aortic leaflets overhanging the prosthesis with resultant residual aortic stenosis. A second prosthesis deployed more aortic ("higher") will correct the residual aortic stenosis but cannot correct the interference with the mitral valve.

Despite the complications of placing the prosthesis too ventricular ("low"), many operators prefer to err in that direction to avoid placing the prosthesis too aortic ("high") since the consequences of an excessively aortic placement include severe aortic regurgitation, a high likelihood of embolization, left coronary obstruction, and damage to the sinotubular ridge if the sinuses of Valsalva are short. Left coronary obstruction can be identified by direct anatomic visualization, high velocity Doppler flow in the left coronary or by ventricular dysfunction commencing shortly after deployment. Figure 34.3 demonstrates deployment of a prosthesis that is too aortic. As is commonly the case, the prosthesis embolized shortly after deployment.

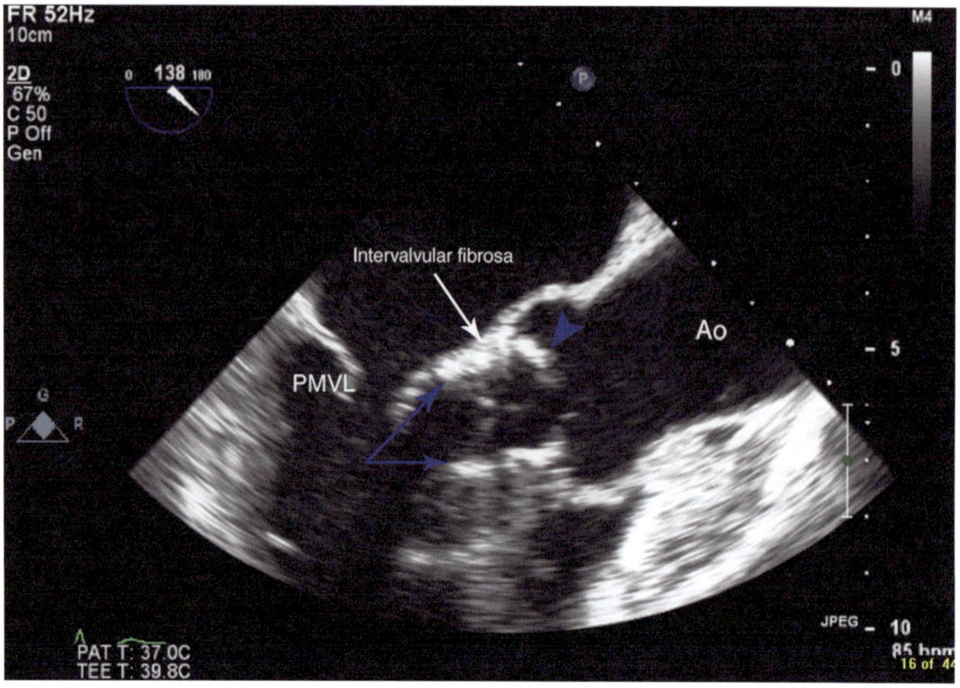

Fig. 34.2 The transcatheter aortic valve is deployed too low. The ventricular ends of the valve stent posts are seen within the left ventricular outflow tract (*blue arrows*) contacting the mobile portion of the anterior mitral leaflet. The aortic end of the valve is seen just aortic to the level of the intervalvular fibrosa (*white arrow*). Native aortic leaflet is seen overhanging the aortic end of the transcatheter aortic valve (*blue arrowhead*). *PMVL* posterior mitral valve leaflet, *Ao* aorta

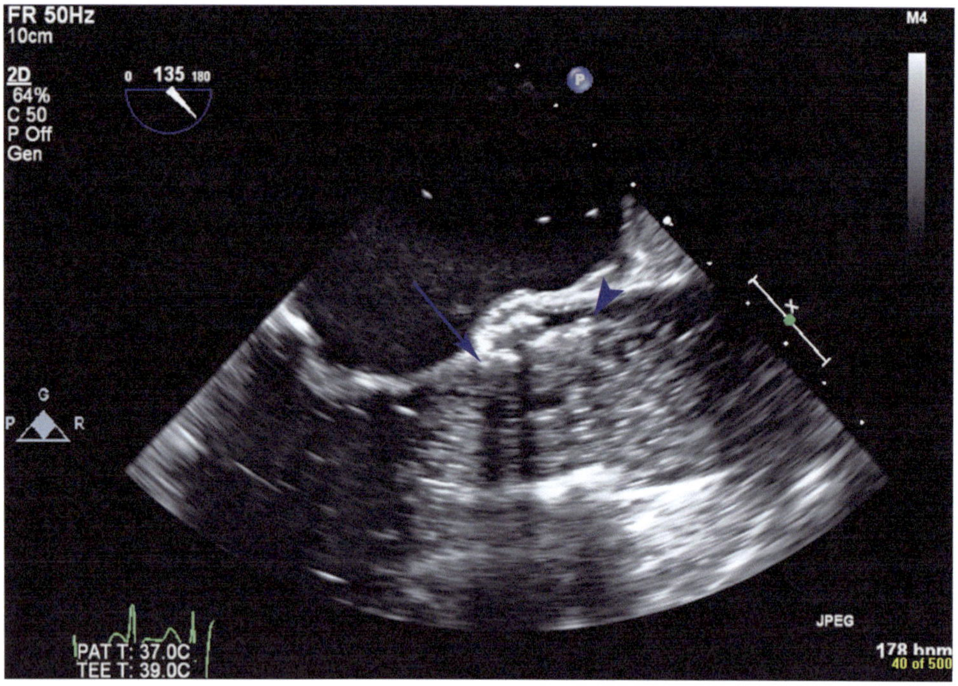

Fig. 34.3 Still frame of aortic valve deployment. A balloon filled with dilute radiopaque contrast is seen within the aortic root and left ventricular outflow tract. The ventricular end of the valve stent is too high, at the level of the native aortic valve annulus (*blue arrow*). The aortic end of the valve stent (*blue arrowhead*) is seen above the sinotubular junction. The valve subsequently embolized

Paravalvular Aortic Regurgitation

Immediately following deployment once the valve is seen to be stable, color Doppler is used to assess for paravalvular regurgitation (Fig. 34.4). At this stage, the guidewire is usually still across the aortic prosthesis, and differentiation between transvalvular and paravalvular aortic regurgitation may be difficult. Assessment of regurgitation is performed in both the short- and long-axis views. Some degree of paravalvular aortic regurgitation is reported in 80–96 % of cases [1]. In most cases, the degree of regurgitation is trivial or mild. Moderate and severe paravalvular regurgitation have been shown to be an independent predictor of short- and long-term mortality [1, 7, 12]. In the case of greater than mild paravalvular regurgitation, the prosthesis may require further balloon dilatation, or implantation of a second, overlapping

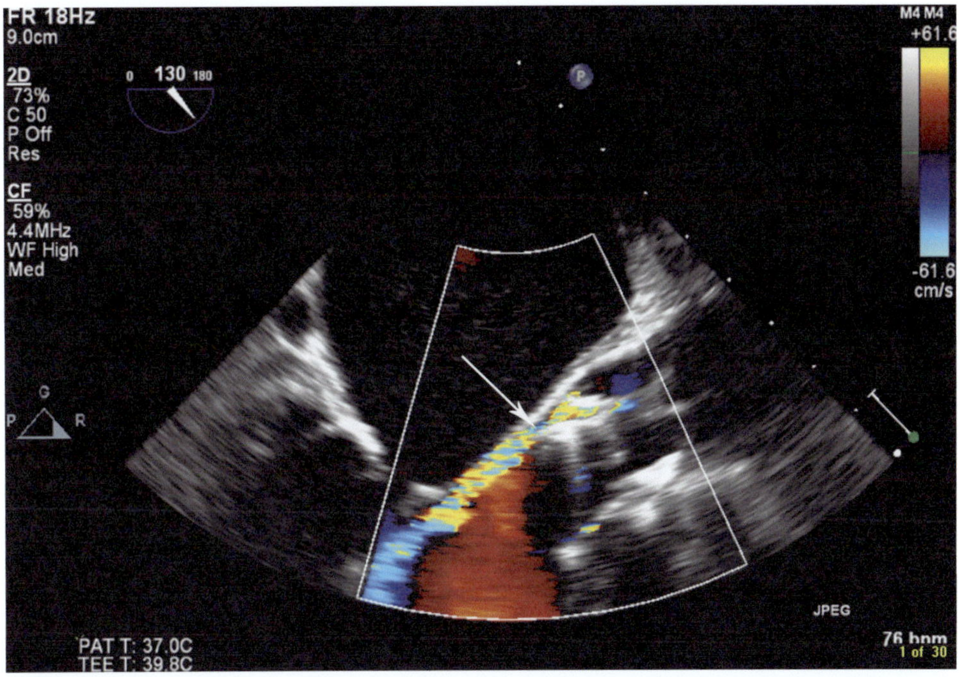

Fig. 34.4 Post-deployment of transcatheter aortic valve, paravalvular aortic regurgitation is seen posteriorly in the area of the noncoronary cusp (*arrow*)

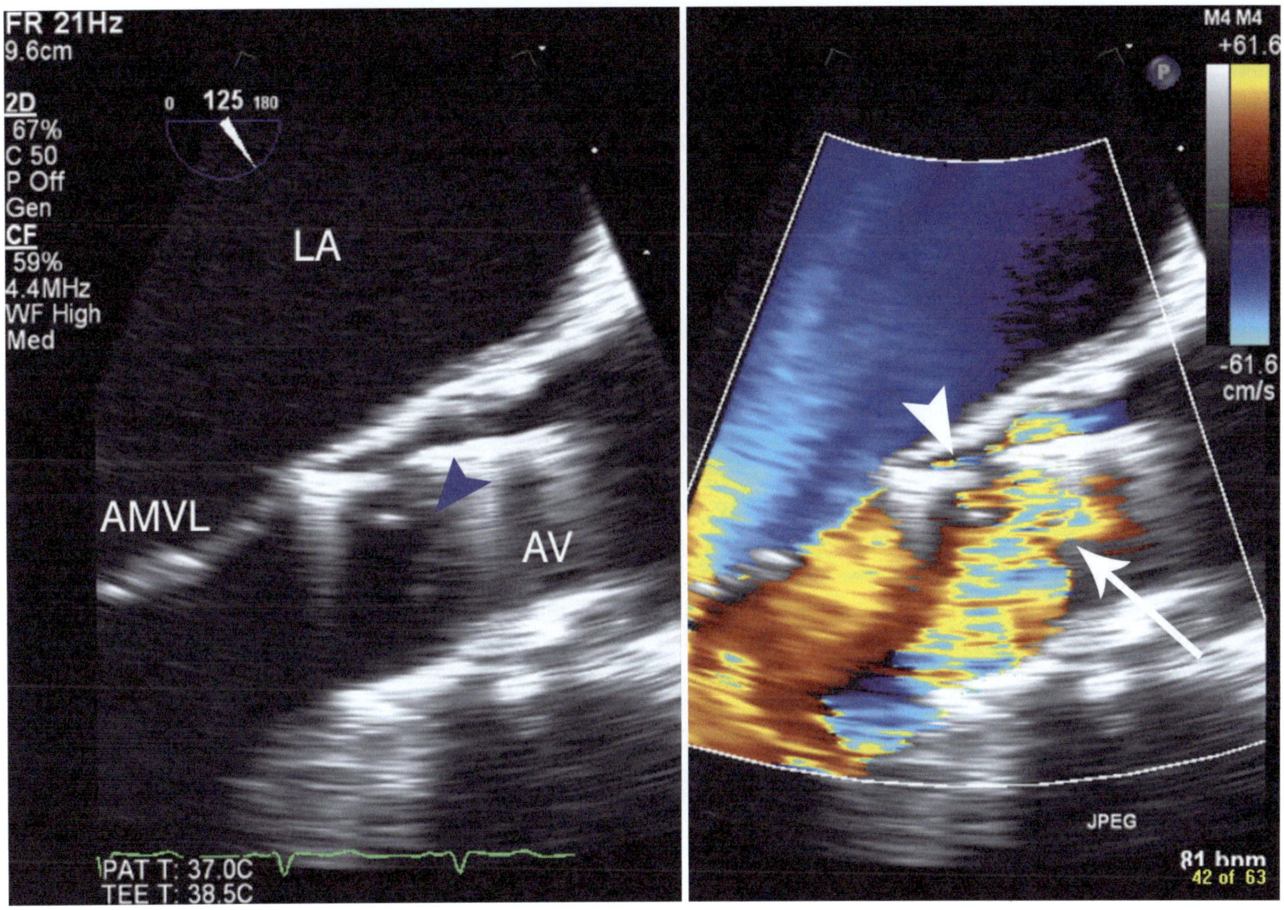

Fig. 34.5 Following deployment of the prosthesis, there are both paravalvular regurgitation (*arrowhead*) and leaflet dysfunction causing transvalvular regurgitation. The two-dimensional image (*left panel*) shows malcoaptation of the prosthesis leaflets (*blue arrowhead*), *LA* left atrium, *AMVL* anterior mitral valve leaflet, *AV* transcatheter aortic valve prosthesis

transcatheter valve [1]. In the case of self-expanding valves, repositioning may improve the regurgitation. Once the guidewire has been withdrawn, a further assessment for any transvalvular regurgitation should be made (Fig. 34.5). Although rare, leaflet dysfunction can occur and requires further intervention [1, 13, 14].

Table 34.1 Prosthetic aortic valve regurgitation criteria (central and paravalvular)

Parameter	Mild	Moderate	Severe
Valve structure and motion			
Mechanical or bioprosthetic	Usually normal	Usually abnormal	Usually abnormal
Structural parameters			
Left ventricular size	Normal	Normal/mildly dilated	Dilated
Doppler parameters (qualitative or semiquantitative)			
Jet width in central jets (% LVO diameter): color[a]	Narrow (≤25 %)	Intermediate (26–64 %)	Large (≥65 %)
Jet density: CW Doppler	Incomplete or faint	Dense	Dense
Jet deceleration rate (PHT, ms): CW Doppler[b]	Slow (>500)	Variable (200–500)	Steep (<200)
LV outflow vs. pulmonary flow: PW Doppler	Slightly increased	Intermediate	Greatly increased
Diastolic flow reversal in the descending aorta			
PW Doppler	Absent or brief early diastolic	Intermediate	Prominent, holodiastolic
Cicumferential extent of paraprosthetic AR (%)[c]	<10	10–20	>20
Doppler parameters (quantitative)			
Regurgitant volume (ml/beat)	<30	30–59	>60
Regurgitant fraction (%)	<30	30–50	>50

Reprinted with permission from Leon et al. [6]
AR aortic regurgitation, *CW* continuous wave, *LVO* left ventricular outflow, *PW* pulsed wave
[a]Parameter applicable to central jets and is less accurate in eccentric jets
[b]Influenced by left ventricular compliance
[c]For paravalvular aortic regurgitation

Assessment of paravalvular regurgitation can prove difficult as there is commonly more than one site of regurgitation and the regurgitant jets are frequently eccentric. Furthermore, the grading system for aortic regurgitation was developed for valvular, not paravalvular jets. In the PARTNER trial echo sub-study, paravalvular aortic regurgitation was graded according to the Valve Academic Research Consortium Criteria (Table 34.1) [6], which adds the circumferential extent of the regurgitation in the short-axis view to traditional assessment criteria. Paravalvular aortic regurgitation that extends less than 10 % of the perimeter is graded mild, 10–20 % is graded moderate, and greater than 20 % is graded severe. Care must be taken to assess the circumferential extent of the regurgitation at the level of the vena contracta, as assessment made toward the left ventricular outflow tract will image the jet of the regurgitation and will overestimate the degree of regurgitation. As in valvular aortic regurgitation, the proportion of the jet width occupying the left ventricular outflow tract (LVOT) suggests mild regurgitation where less than 25 % of the LVOT is occupied and severe regurgitation where greater than 65 % of the LVOT is filled with regurgitant jet. A dense jet on continuous wave Doppler supports moderate or severe regurgitation, and a pressure half time of less than 200 ms is consistent with severe regurgitation. A greatly increased left ventricular outflow tract flow on pulse wave Doppler relative to the pulmonary outflow tract may also support more severe regurgitation. Similarly, holodiastolic flow reversal seen in the descending aorta strongly suggests that the aortic regurgitation is severe. At our institution, we classify trivial jets as those that are extremely narrow, limited to the distal left ventricular outflow tract and judged to be hemodynamically insignificant. Classification into mild, moderate, or severe is then based on the above criteria. The difficulties in accurately determining aortic regurgitation severity have led many investigators to pursue novel techniques of assessment. Some, such as use of three-dimensional color imaging, are promising but not yet commonly used routinely [15]. Sinning has proposed a simple hemodynamic assessment of aortic regurgitation severity called the aortic regurgitation index which can be very useful to resolve ambiguous cases [16].

Paravalvular regurgitation can be multifactorial with selection of an undersized valve, and deployment either too aortic or too ventricular being the most common [17]. Calculation of a cover index, defined as 100×(prosthesis diameter – transesophageal echocardiography annulus diameter)/prosthesis diameter, has also been found to be a predictor of paravalvular aortic regurgitation with a suggestion in the original publication that paravalvular AR did not occur when the cover index was greater than 8 % [18]. However, paravalvular AR has been reported with a cover index greater than 8 % [16] and a greater reliance on three-dimensional imaging to provide an annular area is being used [7]. The use of aortic annular area as measured on multidetector computed tomography has been shown to be predictive of moderate or severe aortic regurgitation. Recent research has shown that by slight oversizing of the prosthesis size using the mean annular area by 5 to 10 %, this may reduce the incidence of significant regurgitation due to an undersized valve [7, 19]. Marked asymmetric calcium distribution has also been associated with regurgitation [17]. Transvalvular regurgitation can result from post-deployment balloon dilatation with increased balloon volume, and there was a suggestion of increased strokes with post-dilatation in one series [12, 20, 21].

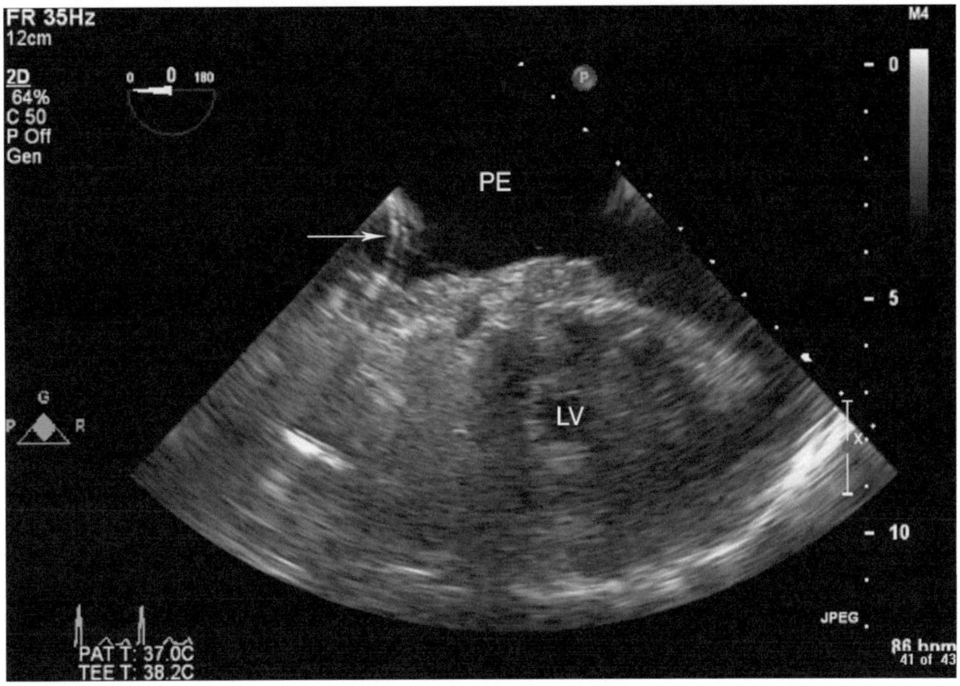

Fig. 34.6 A large pericardial effusion (*PE*) is seen from the transgastric view on transesophageal echo. A catheter (*arrow*) is seen in the pericardial space. *PE* pericardial effusion, *LV* left ventricle

Troubleshooting Hemodynamic Instability

It is not surprising that hypotension occurs fairly frequently during transcatheter aortic valve replacement. The echocardiographer is commonly asked to help determine the cause of the hypotension. A rapid assessment for pericardial fluid, left and right ventricular function, acute valvular complications, and aortic dissection is required. The stage of the procedure during which hypotension occurs frequently points to the likely cause. For example, hypotension which occurs in close proximity to the insertion of the super stiff or extra stiff guidewire into the left ventricular apex is usually caused either by guidewire interference with the mitral leaflets or chordae tendineae or by guidewire perforation of the left ventricle.

Left and Right Ventricular Systolic Dysfunction

Although uncommon, compromise of the coronary arteries can occur with TAVR with emboli or coronary occlusion from extensive calcium displacement. Risk factors for coronary occlusion include a heavy burden of leaflet and aortic root calcification, reduced height of origin of the coronary ostium from the annulus, with a low coronary height to be considered 12 mm from the basal leaflet insertion [1], "flat" aortic sinuses, an oversized prosthesis, or deployment of the prosthesis too aortic . In the setting of acute hypotension, part of the assessment is repeat evaluation of both right and left ventricular systolic function, and assessment for any new regional wall motion changes.

Cardiac Tamponade

Cardiac tamponade can occur at any point during the procedure, from early on at the time of pacing wire insertion to after deployment due to aortic root rupture. The reported incidence of tamponade varies from 0 to 7 % [4]. Left ventricular perforation can occur from a stiff wire causing trauma following a retrograde approach once the aortic valve is crossed. Creation of a large curve on the soft portion of the wire is frequently used in an attempt to minimize the occurrence of this complication [4]. Cardiac tamponade is usually managed with pericardiocentesis and catheter drainage but rarely may require thoracotomy. Figure 34.6 shows a transgastric view of a pericardial effusion following pacing wire insertion.

Aortic Root Rupture

The most feared complication of TAVR is rupture of the aortic annulus or aorta [22]. This results from selection of a prosthesis which is too large for the aortic annulus or failure to recognize that bulky calcium on the native aortic cusp cannot be accommodated in the area of the aortic sinus of Valsalva after the prosthesis has been deployed. Excessive balloon dilation may also increase the risk of rupture [23]. Figure 34.7 shows aortic rupture as it occurs. In Fig. 34.7a, a nodule of calcium on the posterior aortic cusp is just beginning to distort the posterior aortic sinus. Figure 34.7b shows a clear steplike deformity in the posterior sinus, a suggestion of discontinuity of the wall of the sinus and evidence of radiocontrast in the transverse sinus confirming that aortic rupture has occurred.

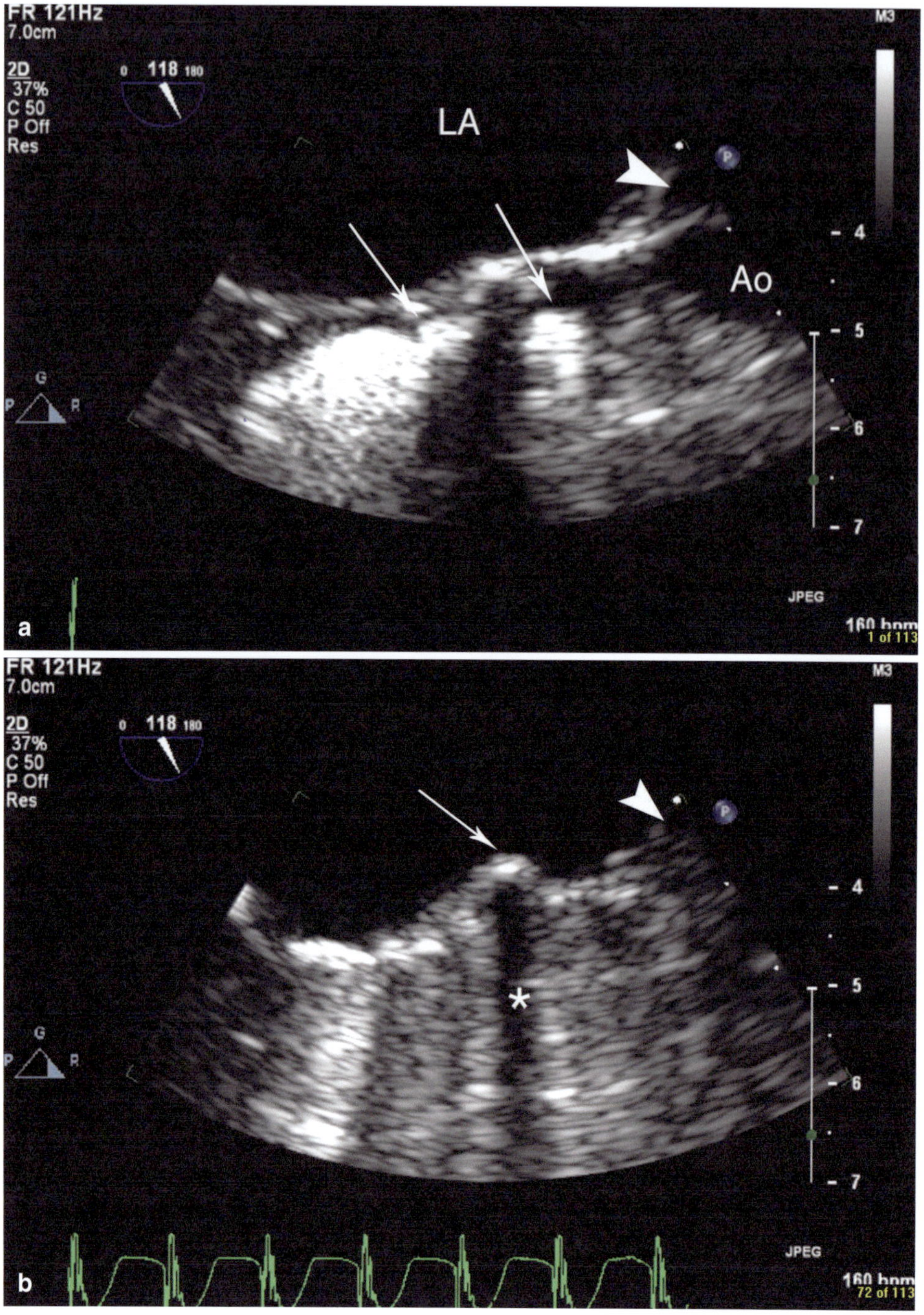

Fig. 34.7 (**a**) Still frame of percutaneous aortic prosthesis deployment. The ventricular and aortic ends of the prosthesis (*arrows*) are seen during balloon inflation. Echo poor pericardial fluid is seen within the transverse sinus (*arrowhead*). (**b**) The balloon is fully expanded within the left ventricular outflow tract and aortic root (*asterisk*). Tenting of the posterior aortic sinus (*arrow*) is seen with full balloon inflation. The echo poor area of the transverse sinus has become echodense (*arrowhead*) as the aortic root and balloon rupture and radiocontrast leaks into the transverse sinus

Aortic Root Hematoma

It is possible to create a less than full thickness tear in the aortic annulus or aortic sinus in which case a hematoma rather than rupture result. A posterior sinus hematoma is delineated in Fig. 34.8. Following both balloon inflation and prosthesis deployment, the echocardiographer should continue to watch for the development of aortic root hematoma, the development of which may be delayed following prosthesis deployment [24].

Ventricular Septal Rupture

Ventricular septal rupture is a rare, but serious, complication of TAVR. A complete understanding of causal factors remains unknown, but it is most likely the same risk factors for aortic root rupture, including oversizing, as well as concentration of calcification toward the membranous septum. Cases of delayed presentation of ventricular septal rupture have been reported [22]. Both ventricular septal rupture and aortic root rupture from TAVR are associated with

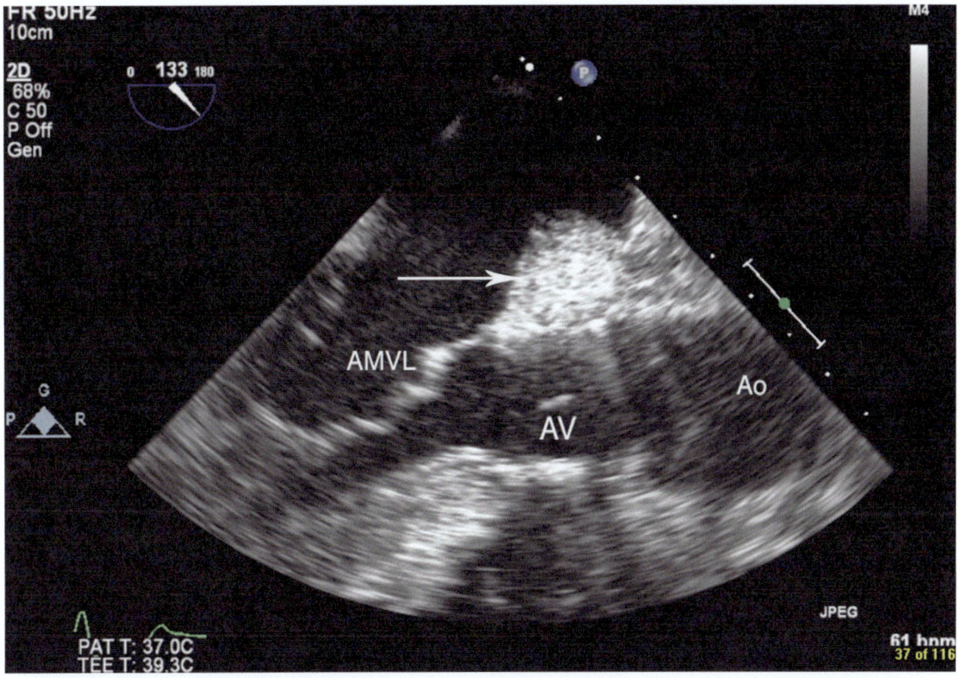

Fig. 34.8 An echodense well-circumscribed hematoma deforms the posterior aortic sinus (*arrow*) following aortic prosthesis deployment. *AV* transcatheter aortic prosthesis with closed leaflets, *AMVL* anterior mitral valve leaflet, *Ao* aorta

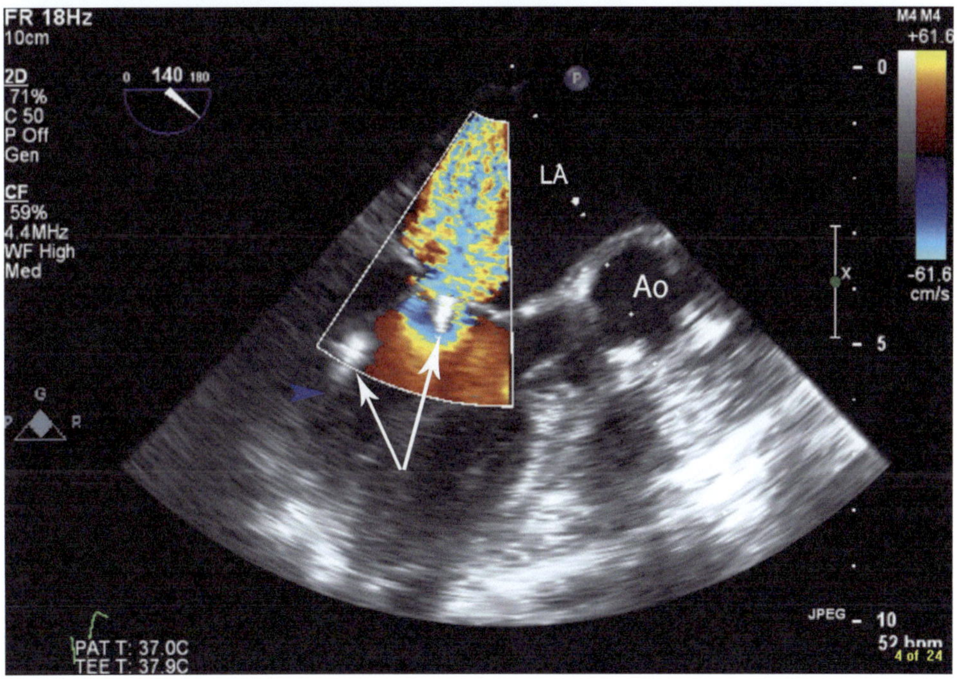

Fig. 34.9 A guidewire extends through the native aortic valve into the left ventricle. The wire (*short white arrow*) is seen at the level of the papillary muscle (*blue arrowhead*), with the tip of the wire entangled in the mitral apparatus (*long white arrow*). Interference with the mitral chordae tendineae has caused severe mitral regurgitation. *LA* left atrium, *Ao* aorta

poor prognosis despite recognition and emergency cardiopulmonary bypass and surgical repair [23].

Acute Severe Mitral Regurgitation

With a retrograde approach, the guidewire is ideally placed in the left ventricular apex prior to proceeding with balloon valvuloplasty and prosthesis delivery. The guidewire can become entangled within the mitral chordae and subvalvular apparatus. This can result in acute severe mitral regurgitation, but with prompt recognition, the guidewire can be repositioned. Figure 34.9 shows the guidewire interfering with the mitral apparatus resulting in severe mitral regurgitation and marked hypotension. We commonly image the wire as it is being laid out and, if interference with the mitral apparatus occurs, attempt to help the interventionalist to select a new catheter position away from the mitral apparatus from which to lay out the guidewire.

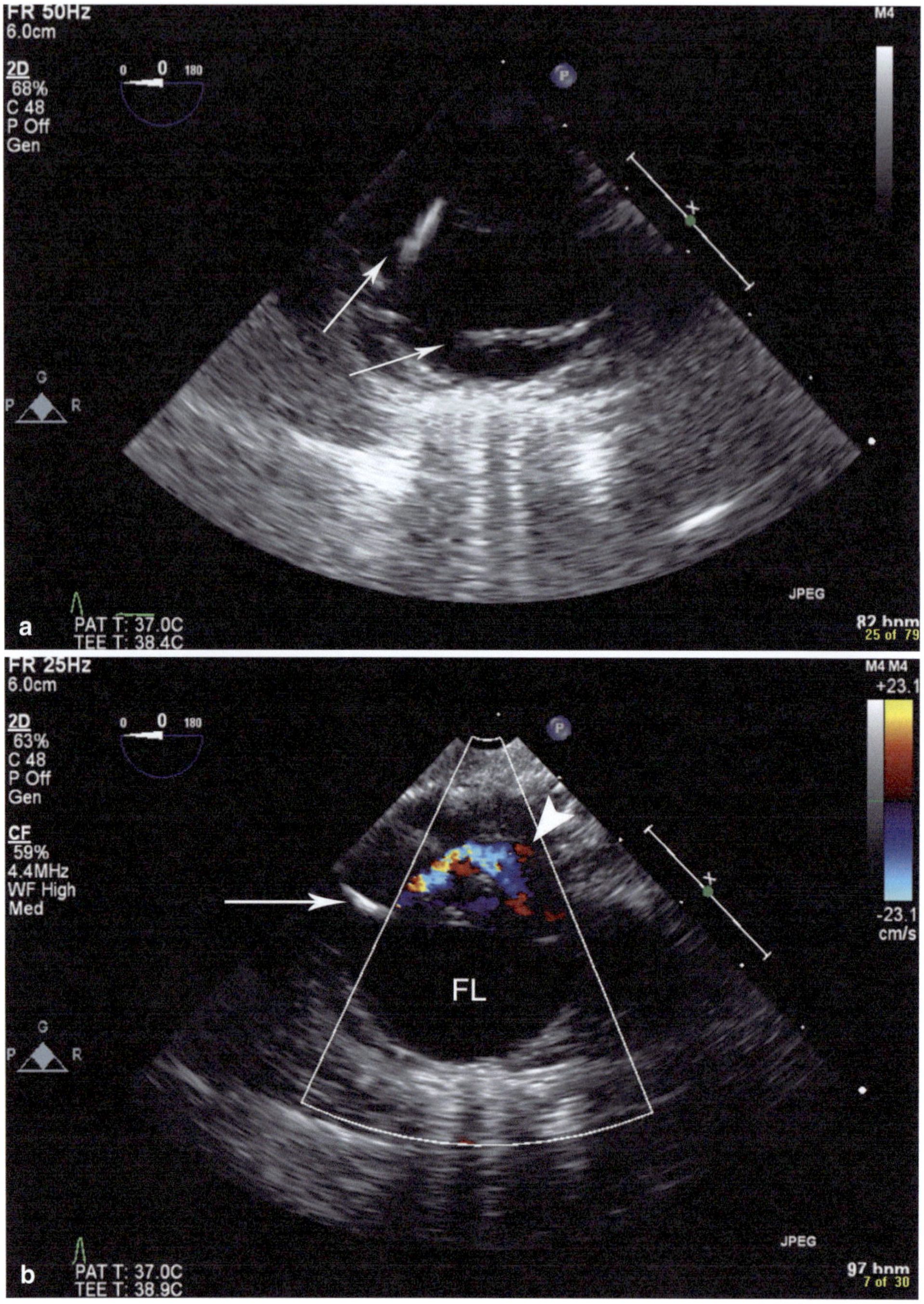

Fig. 34.10 (**a**) A dissection flap (*arrows*) resulting from aortic trauma induced while trying to reposition an embolized prosthesis in the descending thoracic aorta. (**b**) Color flow(*arrowhead*) is seen in the true lumen of the descending aorta following aortic dissection. The dissection flap (*arrow*) separates a large false lumen (*FL*)

Aortic Dissection

Finally, aortic trauma with dissection can occur at many stages of the procedure. Aortic dissection remains a worrisome risk despite the smaller transcatheter delivery systems developed over the years. Aortic assessment is also performed as part of the "troubleshooting" imaging in the setting of hemodynamic instability. Figure 34.10 shows an extensive aortic dissection which occurred during attempts to reposition an embolized prosthesis in the descending aorta. Prior to completing the echocardiographic study after the procedure, the entire aorta is imaged to assess for any

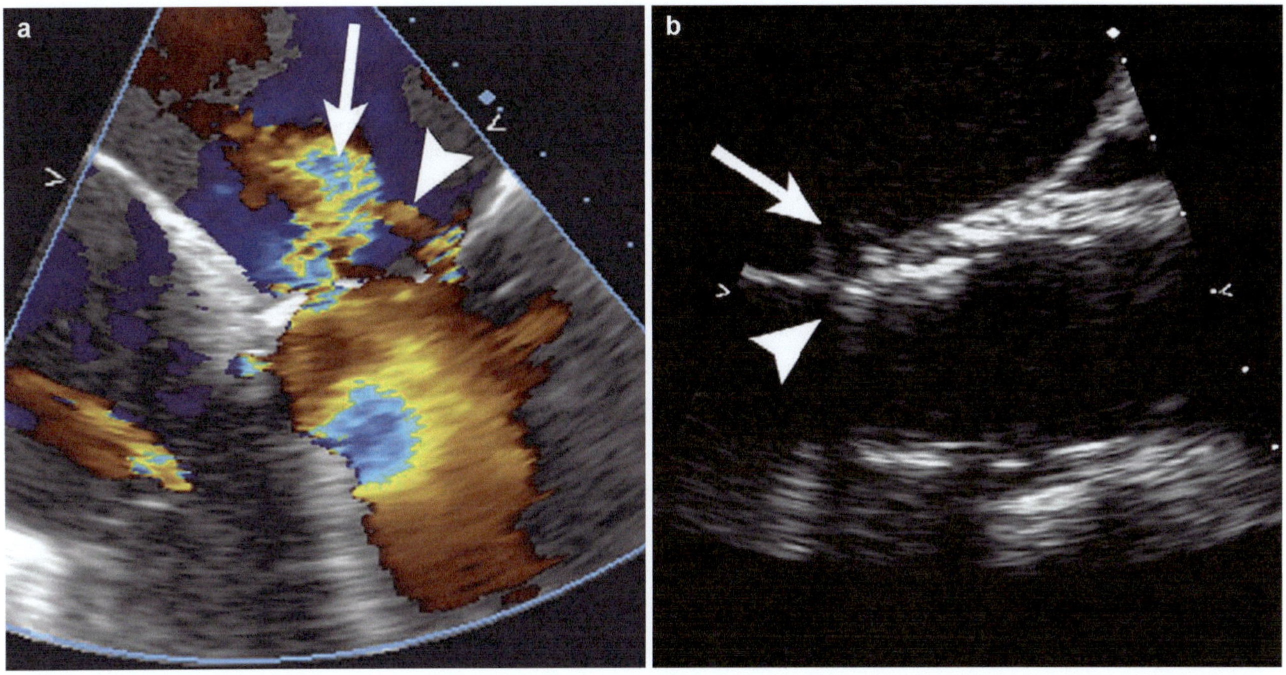

Fig. 34.11 Transesophageal echocardiographic evaluation of severe mitral regurgitation. (**a**) Two regurgitant jets are identified, one transvalvular (*arrow*) and a second through a perforation in the anterior mitral leaflet (*arrowhead*). (**b**) A ruptured aneurysm (*arrow*) of the anterior leaflet of the mitral valve was present adjacent to the ventricular edge (*arrowhead*) of the implanted transcatheter aortic valve (Reprinted with permission from Wong et. al. [29])

intimal tears that may not have become clinically apparent. Importantly, late deaths due to aortic dissection which was not recognized during the procedure have been reported [25].

Stroke

The incidence of stroke following TAVI has been reported to be between 1.7 and 8.4 % [1]. It is useful to include assessment of the descending thoracic aorta and aortic arch as part of the baseline imaging. Cases with more severe atherosclerotic disease are at greater risk of an early neurological event. Other predictors of an early neurological event include a prior neurological event and smaller aortic valve area [1]. It is also always concerning to see highly mobile calcifications attached to the native aortic valve prior to balloon valvuloplasty.

Endocarditis

Endocarditis is a possible late sequela of aortic prosthesis implantation [26–29]. Since a too ventricular ("low") prosthesis position commonly results in contact with the moving portion of the anterior mitral leaflet and with paravalvular regurgitation, there is a setup for infective endocarditis. The repeated contact of the ventricular end of the prosthesis may abrade the surface of the mitral leaflet, while the paravalvular regurgitant jet streams blood and bacteria (if present) onto the abraded surface. Figure 34.11 demonstrates an anterior mitral leaflet aneurysm resulting from infective endocarditis on a prosthesis placed too ventricular.

Complications Unique to Transapical TAVR

Extensive aortic atheroma, a porcelain aorta, or inadequate femoral access is an indication for an alternate approach, usually a transapical approach. Development of an apical pseudoaneurysm is an uncommon complication, usually becoming evident days to months following the procedure (Fig. 34.12) [3, 30, 31]. Friable tissue and difficult visualization at the time of closure have been reported as risk factors for development [3, 31]. Pseudoaneurysms may continue to enlarge requiring surgical intervention although cases of stable defects managed conservatively are also reported (Box 34.1).

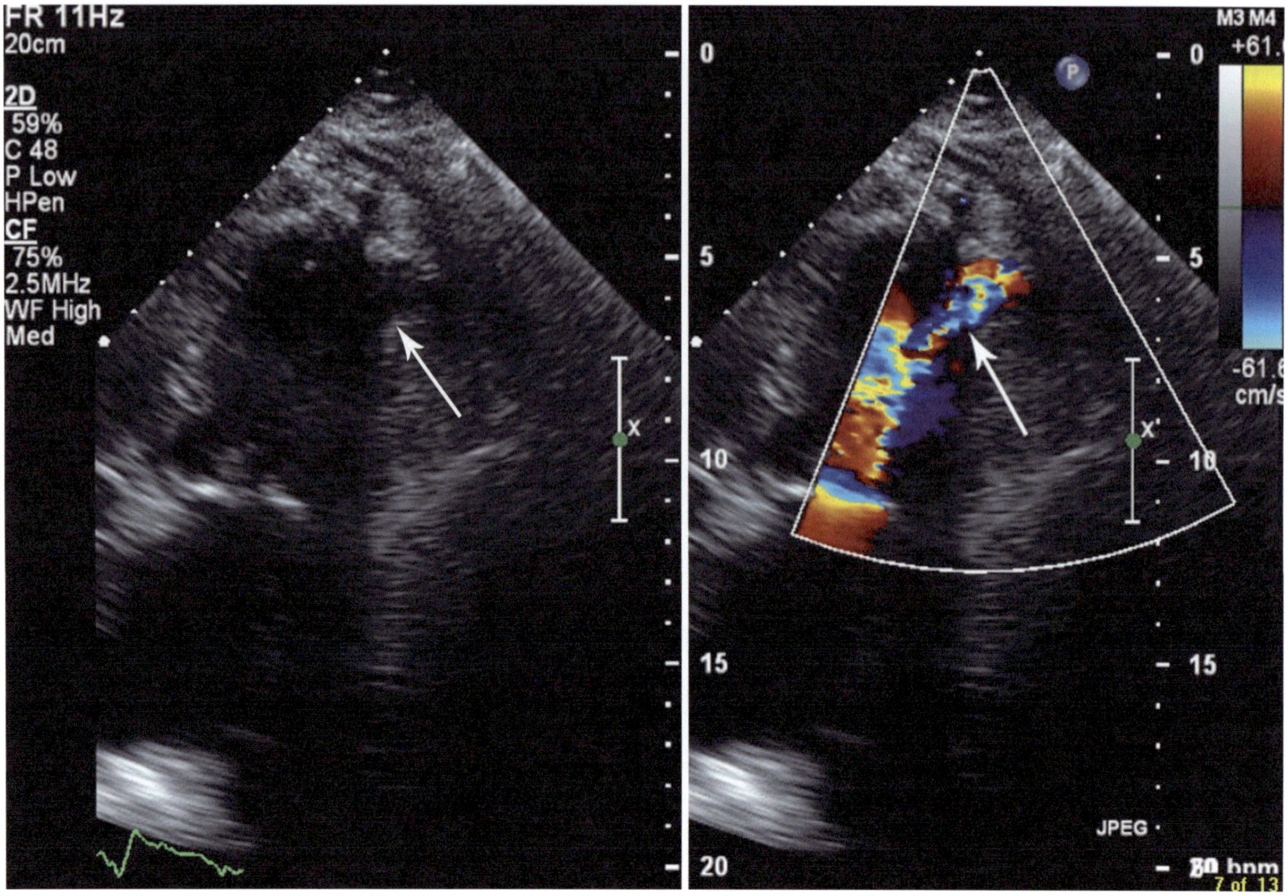

Fig. 34.12 Transthoracic apical four-chamber view demonstrating an apical pseudoaneurysm after transapical TAVR. The neck of the aneurysm is evident on the gray-scale image (*arrow*) with flow out of the neck of the aneurysm in diastole evident on the color flow image (*arrow*)

Box 34.1 Potential Complications Associated with TAVR

- Aortic dissection
- Aortic root hematoma
- Aortic pseudoaneurysm
- Aortic root rupture
- Cardiac tamponade
- Endocarditis
- Improper valve positioning
- Inappropriate valve sizing
- Mitral regurgitation, acute
- Paravalvular aortic regurgitation
- Stroke
- Ventricular function
- Ventricular septal rupture

References

1. Généreux P, Head SJ, Wood DA, Kodali SK, Williams MR, Paradis JM, Spaziano M, Kappetein AP, Webb JG, Cribier A, Leon MB. Transcatheter aortic valve implantation 10-year anniversary: review of current evidence and clinical implications. Eur Heart J. 2012;33: 2388–98.
2. Webb JG, Altwegg L, Boone RH, Cheung A, Ye J, Lichtenstein S, Lee M, Masson JB, Thompson C, Moss R, Carere R, Munt B, Nietlispach F, Humphries K. Transcatheter aortic valve implantation: impact on clinical and valve-related outcomes. Circulation. 2009;119(23):3009–16.
3. Al-Attar N, Ghodbane W, Himbert D, Rau C, Raffoul R, Messika-Zeitoun D, Brochet E, Vahanian A, Nataf P. Unexpected complications of transapical aortic valve implantation. Ann Thorac Surg. 2009;88(1):90–4.
4. Masson J-B, Kovac J, Schuler G, Ye J, Cheung A, Kapadia S, Tuzcu ME, Kodali S, Leon MB, Webb JG. Transcatheter aortic valve implantation. JACC Cardiovasc Interv. 2009;2(9):811–20.

5. Gurvitch R, Tay EL, Wijesinghe N, Ye J, Nietlispach F, Wood DA, Lichtenstein S, Cheung A, Webb JG. Transcatheter aortic valve implantation: lessons from the learning curve of the first 270 high-risk patients. Catheter Cardiovasc Interv. 2011;78(7): 977–84.
6. Leon MB, Piazza N, Nikolsky E, Blackstone EH, Cutlip DE, Kappetein AP, Krucoff MW, Mack M, Mehran R, Miller C, Morel MA, Petersen J, Popma JJ, Takkenberg JJ, Vahanian A, van Es GA, Vranckx P, Webb JG, Windecker S, Serruys PW. Standardized endpoint definitions for transcatheter aortic valve implantation clinical trials: a consensus report from the Valve Academic Research Consortium. J Am Coll Cardiol. 2011;57(3):253–69.
7. Willson AB, Webb JG, LaBounty TM, Achenbach S, Moss R, Wheeler M, Thompson C, Min JK, Gurvitch R, Norgaard BL, Hague CJ, Toggweiler S, Binder R, Freeman M, Poulter R, Poulsen S, Wood DA, Leipsic J. 3-Dimensional aortic annular assessment by multidetector computed tomography predicts moderate or severe paravalvular regurgitation after transcatheter aortic valve replacement a multicenter retrospective analysis. J Am Coll Cardiol. 2012;59(14):1287–94.
8. Wood DA, Tops LF, Mayo JR, Pasupati S, Schalij MJ, Humphries K, Lee M, Al Ali A, Munt B, Moss R, Thompson CR, Bax JJ, Webb JG. Role of multislice computed tomography in transcatheter aortic valve replacement. Am J Cardiol. 2009;103(9):1295–301.
9. Moss RR, Ivens E, Pasupati S, Humphries K, Thompson CR, Munt B, Sinhal A, Webb JG. Role of echocardiography in percutaneous aortic valve implantation. JACC Cardiovasc Imaging. 2008;1(1): 15–24.
10. Jayasuriya C, Moss RR, Munt B. Transcatheter aortic valve implantation in aortic stenosis: the role of echocardiography. J Am Soc Echocardiogr. 2011;24(1):15–27.
11. Webb JG, Chandavimol M, Thompson CR, Ricci DR, Carere RG, Munt BI, Buller CE, Pasupati S, Lichtenstein S. Percutaneous aortic valve implantation retrograde from the femoral artery. Circulation. 2006;113(6):842–50.
12. Gotzmann M, Korten M, Bojara W, Lindstaedt M, Rahlmann P, Mugge A, Ewers A. Long-term outcome of patients with moderate and severe prosthetic aortic valve regurgitation after transcatheter aortic valve implantation. Am J Cardiol. 2012;110:1500–6.
13. Al-Attar N, Himbert D, Vahanian A, Nataf P. Severe intraprosthetic regurgitation by immobile leaflet after trans-catheter aortic valve implantation. Eur J Cardiothorac Surg. 2011;39(4):591–2.
14. Zahn R, Schiele R, Kilkowski C, Zeymer U. Severe aortic regurgitation after percutaneous transcatheter aortic valve implantation: on the importance to clarify the underlying pathophysiology. Clin Res Cardiol. 2010;99(3):193–7.
15. Gonçalves A, Almeria C, Marcos-Alberca P, Feltes G, Hernández-Antolín R, Rodríguez E, Silva Cardoso JC, Macaya C, Zamorano JL. Three-dimensional echocardiography in paravalvular aortic regurgitation assessment after transcatheter aortic valve implantation. J Am Soc Echocardiogr. 2012;25(1):47–55.
16. Sinning J-M, Hammerstingl C, Vasa-Nicotera M, Adenauer V, Lema Cachiguango SJ, Scheer A-C, Hausen S, Sedaghat A, Ghanem A, Müller C, Grube E, Nickenig G, Werner N. Aortic regurgitation index defines severity of peri-prosthetic regurgitation and predicts outcome in patients after transcatheter aortic valve implantation. J Am Coll Cardiol. 2012;59(13):1134–41.
17. Gripari P, Ewe SH, Fusini L, Muratori M, Ng ACT, Cefalu C, Delgado V, Schalij MJ, Bax JJ, Marsan NA, Tamborini G, Pepi M. Intraoperative 2D and 3D transoesophageal echocardiographic predictors of aortic regurgitation after transcatheter aortic valve implantation. Heart. 2012;98(16):1229–36.
18. Détaint D, Lepage L, Himbert D, Brochet E, Messika-Zeitoun D, Iung B, Vahanian A. Determinants of significant paravalvular regurgitation after transcatheter aortic valve implantation. JACC Cardiovasc Interv. 2009;2(9):821–7.
19. Binder RK, Webb JG, Willson AB, Urena M, Hansson NC, Norgaard BL, Pibarot P, Barbanti M, Larose E, Freeman M, Dumont E, Thompson C, Wheeler M, Moss RR, Yang T, Pasian S, Hague C, Nguyen G, Raju R, Toggweiler S, Min JK, Wood DA, Rodés-Cabau J, Leipsic J. The impact of integration of a multidetector computed tomography annulus area sizing algorithm on outcomes of transcatheter aortic valve replacement: A prospective, multicenter, controlled trial. J Am Coll Cardiol. 2013 (Article in Press).
20. Pasupati S, Sinhal A, Humphries K, Ivens E, Moss R, Thompson CR, Muni B, Carere R, Webb J. Re-dilation of balloon expandable aortic valves BEAV: what do we know? Am J Cardiol. 2007;100(8A):57L.
21. Nombela-Franco L, Rodes-Cabau J, DeLarochelliere R, Larose E, Doyle D, Villeneuve J, Bergeron S, Bernier M, Amat-Santos IJ, Mok M, Urena M, Rheault M, Dumesnil J, Cote M, Pibarot P, Dumont E. Predictive factors, efficacy, and safety of balloon post-dilation after transcatheter aortic valve implantation with a balloon-expandable valve. JACC Cardiovasc Interv. 2012; 5(5):499–512.
22. Aminian A, Lalmand J, Dolatabadi D. Late contained aortic root rupture and ventricular septal defect after transcatheter aortic valve implantation. Catheter Cardiovasc Interv. 2012;81:E72–5.
23. Masson JB, Altwegg LA, Al Ali A, Al Bugami S, Boone RH, Carere RG, Lichtenstein SV, Cheung A, Moss R, Munt B, Thompson CR, Ye J, Webb JG, 18. Incidence and management of procedural complications associated with transcatheter aortic valve implantation. Circulation. 2008;118:S808.
24. Généreux P, Reiss GR, Kodali SK, Williams MR, Hahn RT. Periaortic hematoma after transcatheter aortic valve replacement: description of a new complication. Catheter Cardiovasc Interv. 2012;79(5):766–76.
25. Gerber RT, Osborn M, Mikhail GW. Delayed mortality from aortic dissection post transcatheter aortic valve implantation (TAVI): The tip of the iceberg. Catheter Cardiovasc Interv. 2010;76(2): 202–4.
26. Loh PH, Bundgaard H, Sondergaard L. Infective endocarditis following transcatheter aortic valve replacement: diagnostic and management challenges. Catheter Cardiovasc Interv. 2012;81: 623–7.
27. Castiglioni A, Pozzoli A, Maisano F, Alfieri O. Endocarditis after transfemoral aortic valve implantation in a patient with Osler-Weber-Rendu syndrome. Interact Cardiovasc Thorac Surg. 2012;15(3):553–4.
28. Head SJ, Dewey TM, Mack MJ. Fungal endocarditis after transfemoral aortic valve implantation. Catheter Cardiovasc Interv. 2011;78(7):1017–9.
29. Wong DR, Boone RH, Thompson CR, Allard MF, Altwegg L, Carere RG, Cheung A, Ye JA, Lichtenstein SV, Ling H, Webb JG. Mitral valve injury late after transcatheter aortic valve implantation. J Thorac Cardiovasc Surg. 2009;137(6):1547–9.
30. Vanezis AP, Baig MK, Mitchel IM, Shajar M, Naik SK, Henderson RA, Mathew T. Pseudoaneurysm of the left ventricle following apical approach TAVI. J Cardiovasc Magn Reson. 2011;13(1):79.
31. Elhenawy A, Rocha R, Feindel CM, Brister SJ. Persistent left ventricular false aneurysm after transapical insertion of an aortic valve. J Card Surg. 2011;26(1):51–3.

Case-Based Examples of Complications Associated with Transcatheter Aortic Valve Replacement

35

Jorge Castellanos, Robert J. Siegel, Hasan Jilaihawi, Tarun Chakravarty, and Raj Makkar

Abstract

As with any new procedure, the complications associated with transcatheter aortic valve replacement (TAVR) are just as important as its therapeutic clinical benefits. A skilled operator must be able to quickly identify and mitigate any associated complications. The following is a list of the different types of TAVR-related complications an operator can experience before and during valve deployment.

TAVR complications:

- Aortic annulus rupture
- Prosthesis embolization
- Stroke
- Myocardial infarction
- Cardiac tamponade
- Transient left ventricular dysfunction
- Coronary obstruction
- Mitral regurgitation
- Aortic regurgitation
- Complete heart block
- Vascular access problems

We present six cases in which echocardiography was instrumental in identifying TAVR-associated complications. When data was available, we included the incidence, high-risk features, prognosis, and steps the operator took in order to address the complication. In some of the examples, we have included additional images from other patients in order to illustrate more severe forms of the complication.

J. Castellanos, MD, MPP (✉) • T. Chakravarty, MD
Department of Cardiology, Cedars Sinai Medical Center,
8700 Beverly Blvd, Rm 5536B, Los Angeles, CA 90048, USA
e-mail: jorge.castellanos@cshs.org; tarun.chakravarty@cshs.org

R.J. Siegel, MD, FACC, FASE
Department of Cardiology, Cedars Sinai Medical Center,
8700 Beverly Blvd, Rm 523, Los Angeles, CA 90048, USA
e-mail: robertjames.siegel@cshs.org

H. Jilaihawi, MD, MRCP • R. Makkar, MD, FACC
Department of Cardiology, Cedars-Sinai Heart Institute,
Cedars-Sinai Medical Center, 8631 West 3rd St, Ste 415,
Los Angeles, CA 90048, USA
e-mail: hasanjilaihawi@gmail.com; raj.makkar@cshs.org

J.K. Min et al. (eds.), *Multimodality Imaging for Transcatheter Aortic Valve Replacement*,
DOI 10.1007/978-1-4471-2798-7_35, © Springer-Verlag London 2014

Keywords
TAVR • Transcatheter aortic valve replacement • Complications • Aortic regurgitation • Pericardial effusion • Pericardial tamponade • Mitral regurgitation • Root hematoma • Left main • Embolized valve

Case 1: Aortic Regurgitation

Nearly 88 % of patients that undergo TAVR have some form of paravalvular or transvalvular aortic regurgitation [1]. Although the majority of paravalvular aortic regurgitation is mild, recent studies estimate the incidence of moderate-to-severe paravalvular aortic regurgitation post TAVR to be approximately 7–10 % [2–4]. Two-year data from the PARTNER trial, where 699 patients with severe aortic stenosis were randomized to surgical aortic valve replacement versus TAVR, found a 2.11-fold increase in 2-year mortality among patients who underwent TAVR and had mild to severe paravalvular aortic regurgitation relative to patients with non or trace paravalvular aortic regurgitation. These data suggest the importance of attempting to limit the amount of mild to severe paravalvular aortic regurgitation post TAVR [2, 5].

There are several factors that can influence the development of paravalvular aortic regurgitation, including the position of the prosthetic valve, the size of the aortic annulus and the pattern of calcification in the native valve [6–9]. The use of multiple imaging modalities, including TEE, CT, and fluoroscopy, can be used to limit the extent of aortic regurgitation by accurately measuring the size of the aortic valve annulus and by guiding the correct positioning of the bioprosthetic valve.

Reversing anticoagulation and a second balloon inflation, that better approximates the bioprosthetic valve to the aortic valve annulus, may help reduce the extent of paravalvular aortic regurgitation post TAVR. In contrast, when there is transvalvular aortic regurgitation, as in this case presentation, the management can include the delivery of a second bioprosthetic valve within the first valve. Only limited series and case reports have been published using this transcatheter "valve-in-valve" approach [10] and have demonstrated promising results. The following case describes the effective management of severe post TAVR transvalvular aortic regurgitation using this technique.

Case 1: H.R

An 81-year-old male presented with a history of severe aortic valve stenosis, coronary artery disease status post redo CABG, rheumatoid arthritis, myelodysplastic syndrome, and congestive heart failure. TTE showed LVEF 72 %, diastolic dysfunction, a mean AV gradient of 44 mmHg, and an AVA 0.8 cm^2.

Patient Underwent

1. Balloon aortic valvuloplasty with a Z-MED 20 × 40 mm balloon
2. Transcatheter aortic valve implantation using a 23-mm Edwards Sapien valve via femoral approach (Figs. 35.1, 35.2, 35.3, 35.4, 35.5, 35.6, 35.7, 35.8, and 35.9)

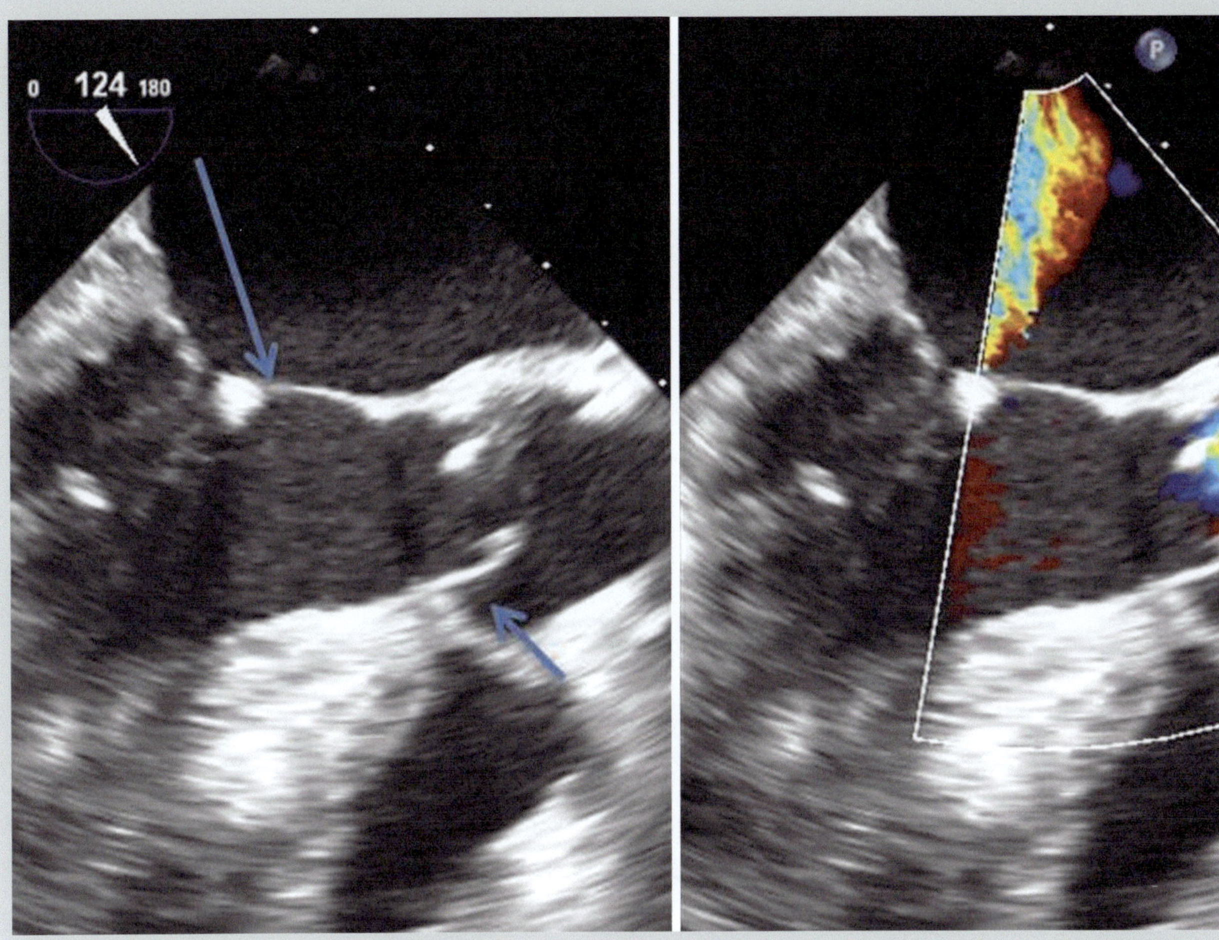

Fig. 35.1 Mitral valve (*long arrow*) and aortic valve (*short arrow*) in view. Note the minimal leaflet excursion of the aortic valve cusps

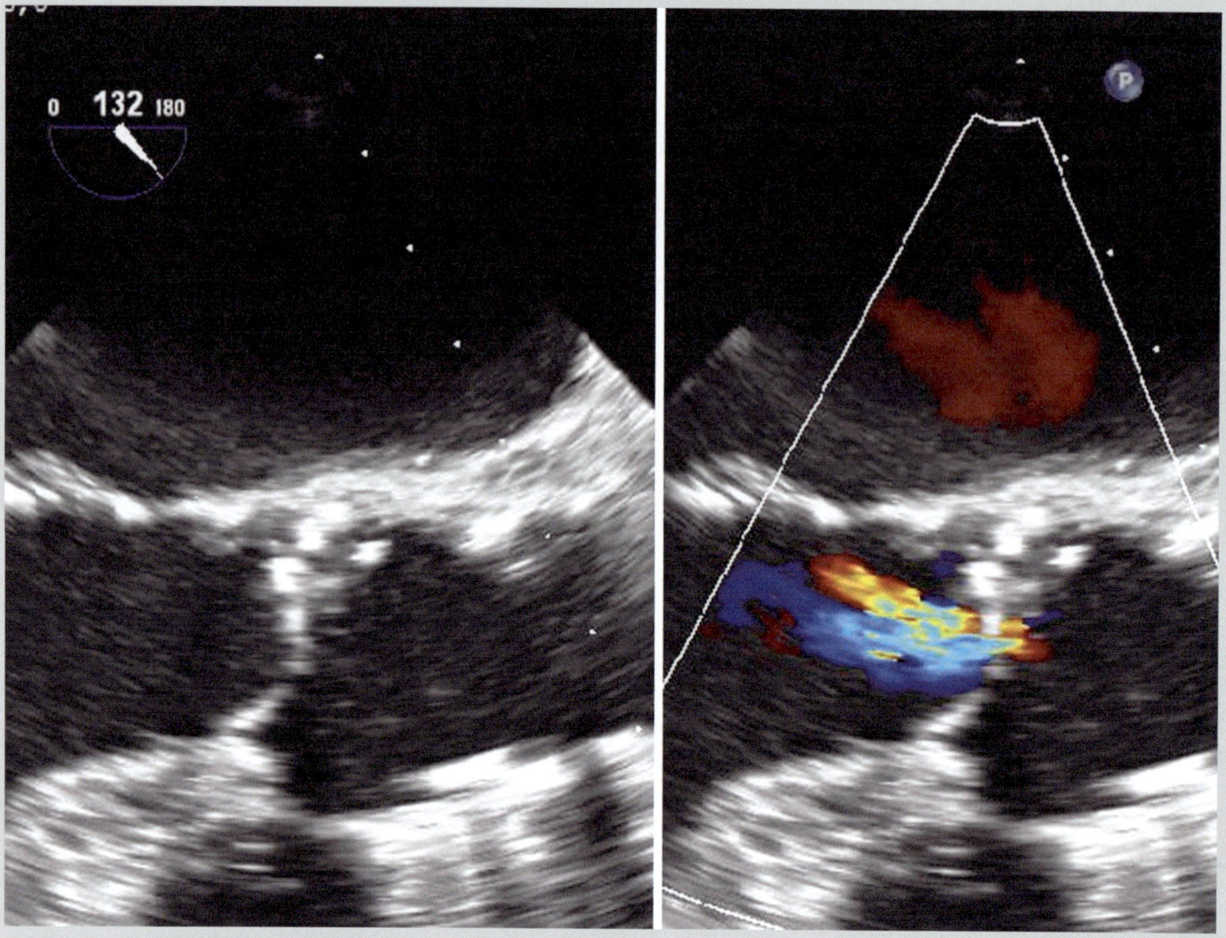

Fig. 35.2 Moderate aortic regurgitation prior to TAVR

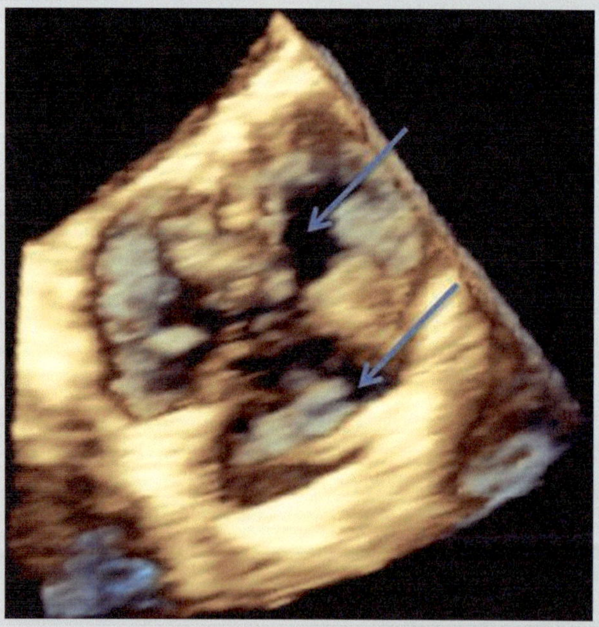

Fig. 35.3 3D TEE of the aortic valve. The extent of calcium deposition can be appreciated from this short axis image. The echolucent areas along the base of the cusp commissures are dropout artifact of the image and do not represent true openings (*arrows*)

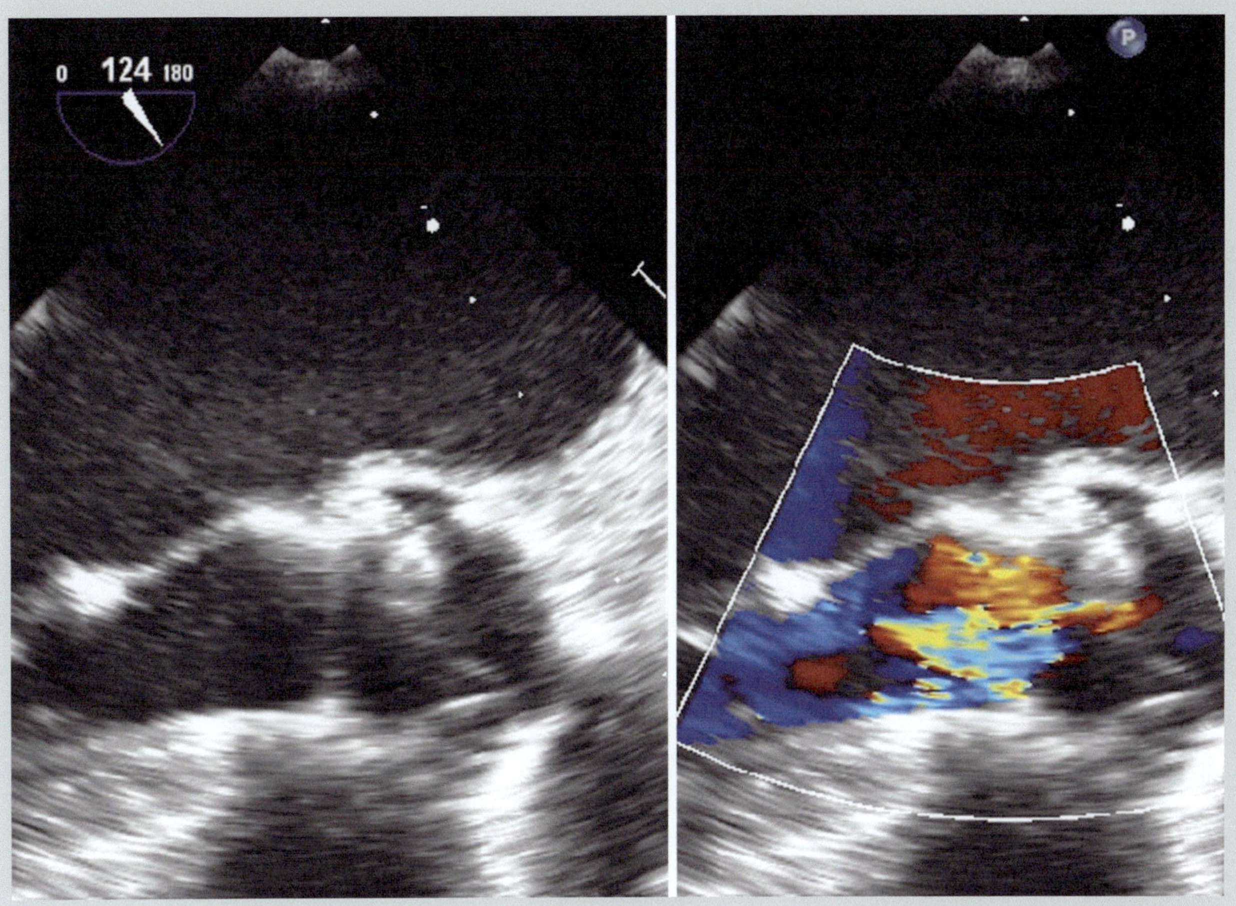

Fig. 35.4 Severe transvalvular aortic regurgitation immediately post TAVR

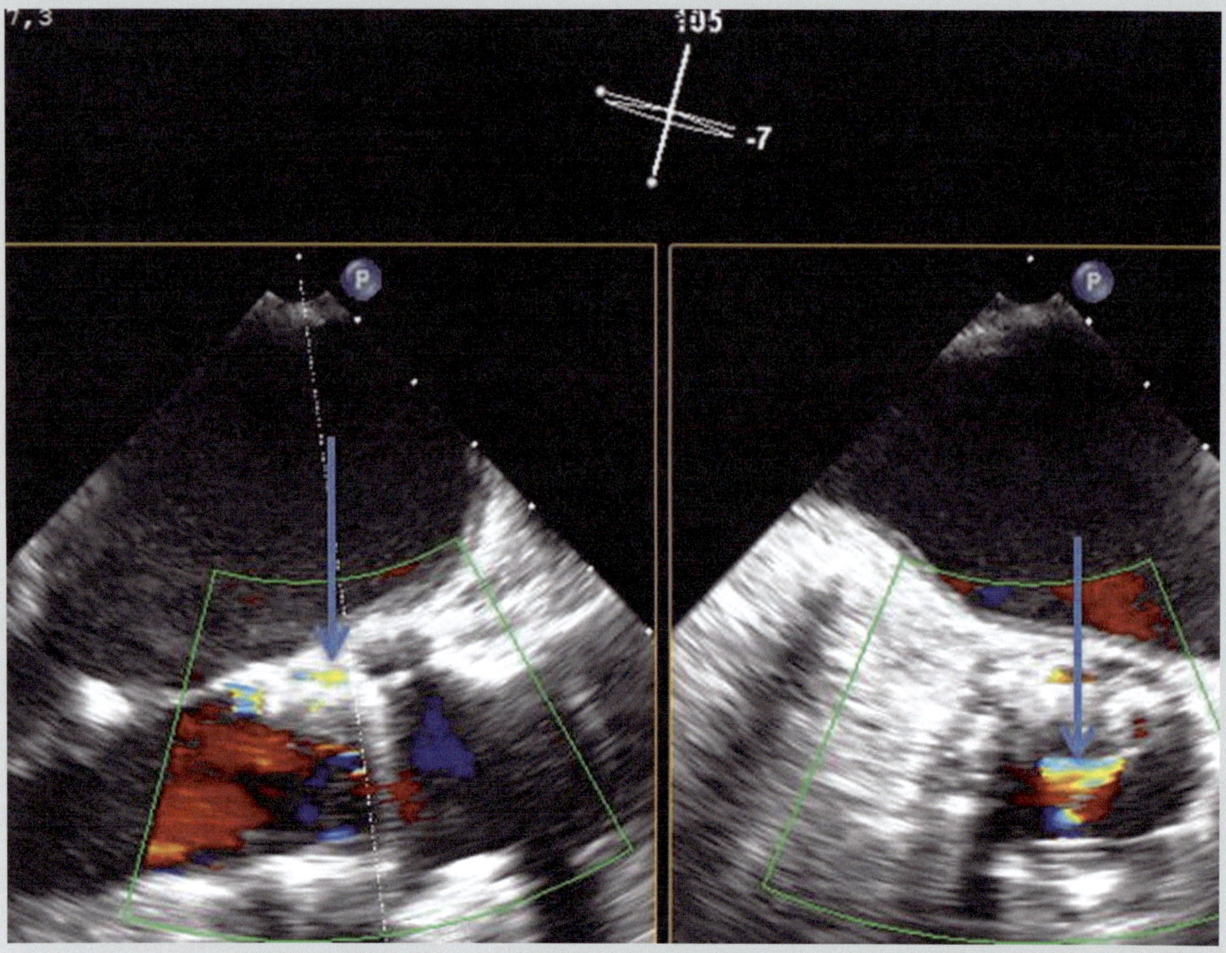

Fig. 35.5 *Arrow* shows trace paravalvular aortic regurgitation (*left*) and severe transvalvular aortic regurgitation (*right*)

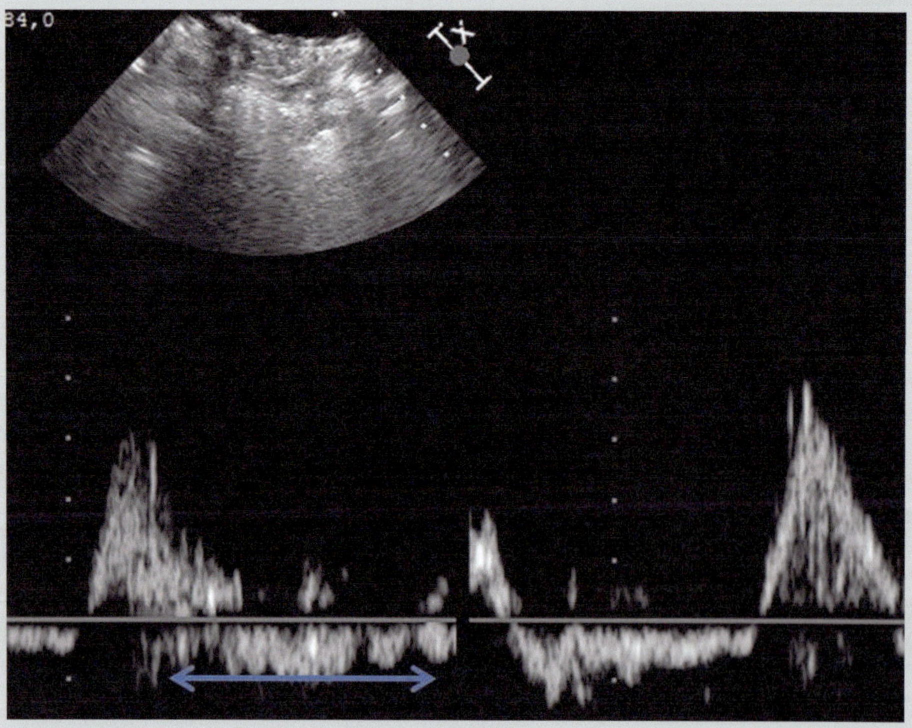

Fig. 35.6 Aortic flow reversal along descending aorta, consistent with severe aortic regurgitation (*arrow* denotes duration of diastolic flow reversal)

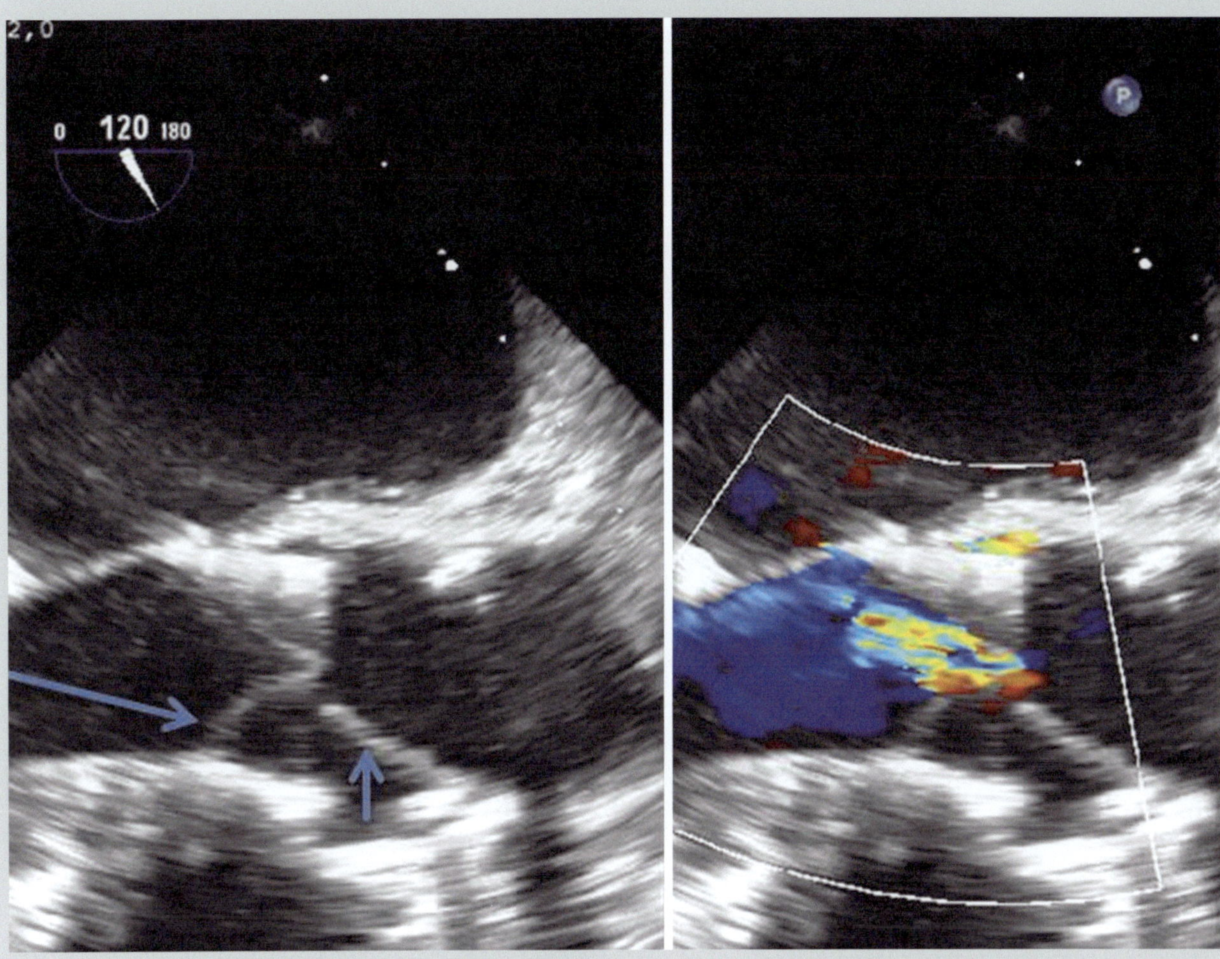

Fig. 35.7 Decision is made to recross the deployed transcatheter valve and place a second transcatheter valve within the first (valve-in-valve). *Arrows* show the guide wire (*short arrow*) and bioprosthetic leaflet (*long arrow*) during diastole

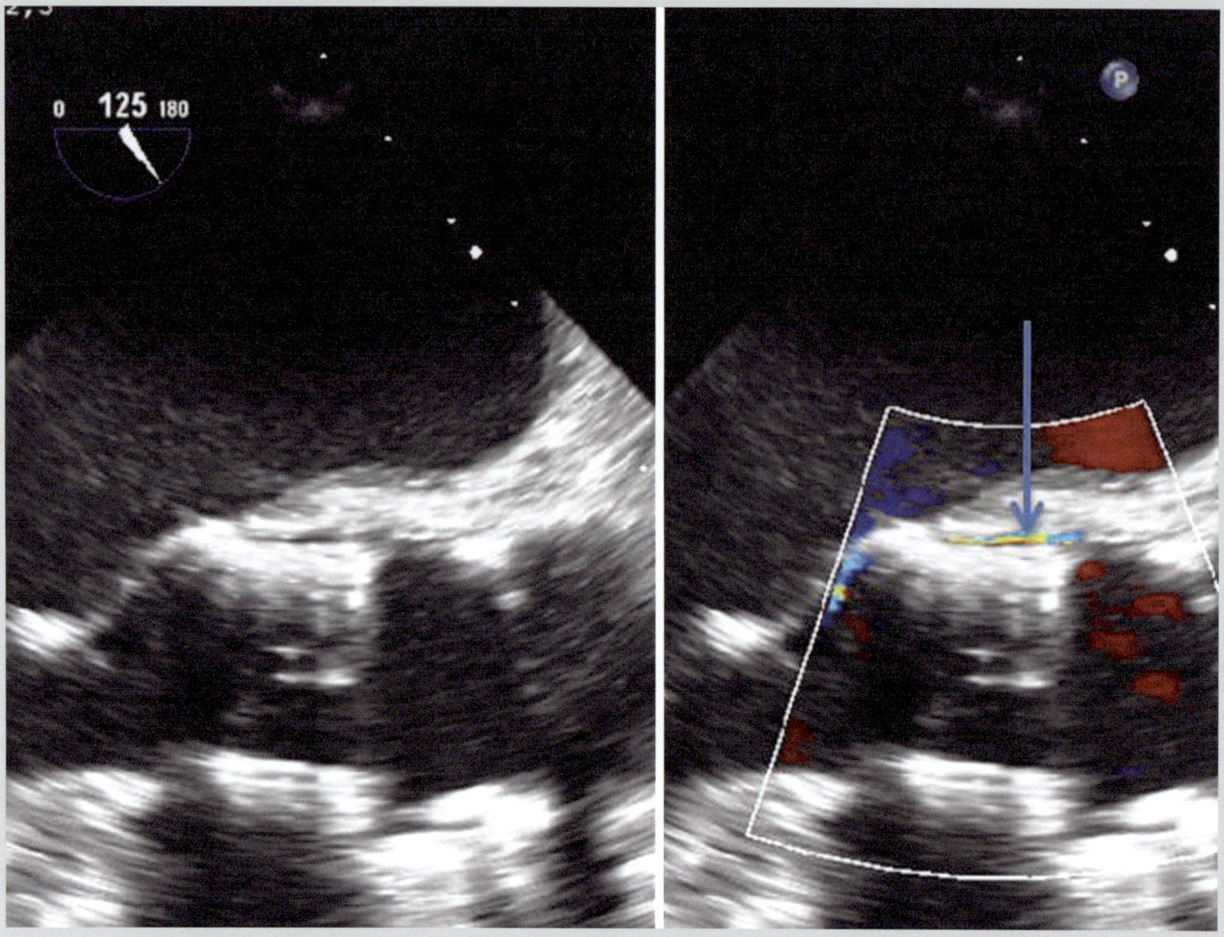

Fig. 35.8 A second bioprosthetic aortic valve has been deployed and there is no longer any transvalvular aortic regurgitation, with trace paravalvular aortic regurgitation (*arrow*)

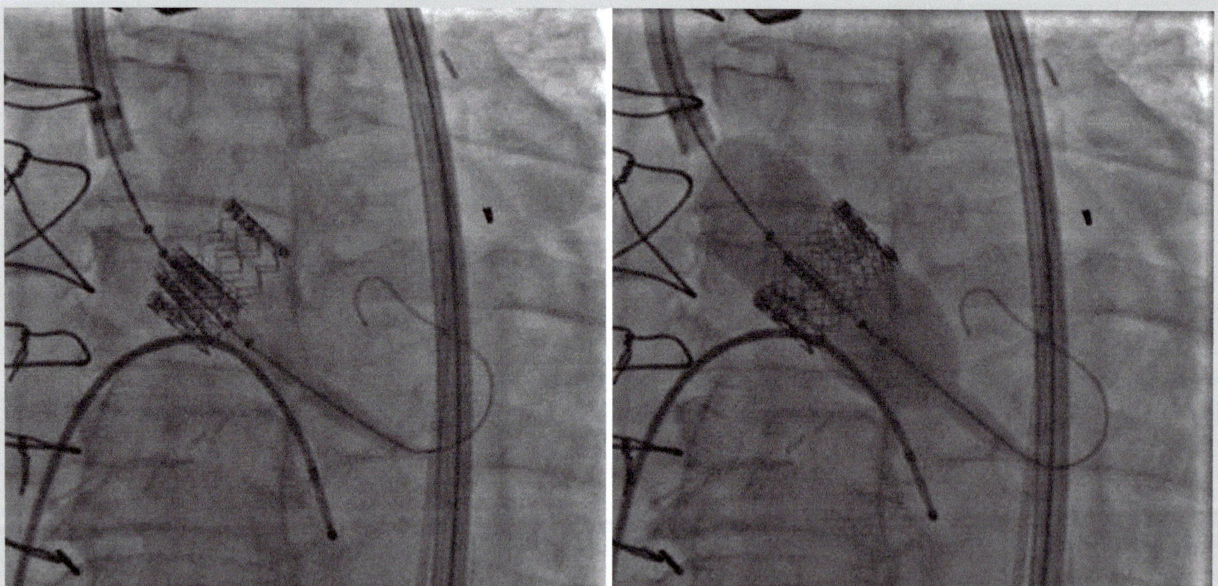

Fig. 35.9 Fluoroscopy of transcatheter valve-in-valve, immediately prior to deployment (*left*) and post deployment (*right*)

Case 2: Mitral Regurgitation

If the valve is deployed too high in the aortic root, it can lead to coronary ostia obstruction or upward valve embolization, but if it is deployed too low in the LVOT, it can lead to downward valve embolization or restriction of the anterior mitral leaflet with resultant mitral regurgitation (MR). One of the major benefits of TEE over other imaging modalities for TAVR is that it can help the operator discern the distance of the bioprosthetic valve to neighboring intracardiac structures in real-time, including the mitral valve. It is unclear what high-risk features can lead to anterior mitral leaflet restriction or how to manage it as there are is a paucity of published cases, but as will become evident by the case that follows, it is a potential complication of TAVR. This is a case of a bioprosthetic aortic valve that was deployed too low in the LVOT, leading to restriction of the anterior mitral leaflet and the development of mitral regurgitation.

Case 2: P.I

An 88-year-old male presented with history of aortic valve stenosis, coronary artery disease status post CABG, hypertension, hyperlipidemia, cerebrovascular disease, and diabetes. TTE showed LVEF 72 %, a mean AV gradient of 48 mmHg, and an AVA 0.8 cm^2.

Patient Underwent

1. Balloon aortic valvuloplasty with a Z-MED 22×40 mm balloon
2. Transcatheter aortic valve implantation using a 26-mm Edwards Sapien valve via femoral approach (Figs. 35.10, 35.11, 35.12, 35.13, and 35.14)

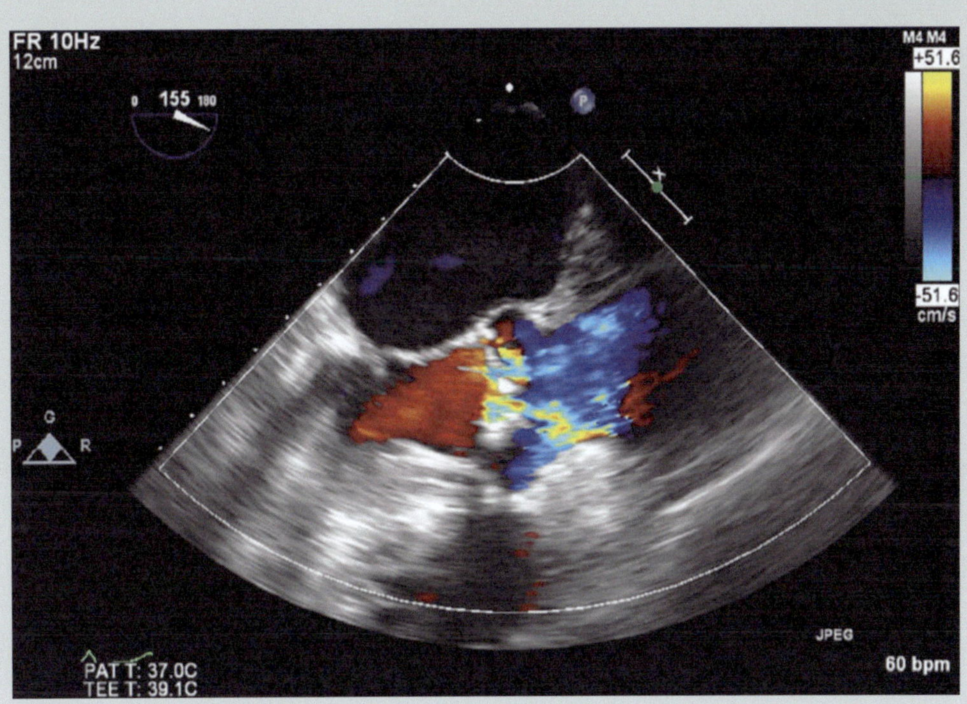

Fig. 35.10 Severe aortic stenosis with no evidence of mitral regurgitation

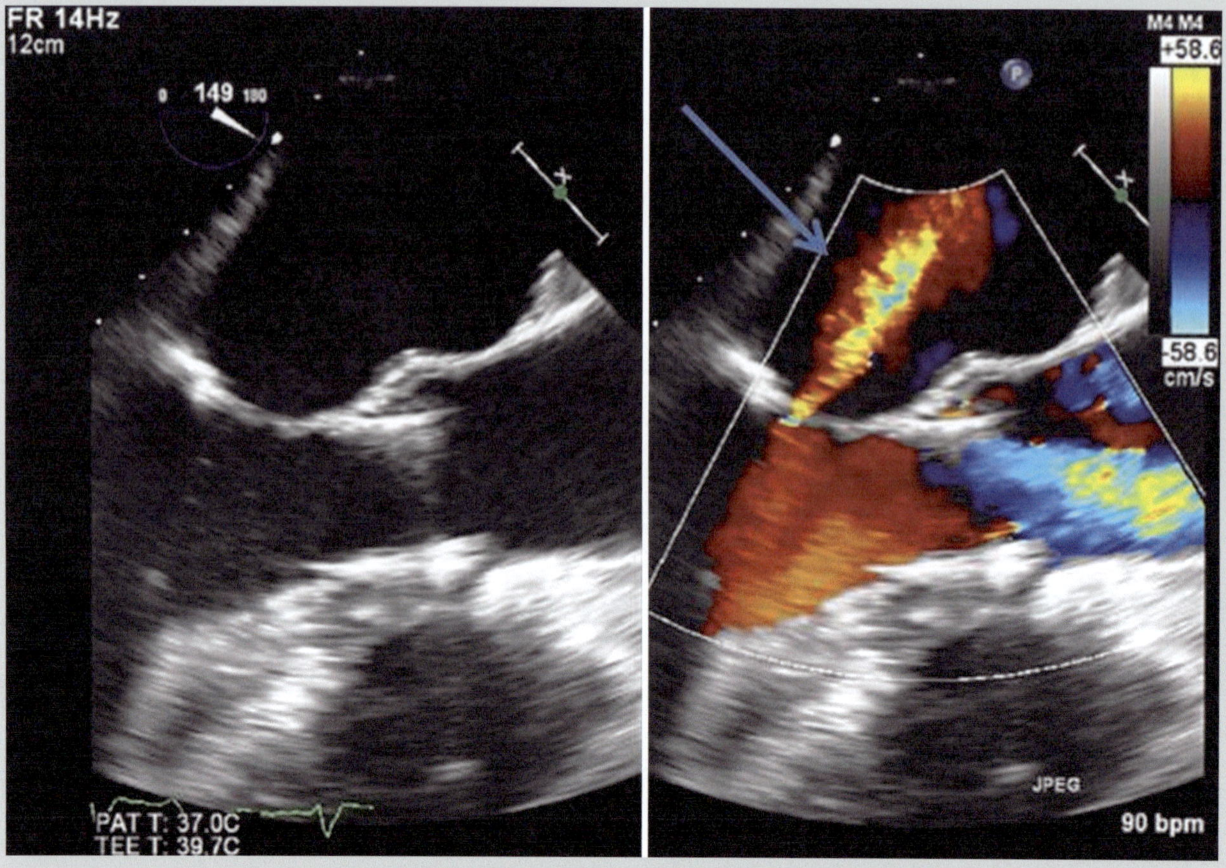

Fig. 35.11 Moderate mitral regurgitation (*arrow*) as a result of a low-lying bioprosthetic aortic valve restricting the movement of the anterior mitral leaflet

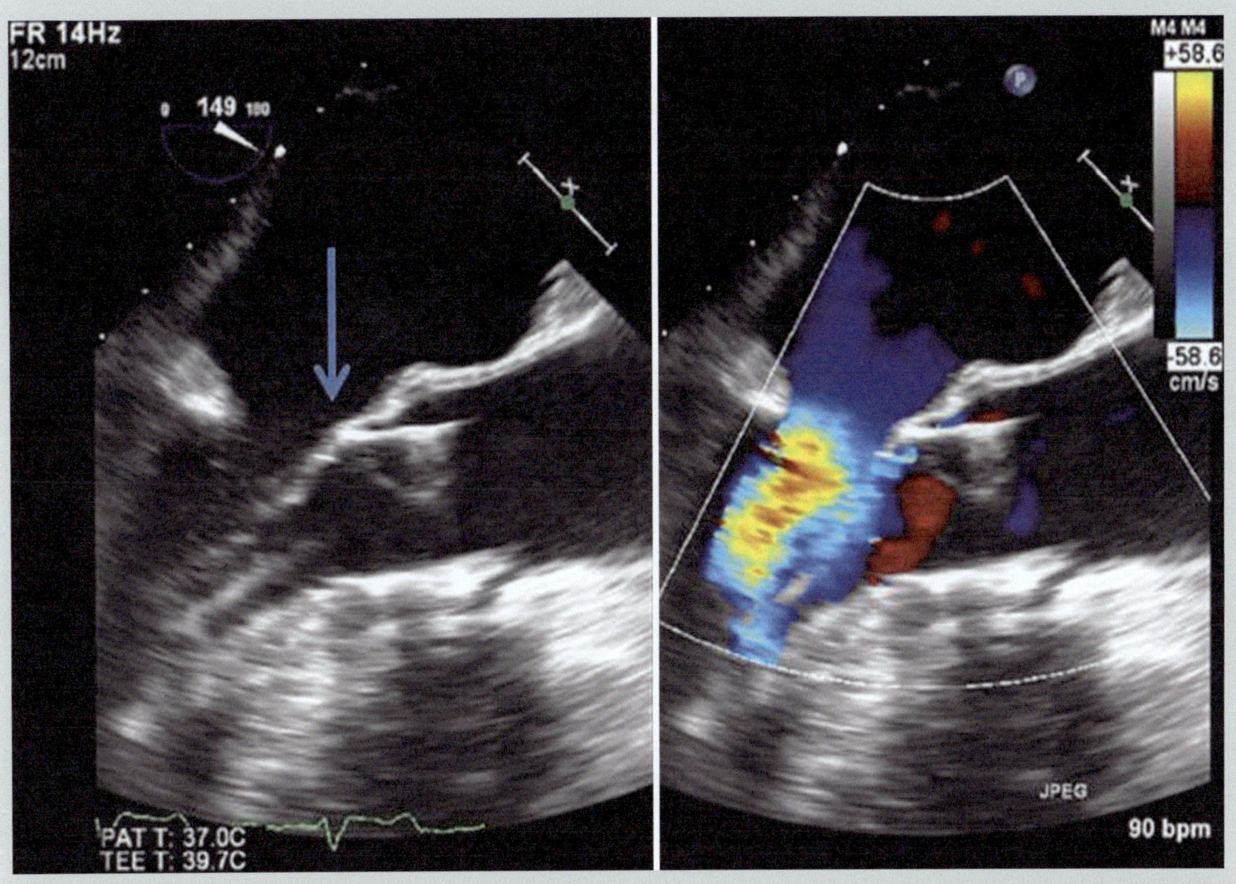

Fig. 35.12 *Arrow* shows where the anterior mitral leaflet comes into contact with the distal portion of the struts on the bioprosthetic aortic valve, restricting its motion

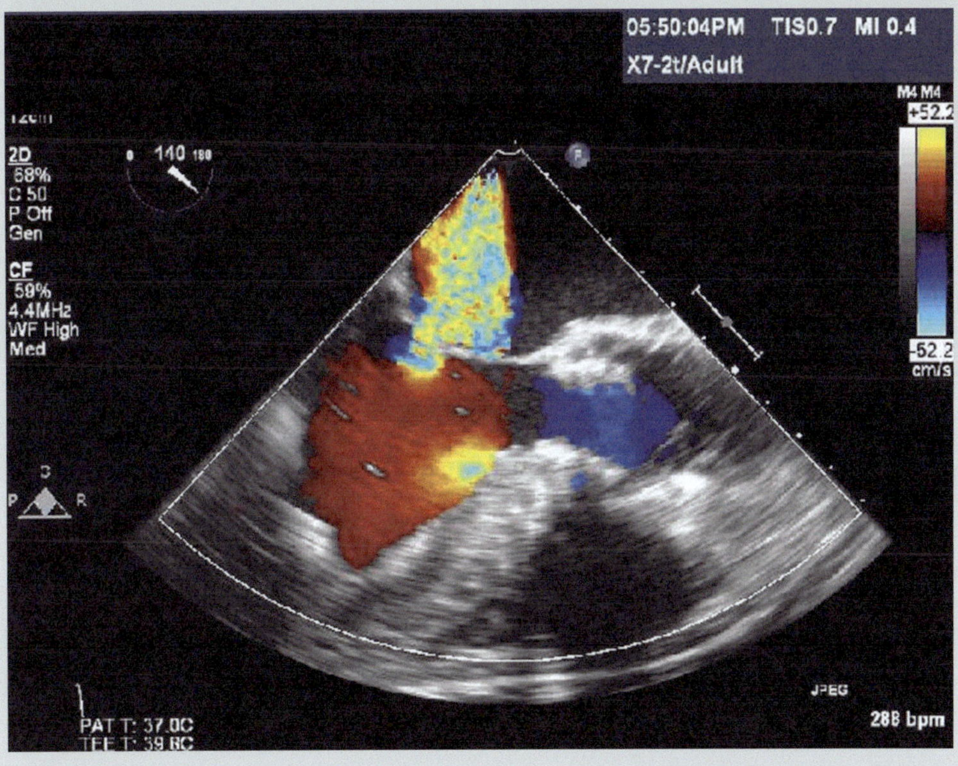

Fig. 35.13 A different patient with severe mitral regurgitation as a result of transient left ventricular dysfunction (stunning) after rapid ventricular pacing required for TAVR deployment

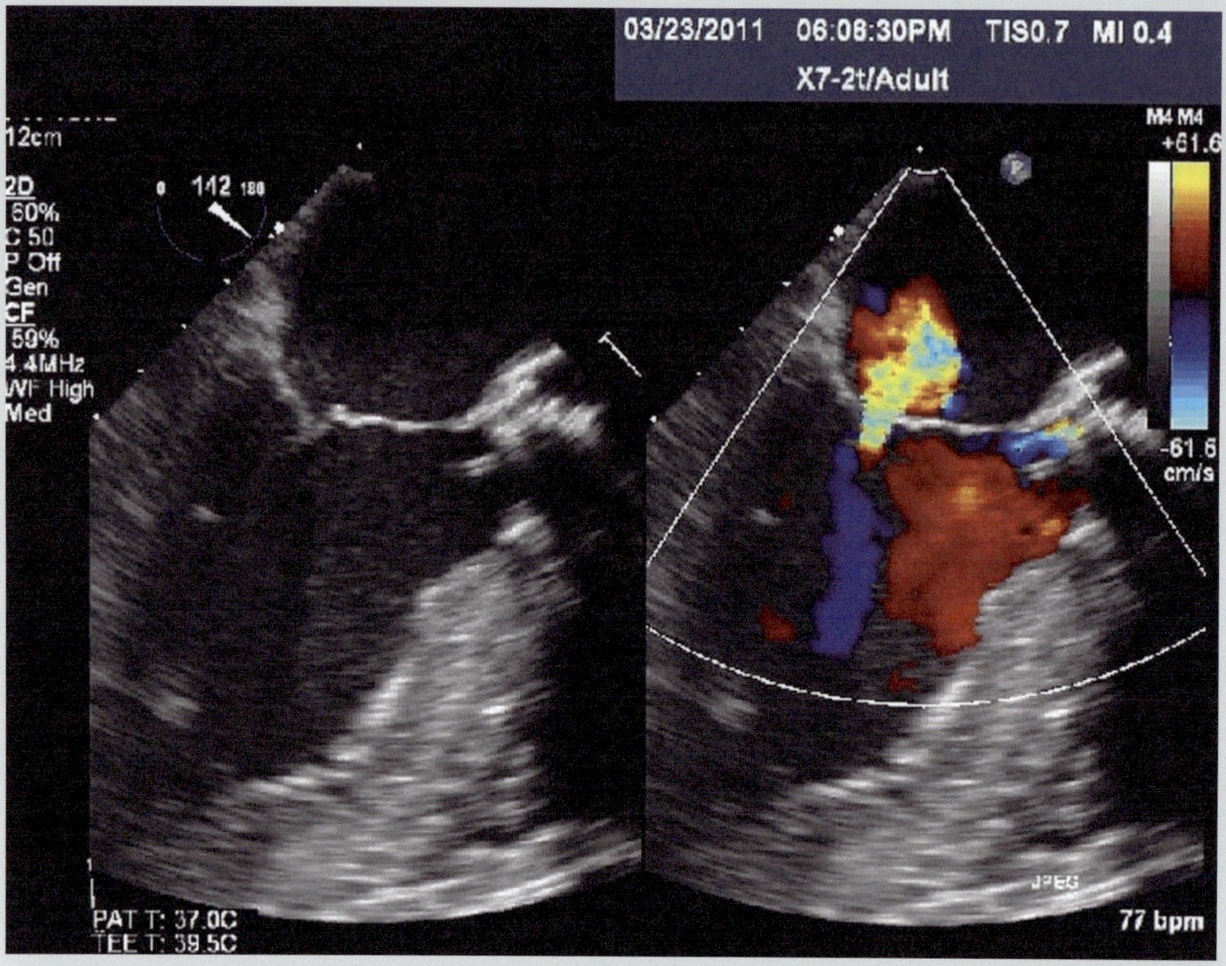

Fig. 35.14 Patient in Fig. 35.13 showing a marked decrease in mitral regurgitation after recovery of left ventricular function

Case 3: Aortic Root Hematoma

An extremely rare but serious complication of TAVR is aortic annulus rupture. This complication usually occurs during balloon valvuloplasty of the aortic valve or during valve deployment, with an incidence of aortic annular rupture of approximately 0.50 % [3, 4]. High-risk features that can predispose patients to aortic annular rupture include a heavily calcified aortic annulus or a narrow sinotubular junction. Correctly sizing these structures is of critical importance in limiting this complication. Efforts must be made to limit overdilating a small and calcified aortic annulus or sinotubular junction.

The consequences of aortic annulus rupture can be devastating, including death. It is possible to manage some of these patients conservatively with blood pressure control and reversing anticoagulation, but there are circumstances when they may need cardiopulmonary bypass in preparation for cardiothoracic surgical repair. This is a case of aortic root hematoma that was quickly noticed by TEE. The operator was able to limit its extent, preventing annular rupture and tamponade by aggressively controlling the patient's blood pressure and reversing anticoagulation.

Case 3: S.C

An 83-year-old female presented with history of severe aortic valve stenosis, coronary artery disease status post CABG, hypertension, hyperlipidemia, atrial fibrillation, and severe mitral regurgitation. TTE showed LVEF 50 %, mean AV gradient of 51 mmHg, AVA 0.5 cm^2, severe mitral regurgitation, and moderate-to-severe tricuspid regurgitation.

Patient Underwent

1. Balloon aortic valvuloplasty using 18 × 50 mm Z-MED II balloon
2. Transcatheter aortic valve replacement using 23-mm Edwards Sapien XT valve via femoral approach (Figs. 35.15, 35.16, and 35.17)

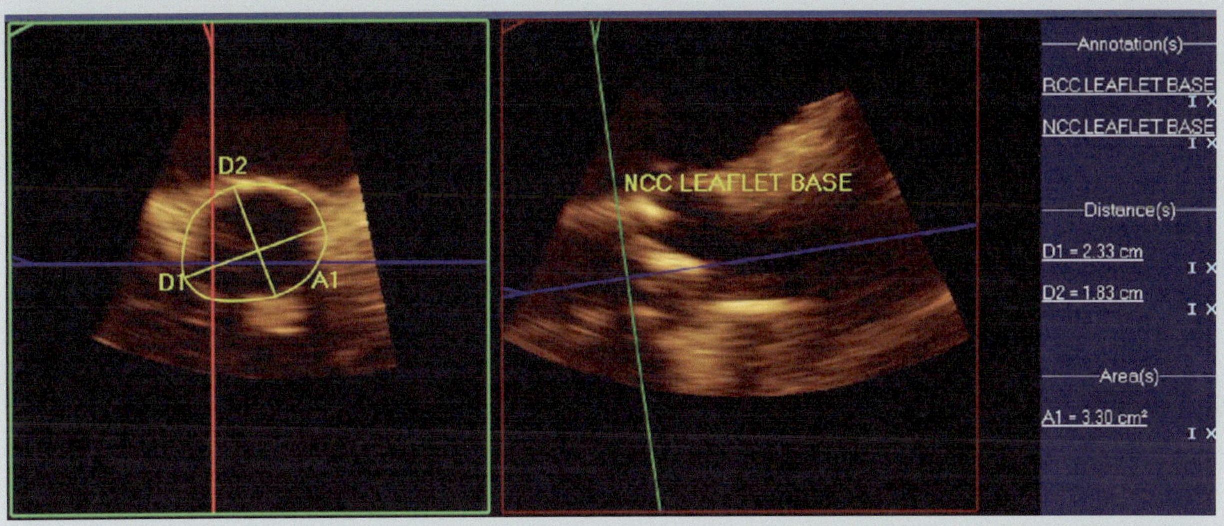

Fig. 35.15 Note the elliptical shape of the aortic annulus. The minor axis measured 1.8 cm and the major axis measured 2.3 cm

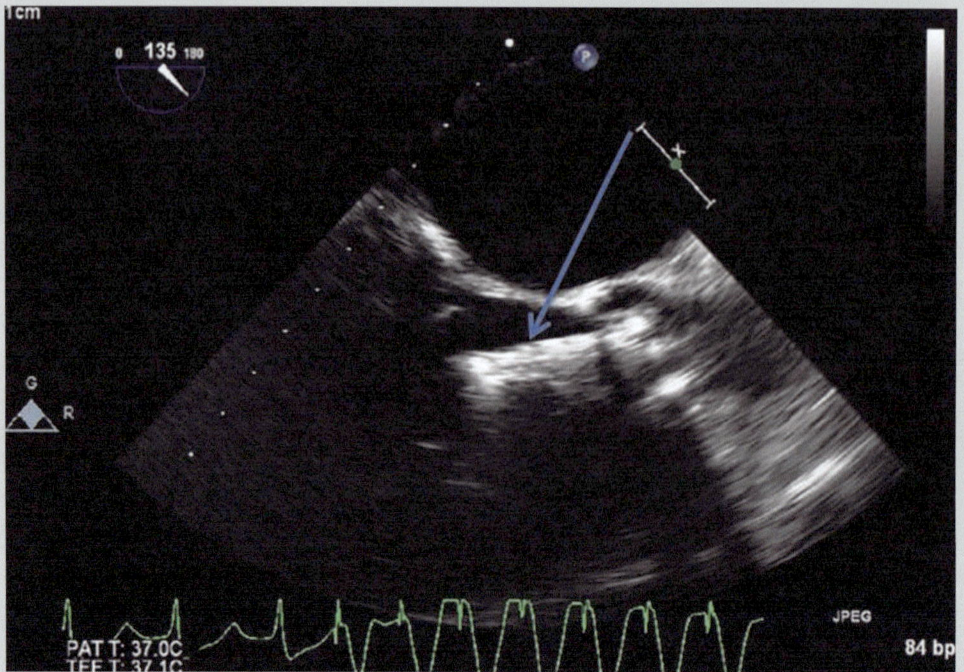

Fig. 35.16 Catheter across the aortic valve, immediately prior to Edwards Sapien valve deployment (*arrow*)

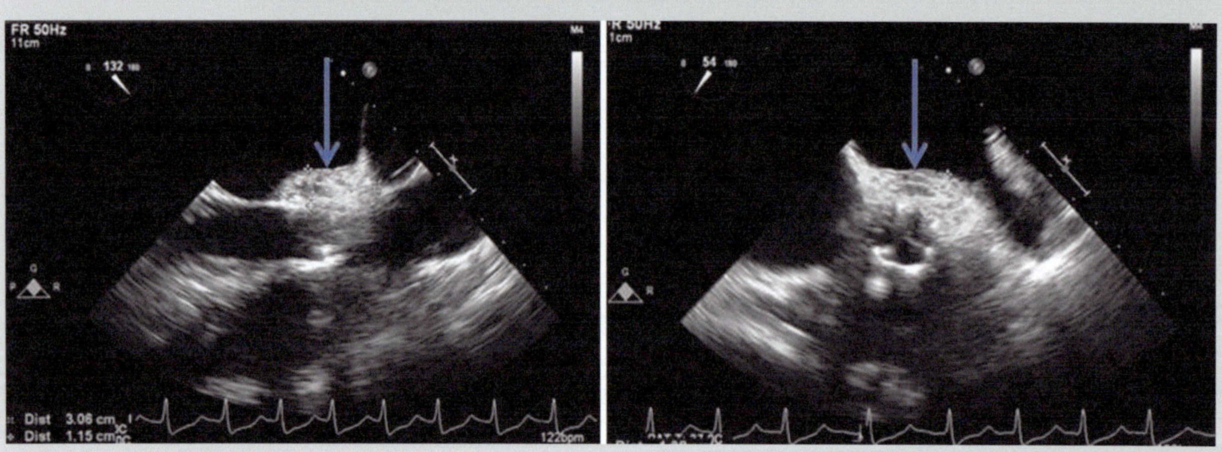

Fig. 35.17 Long axis of the aortic root hematoma (*arrows*), measuring 3.1 cm by 1.2 cm (*left*). Short axis of the aortic annulus (*right*)

Case 4: Left Main

The spatial relationship between the bioprosthetic valve and the coronary ostia is important because native leaflet calcium can be dislodged or displaced during valve deployment and lead to coronary artery obstruction. The incidence of coronary obstruction post TAVR is estimated to be approximately 0.70 %, and for acute myocardial infarction 0.56–1.1 %, depending on the meta-analysis cited [3, 4]. When patients have a preexisting ostial right coronary artery or left main (LM) stent, deployment of the bioprosthetic aortic valve can crush the stent and lead to coronary compromise. Protecting the coronary artery with a guide wire prior to valve deployment can help secure patency of the coronary. Appearance of new electrocardiographic changes, wall motion abnormalities, impaired coronary Doppler flow, or hemodynamic compromise following valve deployment should alert the operator to rule out coronary obstruction. This is a case of a patient with LM stenting who underwent TAVR, but the operator protected the LM stent with guide wires and performed a post TAVR balloon angioplasty of the LM stent.

Case 4: K.D

An 88-year-old female presented with a history of aortic stenosis, coronary artery disease, non-STEMI, status post left main stenting, hypertension, cerebrovascular disease, status post right carotid endarterectomy, hyperlipidemia, hypothyroidism, who underwent transcatheter aortic valve replacement. TTE showed LVEF 45 %, a mean AV gradient of 43 mmHg, and AVA 0.8 cm^2.

Patient Underwent

1. Balloon aortic valvuloplasty with a Z-MED 20×40 mm balloon
2. Transcatheter aortic valve implantation using a 23-mm Edwards Sapien valve via femoral approach
3. Left main balloon angioplasty (Figs. 35.18, 35.19, 35.20, and 35.21)

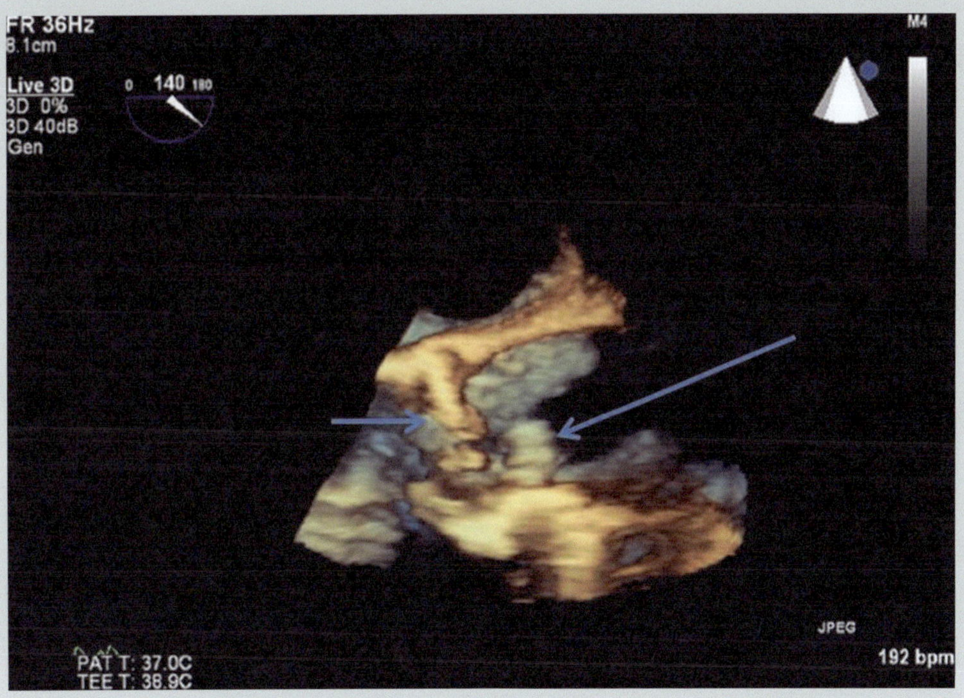

Fig. 35.18 Aortic valve (*short arrow*) and left main stent (*long arrow*)

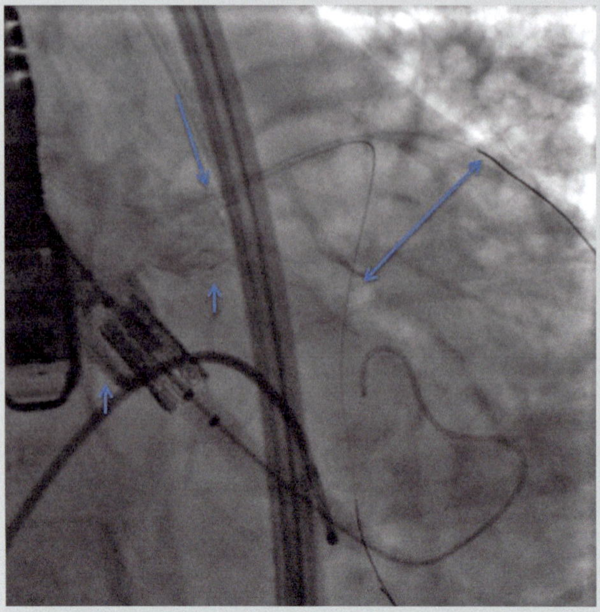

Fig. 35.19 Nonselective aortic root angiography. There are two balance wires advanced into the LAD and LCx coronary arteries (*double arrow heads*). Coronary cusps (*short arrows*) and left main stent (*long arrow*)

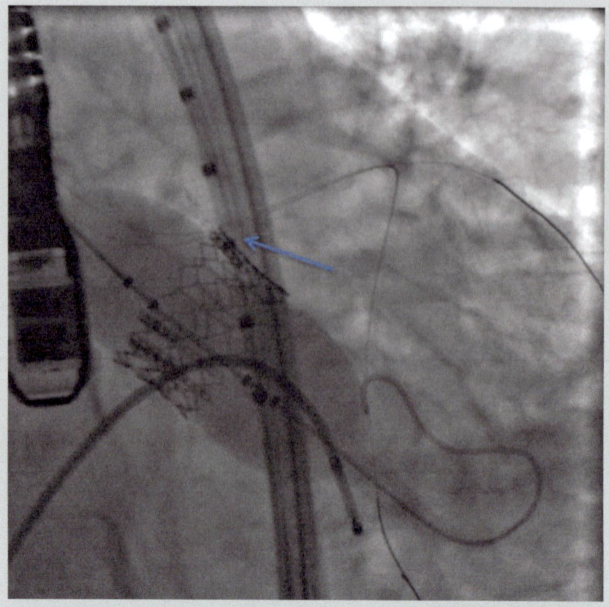

Fig. 35.20 Inferior aspect of left main stent (*arrow*)

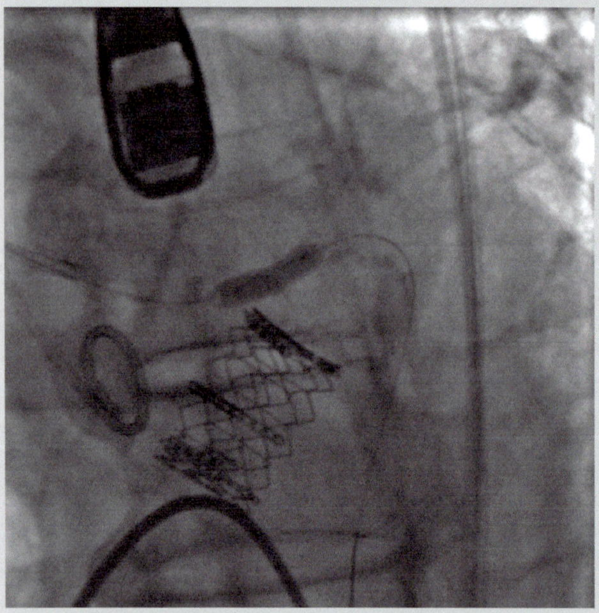

Fig. 35.21 Balloon angioplasty of left main after bioprosthetic valve deployment

Case 5: Embolized Valve

Correctly sizing the aortic annulus is of key importance because oversizing it can lead to aortic annulus rupture as previously noted, but undersizing can lead not only to paravalvular regurgitation but also to valve embolization. The incidence of valve embolization during TAVR can vary among sources, but it is estimated to be 0.56–1.7 % [3, 4]. High-risk features that can predispose to valve embolization include undersizing or malpositioning. This again underscores the importance of correctly measuring the aortic annulus and careful valve positioning using a combination of fluoroscopy and TEE. Once a bioprosthetic valve has embolized, if this is in the upward direction, it can be stabilized in the aorta. In contrast, downward embolization generally requires cardiothoracic surgical removal of the valve. This is an example of a bioprosthetic valve that was underexpanded and subsequently embolized upwards. The operator was able to fully expand the bioprosthetic valve in the aorta, secure it in place with a 10×40 mm Palmaz-Schatz stent, and deploy a second bioprosthetic aortic valve in the correct position.

Case 5: C.D

A 68-year-old female presented with a history of severe aortic stenosis, CHF, breast cancer, status post cobalt radiation and bilateral mastectomy in 1975, TIA, and diabetes mellitus. TTE showed a mean AV gradient of 48 mmHg and an AVA 0.7 cm^2.

Patient Underwent

1. Balloon aortic valvuloplasty with a Z-MED 20×50 mm balloon
2. Transcatheter aortic valve implantation using a 23-mm Edwards Sapien valve via femoral approach ×2 (Figs. 35.22, 35.23, 35.24, and 35.25)

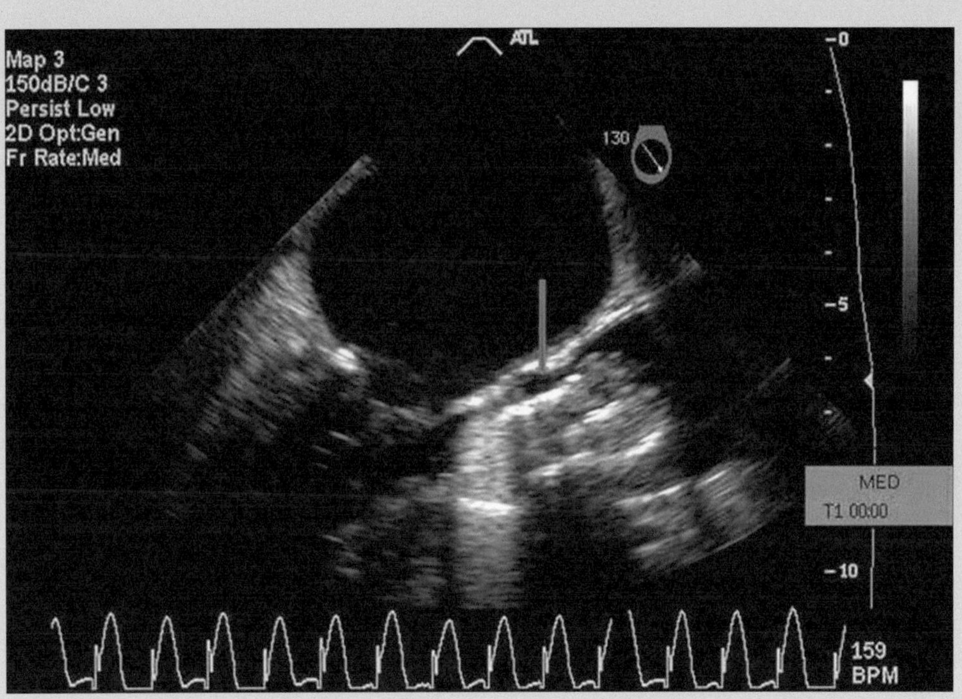

Fig. 35.22 Note the underdeployment of the aortic valve (*arrow*)

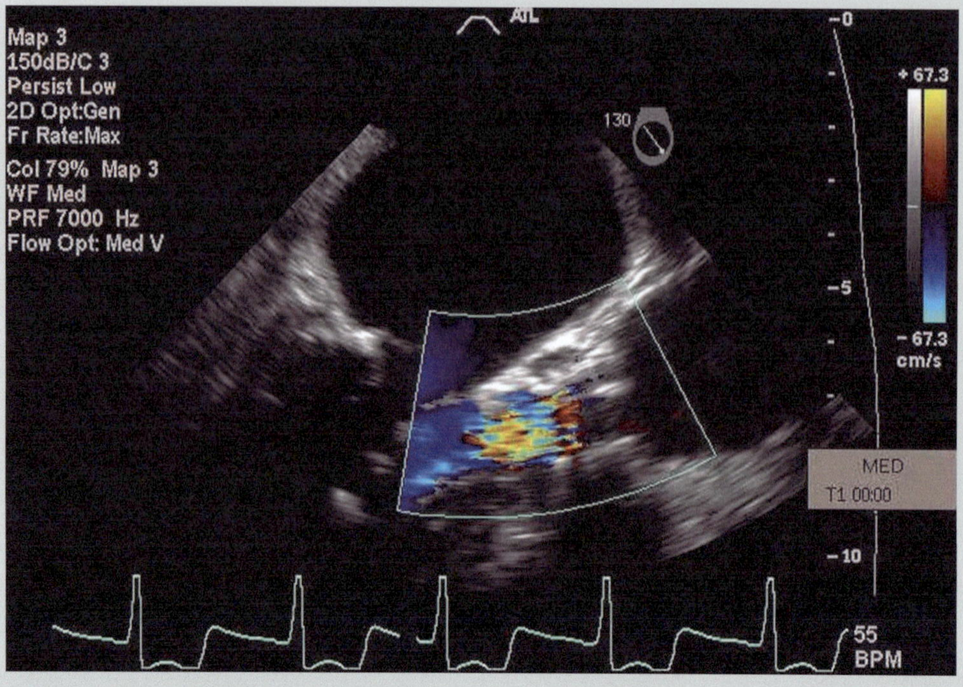

Fig. 35.23 Severe paravalvular aortic regurgitation

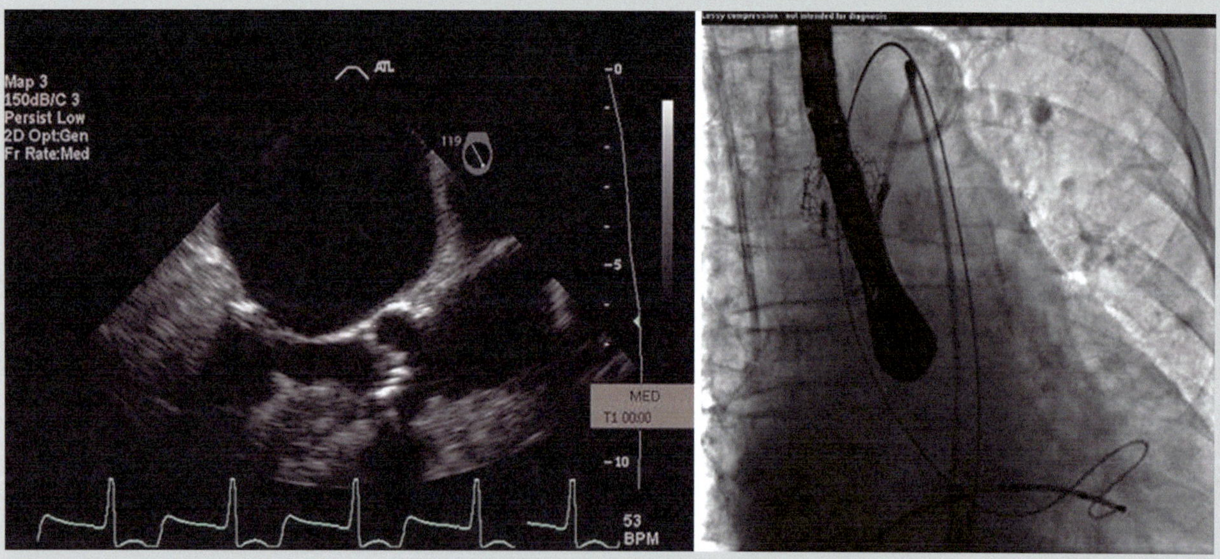

Fig. 35.24 Bioprosthetic is no longer visible as it has embolized (*left*). The fluoroscopic image shows the valve in the ascending aorta (*right*)

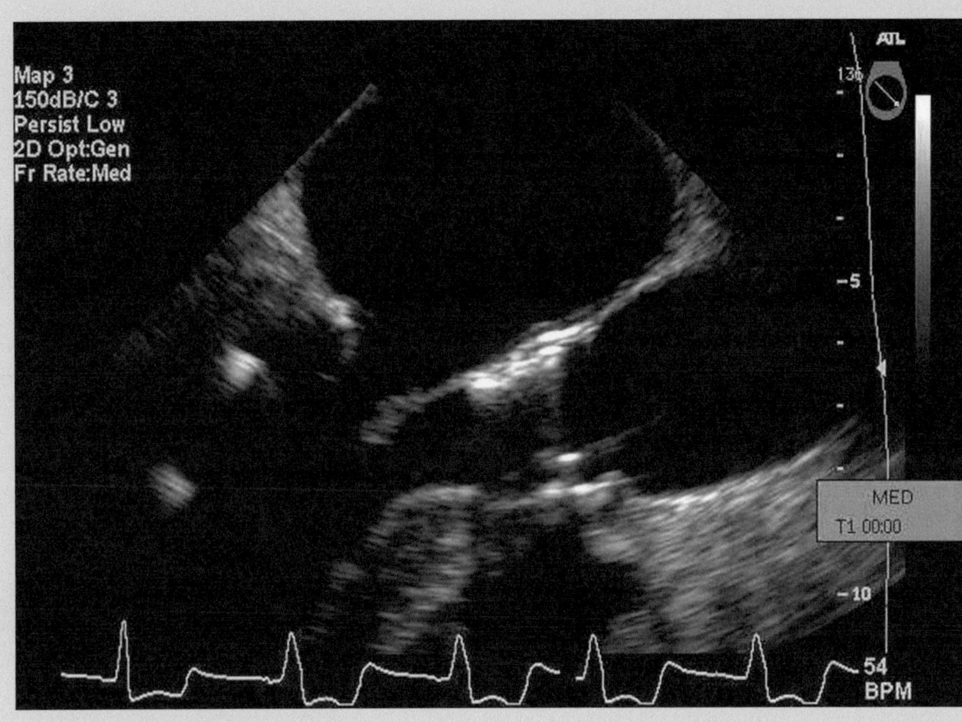

Fig. 35.25 A second bioprosthetic valve is deployed in the aortic annulus without complications

Case 6: Pericardial Tamponade

Another serious complication is the development of pericardial tamponade as a result of a guide wire perforation or from an aortic root dissection. The incidence of pericardial tamponade post TAVR varies among studies, but it is estimated to be 1.4–2.7 % and of aortic dissection 0.17–1.1 % [3, 4]. Putative risk factors for pericardial tamponade include a small left ventricular cavity, a heavily calcified aortic root complex associated with mitral annular calcification, or a small sinotubular junction. Patients that are especially predisposed to rupture appear to include those with radiation-induced aortic stenosis or a porcelain aorta.

Care with guide wire and pacing wire manipulation can reduce the risk of left and right ventricular perforation, respectively. In order to avoid aortic annular and root dissections, the operator avoids overexpanding the aortic annulus or the sinotubular junction. But once either of these complications has occurred, management typically includes reversing anticoagulation, lowering systolic blood pressure (if elevated), autotransfusion if pericardial blood is aspirated, and, if the former maneuvers are unsuccessful, cardiothoracic surgery.

A case of an aortic root dissection at the time of valve deployment is presented. Unfortunately, the patient expired despite the use of emergent cardiopulmonary bypass.

Case 6: S.F

A 66-year-old female presented with history of Hodgkin lymphoma, status post radiation in 1968, hypertension, and hyperlipidemia. TTE showed LVEF 59 %, mean AV gradient of 41 mmHg, and AVA 0.51 cm^2.

Patient Underwent

1. Balloon aortic valvuloplasty using 18×40 mm Z-MED II balloon
2. Transcatheter aortic valve replacement using 23-mm Edwards Sapien XT valve via femoral approach (Figs. 35.26, 35.27, and 35.28)

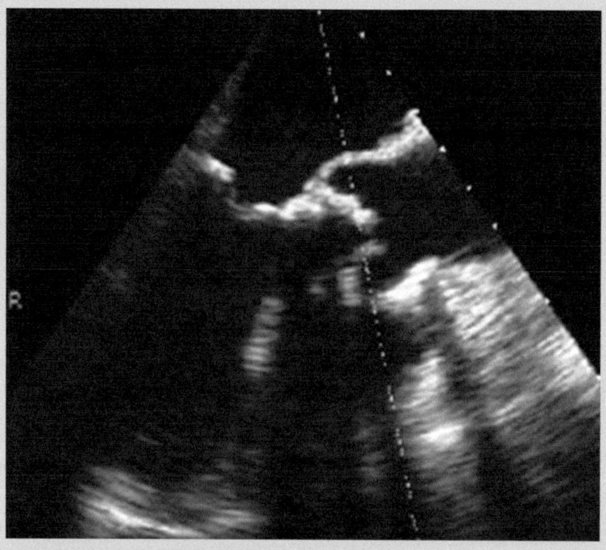

Fig. 35.26 Heavily calcified aortic valve and left ventricular outflow tract prior to valve deployment

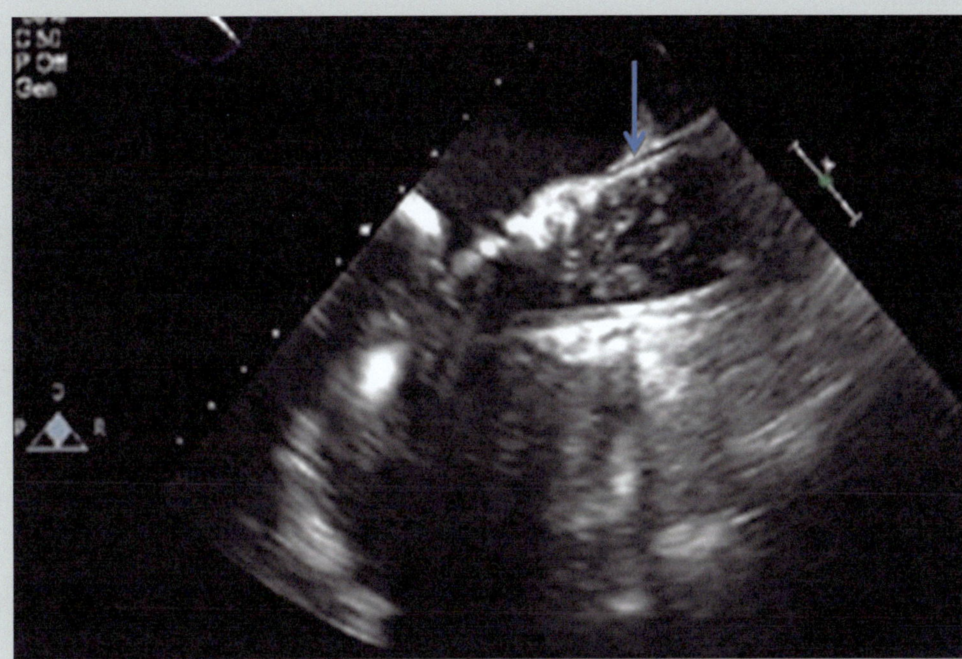

Fig. 35.27 *Arrow* points to a thin *black line* illustrating an aortic annulus rupture that lead to an aortic root dissection after the bioprosthetic valve was deployed

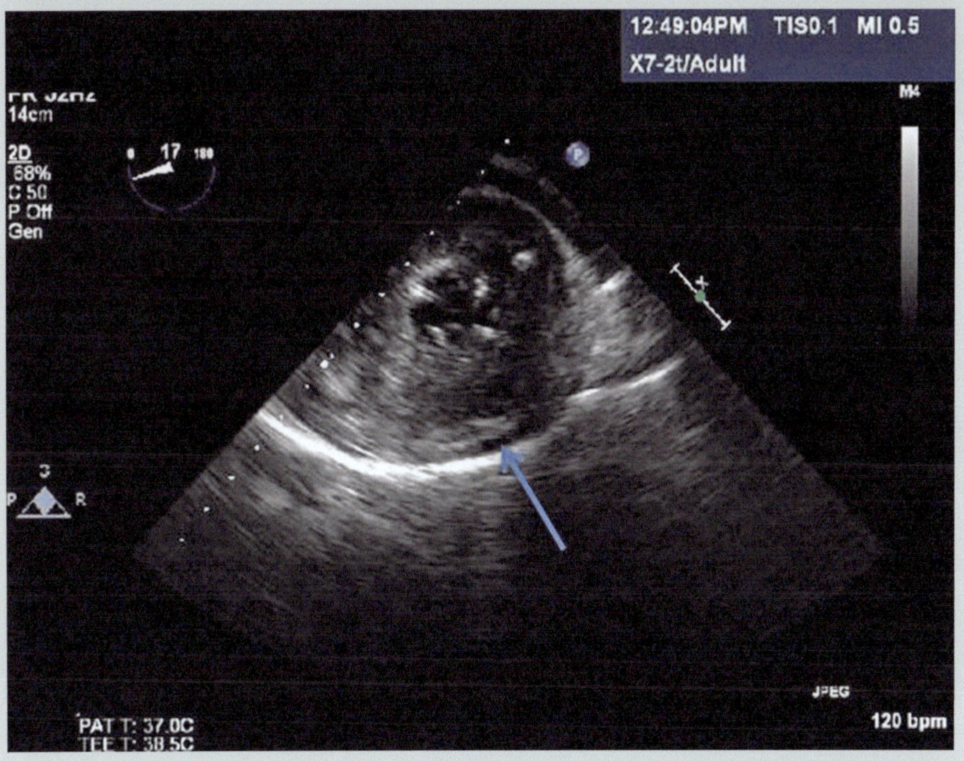

Fig. 35.28 The aortic annulus rupture produced a pericardial effusion (*arrow*) that evolved into pericardial tamponade. Patient could not be resuscitated despite rapid institution of cardiopulmonary bypass

References

1. Moss RR, Ivens E, Pasupati S, Humphries K, Thompson CR, Munt B, et al. Role of echocardiography in percutaneous aortic valve implantation. JACC Cardiovasc Imaging. 2008;1(1):15–24. PubMed PMID: 19356400. Epub 2008/01/01. eng.
2. Kodali SK, Williams MR, Smith CR, Svensson LG, Webb JG, Makkar RR, et al. Two-year outcomes after transcatheter or surgical aortic-valve replacement. N Engl J Med. 2012;366(18):1686–95. PubMed PMID: 22443479. Epub 2012/03/27. eng.
3. Genereux P, Head SJ, Van Mieghem NM, Kodali S, Kirtane AJ, Xu K, et al. Clinical outcomes after transcatheter aortic valve replacement using valve academic research consortium definitions: a weighted meta-analysis of 3,519 patients from 16 studies. J Am Coll Cardiol. 2012;59:2317–26.
4. Jilaihawi H, Chakravarty T, Weiss RE, Fontana GP, Forrester J, Makkar RR. Meta-analysis of complications in aortic valve replacement: comparison of Medtronic-Corevalve, Edwards-Sapien and surgical aortic valve replacement in 8,536 patients. Catheter Cardiovasc Interv. 2012;80(1):128–38. PubMed PMID: 22415849. Epub 2012/03/15. eng.
5. Tamburino C, Capodanno D, Ramondo A, Petronio AS, Ettori F, Santoro G, et al. Incidence and predictors of early and late mortality after transcatheter aortic valve implantation in 663 patients with severe aortic stenosis. Circulation. 2011;123(3):299–308. PubMed PMID: 21220731. Epub 2011/01/12. eng.
6. Koos R, Mahnken AH, Dohmen G, Brehmer K, Gunther RW, Autschbach R, et al. Association of aortic valve calcification severity with the degree of aortic regurgitation after transcatheter aortic valve implantation. Int J Cardiol. 2011;150:142–5.
7. Haensig M, Lehmkuhl L, Rastan AJ, Kempfert J, Mukherjee C, Gutberlet M, et al. Aortic valve calcium scoring is a predictor of significant paravalvular aortic insufficiency in transapical-aortic valve implantation. Eur J Cardiothorac Surg. 2012;41:1234–40; discussion 40–1.
8. Colli A, D'Amico R, Kempfert J, Borger MA, Mohr FW, Walther T. Transesophageal echocardiographic scoring for transcatheter aortic valve implantation: impact of aortic cusp calcification on postoperative aortic regurgitation. J Thorac Cardiovasc Surg. 2011;142:1229–35.
9. Detaint D, Lepage L, Himbert D, Brochet E, Messika-Zeitoun D, Iung B, et al. Determinants of significant paravalvular regurgitation after transcatheter aortic valve: implantation impact of device and annulus discongruence. JACC Cardiovasc Interv. 2009;2:821–7.
10. Rodes-Cabau J, Dumont E, Doyle D. "Valve-in-valve" for the treatment of paravalvular leaks following transcatheter aortic valve implantation. Catheter Cardiovasc Interv. 2009;74(7):1116–9. PubMed PMID: 19626691. Epub 2009/07/25. eng.

Structural and Hemodynamic Integrity of the Implanted TAVR Valve

36

Philippe Pibarot, Rebecca T. Hahn, and Jean G. Dumesnil

Abstract

Careful follow-up of prosthetic valve position, morphology, and function after transcatheter aortic valve replacement (TAVR) is key for early detection and optimal management of complications. The purpose of this chapter is to provide an overview of the current state of knowledge and future perspectives with regard to the role of multimodality imaging in the evaluation of the structural and hemodynamic integrity of the implanted transcatheter heart valve (THV). The goals of post-implant imaging are the following: (1) *structural evaluation*, including assessment of valve stent deployment and position and of valve cusps morphology and mobility; (2) *functional evaluation* including measurement of transprosthetic gradients, valve effective orifice area (EOA), and Doppler velocity index, and quantification of valvular an paravalvular regurgitation; and (3) *detection of late complications* such as migration of the prosthesis, formation of pannus or thrombus, impingement of the mitral valve, perforation of the ventricular septum, and endocarditis.

Keywords

Aortic valve • Transcatheter heart valve • Stenosis • Regurgitation Doppler echocardiography • Computed tomography • Cardiac magnetic resonance

P. Pibarot, DVM, PhD, FACC, FAHA, FASE, FESC (✉)
Department of Cardiology, Institut Universitaire de Cardiologie et de Pneumologie de Québec, Québec Heart and Lung Institute, 2725 Chemin Sainte-Foy, Québec, QC G1V-4G5, Canada
e-mail: philippe.pibarot@med.ulaval.ca

R.T. Hahn, MD, FACC, FASE
Department of Medicine, Columbia University Medical Center, New York-Presbyterian Hospital, 161 Fort Washington Avenue, HIP 6-623, New York 10032, USA
e-mail: rth2@columbia.edu

J.G. Dumesnil, OQ, MD, FRCPC, FACC, FASE (Hon)
Department of Cardiology, Quebec Heart and Lung Institute, Laval University, 2725 Chemin Sainte-Foy, Quebec, QC G1V 4G5, Canada
e-mail: jean.dumesnil@med.ulaval.ca

Abbreviations

CMR	Cardiac magnetic resonance
DVI	Doppler velocity index
EOA	Effective orifice area
LA	Left atrium
LV	Left ventricle
LVOT	Left ventricular outflow tract
MDCT	Multidetector computed tomography
RV	Right ventricle
SAVR	Surgical aortic valve replacement
TAVR	Transcatheter aortic valve replacement
THV	Transcatheter heart valve
TTE	Transthoracic echocardiography
TEE	Transesophageal echocardiography
TVI	Time-velocity integral

J.K. Min et al. (eds.), *Multimodality Imaging for Transcatheter Aortic Valve Replacement*, DOI 10.1007/978-1-4471-2798-7_36, © Springer-Verlag London 2014

Introduction

Careful follow-up of prosthetic valve position, morphology, and function after transcatheter aortic valve replacement (TAVR) is key for early detection and optimal management of complications. The purpose of this chapter is to provide an overview of the current state of knowledge and future perspectives with regard to the role of multimodality imaging in the evaluation of the structural and hemodynamic integrity of the implanted transcatheter heart valve (THV). The goals of post-implant imaging are the following: (1) *structural evaluation*, including assessment of valve stent deployment and position and of valve cusps morphology and mobility; (2) *functional evaluation* including measurement of transprosthetic gradients, valve effective orifice area (EOA), and Doppler velocity index, and quantification of valvular an paravalvular regurgitation; and (3) *detection of late complications* such as migration of the prosthesis, formation of pannus or thrombus, impingement of the mitral valve, perforation of the ventricular septum, and endocarditis.

Owing to its versatile, noninvasive, radiation-free, and low-cost nature, Doppler echocardiography is the method of choice to evaluate prosthetic valve structure and function after surgical or transcatheter aortic valve replacement. The Doppler echocardiographic evaluation of THVs follows the same principles used for the evaluation of native or surgical prosthetic valves with some important specifics and caveats described in this chapter [1–5]. Three-dimensional echocardiography may also provide incremental information for the measurement of the size of the LV outflow tract (LVOT) and the quantification of paravalvular regurgitation [3, 6, 7]. Although Doppler echocardiography is the primary imaging modality to evaluate prosthetic valve morphology and hemodynamic performance after TAVR, other imaging modalities may be useful to detect and quantify valve dysfunction [3, 4]. Multidetector computed tomography (MDCT) may provide superior image quality to assess the position and deployment of the prosthesis stent and to detect the presence of pannus [3, 4, 8–10], whereas cardiac magnetic resonance imaging (CMR) allows accurate quantification of prosthetic valve regurgitation.

Timing of Imaging Follow-Up After TAVR

A baseline postoperative transthoracic echocardiographic (TTE) study should be performed before hospital discharge. In patients who underwent TAVR with the use of the transapical or transaortic approach, it may be preferable to perform the baseline TTE at the first follow-up visit, 3–12 weeks after TAVR, when the chest wound has healed [1, 5, 11]. The acquisition of a baseline TTE at discharge and/or at 3–12 weeks is essential to assess the stability of prosthetic valve position, morphology, and function over time. This baseline echocardiographic exam indeed provides a description of the structural and hemodynamic status of the valve early after TAVR and can be used as a reference to interpret the findings of the subsequent echocardiographic exams at late follow-up.

Given that TAVR is a relatively new technology and that there is very few data about the durability of the morphology and function of THVs [12, 13], it is recommended to perform serial echocardiographic follow-up at 3–6 months after TAVR, 1 year, and then annually [1, 3, 5, 11]. Furthermore, any change in clinical status should prompt the realization of a TTE, regardless of the timing of the planned follow-up.

Multidetector row computed tomography (MDCT) imaging of the valve may be obtained prior to discharge or at 3–12 weeks post-implant. Moreover, MDCT should be performed whenever there is a suspicion of device migration and/or deterioration of valve structure or function during follow-up. Cardiac magnetic resonance (CMR) imaging may be used to corroborate the severity of prosthetic valve regurgitation, especially when a change in the clinical status, a dilation of the LV, and/or a decline in LV systolic function occur during follow-up

Structural Evaluation

The structural evaluation of the THVs should include the assessment of the deployment and position of the prosthesis stent, the evaluation of the morphology and mobility of the valve cusps, and the detection of pannus, thrombus, or masses within or in the vicinity of the prosthesis stent.

Assessment of THV Stent Deployment and Position

The adequacy of the position and deployment of the prosthesis stent can be assessed by TTE in the left parasternal short- and long-axis views. However, MDCT is superior to echocardiography for the assessment of the position, expansion, circularity/eccentricity, and structural integrity of the prosthesis stent [3, 4, 8, 10]. Three-dimensional echocardiographic imaging might be useful for post-THV evaluation, and its value will need be investigated in future studies.

THV Position

The position of the THV relative to the aortic annulus plane is evaluated by measuring the distance between the lower rim of the prosthesis stent and the aortic annulus. In balloon-expandable THVs, the position of the stent relative to the coronary ostia is determined by measuring the distance between the upper rim of the stent and the left and right coronary ostia (Fig. 36.1) [8]. With TTE, it is more difficult to identify the aortic annulus after TAVR as well as the

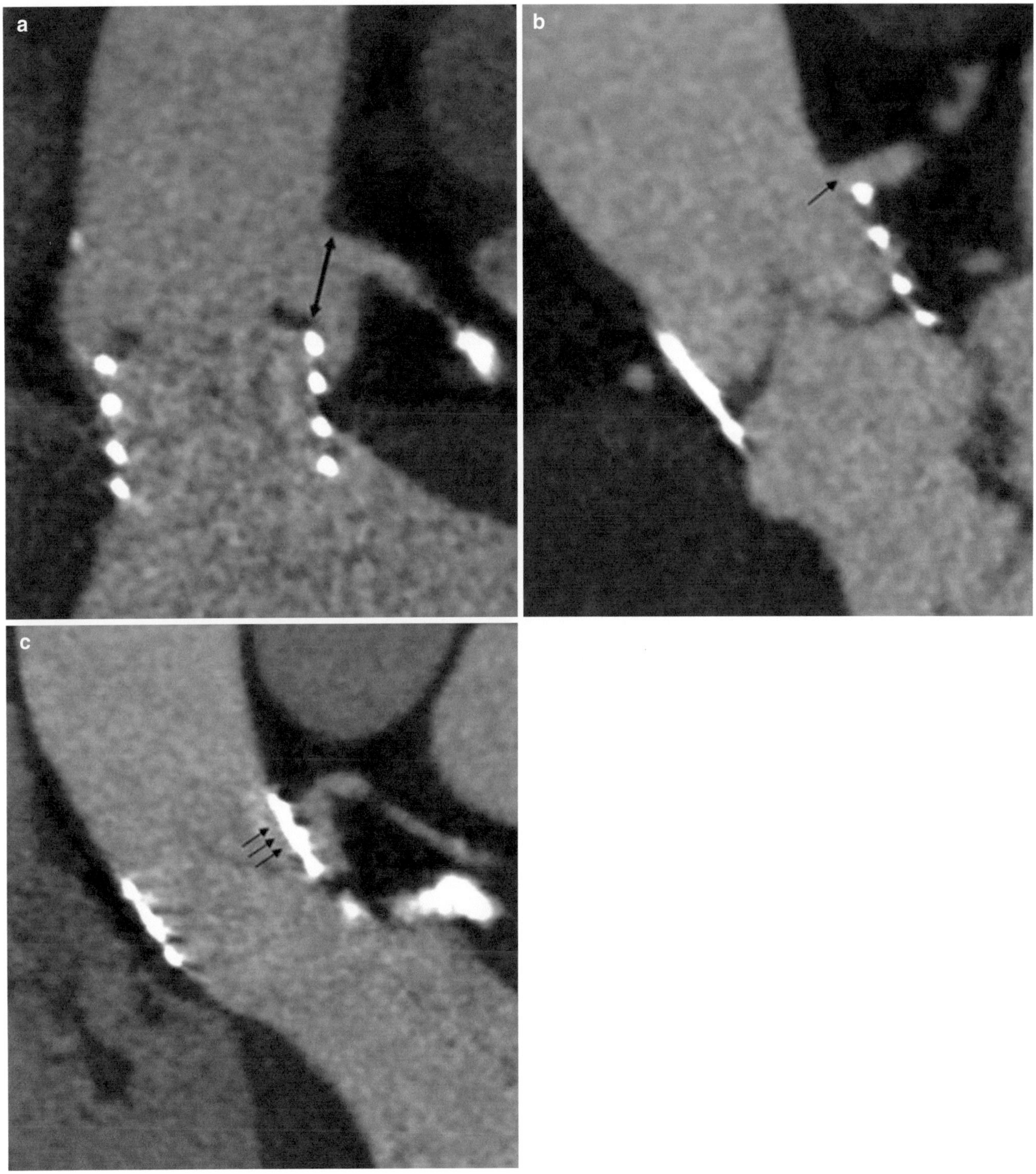

Fig. 36.1 Assessment of prosthesis positioning relative to the left coronary ostium and aortic annulus by MDCT. MDCT enables the visualization of the position of the prosthetic valve in relation to the aortic annulus and left coronary ostium: below the coronary ostium (**a**), at the same level of the coronary ostium (**b**), or overpassing the height of the coronary ostium (Reproduced with permission from [8]) (**c**)

coronary ostia. The position of the stent can be assessed and monitored over time by measuring the distance between the lower rim of the stent and the hinge point of the anterior mitral leaflet in the long-axis view. Rarely, a low-positioned stent may result in native leaflet "overhang" with the uncovered tip of the coronary cusp causing abnormal THV flow (Fig. 36.2). Although very rare, some cases of late migration and embolization of the prosthesis have been reported following TAVR (Fig. 36.3) [14]. The migration may occur toward the LV or toward the aorta (Fig. 36.4).

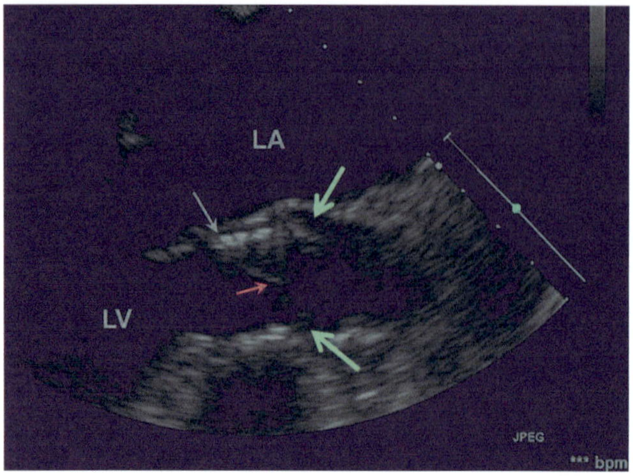

Fig. 36.2 Low-positioned THV with native leaflet "overhang". The TEE long-axis view shows a low position of the THV (*white arrow*) with the uncovered cusps of the native valve (*yellow arrows*) overhanging above the distal rim of the THV stent. *Red arrow* indicates the THV cusp. *LA* left atrium, *LV* left ventricle

Undersizing and/or malpositioning of the THV are thought to predispose to migration/embolization of the valve.

THV Expansion

The adequacy of THV expansion can be assessed by calculating the ratio of the MDCT-derived external area of the valve stent to the nominal external area of the THV, expressed in percent (Fig. 36.5) [8, 10]. An underexpanded valve is defined as having an expansion ratio of ≤90 %. In a recent study, Willson et al. found that 8 % of patients have underexpanded valves following TAVR with balloon-expandable THV. Underexpansion occurred predominantly at the inflow level. Valve underexpansion may be associated with prosthetic valve stenosis or regurgitation [10].

THV Eccentricity or Circularity

The minimum external diameter, maximum external diameter, and external valve area are measured by MDCT at three cross-sectional levels: inflow, mid-stent, and

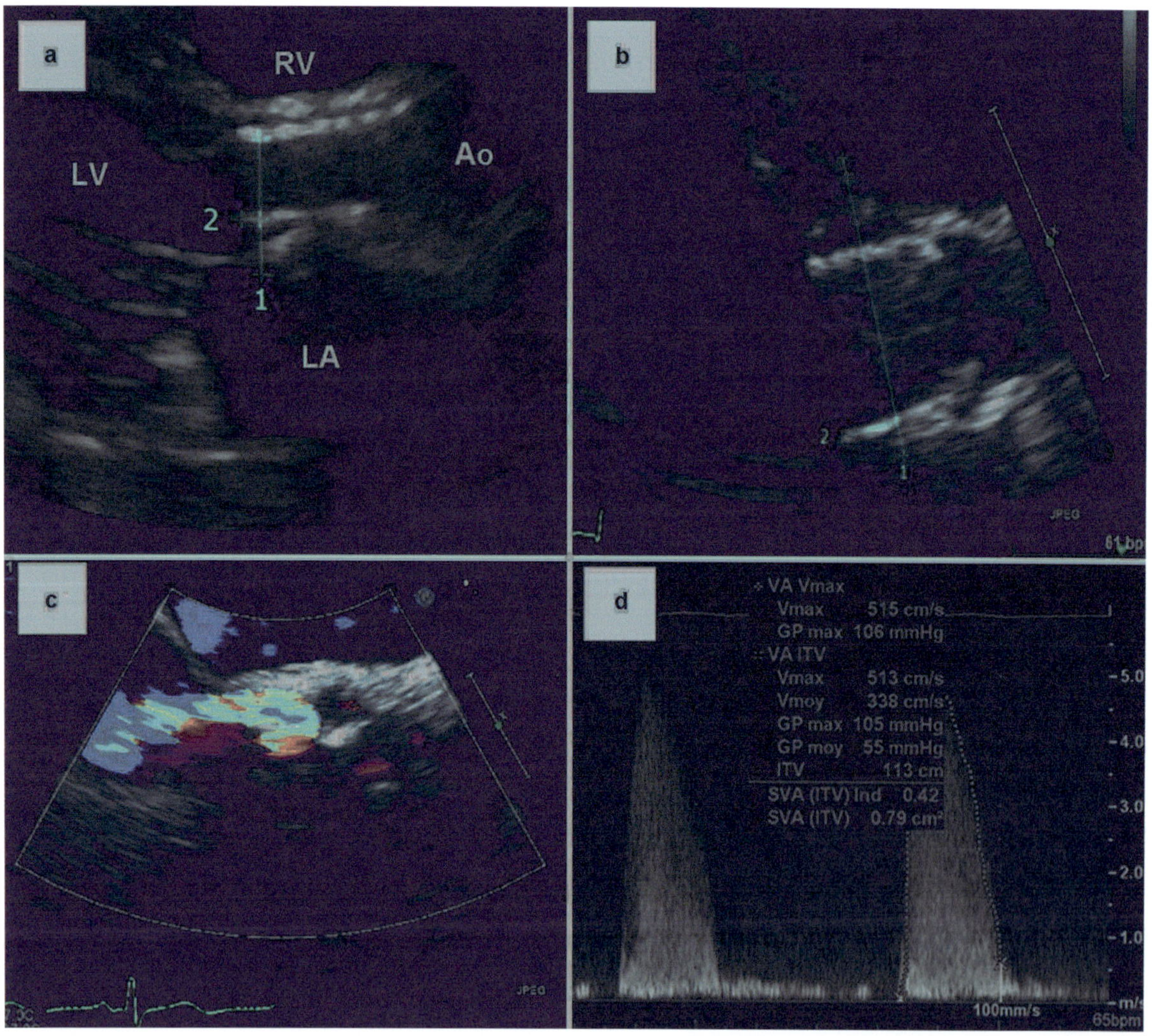

Fig. 36.3 Late migration of a balloon-expandable THV. These Doppler echocardiographic images show the case of a late (4 months post-TAVR) migration of a balloon-expandable SAPIEN THV toward the LV outflow tract. Panels (**a**) and (**b**) show the displacement of the valve predischarge to 4-month follow-up. The distance between the apical end of the stent (*1*) and the hinge point of the anterior mitral leaflet (*2*) increased from 3.2 to 9.6 mm between the two echocardiograms. Other images obtained at 4-month post-TAVR reveal a moderate paravalvular regurgitation (Panel **c**) and a high mean transprosthetic gradient (55 mmHg, Panel **d**). *Ao* aorta, *LA* left atrium, *LV* left ventricle, *RV* right ventricle

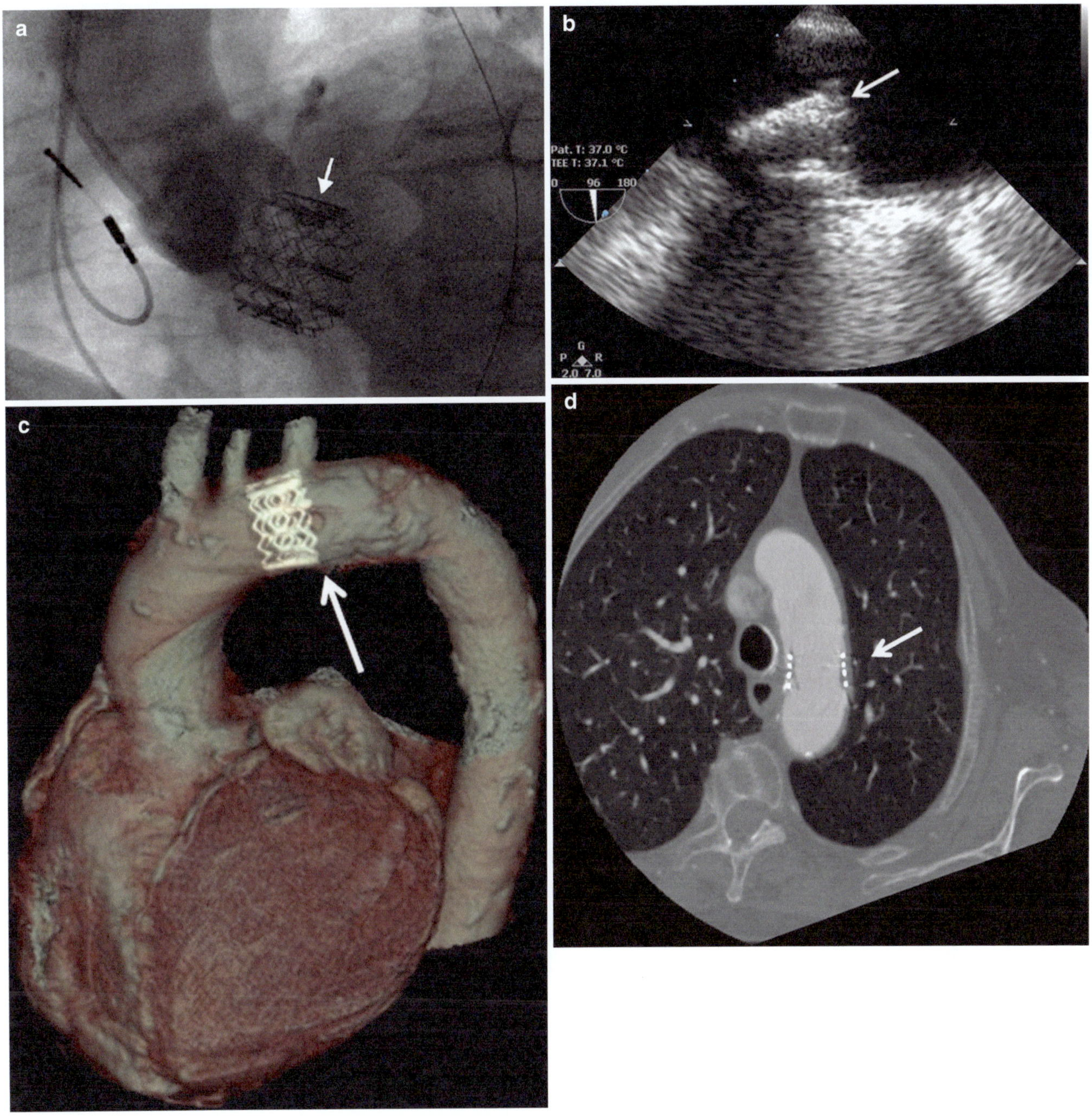

Fig. 36.4 Embolization of THVs assessed by multimodality imaging. Panel (**a**): Cinefluoroscopic image of a THV migration in the LV outflow tract (Reproduced with permission from [14]); Panel (**b**): TTE image of a THV embolization in the proximal descending aorta visualized; Panels (**c**) and (**d**): MDCT images of THV embolization in the aortic arch (Courtesy of Dr Jonathon Leipsic, St Paul Hospital, Vancouver). The *white arrows* indicate the THV

outflow. THV eccentricity is calculated as 100 × (1–minimum external stent diameter/maximum external stent diameter). Noncircular deployment of THV is generally defined as an eccentricity >10 %. In balloon-expandable THVs, earlier studies reported that about 15 % of patients have noncircular deployment [8], whereas more recent studies reported <5 % of THV noncircularity [10]. The patients with noncircular deployment of the stent more often have larger aortic annulus and more calcified native valves (Fig. 36.6) [8]. The presence of large bulky calcifications at the level of the native valve cusps, aortic annulus, or LV outflow tract (LVOT) may predispose to a less circular deployment of the stent and thus to prosthetic valve regurgitation or stenosis (Figs. 36.6 and 36.7). Noncircular deployment of the stent might also reduce the durability of the valve due to increased mechanical stress upon the valve cusps.

Structural Integrity of the THV Stent and Surrounding Structures

Structural integrity of the THV stent can be assessed by MDCT or cinefluoroscopy. Until now, there has been no

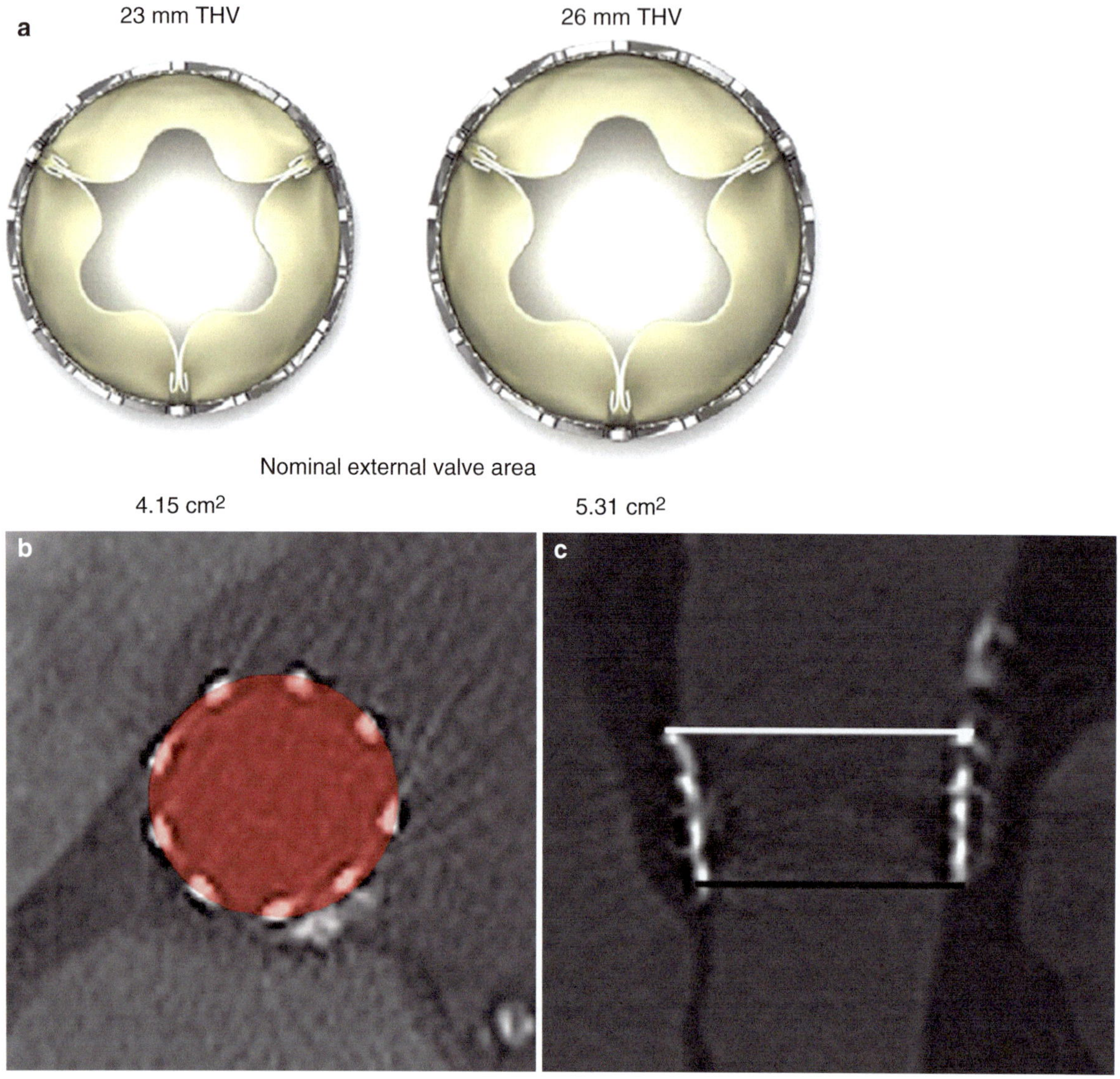

Fig. 36.5 THV expansion as assessed by MDCT. (**a**) Nominal external valve area of the 23- and 26-mm balloon-expandable SAPIEN valves. (**b**) THV expansion is calculated by dividing MDCT-derived external valve area by nominal external valve area. (**c**) A SAPIEN 26-mm valve underexpanded at the inflow with increasing expansion toward the outflow level (inflow external valve area = 460 mm^2, inflow expansion = 86.5 %, outflow external valve area = 597 mm^2, outflow expansion: 112.4 %) (Reproduced with permission from [10])

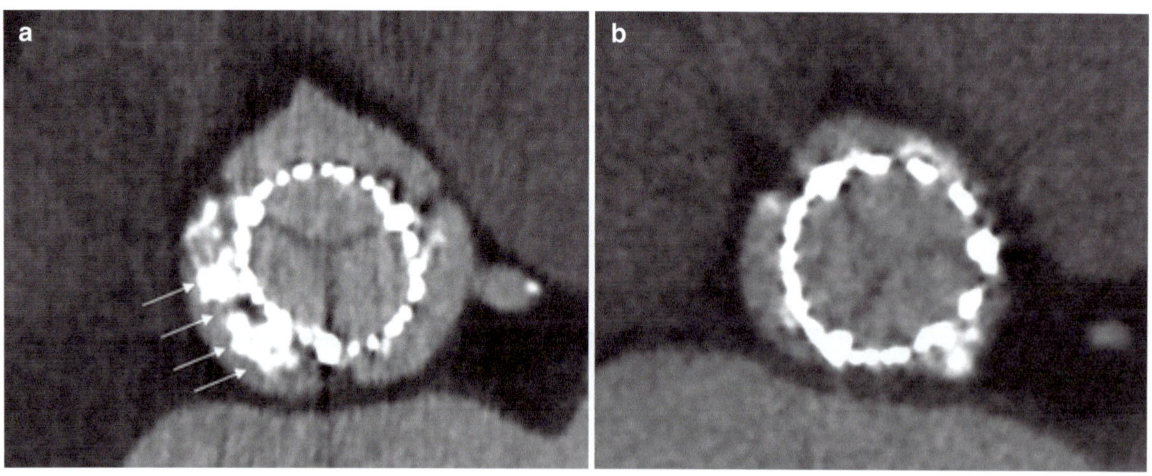

Fig. 36.6 THV deployment as assessed by MDCT. MDCT is helpful to evaluate THV prosthesis deployment. Panel (**a**) should a noncircular deployment of the valve associated with heavily, bulky calcified native aortic cusps. Panel (**b**) shows circular deployment of the valve (Reproduced with permission from [4])

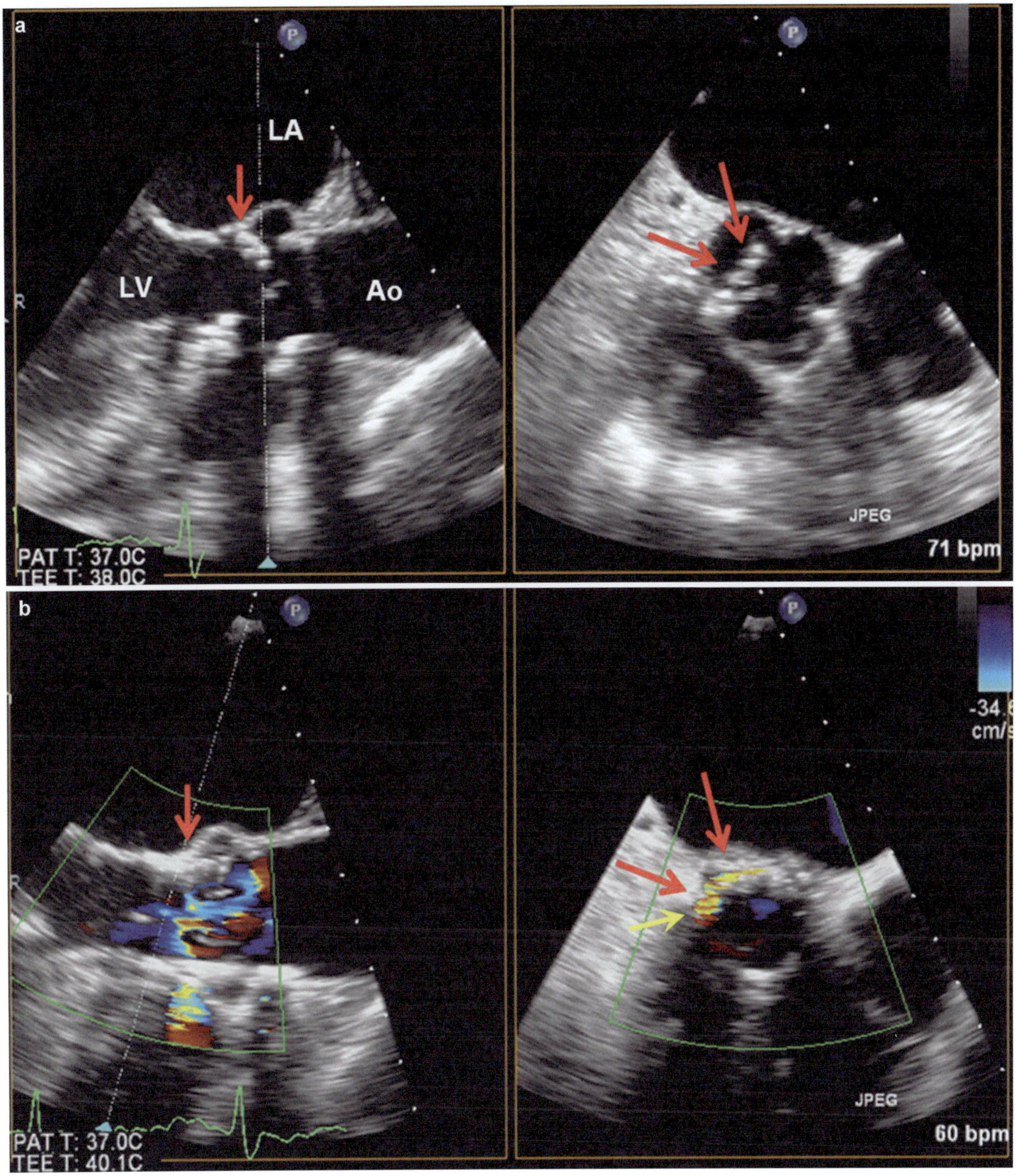

Fig. 36.7 Relation between native valve calcification and THV paravalvular regurgitation. Panels (**a**) and (**b**) show TEE long- and short-axis views of large bulky calcification of native aortic valve cusp (*red arrows*) prior to TAVR (**a**) and ensuing paravalvular regurgitation (*yellow arrow*) after TAVR (**b**). *Ao* aorta, *LA* left atrium, *LV* left ventricle

report of stent fracture with the currently used THVs [3, 4, 10]. The structural evaluation should also include the assessment of the impact of the TAVR procedure and of the THV on the surrounding anatomical structures, i.e., the mitral valve, the aortic root, and the left ventricular wall. In particular, if the landing zone of the stent is low in the LVOT, the apical end of the stent may cause an erosion and perforation of the anterior mitral leaflet or of the membranous septum (Fig. 36.8). Owing to their high performance for anatomical imaging, MDCT or CMR is useful to assess the prosthesis

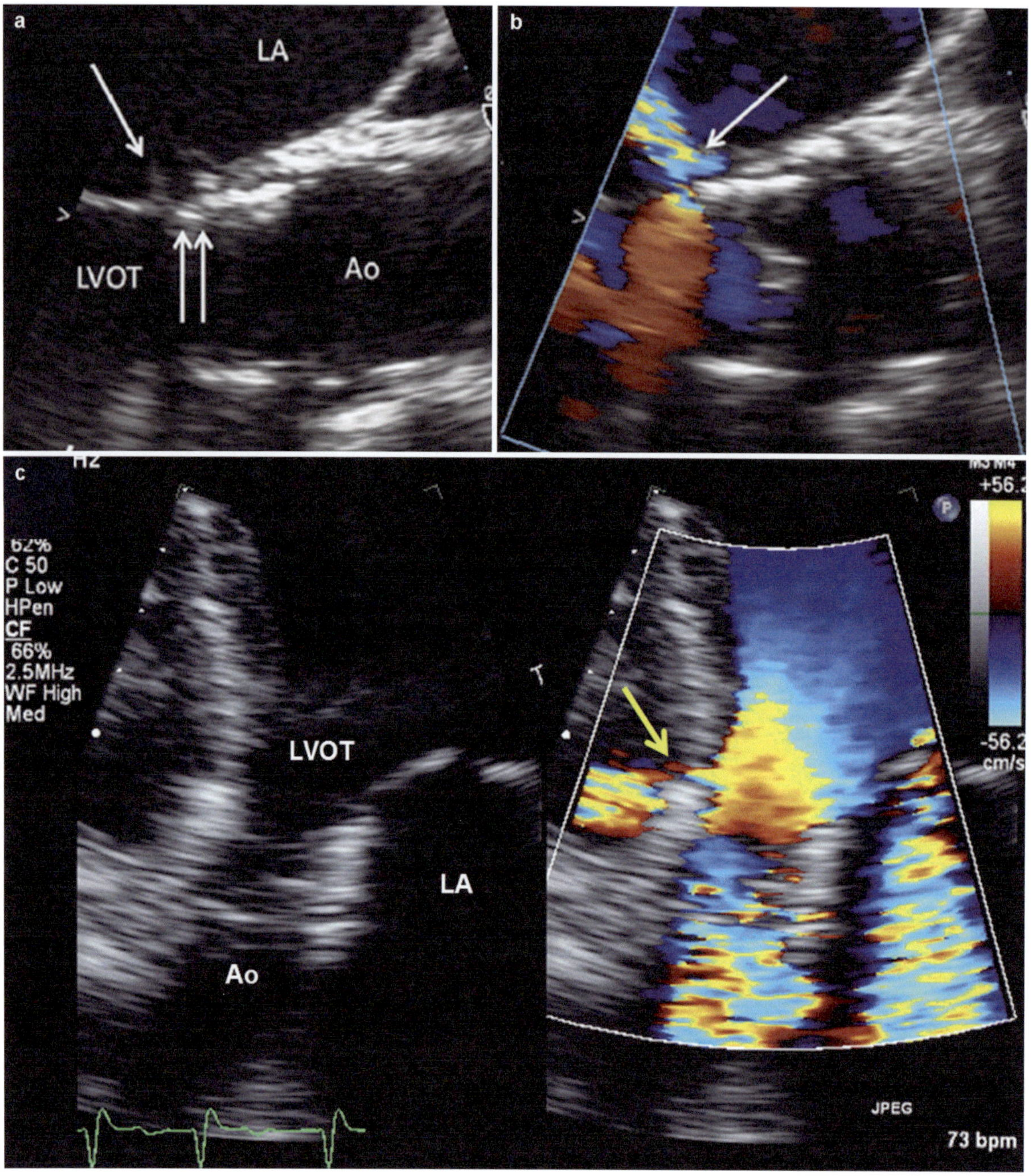

Fig. 36.8 Lesions of septum and mitral valve caused by THV. Panels (**a**) and (**b**) show TEE views of a delayed mitral valve injury (Reproduced with permission from [15]). Panel (**a**): The stent (*double arrow*) is in contact with the anterior mitral leaflet. Prosthetic valve endocarditis 1 year after implantation associated with perforation of the mitral leaflet at the point of contact (*single arrow*). Panel (**b**) Ensuing severe mitral regurgitation. Panel (**c**) shows a perforation of the membranous septum caused by THV stent and ensuing left-to-right shunt (*yellow arrow*). *Ao* aorta, *LV* left ventricle, *LVOT* LV outflow tract, *RV* right ventricle

and its relationship to the native aortic valve, annulus, root, mitral valve, and ventricle as well as detecting pseudoaneurysms of the root or other rare complications (Fig. 36.9).

Assessment of THV Cusps Morphology and Mobility

Meticulous assessment of thickness, calcification, and mobility of valve cusps is key to detect the presence of tissue degeneration of surgical or transcatheter bioprosthetic valves, with echocardiography the method of choice for this purpose. THVs cause less reverberation and acoustic shadowing compared to surgical prostheses. The morphology and mobility of THV cusps can generally be adequately assessed by TTE. In cases where visualization of valve cusps is not feasible or inadequate, transesophageal echocardiography (TEE) can provide improved image quality and thereby improved detection of cusp calcification and thickening, vegetations due to endocarditis, thrombus or pannus,

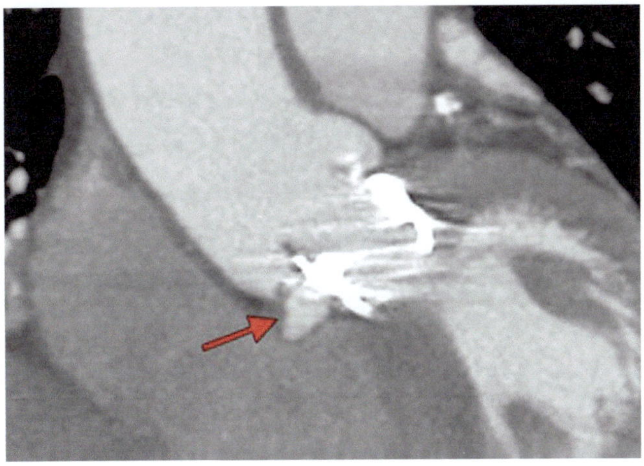

Fig. 36.9 Pseudo-aneurysm of the aortic root visualized by MDCT. Coronal multiplanar reconstruction of the aortic root in an 89-year-old female patient 3 days after transcatheter aortic valve replacement. Difficulties with the rapid ventricular pacing were encountered, resulting in a low deployment, root injury, and a resultant pseudo-aneurysm (*arrow*) (Reproduced with permission from [3])

and reduced cusp mobility. MDCT may be useful to identify pannus or thrombus and to detect the presence of cusp calcification. Given that few patients have follow-up duration longer than 5 years after TAVR, there is very limited data about the structural and functional durability of THVs. However, there has been some reports of calcific degeneration of valve cusps [16].

Functional Evaluation

The evaluation of THV function includes the identification and quantification of prosthesis-patient mismatch (PPM) and acquired dysfunction, that is, stenosis and/or regurgitation. The functional evaluation of THVs is generally much more complex than that of native or surgical bioprosthetic valves because of the pitfalls in the measurement of the valve effective orifice area (EOA) and the high prevalence of paravalvular regurgitation.

Identification and Quantification of Prosthesis-Patient Mismatch

Prosthesis-patient mismatch is not an intrinsic dysfunction of the prosthesis, per se. This problem indeed occurs when the EOA of a normally functioning prosthesis is too small in relation to the patient's body size (and thus cardiac output requirements), resulting in abnormally high postoperative velocities and gradients (Box 36.1) [17]. PPM is defined with the use of the EOA projected from normal reference values or measured early after valve replacement and then indexed for patient's body surface area. Moderate PPM (indexed EOA <0.85 cm^2/m^2) may be quite frequent (20–70 %) following surgical aortic valve replacement (SAVR), whereas the prevalence of severe PPM (indexed EOA <0.65 cm^2/m^2) ranges from 2 to 20 % [17].

Box 36.1 Definitions of Moderate and Severe Patient-Prosthesis Mismatch

Severity	Effective orifice area (cm^2/m^2)
None/Mild	<0.85–0.9
Moderate	<0.85
Severe	<0.65

In SAVR series, PPM, and especially severe PPM, is associated with increased risk of operative mortality, less improvement in symptoms, less regression of LV hypertrophy, more adverse cardiac events, and reduced long-term survival [17]. This detrimental impact of PPM on outcomes is more pronounced in patients with depressed LV systolic function, severe LV hypertrophy, and/or concomitant mitral regurgitation.

Given that there are not yet normal reference values of EOA established for THVs and that these values may vary not only with the model and label size of THV but also with the patient's aortic annulus size [18], the projected indexed EOA of THVs is presently difficult to obtain, and it is thus preferable to use the indexed EOA measured by echocardiography at predischarge or 1-month post-TAVR to detect the presence of PPM. However, the utilization of the indexed EOA measured early after TAVR may yield to overestimation of the degree of PPM in presence of low-flow states (i.e., indexed EOA may be "pseudo-severized") or in presence of obesity (i.e., body surface area may overestimate cardiac output requirements). The incidence of moderate PPM reported in series of patients who received balloon- or self-expandable THVs is between 18 and 32 % and that of severe PPM was between 2 and 9 % [19–24]. Furthermore, PPM was associated with less regression of LV mass, volumes, and diastolic dysfunction as well as less functional improvement following TAVR [24]. It is also important to emphasize that the patient's aortic annulus size in these TAVR series was, on average, much smaller compared to contemporary SAVR series. Accordingly, in a previous study where TAVR and SAVR cohorts were matched for aortic annulus size [19], the incidence of severe PPM was lower with TAVR (6 %) compared to SAVR (28 % with stented bioprostheses and 20 % with stentless bioprostheses). The superiority of TAVR over SAVR for the prevention of PPM was particularly obvious in the subset of patients with a small aortic annulus [19, 23]. However, these encouraging results will have to be further confirmed by randomized clinical trials. In PARTNER-Cohort A trial, TAVR was associated with significantly larger EOAs and lower gradients compared to SAVR [25, 26]

Detection and Quantification of Prosthetic Valve Stenosis

Table 36.1 presents the proposed Doppler echocardiographic parameters and criteria for the detection and quantification of prosthetic valve stenosis following

Table 36.1 Doppler echocardiographic criteria for detection and quantification of transcatheter heart valve stenosis

	Normal	Possible stenosis	Significant stenosis
Structural parameters			
Valve stent and cusps	Usually normal	Normal/abnormal[a]	Usually abnormal[a]
Doppler quantitative parameters			
Peak aortic jet velocity (m/s)[b,c]	<3	3–4	>4
Mean gradient (mmHg)[b,c]	<20	20–35	>35
Doppler velocity index[b,d]	≥0.35	0.25–0.35	<0.25
Effective orifice area (cm^2)[b]	>1.2	0.8–1.2	<0.8
Contour of the transprosthetic jet[e]	Triangular, early peaking	Triangular to intermediate	Rounded, symmetrical
Acceleration time (ms)[e]	<80	80–100	>100
Acceleration time/LV ejection time ratio[e]	–	0.30–0.37	>0.37

[a]In case of significant stenosis there are generally abnormalities of stent position, deployment, and/or circularity or of valve cusps morphology and mobility (thickened cusps with reduced mobility). In the case of possible stenosis, the THV structure may appear normal or abnormal
[b]The criteria proposed for these parameters are valid for near-normal or normal stroke volume (i.e., stroke volume: 50–90 ml)
[c]These parameters are more affected by low- or high-flow states including low cardiac output and concomitant THV regurgitation
[d]This parameter is dependent on the size of the LV outflow tract
[e]These parameters are influenced by chronotropy, LV function, and/or atrioventricular compliance

TAVR. As in patients with surgical bioprosthetic valves, acquired prosthetic valve stenosis is expected to be associated with abnormalities of cusps morphology and mobility (calcification and thickening of the valve cusps with reduced mobility). Quantitative parameters of prosthetic valve function include transprosthetic flow velocity and pressure gradients, valve EOA, and Doppler velocity index (DVI).

Transprosthetic Flow Velocity and Gradient

The principles of interrogation and recording of flow velocity through THVs are similar to those used in evaluating native valve stenosis [1, 3, 5, 11]. However, as in surgical prosthetic valves, high velocity or gradient alone is not proof of intrinsic prosthetic obstruction and may be secondary to PPM, high-flow conditions, prosthetic valve regurgitation, and technical pitfalls. Significant prosthetic valve regurgitation may indeed cause the flow rate across the prosthesis to increase, resulting in increased gradients. This phenomenon may be more frequent in transcatheter than in surgical valves, due to the higher incidence of paravalvular regurgitation in the former. It is also important to keep in mind that several conditions, e.g., PPM and intrinsic dysfunction (stenosis and/or regurgitation) may coexist.

Valve Effective Orifice Area

The EOA of THVs is calculated with the continuity equation, similar to native or surgical prosthetic aortic valve EOA [27, 28]: $EOA = (CSA_{LVOT} \times TVI_{LVOT})/TVI_{THV}$, where CSA_{LVOT} is the cross-sectional area of the LVOT; TVI_{LVOT}, the time-velocity integral obtained by pulse wave (PW) Doppler in the LVOT; and TVI_{THV}, the time-velocity integral obtained by CW Doppler through the THV. This method is also valid in presence of concomitant THV regurgitation.

When measuring the EOA of THVs, it is generally recommended to measure the LVOT diameter and velocity immediately proximal to the lower border of the stent (Figs. 36.10 and 36.11) [3, 11, 18, 29]. There are indeed two levels of flow acceleration in the LVOT: the first one occurs when the flow enters into the lower portion of the stent and the second one when the flow passes through the valve cusps (Fig. 36.10). Hence, an in-stent, pre-cusp positioning of the pulse wave Doppler sample may yield to overestimation of LVOT stroke volume and thus of valve EOA, especially if it is combined to a LVOT diameter measured pre-stent (Figs. 36.10 and 36.11). The EOA estimated by continuity equation with the use of the LVOT stroke volume measured pre-stent has been shown to be more accurate and reproducible than the EOA derived from in-stent measure of stroke volume [18, 29]. However, if

Fig. 36.10 Schematic and examples of spectral Doppler flow acceleration in a SAPIEN THV. Panel (**a**) Schematic presentation of echocardiographic pulse wave (*PW*) Doppler patterns when the sample volume is placed pre-stent, in-stent, but pre-cusps, and continuous wave (*CW*) through the aortic valve. Due to flow acceleration, it is generally recommended that the subvalvular velocities used in either Doppler velocity index or effective orifice area be sampled proximal to the stent. Panel (**b**) The PW Doppler pattern of a sample volume placed before stent. *White arrows* show the extent of the THV in the aortic root. *Red arrow* shows the level of the prosthetic aortic cusps. Panel (**c**) The PW Doppler pattern of sample volume placed within the stent but before cusps. Panel (**d**) The PW Doppler pattern of a sample volume placed at the level of the cusps

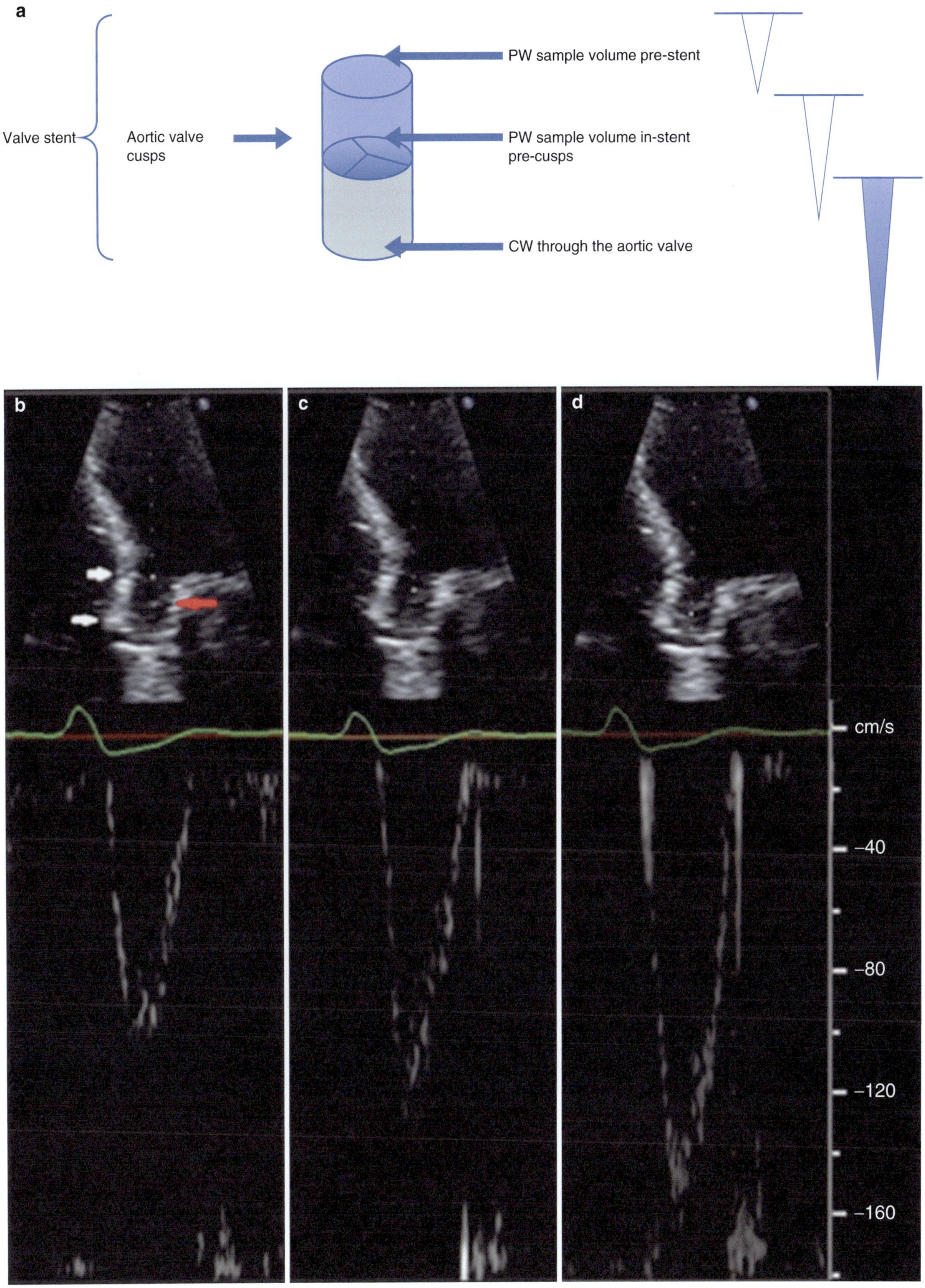
a
Valve stent
Aortic valve cusps
PW sample volume pre-stent
PW sample volume in-stent pre-cusps
CW through the aortic valve
b
c
d
cm/s
–40
–80
–120
–160

the lower border of the stent sits low in the LVOT, which may occur more frequently with self-expandable THVs such as the CoreValve, it may be preferable to measure the LVOT diameter and velocity within the lower portion of the stent at approximately 5–10 mm below the THV cusps (Fig. 36.11). In self-expandable valves, the valve cusps are attached higher within the valve stent compared to balloon-expandable valves, which provides more space for in-stent velocity sampling below the cusps. If the in-stent measure has to be used due to low position of the stent in the LVOT, it is important to measure both the LVOT diameter and velocity at approximately the same location in the stent and not too close to the

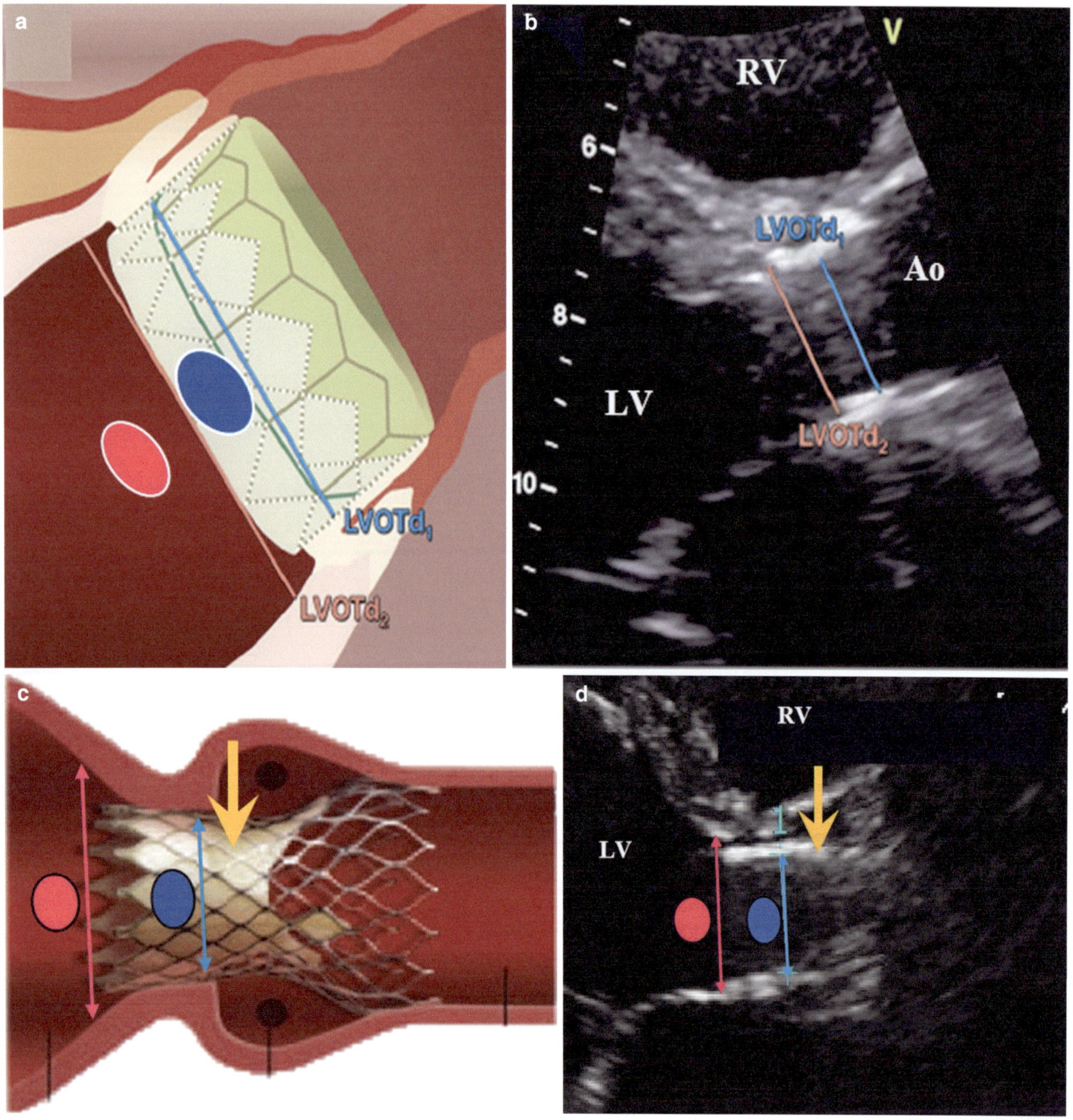

Fig. 36.11 Schematic and examples of spectral Doppler flow acceleration in a SAPIEN THV. This figure shows the positioning of the pulse wave (*PW*) Doppler velocity acquisition and of the LV outflow tract (*LVOT*) diameter measurement at the pre- (*pink oval and line*) and in- (*blue oval and line*) stent locations for balloon- (Panels **a** and **b**) and self- (Panels **c** and **d**) expandable THVs. Panels (**e**) and (**f**) show the PW velocities at pre- and in-stent locations, respectively. It is recommended to measure the LVOT diameter and velocity at the present location except in cases where the position of the apical portion of the THV stent is low in the LVOT, which occurs more frequently with the self-expandable THVs. The *yellow arrows* indicate the location of the prosthetic cusps: the in-stent, pre-cusps segment of the valve is longer in self-expandable than in balloon-expandable THVs (Adapted with permission from [18]). *Ao* aorta, *LV* left ventricle, *RV* right ventricle

Fig. 36.11 (continued)

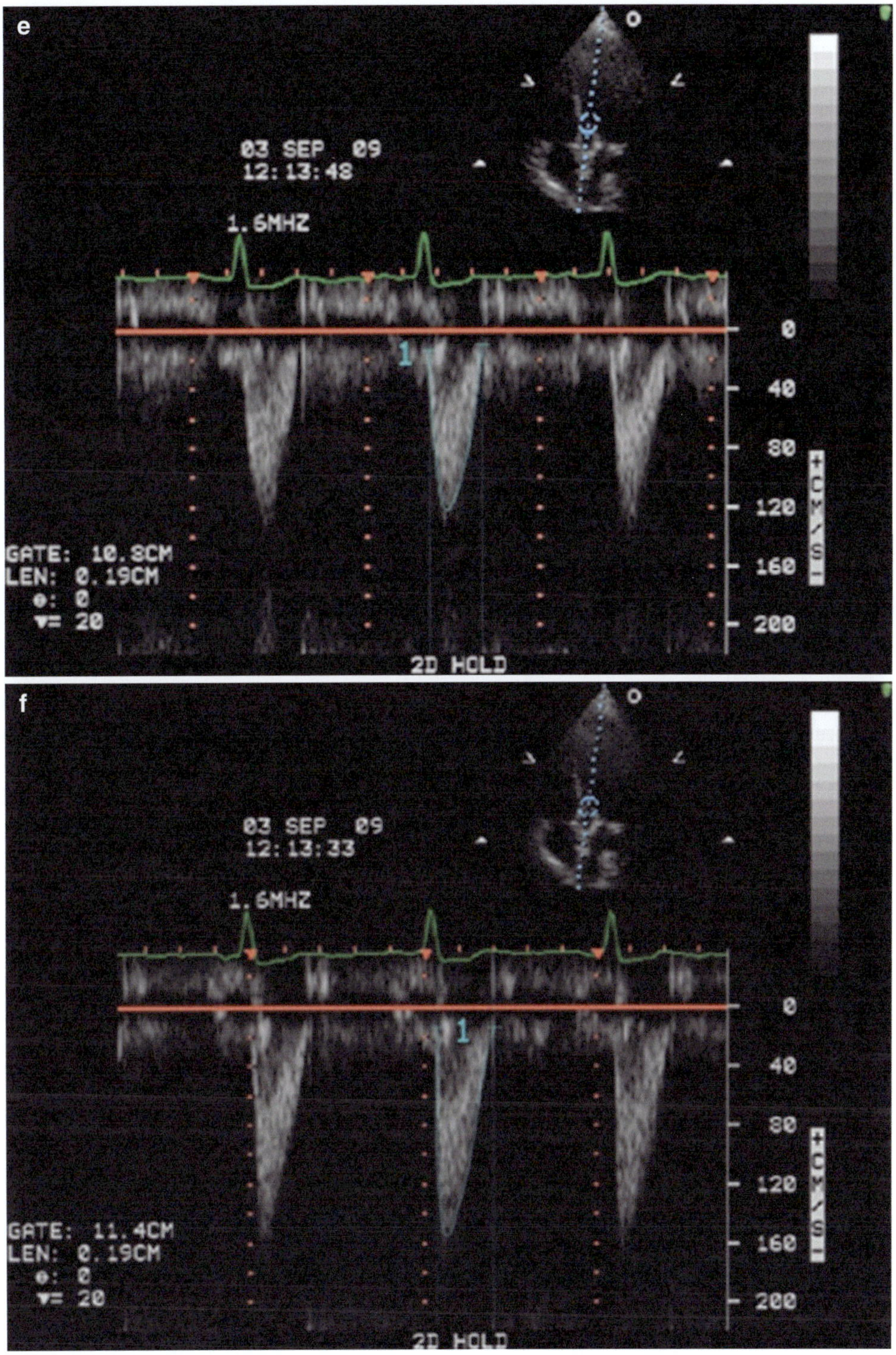

valve cusps (Fig. 36.11). The combination of LVOT velocity measured in the stent with a diameter measured pre-stent or vice versa yields to important errors in the estimation of stroke volume and EOA.

There are a few additional caveats worth mentioning when measuring the LVOT diameter and velocity following TAVR: (1) For the recording of LVOT velocity signal, care should be exercised in locating the PW Doppler sample volume proximal to the prosthesis stent as previously discussed. To well identify the two levels of flow acceleration in the LVOT, one can use a "pull-back" method where the pulse wave sample volume is first placed above the valve cusps and then progressively moved toward the ventricle (Fig. 36.10). A first drop of velocity is generally observed when the sample volume is moved below the valve cusps and a second one when it is moved below the lower border of the stent [3, 29]. (2) The cross-sectional area of the LVOT is derived from the diameter measurement performed just proximal to the prosthesis stent in the parasternal long-axis zoomed view in mid-systole from the white-black interface of the septal endocardium to the anterior mitral leaflet (Fig. 36.11). This method assumes a circular geometry of the LVOT. However, some studies have reported that Doppler echocardiography may underestimate the LVOT diameter and thus the stroke volume and EOA due to the fact that a substantial proportion of patients have a noncircular, i.e., oval, LVOT cross-sectional shape, and that 2D echocardiography view tends to measure the smaller diameter of this noncircular cross section [7]. However, following TAVR, this source of error is less likely to occur because the TAVR procedure tends to circularize the LVOT cross section [8, 30]. The measurement of the LVOT diameter is sometimes technically difficult because of the reverberations and artifacts caused by the prosthesis stent or by the calcific nodules of the native annulus or valve. Particular attention should thus be paid not to mistake the inner border of the prosthesis stent for the inner edge of the LVOT.

The cutoff values of EOA proposed in the American Society of Echocardiography (ASE) guidelines [1] to identify prosthetic valve stenosis (Table 36.1) have important limitations given that they may overlap substantially with the normal values of EOA of small-size THVs, especially if implanted in a small aortic annulus. Hence, a multiparametric approach that also includes the gradient, Doppler velocity index, and valve cusps morphology and mobility should be used to corroborate the presence of prosthetic valve stenosis.

Valve Anatomic Orifice Area

The anatomic orifice area (AOA) measured by planimetry requires high-quality image of the valve orifice, whether it be by TTE, TEE, MDCT, or CMR. From the standpoint of physiology, the AOA and the EOA are however not equivalent. Indeed, the pressure gradient and the associated LV workload are related much more to the EOA than the AOA, and the former is therefore physiologically and clinically more meaningful. Because the flow contracts downstream of the valve orifice, the EOA is always smaller than the AOA. Furthermore, the AOA corresponds to the peak value of valve area measured at peak systole, whereas the EOA represents the mean valve area averaged over the systolic period.

Doppler Velocity Index (DVI)

The DVI is a dimensionless ratio of the proximal flow velocity in the LVOT to the flow velocity through the THV: $DVI = V_{LVOT}/V_{THV}$. Time-velocity time integrals may also be used in place of peak velocities to calculate $DVI = TVI_{LVOT}/TVI_{THV}$. These parameters can be helpful to screen for valve stenosis, particularly when the cross-sectional area of the measurement of the LVOT diameter is technically difficult or not feasible (Table 36.1) [31]. These parameters also provide useful complementary tools to follow the valve hemodynamic function over time in a given patient. For example, if the EOA decreases significant during follow-up in a patient but the DVI and gradient remain stable, one should suspect an error in the measurement of the LVOT diameter.

Transprosthetic Jet Contour and Acceleration Time

In a normal native or prosthetic valve, the contour of the continuous wave (CW) flow velocity through the prosthesis generally has triangular shape, with early peaking of the velocity and a short acceleration time (i.e., the time from the onset of flow to maximal velocity (Table 36.1). With prosthetic valve obstruction, a more rounded velocity contour is expected, with the velocity peaking almost in mid-ejection, prolonged acceleration time (>100 ms) [1]. These parameters present the advantage of being angle-independent as opposed to transprosthetic velocities and gradients, EOA, or DVI. However, they should be interpreted with caution as they are also highly influenced by LV chronotropy and function. The heart-rate dependency of the acceleration time may be, at least in part, reduced by indexing this parameter for the LV ejection time; an acceleration time/ejection time ratio >0.37 being suggestive of prosthetic valve stenosis [32]. However, this new parameter has not been validated in the patients with depressed LV systolic function, who represent an important proportion of patients undergoing TAVR.

Resolving Difficult Situations

In presence of high gradient (mean gradient ≥20 mmHg) across a THV, it is important to make the differential diagnosis between PPM versus acquired THV stenosis. PPM is identified with the use of the indexed EOA measured early (predischarge or 1 month echo) after TAVR. Deterioration of parameters of valve structure (i.e., stent position and shape, cusp morphology and mobility, visualization of thrombus, pannus, or vegetation) and function (i.e., gradient, EOA, and DVI) since early post-TAVR echocardiogram suggests the presence of acquired THV dysfunction. PPM and THV dysfunction may often coexist.

In case of discordance between EOA (i.e., <1.0 cm^2) and gradient (i.e., <20 mmHg), one can first calculate the indexed EOA, and if it is >0.85 cm^2/m^2, the presence of a low gradient despite a small EOA is most likely due to small patient's body size. The next step is to determine the DVI; if it is >0.35, one should suspect an error in the measurement of the LVOT diameter. If the DVI is low, the discordance between EOA and gradient is most likely due to a low-flow state.

Detection and Quantification of THV Regurgitation

Assessment of severity of THV regurgitation is much more complex than in native or surgical prosthetic valves because of the high prevalence of paravalvular regurgitation and eccentric jets. Paravalvular aortic valvular regurgitation (PAR) is indeed much more common following

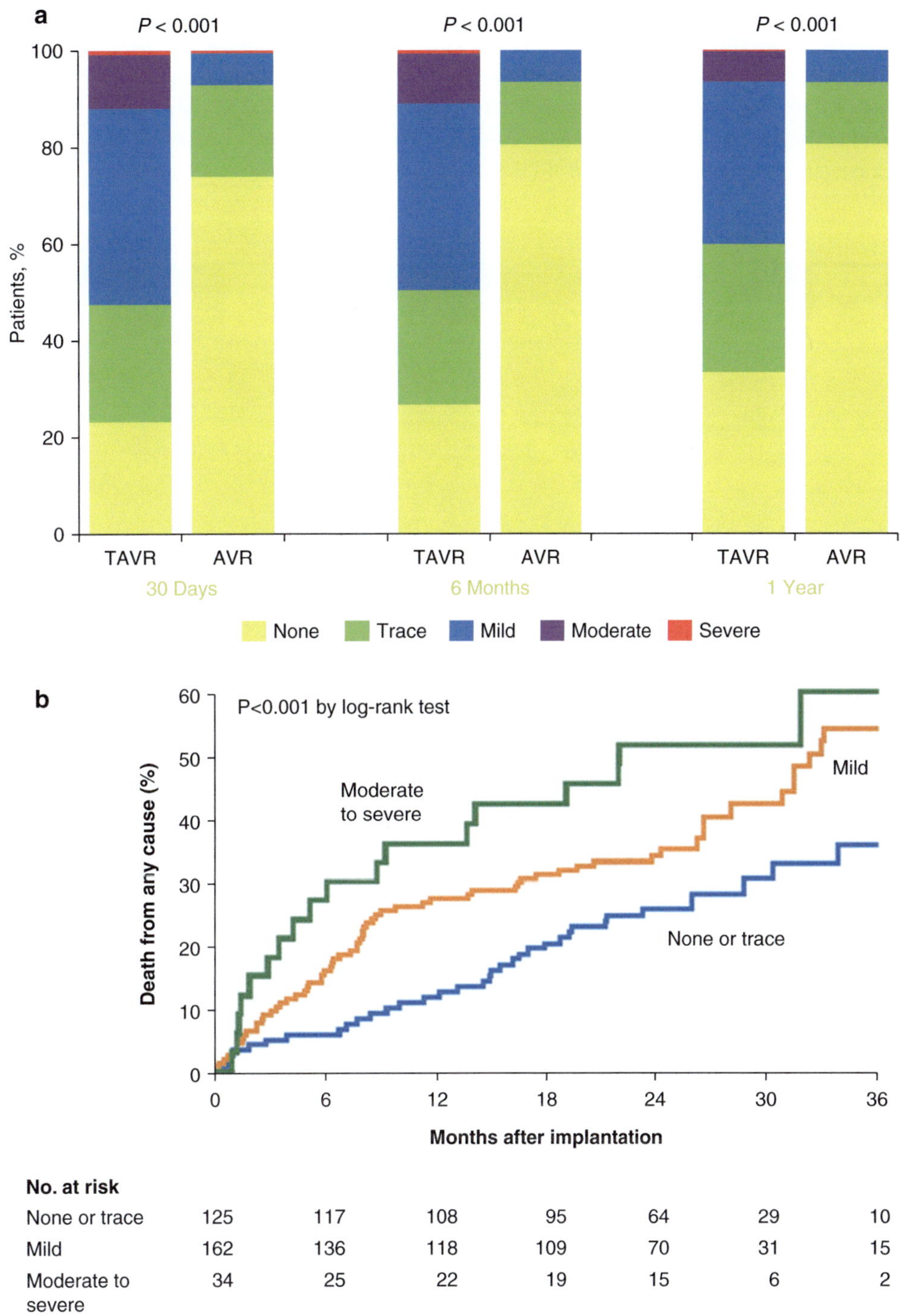

Fig. 36.12 Incidence and impact on survival of prosthetic regurgitation in the PARTNER-A trial. Panel (**a**): Comparison of the percentages of patients with no, trace, mild, moderate, or severe prosthetic regurgitation in the transcatheter and surgical AVR groups of the PARTNER-IA trial at 30 days, 6 months, and 1 year post-AVR. Panel (**b**): Impact of mild and moderate-to-severe prosthetic regurgitation on all-cause mortality in the TAVR group. Reproduced with permission [26]

TAVR versus SAVR [19, 25, 26]. Although the severity of post-TAVR regurgitation has been assessed by a variety of methods, the reported incidence of regurgitation ranges from 30 to 80 % with 5–20 % being moderate or severe [19, 33–36]. The incidence and severity of PAR appear to remain stable during follow-up, but there is very limited data in this regard [12, 26]. The PARTNER-IA trial as well as several large registries have shown that THV regurgitation, even mild, is associated with increased late mortality following TAVR (Fig. 36.12) [25, 26, 34, 35]. However, it remains unclear if this association solely reflects a direct and independent contribution of the regurgitation per se and/or if it is due, at least in part, to other causal risk factors. Indeed, previous studies [36–40] have identified several risk factors for the occurrence of PAR following TAVR including (1) inappropriate THV sizing and positioning (Fig. 36.3), (2) severe/bulky/asymmetrical calcifications of native valve cusps (Fig. 36.7), and (3) more pronounced angle of LVOT to ascending aorta (for self-expandable THVs). Nonetheless, identification, localization, and quantification of THV regurgitation remain crucial for optimal risk stratification and follow-up after TAVR.

Doppler Echocardiographic Assessment of THV Regurgitation Severity

TTE generally provides a good visualization of the LVOT and of THV regurgitation (Fig. 36.13). TEE may be useful to identify the origin (paravalvular vs. central) of the regurgitant jets in technically difficult TTE studies (Figs. 36.3, 36.7 and 36.13). The same principles and methods used for grading severity of native or surgical prosthetic valve regurgitation can be used for THV regurgitation (Table 36.2) [1, 5]. It must be remembered, however, that there is very limited data on the application and validation of quantitative parameters such as the width of the regurgitant jet or of the vena contracta, the effective regurgitant orifice area, and the regurgitant volume in the context of THVs. Given that

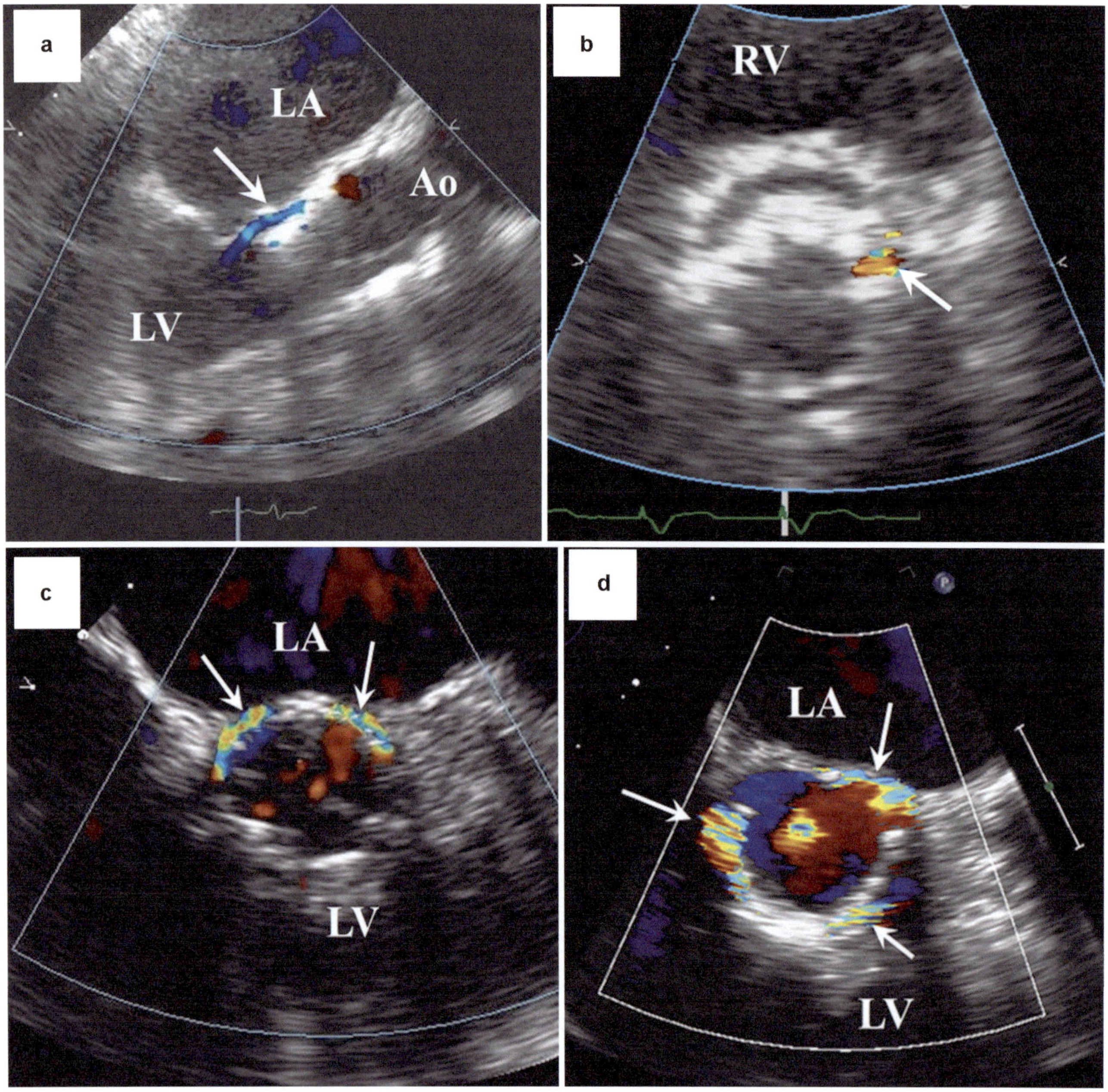

Fig. 36.13 Color Doppler echocardiographic images of paravalvular regurgitation. Panel (**a**): TEE long-axis view of mild paravalvular regurgitation. Paravalvular aortic regurgitation can be graded according to the circumferential extent of the regurgitant jet on the TTE or TEE short-axis view: mild (~8 % circumferential extent; Panel **b**), moderate (~29 % circumferential extent; Panel **c**), and severe (~42 % circumferential extent; Panel **d**) paravalvular regurgitation. The *white arrows* indicate the regurgitant jets (Panels **a**, **b**, and **c** are reproduced with permission from [5]). *LA* left atrium, *LV* left ventricle, *RV* right ventricle

Table 36.2 Doppler echocardiographic criteria for severity of transcatheter heart valve regurgitation (central and paravalvular)

	Mild	Moderate	Severe
Structural parameters			
Valve stent and cusps	Usually normal	Normal/abnormal[a]	Usually abnormal[a]
LV size[b]	Normal	Normal/mildly dilated	Dilated
Doppler parameters (qualitative or semiquantitative)			
Vena contracta width (mm)[c]	<3	3–6	>6
Jet width in central jets (%LVOT diameter): color Doppler[c]	Narrow (≤25)	Intermediate (26–64)	Large (≥65)
Jet density: CW Doppler	Incomplete or faint	Dense	Dense
Jet deceleration rate (PHT, ms): CW Doppler[d]	Slow (>500)	Variable (200–500)	Steep (<200)
LV to RV outflow VTI ratio: PW Doppler	Slightly increased	Intermediate	Greatly increased
(ratio of time-velocity integrals)	(>1.2)	(>1.5)	(>1.8)
Diastolic flow reversal in the descending aorta: PW Doppler	Absent or brief early diastolic	Intermediate	Prominent holodiastolic (end-diast. vel. > 18 cm/s)
Circumferential extent of paravalvular regurgitation (%)[e]	<10	10–30	>30
Doppler parameters (quantitative)			
Regurgitant volume (ml/beat)	<30	30–59	≥60
Regurgitant fraction (%)	<30	30–49	≥50

Adapted with permission in part from references [1] and [5]

PHT pressure half time, *end-diast. vel.* end-diastolic velocity, *CW* continuous wave, *LV* left ventricular, *LVOT* LV outflow tract, *PHT* pressure half time, *PW* pulse wave, *RV* right ventricular

[a]In case of severe regurgitation, there are often (but not always) abnormalities of stent position, deployment, and/or circularity or of valve cusps morphology and mobility (teared cusp or cusp fixed in open position). In the case of moderate regurgitation, the THV structure may appear normal or abnormal

[b]Applies to chronic THV regurgitation in the absence of other etiologies

[c]Parameter applicable to central jets and is less accurate in paravalvular jets

[d]This parameter is influenced by LV compliance

[e]Applies only to paravalvular regurgitation. Has not been well validated. The cut-point value of circumferential extent proposed in the American Society of Echocardiography for severe regurgitation is 20 %, but a value of 30 % has been used in the PARTNER-I trial

all parameters of prosthetic valve regurgitation have important limitations and may be subject to measurement errors, a comprehensive, multiparametric approach is highly recommended (Table 37.2) [1, 5, 11].

Central Regurgitation

The width of the vena contracta and the ratio of the regurgitant jet width to the LVOT diameter measured in the long-axis and short-axis views may be used to assess the severity of central regurgitation. For the calculation of this ratio the measurements should be made just underneath the insertion of the THV cusps, which implies that both the jet width and LVOT diameter are measured within the lower portion of the stent. The vena contracta width and the jet width/LVOT diameter may however underestimate the regurgitation severity in the case of eccentric or crescent-shaped jets and overestimate severity in the case of jets impinging the wall of the LVOT or of anterior mitral valve. Hence, these parameters are generally not suitable for the assessment of paravalvular regurgitation.

Paravalvular Regurgitation

The circumferential extent of the regurgitant jet(s) estimated in the short-axis view has been proposed for semiquantitative evaluation of the severity of paravalvular regurgitation (Fig. 36.13, Table 36.2) [1, 3, 5, 11]. However, this parameter has not been validated either in the context of surgical prostheses or in that of THVs, and pending further validation, its use must be viewed as arbitrary and at best semiquantitative in the context of a multiparametric and multiwindow evaluation. For the assessment of this parameter, it is important to use a short-axis plane cutting the LVOT just underneath the stent. An image plane at the level of the stent may over- or underestimate the regurgitation because the jet is confined between the stent and the native tissues. On the other hand, a plane that is too low in the LVOT may overestimate the regurgitation severity due to rapid broadening of the jet after the vena contracta. The circumferential extent of the jet becomes even more complex and less reliable when multiple jets are present (Fig. 36.13).

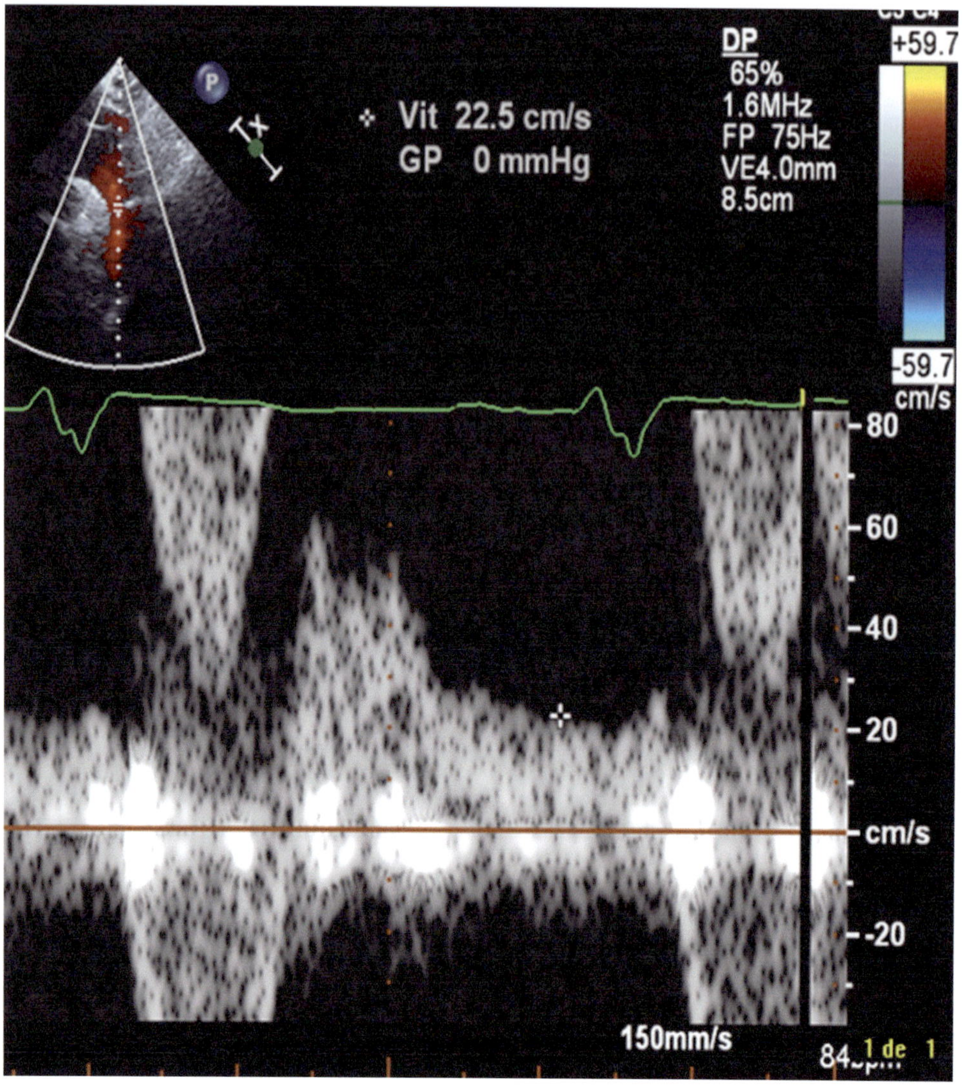

Fig. 36.14 Diastolic flow reversal in the ascending aorta associated with severe aortic regurgitation. Holodiastolic flow reversal in the ascending aorta with end-diastolic velocity of 22.5 cm/s (*white cross*) indicating the presence of severe aortic regurgitation

Because THV regurgitation is often characterized by paravalvular, eccentric, and/or multiple jets (Fig. 36.13), the proximal isovolumic surface area (PISA) method is often impossible to achieve, and the Doppler volumetric method can be used for regurgitation quantitation [1]. With this latter method, the regurgitant volume is estimated by calculating the difference between the stroke volume measured in the LVOT and the mitral inflow volume, providing that there is no mitral stenosis or regurgitation. In the absence of significant pulmonic regurgitation, the stroke volume measured in the right ventricular outflow tract may alternately be used in place of the mitral inflow volume and a semiquantitative evaluation of the regurgitation may also be provided by calculating the LVOT to RV outflow tract time-velocity integrals ratio (Table 36.2). Other Doppler parameters may also be determined to corroborate THV regurgitation severity, including the signal intensity of the continuous wave envelope of the regurgitant jet and the diastolic flow reversal in the descending aorta (Fig. 36.14, Table 36.2).

The consideration of the size of LV cavity is also important to consider in the context of chronic THV regurgitation (Table 36.2). In particular, notwithstanding the immediate postoperative period, the presence of either moderate-to-severe or severe aortic regurgitation is expected to be associated with significant LV dilation during follow-up, and its absence should in most situations preclude the diagnosis of significant regurgitation whereas its presence should increase the level of suspicion.

Total Aortic Regurgitation

In THVs, paravalvular and central regurgitation are often present concomitantly, and it is thus important to assess the total (central and paravalvular) amount of regurgitation. In most cases, the severity of total regurgitation will be equal to the most severe degree of either transvalvular or paravalvular regurgitation [3]. However, in some cases, the addition of the two regurgitations will push the grading to the next level of severity (e.g., mild transvalvular regurgitation plus mild moderate paravalvular regurgitation will be graded as moderate total regurgitation).

The analysis of 3D color Doppler images and/or of the backscattered Doppler power analysis may provide interesting new avenues for quantification of THV regurgitation. Some recent studies indeed suggest that 3D color Doppler echocardiography may improve the assessment of the severity of paravalvular regurgitation in THVs [6]. However, further studies are needed to confirm the feasibility and accuracy of this new method.

CMR Assessment of THV Regurgitation Severity

As described above, quantification of THV regurgitation by echocardiography remains a difficult challenge. CMR may help to corroborate the severity of regurgitation in cases where echocardiography remains inconclusive. For this purpose, phase contrast imaging is obtained in a short-axis plane cutting the aorta just above the THV stent to measure the antegrade and retrograde aortic flows and then to calculate the regurgitant volume and fraction. With this method, regurgitant fraction (RF) of ≥1–15 % is generally graded as mild, 16–30 % as mild-to-moderate, 31–50 % as moderate-to-severe, and >50 % as severe regurgitation. The repercussion of the THV regurgitation on LV volumes and function can also be assessed using standard cine CMR sequences. Further studies are needed to establish the diagnostic and prognostic values of CMR for the assessment of THV regurgitation.

Identification of Other THV Complications

There have been a few reports of THV thrombosis early after TAVR despite dual antiplatelet therapy (Fig. 36.15) [41]. If THV thrombosis is suspected, a comprehensive TTE should be performed first, with particular attention directed at evaluation of cusp mobility and valve hemodynamic function and identification of thrombus and/or pannus. TEE often provides important incremental diagnostic information and may be useful to monitor the response to therapy. Although there is until now no data in the context of TAVR, MDCT may likely be helpful to differentiate thrombi from a fibrous pannus.

A few cases of valve infective endocarditis have been reported following TAVR (Fig. 36.15) [42, 43]. Although rare, prosthetic valve endocarditis is often associated with high rates of morbidity and mortality and early diagnosis is key to successful therapy [17]. However, the sensitivity and specificity of both TTE and TEE are lower in surgical prosthetic valve endocarditis compared to native valve endocarditis [44]. There is not yet any data available with regard to the accuracy of echocardiography for the detection of THV endocarditis. Pending further data, we would recommend repeating TEE within 5–7 days and/or using alternative imaging modality if the initial TEE is negative but suspicion for infective THV endocarditis remains. In this regard, MDCT might be useful to detect the presence of THV infective endocarditis as well as to assess the extension of the pathologic process toward the surrounding structures [17].

Conclusion

Multimodality imaging combining echocardiography and MDCT is key to evaluate the structural integrity of THVs. Doppler echocardiography is the method of choice for the evaluation and follow-up of THV hemodynamic function. However, the particular context of THVs poses some major challenges in terms of estimation of EOA and quantification of paravalvular regurgitation. A comprehensive approach that integrates several direct and indirect parameters of valve function measured by TTE and TEE is key to appropriately assess THV function, and other imaging modalities, including MDCT, are useful to complement or confirm the information obtained by Doppler echocardiography. The role of echocardiography and CMR imaging in quantitating paravalvular prosthetic regurgitation is promising and needs further investigation.

Acknowledgement Dr. Pibarot holds the Canada Research Chair in Valvular Heart Diseases, Canadian Institutes of Health research, Ottawa, Ontario.

Competing Interests The authors have no interests to disclose with regard to this work.

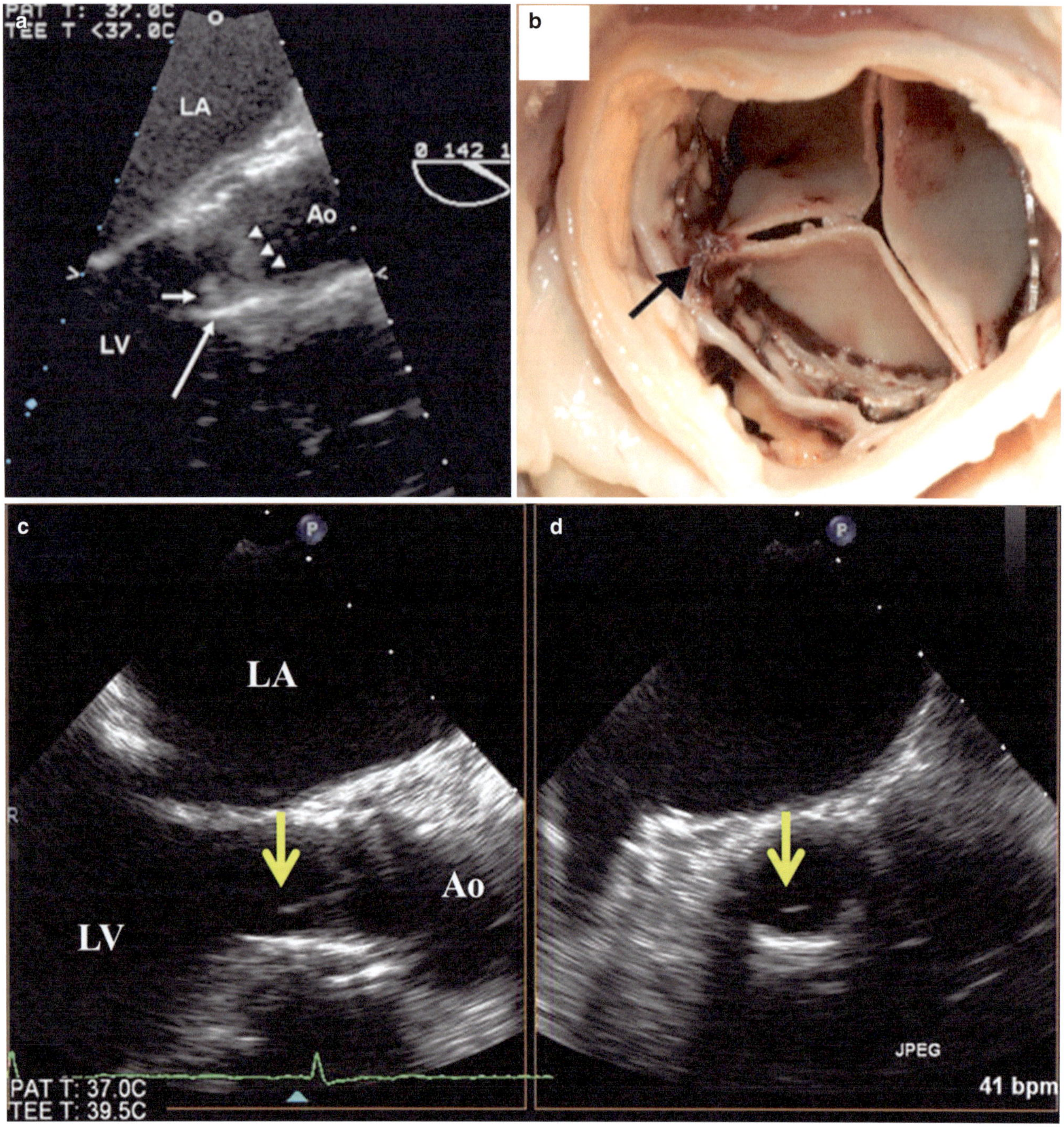

Fig. 36.15 Thrombosis and Endocarditis in Transcatheter Heart Valves Panel (**a**): TEE long-axis view of the LV outflow tract showing a thrombus on the stent (*short white arrow*) and the thickened valve leaflets (*white arrow heads*). Panel (**b**): Postmortem image of thrombi on the outflow stent frame of the THV (*black arrow*) (Panels **a** and **b** are reproduced with permission from [41]). Panels (**c**) and (**d**): small vegetation attached to the THV cusps in a patient with hyperthermia, high white blood cell count, and multiple positive blood cultures. *LA* left atrium, *Ao* aorta, *LV* left ventricle

References

1. Zoghbi W, Chambers J, Dumesnil J, et al. Recommendations for evaluation of prosthetic valves with echocardiography and Doppler ultrasound: a report from the American Society of Echocardiography's Guidelines and Standards Committee and the Task Force on Prosthetic Valves, developed in conjunction with the American College of Cardiology Cardiovascular Imaging Committee, Cardiac Imaging Committee of the American Heart Association, the European Association of Echocardiography, a registered branch of the European Society of Cardiology, the Japanese Society of Echocardiography and the Canadian Society of Echocardiography, endorsed by the American College of Cardiology Foundation, American Heart Association, European Association of Echocardiography, a registered branch of the European Society of Cardiology, the Japanese Society of Echocardiography, and Canadian Society of Echocardiography. J Am Soc Echocardiogr. 2009;22:975–1014.
2. Zamorano J, Badano L, Bruce C, et al. Eae/Ase recommendations for the Use of echocardiography in new transcatheter interventions for valvular heart disease. J Am Soc Echocardiogr. 2011;24: 937–65.
3. Bloomfield G, Gillam L, Hahn R, et al. A practical guide to multimodality imaging of transcatheter aortic valve replacement. JACC Cardiovasc Imaging. 2012;5:441–55.
4. Delgado V, Kapadia S, Schalij M, Schuijf J, Tuzcu E, Bax J. Transcatheter aortic valve implantation: and implications of multimodality imaging in patient selection, procedural guidance, outcomes. Heart. 2012;98:743–54.
5. Pibarot P, Dumesnil J. Doppler echocardiographic evaluation of prosthetic valve function. Heart. 2012;98:69–78.
6. Goncalves A, Almeria C, Marcos-Alberca P, et al. Three-dimensional echocardiography in paravalvular aortic regurgitation assessment after transcatheter aortic valve implantation. J Am Soc Echocardiogr. 2012;25:47–55.
7. Gaspar T, Adawi S, Sachner R, et al. Three-dimensional imaging of the left ventricular outflow tract: impact on aortic valve area estimation by the continuity equation. J Am Soc Echocardiogr. 2012; 25:749–57.
8. Delgado V, Ng A, Van De Veire N, et al. Transcatheter aortic valve implantation: role of multi-detector row computed tomography to evaluate prosthesis positioning and deployment in relation to valve function. Eur Heart J. 2010;31:1114–23.
9. Leipsic J, Gurvitch R, Labounty T, et al. Multidetector computed tomography in transcatheter aortic valve implantation. JACC Cardiovasc Imaging. 2011;4:416–29.
10. Willson A, Webb J, Gurvitch R, et al. Structural integrity of balloon-expandable stents after transcatheter aortic valve replacement: assessment by multidetector computed tomography. J Am Coll Cardiol Intv. 2012;5:525–32.
11. Zamorano J, Badano L, Bruce C, et al. Eae/Ase recommendations for the Use of echocardiography in new transcatheter interventions for valvular heart disease. Eur Heart J. 2011;32:2189–214.
12. Gurvitch R, Wood D, Tay E, et al. Transcatheter aortic valve implantation. Durability of clinical and hemodynamic outcomes beyond 3 years in a large patient cohort. Circulation. 2010;122: 1319–27.
13. Ussia G, Barbanti M, Petronio A, et al. Transcatheter aortic valve implantation: 3-year outcomes of self-expanding corevalve prosthesis. Eur Heart J. 2012;33:969–76.
14. Clavel M, Dumont E, Pibarot P, et al. Severe valvular regurgitation and late prosthesis embolization after percutaneous aortic valve implantation. Ann Thorac Surg. 2009;87:618–21.
15. Masson J, Kovac J, Schuler G, et al. Transcatheter aortic valve implantation: review of the nature, management, and avoidance of procedural complications. JACC Cardiovasc Interv. 2009;2: 811–20.
16. Ong S, Mueller R, Iversen S. Early calcific degeneration of a corevalve transcatheter aortic bioprosthesis. Eur Heart J. 2012;33: 586.
17. Pibarot P, Dumesnil J. Prosthetic heart valves: selection of the optimal prosthesis and long-term management. Circulation. 2009; 119:1034–48.
18. Clavel M, Rodés-Cabau J, Dumont E, et al. Validation and characterization of transcatheter aortic valve effective orifice area measured by Doppler echocardiography. J Am Coll Cardiol Img. 2011; 4:1053–62.
19. Clavel M, Webb J, Pibarot P, et al. Comparison of the hemodynamic performance of percutaneous and surgical bioprostheses for the treatment of severe aortic stenosis. J Am Coll Cardiol. 2009;53:1883–91.
20. Clavel M, Webb J, Rodés-Cabau J, et al. Comparison between transcatheter and surgical prosthetic valve implantation in patients with severe aortic stenosis and reduced left ventricular ejection fraction. Circulation. 2010;122:1928–36.
21. Jilaihawi H, Chin D, Spyt T, et al. Prosthesis-patient mismatch after transcatheter aortic valve implantation with the medtronic-corevalve bioprosthesis. Eur Heart J. 2010;31:857–64.
22. Tzikas A, Piazza N, Geleijnse M, et al. Prosthesis-patient mismatch after transcatheter aortic valve implantation with the Medtronic corevalve system in patients with aortic stenosis. Am J Cardiol. 2010;106:255–60.
23. Kalavrouziotis D, Rodés-Cabau J, Bagur R, et al. Transcatheter aortic valve implantation in patients with severe aortic stenosis and small aortic annulus. J Am Coll Cardiol. 2011;58: 1016–24.
24. Ewe S, Muratori M, Delgado V, et al. Hemodynamic and clinical impact of prosthesis-patient mismatch after transcatheter aortic valve implantation. J Am Coll Cardiol. 2011;58:1910–9.
25. Smith C, Leon M, Mack M, et al. Transcatheter versus surgical aortic-valve replacement in high-risk patients. N Engl J Med. 2011;364:2187–98.
26. Kodali S, Williams M, Smith C, et al. Two-year outcomes after transcatheter or surgical aortic-valve replacement. N Engl J Med. 2012;366:1686–95.
27. Chafizadeh E, Zoghbi W. Doppler echocardiographic assessment of the St-Jude medical prosthetic valve in the aortic position using the continuity equation. Circulation. 1991;83:213–23.
28. Dumesnil J, Honos G, Lemieux M, Beauchemin J. Validation and applications of indexed aortic prosthetic valve areas calculated by Doppler echocardiography. J Am Coll Cardiol. 1990; 16:637–43.
29. Shames S, Koczo A, Hahn R, Jin Z, Picard M, Gillam L. Flow characteristics of the Sapien aortic valve: the importance of recognizing in-stent flow acceleration for the echocardiographic assessment of valve function. J Am Soc Echocardiogr. 2012;25:603–9.
30. Willson A, Webb J, Labounty T, et al. 3-Dimensional aortic annular assessment by multidetector computed tomography predicts moderate or severe paravalvular regurgitation after transcatheter aortic valve replacement. A multicenter retrospective analysis. J Am Coll Cardiol. 2012;59:1287–94.
31. Fernandes V, Olmos L, Nagueh S, Quinones M, Zoghbi W. Peak early diastolic velocity rather than pressure half-time is the best index of mechanical prosthetic mitral valve function. Am J Cardiol. 2002;89:704–10.
32. Sb Z, Rm S, Ozkan M, et al. Flow acceleration time and ratio of acceleration time to ejection time for prosthetic aortic valve function. JACC Cardiovasc Imaging. 2011;4:1161–70.
33. Leon M, Smith C, Mack M, et al. Transcatheter aortic-valve implantation for aortic stenosis in patients who cannot undergo surgery. N Eng J Med. 2010;363:1597–607.
34. Gilard M, Eltchaninoff H, Iung B, et al. Registry of transcatheter aortic-valve implantation in high-risk patients. N Eng J Med. 2012; 366:1705–15.

35. Abdel-Wahab M, Zahn R, Horack M, et al. Aortic regurgitation after transcatheter aortic valve implantation: incidence and early outcome. Results from the German transcatheter aortic valve interventions registry. Heart. 2011;97:899–906.
36. Sinning J, Hammerstingl C, Vasa-Nicotera M, et al. Aortic regurgitation index defines severity of peri-prosthetic regurgitation and predicts outcome in patients after transcatheter aortic valve implantation. J Am Coll Cardiol. 2012;59:1134–41.
37. Ewe S, Ng A, Schuijf J, et al. Location and severity of aortic valve calcium and implications for aortic regurgitation after transcatheter aortic valve implantation. Am J Cardiol. 2011;108:1470–7.
38. Haensig M, Lehmkuhl L, Rastan A, et al. Aortic valve calcium scoring is a predictor of significant paravalvular aortic insufficiency in transapical-aortic valve implantation. Eur J Cardiothorac Surg. 2012;41:1234–40.
39. Unbehaun A, Pasic M, Dreysse S, et al. Transapical aortic valve implantation: incidence and predictors of paravalvular leakage and transvalvular regurgitation in a series of 358 patients. J Am Coll Cardiol. 2012;59:211–21.
40. Sherif M, Abdel-Wahab M, Stocker B, et al. Anatomic and procedural predictors of paravalvular aortic regurgitation after implantation of the Medtronic core valve bioprosthesis. J Am Coll Cardiol. 2010;56:1623–9.
41. Tay E, Gurvitch R, Wijeysinghe N, et al. Valve thrombosis after transcatheter heart valve implantation. EuroIntervention. 2011;7:170–1.
42. Chrissoheris M, Ferti A, Spargias K. Early prosthetic valve endocarditis complicating repeated attempts at corevalve implantation. J Invasive Cardiol. 2011;23:E291–2.
43. Loh P, Bundgaard H, Sondergaard L. Infective endocarditis following transcatheter aortic valve replacement: diagnostic and management challenges. Catheter Cardiovasc Interv. 2012;81:623–7.
44. Habib G, Badano L, Tribouilloy C, et al. Recommendations for the practice of echocardiography in infective endocarditis. Eur J Echocardiogr. 2010;11:202–19.

How Can Imaging Preclinical Models Help Us with TAVR?

37

Juan F. Granada and Piotr P. Buszman

Abstract

The successful clinical introduction of transcatheter aortic valve replacement (TAVR) technologies among inoperable high-risk patients with calcified aortic valve stenosis (CAVS) is a major milestone in cardiovascular disease therapeutics of recent years [1]. The rapid pace of growth of this field has created new opportunities for the development of new devices, techniques, and ancillary tools. In addition, it has created the need for the development of a multidisciplinary physician team approach and the redesign of the catheterization laboratory environment including imaging integration as a key component.

Keywords

Transcatheter aortic valve replacement • Animal models • Imaging • Calcific aortic valve stenosis

Introduction

The successful clinical introduction of transcatheter aortic valve replacement (TAVR) technologies among inoperable high-risk patients with calcified aortic valve stenosis (CAVS) is a major milestone in cardiovascular disease therapeutics of recent years [1]. The rapid pace of growth of this field has created new opportunities for the development of new devices, techniques, and ancillary tools. In addition, it has created the need for the development of a multidisciplinary physician team approach and the redesign of the catheterization laboratory environment including imaging integration as a key component.

J.F. Granada, MD (✉)
The Skirball Center for Cardiovascular Research, Cardiovascular Research Foundation, 8 Corporate Dr, Orangeburg, NY 10962, USA
e-mail: jgranada@crf.org

P.P. Buszman, MD, PhD
The Skirball Center for Cardiovascular Research, Cardiovascular Research Foundation, 8 Corporate Dr, Orangeburg, NY 10962, USA

American Heart of Poland, Center for Cardiovascular Research and Development, Katowice, Poland
e-mail: pbuszman@crf.org, pbuszman@gmail.com

The successful development of TAVR technologies has relied, in part, on the extensive experimental work performed over two decades ago [2, 3]. Despite inherent limitations of animal models, these early studies demonstrated the feasibility of the technique and assisted in the refinement of the early TAVR concepts. In addition, these studies assisted to develop the basic implantation methods and imaging principles utilized in the first in human clinical study with a TAVR device in 2002 [4] and future clinical trials. Although most of the validation process of TAVR devices is performed in vitro, the experimental validation of emerging TAVR devices plays an important role in the technological refinement of these devices and other ancillary tools. In the following review, we describe currently available preclinical models for TAVR validation and testing, explain the role of imaging in these experiments, and offer a perspective of future development in this field.

Experimental Models and TAVR Validation

The most common experimental models used in TAVR validation are the sheep and swine. The main limitations of these models are the lack of a basic pathological condition (absence of stenosis and calcification) and the anatomical differences compared to humans. Subsequently, no anchoring mechanism

J.K. Min et al. (eds.), *Multimodality Imaging for Transcatheter Aortic Valve Replacement*, DOI 10.1007/978-1-4471-2798-7_37, © Springer-Verlag London 2014

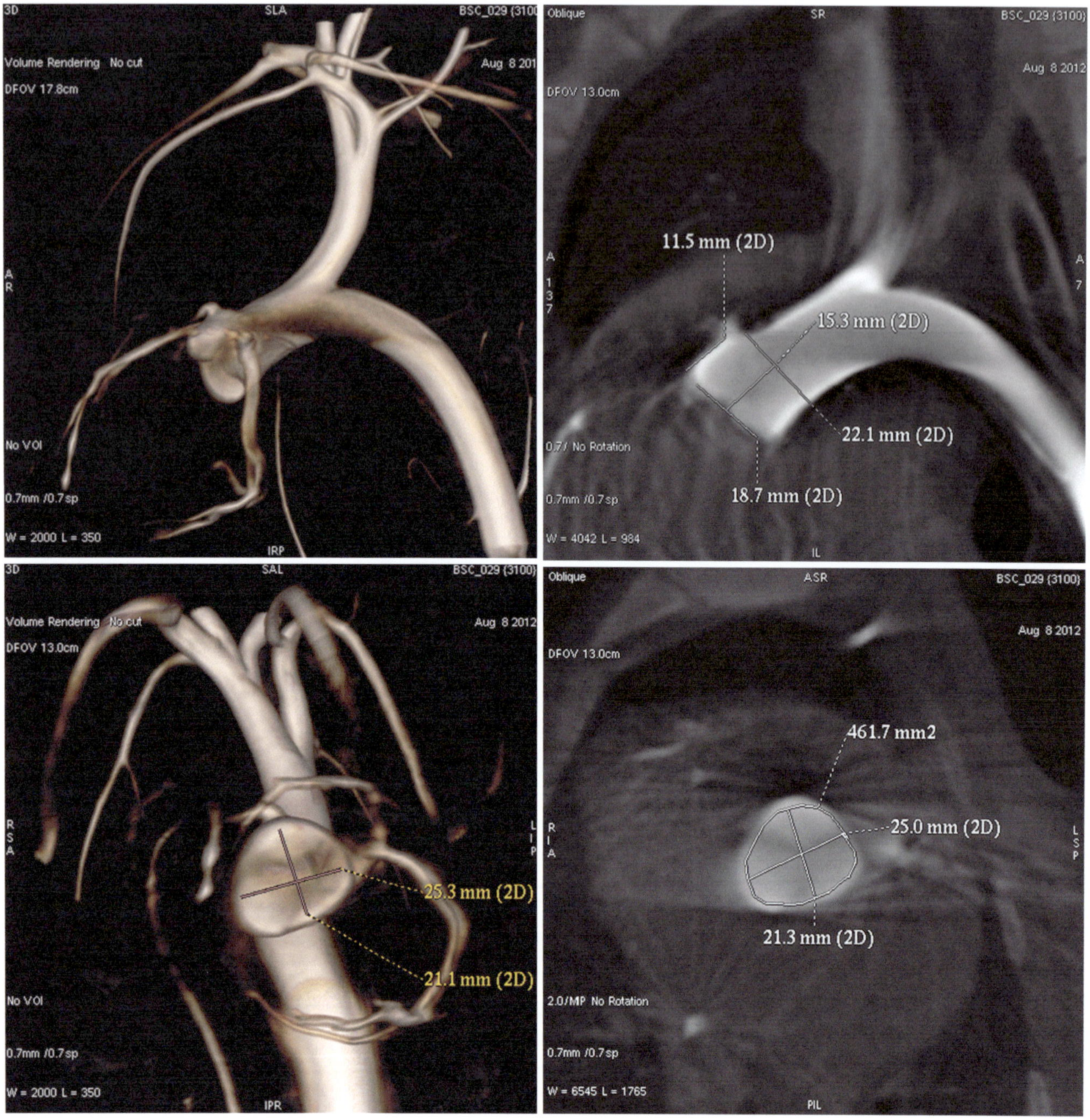

Fig. 37.1 Cone beam angiography with three-dimensional reconstruction of sheep arch anatomy in contralateral projections

for the TAVR device is present, making difficult the performance of long-term retention studies due to device dislodgment. Figure 37.1 shows a CT angiogram and 3D reconstruction of the aortic arch of an adult sheep and the basic measurements at the aortic root level of both models. Nevertheless, assessment of device delivery system performance and the long-term biocompatibility of several valve components is feasible by the use of these models (summarized in Table 37.1). Utilization of multiple imaging methods is crucial for the acute and long-term evaluation of these devices.

Experimental Models and Vascular Access

Several routes of implantation of TAVR devices have been reported in humans; however, the transfemoral and trans-apical approaches are the most commonly used. Due to the importance of vascular access to procedural success and clinical outcomes, emerging TAVR concepts are usually tested for safety at the experimental setting. The vascular anatomy in the porcine and ovine models is generally similar to humans. Contrary to humans, both animal models lack a common femoral artery

(CFA) and thus, the usual access site is located within the proximal segment of the superficial femoral artery (SFA) or external iliac artery (EIA). Based upon our data, the mean vessel diameters are 5.3 ± 0.5 mm for the SFA and 5.85 ± 0.9 mm for the EI in sheep and slightly smaller in swine (SFA = 5.2 ± 0.5 mm, EIA = 5.63 ± 0.7 mm) (Fig. 37.2a–d). In comparison, the mean human CFA diameters (8.17 ± 1.14 mm) tend to be larger than both animal models [5]. In consequence, these vessel diameter

Table 37.1 Current indications for preclinical TAVR evaluation

Delivery system evaluation (acute studies: nonpermanent implant)		
	Safety of access (femoral versus trans-apical)	
	Delivery system	
		Profile evaluation (vascular compatibility)
		Aortic arch trackability
	Valve component	
		Delivery mechanism
		Retention and anchoring
		Retrieval
Valve component evaluation (chronic studies: implantable)		
	Stent frame	
		Material biocompatibility
		Biomechanics (fatigability)
	Tissue valve	
		Valve biocompatibility and healing
		Short (post-implant) and long-term performance
		Others: sutures + adhesive components (polymers)

ranges permit the validation of devices within the 22–24 F diameter ranges. Although the basic femoral vessel animal anatomy is similar to humans, the most important difference is the lack of a disease state (i.e., calcification), no significant tortuosity or vessel pathology (i.e., calcifications); the absence of these pathologies mitigates the trackability of the delivery system and renders a smoother delivery in the experimental setting (Fig. 37.2d–e). However, basic safety features can be successfully tested by the use of the experimental models. In addition, the acute and long-term safety and efficacy of large bore closure devices can also be tested at the experimental setting.

The trans-apical approach can also be successfully evaluated in the preclinical setting. Vascular access is gained through a limited sternotomy or lateral thoracotomy to reach apex of the beating heart [6]. Full sternotomy may be also performed in order to facilitate direct aortic ultrasound imaging. Advanced tools, like MRI, could be potentially used not only for imaging (Fig. 37.3a) but also for procedural guidance (Fig. 37.3b). The porcine heart is an ideal model due to comparable human anatomy and physiology including wall geometry, myocardial wall thickness, ventricular wall motion, and hemodynamics. However, due to the fact that larger hearts are needed in some circumstances, the ovine model may be an acceptable alternative, particularly for displaying thin walled ventricles, similar to end-stage left ventricle remodeling due to CAVS. Similarly to the peripheral vascular approach, the testing of devices utilizing the apical approach (access and closure, Fig. 37.3b) can be performed [7, 8].

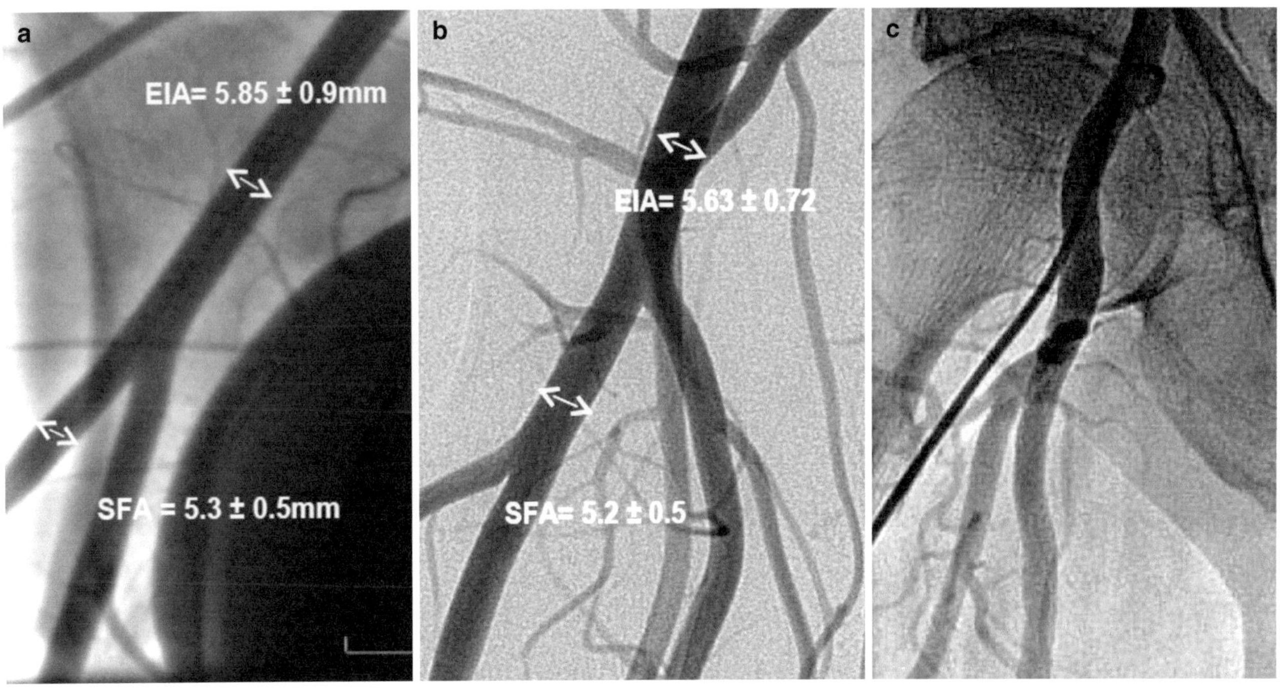

Fig. 37.2 Vascular angiography of ovine (**a**), porcine (**b**), and human (**c**) vascular access. Ovine (cone beam angiography) and human iliofemoral arteries (3D CT) are presented on picture (**d**) and (**e**). Average length 60–70 mm and diameter ~6 mm allows testing for devices that are within 22–24 F (Images **a**, **b**, and **d**, courtesy of Skirball Center for Cardiovascular Research. Images **c** and **e**, courtesy of American Heart of Poland)

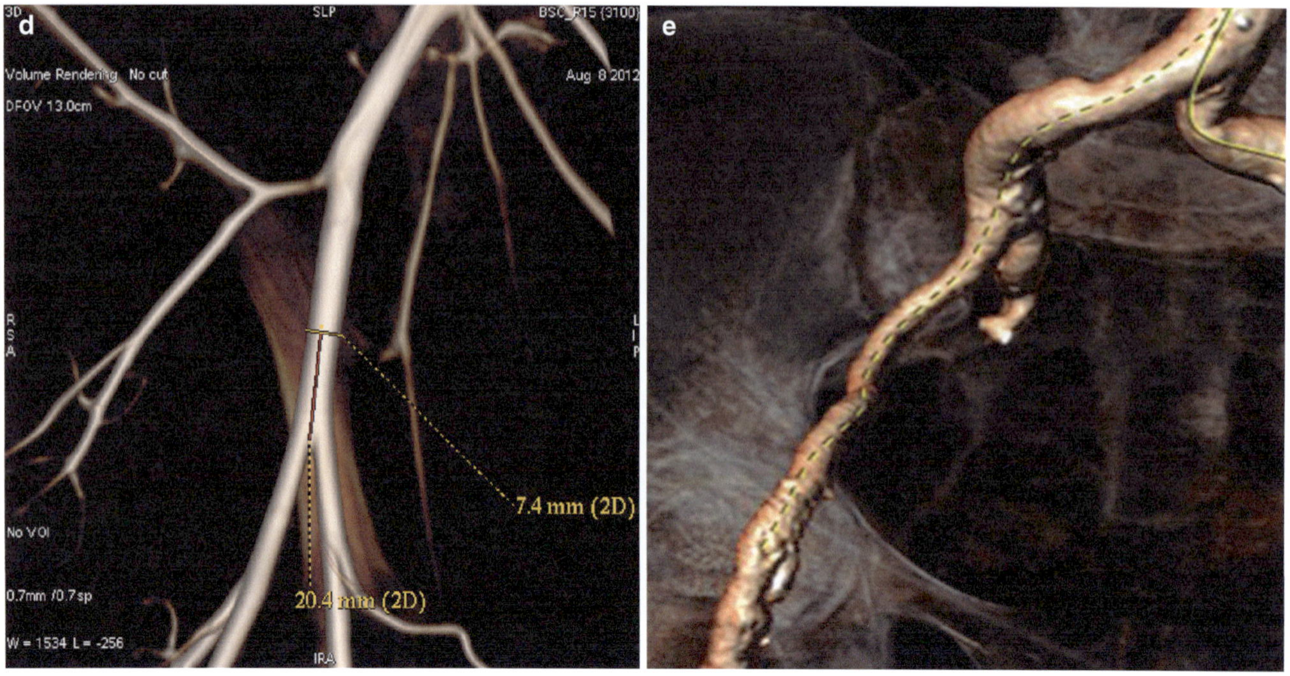

Fig. 37.2 (continued)

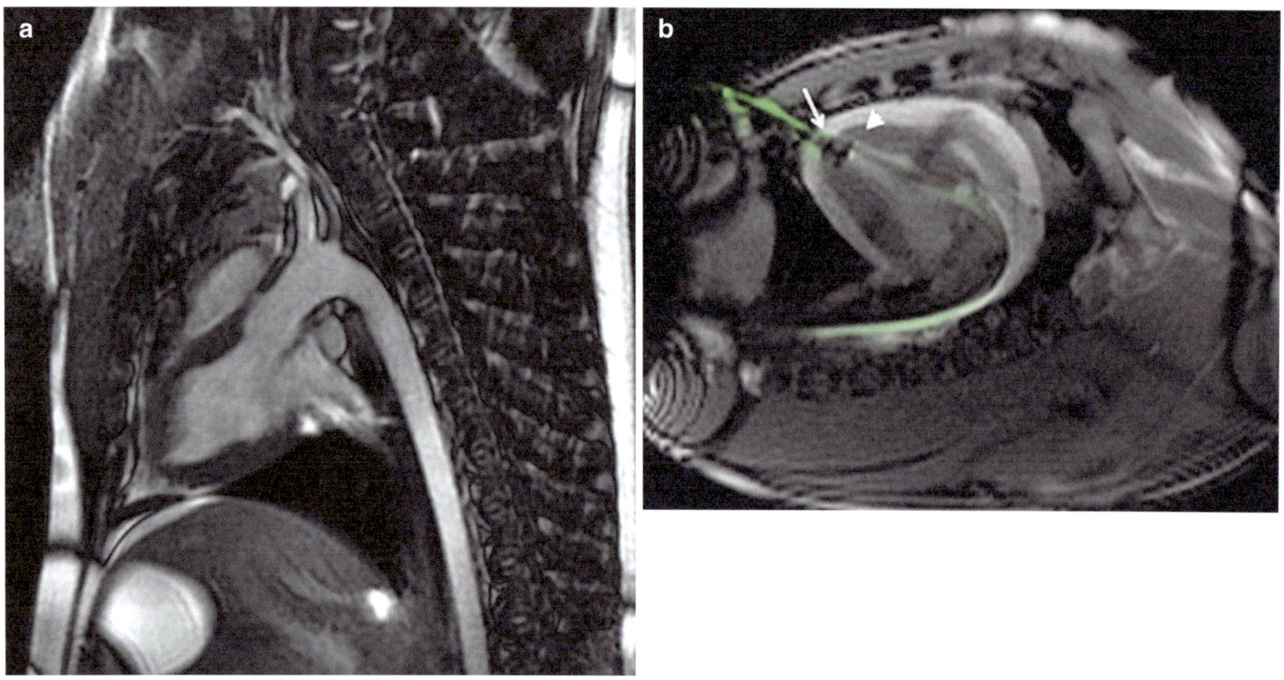

Fig. 37.3 MRI of aortic TAVR route (Image **a**, courtesy of American Heart of Poland) and guided placement of apical closure (*arrow*) displays the apex device in swine (*arrowhead*) (Image **b**, courtesy of I.M. Barbash [4])

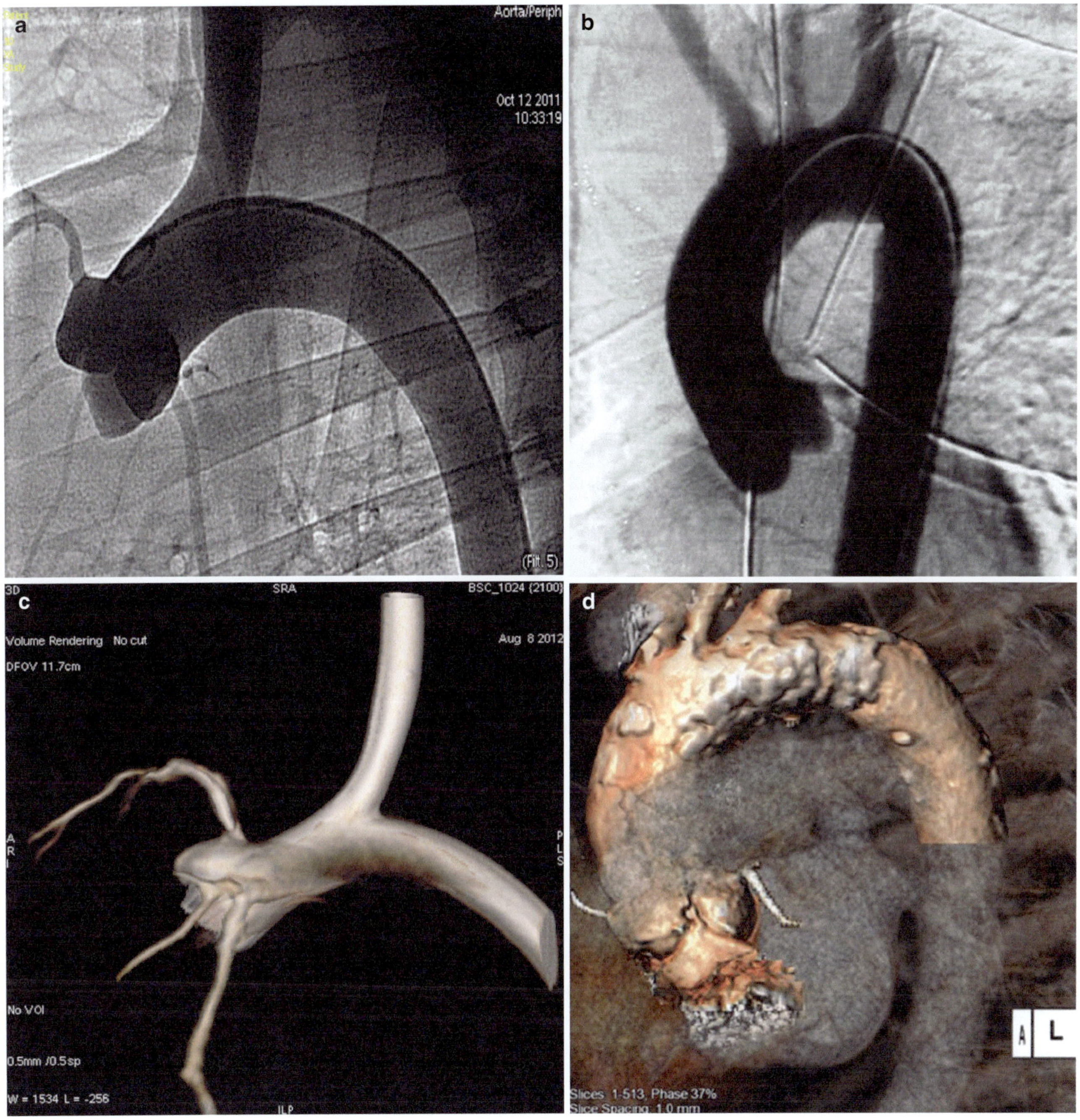

Fig. 37.4 Delivery system trackability and anatomic resemblance (A-ovine, C-human). Images (**a**) and (**b**) conventional vascular angiography. Image (**c**) cone beam angiography with three-dimensional reconstruction. Image (**d**) CT with three-dimensional reconstruction (Images **b** and **d** courtesy of American Heart of Poland)

Aortic Arch Anatomy and Delivery System Trackability

One of the most important components during the validation process of TAVR devices is the testing of delivery system tracking throughout the aortic arch. This is a particularly important feature as some neurovascular complications with TAVR are associated with interaction of the device to a diseased and highly calcific aorta. Although, in general terms, the basic anatomic landmarks are present in all large experimental models, major differences occur in the ascending and descending aortae compared to humans (Figs. 37.3a and 37.4a–d). Experimental models display a less angulated arch compared to humans, making it easier for devices to track throughout the process of valve delivery. In addition, the short length of the ascending aorta, a common feature of

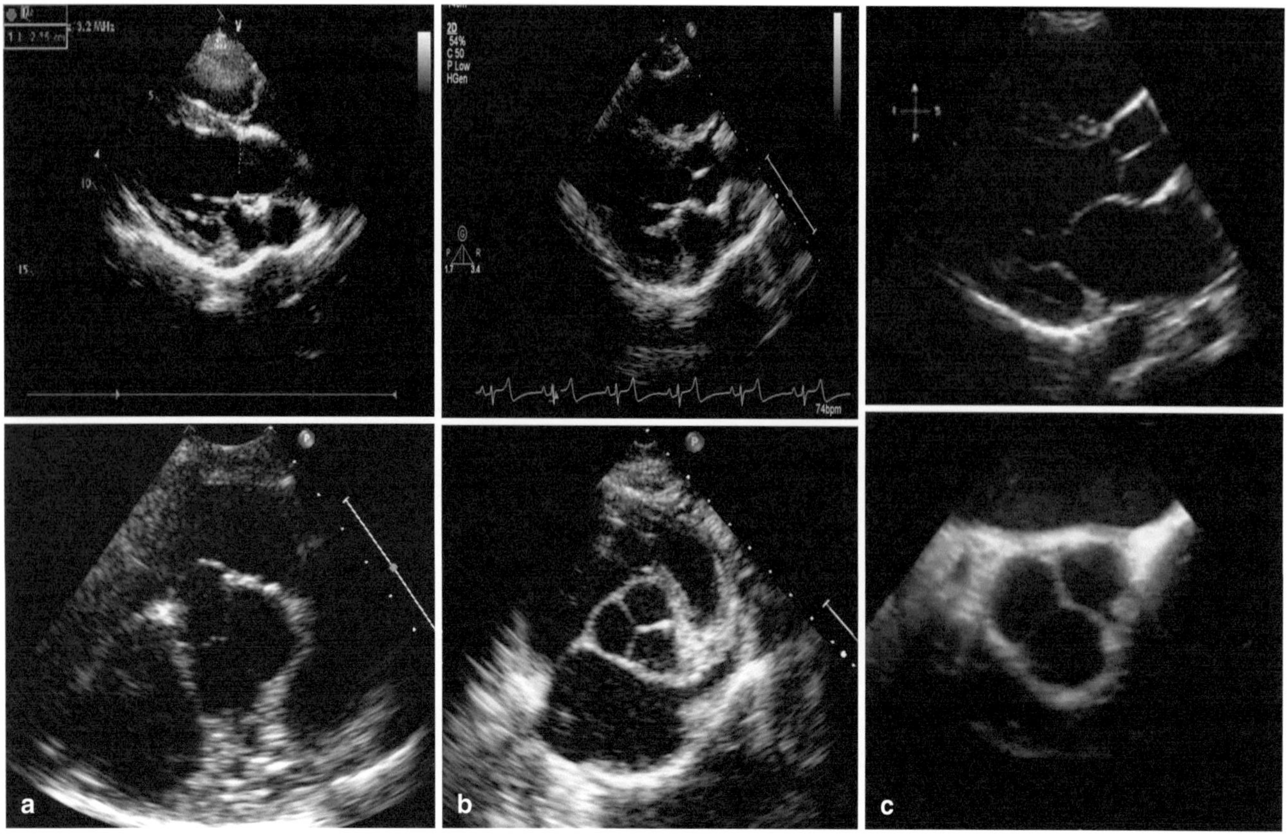

Fig. 37.5 Comparative heart and valvular anatomy in long (*top*) and short axis (*bottom*) in echocardiography: (**a**) sheep, (**b**) swine, (**c**) human

cloven-footed animals (calves, sheep, goats), gives way to the aortic bifurcation a short way downstream of the aortic valve. The decreased angulation of aortic arch makes the wire placement through the aortic valve and valve system positioning non-coaxial to annulus long axis. Consequently, these anatomical features make the transcatheter valve delivery technically challenging.

An important difference in experimental models is the anatomical variants of the large vessels derived from the aorta compared to humans. In sheep, both carotid arteries arise from brachiocephalic trunk, whereas in swine the anatomy of aortic arch is similar to human with the brachiocephalic trunk and common carotid artery arising from the aortic arch (Figs. 37.1 and 37.4). This feature is particularly important in the testing of embolic protection devices.

Acute Evaluation of Valve Delivery and Deployment

For experimental models, the aortic root, valve architecture, and its components (leaflets, sinutubular junction, and coronary ostia annulus) present identical morphological features compared to humans (Figs. 37.1, 37.4, and 37.5). Due to its size and anatomical configuration, the sheep model is the most common model used for TAVR testing today. In this model, the aortic annulus size is comparable to humans except at the level of the sinutubular junction, where it is significantly bigger. In the ovine, the coronary ostia are located usually lower when compared to human and the right ostium is higher than the left. Basing on our experience the average distance from the annulus to right coronary ostium is 9.2 ± 1.9 and 8.4 ± 1.7 mm to the left coronary ostium. In the clinical setting this origins are considered low and at increased risk of coronary occlusion [9]; however, in the preclinical setting this is a very unusual event.

One major difference in the sheep is the absence of space between the aortic and mitral valve annulus, the so-called intervalvar septum or membranous septum, which is commonly present in humans (1.0–1.5 cm). The anatomical variant may limit the use of some TAVR devices as they may potentially impinge on the mitral leaflets leading to periprocedural complications. The swine model displays similar features except for its overall size—which is smaller—when compared to the sheep heart (Table 37.2).

The acute evaluation of valve delivery and anchoring is one of the most important components of the evaluation of TAVR safety. Most of TAVR devices developed to date rely on the presence of valve thickening and calcification as the primary mechanism for valve retention. Therefore, the most

Table 37.2 Comparative anatomy of the normal aortic annulus and STJ

	Aortic annulus basal diameter (mm) Pathology		
	Human	**Sheep**	**Pig**
Laizzo PA. *Handbook of Cardiac Anatomy, Physiology, and Devices* (2009)	30.0 ± 2.6 (*n* = 8)	28.9 ± 5.4 (*n* = 10)	25.1 ± 3.2 (*n* = 10)
Sands MP. *Ann Thorac Surg* (1969)	26.4 ± 3.15 (*n* = 7)	25.8 ± 0.29 (*n* = 9)	26.6 ± 1.84 (*n* = 10)
Sim EK. *Clin Anat* (2003)	25.5 ± 1.3 (*n* = 12)		22.0 ± 3.2 (*n* = 12)
Combined	27.3 ± 2.3	27.3 ± 2.8	24.6 ± 2.7
SCCR		23.5 ± 3.7 (*n* = 10)	
	Echocardiography		
1. Yankah AC. *Aortic Root Surgery* 2. Falkner, OJVR (2005) 3. Dewey TM, ATS (2006)	22.6 ± 1.5 (*n* = 665) [1]	23 ± 4 (*n* = 30) [2]	19 ± 3.5 (*n* = 34) [3]
	Sinutubular junction diameter (mm)		
Sands MP (1969)	26.4	20.4	21.4
SCCR		25.1 ± 4.8	

important limitation of all experimental models is the absence of leaflet calcification and thickening, thus limiting long-term anchoring of the implanted device. In consequence, the majority of these experimental models are used to test the short-term technical features of valve delivery and deployment (Fig. 37.6). All experimental models allow the use of most currently available TAVR devices clinically available (18–24 mm). However, the use of very large devices (>27 mm) may be challenging. Experimental data in regard to the long-term evaluation of the biological response to TAVR devices implanted in the native aortic position is limited. However, latest generation TAVR devices equipped with different anchoring mechanisms have permitted the evaluation of valve performance in the aortic position.

Evaluation of Valve Healing and Performance

Long-term TAVR implants at the experimental setting are used to test material durability, biocompatibility, healing, and valve performance. However, due to the pathological differences described above, most of this testing is performed in heterotopic locations such as the brachiocephalic trunk or descending aorta, with creation of forced aortic valve regurgitation to achieve the necessary gradient to enable valve opening and closure. In an experiment by Eltchaninoff et al. [10], moderate-to-severe aortic insufficiency was created in juvenile sheep using a bioptome device when a valve was implanted distal to the left subclavian artery. This enabled intermediate testing of the valve for 5 months for measures of healing and performance. Also, other non-orthotopic positions (i.e., mitral) have been used for the long-term evaluation of TAVR devices (Fig. 37.7). At long-term follow-up, imaging reconstruction of the valve allows the evaluation of material fatigability (i.e., fractures) and valve functionality (Fig. 37.7d, e).

Diseased Models of Aortic Valve Disease

Although CAVS with significant hemodynamic gradient is inducible in mice and rabbits by genetic knockout with or without additional hypercholesterolemic diet [11, 12], large animal models of CAVS enabling long-term testing of TAVR devices in the aortic position are not available. Some anecdotal reports have described that swine fed with high-cholesterol diet develop aortic valve thickening and lipid deposits on the aortic side of leaflets (Fig. 37.8); however, no significant calcifications and subsequent hemodynamic changes typical for CAVS have been reported. Early work developed in our laboratory has confirmed these findings in a familial hypercholesterolemic swine model (FHS). This model lacks the liver LDL receptor and bears a homozygous mutation in one allelic mutant gene, Lpb5 at the apo B locus and, as a consequence, naturally develop hypercholesterolemia (>240 mg/dl) and atherosclerosis even if maintained under low-cholesterol, low-fat diet [13, 14]. By 2 years, these animals develop eccentric coronary lesions that consist predominantly of macrophage derived foam cells with admixed smooth muscle cells. By the third year, large areas of necrosis, fibrous cap formation, mononuclear cell infiltration and intra-plaque hemorrhage are commonly seen in these lesions [15]. This animal model also develops significantly more pronounced neointimal proliferation after coronary stent implantation when compared to domestic swine, therefore enhancing the ability for device efficacy testing [16]. Furthermore at 2 years, aortic valves of these animals

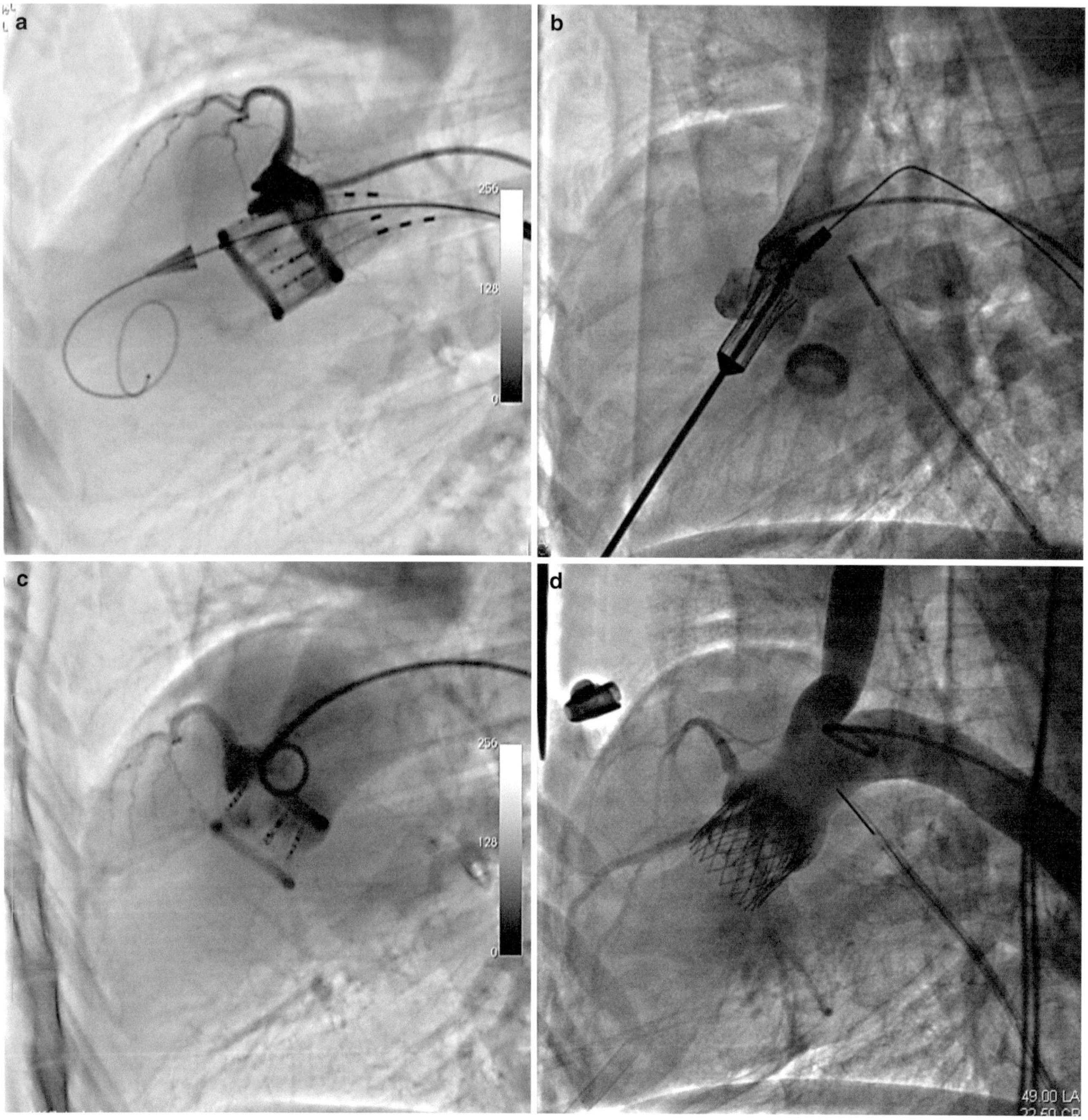

Fig. 37.6 Transcatheter valve positioning under fluoroscopic guidance (**a**, **b**) and acute outcome after delivery system retrieval in the sheep model (**c**, **d**) (**a**, **c** Direct Flow Medical and **c**, **d** Thubrikar Aortic Valve, Inc.)

develop lipid depositions, macrophage infiltrations, and macroscopically visible calcific nodules (Fig. 37.8). Further development of this experimental model is underway aiming to accelerate the process of calcification and leaflet thickening for TAVR study.

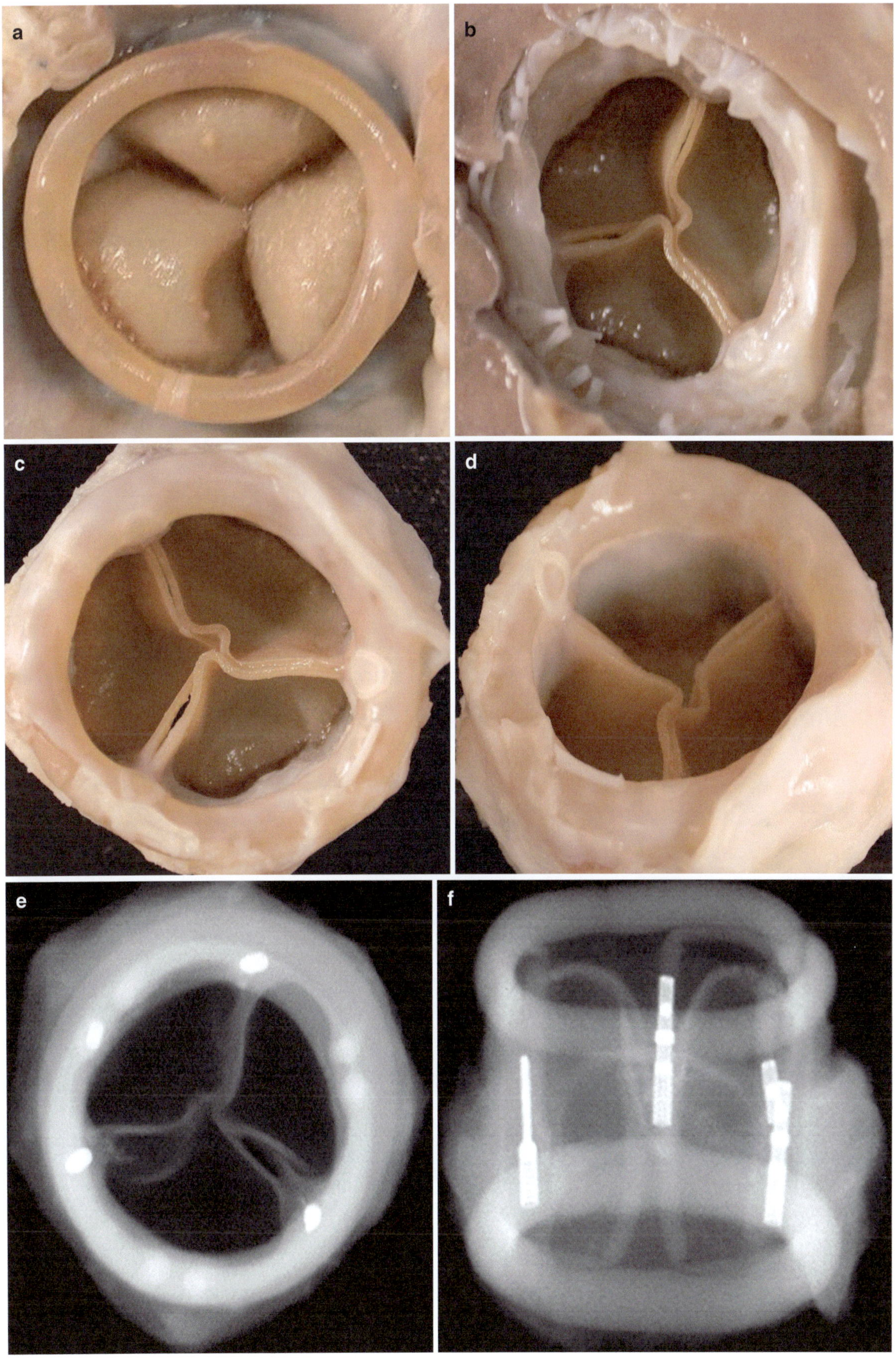

Fig. 37.7 Long-term healing (90 Days) of the transcatheter valve implanted surgically in the mitral position in sheep: (**a**) left atrial view, (**b**) LV apical view, (**c**) aortic root view, (**d**) cusp view, (**e**) lateral view. Images (**d**) and (**f**) faxitron radiography

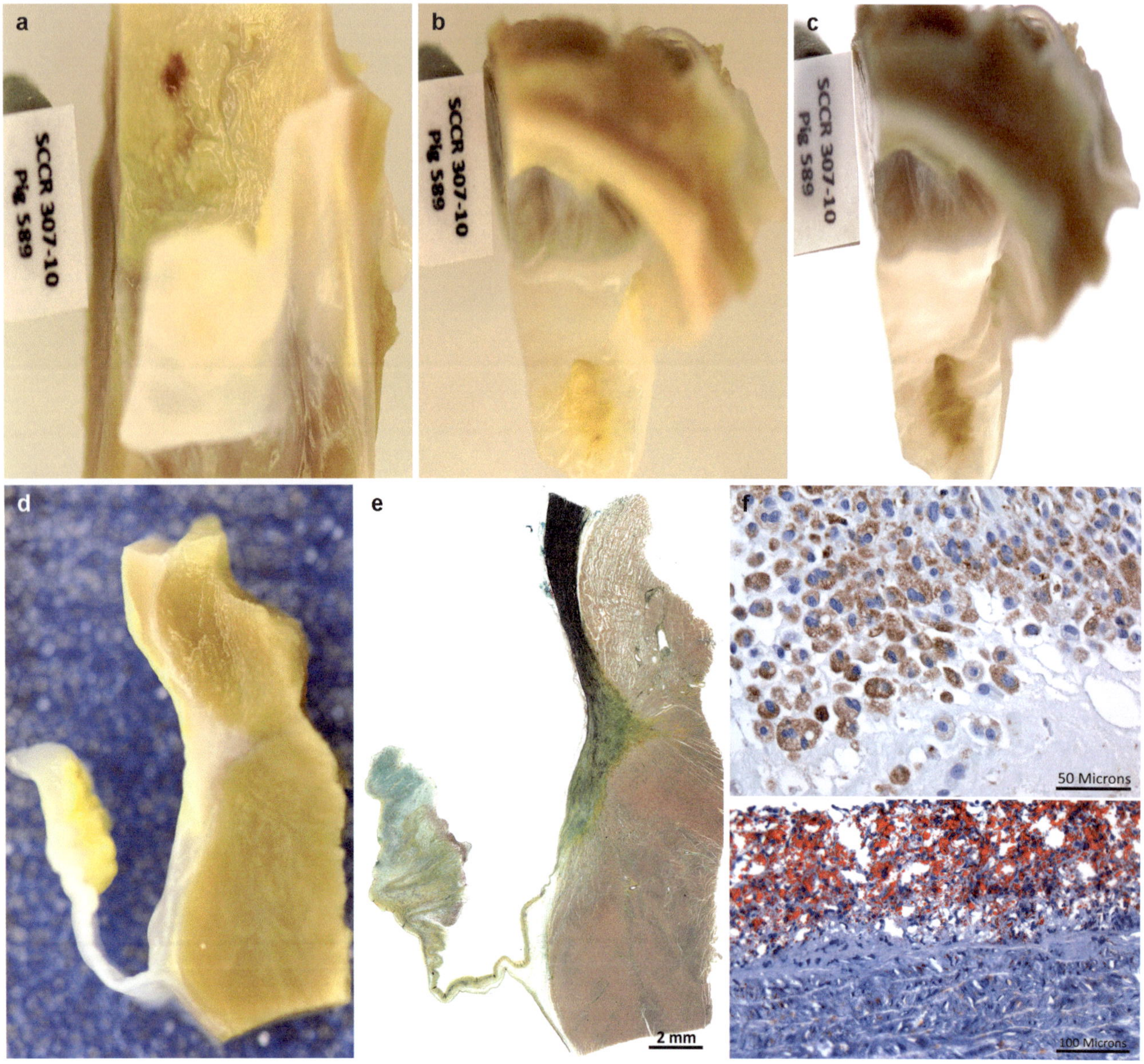

Fig. 37.8 Aortic valve thickening, fibrosis, and inflammation in the FHS model at 18 months. (**a**–**c**) Macroscopically visible calcific nodulues, (**d**, **e**) sagittal cross section of aortic root and valve leaflet, (**f**) CD107+ staining represents visible lipid deposition

Conclusion

Experimental animal models provide a similar anatomical environment compared to humans and allow the evaluation of safety features and performance of TAVR devices. Furthermore, the generally comparable peripheral vascular anatomy exhibited by these models permit the evaluation of safety features on access, trackability, and closure. Due to the lack of a primary disease state (i.e., calcification), the evaluation of long-term biocompatibility, tissue response, and healing of TAVR devices placed in the native aortic valve position is limited. However, innovative experimental models and techniques of TAVR implantation in other anatomical locations have shown to be effective for these chronic studies. Emerging diseased models of CAVS are under development and may facilitate the study of long-term healing and device integrity of devices placed at the aortic position.

References

1. Leon MB, Smith CR, Mack M, Miller DC, Moses JW, Svensson LG, Tuzcu EM, Webb JG, Fontana GP, Makkar RR, Brown DL, Block PC, Guyton RA, Pichard AD, Bavaria JE, Herrmann HC, Douglas PS, Petersen JL, Akin JJ, Anderson WN, Wang D, Pocock S. Transcatheter aortic-valve implantation for aortic stenosis in patients who cannot undergo surgery. N Engl J Med. 2010;363:1597–607.
2. Knudsen LL, Andersen HR, Hasenkam JM. Catheter-implanted prosthetic heart valves. Transluminal catheter implantation of a new

expandable artificial heart valve in the descending thoracic aorta in isolated vessels and closed chest pigs. Int J Artif Organs. 1993;16:253–62.

3. Andersen HR, Knudsen LL, Hasenkam JM. Transluminal implantation of artificial heart valves. Description of a new expandable aortic valve and initial results with implantation by catheter technique in closed chest pigs. Eur Heart J. 1992;13:704–8.
4. Cribier A, Eltchaninoff H, Bash A, Borenstein N, Tron C, Bauer F, Derumeaux G, Anselme F, Laborde F, Leon MB. Percutaneous transcatheter implantation of an aortic valve prosthesis for calcific aortic stenosis: First human case description. Circulation. 2002; 106:3006–8.
5. Hayashida K, Lefevre T, Chevalier B, Hovasse T, Romano M, Garot P, Mylotte D, Uribe J, Farge A, Donzeau-Gouge P, Bouvier E, Cormier B, Morice MC. Transfemoral aortic valve implantation new criteria to predict vascular complications. JACC Cardiovasc Interv. 2011;4:851–8.
6. Dewey TM, Walther T, Doss M, Brown D, Ryan WH, Svensson L, Mihaljevic T, Hambrecht R, Schuler G, Wimmer-Greinecker G, Mohr FW, Mack MJ. Transapical aortic valve implantation: an animal feasibility study. Ann Thorac Surg. 2006;82:110–6.
7. Kappetein AP, Piazza N, Laborde JC, de Jaegere PP, Serruys PW. Transapical implantation of a self-expanding aortic valve bioprosthesis – animal feasibility study. Eur J Cardiothorac Surg. 2009;36:813–7.
8. Barbash IM, Saikus CE, Faranesh AZ, Ratnayaka K, Kocaturk O, Chen MY, Bell JA, Virmani R, Schenke WH, Hansen MS, Slack MC, Lederman RJ. Direct percutaneous left ventricular access and port closure: pre-clinical feasibility. JACC Cardiovasc Interv. 2011;4:1318–25.
9. Webb JG, Wood DA. Current status of transcatheter aortic valve replacement. J Am Coll Cardiol. 2012;60:483–92.
10. Eltchaninoff H, Nusimovici-Avadis D, Babaliaros V, Spenser B, Felsen B, Cribier A. Five month study of percutaneous heart valves in the systemic circulation of sheep using a novel model of aortic insufficiency. EuroIntervention. 2006;1:438–44.
11. Weiss RM, Ohashi M, Miller JD, Young SG, Heistad DD. Calcific aortic valve stenosis in old hypercholesterolemic mice. Circulation. 2006;114:2065–9.
12. Miller JD, Weiss RM, Heistad DD. Calcific aortic valve stenosis: methods, models, and mechanisms. Circ Res. 2011;108:1392–412.
13. Hasler-Rapacz J, Ellegren H, Fridolfsson AK, Kirkpatrick B, Kirk S, Andersson L, Rapacz J. Identification of a mutation in the low density lipoprotein receptor gene associated with recessive familial hypercholesterolemia in swine. Am J Med Genet. 1998;76: 379–86.
14. Prescott MF, McBride CH, Hasler-Rapacz J, Von Linden J, Rapacz J. Development of complex atherosclerotic lesions in pigs with inherited hyper-ldl cholesterolemia bearing mutant alleles for apolipoprotein b. Am J Pathol. 1991;139:139–47.
15. Granada JF, Kaluza GL, Wilensky RL, Biedermann BC, Schwartz RS, Falk E. Porcine models of coronary atherosclerosis and vulnerable plaque for imaging and interventional research. EuroIntervention. 2009;5:140–8.
16. Tellez A, Krueger CG, Seifert P, Winsor-Hines D, Piedrahita C, Cheng Y, Milewski K, Aboodi MS, Yi G, McGregor JC, Crenshaw T, Reed JD, Huibregtse B, Kaluza GL, Granada JF. Coronary bare metal stent implantation in homozygous LDL receptor deficient swine induces a neointimal formation pattern similar to humans. Atherosclerosis. 2010;213:518–24.

What Future Studies Are Needed for TAVR Imaging?

38

James K. Min, Jonathon Leipsic, and Paul Schoenhagen

Abstract

The development of transcatheter valve procedures has been revealed an ever-increasing importance of pre-, peri-, and post-procedural imaging. Extensive imaging evaluation of the aortic valve, aortic root, aorta, and iliac arteries has contributed to the evolution and optimization the procedure. The initial approach has been focused towards obtaining a maximum amount of information, often times with multiple imaging modalities. Eventually, it will be necessary to consolidate the accumulating data into standardized imaging approaches, which can be recommended only to operators in the presence of high-quality scientific evidence.

Keywords

Aortic valve • Transcatheter heart valve • Stenosis • Post-procedural evaluation • Procedural simulation • Stroke

Introduction

The development of transcatheter valve procedures has been revealed an ever-increasing importance of pre-, peri-, and post-procedural imaging. Extensive imaging evaluation of the aortic valve, aortic root, aorta, and iliac arteries has contributed to the evolution and optimization the procedure. The initial approach has been focused towards obtaining a maximum amount of information, often times with multiple imaging modalities. Eventually, it will be necessary to consolidate the accumulating data into standardized imaging approaches, which can be recommended only to operators in the presence of high-quality scientific evidence. Following the other chapter in this book, which describe the current status of the transcatheter aortic valve replacement (TAVR) experience, the goal of this chapter is to consider what future imaging clinical research studies are most needed to provide the basis for evidence-based consensus guidelines.

Annulus and Aortic Valve

Optimal adaptation of the aortic valve prosthesis to the aortic annulus is a prerequisite for long-term durability of the transcatheter valve. During surgical aortic valve replacement, the size of the annulus is measured with dilaters, matching common size valve prostheses. After choosing the appropriate size valve, suturing the valve ring to the aortic annulus provides tight circumferential adaptation. In contrast, during TAVR, the stent anchors and adapts to the anatomy of the aortic annulus and root. This process is dependent on details of deployment,

J.K. Min, MD, FACC, FSCCT (✉)
Weill Cornell Medical College, NewYork-Presbyterian Hospital, New York, NY, USA
e-mail: jkm2001@med.cornell.edu

J. Leipsic, MD, FRCPC, FSCCT
Division of Cardiology, Department of Radiology, University of British Columbia, St. Paul's Hospital, Vancouver, BC, Canada

P. Schoenhagen, MD
Departments of Cardiovascular Medicine and Radiology, Imaging Institute and Heart and Vascular Institute, Cleveland Clinic, 9500 Euclid Avenue, Cleveland, OH 44195, USA
e-mail: schoenp1@ccf.org

J.K. Min et al. (eds.), *Multimodality Imaging for Transcatheter Aortic Valve Replacement*, DOI 10.1007/978-1-4471-2798-7_38, © Springer-Verlag London 2014

size, geometry, and tissue composition of the landing zone. Therefore, as describe in other chapters of this book, assessment of the complex anatomy of the aortic annulus (virtual basal ring), aortic valve, and aortic root is critical for successful TAVR. Anatomically, the aortic valve leaflets are attached to the aortic root in a crown-shaped manner along the commissures and often referred to as a coronet [1]. By imaging, the annulus (or better inferior virtual basal ring) is defined by the level of basal attachment of the leaflets.

Multiple studies have examined differences in aortic annulus measurements between echocardiography and multidetector row computed tomography (MDCT) and have demonstrated an ovoid shape of the annulus with significant differences in diameters between modalities [2–7]. The mean MDCT diameter is significantly larger than the echocardiographic measurements, although the differences are small. Current clinical experience and recommendations are based on echocardiographic measurements. Using a decision model for the TAVR strategy with the TEE measurement as the gold standard, Messika-Zeitoun et al. [2] demonstrated that more patients would have been denied the procedure based on the MDCT measurements, despite good results with the standard TEE-based strategy. These data demonstrate that the increased precision of three-dimensional measurements with MDCT do not necessarily translate to improved clinical outcome without the appropriate development of MDCT transcatheter heart valve sizing guidelines. These limitations serve to define the need for future studies correlating imaging findings with clinical outcome.

The distance between the annulus and the ostia of the coronary arteries in relationship to the length of the coronary leaflets can be derived from MDCT scans [3–7]. In a small minority of patients, a particularly low origin (<10 mm) has been associated with coronary complication during the procedure. However, based on current experience, this is an infrequent event and careful assessment during routine cardiac catheterization or on standard MDCT scans can provide reliable information. While some studies suggest remodeling of the root including the origin of the coronary arteries in patients with AS, it is unlikely that more detailed description will have significant clinical impact.

What Future Studies Are Needed to Assess the Annulus and Valve?

Previously published data demonstrate that the increased precision of three-dimensional measurements by MDCT do not automatically correspond with better clinical outcome and define the need for future comparative studies correlating imaging findings with clinical outcome. Areas where data is still incomplete and future studies appear necessary are manifold.

Appropriate device sizing is most likely dependent on not only pre-procedural dimensions but also tissue composition and distribution of disease. As the hinge points of the valve leaflets provide the anchor point to the valve, differences in the characteristics of the sub-leaflet tissue (muscular septum, membranous septum, or aortomitral curtain) will determine distortion at the time of stent valve deployment. Understanding how an aortic valve prosthesis interacts with the aortic root anatomy and the left ventricular outflow tract will allow prediction the final shape of the prosthetic valve, displacement of the native calcified leaflets, and sealing around the prosthesis [8]. Of particular interest is the extent and distribution of the aortic valve and root calcification, including extension of calcification along the LVOT [9, 10] and mitral annular calcification (MAC). This information may facilitate proper placement and subsequent aortic regurgitation, dysfunction of the conduction system, and mitral valve function.

The impact of more detailed assessment of the aortic annulus and root requires examination in future clinical outcome trials. In such studies, echocardiographic outcomes should be compared to other modalities for measures of post-procedural aortic regurgitation and other imaging complications. Clinical endpoints should invariably be assessed as well and include conduction abnormalities (with subsequent need for permanent pacemaker implantation), morbidity, and mortality. Such data will need to be derived from emerging large registries and eventually from prospective trials.

Discordance of Aortic Stenosis Severity

Grading of AS with echocardiography is well standardized for the majority of patients. However, there is a non-negligible portion of patients who exhibit discrepancies between aortic valve area (AVA) and transvalvular gradient for measures of AS severity. In fact, for as many as 30 % of patients with a calculated AVA in the severe range, other parameters suggest only mild or moderate disease (e.g., mean gradient 30 mmHg) [11]. These patients with low-flow low-gradient AS (LF-LGAS) may truly have severe AS with resultant myocardial failure (true AS) or may have more moderate degrees of AS and unrelated myocardial dysfunction (pseudo-AS). In the latter setting, the aortic valve may appear severely stenotic as a result of the flow-dependent nature of the valve area calculation by either invasive or non-invasive techniques [12] and the inability of the myopathic ventricle to generate adequate force to fully open the valve. Distinguishing between these possibilities has important clinical implications with regard to prognosis and management options, as patients with true AS will likely benefit from corrective valve surgery, whereas patients with pseudo-AS may not.

While the majority of patients with LF-LGAS have reduced left ventricular systolic function (LVEF <40 %), a number of patients have paradoxically low flow, defined as a stroke volume index of 35 mL/m², despite preserved LVEF >50 % [13]. These patients have lower peak transaortic velocities (3.5 vs. 4.0 m/s) and lower mean gradients (32 vs. 40 mmHg) compared to patients who have normal transaortic flow rates, despite having similar AVA (0.76 vs. 0.84 cm²), similar dimensionless index (0.24 vs. 0.23), and similar LVEF (65 % vs. 69 %). These features predispose diagnosis to an underestimation of the severity of AS in these patients and delay in pursuing appropriate care. The mechanism of the paradoxically low flow in the face of preserved LVEF likely relates to high afterload, and the reduced stroke volume in this setting is probably an early marker of intrinsic myocardial dysfunction.

The prognosis of patients with LF-LGAS with preserved LVEF depends, in part, on the presence of symptoms [11, 13]. In a series of symptomatic patients, those with low transaortic flow experienced a worse prognosis compared with their counterparts with normal flow (3-year survival 76 % vs. 86 %); however, they obtained similar mortality benefits from AVR [13]. In contrast, in a larger and more contemporary report, asymptomatic patients with LF-LGAS with preserved LVEF had a prognosis similar to that of patients with more moderate AS (92.2 % vs. 95.1 % survival at 46 months) [11].

Determining which patients with LF-LGAS will benefit from AVR can be challenging [14–17]. The utility of a dobutamine challenge in the evaluation of LF-LGAS during either cardiac catheterization or stress echocardiography has been well documented [18–22], but differentiation between true from pseudo-AS in patients with no contractile reserve remains challenging.

What Future Studies Are Necessary in AS Grading?

Other imaging modalities may aid in the identification of severe AS in this setting. Recent small studies have demonstrated good correlation between the aortic valve calcium score as measured by multidetector computed tomography and the severity of AS as assessed by echocardiography [23, 24].

Another study correlated delayed enhancement by preoperative cardiac magnetic resonance (MR) with the presence of myocardial fibrosis on surgical biopsy in patients with severe AS [25, 26]. Although the utility of MR for determining the prognosis of patients with LF-LGAS is unclear, it is likely that the lack of contractile reserve in some patients with LF-LGAS is mediated, in part, by the presence of irreversible cardiac fibrosis. While these modalities may help to further risk stratify these patients, data is incomplete and correlation with clinical outcome is missing. Large registries and future randomized studies will provide answers.

Stroke, Aorta, and Plaque

A concern based on the initial randomized trials of TAVR is the higher initial stroke rate with TAVR. In the PARTNER trial [27] at 1 year, the rate of death from any cause was 30.7 % with TAVR, as compared with 50.7 % with standard therapy (hazard ratio with TAVR, 0.55; 95 % confidence interval [CI], 0.40 to 0.74; $p<0.001$). However, at 30 days, TAVR—when compared with standard therapy—was associated with a higher incidence of major strokes (5.0 % vs. 1.1 %, $p=0.06$). Randomized trials have also identified a higher incidence of CVI with TAVR compared to surgical treatment [28]. A recent study described a prospective investigation of silent and clinically apparent cerebral embolic events and neurological impairment after TAVR [29]. The authors investigated peri-interventional cerebral embolism with diffusion-weighted magnetic resonance imaging (DW-MRI) and its relationship to clinical and serologic parameters of brain injury. Cerebral DW-MRI was performed before, directly, and 3 months after TAVR with the current third-generation self-expanding CoreValve (Medtronic, Minneapolis, Minnesota) prosthesis. At the time points of these serial MRI studies, focal neurological impairment was assessed according to the National Institutes of Health Stroke Scale (NIHSS), and serum concentration of neuron-specific enolase (NSE), a marker of the volume of brain tissue involved in an ischemic event, was determined. Thirty patients were enrolled and 22 completed the imaging protocol. Three patients (10 %) had new neurological findings after TAVR, of whom only 1 (3.6 %) had a permanent neurological impairment. Of the 22 TAVR patients with complete imaging data, 16 (72.7 %) had 75 new cerebral lesions after TAVR presumed to be embolic. The NIHSS and NSE were not correlated with DW-MRI lesions. While the incidence of clinically silent peri-interventional cerebral embolic lesions after TAVR was high, the incidence of persistent neurological impairment was low.

It remains unclear if stroke rates continue to remain high in the early and intermediate-term period after TAVR, and, consequently, the optimal dose and duration of anticoagulation in the post-TAVR period is unclear. A recent study examined whether there exists a high-risk period for cerebrovascular events (CVE) after TAVR [30]. Patients who underwent TAVR were evaluated at baseline, at discharge, at 1 and 6 months, and yearly. Outcomes assessed were CVE events and death. The timing of such events, predictors, and impact on survival were analyzed in a total of 253 patients with a median age was 85 years. During a follow-up of 455 days, 23 patients experienced a CVE event. The incidence was highest in the first 24 h but remained high for 2 months. In-hospital mortality rate after a CVE event was 21 %. A prior history of CVE disease was an independent predictor of an event (hazard ratio, 4.23; 95 % CI, 1.60–11.11; $p=0.004$).

The pathophysiologic mechanisms underlying the increased CVE event rate remains incompletely understood, but aortic plaque burden may play a significant role. In population-based studies of asymptomatic individuals and persons with suspected coronary artery disease, calcified aortic atheroma has been shown to be associated with increased risk of major cardiovascular events [31, 32]. In population-based asymptomatic individuals, based on non-contrast enhanced CT studies, there is a relationship between calcified aortic atheroma [33] and all-cause mortality, independent of conventional CVD risk factors [34, 35]. In patients evaluated for conventional cardiothoracic surgery, calcified and non-calcified aortic atheromas have also been established as a predictor of postoperative complications, as well as of adverse long-term outcome [36–40].

One explanation for the role of aortic plaque invokes a dominant role of embolic complications, in particular, in the context of manipulations of the aorta during the procedure. An alternative hypothesis suggests a more systemic effect of the diffuse atherosclerotic disease process, with aortic plaque burden a marker of atherosclerotic disease and complications in other vascular regions. Importantly, the relationship of plaque extent to mortality is independent of distribution along the aorta, which is evidence that mortality is related to the systemic atherosclerotic disease process rather than focal or embolic complications alone [40]. This is further supported by recent studies in the carotid circulation and previous data describing a relationship between coronary and aortic calcifications [41]. Recent data from patients evaluated for transcatheter aortic valve implantation (TAVR), a population with very high mortality, reveal extensive atherosclerotic disease of the aorta [42]. Together, these results identify the extent of thoracic atheroma burden as a risk factor for cerebral complications of TAVR.

What Future Studies Are Needed?

Based on these data, studies examining aortic plaque burden and composition in a volumetric fashion in relationship to CVE are necessary. Such studies should employ imaging endpoints such as intracranial Doppler, MDCT, and diffuse weighted MRI along with clinical endpoints.

Vascular Access Site

There is a spectrum of arterial access strategies for TAVR, ranging from a percutaneous transfemoral, transapical, transaxillary, to open iliofemoral approaches [43–47]. Because of the large device size of current generation systems, the transfemoral approach requires favorable iliofemoral arterial anatomy [48]. In the setting of insufficient luminal diameter, extensive calcification, or excess tortuosity of the iliofemoral arteries, the transfemoral approach is associated with a higher incidence of arterial injury [49]. The prevalence of significant peripheral arterial disease (PAD) in the high-risk population currently undergoing assessment for TAVR is high. Limited angiographic assessment of the iliofemoral anatomy is routinely performed during pre-procedural coronary angiography. However, dedicated three-dimensional evaluation of infrarenal aortic and iliofemoral arterial anatomy by MDCT provided more precise cross-sectional diameter measurements, assessment of the extent and distribution of calcification, and three-dimensional course and tortuosity of the iliofemoral arteries. This may allow identification of patients with unsuitable iliofemoral anatomy for a transfemoral approach to TAVR and eventually pre-procedural planning of arterial access [42]. Using MDCT of the infrarenal abdominal aorta and iliofemoral arteries, our group described [42] that one third of patients with severe aortic stenosis evaluated for TAVR had anatomic criteria of unfavorable atherosclerotic iliofemoral disease. Of these patients, a majority (77 %) demonstrated small luminal narrowing (<8 mm) of the iliofemoral arteries; the remaining 23 % showed other criteria of advanced disease, including circumferential calcification and severe tortuosity, despite sufficient luminal diameter. Comparison between the groups of patients with and without any of these criteria demonstrated that the presence of any one of these criteria identifies a high-risk group of patient with significantly higher clinical risk profile and more unfavorable anatomy of the entire infrarenal and iliofemoral arteries. Because of the known overlap of etiology and risk factors for atherosclerotic vascular disease and aortic stenosis, it is not surprising to find a high number of patients with significant peripheral arterial disease in this population.

Pre-procedural interventional planning is widely established and routinely performed in the context of aortic endovascular stent procedures [50, 51]. The importance for planning of vascular access may diminish with the development of TAVR valve delivery systems with small diameters. However, previous data suggest that the identification of unfavorable iliofemoral anatomy may identify a high-risk group of patients in whom careful planning of access strategy may be of particular importance.

What Future Studies Are Needed?

With recent developments of new TAVR techniques, direct head-to-head randomized studies of transaortic and transapical approaches are warranted to provide further evidence required for decision making for the optimal approach in a particular patient. As well, head-to-head randomized trials will be necessary to evaluate new valve and delivery device designs to assess their comparative effectiveness as treatments for aortic stenosis. The currently underway PARTNER IIB trial which randomizes patients between the Sapien and XT valves and their delivery systems is an example of one such trial that is essential to move the field forward.

Post-procedural Imaging

Post-procedural imaging relies on echocardiography. However, different methods for the measurement of the valve effective orifice area (EOA) following TAVR have been described, and factors influencing the EOA of transcatheter valves are unknown. A recent study [52] compared different Doppler echocardiographic methods for the measurement of prosthetic valve EOA following TAVR and to determine the factors influencing the EOA of transcatheter balloon expandable valves. In 122 patients who underwent TAVR with the use of the Edwards SAPIEN valve, the EOA was measured by transthoracic echocardiography at hospital discharge, 6 months, and 1 year after TAVR with the use of 2 methods as described in previous studies. By the first method for EOA calculation [1], LVOT diameter (LVOTd) entered in the continuity equation was measured at the base of prosthesis cusps, whereas in the second method EOA[2], LVOTd was measured immediately proximal to the prosthesis stent. The average EOA was larger by the second method compared to the first method (1.57 ± 0.41 cm^2 vs. 1.21 ± 0.38 cm^2, $p<0.01$) [1]. Accordingly, incidence of severe patient prosthesis mismatched, with an indexed EOA ≤ 0.65 cm^2/m^2, was 3-fold lower with the use of the second method compared to the first (9 % vs. 33 %; $p<0.001$). Mean transprosthetic gradient also correlated better with the second method compared to the first ($r=-0.70$ vs. $r=-0.58$, $p=0.03$). The authors thus recommend to use the LVOT diameter and velocity measured immediately proximal to the stent when estimating the EOA of Edwards SAPIEN valves by Doppler echocardiography.

Future Considerations

Cardiovascular Magnetic Resonance (CMR)

CMR is a conceptually attractive alternative for real-time guidance of transarterial aortic valve implantation (TAVR). It allows unlimited scan plane orientation, excellent soft-tissue contrast without the administration of intravenous contrast medium, and radiation exposure [53]. However, the complexity of CMR pulse sequences and the limited dissemination of the technology have prevented its widespread implementation thus far. In addition, the composition of some of the currently available transcatheter heart valves result in significant susceptibility artifact when imaged by MRI, thereby significantly limiting image quality. Future technological advances employing CMR are underway, including dedicated delivery devices and CMR-compatible delivery device for real-time CMR-guided TAVR [54]. The devices have been examined in phantom models on a 1.5-T scanner using high-resolution T1-weighted 3D FLASH, real-time TrueFISP, and flow-sensitive phase-contrast sequences. Images were analyzed for device visualization quality, device-related susceptibility artifacts, and radiofrequency signal shielding. CMR revealed major susceptibility artifacts for the two commercial delivery devices caused by considerable metal braiding and precluding in vivo application. The stainless steel-based Edwards SAPIEN™ prosthesis was also regarded not suitable for CMR-guided TAVR due to susceptibility artifacts exceeding the valve's dimensions and hindering an exact placement. In contrast, the nitinol-based Medtronic CoreValve prosthesis was excellently visualized with delineation even of small details and, thus, regarded suitable for CMR-guided TAVR, particularly since reengineering of its delivery device toward CMR-compatibility resulted in artifact elimination and excellent visualization during catheter movement and valve deployment on real-time TrueFISP imaging. Reliable flow measurements could be performed for both stent valves after deployment using phase-contrast sequences. The present study shows that the Medtronic CoreValve prosthesis is potentially suited for real-time CMR-guided placement in vivo after suggested design modifications of the delivery system. If proven to be an effective means for device delivery, further adaptations of transcatheter heart valve designs may encourage further investigation and incorporation of advanced MR guidance for the procedure.

Procedural Simulations

An exciting use of four-dimensional data incorporating volumetric heart images over time is the use of this data for patient-specific analyses and simulation. Small feasibility studies have described this approach in the context of TAVR [55]. In a small study of four patients with failed bioprosthetic aortic valves and one patient with an incompetent, native aortic valve, imaging models of implantation sites were reconstructed from MDCT images. TAVR with an Edwards Sapien stent was then simulated using finite element modeling, with outcome variables including stress distribution and geometric orifice areas. The authors suggest that fine element analyses can in the future both refine patient selection and characterize device mechanical performance in TAVR.

Conclusion

Aortic stenosis (AS) is one of the most common valve disorders encountered in clinical practice and one of the most frequent indications for valve replacement surgery.

Based on extensive research and clinical experience, clinical evidence-based guidelines provide an approach to the management of patients with AS. The early rapid evolution of any new technique is commonly associated with a lack of standardized approaches and a lack of evidence-based clinical data. TAVR investigators have generated considerable high-quality data through well-designed randomized trials, and consensus recommendations are emerging to guide appropriate practice [56, 57]. Still, boundless questions remain, particularly with respect to imaging. While the role of imaging has evolved alongside the procedural aspects of TAVR, randomized trials and large-scale observational data are still lacking. Ongoing research to advance the proper role of imaging in the pre-, intra-, and post-procedural evaluation of patients undergoing TAVR will be invariably needed, and the questions posed in this chapter represent only an initial step in the full understanding of imaging for TAVR.

References

1. Piazza N, de Jaegere P, Schultz C, et al. Anatomy of the aortic valvar complex and its implications for transcatheter implantation of the aortic valve. Circ Cardiovasc Interv. 2008;1:74–81.
2. Messika-Zeitoun D, Serfaty J-M, Brochet E, et al. Multimodal assessment of the aortic annulus diameter: implications for transcatheter aortic valve implantation. J Am Coll Cardiol. 2010;55:186–94.
3. Tops LF, Wood DA, Delgado V, et al. Noninvasive evaluation of the aortic root with multislice computed tomography: implications for transcatheter aortic valve replacement. J Am Coll Cardiol Img. 2008;1:321–30.
4. Knight J, Kurtcuoglu V, Muffly K, et al. Ex vivo and in vivo coronary ostial locations in humans. Surg Radiol Anat. 2009;31:597–604.
5. Akhtar M, Tuzcu EM, Kapadia SR, et al. Aortic root morphology in patients undergoing percutaneous aortic valve replacement. Evidence of aortic root remodeling. J Thorac Cardiovasc Surg. 2009;137:950–6.
6. Stolzmann P, Knight J, Desbiolles L, et al. Remodelling of the aortic root in severe tricuspid aortic stenosis: implications for transcatheter aortic valve implantation. Eur Radiol. 2009;19:1316–23.
7. Wood DA, Tops LF, Mayo JR, et al. Role of multislice computed tomography in transcatheter aortic valve replacement. Am J Cardiol. 2009;103:1295–301.
8. Kronzon I, Sugeng L, Perk G, et al. Real-time 3-dimensional transesophageal echocardiography in the evaluation of post-operative mitral annuloplasty ring and prosthetic valve dehiscence. J Am Coll Cardiol. 2009;53:1543–7.
9. Latsios G, Gerckens U, Buellesfeld L, Mueller R, John D, Yuecel S, Syring J, Sauren B, Grube E. "Device landing zone" calcification, assessed by MSCT, as a predictive factor for pacemaker implantation after TAVR. Catheter Cardiovasc Interv. 2010;76:431–9.
10. John D, Buellesfeld L, Yuecel S, Mueller R, Latsios G, Beucher H, Gerckens U, Grube E. Correlation of device landing zone calcification and acute procedural success in patients undergoing transcatheter aortic valve implantations with the self-expanding CoreValve prosthesis. J Am Coll Cardiol Intv. 2010;3:233–43.
11. Jander N, Minners N, Holme I, Gerdts E, Boman K, Brudi P, Chambers JB, Egstrup K, Kesaniemi YA, Malbecq W, Nienaber CA, Ray S, Rossebø A, Pedersen TR, Skjærpe T, Willenheimer R, Wachtell K, Neumann FJ, Gohlke-Ba¨rwolf C. Outcome of patients with low-gradient "severe" aortic stenosis and preserved ejection fraction. Circulation. 2011;123:887–95.
12. Burwash IG, Thomas DD, Sadahiro M, Pearlman AS, Verrier ED, Thomas R, Kraft CD, Otto CM. Dependence of Gorlin formula and continuity equation valve areas on transvalvular volume flow rate in valvular aortic stenosis. Circulation. 1994;89:827–35.
13. Hachicha Z, Dumesnil JG, Bogaty P, Pibarot P. Paradoxical low-flow, low-gradient severe aortic stenosis despite preserved ejection fraction is associated with higher afterload and reduced survival. Circulation. 2007;115:2856–64.
14. Levy F, Laurent M, Monin JL, Maillet JM, Pasquet A, Le Tourneau T, Petit Eisenmann H, Gori M, Jobic Y, Bauer F, Chauvel C, Leguerrier A, Tribouilloy C. Aortic valve replacement for low-flow/low-gradient aortic stenosis operative risk stratification and long-term outcome: a European multicenter study. J Am Coll Cardiol. 2008;51:1466–72.
15. Clavel MA, Fuchs C, Burwash IG, Mundigler G, Dumesnil JG, Baumgartner H, Bergler-Klein J, Beanlands RS, Mathieu P, Magne J, Pibarot P. Predictors of outcomes in low-flow, low-gradient aortic stenosis. Results of the multicenter TOPAS Study. Circulation. 2008;118 Suppl 1:S234–42.
16. Tribouilloy C, Le´vy F, Rusinaru D, Gue´ret P, Petit-Eisenmann H, Baleynaud S, Jobic Y, Adams C, Lelong B, Pasquet A, Chauvel C, Metz D, Que´re´ JP, Monin JL. Outcome after aortic valve replacement for low-flow/low-gradient aortic stenosis without contractile reserve on dobutamine stress echocardiography. J Am Coll Cardiol. 2009;53:1865–73.
17. Kulik A, Burwash IG, Kapila V, Mesana TG, Ruel M. Long-term outcomes after valve replacement for low-gradient aortic stenosis: impact of prosthesis- patient mismatch. Circulation. 2006;114(Suppl I):I553–8.
18. Nishimura RA, Grantham JA, Connolly HM, Schaff HV, Higano ST, Holmes Jr DR. Low-output, low-gradient aortic stenosis in patients with depressed left ventricular systolic function: the clinical utility of the dobutamine challenge in the catheterization laboratory. Circulation. 2002;106:809–13.
19. Monin JL, Monchi M, Gest V, Duval-Moulin AM, Dubois-Rande JL, Gueret P. Aortic stenosis with severe left ventricular dysfunction and low transvalvular pressure gradients: risk stratification by low-dose dobutamine echocardiography. J Am Coll Cardiol. 2001;37:2101–7.
20. Quere JP, Monin JL, Levy F, Petit H, Baleynaud S, Chauvel C, Pop C, Ohlmann P, Lelguen C, Dehant P, Gueret P, Tribouilloy C. Influence of preoperative left ventricular contractile reserve on postoperative ejection fraction in low-gradient aortic stenosis. Circulation. 2006;113:1738–44.
21. Monin J, Que´re´ J, Monchi M, Petit H, Baleynaud S, Chauvel C, Pop C, Ohlmann P, Lelguen C, Dehant P, Tribouilloy C, Gue´ret P. Low-gradient aortic stenosis operative risk stratification and predictors for long-term outcome: a multicenter study using dobutamine stress hemodynamics. Circulation. 2003;108:319–24.
22. Blais C, Burwash IG, Mundigler G, Dumesnil JG, Loho N, Rader F, Baumgartner H, Beanlands RS, Chayer B, Kadem L, Garcia D, Durand LG, Pibarot P. Projected valve area at normal flow rate improves the assessment of stenosis severity in patients with low-flow, low-gradient aortic stenosis: the multicenter TOPAS (Truly or Pseudo-Severe Aortic Stenosis) study. Circulation. 2006;113:711–21.
23. Messika-Zeitoun D, Aubry MC, Detaint D, Bielak LF, Peyser PA, Sheedy PF, Turner ST, Breen JF, Scott C, Tajik AJ, Enriquez-Sarano M. Evaluation and clinical implications of aortic valve calcification measured by electron-beam computed tomography. Circulation. 2004;110:356–62.
24. Cueff C, Serfaty J, Cimadevilla C, Laissy JP, Himbert D, Tubach F, Duval X, Iung B, Enriquez-Sarano M, Vahanian A, Messika-Zeitoun D. Measurement of aortic valve calcification using

multislice computed tomography: correlation with haemodynamic severity of aortic stenosis and clinical implication for patients with low ejection fraction. Heart. 2011;97:721–6.
25. Weidemann F, Herrmann S, Sto¨rk S, Niemann M, Frantz S, Lange V, Beer M, Gattenlo¨hner S, Voelker W, Ertl G, Strotmann JM. Impact of myocardial fibrosis in patients with symptomatic severe aortic stenosis. Circulation. 2009;120:577–84.
26. Dweck MR, Joshi S, Murigu T, Alpendurada F, Jabbour A, Melina G, Banya W, Gulati A, Roussin I, Raza S, Prasad NA, Wage R, Quarto C, Angeloni E, Refice S, Sheppard M, Cook SA, Kilner PJ, Pennell DJ, Newby DE, Mohiaddin RH, Pepper J, Prasad SK. Midwall fibrosis is an independent predictor of mortality in patients with aortic stenosis. J Am Coll Cardiol. 2011;58:1271–9.
27. Leon MB, Smith CR, Mack M, Miller DC, Moses JW, Svensson LG, Tuzcu EM, Webb JG, Fontana GP, Makkar RR, Brown DL, Block PC, Guyton RA, Pichard AD, Bavaria JE, Herrmann HC, Douglas PS, Petersen JL, Akin JJ, Anderson WN, Wang D, Pocock S. Transcatheter aortic-valve implantation for aortic stenosis in patients Who cannot undergo surgery. N Engl J Med. 2010;363:1012–5.
28. Smith CR, Leon MB, Mack MJ, Miller DC, Moses JW, Svensson LG, Tuzcu EM, Webb JG, Fontana GP, Makkar RR, Williams M, Dewey T, Kapadia S, Babaliaros V, Thourani VH, Corso P, Pichard AD, Bavaria JE, Herrmann HC, Akin JJ, Anderson WN, Wang D, Pocock SJ, PARTNER Trial Investigators. Transcatheter versus surgical aortic-valve replacement in high-risk patients. N Engl J Med. 2011;364:2187–98.
29. Ghanem A, Müller A, Nähle CP, Kocurek J, Werner N, Hammerstingl C, Schild HH, Schwab JO, Mellert F, Fimmers R, Nickenig G, Thomas D. Risk and fate of cerebral embolism after transfemoral aortic valve implantation: a prospective pilot study with diffusion-weighted magnetic resonance imaging. J Am Coll Cardiol. 2010;55:1427–32.
30. Tay EL, Gurvitch R, Wijesinghe N, Nielispach F, Wood D, Cheung A, Ye J, Lichtenstein SV, Carere R, Thompson C, Webb JG. A high-risk period for cerebrovascular events exists after transcatheter aortic valve implantation. JACC Cardiovasc Interv. 2011;4:1290–7.
31. Iribarren C, Sidney S, Sternfeld B, Browner WS. Calcification of the aortic arch: risk factors and association with coronary heart disease, stroke, and peripheral vascular disease. JAMA. 2000;283:2810–5.
32. Eisen A, Tenenbaum A, Koren-Morag N, et al. Calcification of the thoracic aorta as detected by spiral computed tomography among stable angina pectoris patients: association with cardiovascular events and death. Circulation. 2008;118:1328–34.
33. Takasu J, Katz R, Nasir K, et al. Relationships of thoracic aortic wall calcification to cardiovascular risk factors: the Multi-Ethnic Study of Atherosclerosis (MESA). Am Heart J. 2008; 155:765–71.
34. Santos RD, Rumberger JA, Budoff MJ, et al. Thoracic aorta calcification detected by electron beam tomography predicts all-cause mortality. Atherosclerosis. 2010;209:131–5.
35. Wong ND, Gransar H, Shaw L, et al. Thoracic aortic calcium versus coronary artery calcium for the prediction of coronary heart disease and cardiovascular disease events. JACC Cardiovasc Imaging. 2009;2:319–26.
36. van der Linden J, Hadjinikolaou L, Bergman P, Lindblom D. Postoperative stroke in cardiac surgery is related to the location and extent of atherosclerotic disease in the ascending aorta. J Am Coll Cardiol. 2001;38:131–5.
37. Mitusch R, Doherty C, Wucherpfennig H, et al. Vascular events during follow-up in patients with aortic arch atherosclerosis. Stroke. 1997;28:36–9.
38. Davila-Roman VG, Murphy SF, Nickerson NJ, Kouchoukos NT, Schechtman KB, Barzilai B. Atherosclerosis of the ascending aorta is an independent predictor of long-term neurologic events and mortality. J Am Coll Cardiol. 1999;33:1308–16.
39. Thambidorai SK, Jaffer SJ, Shah TK, Stewart WJ, Klein AL, Lauer MS. Association of atheroma as assessed by intraoperative transoesophageal echocardiography with long-term mortality in patients undergoing cardiac surgery. Eur Heart J. 2007;28:1454–61.
40. Kurra V, Lieber ML, Sola S, Kalahasti V, Hammer D, Gimple S, Flamm SD, Bolen MA, Halliburton SS, Mihaljevic T, Desai MY, Schoenhagen P. Extent of thoracic aortic atheroma burden and long-term mortality after cardiothoracic surgery: a computed tomography study. JACC Cardiovasc Imaging. 2010;3(10):1020–9.
41. Hellings WE, Peeters W, Moll FL, et al. Composition of carotid atherosclerotic plaque is associated with cardiovascular outcome. A prognostic study. Circulation. 2010;121:1941–5.
42. Kurra V, Schoenhagen P, Roselli EE, et al. Prevalence of significant peripheral artery disease in patients evaluated for percutaneous aortic valve insertion: preprocedural assessment with multidetector computed tomography. J Thorac Cardiovasc Surg. 2009; 137:1258–64.
43. da Gama Ribeiro V, Vouga L, Markowitz A, Bezerra HG, Braga P, Ansari M, Leite D, Rocha J, Carvalho M, Simon DI, Costa MA. Vascular access in transcatheter aortic valve implantation. Int J Cardiovasc Imaging. 2011;27(8):1235–43.
44. Petronio AS, De Carlo M, Bedogni F, Marzocchi A, Klugmann S, Maisano F, Ramondo A, Ussia GP, Ettori F, Poli A, Brambilla N, Saia F, De Marco F, Colombo A. Safety and efficacy of the subclavian approach for transcatheter aortic valve implantation with the CoreValve revalving system. Circ Cardiovasc Interv. 2010;3(4): 359–66.
45. Svensson LG, Dewey T, Kapadia S, Roselli EE, Stewart A, Williams M, et al. United States feasibility study of transcatheter insertion of a stented aortic valve by the left ventricular apex. Ann Thorac Surg. 2008;86:46–54.
46. Lichtenstein SV, Cheung A, Ye J, Thompson CR, Carere RG, Pasupati S, et al. Transapical transcatheter aortic valve implantation in humans: initial clinical experience. Circulation. 2006;114: 591–6.
47. Ye J, Cheung A, Lichtenstein SV, Pasupati S, Carere RG, Thompson CR, et al. Six-month outcome of transapical transcatheter aortic valve implantation in the initial seven patients. Eur J Cardiothorac Surg. 2007;31:16–21.
48. Tops LF, Kapadia SR, Tuzcu EM, Vahanian A, Alfieri O, Webb JG, et al. Percutaneous valve procedures: an update. Curr Probl Cardiol. 2008;33:417–57.
49. Murray D, Ghosh J, Khwaja N, Murphy MO, Baguneid MS, Walker MG. Access for endovascular aneurysm repair. J Endovasc Ther. 2006;13:754–61.
50. Roselli EE, Greenberg RK, Pfaff K, Francis C, Svensson LG, Lytle BW. Endovascular treatment of thoracoabdominal aortic aneurysms. J Thorac Cardiovasc Surg. 2007;133:1474–82.
51. Peterson BG, Longo GM, Matsumura JS, Kibbe MR, Morasch MD, Cardeira KR, et al. Endovascular repair of thoracic aortic pathology with custom-made devices. Surgery. 2005;138:598–605.
52. Clavel MA, Rodés-Cabau J, Dumont É, Bagur R, Bergeron S, De Larochellière R, Doyle D, Larose E, Dumesnil JG, Pibarot P. Validation and characterization of transcatheter aortic valve effective orifice area measured by Doppler echocardiography. JACC Cardiovasc Imaging. 2011;4(10):1053–62.
53. Kurra V, Kapadia SR, Tuzcu EM, Halliburton SS, Svensson L, Roselli EE, Schoenhagen P. Pre-procedural imaging of aortic root orientation and dimensions: comparison between X-ray angiographic planar imaging and 3-dimensional multidetector row computed tomography. JACC Cardiovasc Interv. 2010; 3:105–13.
54. Kahlert P, Eggebrecht H, Plicht B, Kraff O, McDougall I, Decker B, Erbel R, Ladd ME, Quick HH. Towards real-time cardiovascular magnetic resonance-guided transarterial aortic valve implantation: in vitro evaluation and modification of existing devices. J Cardiovasc Magn Reson. 2010;12:58.

55. Capelli C, Bosi GM, Cerri E, Nordmeyer J, Odenwald T, Bonhoeffer P, Migliavacca F, Taylor AM, Schievano S. Patient-specific simulations of transcatheter aortic valve stent implantation. Med Biol Eng Comput. 2012;50(2):183–92.
56. Vahanian A, Alfieri O, Al-Attar N, et al. Transcatheter valve implantation for patients with aortic stenosis: a position statement from the European Association of Cardio-Thoracic Surgery (EACTS) and the European Society of Cardiology (ESC), in collaboration with the European Association of Percutaneous Cardiovascular Interventions (EAPCI). Eur Heart J. 2008; 29:1463–70.
57. Leon MB, Piazza N, Nikolsky E, Blackstone EH, Cutlip DE, Kappetein AP, Krucoff MW, Mack M, Mehran R, Miller C, Morel MA, Petersen J, Popma JJ, Takkenberg JJM, Vahanian A, van Es GA, Vranckx P, Webb JG, Windecker S, Serruys PW. Standardized endpoint definitions for transcatheter aortic valve implantation clinical trials: a consensus report from the Valve Academic Research Consortium. Eur Heart J. 2011;32(1):134–5.

Index

J.K. Min et al. (eds.), *Multimodality Imaging for Transcatheter Aortic Valve Replacement*,
DOI 10.1007/978-1-4471-2798-7, © Springer-Verlag London 2014

MIX
Papier aus verantwortungsvollen Quellen
Paper from responsible sources
FSC® C105338

If you have any concerns about our products,
you can contact us on
ProductSafety@springernature.com

In case Publisher is established outside the EU,
the EU authorized representative is:
Springer Nature Customer Service Center GmbH
Europaplatz 3, 69115 Heidelberg, Germany

Printed by Libri Plureos GmbH
in Hamburg, Germany